Stedman's

PATHOLOGY & LAB MEDICINE
WORDS

INCLUDES
HISTOLOGY
Fifth Edition

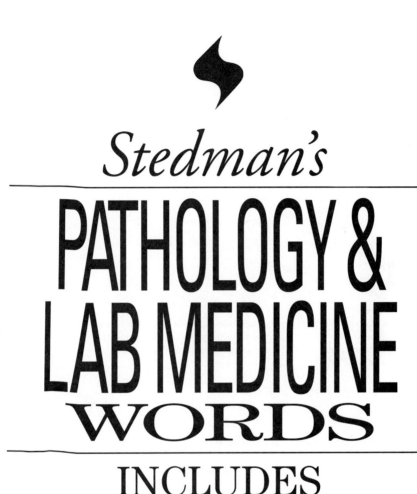

Stedman's
PATHOLOGY & LAB MEDICINE
WORDS

INCLUDES
HISTOLOGY
Fifth Edition

 Wolters Kluwer | Lippincott Williams & Wilkins
Health

Philadelphia • Baltimore • New York • London
Buenos Aires • Hong Kong • Sydney • Tokyo

Publisher: Julie K. Stegman
Editorial Manager: Eric Branger
Associate Managing Editor: Erin M. Cosyn
Manufacturing Coordinator: Margie Orzech-Zeranko
Typesetter: Aptara, Inc.
Printer & Binder: Data Reproductions Corporation

Copyright © 2009 Lippincott Williams & Wilkins
351 West Camden Street
Baltimore, Maryland 21201-2436

Printed in the United States of America

2009

Library of Congress Cataloging-in-Publication Data

Stedman's pathology & lab medicine words : includes histology. – 5th ed.
   p. ; cm. – (Stedman's word book series)
   Includes bibliographical references.
   ISBN 978-0-7817-8995-0
1. Pathology–Terminology. 2. Diagnosis, Laboratory–Terminology.   I. Stedman, Thomas Lathrop, 1853–1938. II. Title: Pathology & lab medicine words.   III. Title: Stedman's pathology and lab medicine words.   IV. Series: Stedman's word books.
   [DNLM: 1. Pathology–Terminology–English. 2. Laboratory Techniques and Procedures–Terminology–English. QZ 15 S8123 2009]
  RB115.S73 2009
  616.07–dc22   2008008837

09 10 11 12
1 2 3 4 5 6 7 8 9 10

Contents

Acknowledgments

An important part of our editorial process is the involvement of medical transcriptionists—as advisors, reviewers, and editors.

We extend special thanks to Sue Dickinson and independent medical transcriptionist Erin J. Graczyk, RN (inactive), BSN for editing the manuscript and helping to resolve many difficult questions; to Janet West for helping to revise and develop the appendices; and to Jo-Ann Clarke for her assistance with the sample reports. We are grateful to advisory board members Kristine Krafts, Beth Pessetto, Terry B. Lary, CMT, Suzanne Taubert, CMT, AHDI-F, and Carol Ferdinand, who shared their valuable judgment, insight, and perspective.

Our appreciation goes to the following reviewers who helped to enhance the A-to-Z content for this edition: Jeanne Bock, CSR, MT; Kimberly Adams; Tamara Dicks, CMT; Kristine Krafts; Carol Ferdinand; Beth Pessetto; Rhonda S. Hase; Shemah Fletcher; and Robin Koza. We thank Lisa Koepenick, who played an integral role in the process by reviewing the content files for format and updating the manuscript. We also extend thanks to Helen Littrell, IMT for performing the final prepublication review.

As with all our *Stedman's* word references, this resource incorporates the suggestions and expertise of our many contacts in the medical transcriptionist community. Thanks to all of our advisory board participants, reviewers, and editors; AAMT meeting attendees; and others who have written us with requests and comments—keep talking, and we'll keep listening.

Editor's Preface

Pathology has deep roots in research and is the dedicated discipline to studying and understanding human diseases. The global emergence of new viruses, molecular pathology gene targeting of hereditary diseases, age of revolutionary "omics," bioterrorism, and new immunohistochemical assays produce an overabundance of hard-to-find pathological terms and investigative tools. Contemporary diagnostic processes used routinely for patient care like flow cytometry, DNA sequencing, or electron microscopy were at one time breakthrough technology found only in research laboratories.

Medical language professionals experiencing these rapid specialty terminology evolutions have been challenged to maintain current, comprehensive references as well as have quick access to a broad spectrum of new terms. *Stedman's Pathology & Lab Medicines Words, Includes Histology, Fifth Edition* includes hundreds of new terms that support basic science and clinical treatments as well as cutting-edge technology that has evolved since publication of the 4th edition.

There were many pathology and medical transcription healthcare professionals involved in the preparation of this book. During the editing process we also refined, eliminated, and/or reorganized many words and phrases to make this edition a more efficient and "ready" reference.

Thank you to the remarkable Lippincott Williams & Wilkins, Stedman's Word Book series managing editors, Erin Cosyn and Eric Branger, for your patient guidance as our teams worked through our new standardized database formats. The Stedman's editorial advisory board, review, and research teams deserve special recognition for their immeasurable contributions of hundreds of new verified terms at the outset of our path and lab word journey.

My heartfelt thanks goes to second editor, Erin Graczyk, for her countless hours of work on both the first and second passes and for being my second pair of eyes as well as my right arm. It was a joy being teamed with you.

I am also grateful to Janet West for her diligent work as appendiceal editor. There are many new appendices in this edition based on your requests that were supplemented and enhanced by her experienced editing.

During the editorial progression of this book, I lost my mother, Mollie Lucas, who enjoyed many of my sleuthing yarns about the text while it was still in manuscript form. This book is also devoted to your memory, Mama. I am most grateful to my husband, Dennis, who sustained me through those difficult times, copied and mailed my edits, and kept me within deadlines.

My decades-long love affair of medical "word hunts" was rejuvenated when I began editing this specialty terminology book in particular. With respect and admiration for their many skills, I dedicate this edition to my fellow medical transcriptionists and students. Your continuing requests and support of the Stedman's Word Book series inspires commitment to standardization and excellence.

I hope this reference becomes one of your favorites.

Sue Dickinson, CMT
February 26, 2008

Publisher's Preface

Stedman's Pathology & Lab Medicine Words, Includes Histology, Fifth Edition offers an authoritative assurance of quality and exactness to the wordsmiths of the healthcare professions—medical transcriptionists, medical editors and copyeditors, health information management personnel, court reporters, and the many other users and producers of medical documentation.

Users will find an extensive array of clinical pathology, anatomical pathology, hematology, medical technology, blood banking, clinical chemistry, histology, bacteria, fungi, parasites, viruses, and bioterrorism terminology. The appendix sections in this edition include labeled anatomical illustrations; culture media; stains, dyes, and fixatives; sample reports; the Greek alphabet; and common terms by procedure; plus, new to this edition, common pathology report terms & guidelines, and classification by system including grades & stages.

This new edition, with more than 100,000 entries, includes the *Stedman's Word Book Series* trademarks: cross-indexing by first and last word, A-Z format with main entries and subentries, and appendix material for additional comprehension and application of the terminology.

We at Lippincott Williams & Wilkins strive to provide you with the most up-to-date and accurate word references available. Your use of this Word Book will prompt new editions, which we will publish as often as updates and revisions justify. We welcome your suggestions for improvements, changes, corrections, and additions—whatever will make this *Stedman's* product more useful to you. Please send us your suggestions and recommendations online at www.stedmans.com.

Explanatory Notes

Medical transcription is an art as well as a science. Both approaches are needed to correctly interpret the dictation of a physician, whose language is a product of education, training, and experience. This variety in medical language means that there are several acceptable ways to express certain terms, including jargon. *Stedman's Pathology & Lab Medicine Words, Includes Histology, Fifth Edition* provides variant spellings and phrasings for many terms. These elements, in addition to complete cross-indexing, make *Stedman's Pathology & Lab Medicine Words, Includes Histology, Fifth Edition* a valuable resource for determining the validity of terms as they are encountered.

Alphabetical Organization

Alphabetization of main entries is letter by letter as spelled, ignoring punctuation, spaces, prefixed numbers, or other characters. For example:

1-adamantanamine sulfate
albumose-free tuberculin (TAF)
ameloblast
amylase/creatinine clearance

Terms beginning or ending with Greek letters show the Greek letters spelled out and listed alphabetically. For example:

alpha
   a. decay
   a. interferon therapy
   a. smooth muscle actin (ASMA)
   a. tropomyosin

In subentry alphabetization, the abbreviated singular form or the spelled-out plural form of the noun main entry word is ignored.

Format and Style

All main entries are in **boldface** to expedite locating a sought-after term, to enhance distinction between main entries and subentries, and to relieve the textual density of the pages.

Irregular plurals and variant spellings are shown on the same line as the singular or preferred form of the word. For example:

lentigo, pl. lentigines
precipitinogen, precipitogen

Capitalization

Trade/brand names (proprietary) and proper names (eponyms) begin with a capital letter.

Chagres virus
Gram stain
Monsel solution
Walker carcinoma
Zenker fluid

However, word formations using a proper name are not capitalized.

gram-negative bacillus

Product names that are represented in all uppercase by the manufacturer are represented with an initial uppercase in this book as shown in bold below.

Binax NOW Legionella test = **Binax Now Legionella test**

An all uppercase product name that is an acronym remains all uppercase.

LUA ELISA test

Irregular capitalization used by the manufacturer is maintained as shown below.

FLx/TDx immunoassay analyzer
HercepTest assay
StatSpin centrifuge

In the formal representation of bacteria genus and species names, the genus is capitalized and both genus and species are italicized. A general reference is not capitalized or italicized.

Mycoplasma fermentans
mycoplasma culture

Hyphenation

As a rule of style, multiple eponyms (e.g., **Weber-Rendu-Osler disease**) are hyphenated. Terms combining an eponym and a manufacturer's name may be hyphenated (e.g., **Abbé-Zeiss counting chamber**). Some eponyms are actually first and last names and thus not hyphenated (e.g., **Austin Moore prosthesis**). Please note that in many cases, hyphenation is a question of style, not of accuracy, and thus is a matter of choice.

Possessives

Possessive forms have been dropped in this reference for the sake of consistency and conformance with the guidelines of the Association for Healthcare Documentation Integrity (AHDI) and other groups. Please note, however, that in many cases, retaining the possessive, like hyphenating, is a question of style, not of accuracy, and thus is a matter of choice. To form the possessive of a word, simply add the apostrophe or apostrophe "s" to the end of the word.

Cross-indexing

The word list is in an index-like main entry-subentry format that contains two combined alphabetical listings:

(1) A *noun* main entry-subentry organization, which is typical of the A-Z section of medical dictionaries like *Stedman's*:

goiter
  endemic g.
  lingual g.

plate
  lingual p.
  microtiter p.

(2) An *adjective* main entry-subentry organization, which lists words and phrases as you hear them. The main entries are the adjectives or modifiers

in a multiword term. The subentries are the nouns around which the terms are constructed and to which the adjectives or modifiers pertain:

melanotic
   m. pigment
   m. schwannoma

scarlet
   s. fever
   s. red stain

This format provides the user with more than one way to locate and identify a multiword term. For example:

metabolic
   m. acidosis

acidosis
   metabolic a.

endolymphatic
   e. duct

duct
   endolymphatic d.

It also allows the user to see together all terms that contain a particular descriptor, as well as all types, kinds, or variations of a noun entity. For example:

fungal
   f. hyphae
   F. Prions
   f. skin testing

mucosa
   intestinal m.
   neisseria m.
   tunica m.

Wherever possible, abbreviations are separately defined and cross-referenced. For example:

AAA
   abdominal aortic aneurysm

abdominal
   a. aortic aneurysm (AAA)

aneurysm
   abdominal aortic a. (AAA)

References

In addition to the manufacturers' literature we gather at various medical meetings, scientific reports from hospitals, and the lists of our MT Editorial Advisory Board members (from their daily transcription work), we used the following sources for new terms in *Stedman's Pathology & Lab Medicine Words, Includes Histology, Fifth Edition.*

Books

Anderson WR. *Forensic Sciences in Clinical Medicine: A Case Study Approach.* Philadelphia: Lippincott-Raven, 1998.

Baggish MS, Valle RF, Guedi H. *Hysteroscopy: Visual Perspectives of Uterine Anatomy, Physiology, and Pathology, Third Edition.* Baltimore: Lippincott Williams & Wilkins: 2007.

Bishop ML, Duben-Engelkirk JL, Fody EP (eds.). *Clinical Chemistry: Principles, Procedures, Correlations, Fourth Edition.* Philadelphia: Lippincott Williams & Wilkins, 2000.

Chernecky CC, Berger BJ. *Laboratory Tests & Diagnostic Procedures, Fifth Edition.* Philadelphia: Saunders, 2007.

Clinical Laboratory Tests: Values and Implications, Third Edition. Springhouse, PA: Springhouse, 2001.

Damjanov I. *High-Yield Pathology, Second Edition.* Baltimore: Lippincott Williams & Wilkins: 2005.

Desai SP. *Clinician's Guide to Laboratory Medicine: A Practical Approach.* Hudson, OH: Lexi-Comp, 2004.

Desai SP. *Clinician's Guide to Laboratory Medicine Pocket.* Hudson, OH: Lexi-Comp, 2004.

Dorland's Laboratory/Pathology Word Book for Medical Transcriptionists. St. Louis: Saunders, 2002.

Drake E. *Sloane's Medical Word Book, Fourth Edition.* Philadelphia: Saunders, 2002.

Dudek RW. *High-Yield Histology, Third Edition.* Baltimore: Lippincott Williams & Wilkins, 2004.

Eroschenko VP. *diFiore's Atlas of Histology with Functional Correlations, Tenth Edition.* Baltimore: Lippincott Williams & Wilkins, 2005.

Fenderson B, Rubin R (eds.). *Lippincott's Review of Pathology: Illustrated Interactive Q&A.* Baltimore: Lippincott Williams & Wilkins, 2006.

Fischbach F. *A Manual of Laboratory and Diagnostic Tests, Seventh Edition.* Philadelphia: Lippincott Williams & Wilkins, 2004.

Goljan EF (ed.). *Rapid Review Series: Pathology.* Philadelphia: Mosby, 2004.

References

Handbook of Diagnostic Tests, Third Edition. Springhouse, PA: Lippincott Williams & Wilkins, 2003.

Jacobs DS, DeMott WR, Oxley DK (eds.). *Laboratory Test Handbook, Fifth Edition.* Hudson, OH: Lexi-Comp, 2001.

Jakob M. *Normal Values Pocket.* Hermosa Beach, CA: Börm Bruckmeier, 2002.

Jones SL (ed.). *Clinical Laboratory Pearls.* Philadelphia: Lippincott Williams & Wilkins, 2001.

Keyes DC, Burstein JL, Schwartz RB, Swienton RE. *Medical Response to Terrorism: Preparedness and Clinical Practice.* Philadelphia: Lippincott Williams & Wilkins, 2005.

McClatchey KD (ed.). *Clinical Laboratory Medicine, Second Edition.* Philadelphia: Lippincott Williams & Wilkins, 2002.

McConnell HC. *The Nature of Disease: Pathology for the Health Professions.* Baltimore: Lippincott Williams & Wilkins: 2006.

Michota FA (ed.). *Diagnostic Procedures Handbook, Second Edition.* Hudson, OH: Lexi-Comp, 2001.

Mills SE, Carter D, Greenson JK, Oberman HA, Reuter VE (eds.). *Diagnostic Surgical Pathology, Fourth Edition.* Philadelphia: Lippincott Williams & Wilkins, 2004.

Mills SE (ed.). *Histology for Pathologists, Third Edition.* Baltimore: Lippincott Williams & Wilkins, 2006.

Professional Guide to Diagnostic Tests. Ambler, PA: Lippincott Williams & Wilkins, 2005.

Raab SS, Grzybicki DM. *Year Book of Pathology and Laboratory Medicine 2007.* Philadelphia: Mosby, 2007.

Rosen PP, Hoda SA (eds.). *Breast Pathology: Diagnosis by Needle Core Biopsy, Second Edition.* Baltimore: Lippincott Williams & Wilkins, 2005.

Rubin E, Farber JL (eds.). *Pathology, Third Edition.* Philadelphia: Lippincott Williams & Wilkins, 1999.

Rubin R, Strayer DS (eds.). *Rubin's Pathology: Clinicopathologic Foundations of Medicine, Fifth Edition.* Baltimore: Lippincott Williams & Wilkins, 2007.

Schneider AS, Szanto PA. *Board Review Series Pathology, Second Edition.* Baltimore: Lippincott Williams & Wilkins, 2002.

Sloane SB, Dusseau JL. *A Word Book in Pathology & Laboratory Medicine, Second Edition.* Philadelphia: Saunders, 1995.

Stedman's Medical Dictionary, 28th Edition. Baltimore: Lippincott Williams & Wilkins, 2006.

Turgeon ML. *Clinical Hematology, Theory and Procedures, Fourth Edition.* Philadelphia: Lippincott Williams & Wilkins, 2004.

Vera Pyle's Current Medical Terminology, Tenth Edition. Modesto, CA: Health Professions Institute, 2005.

Wahl CE. *The Hardcore Pathology, Second Edition.* Baltimore: Lippincott Williams & Wilkins: 2006.

Journals

ADVANCE for Health Information Professionals. King of Prussia, PA: Merion, 2003–2004.

Advances in Anatomic Pathology. Philadelphia: Lippincott Williams & Wilkins, 1999–2007.

American Journal of Clinical Pathology. Philadelphia: Lippincott Williams & Wilkins, 2004.

The American Journal of Forensic Medicine and Pathology. Philadelphia: Lippincott Williams & Wilkins, 2003–2007.

The American Journal of Pathology. Bethesda, MD: American Society for Investigative Pathology, 2003.

American Journal of Surgical Pathology. Philadelphia: Lippincott Williams & Wilkins, 1998–2007.

Applied Immunohistochemistry & Molecular Morphology. Philadelphia: Lippincott Williams & Wilkins, 2003–2007.

Archives of Pathology & Lab Medicine. Northfield, IL: College of American Pathologists, 2003.

Blood. Washington, DC: The American Society of Hematology, 2003.

Clinical Lab Products. Amherst, NH: Clinical Lab Products, 2000–2002.

The Endocrinologist. Baltimore: Lippincott Williams & Wilkins, 2000–2007.

Internal Medicine. Montvale, NJ: Medical Economics, 2000.

JAAMT. Modesto, CA: American Association for Medical Transcription, 2001–2003.

Journal of Clinical Pathology. London: BMJ Publishing Group, 2003.

The Journal of Pathology. Hoboken, NJ: John Wiley & Sons, 2003.

Laboratory Medicine. Chicago: American Society of Clinical Pathologists, 1998.

The Latest Word. Philadelphia: Saunders, 1999, 2002–2004.

Modern Pathology. Baltimore: Lippincott Williams & Wilkins, 1999–2000.

Pathology Case Reviews. Philadelphia: Lippincott Williams & Wilkins, 2003–2007.

Pathology Patterns. Chicago: American Society of Clinical Pathologists, 1994, 1997.

Perspectives. Modesto, CA: Health Professions Institute, 2001–2004.

Images

Hardy NO, Westport CT. *Stedman's Medical Dictionary, 27th ed.* Baltimore: Lippincott Williams & Wilkins, 2000.

LifeART Nursing 1, CD-ROM. Baltimore: Lippincott Williams & Wilkins.

LifeART Nursing 2, CD-ROM. Baltimore: Lippincott Williams & Wilkins.

LifeART Nursing 3, CD-ROM. Baltimore: Lippincott Williams & Wilkins.

LifeART Pediatricts 1, CD-ROM. Baltimore: Lippincott Williams & Wilkins.

LifeART Super Anatomy Collection 2, CD-ROM. Baltimore: Lippincott Williams & Wilkins.

LifeART Super Anatomy Collection 5, CD-ROM. Baltimore: Lippincott Williams & Wilkins.

MediClip Clinical Cardiopulmonary, CD-ROM. Baltimore: Lippincott Williams & Wilkins.

MediClip Clinical OB/GYN, CD-ROM. Baltimore: Lippincott Williams & Wilkins.

Smeltzer SC, Bare BG. *Textbook of Medical-Surgical Nursing, Ninth Edition.* Philadelphia: Lippincott Williams & Wilkins, 2000.

Ward L. Salt Lake City, UT. Fuller J, Schaller-Ayers J. *Health Assessment: A Nursing Approach, Second Edition.* Philadelphia: J.B. Lippincott Company, 1994.

Willis MC. *Medical Terminology: A Programmed Learning Approach to the Language of Health Care.* Baltimore: Lippincott Williams & Wilkins, 2002.

Websites

http://arpa.allenpress.com

http://jama.ama-assn.org

http://menopause.home.test.biolifedynamics.com

http://perso.wanadoo.fr/alzheimer.lille/pdf/2000/2000DelacourteBueeCOIN.pdf

http://quickmedical.com

http://us.labsystem.roche.com

http://www.abbottdiagnostics.com

http://www.abbottdiagnostics.com

http://www.accutech-llc.com

http://www.acrometrix.com

http://www.aerocrine.com

http://www.afip.org

http://www.ascp.org
http://www.bacterio.cict.fr/allnamestwo.html
http://www.beckman.com
http://www.brinkmann.com
http://www.cap.org
http://www.ciphergen.com
http://www.compumed.net
http://www.dakocytomation.us
http://www.dpcweb.com
http://www.e-perspectives
http://www.fda.gov
http://www.hemametrics.com
http://www.hematology.org
http://www.hpisum.com
http://www.jimro.com
http://www.medtox.com
http://www.mtdesk.com
http://www.mtmonthly.com
http://www.orasure.com
http://www.orthoclinical.com
http://www.prometheuslabs.com
http://www.quidel.com
http://www.quidel.com
http://www.responsebio.com
http://www.roche-diagnostics.com
http://www.spectraldx.com
http://www.stanford.edu/group/hopes/sttools/gloss
http://www.statspin.com
http://www.tapestrypharma.com
http://www.thelatestword.com
http://www.thermo.com
http://www.vielle.info/menopause
http://www.vysis.com

A
  adenine
  ampere
    A antigen
    A band
    A cell
    A disc
    A fiber
a
    a disintegrin and metalloprotease
      (ADAM)
    a disintegrin and metalloproteinase
      with thrombospondin domain 13
      (ADAMTS 13)
    a hypotonic environment
Å
  angstrom
A1
  angiotensin 1
A2
  angiotensin 2
    A2 MicroArray system
A3
  angiotensin 3
AA
  amyloid A
  arachidonic acid
    AA amyloidosis
aA
  azure A
AAA
  abdominal aortic aneurysm
  androgenic anabolic agent
A1AC
  alpha-1 antichymotrypsin
AAC
  antibiotic-associated colitis
AAD
  antibiotic-associated diarrhea
AADC
  aromatic l-amino acid
    decarboxylase
AAH
  atypical adenomatous hyperplasia
AAN
  amino acid nitrogen
    AAN test
AAO
  automated assay optimization
Aarskog-Scott syndrome
Aarskog syndrome
AAS
  aminoalkylsilane
  atomic absorption spectrophotometer
  atomic absorption spectrophotometry

A1AT
  alpha$_1$ antitrypsin
    A1AT deficiency
    A1AT deficiency panniculitis
AAT
  alpha antitrypsin
AAV
  adeno-associated virus
A:B
  acid-base ratio
AB
  abortion
  Alcian blue
  asbestos body
  asthmatic bronchitis
    AB decalcification
Ab
  antibody
aB
  azure B
ab initio
abacterial thrombotic endocarditis
abarticular gout
abarticulation
abattoir worker
ABB
  acute bronchitis/bronchiolitis
abbau
Abbé
    A. condenser
    A. test plate
Abbé-Zeiss
    A.-Z. apparatus
    A.-Z. counting chamber
ABBI
  advanced breast biopsy
    instrumentation
Abbott
    A. AxSYM Prizm HCV assay
    A. Cell-Dyn hematology analyzer
ABC
  aneurysmal bone cyst
  aspiration biopsy cytology
  ATP-binding cassette
  avidin-biotin peroxidase complex
    ABC immunodetection system
    ABC staining method
    ABC technique
abdominal
    a. anthrax
    a. aortic aneurysm (AAA)
    a. ascites
    a. dropsy
    a. fibromatosis
    a. fistula

abdominal (*continued*)
    a. muscle deficiency syndrome
    a. viscera
abdominis
    hydrops a.
Abell-Kendall method
Abelson
    A. murine leukemia virus (AbMLV)
    A. oncogene
abequose
Abercrombie syndrome
aberrans
    Haller vas a.
aberrant
    a. angiogenesis
    a. crypt focus
    a. duct
    a. ductule
    a. ganglion
    a. germ
    a. goiter
    a. hemoglobin
    a. pancreas
    a. renal vessel
    a. rest
    a. ribonucleic acid
    a. tissue
aberrantes
    ductuli a.
    ductus a.
aberrantia
    Ferrein vasa a.
    vasa a.
aberrata
    struma a.
aberration
    chromatic a.
    chromosomal a.
    chromosome a.
    heterosomal a.
    interchromosomal a.
    intrachromosomal a.
    karyotype a.
    tetra-X chromosomal a.
    triple-X chromosomal a.
abetalipoproteinemia (ABL)
ABG
    arterial blood gas
ABH antigen
abietic acid
ability
Abiotrophia
abiotrophy
ABI Prism 3100 Genetic Analyzer
abiuret
abiuretic
ABL
    abetalipoproteinemia
ablastin

ablatio
    a. placentae
    a. retinae
ablative chemotherapy
ablepharon
abluminal surface
ABMA
    antibasement membrane antibody
AbMLV
    Abelson murine leukemia virus
A5B7 monoclonal antibody
ABMT
    autologous blood and marrow
      transplantation
    autologous bone marrow transplantation
ABN
    abnormal
abnormal (ABN)
    a. banding region
    a. beta cell function
    a. chorion
    a. chorionic villus
    a. clinical manifestation
    a. flow
    a. mitosis
    a. shortening
abnormality
    bell-clapper a.
    chromosomal a.
    cytologic a.
    fetal a.
    gain-of-function a.
    genetic a.
    morphologic a.
    no histopathologic a. (NHPA)
    nonspecific hepatocellular a. (NHA)
    no serious a. (NSA)
    no significant a. (NSA)
    sex chromosome a.
    transient enzyme a.
    traumatic a.
    wire-loop a.
abnormally localized immature precursor (ALIP)
ABO
    blood group systems
    ABO antibody
    ABO antigen
    ABO compatibility
    ABO factor
    ABO hemolytic disease of the
      newborn
    ABO incompatibility
    ABO typing
ABO-Rh typing
aborted ectopic pregnancy
abortion (AB)
    afebrile a.
    ampullar a.

artificial a.
cervical a.
complete a.
criminal a.
habitual a.
imminent a.
incomplete a.
induced a.
inevitable a.
infected a.
justifiable a.
missed a.
placenta previa a.
septic a.
spontaneous a.
therapeutic a. (TA)
threatened a.
tubal a.

abortive
a. infection
a. neurofibromatosis
a. transduction
a. viral disease

abortus
Brucella a.
Chlamydophila a.
a. fever
hydropic a.

ABP
androgen-binding protein

ABPA
allergic bronchopulmonary aspergillosis

ABPM
allergic bronchopulmonary mycosis

Abrams test

abrasion
a. collar
muzzle a.
punctate a.
a. rim
a. ring
tattooing a.

abrasive cytology

Abrikosov tumor

abrin

abruption
placental a.

abruptio placentae

Abrus precatorius

ABS
alkylbenzene sulfonate

abscess
acute a.
a. aerobic culture
alveolar a.
amebic brain a.
apical a.
appendiceal a.
Bartholin a.

Bezold a.
bicameral a.
bone a.
brain a.
Brodie a.
bursal a.
caseous a.
cerebral epidural a.
cholangitic a.
chronic a.
cold a.
collar button a.
crypt a.
diffuse a.
Douglas a.
dry a.
Dubois a.
embolic a.
eosinophilic a.
epidural a.
fecal a.
follicular a.
gas a.
gravitation a.
gummatous a.
hematogenous a.
hepatic a.
hot a.
hypostatic a.
ischiorectal a.
Kogoj a.
lacunar a.
metastatic a.
migrating a.
miliary a.
Munro a.
mycotic a.
otitic a.
Pott a.
premammary a.
psoas a.
pyemic a.
pylephlebitic a.
pyogenic a.
residual a.
satellite a.
septicemic a.
shirt-stud a.
stellate a.
stercoral a.
sterile a.
stitch a.
subacute a.
sudoriferous a.
sudoriparous a.
syphilitic a.
Tornwaldt a.
tropical a.
trunk a.

abscess (*continued*)
    tuberculous a.
    tuboovarian a. (TOA)
    verminous a.
    wandering a.
    worm a.
abscessus
    Mycobacterium chelonae subsp. *a.*
    Nocardia a.
absence
    congenital a.
absent regression
Absidia
    A. corymbifera
    A. ramosa
absolute
    a. alcohol
    atmosphere a.
    a. cell increase
    a. eosinophil count
    a. erythrocytosis
    a. granulocyte count (AGC)
    a. iodine uptake (AIU)
    a. leukocytosis
    a. neutrophil count (ANC)
    a. polycythemia
    a. retention time (ART)
    a. system of units
    a. temperature scale
    a. terminal innervation ratio
    a. value
    a. viscosity
    a. zero
absorbed
    anthrax vaccine a.
    a. dose
absorbefacient
absorbency index
absorbent
    carbon dioxide a.
absorber
absorptiometer
absorption
    atomic a.
    a. cavity
    a. cell
    a. coefficient
    a. constant
    disjunctive a.
    d-xylose a.
    fat a.
    guinea pig kidney a. (test) (GPKA)
    intestinal a.
    a. of erythrocyte antibody
    a. peak
    a. spectrum
absorptive
    a. cell
    a. disorder

    a. lipemia
    a. state
absorptivity
    molar a.
    specific a.
abstinence
    alimentary a.
abstriction
abundant cytoplasm
abuse
    drugs of a. (DOA)
    InstaCheck Med+ immunoassay for
      drugs of a.
ABx
    antibiotic
abyssalis
    Idiomarina a.
abyssi
    Caldithrix a.
    Deferribacter a.
    Moritella a.
A:C
    amylase/creatinine clearance ratio
AC
    adenocarcinoma
    anticoagulant
    anticomplementary
    antiinflammatory corticoid
    autoclave
    NATO code for HCN
Ac
    actinium
A1c
    A1c At·Home testing kit
aC
    azure C
ACA
    acrodermatitis chronica atrophicans
    adenocarcinoma
    anticardiolipin antibody
acalculous cholecystitis
acanthamebiasis
Acanthamoeba
    A. astronyxis
    A. castellanii
    A. culbertsoni
    A. hatchetti
    A. keratitis
    A. medium
    A. polyphaga
    A. rhysodes
Acanthella
Acanthia lectularia
Acanthobdella
Acanthocephala
acanthocephaliasis
Acanthocheilonema
    A. perstans
    A. streptocerca

acanthocyte
acanthocyte-associated hemolytic anemia
acanthocytosis
    hereditary a.
acanthoid cell
acantholysis
acantholytic dermatosis
acanthoma
    a. adenoides cysticum
    basal cell a.
    clear cell a.
    large-cell a.
    pilar sheath a.
    a. verrucosa seborrheica
acanthomatous ameloblastoma
acanthopodia
acanthor
acanthorrhexis
acanthosis
    glycogen a.
    glycogenic a.
    a. nigricans
    verrucous a.
acanthotic
acanthrocytosis
acapnia
acapnial alkalosis
acarbia
acardiacus
acardius
    fetus a.
acariasis
acaricide
acarid
Acaridae
acaridan, acaridean, acaridian
acaridean (*var. of* acaridan)
acaridian (*var. of* acaridan)
acaridiasis
Acarina
acarine
acarinosis
acarodermatitis
acaroid
acarology
Acarus
    A. folliculorum
    A. gallinae
    A. hordei
    A. rhizoglypticus hyacinthi
    A. scabiei
    A. siro
acaryote (*var. of* akaryocyte)
ACAT
    acyl-CoA acyltransferase
acatalasemia
acatalasia, acatalasemia
acathectic

acathexia
Acaulium
ACB
    albumin cobalt binding
    ACB test
ACC
    acinar cell carcinoma
    adenoid cystic carcinoma
acceava
    A. hCG Basic
    A. hCG Combo
    A. *Helicobacter pylori*
    A. Mono
    A. Strep A
accelerant
accelerated
    a. reaction
    a. rejection
    a. villous maturation
acceleration
    angular a.
    growth a.
    linear a.
    serum prothrombin conversion a. (SPCA)
accelerator
    a. factor
    a. globulin (AcG)
    proserum prothrombin conversion a. (PPCA)
    prothrombin a.
    serum prothrombin conversion a. (SPCA)
    serum thrombotic a. (STA)
    thromboplastin generation a.
accelerin
Accelon Combi biosampler
accentuator
acceptor
    hydrogen a.
    oxygen a.
    proton a.
access
    A. AccuTnI test
    A. AFP immunoassay analyzer
    exit a.
    A. Hybritech PSA test
    A. 2 immunoassay system
    multiple a.
    A. Ostase test
    sequential a.
    A. testosterone assay
    a. time
accessible antigen
accessoria, *pl.* **accessoriae**
    glandulae areolares accessoriae
    glandulae buccales accessoriae
    glandulae ceruminosae accessoriae

accessoria (*continued*)
    glandulae cervicales uteri accessoriae
    glandulae ciliares accessoriae
    glandulae circumanales accessoriae
    glandulae conjunctivales accessoriae
    glandulae cutis accessoriae
    glandulae duodenales accessoriae
    glandulae endocrinae accessoriae
    glandulae esophageae accessoriae
    glandulae gastricae accessoriae
    glandulae lacrimales accessoriae
    glandulae suprarenales accessoriae
    glandula parotidea a.
    glandula parotis a.
    glandula thyroidea a.
    glandulae glomiformes accessoriae
    glandulae intestinales accessoriae
    glandulae labiales accessoriae
    glandulae laryngeae accessoriae
    glandulae mucosae biliosae accessoriae
    glandulae nasales accessoriae
    glandulae olfactoriae accessoriae
    glandulae oris accessoriae
    glandulae palatinae accessoriae
    glandulae pharyngeales accessoriae
    glandulae preputiales accessoriae
    glandulae pyloricae accessoriae
    glandulae sebaceae accessoriae
    glandulae sine ductibus accessoriae
    glandulae sudoriferae accessoriae
    glandulae tarsales accessoriae
    thyroidea a.
    glandulae tracheales accessoriae
    glandulae tubariae accessoriae
    glandulae urethrales femininae accessoriae
    glandulae urethrales masculinae accessoriae
    glandulae uterinae accessoriae
    glandulae vestibulares minores accessoriae
accessorius
    ductus pancreaticus a.
    lien a.
    splen a.
accessory
    a. adrenal
    a. atrium
    a. cell
    a. chromosome
    a. gland
    a. molecule
    a. organ
    a. pancreas
    a. pancreatic duct
    a. spleen
    a. thyroid

accident
    cerebrovascular a. (CVA)
    neonatal cerebrovascular a.
    serum a.
accidental
    a. host
    a. parasite
acclimation
accolé form
accommodation
    histologic a.
    spasm of a.
account
    dose a.
accreta
    placenta a.
accretionary growth
accretion line
AccuDx test
accumbens
    nucleus a.
AccuMeter
    A. fructosamine
    A. HDL
    A. theophylline
accumulation
    a. disease
    extensive a.
    forskolin-stimulated intracellular cAMP a.
    intracellular a.
    lipofuscin a.
    a. of complex lipids
    a. of protein
    pulmonary a.
accumulator
AccuProbe method
accuracy
    Standards for Reporting of Diagnostic A. (STARD)
    wavelength a.
Accurun 515 drug resistant mutant control series
AccuTnI test
ACD
    acid-citrate-dextrose
ACE
    adrenocortical extract
acellular
    a. basement membrane
    a. mucus lake
    a. tumor
acelom
acelomate, acelomatous
acelomatous (*var. of* acelomate)
acentric
acephalia (*var. of* acephaly, acephalus)
acephaline
acephalocyst

acephalous
acephalus, acephalia
    holoacardius a.
acephaly, acephalia
acerina
    Centrospora a.
    Mycocentrospora a.
acervulus
acestoma
acetal
acetaldehydase
acetaldehyde
acetamide
acetaminophen
    a. assay
    a. hepatic toxicity
acetanilid poisoning
acetarsol
    sodium a.
acetate
    aqueous uranyl a.
    cellulose a.
    cresyl violet a.
    deoxycorticosterone a. (DOCA)
    ethyl a.
    fluorescein mercuric a.
    leuprolide a.
    methyl a.
    potassium a.
    sodium a.
acetazolamide
    sodium a.
Acetest
aceti
    Acetobacter a.
    Turbatrix a.
acetic
    a. acid-alcohol-formalin
    a. acid and potassium ferrocyanide
      test
    a. acid-induced writhing test
    a. aldehyde
    a. anhydride
    a. orcein
aceticus
    Acidilobus a.
acetigenes
    Sporanaerobacter a.
acetiphilus
    Denitrovibrio a.
acetoacetate
acetoacetic
    a. acid
    a. acid test
    a. aciduria
acetoacetyl
acetoacetyl-CoA
    a.-C. reductase
    a.-C. thiolase

Acetobacter
    A. aceti
    A. cerevisiae
    A. cibinongensis
    A. estunensis
    A. indonesiensis
    A. lovaniensis
    A. malorum
    A. orientalis
    A. orleanensis
    A. syzygii
    A. tropicalis
    A. xylinus
Acetobacterium tundrae
acetobutylicum
    Clostridium a.
acetocarmine
acetoin test
acetolysis
acetonation
acetone
    a. body
    a. compound
    a. fixative
    a. methylbenzoate, xylene (AMeX)
    a. test
acetone-insoluble antigen
acetonemia
acetonemic
acetonitrile
acetonuria
acetoorcein stain
acetosoluble albumin
acetous
acetowhite test
acetoxidans
    Desulfobacca a.
aceturate
    diminazene a.
acetyl
    a. group
    a. value
acetylated low-density lipoprotein (AcLDL)
acetylation
acetylator
acetylcholine receptor antibody (AChRAb)
acetylcholinesterase
    a. assay
acetyl-CoA
    acetylcoenzyme A
      acetyl-CoA acetyltransferase
      acetyl-CoA acyltransferase
      acetyl-CoA carboxylase
      acetyl-CoA hydrolase
      acetyl-CoA synthetase
acetylcoenzyme A (acetyl-CoA)
acetylene trichloride
acetylhydrolase
    platelet-activating factor a. (PAF-AH)

acetylization
acetylmethylcarbinol
acetylsalicylic acid (ASA)
acetylsulfadiazine
acetylsulfaguanidine
acetylsulfathiazole
acetyltransferase
    acetyl-CoA a.
    choline a.
    histone a. (HAT)
AcG
    accelerator globulin
aCGH
    array-based comparative genomic
    hybridization
ACH
    adrenocortical hormone
Achaetomium
achalasia
    biliary a.
    esophageal a.
    sphincteral a.
Achard syndrome
Achard-Thiers syndrome
Achatina
Achenbach syndrome
Achillea
achiral
achlorhydria
    watery diarrhea, hypokalemia, a.
    (WDHA)
achlorhydric anemia
achlorophyllous
Acholeplasma
    A. axanthum
    A. granularum
    A. laidlawii
    A. vituli
Acholeplasmataceae
Acholeplasmatales
acholic stool
acholuria
acholuric jaundice
achondrogenesis
achondroplasia
    homozygous a.
achondroplastic
    a. dwarf
    a. dwarfism
Achorion
AChRAb
    acetylcholine receptor
    antibody
achrestic anemia
achroacyte
achroacytosis
achromasia
achromate
Achromatiaceae

achromatic
    a. apparatus
    a. lens
    a. objective
    a. spindle
achromatin, achromin
achromatinic
achromatism
achromatize
achromatocyte
achromatolysis
achromatophil, achromophilic,
   achromophilous
achromatophilia
achromatopsia, achromatopsy
achromatopsy (*var. of* achromatopsia)
achromatosis
achromatous
achromaturia
achromia
    central a.
    congenital a.
    cortical a.
    a. parasitica
    a. unguium
achromians
    incontinentia pigmenti a.
achromic
achromin (*var. of* achromatin)
Achromobacter
    A. denitrificans
    A. insolitus
    A. lwoffii
    A. spanius
Achromobacteraceae
achromocyte
achromophilic (*var. of* achromatophil)
achromophilous (*var. of* achromatophil)
achrooamyloid
achroodextrin
achrotrichium
Achucarro stain
achylia
Aciculoconidium
acid
    aberrant ribonucleic a.
    abietic a.
    acetoacetic a.
    acetylsalicylic a. (ASA)
    acrylic a.
    adenylic a.
    agaric a.
    a. agglutination
    a. albumin
    a. alcohol
    alcohol-formaldehyde-acetic a. (AFA)
    aldaric a.
    aldonic a.
    alginic a.

aliphatic a.
allantoic a.
all-*trans*-retinoic a. (ATRA)
alpha amino a.
alpha ketoglutaric a.
alpha-linolenic a. (ALA)
amino a.
aminoacetic a.
aminocaproic a.
aminoglutaric a.
aminolevulinic a. (ALA)
aminopenicillanic a. (APA)
aminosuccinic a.
a. anhydride method
anthranilic a.
apurinic a.
arachidonic a. (AA)
argininosuccinic a.
aromatic amino a.
ascorbic a.
asparaginic a.
aspartic a. (Asp)
aurin tricarboxylic a.
basic amino a.
behenic a.
benzoic a.
benzoylaminoacetic a.
bile a.
binary a.
boric a.
branched-chain amino a. (BCAA)
branched-chain keto a. (BCKA)
Brönsted-Lowry a.
butanoic a.
butyric a. (BA)
cacodylic a.
carbolic a.
carbonic a.
carboxylic a.
carminic a.
catechinic a.
catechuic a.
a. cell
cerebronic a.
a. challenge test
chenodeoxycholic a. (CDC)
chloracetic a.
chloranilic a.
cholic a.
chromic a.
chromotropic a.
citric a.
a. clearance test (ACT)
conjugate a.
cytidylic a.
decanoic a.
dehydroascorbic a.
delta ALA a.
deoxyadenylic a.

deoxycholic a.
deoxycytidylic a.
deoxyguanylic a.
deoxyribonucleic a. (DNA)
deoxyuridylic a.
d-glucaric a.
diacetic a.
dibasic a.
dicarboxylic a.
dichlorophenoxy acetic a.
diethylenetriaminepentaacetic a.
dihomogammalinolenic a. (DGLA)
dihydrofolic a.
dihydroxymandelic a. (DHMA, DOMA)
dihydroxyphenylacetic a. (DOPAC)
1-dimethylaminonaphthalene-5-sulfonic a. (DANS)
dimethylarsinic a. (DMA)
dinitrobenzoic a.
dipicolinic a.
docosahexaenoic a. (DHA)
a. dye
edetic a.
eicosapentaenoic a. (EPA)
elaidic a.
a. electrophoresis
a. elution test
epoxyeicosatrienoic a.
epsilon a.
essential fatty a. (EFA)
ethacrynic a. (ECA)
ethanoic a.
ethylenediaminetetraacetic a. (EDTA)
ethylene glycol tetraacetic a. (EGTA)
ethylene tetraacetic a.
fatty a. (FA)
ferric chloride, perchloric acid, nitric a. (FPN)
flavianic a.
folic a.
folinic a.
a. formaldehyde hematin
formic a.
formiminoglutamic a. (FIGLU)
free fatty a. (FFA)
a. fuchsin
fumaric a.
galacturonic a.
gamma aminobutyric a. (GABA)
gastric a.
genomic deoxyribonucleic a. (gDNA)
Gerhardt test for acetoacetic a.
germ cell deoxyribonucleic a. (germ cell DNA)
glacial acetic a.
a. gland
glucogenic amino a.
glucuronic a.

acid (*continued*)
    glutamic a. (E, Glu)
    glutaric a.
    glycochenodeoxycholic a.
    glycocholic a.
    glycodeoxycholic a.
    glycolic a.
    glycolithocholic a.
    a. glycoprotein
    guanidino-aminovaleric a.
    guanylic a.
    a. hemolysin test
    a. hemolysis test
    heparinic a.
    hexanoic a.
    hexuronic a.
    hippuric a.
    homogentisic a. (HGA)
    homovanillic a. (HVA)
    hyaluronic a. (HA)
    hydrochloric a. (HCl)
    hydrocyanic a.
    hydrofluoric a.
    a. hydrolase
    5-hydroxyindoleacetic a. (5-HIAA)
    hydroxyphenylpyruvic a. (HPPA)
    hypobromous a.
    hypochlorous a.
    iduronic a.
    imidazolepyruvic a.
    imino a.
    iminodiacetic a. (IDA)
    indolacetic a.
    indolaceturic a.
    indolelactic a.
    infectious nucleic a.
    inorganic a.
    inosinic a.
    a. intoxication
    iodic a.
    a. ionization constant
    isobutyric a.
    isocitric a.
    isolation of nucleic a.
    isovaleric a.
    keto a.
    ketogenic amino a.
    a. lability test
    lactic a.
    lauric a.
    leukocyte ascorbic a. (LAA)
    Lewis a.
    lignoceric a.
    linoleic a.
    linolenic a.
    linolic a.
    lipid-associated sialic a. (LASA)
    lipoic a.
    lithic a.

lithocholic a.
long-chain fatty a. (LCFA)
long-chain polyunsaturated fatty a. (LCPUFA)
lysergic a.
lysophosphatidic a. (LPA)
a. magenta
malic a.
Mallory phosphotungstic a.
malonic a.
a. maltase deficiency
medium-chain fatty a. (MCFA)
mercaptoacetic a.
messenger ribonucleic a. (mRNA)
metaphosphoric a.
methoxyhydroxymandelic a. (MOMA)
methylmalonic a.
mitochondrial deoxyribonucleic a. (mDNA, mtDNA)
modified amino a.
monoaminodicarboxylic a.
monoaminomonocarboxylic a.
monobasic a.
monoenoic fatty a.
monomethylarsonic a. (MMA)
^{99m}Tc pentetic a.
a. mucopolysaccharide (AMP)
muramic a.
muriatic a.
mycolic a.
myristic a.
N-acetylaspartate a. (NAA)
N-acetylmuramic a.
nalidixic a.
neuraminic a.
nicotinic a.
nitric a.
3-nitroproprionic a. (3NP)
nitrous a.
nonesterified fatty a.
n-tetracosanoic a.
a. number
octanoic a.
octulosonic a.
o-hydroxyphenylacetic a.
oleic a.
oleic a. I 125
a. orcein
organic a.
orotic a.
orthophosphoric a.
osmic a.
oxalic a.
oxaloacetic a.
oxo a.
oxobutyric a.
oxoglutaric a.
oxolinic a.
p-aminobenzoic a. (PAB, PABA)

p-aminohip
p-aminosal
a. perfusion te
peroxyacetic a.
a. phosphatase (ACP,
a. phosphatase assay
a. phosphatase serum
a. phosphatase stain
a. phosphatase staining
a. phosphatase test
a. phosphatase test for semen
a. phosphate
p-hydroxybenzoic a.
p-hydroxyphenyllactic a.
p-hydroxyphenylpyruvic a.
p-nitrophenylic a.
polyadenylic a. (polyA)
polybasic a.
polycytidylic a. (polyC)
polyenoic a.
polyphosphoric a.
polysialic a.
polyunsaturated fatty a. (PUFA)
polyuridylic a. (polyU)
pristanic a.
propanoic a.
propionic a.
p-rosolic a.
prostanoic a.
proton a.
prussic a.
pteroic a.
pteroylglutamic a.
pyridoxic a.
pyrophosphoric a.
pyroracemic a.
pyruvic a.
quinolinic a.
radioiodinated fatty a. (RIFA)
a. reaction
a. red 87, 91
a. reflux test
respiratory syncytial virus nucleic a.
retinoic a.
rhodanic a.
ribonucleic a. (RNA)
ribothymidylic a. (rTMP, TMP)
ricinoleic a.
rubeanic a.
saccharic a.
salicylic a.
salicylsalicylic a.
salicylsulfonic a.
salicyluric a.
saturated fatty a.
a. secretion rate
a. seromucoid
serum uric a. (SUA)
sialic a.

silicic a.
sodium p-aminohippuric a.
soluble ribonucleic a. (sRNA)
somatic cell deoxyribonucleic a.
(somatic cell DNA)
sorbic a.
stearic a.
cinic a.
a.
sic a.
tic a.
sulfos
sulfur-con
sulfuric a. (SSA)
sulfurous a. mino a.
tannic a.
tartaric a.
taurochenodeoxycholic a.
taurocholic a.
taurodeoxycholic a.
taurolithocholic a.
teichoic a.
ternary a.
tetrahydrofolic a.
thioctic a.
thioglycolic a.
thiolaminopropionic a.
thymidylic a.
a. tide
titratable a. (TA)
toluic a.
total fatty a. (TFA)
tribasic a.
tricarboxylic a. (TCA)
trichloroacetic a.
trichlorophenoxy acetic a.
tuberculostearic a.
tungstic a.
UDP-glucuronic a.
UDP-iduronic a.
uncoded amino a.
unesterified fatty a. (UFA)
uric a. (UA)
uridylic a.
urine alpha hydroxybutyric a.
urine amino a.
urine argininosuccinic a.
urine 2,5-dihydroxyphenylacetic a.
urine homogentisic a.
urine 5-hydroxyindoleacetic a. (urine
5-H1AA)
urine uric a.
urine vanillylmandelic a.
urobenzoic a.
urocanic a.
uronic a.
ursodeoxycholic a. (UDCA)

acid (*continued*)
    vaccenic a.
    valeric a.
    valproic a.
    a. value
    vanillic a.
    vanillylmandelic a. (VM
    vinegar a.
    viral nucleic a.
    a. wave
    xanthurenic a.
    xanthylic a.
acidalbumin
acid-alcohol-forma
    acetic a.-
acidaminiphila *monas* a.
    *Stenotr*as *fermentans*
Acidaminoc
acidami. *rans*
    Dethiosulfovibrio a.
    Thermanaerovibrio a.
    Thermococcus a.
acidaminuria
acid-base
    a.-b. balance
    a.-b. diagram
    a.-b. disorder
    a.-b. indicator
    a.-b. nomogram
    a.-b. ratio (A:B)
acid-citrate-dextrose (ACD)
acid-concanavalin
acidemia
    argininosuccinic a.
    glutaric a.
    hydroxy-3-methylglutaric a.
    lactic a.
    methylmalonic a.
    propionic a.
acid-fast
    a.-f. bacillus (AFB)
    a.-f. bacterium
    a.-f. culture (AFC)
    a.-f. smear
    a.-f. stain
    a.-f. staining histopathology
    a.-f. staining method
acid-forming
Acidianus
acidic
    a. dye
    a. isoferritin
acidifaciens
    Bacteroides a.
acidifiable
acidified
    a. phagolysosome
    a. prelysosomal compartment
    a. serum lysis test

    aceticus
    ry
    microbiaceae
    dimicrobiales
Acidimicrobidae
acidiphilum
    Ferroplasma a.
acidiphilus
    Alicyclobacillus a.
acidipiscis
    Lactobacillus a.
acidisoli
    Clostridium a.
Acidisphaera rubrifaciens
Acidithiobacillus
    A. albertensis
    A. caldus
    A. ferrooxidans
    A. thiooxidans
aciditrophicus
    Syntrophus a.
acidity
    a. reduction test
    total a.
Acidobacteria
Acidobacteriales
acidocyte
acidocytopenia
acidocytosis
acidogenic
acidophil, acidophile
    a. adenoma
    alpha a.
    a. body
    a. cell
    a. granule
acidophile (*var. of* acidophil)
acidophilic
    a. adenoma
    a. body
    a. dye
    a. index
    a. leukocyte
    a. necrosis
    a. normoblast
    a. yolk globule
acidophilum
    Hydrogenobaculum a.
    Thermoplasma a.
acidophilus
    Lactobacillus a.
    a. milk
    Rhodoblastus a.
acidosis
    carbon dioxide a.
    compensated a.
    diabetic a.

D-lactic a.
high anion gap a.
hypercapnic a.
hyperchloremic metabolic a.
hypochloremic metabolic a.
lactic a.
metabolic a.
normal-AG metabolic a.
normal anion gap a.
potassium a.
primary renal tubular a.
renal tubular a. (RTA)
respiratory a.
secondary renal tubular a.
a. test
uncompensated a.
Acidothermaceae
acidotic
acidovorans
Delftia a.
Pseudomonas a.
Acidovorax
A. anthurii
A. valerianellae
acidristocetin
arachidonic a.
acid-Schiff
diastase-periodic a.-S. (D-PAS)
a.-S. stain
acidulated
aciduria
acetoacetic a.
beta-aminoisobutyric a.
glutamic a.
glycolic a.
hereditary orotic a.
l-glyceric a.
methylmalonic a.
orotic a.
propionic a.
xanthurenic a.
aciduric
acificus
Caldanaerobacter subterraneus subsp. a.
acinar
a. adenocarcinoma
a. cell
a. cell carcinoma (ACC)
a. cell tumor
a. lumen
a. pattern
a. unit
Acinetobacter
A. baumannii
A. baylyi
A. bouvetii
A. calcoaceticus
A. calcoaceticus anitratus
A. calcoaceticus lwoffi
A. gerneri
A. grimontii
A. parapertussis
A. parvus
A. pneumonia
A. radioresistens
A. schindleri
A. tandoii
A. tjernbergiae
A. towneri
A. ursingii
acini (*pl. of* acinus)
acinic
a. cell adenocarcinoma
a. cell carcinoma
a. cell tumor
a. cell tumor of lung
aciniform
acinitis
acinose (*var. of* acinous)
a. carcinoma
acinotubular gland
acinous, acinose
a. carcinoma
a. cell
a. gland
acinus, *pl.* **acini**
hepatic a.
liver a.
mucous a.
pulmonary a.
Rappaport a.
secretory a.
serous a.
ACIS
automated cellular imaging system
ACIT
allogeneic cellular immune therapy
ACIT system
ackee, akee
ACL
ACL 100, 1000, 7000, 8000, 9000, 10000 Advance coagulation analyzer
ACL Advance coagulation testing system
ACL 1000 coagulation testing system
ACL Elite coagulation testing system
ACL Top coagulation testing system
ACLA
anticardiolipin antibody
Acladium
aclasis
diaphysial a.
tarsoepiphyseal a.

AcLDL
acetylated low-density lipoprotein
ACM
albumin-calcium-magnesium
aCML
atypical chronic myeloid
leukemia
acne
a. atrophia
a. conglobata
a. rosacea
a. rosacea keratitis
a. vulgaris
acneform (*var. of* acneiform)
acneiform, acneform
acnes
Propionibacterium a.
aconitase
aconitate hydratase
aconitine
Aconitum
aconitus
Anopheles a.
acormus
holoacardius a.
Acosta disease
acoustic
a. cell
a. coupler
a. crest
a. micrograph
a. microscope
a. neurilemmoma
a. neurinoma
a. neuroma
a. papilla
a. schwannoma
a. spot
ACP
acid phosphatase
ACPA
anticytoplasmic antibody
ACPA test
acquired
a. agammaglobulinemia
a. atrophy
a. C1EInh deficiency
a. character
a. defect
a. deformity
a. dysplasia
a. fibrokeratoma
a. genetic factor
a. hemolytic anemia (AHA)
a. hemolytic icterus
a. hepatic porphyria
a. hypogammaglobulinemia
a. ichthyosis
a. immunity

a. immunodeficiency syndrome
(AIDS)
a. leukoderma
a. leukopathia
a. methemoglobinemia
a. nevus
a. qualitative disorders of
platelets
a. renal cystic disease (ARCD)
a. sensitivity
a. sideroblastic anemia
a. tufted angioma
a. von Willebrand disease
acquisita
epidermolysis bullosa a.
hypertrichosis lanuginosa a.
acquisitum
keratoderma a.
acral
a. lentiginous melanoma
a. nevus
acrania
Acrel ganglion
Acremoniella
Acremonium
acridine
a. dye
a. hydrochloride
a. orange (AO)
a. orange method
a. orange stain
tetramethyl a.
a. yellow
acridinium ester
acriflavine
acroasphyxia
acroblast
acrobrachycephaly
acrobystitis
Acrocarpospora
A. corrugata
A. macrocephala
A. pleiomorpha
acrocentric chromosome
acrocephalia (*var. of* acrocephaly)
acrocephalic
acrocephalosyndactylia (*var. of*
acrocephalosyndactyly)
acrocephalosyndactyly,
acrocephalosyndactylia
acrocephalous
acrocephaly, acrocephalia
acrochordon
acrocyanosis
Acrocylindrium
acrodermatitis
a. chronica atrophicans
a. continua
a. enteropathica

a. enteropathy
a. perstans
acrodolichomelia
Acrodontium salmoneum
acroedema
acrofacial
a. dysostosis
a. syndrome
acrogenous
acrokeratoelastoidosis
acrokeratosis verruciformis
acrolein
acromegalia (*var. of* acromegaly)
acromegalic
acromegalogigantism
acromegaloidism
acromegaly, acromegalia
acromelia
acromelic dwarfism
acromesomelia
acromicria
acroosteolysis
acroosteolytica
osteopetrosis a.
acropachy
acropachyderma
acropathy
acropetal
Acrophialophora fusispora
acropleurogenous
acroposthitis
acroscleroderma (*var. of*
acrosclerosis)
acrosclerosis, acroscleroderma
acrosomal
a. cap
a. complex
a. granule
a. vesicle
acrosome
a. granule
a. reaction
acrospiroma
eccrine a.
Acrosporium
acrostealgia
acrosyringium
acroterica
morphea a.
Acrotheca pedrosoi
Acrothesium floccosum
acrotrophoneurosis
acrylamide gel electrophoresis
acrylate
acrylic acid
acrylonitrile
ACS
acute coronary syndrome
American Chemical Society

antireticular cytotoxic serum
ACS grade
ACS 180 SE automated
chemiluminescent immunoassay
system
ACS:180 CK/MB analyzer
ACT
acid clearance test
activated clotting time
activated coagulation time
alpha antichymotrypsin
anticoagulant therapy
act
Bayh-Dole A.
Emergency Medical Treatment and
Labor A. (EMTALA)
Health Insurance Portability and
Accountability A. (HIPAA)
Resource Conservation and Recovery
A.
Ac·T
Ac·T diff, Ac·T diff2 hematology
analyzer
Ac·T 5 diff AL auto loader
hematology analyzer
Ac·T 5 diff CP cap pierce
hematology analyzer
Ac·T 5 diff OV open vial
hematology analyzer
Ac·T series hematology analyzer
Actaea
Actalyke test
ACTH
adrenocorticotropic hormone
ACTH stimulation test
ACTH-producing adenoma
ACTH-RF
adrenocorticotropic hormone-releasing
factor
actin
alpha cardiac a.
alpha skeletal a.
alpha smooth muscle a. (ASMA)
antisarcomeric a.
antismooth muscle a.
a. cytoskeleton
a. distribution
a. filament
monomeric a.
muscle a. (MA)
muscle-specific a. (MSA)
sarcomeric a.
smooth muscle a. (SMA)
actin-filament polymerization
actinic
a. dermatitis
a. keratosis
a. porokeratosis
a. reticuloid

actinide
actinin
    alpha a.
actinium (Ac)
actin-myosin web
Actinoalloteichus cyanogriseus
Actinobacillus
    A. *actinomycetemcomitans*
    A. *arthritidis*
    A. *equuli*
    A. *lignieresii*
    A. *mallei*
    A. *pseudomallei*
Actinobacteria
Actinobacteridae
Actinobaculum urinale
Actinocorallia
    A. *aurantiaca*
    A. *glomerata*
    A. *libanotica*
    A. *longicatena*
actinohematin
actinoides
    Thysanosoma a.
Actinokineospora
    A. *auranticolor*
    A. *enzanensis*
Actinomadura
    A. *africana*
    A. *catellatispora*
    A. *glauciflava*
    A. *latina*
    A. *madurae*
    A. *mexicana*
    A. *meyerae*
    A. *namibiensis*
    A. *pelletieri*
    A. *viridilutea*
Actinomucor
Actinomyces (A)
    A. *bovis*
    A. *canis*
    A. *cardiffensis*
    A. *catuli*
    A. *coleocanis*
    A. *congolensis*
    A. *culture*
    A. *eriksonii*
    A. *funkei*
    A. *hongkongensis*
    A. *israelii*
    Mallory stain for *A.*
    A. *marimammalium*
    A. *muris*
    A. *muris-ratti*
    A. *naeslundii*
    A. *nasicola*
    A. *necrophorus*
    A. *odontolyticus*

A. *oricola*
A. *radicidentis*
A. *rhusiopathiae*
A. *suimastitidis*
A. *urogenitalis*
A. *vaccimaxillae*
A. *vinaceus*
A. *viscosus*
Weigert stain for *A.*
Actinomycetaceae
Actinomycetales
actinomycete
    nocardioform a.
    thermophilic a.
actinomycetemcomitans
    Actinobacillus a.
    Haemophilus a.
actinomycetic
actinomycetin
actinomycetoma
actinomycin
actinomycosis
    genital tract a.
    mammary a.
    oral a.
    pulmonary a.
    thoracic a.
actinomycotic
    a. appendicitis
    a. mycetoma
actinomyoma
Actinomyxidia
actinophage
actinophytosis
Actinoplanaceae
Actinoplanales
Actinoplanes
    A. *capillaceus*
    A. *friuliensis*
Actinopoda
Actinopolymorpha singaporensis
actinosclerus
    Hymenobacter a.
Actinosynnemataceae
action
    buffer a.
    calorigenic a.
    capillary a.
    cumulative a.
    diastasic a.
    law of mass a.
    opsonic a.
    a. potential synaptic
        cleft
    specific dynamic a.
    spectrum a.
    a. spectrum
    thermogenic a.
    vitaminoid a.

activated
- a. charcoal
- a. clotting factor
- a. clotting time (ACT)
- a. coagulation time (ACT)
- a. complex
- a. lymphocyte
- a. macrophage
- a. microglia
- a. partial thromboplastin substitution test
- a. partial thromboplastin time (aPTT, APTT)
- a. protein C (APC)
- a. protein C cofactor (APC cofactor)
- a. protein C resistance (APCR)

activating
- a. agent
- a. enzyme

activation
- allosteric a.
- a. analysis
- B cell a.
- cis a.
- complement a.
- cross a.
- a. energy
- ergoreceptor a.
- lymphocyte a.
- a. of the coagulation pathways
- oncofetal a.
- plasma a.
- trans a.
- very late a. (VLA)
- washed platelet a.

activation-induced cell death (AICD)

activator
- glucokinase a. (GKA)
- plasminogen a.
- polyclonal a.
- a. protein 1 (AP1)
- urokinase plasminogen a. (uPA)

active
- a. anaphylaxis
- a. chronic hepatitis
- a. chronic inflammation
- a. electrode
- endocytotically a.
- a. immunity
- a. immunization
- a. medium
- a. prophylaxis
- a. protein expression
- a. range of motion (AROM)
- a. rosette test
- a. sensitization
- a. total PSA ELISA kit
- a. transport

Activin AB free beta-HCG ELISA test

activity
- altered lipid-peroxidation a.
- antiatherogenic a.
- blood granulocyte-specific a. (BGSA)
- chemotactic a.
- c-kit a.
- Clinician Outreach and Communication A. (COCA)
- colony-stimulating a. (CSA)
- a. determination
- endogenous avidin-binding a. (EABA)
- erythrocyte aspartate aminotransferase a. (eAST)
- gelatinolytic a.
- general gonadotropic a. (GGA)
- a. index
- insertional a.
- insulinlike a. (ILA)
- leukemia-associated inhibitory a. (LIA)
- mean dose per unit cumulated a.
- neutrophil killing a.
- nonsuppressible insulinlike a. (NSILA)
- plasma insulin a. (PIA)
- plasma renin a. (PRA)
- postheparin lipolytic a. (PHLA)
- proliferative a.
- protein tyrosine kinase a.
- a. ratio
- relative specific a. (RSA)
- renal vein renin a. (RVRA)
- rheumatoid factor-like a. (RFLA)
- surface-oriented pinocytic a.
- telomerase a.
- thyroxine-specific a. (T_4SA)
- total antitryptic a. (TAT)
- tryptic a.
- unit of luteinizing a. (international)
- unit of progestational a. (international)
- unit of thyrotrophic a.

actodigin

actomyosin
- a. D
- platelet a.

Actonia

ACTP
- adrenocorticotropic polypeptide

actuate

Acuaria spiralis

aculeate

aculeatum
- stratum a.

acuminata (*pl. of* acuminatum)

acuminate

acuminatum, *pl.* **acuminata**
    condyloma a.
    giant anorectal condyloma a.
    verruca acuminata
acustica
    tuba a.
acustici
    dentes a.
acuta
    pityriasis lichenoides et varioliformis
      a. (PLEVA)
    polyarthritis rheumatica a.
    pustulosis vacciniformis a.
acute
    a. abscess
    a. and chronic inflammation
    a. anterior poliomyelitis
    a. atrophic paralysis
    a. bacterial endocarditis
    a. biphenotypic leukemia
    a. bleed
    a. bronchitis
    a. bronchitis/bronchiolitis (ABB)
    a. bulbar poliomyelitis
    a. cardiovascular disease (ACVD)
    a. cellular rejection
    a. compression triad
    a. contagious conjunctivitis
    a. coronary syndrome (ACS)
    a. crescentic glomerulonephritis
    a. cryptitis
    a. disseminated encephalomyelitis
      (ADEM)
    a. disseminated lupus erythematosus
    a. epidemic conjunctivitis
    a. epidemic infectious adenitis
    a. epidemic leukoencephalitis
    a. erythroleukemia (M6)
    a. exudative glomerulonephritis
    a. fatty liver of pregnancy
    a. febrile jaundice
    a. fibrinous pleuritis
    a. focal hepatitis
    a. follicular conjunctivitis
    a. fulminating meningococcal
      septicemia
    a. fulminating primary amebic
      meningoencephalitis
    a. gangrenous appendicitis
    a. gelatinous pneumonia
    a. glomerulonephritis (AGN)
    a. goiter
    a. graft-versus-host disease
      (aGVHD)
    a. granulocytic leukemia (AGL)
    a. hemolytic transfusion reaction
    a. hemorrhagic bronchopneumonia
    a. hemorrhagic cholecystitis
    a. hemorrhagic cystitis

    a. hemorrhagic encephalitis
    a. hemorrhagic erosive gastritis
    a. hemorrhagic glomerulonephritis
    a. hemorrhagic inflammation
    a. hemorrhagic leukoencephalitis
      (AHLE)
    a. hemorrhagic pancreatitis
    a. hemorrhagic ulceration
    a. humoral rejection
    a. hyperemia
    a. idiopathic polyneuritis
    a. infarct
    a. infectious disease (AID)
    a. infectious nonbacterial
      gastroenteritis
    a. infective endocarditis
    a. inflammatory infiltrate
    a. inflammatory necrosis
    a. inflammatory transudate
    a. intermittent porphyria (AIP)
    a. interstitial nephritis (AIN)
    a. interstitial pneumonia (AIP)
    a. lymphoblastic leukemia (ALL)
    a. lymphoblastic leukemia in older
      children
    a. lymphoblastic leukemia secondary
      to Burkitt lymphoma
    a. lymphocytic leukemia (ALL)
    a. massive liver necrosis
    a. mastitis
    a. megakaryoblastic leukemia
    a. megakaryocytic leukemia (M7)
    a. mesenteric adenitis
    a. miliary tuberculosis
    a. monoblastic leukemia (AMoL)
    a. monocytic leukemia
      (AMoL, M5)
    a. monocytic leukemia with
      differentiation (M5b)
    a. monocytic leukemia without
      differentiation (M5a)
    a. myeloblastic leukemia with
      maturation (M2)
    a. myeloblastic leukemia without
      localized differentiation (M0)
    a. myeloblastic leukemia without
      maturation (M1)
    a. myelocytic leukemia (AML)
    a. myelogenous leukemia
    a. myeloid leukemia (AML)
    a. myelomonocytic leukemia
      (AMML, M4)
    a. myocardial infarction (AMI)
    a. necrotizing encephalitis
    a. necrotizing enterocolitis
    a. necrotizing hemorrhagic
      encephalomyelitis
    a. necrotizing myelitis
    a. necrotizing ulcerative gingivitis

a. necrotizing ulcerative tonsillitis
a. nephrosis
a. nonlymphocytic leukemia (ANLL)
a. normovolemic hemodilution (ANH)
otitis media, purulent, a. (OMPA)
a. parenchymatous hepatitis
a. paroxysmal myoglobinuria
a. phase protein
a. phase reactant (APR)
a. phase reaction
A. Physiology and Chronic Health Evaluation (APACHE)
a. posthemorrhagic anemia
a. poststreptococcal glomerulonephritis
a. primary hemorrhagic meningoencephalitis
a. proliferative
a. proliferative glomerulonephritis
a. promyelocytic leukemia (APL)
a. pulmonary alveolitis
a. pyelonephritis
a. radiation syndrome (ARS)
a. recurrent rhabdomyolysis
a. renal failure (ARF)
a. respiratory disease
a. respiratory distress syndrome (ARDS)
a. respiratory failure (ARF)
a. rheumatic arthritis
a. rheumatic fever (ARF)
a. rhinitis
a. rickets
a. salivary adenitis
a. self-limited hemolytic anemia
a. serous synovitis
a. splenic tumor
a. splenitis
a. suppurative appendicitis
a. suppurative lymphadenitis
a. thyroiditis
a. transverse myelitis
a. tubular necrosis (ATN)
a. ulcerative colitis
a. undifferentiated leukemia (AUL)
a. urethral syndrome
a. uric acid nephropathy
a. vascular rejection
a. viral hepatitis (AVH)
a. yellow atrophy
acutum
ulcus vulvae a.
ACVD
acute cardiovascular disease
acyl
a. carrier protein
a. coenzyme A (acyl-CoA)

a. enzyme
a. peroxide
acylation
acyl-CoA
acyl coenzyme A
a. acyltransferase (ACAT)
a. dehydrogenase
a. desaturase
a. synthetase
acyloxy group
acylsphingosine deacylase
acyltransferase
acetyl-CoA a.
acyl-CoA a. (ACAT)
cholesterol a.
lecithin-cholesterol a. (LCAT)
ADA
adenosine deaminase
ADA deficiency
adactylia (*var. of* adactyly)
adactyly, adactylia
Adair-Dighton syndrome
ADAM
a disintegrin and metalloprotease
ADAM protein
1-adamantanamine sulfate
adamantina
prismata a.
substantia a.
adamantine prism
adamantinoma
a. of long bones
pituitary a.
adamantoblast
Adamkiewicz test
adamsite
Adams-Stokes (AS)
A.-S. attack (ASA)
A.-S. disease
ADAMTS 13
a disintegrin and metalloproteinase with thrombospodin domain 13
ADAMTS 13 protein
Adansonia
adaptation
cellular a.
enzymatic a.
genetic a.
adapter, adaptor
adaptive
a. enzyme
a. hormone
a. hypertrophy
a. immunity
adaptor (*var. of* adapter)
AD7C Alzheimer test
ADCC reaction
antibody-dependent cell-mediated cytotoxicity

ADD1
    adipocyte determination and
       differentiation factor 1
Addis
    A. count
    A. test
Addison
    A. anemia
    A. disease
    A. keloid
Addison-Biermer disease
addisonia
    encephalopathia a.
addisonian
    a. anemia
    a. crisis
    a. syndrome
addisonism
addition
    binary a.
    a. polymer
    a. reaction
addition-deletion mutation
additive
    POES a.
addressin
    vascular a.
addressing
    indirect a.
    a. ligand
adducin gene
adduct removal
adecarboxylata
    Escherichia a.
adelomorphic
adelomorphous
ADEM
    acute disseminated encephalomyelitis
adendric (*var. of* adendritic)
adendritic, adendric
adenectopia
Aden fever
adenine (A)
    a. arabinoside
    a. deaminase
adenine-thymine/guanine-cytosine ratio
adeninivorans
    Arxula a.
adenitis
    acute epidemic infectious a.
    acute mesenteric a.
    acute salivary a.
    cervical a.
    mesenteric a.
    a. tropicalis
adenoacanthoma
adenoameloblastoma
adeno-associated virus (AAV)
adenoblast

adenocarcinoma (AC, ACA)
    acinar a.
    acinic cell a.
    alveolar a.
    anaplastic a.
    Barrett a. (BCA)
    Barrett-associated a.
    bronchial gland cell a.
    bronchial surface cell a.
    bronchiolar a.
    bronchioloalveolar a.
    Clara cell a.
    clear cell a.
    colloid a.
    dedifferentiated low-grade a.
    endometrial a.
    enteric-type a.
    fetal a.
    follicular and papillary a.
    fungating a.
    gelatinous a.
    goblet cell a.
    Hürthle cell a.
    indeterminate cell a.
    infiltrating duct a.
    inflammatory a.
    a. in situ (AIS)
    lobular a.
    Lucké a.
    medullary a.
    mesonephric a.
    metastatic a. (MA)
    mucinous a.
    mucoid a.
    nonmucinous a.
    a. of Moll
    oxyphilic endometrioid a.
    a. phenotype
    polymorphous low-grade a. (PLGA)
    polypoid a.
    por1 a.
    por2 a.
    prostatic a. (PCA)
    renal a.
    scirrhous a.
    sebaceous a.
    signet ring a.
    solid a.
    sweat gland a.
    terminal duct a.
    trabecular a.
    tub1 a.
    tub2 a.
    tubular a.
    type II alveolar epithelial cell a.
    undifferentiated a.
    vaginal clear cell a.
    villoglandular a. (VGA)
    well-differentiated fetal a. (WDFA)

adenocarinoma
adenocellulitis
adenochondroma
adenocystic carcinoma
adenocystoma lymphomatosum
adenocyte
adenodiastasis
adenoepithelioma
adenofibroma
    metanephric a. (MAF)
adenofibromyoma
adenofibrosis
adenohypophyseal (*var. of*
  adenohypophysial)
adenohypophyseos
adenohypophysial, adenohypophyseal
    a. hormone
adenohypophysis
adenohypophysitis
    lymphocytic a.
adenoid (adn)
    a. cystic carcinoma (ACC)
    a. face
    a. facies
    a. hyperplasia
    a. hypertrophy
    a. squamous cell carcinoma
    a. tissue
    a. tumor
adenoidal-pharyngeal-conjunctival (A-P-C,
APC)
adenoleiomyofibroma
adenolipoma
adenolipomatosis
    symmetric a.
adenolymphocele
adenolymphoma
adenolysis
adenoma (A), *pl.* **adenomas, adenomata**
    acidophil a.
    acidophilic a.
    ACTH-producing a.
    adnexal a.
    adrenal cortical a.
    adrenocortical a.
    adrenocorticotropic hormone-
      producing a.
    aldosterone-producing a. (APA)
    angioinvasive a.
    apocrine a.
    basal cell a.
    basophil a.
    bile duct a.
    black thyroid a.
    bronchial a.
    canalicular a.
    carcinoma ex pleomorphic a.
    ceruminous a.
    chief cell a.

chromophil a.
chromophobe a.
chromophobic a.
clear cell a.
colloid a.
corticotrope a.
depressed a.
diploid a.
ductal a.
embryonal a.
eosinophil a.
fetal a.
fibroid a.
a. fibrosum
follicular a.
Fuchs a.
gastric tubular a.
gonadotrope a.
gonadotropin-producing a.
growth hormone-producing a.
hepatic a.
hepatocellular a. (HCA)
Hürthle cell a.
islet cell a.
lactating a.
lactotrope a.
Leydig cell a.
liver cell a.
macrofollicular a.
malignant a.
mammosomatotropic a.
metanephric a.
microfollicular a.
middle ear a.
monomorphic a. (MA)
mucinous a.
multiple a.
multiploid a.
nephrogenic a.
neuroendocrine-type feature in
  adrenal cortical a.
nipple a.
null cell a.
oncocytic a.
ovarian tubular a.
oxyphil a.
pituitary a.
pleomorphic a. (PA)
Plummer a.
plurihormonal a.
polypoid a.
primary pulmonary a. (PPA)
prolactin-producing a.
prostatic a.
renal cortical a.
sebaceous a.
a. sebaceum
serrated a.
sessile serrated a.

adenoma (*continued*)
    somatotroph a.
    somatotropic a.
    sweat duct a.
    sweat gland a.
    syringomatous a.
    testicular tubular a.
    thyroid a.
    thyrotrope a.
    thyrotroph cell a.
    thyrotropin-producing a.
    toxic a.
    trabecular a.
    tubovillous a.
    tubular a.
    undifferentiated cell a.
    villous a.
adenomas (*pl. of* adenoma)
adenomata (*pl. of* adenoma)
adenomatoid
    a. cystic papillary nodule
    a. odontogenic tumor
adenomatosis
    endocrine a.
    fibrosing a.
    multiple endocrine a.
     (MEA)
    pluriglandular a.
    polyendocrine a.
    pulmonary a.
adenomatous
    a. crypt
    a. epithelium
    a. goiter
    a. hyperplasia
    a. polyp
    a. polyposis coli (APC)
adenomere
adenomyoepithelial adenosis
adenomyoepithelioma
adenomyofibroma
    atypical polypoid a. (APA)
adenomyoma
    atypical polypoid a. (APA)
adenomyosarcoma
adenomyosis uteri
adenopathy (ADP)
adenophlegmon
Adenophorasida
Adenophorea
adenophyma
adenosalpingitis
adenosarcoma
    metanephric a.
    müllerian a.
adenosatellite virus
adenosine
    a. 3′,5′-cyclic monophosphate
     (cAMP)

    a. 3′,5′-cyclic phosphate (cAMP)
    a. deaminase (ADA)
    a. deaminase assay
    a. deaminase deficiency
    a. 5′-diphosphate (ADP)
    a. diphosphate
    a. 5′-diphosphate/adenosine
     triphosphate (ADP/ATP)
    a. 5′-diphosphate/adenosine
     triphosphate ratio
    a. kinase
    a. monophosphate (AMP)
    a. triphosphatase (ATPase)
    a. triphosphate (ATP)
adenosis
    adenomyoepithelial a.
    apocrine a.
    blunt duct a.
    fibrosing a.
    florid a.
    microglandular a.
    nodular a.
    sclerosing polycystic a.
    sclerosis a.
    secretory a.
    simple a.
    tubular a.
    vaginal a.
adenosquamous cell carcinoma
 (ADSQC)
adenotonsillar
adenoviral transduction
Adenoviridae
adenovirus
    alpha antigen of a.
    beta antigen of a.
    canine a. 1
    a. culture
    a. immunofluorescence
    porcine a.
    a. test kit
adenylate
    a. cyclase
    a. deaminase
    a. kinase
    a. kinase deficiency
adenyl cyclase
adenylic
    a. acid
    a. acid deaminase
adenylosuccinate lyase
adenylpyrophosphatase
adenylylation
adenylyl transferase
Adeza TLi fetal fibronectin analysis
 system
ADH
    alcohol dehydrogenase
    antidiuretic hormone

atypical ductal hyperplasia
    ADH assay
    ADH deficiency
adhaerens
    Hyphomonas a.
adherence
    bacterial a.
    immune a.
    Treponema pallidum immobilization
    (immune) a. (TPIA)
adherens
    fascia a.
    a. junction-associated catenin
    macula a.
    zonula a.
adherent
    a. pericarditis
    a. pericardium
    a. plug
adhering junction
adhesin
adhesiolysis
adhesion
    amniotic a.
    a. assay
    fibrinous a.
    fibrous a.
    intraabdominal a.
    joint a.
    a. molecule
    pelvic a.
    a. phenomenon
    plaque a.
    sublabial a.
    a. test
    wispy a.
adhesive
    albumin slide a.
    a. arachnoiditis
    a. capsulitis
    a. chronic pachymeningitis
    a. extracellular domain
    gelatin slide a.
    a. inflammation
    a. pericarditis
    a. peritonitis
    a. phlebitis
    a. pleurisy
    a. vaginitis
adiacens
    Granulicatella a.
adiadochokinesia
Adiantum
adiaspiromycosis
adiaspirosis
adiaspore
Adie
    A. pupil
    A. syndrome

Adinida
adiphenine hydrochloride
adipic
adipica
    Desulfovirga a.
adipocele
adipocellular
adipoceratous
adipocere
adipocyte
    a. determination and differentiation
    factor 1 (ADD1)
    a. differentiation
    mature a.
    necrotic a.
adipocytic neoplasm
adipoid
adipokinesis
adipokinetic hormone
adipolysis
adipolytic
adiponecrosis
adipose
    a. capsule
    a. cell
    a. degeneration
    a. fossa
    a. infiltration
    a. tissue
    a. tissue extract
    a. tumor
adiposis
    a. cardiaca
    a. cerebralis
    a. dolorosa
    a. hepatica
    a. orchica
    a. tuberosa
      simplex
    a. universalis
adiposity
adiposogenital dystrophy
adiposum
    cor a.
    sclerema a.
adiposuria
adiposus
    ascites a.
aditus
adjunct
    anesthesia a.
adjuvant
    a. chemotherapy
    Freund complete a.
    Freund incomplete a.
    mycobacterial a.
    a. vaccine
Adler test
admaxillary gland

administration
>Health Resources and Services A. (HRSA)
>Occupational Safety and Health A. (OSHA)

admix

admixture

ADN-B
>antideoxyribonuclease B
>ADN-B assay

adnexal
>a. adenoma
>a. carcinoma
>a. neoplasm

adnexitis

ADO2
>autosomal dominant osteopetrosis type 2

adolescent
>a. albuminuria
>a. round back

adolescentium
>apophysitis tibialis a.

adoptive
>a. immunity
>a. immunotherapy

ADP
>adenosine 5′-diphosphate

ADP/ATP
>adenosine 5′-diphosphate/adenosine triphosphate

adrenal
>accessory a.
>androgen-secreting a.
>a. antibody
>a. ascorbic acid depletion test
>a. body
>a. cancer
>a. capsule
>a. cortex
>a. cortex cell
>a. cortical adenoma
>a. cortical hyperplasia
>a. crisis
>a. disease
>a. epithelioid angiosarcoma
>a. failure
>feminization syndrome, a.
>a. feminizing syndrome
>a. function test
>a. gland
>a. gland virilizing syndrome
>a. hypofunction
>a. insufficiency
>Marchand a.
>a. medulla
>a. neoplasm
>a. rest

adrenalectomized

adrenaline test

adrenalitis

adrenalopathy

adrenarche
>delayed a.
>precocious a.

adrenergic
>a. neuron blockade
>a. neuron blocking agent

adrenochrome

adrenocortical
>a. adenoma
>a. carcinoma
>a. extract (ACE)
>a. hormone (ACH)
>a. hyperplasia
>a. inhibition test
>a. insufficiency
>a. rest tumor

adrenocorticosteroid

adrenocorticotrophic (*var. of* adrenocorticotropic)

adrenocorticotropic, adrenocorticotrophic
>a. cell
>a. hormone (ACTH)
>a. hormone assay
>a. hormone-producing adenoma
>a. hormone-releasing factor (ACTH-RF)
>a. hormone suppression test
>a. polypeptide (ACTP)

adrenocorticotropin

adrenodoxin

adrenogenital syndrome (AGS)

adrenoleukodystrophy (ALD)

adrenomedullary
>a. catecholamine
>a. hormone
>a. triad

adrenomegaly

adrenomyeloneuropathy

adrenopathy

adrenoreceptor

ADS
>antibody deficiency syndrome
>antidiuretic substance
>autonomous detection system

adsorb

adsorbate

adsorbed plasma

adsorbent
>gastrointestinal a.

adsorption
>agglutinin a.
>chemical a.

a. tumor
a. virilism
a. virilization

a. chromatography
immune a.
ADSQC
adenosquamous cell carcinoma
adult
a. celiac disease
a. cystic teratoma
a. gonococcal conjunctivitis
a. granulosa cell tumor (AGCT)
a. hemoglobin
a. medulloepithelioma
a. polycystic kidney disease
a. respiratory distress syndrome
(ARDS)
a. rickets
a. stem cell
a. stem cell plasticity
a. T-cell leukemia/lymphoma (ATLL)
a. T-cell lymphoma (ATL)
a. T-cell lymphoma/leukemia
a. thymectomy
a. tuberculosis
adulteration
adult-onset diabetes
adultorum
blennorrhea a.
scleredema a.
adult-type xanthogranuloma
advanced
a. breast biopsy instrumentation
(ABBI)
a. glycation end product (AGE)
A. Instruments conductivity analyzer
adventitia
aortic tunica a.
membrana a.
tunica a.
adventitial
a. dermis
a. neuritis
a. reticular cell
adventitious
a. albuminuria
a. cyst
Advia
A. 60, 120 automated cell counting
instrument
A. Centaur anti-HBs calibrator
A. Centaur anti-HBs reagent
A. Centaur HBc IgM control
material
A. Centaur HBc IgM reagent
A. Centaur HBc Total immunoassay
A. 1650 chemistry analyzer
A. 120 hematology system
advice
against medical a. (AMA)
adynamia
hereditary a.

adynamic ileus
AE
antitoxin Einheit
AE1
anion exchanger 1
AE1 antibody
AE1 immunoperoxidase stain
AE1 plus CAM
AE3
AE3 antibody
AE1:AE3 antibody ratio
AEC
3-amino-9-ethylcarbazole
5-amino-9-ethylcarbazole
AEC chromogen
AEC detection system
Aedes
A. aegypti
A. albopictus
A. atlanticus
A. cinereus
A. dorsalis
A. flavescens
A. leucocelaenus
A. melanimon
A. mitchellae
A. nigromaculis
A. polynesiensis
A. scutellaris pseudoscutellaris
A. sollicitans
A. spencerii
A. taeniorhynchus
A. triseriatus
A. trivittatus
A. variegatus
A. vexans
aegaeus
Thermococcus a.
aegypti
Aedes a.
aegyptia
Natrialba a.
Nocardiopsis a.
aegyptiaca
Hirudo a.
aegyptius
Haemophilus a.
Thermicanus a.
Aelurostrongylus
AEM
analytical electron microscope
aeolius
Bacillus a.
AEq
age equivalent
aequorin recombinant method
Aequorivita
A. antarctica
A. crocea

Aequorivita (*continued*)
    A. lipolytica
    A. sublithincola
AER
    albumin excretion rate
    aldosterone excretion rate
aerated
aeration
aeria
    Rothia a.
aerial mycelium
aeriphila
    Aeriscardovia a.
Aeriscardovia aeriphila
aerivorans
    Sporomusa a.
Aerobacter
    A. aerogenes
    A. cloacae
    A. liquefaciens
    A. subgroup A, B, C
aerobe
    obligate a.
aerobic
    a. and anaerobic blood
      culture
    a. bacterium
    a. coccobacillus
    a. diphtheroid
    a. metabolism
    a. respiration
aerobiological property
aerobiology
aerobiosis
aerobiotic
aerocele
Aerococcus
    A. urinaehominis
    A. viridans
aerodermectasia
aeroembolism
aerofaciens
    Collinsella a.
    Eubacterium a.
aerogen
aerogenes
    Aerobacter a.
    Enterobacter a.
    Vibrio a.
aerogenesis
aerogenic, aerogenous,
  aerogenous
aerogenoides
aerogenosum
    sputum a.
aerogenous (*var. of* aerogenic)
aerolata
    Promicromonospora a.
    Sphingomonas a.

Aeromicrobium marinum
Aeromonadaceae
Aeromonas
    A. culicicola
    A. hydrophila
    A. hydrophila subsp. *dhakensis*
    A. hydrophila subsp. *ranae*
    A. liquefaciens
    A. (*Plesiomonas*) *shigelloides*
    A. punctata
    A. salmonicida
    A. salmonicida subsp. *pectinolytica*
    A. simiae
    A. sobria
aerophil, aerophile
aerophila
    Caldilinea a.
aerophile (*var. of* aerophil)
aerophilic, aerophilous
aerophilous (*var. of* aerophilic)
aerophilum
    Thialkalimicrobium a.
aerophilus
    Hymenobacter a.
    Thominx a.
aeroplankton
Aeropyrum camini
Aeroset
    A. abused drugs/toxicology test
    A. chemical analyzer
    A. clinical chemistry system
aerosis
aerosol
    a. generator
    lethal anthrax a.
    plague a.
    racemic a.
    A. Resistant Tips (ART)
aerosolization
    secondary a.
aerosolized plague weapon
Aerospray
    A. acid-fast bacteria slide
      stainer/cytocentrifuge
    A. cytocentrifuge
    A. hematology slide
      stainer/cytocentrifuge
aerotaxis
aerotitis media
aerotolerant
aerotonometer
aerotropism
aertrycke
    Bacillus a.
aeruginosa
    Microcystis a.
    Pseudomonas a.
aeschlimannii
    Rickettsia a.

Aessosporon
aestivale
 hydroa a.
aestivalis
 prurigo a.
aestivoautumnal fever
aestuarianus
 Vibrio a.
aestuarii
 Nitrosomonas a.
Aestuariibacter
 A. halophilus
 A. salexigens
AET
 aminoethylisothiouronium
 bromide
aetherivorans
 Rhodococcus a.
aethiopica
 Leishmania a.
aethiopicum
 Plasmodium a.
AF
 aldehyde fuchsin
AFA
 alcohol-formaldehyde-acetic
 acid
 AFA fixative
AFB
 acid-fast bacillus
 AFB smear
 AFB stain
AFC
 acid-fast culture
afebrile abortion
affected
afferens
 vas a.
affinis
 Shewanella a.
affinity
 a. antibody
 a. chromatography
 a. constant
 functional a.
 a. label
 A. multimode plate
 reader
 a. purified
 selective a.
 testosterone-binding a.
 (TBA)
Affymetrix
 A. GeneChip HU'95 array
 A. GeneChip system
 A. human cancer chip
 A. U133A oligonucleotide
 microarray
afibrillar cementum

afibrinogenemia
 congenital a.
AFIP
 Armed Forces Institute of
 Pathology
Afipia
 A. birgiae
 A. felis
 A. massiliensis
aflatoxicosis
aflatoxin B
AFLH
AFM
 atomic force microscopy
AFP
 alpha fetoprotein
 AFP test
africae
 Rickettsia a.
African
 A. hemorrhagic fever
 A. histoplasmosis
 A. horse sickness
 A. horse sickness virus
 A. sleeping sickness
 A. swine fever
 A. swine fever virus
 A. tick-borne fever
 A. trypanosomiasis
africana
 Actinomadura a.
 Nocardia a.
 Taenia a.
africanum
 Mycobacterium a.
africanus
 Streptomyces a.
aftercataract
afterchroming
aftergilding
afterload-reducing drug
aftosa
AFX
 atypical fibroxanthoma
afzelii
 Borrelia a.
A:G
 albumin-globulin
Ag
 antigen
 silver
AGA
 appropriate for gestational
 age
against medical advice (AMA)
agalactiae
 Streptococcus a.
agamete
agamic, agamous

agammaglobulinemia
    acquired a.
    Bruton type a.
    Bruton X-linked a.
    congenital a.
    primary a.
    secondary a.
    Swiss-type a.
    transient a.
    X-linked a. (XLΛ)
agamocytogeny
Agamodistomum ophthalmobium
Agamofilaria
agamogenesis
agamogenetic
agamogony
Agamomermis culicis
Agamonema
Agamonematodum migrans
agamont
agamous (*var. of* agamic)
aganglionic megacolon
aganglionosis
    congenital a.
    total colonic a. (TCA)
    zonal a.

agar
    a. agar
    ascitic a.
    bacteriostasis a.
    a. bead
    bile esculin a.
    bile salt a.
    birdseed a.
    bismuth-sulfite a. (BSA)
    blood a.
    Bordet-Gengou potato blood a.
    brain-heart infusion a.
    brilliant green bile salt a.
    Brucella a.
    Campylobacter selective a.
    casein a.
    CB a.
    cefsulodin-Irgasan-novobiocin a.
    cetrimide a.
    charcoal yeast extract a.
    chocolate blood a.
    Christensen urea a.
    CIN a.
    citrate a.
    clostrisel a.
    Columbia blood a.
    cornmeal a.
    a. cutter
    cycloserine cefoxitin fructose a.
    cycloserine mannitol a.
    cystine trypticase a.
    Czapek-Dox a.
    Czapek solution a.

    deep a.
    deoxycholate-citrate a. (DCA)
    deoxyribonuclease a.
    dextrose a.
    a. diffusion method
    DNase a.
    egg-yolk a.
    EMB Levine a.
    Emmon modification of Sabouraud
      dextrose a.
    Endo a.
    French proof a.
    GC a.
    gelatin a.
    a. gel electrophoresis
    heart infusion a.
    Hektoen enteric a.
    inhibitory mold a.
    Kliger iron a. (KIA)
    Krumwiede triple sugar a.
    laked blood a.
    Levine EMB a.
    Löffler serum a.
    Lowenstein-Jensen a.
    lysine-iron a.
    MacConkey a.
    malt a.
    Martin-Lester a.
    Middlebrook a.
    modified TM a.
    Mueller-Hinton a.
    mycobiotic a.
    Mycoplasma a.
    neomycin assay a.
    nitrate a.
    nutrient a.
    nystatin assay a.
    oatmeal-tomato paste a.
    a. plate count
    polymyxin test a.
    potato-blood a.
    potato dextrose a.
    Pseudomonas selective a.
    rabbit blood a.
    rice-Tween a.
    Russell double-sugar a.
    Sabhi a.
    Sabouraud dextrose and brain heart
      infusion a.
    saccharose-mannitol a.
    Salmonella-Shigella a.
    Schaedler blood a.
    seed a.
    serum a.
    sheep blood a.
    Simmons citrate a.
    standard method a.
    sulfite a.
    TCBS a.

tellurite glycine a.
Thayer-Martin a.
thistle seed a.
Trichophyton a.
triple sugar iron a.
trypticase soy a. (TSA)
tryptic soy a.
TSI a.
urea a.
Wilkins-Chilgren a.
XLD a.
yeast extract a.
Zein a.

Agarbacterium
agarexedens
    Paenibacillus a.
agaric
    a. acid
    deadly a.
    fly a.
Agaricus
agaridevorans
    Paenibacillus a.
Agar-IF
agariperforans
    Reibachia a.
agarivorans
    A. albus
    Pseudoalteromonas a.
    Vibrio a.
agarose gel electrophoresis
Ag-AS
    silver-acidified serum
    Ag-AS stain
agassizii
    Mycoplasma a.
AGC
    absolute granulocyte count
AGCT
    adult granulosa cell tumor
AGE
    advanced glycation end product
age
    appropriate for gestational a. (AGA)
    bone a.
    chronological a. (CA)
    a. equivalent (AEq)
    gestational a. (GA)
    maternal a. (MA)
age-adjusted rate
aged serum
ageing (hippocampal region, patients over 75 years), tau pathology class I
agency
    Environmental Protection A. (EPA)
    A. for Toxic Substances Disease
      Registry (ATSDR)
agenesis
    cerebellar a.

gonadal a.
ovarian a.
pure red cell a.
renal a.
testicular a.
thymic a.
unilateral renal a.

agent
A. 15
activating a.
adrenergic neuron blocking a.
airborne a.
alkylating a.
androgenic anabolic a. (AAA)
antibacterial a.
antifungal a.
antiretroviral a.
antiviral a.
bacteriostatic a.
beta-adrenergic blocking a.
biological alkylating a.
Bittner a.
blister a.
blocking a.
blood a.
calmative a.
category A, B, C a.
caudalizing a.
CDC Category A biological a.'s
  (the highest risk)
CDC Category B biological a.'s
  (next highest risk)
CDC Category C biological a.'s
  (third highest risk)
CDC category of biological a.
chelating a.
chemical a.
chimpanzee coryza a. (CCA)
choking a.
cholinergic blocking a.
convulsant antidote for nerve a.
  (CANA)
Coulter Clenz cleaning a.
CW a.
delta a.
disclosing a.
droplet-borne a.
drying a.
Eaton a.
embedding a.
etiologic a.
F a.
fertility a.
fluid-borne a.
foamy a.
G a.
ganglionic blocking a. (GBA)
gonadotropin-releasing a. (GRA)
Gordon a.

agent (*continued*)
    Hawaii a.
    iatrogenic a.
    immunomodulatory a.
    incapacitating chemical a.
    infectious a.
    initiating a.
    injurious a.
    a. in question
    lysing a.
    Marburg a.
    Marcy a.
    mechanical a.
    military nerve a.
    mobilizing a.
    MS-1 a.
    MS-2 a.
    NATO code for an extremely toxic persistent nerve a. (no common chemical name)
    NATO code for nonpersistent nerve a.
    NATO code for persistent nerve a.
    natriuretic a.
    nerve a.
    nitrosourea a.
    nonpersistent a.
    Norwalk a.
    oxidizing a.
    Pittsburgh pneumonia a.
    progestational a.
    promoting a.
    pulmonary a.
    radiological a.
    reducing a.
    reovirus-like a.
    riot control a.
    splatter-borne a.
    a., state, body site, effects, severity, time course, other (diagnoses), synergism (ASBESTOS)
    surface-active a.
    thermo a.
    thrombolytic a.
    tocolytic a.
    toxic chemical a.
    transforming a.
    urticating a.
    V a.
    vacuolating a.
    vesicating a.
    virus-inactivating a. (VIA)
    volatile nerve a.
    vomiting a.
    wetting a.
age-specific rate
agglomerans
    Enterobacter a.
agglomerate, agglomerated

agglomerated (*var. of* agglomerate)
agglomeration
agglutinable
agglutinant
agglutinate
agglutinating antibody
agglutination
    acid a.
    alpha a.
    bacterial a. (BA)
    bacteriogenic a.
    beta a.
    chick-cell a. (CCA)
    cold a.
    cross a.
    direct a.
    false a.
    febrile a.
    flagellar a.
    group a.
    H a.
    immune a.
    a. immunoassay
    indirect a.
    a. inhibition assay
    intravascular a.
    latex a. (LA)
    macroscopic a.
    mediate a.
    microscopic a.
    mixed a.
    nonimmune a.
    O a.
    platelet a.
    reverse a.
    reverse passive latex a. (RPLA)
    salt a.
    slide latex a. (SLA)
    spontaneous a.
    T a.
    a. test
    a. titer
    Treponema pallidum a. (TPA)
    tube a. (TA)
    Vi a.
    warm a.
agglutinative thrombus
agglutinator
    rheumatoid a.
agglutinin
    a. adsorption
    alpha a.
    anti-A a.
    anti-B a.
    anti-M a.
    anti-N a.
    anti-P a.
    anti-Rh a.
    anti-S a.

beta a.
blood group a.
brucellosis a.
chief a.
cold a.
cross-reacting a.
febrile a.
flagellar a.
group a.
H a.
heterophil a.
immune a.
incomplete a.
latex a.
lectin Ulex europaeus a. I
leukocyte a.
major a.
Mg a.
minor a.
natural a.
O a.
plant a.
platelet a.
Rh a.
saline a.
salmonella a.
serum a.
somatic a.
tularemia a.
Ulex europaeus a.
warm a.
Weil-Felix a.
wheat germ a. (WGA)
agglutinogen
blood group a.
T a.
agglutinogenic, agglutogenic
agglutinophilic
agglutinoscope
agglutogen
agglutogenic (*var. of* agglutinogenic)
aggregans
Eubacterium a.
aggregate
a. anaphylaxis
cytoplasmic crystalline a.
cytoplasmic lipid a.
cytoplasmic macromolecule a.
extracellular lipid a.
extracellular macromolecule a.
a. gland
insoluble complement-bound a.
lymphoid a.
lymphoreticular a.
nuclear crystalline a.
nuclear lipid a.
proteoglycan a.
sheetlike a.
transmural lymphoid a.

tubular a.
tubuloreticular a.
aggregated
a. albumin
a. human immunoglobulin G
(AHuG)
a. lymphatic nodule
a. microsphere
aggregati
folliculi lymphatici a.
aggregation
cell a.
mitochondrial a.
platelet a.
aggregometer
aggregometry
turbidimetric a.
aggresome
aggressin
aggressive
a. angiomyxoma
a. follicular variant
a. infantile fibromatosis
a. thyroid carcinoma (ATC)
agitata
Dechloromonas a.
AGL
acute granulocytic leukemia
aglandular
aglobuliosis
aglobulism
aglomerular
aglutition
aglycemia
aglycogenosis
aglycone
aglycosuria
aglycosuric
agmen peyerianum
agminate, agminated
a. gland
a. nevus
agminated (*var. of* agminate)
agmination
AGN
acute glomerulonephritis
agnathus
agnogenic myeloid metaplasia
AgNOR
argyrophilic nucleolar organizer region
silver-stained nucleolar organizer region
silver-stained nucleolar organizing
region
AgNOR banding
AgNOR method
agona
Salmonella enteritidis serotype *a.*
agonadal
agonadism

agonal
>   a. leukocytosis
>   a. thrombosis
>   a. thrombus

agonist
>   calcium channel a.
>   KOR a.
>   NMDA receptor a.

agonist-induced activation of PLA2

agranular
>   a. cell
>   a. cortex
>   a. endoplasmic reticulum
>   (AER)
>   a. leukocyte

agranulocyte

agranulocytic angina

agranulocytosis
>   feline a.
>   Kostmann a.

agranuloplasia

agranuloplastic

agreement
>   level of a.

Agreia
>   *A. bicolorata*
>   *A. pratensis*

agretope

agria
>   prurigo a.

agricultural terrorism

agrin proteoglycan

Agrobacterium
>   *A. larrymoorei*
>   *A. meteori*

Agrococcus baldri

Agrocybe

Agromyces
>   *A. albus*
>   *A. aurantiacus*
>   *A. bracchium*
>   *A. hippuratus*
>   *A. luteolus*
>   *A. rhizospherae*

agroterrorist
>   a. attack
>   a. event

AGS
>   adrenogenital syndrome

AGT
>   antiglobulin test

ague

AGUS
>   atypical glandular cell of undetermined
>   significance
>   atypical glandular cell of unknown
>   significance

AGV
>   aniline gentian violet

aGVHD
>   acute graft-versus-host disease

agyria

agyric

AH
>   antihyaluronidase
>   AH assay
>   AH titer

AHA
>   acquired hemolytic anemia
>   autoimmune hemolytic anemia

ahangari
>   *Geoglobus a.*

ahaptoglobinemia
>   congenital a.

ahaustral

AHBC
>   hepatitis B core antibody

AHD
>   arteriosclerotic heart disease
>   atherosclerotic heart disease

AHF
>   antihemophilic factor

AHG
>   antihemophilic globulin
>   antihuman globulin
>   AHG factor

AHH
>   analog of histidine

AHLE
>   acute hemorrhagic leukoencephalitis

AHLS
>   antihuman lymphocyte serum

Ahrensia kielensis

A-HRP

AHT
>   antihyaluronidase titer
>   augmented histamine test

AHuG
>   aggregated human
>   immunoglobulin G

Ahumada-Del Castillo syndrome

A549 human lung carcinoma cell

AI
>   aortic incompetence

Aicardi syndrome

AICD
>   activation-induced cell death

aichiensis
>   *Gordonia a.*

AID
>   acute infectious disease

aid
>   cryostat frozen sectioning a.

AIDS
>   acquired immunodeficiency syndrome
>   AIDS serology

AIDS-KS
>   AIDS-related Kaposi sarcoma

AIDS-related
>AIDS-r. complex (ARC)
>AIDS-r. Kaposi sarcoma (AIDS-KS)
>AIDS-r. virus (ARV)

AIH
>artificial insemination homologous
>autoimmune hepatitis

AIHA
>autoimmune hemolytic anemia

AIL
>angiocentric immunoproliferative lesion
>angioimmunoblastic lymphoma
>angioimmunoblastic T-cell lymphoma
>angioimmunoproliferative lesion

AILD
>angioimmunoblastic lymphadenopathy
>with dysproteinemia

AIN
>acute interstitial nephritis
>allergic interstitial nephritis

ainhum

AIO
>amyloid of immunoglobulin origin

AIP
>acute intermittent porphyria
>acute interstitial pneumonia
>automated immunoprecipitation

AIPC
>androgen independent prostate cancer

air
>alveolar a.
>a. bleb assay
>a. bleb membrane
>a. cell
>a. cell of Mosher
>a. core
>a. dose
>a. embolism
>a. embolus
>a. foil
>high-efficiency particulate a. (HEPA)
>intraperitoneal a.
>a. monitor
>a. powered forceps
>a. quality standard
>residual a.
>a. sac
>a. sampler
>a. thermometer
>tidal a.
>a. vesicle

airborne
>a. agent
>a. infection

air-displacement pipette
air-dried smear
Aire
>autoimmune regulator
>Aire gene

air-filled tubular space
Airfuge ultracentrifuge
air-liquid interface
air-purifying respirator (APR)
airway
>a. obstruction disease
>a. resistance

AIS
>adenocarcinoma in situ
>androgen insensitivity syndrome
>antinsulin serum
>AIS of the cervix

AITT
>arginine insulin tolerance test

AIU
>absolute iodine uptake

AJCC
>American Joint Committee on Cancer
>AJCC classification
>AJCC staging modification on
>prostate cancer

AJCCS
>American Joint Committee on Cancer
>Staging

ajelloi
>*Trichophyton a.*

Ajellomyces
>*A. capsulatum*
>*A. dermatitidis*
>*A. dermatitis*

Akabane virus
akagii
>*Clostridium a.*

akamushi
>a. disease
>*Leptotrombidium a.*
>*Trombicula a.*

akari
>*Dermacentroxenus a.*
>*Rickettsia a.*

akaryocyte, akaryote, acaryote
akaryote (*var. of* akaryocyte)
akee (*var. of* ackee)
akeratosis
Akkermansia muciniphila
AKT8 retrovirus
AKT1 virus
Akureyri disease
AL
>primary amyloidosis
>AL protein

ALA
>alpha-linolenic acid
>aminolevulinic acid
>ALA test

alactolyticum
>*Eubacterium a.*

alactolyticus
>*Pseudoramibacter a.*

ALAD
aminolevulinic acid dehydrase
Alagille syndrome
alanine
a. aminotransferase (ALT)
a. aminotransferase:aspartate
aminotransferase ratio
a. aminotransferase assay
alaninemia
alaniniphila
Pseudonocardia a.
alaninuria
alanyl
alanyl-ribonucleic acid
synthetase
alanyl-RNA synthetase
alar chest
alaskensis
Desulfovibrio a.
Sphingomonas a.
Sphingopyxis a.
AlaSTAT latex allergy test
alastrim
alata
Ascaris a.
alba, *pl.* **albae**
Brevundimonas a.
morphea a.
Nocardia a.
pityriasis a.
Prauserella a.
Streptomonospora a.
substantia a.
Zimmermannella a.
albae (*pl. of* alba)
Albarrán
A. disease
A. y Dominguez tubule
Albers-Schönberg disease
Albert
A. diphtheria stain
A. disease
albertensis
Acidithiobacillus a.
albertii
Escherichia a.
Albert-Linder bone sectioning
Albibacter methylovorans
albicans
Candida a.
corpus a.
Endomyces a.
Monilia a.
Saccharomyces a.
Syringospora a.
albicantes
lineae a.
albida
Lentzea a.

Longispora a.
macula a.
albidocapillata
Lentzea a.
Saccharothrix a.
albidoflavus
Amycolatopsis a.
Albidovulum inexpectatum
albidum
atrophoderma a.
albiduria, albinuria
albidus
Cryptococcus a.
albimanus
Anopheles a.
albinism
oculocutaneous a.
albino
albinuria, albiduria
albirubida
Nocardiopsis dassonvillei
subsp. *a.*
albitarsus
Anopheles a.
alboatrum
Verticillium a.
albopictus
Aedes a.
Dermacentor a.
alboprecipitans
Pseudomonas a.
Albright
A. disease
A. hereditary osteodystrophy
A. syndrome
Albright-McCune-Sternberg
syndrome
albuginea
tunica a.
albugineous
album
Engyodontium a.
albumin
a. A, B
acetosoluble a.
acid a.
aggregated a.
alkali a.
a. assay
Bence Jones a.
blood a.
bovine serum a. (BSA)
cerebrospinal fluid a.
a. clearance
coagulated a.
a. cobalt binding (ACB)
a. cobalt binding test
crystalline egg a. (CEA)
delipidated a.

derived a.
a. excretion rate (AER)
a. Ghent
hematin a.
human serum a. (HSA)
I-125 iodinated human serum a.
I-131 iodinated human serum a.
iodinated human serum a.
  (IHSA)
iodinated macroaggregated a.
  (IMAA)
macroaggregated a. (MAA)
a. Mexico
^{99m}Tc labeled human serum a.
a. Naskapi
native a.
normal human serum a.
a. quotient
radioactive iodinated human serum
  a. (RIHSA)
radioactive iodinated serum a.
  (RISA)
radioiodinated serum a.
a. reading
serum a. (SA)
a. slide adhesive
a. suspension test
a. tannate
thyroxine-binding a. (TBA)
triphenyl a.
albumin-agglutinating antibody
albuminate
albuminaturia
albumin-calcium-magnesium
  (ACM)
albuminemia
double a.
albumin-globulin (A:G)
albuminiferous
albuminimeter
albuminimetry
albuminiparous
albuminocytologic dissociation
albuminogenous
albuminoid degeneration
albuminolysis
albuminoptysis
albuminoreaction
albuminorrhea (*var. of* albuminuria)
albuminous
a. cell
a. degeneration
a. gland
a. swelling
albuminuria, albuminorrhea
adolescent a.
adventitious a.
Bamberger a.
Bence Jones a.

benign a.
cardiac a.
colliquative a.
cyclic a.
dietetic a.
digestive a.
essential a.
false a.
febrile a.
functional a.
intermittent a.
lordotic a.
march a.
neuropathic a.
orthostatic a.
postrenal a.
postural a.
prerenal a.
recurrent a.
regulatory a.
transient a.
albuminuric
albumose-free tuberculin
  (TAF)
albumosuria
Bence Jones a.
albus
  Agarivorans a.
  Agromyces a.
  Bulleromyces a.
  Leucobacter a.
  Nocardioides a.
  Staphylococcus pyogenes a.
  Streptacidiphilus a.
  Streptomyces a.
  Thermocrinis a.
Albustix reagent strip
ALC
approximate lethal concentration
alcalescens
  Veillonella alcalescens
    subsp. a.
alcalifaciens
  Providencia a.
Alcaligenaceae
alcaligenes
  Bacillus faecalis a.
  A. bookeri
  A. bronchisepticus
  A. denitrificans
  A. faecalis
  A. faecalis subsp. *parafaecalis*
  A. marshalli
  A. odorans
  Pseudomonas a.
alcaliphila (*pl. of* alcaliphilus)
alcaliphilus, *pl.* **alcaliphila**
  Pseudomonas alcaliphila
  Thermococcus a.

Alcanivorax
>A. *borkumensis*
>A. *jadensis*
>A. *venustensis*

alcaptonuria, alkaptonuria

Alcian
>A. blue (AB)
>A. blue stain

alcianophilic

ALCL
>anaplastic large cell lymphoma

alcohol
>absolute a.
>acid a.
>aliphatic a.
>allyl a.
>anhydrous a.
>a. assay
>benzyl a.
>blood a.
>butyl a.
>a. consumption
>dehydrated a.
>a. dehydrogenase (ADH)
>dihydric a.
>ethyl a.
>a. fixation
>a. fixed smear
>a. intoxication
>isobutyl a.
>isopropyl a. (IPA)
>monohydric a.
>polyhydric a.
>polyvinyl a. (PVA)
>propyl a.
>a. thermometer

alcohol-formaldehyde-acetic acid (AFA)

alcohol-glycerin fixative

alcoholic (alc)
>a. cardiomyopathy
>a. cirrhosis
>a. coma
>a. formalin
>a. hepatitis
>a. hyalin
>a. hyaline
>a. hyaline body
>a. ketoacidosis
>a. myopathy
>a. pneumonia
>a. polymyopathy
>severely malnourished a.

alcoholivorans
>*Desulfovibrio a.*

alcohol-soluble eosin

alcoholuria

AlcoSCRUB instant antiseptic hand cleanser

Alco-Sensor

ALD
>adrenoleukodystrophy

aldaric acid

Aldecount Progenitor Cell Enumeration kit

Aldefluor reagent system

aldehyde
>acetic a.
>a. dehydrogenase
>a. fixative
>formic a.
>a. fuchsin (AF)
>methyl a.
>a. oxidase
>vitamin A_1 a.

Alder
>A. anomaly
>A. body

Alder-Reilly
>A.-R. anomaly
>A.-R. body

aldicarb

aldimine

aldofuranose

aldohexose

aldolase
>alpha hydroxyprogesterone a.
>a. assay
>fructose-bisphosphate a.
>a. test

aldonic acid

aldopentose

aldopyranose

aldose

aldosterone
>a. assay
>a. excretion rate (AER)
>a. secretion
>a. secretion defect (ASD)
>a. secretion rate (ASR)
>a. secretory rate (ASR)
>a. stimulation test
>a. suppression test

aldosterone-producing adenoma (APA)

aldosteronism
>glucocorticoid suppressible a.

aldotriose

Aldrich syndrome

aldrin

Alectorobius talaje

alemmal

ALERT
>antibody-based lateral flow economical recognition ticket

alert check

alesleukin

Aletris
aleukemia
aleukemic
    a. granulocytic leukemia
    a. lymphocytic leukemia
    a. monocytic leukemia
    a. myelosis
aleukemoid
aleukia
aleukocytic
aleukocytosis
aleurioconidium
aleuriospore
Aleurodiscus
Aleurostrongylus
Aleutian
    A. mink disease
    A. mink disease virus
Alexander
    A. disease
    A. leukodystrophy
alexandrii
    Oceanicaulis a.
alexandrinus
    Haloferax a.
alexin unit
aleydigism
Alezzandrini syndrome
Alfamovirus
alfentanil
alfreddugesi
    Eutrombicula a.
    Trombicula a.
ALG
    antilymphocyte globulin
alga, *pl.* algae
    Formosa algae
algae (*pl. of* alga)
algal filament
algens
    Gelidibacter a.
algeriensis
    Saccharothrix a.
algesidystrophy
Algibacter lectus
algicida
    Kordia a.
algicola
    Bacillus a.
    A. bacteriolytica
    Cellulophaga a.
    Ruegeria a.
algid
    a. malaria
    a. stage
algidixylanolyticum
    Clostridium a.
algidus
    Lactobacillus a.

algin
alginate
    sodium a.
alginic acid
alginolyticus
    Vibrio a.
Alginomonas
algodystrophy
algoid cell
Algoriphagus
    A. aquimarinus
    A. chordae
    A. halophilus
    A. ratkowskyi
    A. winogradskyi
algorithm
    biopsy a.
    genetic a. (GA)
    linear discriminant a.
algoscopy
ALH
    atypical lobular hyperplasia
alicyclic hydrocarbon
Alicycliphilus denitrificans
Alicyclobacillus
    A. acidiphilus
    A. acidocaldarius subsp.
     rittmannii
    A. herbarius
    A. hesperidum
    A. pomorum
    A. sendaiensis
    A. vulcanalis
aliena
    Pseudoalteromonas a.
alienia
aliesterase
aligned grid
alignment chart
A-like antigen
alimentaria
    Halomonas a.
alimentarius
    Jeotgalibacillus a.
alimentary
    a. abstinence
    a. canal
    a. diabetes
    a. glycosuria
    a. hypoglycemia
    a. lipemia
    a. osteopathy
    a. pentosuria
    a. tract
    a. tract smear
alinjection
ALIP
    abnormally localized immature
    precursor

aliphatic
>a. acid
>a. alcohol
>a. saturated hydrocarbon
>a. unsaturated hydrocarbon

aliphaticivorans
>*Desulfatibacillum a.*

aliquant

aliquot

Alishewanella fetalis

Alistipes
>*A. finegoldii*
>*A. putredinis*

Alius-Grignaschi anomaly

alive
>a. and well (A&W)
>a. with disease
>(AcD, AWD)
>a. without disease
>(AWOD)

alizarin
>a. cyanin
>a. indicator
>a. purpurin
>a. red
>a. red S
>a. red stain
>a. test
>a. yellow

alizarinsulfonate
>sodium a.

ALK
>anaplastic lymphoma kinase
>ALK protein
>ALK gene

alkalemia

alkalescence

alkali
>a. albumin
>a. denaturation test
>a. metal
>a. tolerance test

Alkalibacterium olivapovliticus

Alkalilimnicola halodurans

alkalimeter

alkalimetry

alkaline
>a. denaturation test
>a. earth metal
>a. intoxication
>a. phosphatase (alk phos, AP)
>a. phosphatase antialkaline
>phosphatase (APAAP)
>a. phosphatase antialkaline
>phosphatase antibody test
>a. phosphatase antialkaline
>phosphatase technique
>a. phosphatase assay
>a. phosphatase isoenzyme

>a. phosphatase isoenzyme
>electrophoresis
>a. phosphatase method
>a. phosphatase stain
>a. phosphatase staining
>a. phosphatase, tissue-nonspecific
>isozyme protein precursor
>(AP-TNAP)
>a. reaction
>a. RNase
>a. tide
>a. toluidine blue O
>a. tuberculin (TA)
>a. wave

alkalinuria, alkaluria

alkaliphila
>*Nocardiopsis a.*

alkaliphilum
>*Desulfotomaculum a.*

alkaliphilus
>*A. crotonatoxidans*
>*Salinicoccus a.*
>*A. transvaalensis*

alkali-resistant hemoglobin

alkali-soluble nitrogen
(ASN)

Alkalispirillum mobile

alkaloid test

alkalosis
>acapnial a.
>compensated a.
>hypokalemic a.
>metabolic a.
>nonrespiratory a.
>potassium a.
>respiratory a.
>uncompensated a.

alkalotic

alkaluria (*var. of* alkalinuria)

alkane

alkanet

Alkanindiges illinoisensis

alkannin paper

alkanoclasticus
>*Planococcus a.*

ALK1 antibody

alkapton body

alkaptonuria (*var. of* alcaptonuria)
>a. test

alkene

alkenivorans
>*Desulfatibacillum a.*

alkenyl

alkoxide ion

alkoxy

alkyl
>a. group
>a. peroxide

alkylate

alkylating agent
alkylation
alkylbenzene sulfonate (ABS)
alkyne
ALL
    acute lymphoblastic
      leukemia
    acute lymphocytic leukemia
      B-cell ALL
      CALLA-positive ALL
      T-cell ALL
allachesthesia
    optical a.
allantoic
    a. acid
    a. cyst
    a. duct remnant
allantoin
allantoinuria
allantois
Allegra
    A. 64R high-speed refrigerated
      benchtop centrifuge
    A. 25R refrigerated benchtop
      centrifuge
    A. X-12, X-15R, X-22 benchtop
      centrifuge
allele
    full-mutation a.
    HLA a.
    a. imbalance analysis
    multiple a.
    null a.
    premutation a.
    wild-type a.
allele-specific
    a.-s. loss
    a.-s. oligomer
    a.-s. oligonucleotide
    a.-s. PCR (A-PCR)
allelic
    a. exclusion
    a. gene
    a. imbalance
    a. loss
allelism
allelochemics
allelotyping
    molecular a.
Allen
    A. correction
    A. test
Allen-Doisy
    A.-D. test
    A.-D. unit
Allen-Masters syndrome
allergen
    atopic a.
    a. challenge test

allergenic
    a. extract
    a. protein preparation
allergen-specific IgE antibody
allergic
    a. airways disease
    a. alveolitis
    a. asthma
    a. bronchopulmonary aspergillosis
      (ABPA)
    a. bronchopulmonary mycosis
      (ABPM)
    a. conjunctivitis
    a. coryza
    a. dermatitis
    a. eczema
    a. encephalitis
    a. encephalomyelitis
    a. extract
    a. fungal sinusitis
    a. granulomatosis
    a. granulomatosis of Churg and
      Strauss
    a. granulomatous angiitis
    a. granulomatous prostatitis
    a. inflammation
    a. interstitial nephritis (AIN)
    a. mucin
    a. neuritis
    a. proctitis
    a. pulmonary edema
    a. purpura
    a. rhinitis
    a. transfusion reaction
allergization
allergized
allergoid
allergosis
allergy
    atopic a.
    bacterial a.
    cold a.
    contact a.
    delayed a.
    drug a.
    food a.
    immediate a.
    latent a.
    latex a.
    polyvalent a.
Allescheria boydii
allescheriosis
Allexivirus
alligatoris
    Mycoplasma a.
alligator skin
Allisonella histaminiformans
Allison-Ghormley body
alloagglutinin

alloalbuminemia
alloantibody
    anti-HLA a.
    a. inhibitor
    leukocyte alloantibodies
alloantigen
alloantin-D antibody
allo-BMT
    allogeneic bone marrow transplantation
allocation
    dynamic storage a.
    static storage a.
    storage a.
allochroic
allochroism
Allodermanyssus sanguineus
alloepitope
Allofustis seminis
allogeneic, allogenic
    a. antigen
    a. bone marrow transplantation
    (allo-BMT)
    a. cellular immune therapy (ACIT)
    a. graft
    a. inhibition
    a. transplantation
allogenic (*var. of* allogeneic)
allograft rejection
allogroup
alloimmune
    a. HDN
    a. hemolytic anemia
    a. hemolytic disease of newborn
    a. thrombocytopenia
alloimmunization
    leukocyte a.
    transfusion-related a.
Alloiococcus otitis
Allolevivirus
allometric
allometry
Allomonas
allomorphism
Allomyces
allophanamide
allophenic
allophore
allophycocyanin (APC)
alloplasia
alloplast
alloploidy
allopolyploidy
allopregnanediol
alloreactivity
allorecognition
allosensitization
allosome
allosteric
    a. activation

    a. effector
    a. enzyme
    a. inhibition
    a. site
allostery
allothreonine
allotope
allotopia
allotoxin
allotransplantation
allotrope
allotropic
allotropy
allotype
    InV a.
    Km a.
allotypic
    a. determinant
    a. marker
alloxan
alloxan-Schiff reaction
alloxuremia
alloxuria
alloy
all-*trans*-retinoic acid (ATRA)
allyl alcohol
Almeida disease
Almén test for blood
ALMI
    anterior lateral myocardial infarct
alni
    Pseudonocardia a.
Alocinma
alocis
    Filifactor a.
alopecia
    a. areatus
    congenital sutural a.
    a. mucinosa
    a. universalis
ALP
    antilymphocyte plasma
Alpers disease
alpha
    a. acid glycoprotein
    a. acidophil
    a. actinin
    a. adrenergic blockade
    a. adrenergic receptor
    a. agglutination
    a. agglutinin
    a. amino acid
    a. amino nitrogen
    a. amino nitrogen test
    a. amylose
    a. antichymotrypsin (ACT)
    a. antigen of adenovirus
    a. 2 antiplasmin
    a. antitrypsin (AAT)

a. band
a. cardiac actin
a. catenin
a. cell
a. cell of hypophysis
a. chain
a. 3, 4, 5 chain collagen stain
a. chain disease
a. contamination
a. decay
a. dextrinase
A. Dx point-of-need test system
a. dystroglycan
estrogen receptor a.
factor a.
a. fetoprotein (AFP)
a. fodrin protein
a. galactosidase A
a. galactosidase A deficiency
a. globin gene
a. globulin
a. globulin antibody
a. glucan-branching enzyme
a. glucan-branching
  glycosyltransferase
a. 1,4-glucosidase
a. glucosidase
a. granule
a. heavy-chain disease
a. helix
a. hemolysin
a. hemolysis
hepatocyte nuclear factor 1 a.
HIF-1 a.
a. hydrazine
a. hydroxyprogesterone
a. hydroxyprogesterone aldolase
interferon a. (IFN-alpha)
a. interferon therapy
a. internexin
a. ketoglutarate
a. ketoglutaric acid
a. lipoprotein
a. macroglobulin
a. mannosidase
a. melanocytic-stimulating hormone
a. metachromasia
a. methyldopa
a. motor neuron
a. naphthol
NRG1 a.
NRG2 a.
a. particle
a. particle detector
alpha, PI
a. porphyrin
a. probe
prostaglandin F_1 a.
prostaglandin F_2 a.

a. radiation
retinoid X receptor a.
RXR a.
a. seromucoid
a. skeletal actin
a. smooth muscle actin (ASMA)
a. source
a. staphylolysin
a. storage pool disease
a. streptococcus
a. substance
a. synuclein
a. thalassemia
a. thalassemia intermedia
TNF a.
a. tropomyosin
tumor necrosis factor a.
a. unit

alpha-1
a.-1 acid glycoprotein
a.-1 antichymotrypsin (A1AC)
a.-1 antitrypsin (A1AT)
a.-1 antitrypsin deficiency
a.-1 antitrypsin deficiency
  panniculitis
a.-1 antitrypsin phenotyping
a.-1 band
a.-1 fetoglobulin
a.-1 fetoprotein
a.-1 fetoprotein assay
a.-1 globulin
a.-1 protease inhibitor
a.-1 seromucoid
a.-1 trypsin inhibitor

alpha-2
a.-2 antiplasmin functional
  assay
a.-2 globulin
a.-2 macroglobulin
a.-2 macroglobulin inhibitor
a.-2 neuraminoglycoprotein

Alphabacteria
alpha$_1$-beta$_1$
  integrin a.-b.
alpha-beta variation
Alphacryptovirus
alpha-d-glucohydrolase
  sucrose a.-d-g.
alpha-dinitrophenol
alpha-estradiol
alpha-fetoprotein (AFP)
  amniotic fluid a.-f.
  maternal serum a.-f. (MSAFP)
alpha-inhibin
alpha-keto acid dehydrogenase
alpha-lactalbumin
  human a.-l.
alpha-L-fucosidase
alpha-L-iduronidase

alpha-linolenic acid (ALA)
alphalipoprotein deficiency
alpha-2-macroglobulin
alpha-methane bridge
alpha-methylacetoacetyl CoA thiolase
alpha-N-acetylgalactosaminidase
alpha-N-acetylglucosaminidase
alpha-naphthol thiourea
alpha-naphthyl acetate esterase
  (ANAE)
Alphanodavirus
Alpharetrovirus
Alpha-TFEB gene fusion
Alphavirus
alpinus
  Microanthomyces a.
Alport
  A. hereditary nephropathy
  A. syndrome
ALPS
  autologous leukapheresis, processing, and storage
  ALPS container
ALS
  amyotrophic lateral sclerosis
  antilymphocyte serum
Alsberg
  A. angle
  A. triangle
Alstonia
Alström syndrome
ALT
  alanine aminotransferase
  ALT test
alteplase
alteration
  bone matrix a.
  cartilage matrix a.
  chromosome a.
  crystalline macromolecule a.
  cyclic tissue a.
  cytologic a.
  cytoplasmic fiber a.
  cytoplasmic fibril a.
  cytoplasmic filament a.
  cytoplasmic lipid droplet a.
  cytoplasmic matrix a.
  decidual a.
  dentin crystal a.
  endometrial gestational a.
  exfoliative cytologic a.
  extracellular fibril a.
  extracellular matrix a.
  extracellular structural a.
  fibrocartilage matrix a.
  gestational a.
  Golgi cavity a.
  Golgi membrane a.
  Golgi vacuole a.

Golgi vesicle a.
growth a.
hematopoietic cell cytoplasmic a.
hematopoietic maturation a.
keratohyaline a.
leukocytic maturation a.
mitochondrial crista a.
mitochondrial matrix a.
mitochondrial membrane a.
Nissl substance a.
nuclear-cytoplasmic ratio a.
nuclear membrane a.
nuclear pore a.
nuclear sap a.
nuclear shape a.
nuclear size a.
predecidual a.
RB1 a.
syncytial a.
verrucopapillary a.
alterative inflammation
altered
  a. intravascular hydrostatic pressure
  a. intravascular osmotic pressure
  a. lipid-peroxidation activity
alternant
  trace a.
Alternaria tenuis
alternata
  Psychoda a.
alternate host
alternating current
alternation of generations
alternative
  a. complement pathway
  a. hypothesis
  a. inheritance
  one-sided a.
  two-sided a.
Alteromonadaceae
Alteromonas
  A. litorea
  A. marina
  A. putrefaciens
  A. stellipolaris
altitude
  a. anoxia
  a. disease
  a. sickness
Altmann
  A. anilin-acid fuchsin stain
  A. fixative
  A. fluid
  A. granule
  A. liquid
  A. theory

Altmann-Gersh method
alum
    a. carmine
    chrome a.
    Einarson gallocyanin-chrome a.
    a. hematoxylin
    potassium a.
    a. precipitate
alumina
    hydrated a.
aluminal tubule
aluminosilicate glassware
aluminosis
aluminum
    a. hydroxide
    a. hydroxide gel
    a. oxide
    a. phosphate
alum-precipitated
    a.-p. antigen
    a.-p. pyridine (APP)
    a.-p. toxoid (APT)
alvei (*pl. of* alveus)
alveolar
    a. abscess
    a. adenocarcinoma
    a. air
    a. air equation
    a. asthma
    a. bone resorption
    a. bony crypt
    a. cell
    a. cell carcinoma
    a. duct
    a. edema
    a. fenestra
    a. gland
    a. hydatid
    a. hydatid cyst
    a. hydatid disease
    a. macrophage
    a. periosteum
    a. phagocyte
    a. pneumocyte hyperplasia
    a. pore
    a. proteinosis
    a. rhabdomyosarcoma
     (ARMS)
    a. sac
    a. septum
    a. soft-part sarcoma
     (ASPS)
alveolar-arterial
    a.-a. carbon dioxide
     difference
    a.-a. oxygen
    a.-a. oxygen difference
alveolar-capillary interface
alveolare

alveolaris
    ductulus a.
    sacculus a.
alveoli (*pl. of* alveolus)
alveolitis
    acute pulmonary a.
    allergic a.
    extrinsic allergic a. (EAA)
    fibrosing a.
alveoloclasia
alveolodental membrane
alveolus, *pl.* **alveoli**
    a. dentalis
    pulmonary a.
    alveoli pulmonis
    tubuli dentales
alveus, *pl.* **alvei**
    Bacillus alvei
    Enterobacter alvei
    Hafnia alvei
    a. hippocampi
    a. of hippocampus
alvinolith
ALW
    arch-loop-whorl
alymphia
alymphocytosis
alymphoplasia
    Nezelof type of thymic
     a.
    thymic a. (TAL)
Alzheimer
    A. cell
    A. disease
    A. disease familial and
     sporadic
    A. fibril
    A. fibrillary degeneration
    A. sclerosis
    A. stain
    A. type I, II astrocyte
Am
    americium
    arabinomannan
AMA
    against medical advice
    antimitochondrial antibody
AMACR antibody
amacrine cell
amalonatica
    Citrobacter a.
    Levinea a.
Amanita
    A. muscaria
    A. pantherina
    A. phalloides
    A. rubescens
    A. verna
    A. virosa

amanitiforme
　　Angulomicrobium a.
amanitin
Am antigen
amarae
　　Gordonia a.
　　Rothia a.
amaranth, amaranthum
amaranthum (*var. of* amaranth)
amastia
amastigote
Amauroascus
amaurosis fugax
amaurotic familial idiocy
amazia
amazonae
　　Volucribacter a.
amazonensis
　　Leishmania mexicana a.
Ambard
　　A. constant
　　A. laws
Amberlite
amber mutation
ambient
　　a. temperature
　　a. temperature and pressure,
　　　saturated (ATPS)
ambifaria
　　Burkholderia a.
ambiguity
　　ribosomal a.
　　somatosexual a.
ambiguous external genitalia
ambiguus
　　Bacillus a.
amblychromasia
amblychromatic
Amblyomma
　　A. americanum
　　A. cajennense
　　A. hebraeum
　　A. maculatum
　　A. variegatum
amblyopia
　　a. neuropathy
　　tobacco a.
amboceptor
　　bacteriolytic a.
　　Bordet a.
　　hemolytic a.
　　a. unit
ambroisiodes
　　Chenopodium a.
Ambrosia
Ambrosiella
Ambrosiozyma cicatricosa
ambulans
　　ulcus a.

ameba, *pl.* **amebae, amebas**
　　coprozoic a.
amebacide
amebae (*pl. of* ameba)
amebas (*pl. of* ameba)
amebiasis
　　intestinal a.
amebic
　　a. brain abscess
　　a. colitis
　　a. dysentery
　　a. granuloma
　　a. meningitis
　　a. meningoencephalitis
　　a. prevalence rate (APR)
　　a. ulcer
amebicidal
amebicide
amebiform
amebiosis
amebism
amebocyte
ameboflagellate
ameboid
　　a. cell
　　a. movement
ameboididity
ameboidism
ameboma, amoeboma
amebula
amebule
ameburia
amegakaryocytic thrombocytopenia
amegakaryocytosis
amelanotic mucosal melanoma
amelia
ameloblast
ameloblastic
　　a. adenomatoid tumor
　　a. fibroma
　　a. fibroodontoma
　　a. fibrosarcoma
　　a. hemangioma
　　a. layer
　　a. neurilemmoma
　　a. odontoma
　　a. sarcoma
ameloblastoma
　　acanthomatous a.
　　basal cell a.
　　calcifying a.
　　cystic a.
　　desmoplastic a.
　　extraosseous a.
　　follicular a.
　　granular cell a.
　　malignant a.
　　melanotic a.
　　multicystic a.

pituitary a.
plexiform unicystic a.
solid a.
unicystic a.
ameloblastomatous craniopharyngioma
amelogenesis imperfecta
amelogenin
amendment
Clinical Laboratory Improvement A.
(CLIA)
amenorrhea
a. and hirsutism
primary a.
secondary a. (SA)
amenorrhea-galactorrhea syndrome
amentia
amentoflavone
American
A. Chemical Society (ACS)
A. Clinical Laboratory Association
A. hookworm
A. Joint Committee on Cancer
(AJCC)
A. Joint Committee on Cancer
Staging (AJCCS)
A. leech
A. leishmaniasis
A. National Standards Institute
(ANSI)
A. rat flea
A. trypanosomiasis
A. Type Culture Collection
(ATCC)
A. Urological Association (AUA)
americana
Cochliomyia a.
leishmaniasis a.
Scopulariopsis a.
Spirochaeta a.
Uncinaria a.
americanum
Amblyomma a.
americanus
Necator a.
americium (Am)
amerism
ameristic
Amersham
A. Biosciences
A. International ECL gene detection
system
A. Life Science PCR product
presequencing kit
A. Life Science Thermo Sequenase
sequencing kit
Ames
A. assay
A. Lab-Tek cryostat
A. test

amethyst violet
AMeX
acetone, methylbenzoate, xylene
AMeX fixation
AMeX processing and embedding
method
AMF
autocrine motility factor
AMFR
autocrine motility factor receptor
AMG
antimacrophage globulin
autometallography
AMH
antimüllerian hormone
AMI
acute myocardial infarction
amiantacea
tinea a.
amianthoid collagen fibers
amicalis
Gordonia a.
Amici
A. disc
A. line
A. stria
amicrobic
amicroscopic
Amicus separator
amidase
amide
primary a.
secondary a.
tertiary a.
amidinotransferase
amido black 10B
amidobenzene
amidohydrolase method
amidonaphthol red
Amidostomum anseris
amiense
Sphingobium a.
amine
aromatic a.
a. precursor uptake and
decarboxylation (APUD)
pressor a.
primary a.
quaternary a.
secondary a.
tertiary a.
vasoactive a.
amino
a. acid
a. acid-activating enzyme
a. acid analyzer
a. acid disorder
a. acid fractionation assay
a. acid nitrogen (AAN)

amino (*continued*)
    a. acid residue
    a. acid screen
    a. acid screening
    a. acid sequencer
    a. acid transporter E16 gene
    a. terminal
aminoacetic acid
aminoacidemia
aminoacidopathy
aminoaciduria
    branched-chain a.
    dibasic a.
aminoacridine hydrochloride
aminoacyl-histidine dipeptidase
aminoacyl-tRNA hydrolase
aminoalkylsilane (AAS)
aminoanthraquinone dye
aminoaromatica
    Thauera a.
Aminobacterium
    A. colombiense
    A. mobile
aminobenzene
aminobutyrate aminotransferase
aminocaproic acid
3-amino-9-ethylcarbazole (AEC)
    3-a.-9-e. stain
5-amino-9-ethylcarbazole
amino-9-ethylcarbazole
aminoethylcysteine ketimine
aminoethylisothiouronium bromide (AET)
aminoglutaric acid
aminoglycoside ototoxicity
aminoguanidine
aminoketone dye
aminolevulinic
    a. acid (ALA)
    a. acid dehydrase (ALAD)
aminomethane
    tris(hydroxymethyl) a.
aminopenicillanic acid (APA)
aminopeptidase (AP)
    a. cytosol
    leucine a. (LAP)
aminophenol
aminophilus
    Desulfovibrio a.
aminopropyltriethoxysilane (APES)
aminopropyltriethyoxysilane-coated glass slide
aminopurine
aminopyrine breath test
aminosuccinic acid
amino-terminal domain
aminoterminus
aminotransferase
    alanine a. (ALT)

    aminobutyrate a.
    aspartate a. (AST)
    ornithine a.
    ornithine-oxo-acid a.
    valine a.
aminoxidans
    Xanthobacter a.
aminuria
amitosis
amitotic
amitriptyline and nortriptyline assays
AML
    acute myeloid leukemia
    angiomyolipoma
AMLS
    antimouse lymphocyte serum
AMLV-RT
    avian myeloblastosis leukemia virus reverse transcriptase
AMM
    ammonia
ammeter
AMML
    acute myelomonocytic leukemia
Ammon
    A. filament
    A. fissure
    A. horn
ammonemia, ammoniemia, hyperammonemia
ammonia (AMM)
    a. assay
    plasma a.
ammoniacal
    a. silver nitrate test
    a. silver solution
    a. urine
ammonia-lyase
    l-histidine a.-l.
ammoniemia (*var. of* ammonemia)
ammonificans
    Thermovibrio a.
ammonium
    a. biurate crystal
    a. chloride
    a. chloride loading test
    a. magnesium phosphate
    a. magnesium phosphate stone
    a. molybdate
    a. nitrate bomb
    a. oxalate
    a. oxalate crystal violet
    a. peroxydisulfate
    a. silver carbonate stain
    a. sulfate
ammoniuria
AMN
    atypical melanocytic nevus

AMNGT
> atypical melanocytic nevi of genital type

amnii
> hydrops a.

amniocentesis
amniocyte
amniogenic cell
amnioma
amnion
> a. cell
> incomplete a.
> a. nodosum
> squamous metaplasia of a.

amnionic (*var. of* amniotic)
> a. corpuscle

amnionitis
amniorrhea
amniotic, amnionic
> a. adhesion
> a. band syndrome
> a. corpuscle
> a. fluid
> a. fluid alpha-fetoprotein
> a. fluid analysis
> a. fluid bilirubin
> a. fluid bilirubin optical density
> a. fluid color
> a. fluid creatinine
> a. fluid desaturated phosphatidylcholine
> a. fluid embolism
> a. fluid embolus
> a. fluid fern test
> a. fluid foam stability index
> a. fluid foam stability test
> a. fluid lecithin/sphingomyelin ratio
> a. fluid primary phospholipid
> a. fluid pulmonary surfactant
> a. fluid shake test
> a. fluid surfactant
> a. fluid total volume
> a. fluid unsaturated lecithin
> a. infection syndrome of Blane

amobarbital
> a. poisoning
> sodium a.

amodiaquine
Amoeba
> *A. buccalis*
> *A. coli*
> *A. dentalis*
> *A. dysenteriae*
> *A. histolytica*
> *A. meleagridis*
> *A. proteus*
> *A. urogenitalis*
> *A. verrucosa*

amoeboma (*var. of* ameboma)
Amoebotaenia
AMOL
> acute monoblastic leukemia
> acute monocytic leukemia

amorph
amorpha
amorphia, amorphism
amorphic
amorphism (*var. of* amorphia)
amorphous
> a. eosinophilic appearance
> a. eosinophilic debris
> a. fraction of adrenal cortex
> a. phosphate crystal

amorphus
> fetus a.
> holoacardius a.

Amoss sign
amoxapine
AMP
> acid mucopolysaccharide
> adenosine monophosphate
> AMP deaminase

amp
> ampule

Ampelomyces
Ampelovirus
amperage (amp)
ampere (A)
> kilovolt a. (kVA)

ampere-second per volt (As/V)
amperometric-coulometric titration
amperometry
amphetamine assay
Amphibacillus
> *A. fermentum*
> *A. tropicus*

amphibolic
> a. fistula
> a. pathway

amphibolous fistula
amphichroic
amphichromatic
amphicrine
> a. cell
> a. differentiation

amphicyte
amphigenous inheritance
amphikaryon
amphileukemic
Amphimerus
amphimicrobe
amphinucleolus
amphipath
amphipathic
amphiphile
amphiphilic

Amphiporthe
amphiprotic
amphistome
amphitrichate, amphitrichous
amphitrichous (*var. of* amphitrichate)
amphixenosis
amphochromatophil, amphochromatophile
amphochromatophile (*var. of*
  amphochromatophil)
amphochromophil, amphochromophile
amphochromophile (*var. of*
  amphochromophil)
amphocyte
ampholyte
amphophil, amphophile
  a. cell
  a. granule
amphophile (*var. of* amphophil)
amphophilic, amphophilous
  a. cytoplasm
  a. homogenization
amphophilous
amphoteric
  a. dye
  a. electrolyte
  a. reaction
amphotericin B
amphotropic virus
ampicillin
AmpliChip CYP450 genotyping test
amplicon
Amplicor
  A. Chlamydia assay
  A. CMV Monitor
  A. CT/NG test
  A. HIV-1 monitor test
amplifiable DNA
amplification
  Chelex DNA a.
  c-myc a.
  a. factor
  gas a.
  gene a.
  group specific a. (GSA)
  ligation-dependent a.
  multiple biotin-avidin a.
  multiple displacement a. (MDA)
  N-myc a.
  nucleic acid sequence based a.
    (NASBA)
  polymerase chain reaction a.
  polymerization-dependent a.
  signal a.
  strand displacement a. (SDA)
  target a.
  transcription-dependent a.
  transcription-mediated a. (TMA)
  tyramide signal a. (TSA)
  whole genome a. (WGA)

amplified probe
amplifier
  audio a.
  buffer a.
  complementary symmetry a.
  Darlington a.
  difference a.
  direct-coupled a.
  electrometer a.
  a. host
  linear a.
  lock-in a.
  logarithmic a.
  operational a.
  power a.
  push-pull a.
amplitude
  wave a.
ampoule (*var. of* ampule)
ampul (*var. of* ampule)
ampule (amp), ampul, ampoule
ampulla, *pl.* ampullae
  a. of uterine tube
  a. tubae uterinae
ampullae (*pl. of* ampulla)
ampullar abortion
ampullaris
  crista a.
  cupula a.
ampullary
  a. aneurysm
  a. carcinoma
  a. crest
  a. cupula
  a. tumor
ampullitis
ampullula
amputating ulcer
amputation
  incomplete a.
  a. neuroma
  spontaneous a.
AMS
  antimacrophage serum
  automated multiphasic screening
Amsterdam syndrome
amu
  atomic mass unit
AMuLV
  Abelson murine leukemia virus
amurskyense
  Salinibacterium a.
amurskyensis
  Zobellia a.
Amussat
  A. valve
  A. valvula
AMV2
  avian myelocytomatosis virus

Amycolatopsis
  A. albidoflavus
  A. balhimycina
  A. decaplanina
  A. eurytherma
  A. fastidiosa
  A. japonica
  A. kentuckyensis
  A. keratiniphila
  A. keratiniphila subsp.
    keratiniphila
  A. keratiniphila subsp.
    nogabecina
  A. lexingtonensis
  A. mediterranei
  A. orientalis subsp.
    lurida
  A. palatopharyngis
  A. pretoriensis
  A. rifamycinica
  A. rubida
  A. sacchari
  A. tolypomycina
  A. vancoresmycina
amycolatum
  Corynebacterium a.
amyctic
amyelencephalia
amyelia
amyelinated
amyelination
amyelinic
amyeloic, amyelonic
amyelonic (*var. of* amyeloic)
amygdala, *pl.* **amygdalae**
amygdalae (*pl. of* amygdala)
amygdalase
amygdalin
amygdaline
amygdalinum
  Clostridium a.
amyl
  a. nitrite pearls
  a. nitrite perles
  a. nitrite popper
  a. nitrite, sodium nitrite, and
    sodium thiosulfate
amylaceous corpuscle, amyloid
  corpuscle
amylaceum
  corpus a. (CA)
amylase
  a. assay
  a. clearance (C_{am}, C_{Am})
  salivary a.
  serum a.
  a. test
  urinary a.
  urine a.

amylase/creatinine
  a. clearance
  a. clearance ratio (A:C)
amylasuria
amylemia
amylin polypeptide
amyloclast
amylo-1,6-glucosidase
amyloid
  a. A (AA)
  a. angiopathy
  a. beta protein
  a. corpuscle
  a. degeneration
  a. fibril
  Highman method for a.
  a. kidney
  a. light chain
  a. nephrosis
  a. neuropathy
  a. of immunoglobulin origin
    (AIO)
  a. of unknown origin
    (AUO)
  a. P component
  a. plaque
  a. precursor protein (APP)
  a. protein A
  serum a. A (SAA)
  a. stain
  a. staining
  a. tumor
amyloidogenic potential
amyloidoma
  nodular a. (NA)
amyloidosis
  AA a.
  cardiac a.
  cutaneous a.
  a. cutis
  diffuse a.
  familial primary systemic a.
  focal a.
  lichen a.
  macular a.
  nodular a.
  primary a. (AL)
  renal a.
  secondary a.
  senile a.
  systemic familial primary a.
  tracheobronchial a.
amyloid-β peptide
amylolytic enzyme
amylolyticum
  Tenacibaculum a.
amylolyticus
  Desulfurococcus a.
  Lactobacillus a.

amylopectin
amylopectinosis
amylorrhea
amylose
    alpha a.
    crystalline a.
Amylostereum
amylovora
    Erwinia a.
amyopathic dermatomyositis
amyoplasia congenita
amyotonia congenita
amyotrophia (*var. of* amyotrophy)
amyotrophic
    a. lateral sclerosis (ALS)
    a. lateral
      sclerosis/parkinsonism±dementia
    complex of Guam
amyotrophy, amyotrophia
    diabetic a.
    neuralgic a.
amyous
ANA
    antinuclear antibody
Anabaena
anabiotic cell
anabolic steroid
anabolism-promoting factor (APF)
anabolite
anacidity
anacmesis
anacrotism
anadenia ventriculi
ANAE
    alpha-naphthyl acetate esterase
anaemicus (*var. of* anemicus)
Anaeroarcus burkinensis
Anaerobacter polyendosporus
Anaerobaculum
    A. mobile
    A. thermoterrenum
anaerobe
    facultative a.
    obligate a.
anaerobian
anaerobic, anaerobiotic
    a. bacteria culture
    a. bacterium
    a. chamber
    a. diphtheroid
    a. glycolysis
    a. jar
    a. metabolism
    a. *Neisseria*
    a. pneumonia
    a. respiration
    a. rod
    a. specimen collector
    a. streptococcus

anaerobiosis
Anaerobiospirillum
    A. succiniciproducens
    A. thomasii
anaerobiotic (*var. of* anaerobic)
anaerobius
    Streptococcus a.
Anaerobranca
    A. californiensis
    A. gottschalkii
Anaerococcus
    A. hydrogenalis
    A. lactolyticus
    A. octavius
    A. prevotii
    A. tetradius
    A. vaginalis
Anaerofustis stercorihominis
anaerogenic
Anaeroglobus geminatus
Anaerolinea thermophila
Anaeromyxobacter dehalogenans
Anaerophaga thermohalophila
Anaeroplasmataceae
Anaeroplasmatales
Anaerostipes caccae
Anaerotruncus colihominis
Anaerovorax odorimutans
anagen
anagenesis
anagenetic
anákhré
anakmesis
anal
    a. atresia
    a. column
    a. duct
    a. fissure
    a. fistula
    a. gland
    a. gland carcinoma
    a. papillitis
    a. sinus
    a. skin tag
    a. verge
anal.
    analysis
analbuminemia
analeptic
anales
    columnae a.
analgesic, analgetic
    a. nephritis
    a. nephropathy
analgetic (*var. of* analgesic)
analis
    linea pectinata canalis a.
anallergenic serum
anallergic

analog (*var. of* analogue)
    a. data
    a. of histidine (AHH)
    a. signal
analogous structure
analogue, analog
    purine a.
analyses (*pl. of* analysis)
analysis (anal.), *pl.* **analyses**
    activation a.
    allele imbalance a.
    amniotic fluid a.
    antigenic a.
    arterial blood gas a.
    automated cell image a.
    blood acylcarnitine a.
    blood gas a.
    bloodstain pattern a.
    body fluid a.
    breakpoint a.
    breath hydrogen a.
    cell lineage a.
    cell sorting a.
    cerebrospinal fluid a.
    chemical a.
    chromosome a.
    clinicopathologic a.
    compartmental a.
    computer-assisted image a.
    computer linkage a.
    Cox regression a.
    critical path a.
    cytofluorimetric a.
    cytogenetic a.
    cytometric image a.
    cytospin a.
    DDD a.
    discriminant function a.
    displacement a.
    DNA array a.
    DNA melting a.
    Dpc4 immunohistochemical
      pancreatic cancer a.
    electroblot a.
    energy dispersed x-ray a.
      (EDS)
    fecal porphyrin a.
    fiber FISH a.
    flow cytometric reticulocyte a.
    Fourier a.
    gastric a.
    genetic abnormality a.
    genetic linkage a.
    graphic a.
    hair a.
    head space a.
    heteroduplex a. (HDA)
    hierarchical clustering a.
    image display and a. (IDA)

    immunohistochemical a.
    intracellular receptor a.
    kidney stone a.
    Ki-67 immunohistochemical
      well-differentiated gastric
      carcinoma a.
    leave-one-out cross-validation a.
    linkage a.
    membrane-bound receptor a.
    microanalytical EDS a.
    microdiffusion a.
    microsatellite a.
    molecular cytogenetic a.
    morphological a.
    morphometric a.
    multicolor FISH a.
    multilocus variable number (tandem
      repeat) a.
    multipixel spectral a.
    multivariate a.
    mutational a.
    Northern blot a.
    nucleic acid sequence based a.
      (NASBA)
    a. of variance (ANOVA)
    optimized robot for chemical a.
      (ORCA)
    p53 immunohistochemical breast
      cancer a.
    ploidy a.
    proteome a.
    qualitative a.
    quantitative a.
    random amplified polymorphic DNA
      a. (RAPD)
    rapid microsatellite a.
    restriction endonuclease a. (REA)
    RFLP Southern hybridization a.
    saturation a.
    semen a.
    semiquantitative a.
    sequential a.
    simkin a.
    Southern blot a.
    stool a.
    sucrose density gradient a.
    synovial fluid a.
    tandem repeat a.
    tetramer a.
    transcriptome a.
    tubeless gastric a.
    univariate a.
    Western blot a.
    zymographic a.
analyte-specific reagent (ASR)
analytic, analytical
    a. cytology
    a. method
    a. ultracentrifuge

analytical (*var. of* analytic)
- a. balance
- a. chemistry
- a. electron microscope (AEM)
- a. immunofiltration
- a. reagent (AR)
- a. reagent grade
- a. sensitivity
- a. specificity
- a. toxicology

analyzer, analyzor
- Abbott Cell-Dyn hematology a.
- ABI Prism 3100 Genetic A.
- Access AFP immunoassay a.
- ACL 100, 1000, 7000, 8000, 9000, 10000 Advance coagulation a.
- ACS:180 CK/MB a.
- Ac·T diff, Ac·T diff2 hematology a.
- Ac·T 5 diff AL auto loader hematology a.
- Ac·T 5 diff CP cap pierce hematology a.
- Ac·T 5 diff OV open vial hematology a.
- Ac·T series hematology a.
- Advanced Instruments conductivity a.
- Advia 1650 chemistry a.
- Aeroset chemical a.
- amino acid a.
- Apec glucose a.
- Aution Max AX-4280 automated urine chemistry a.
- automatic clinical a.
- automatic fluorescent image a.
- AxSYM a.
- batch a.
- Bayer Technicon H-2 a.
- Beckman Synchron CX-7 cholesterol a.
- Careside a.
- centrifugal fast a.
- Cobas Fara H centrifugal a.
- Cobas Helios differential a.
- Cobra Amplicor a.
- continuous flow a.
- Coulter LH 500, 700, 750, 755, 1500 Series hematology a.
- Coulter MAXM hematology a.
- Coulter STKS hematology a.
- CyAn ADP a.
- Delsa 440 SX Zeta potential a.
- Dimension chemical a.
- discrete a.
- Elecsys 2010 modular immunoassay a.
- enzyme a.
- ESRA-10 erythrocyte sedimentation rate a.
- ESR-Auto Plus sedimentation rate a.
- FLx/TDx immunoassay a.
- GenePhor DNA fragment a.
- Gen-S hematology a.
- HemoCue B-Glucose a.
- Hitachi 704, 736, 911 a.
- Hitachi 747-100 cholesterol a.
- Hitachi 747 CK/MB a.
- HmX hematology a.
- IiQ 200 automated urine microscopy a.
- Immulite 2000 chemiluminescent a.
- Immulite Dynamic Duo a.
- IMx a.
- infrared CO_2 a.
- Integra chemical a.
- KC1 Delta coagulation a.
- kinetic a.
- Kodak Ektachem DT-60 cholesterol a.
- Kodak Ektachem Vitros 250, 750, 950 cholesterol a.
- LH 500, 750, 1500 series hematology a.
- LS 100Q/200/230 series laser diffraction particle size a.
- LS 13 320 series laser diffraction particle size a.
- multichannel a. (MCA)
- Nova Celltrak 12 hematology a.
- N5 submicron particle size a.
- Olympus AU5200 cholesterol a.
- Oncometrics Imaging Cyto-Savant image a.
- oxygen a.
- platelet function a. (PFA)
- PocketChem UA a.
- pulse height a. (PHA)
- RapidVUE particle shape and size a.
- SA 3100 surface area and pore size a.
- sequential multiple a. (SMA)
- simultaneous multiple a. (SMA)
- spectrum a.
- Stat Profile pHOx blood gas a.
- Stratus II automatic a.
- SureStep Pro glucose a.
- Sweat-Chek conductivity a.
- Sysmex NE-8000 CBC a.
- Sysmex XE-2100 hematology a.
- Sysmex XT-2000i automated hematology a.
- TDxFlx a.
- Triturus automated ELISA immunoassay a.

Urisys 2400 urine a.
Vi-CELL series cell viability a.
Vitros a.
Viva-E drug testing a.
V-Twin drug testing a.
wave a.
Wescor Sweat-Chek conductivity a.
YSI 2300 STAT glucose and
  lactate a.
analyzor (*var. of* analyzer)
anamnesis
anamnestic
  a. reaction
  a. response
anamorph
ananaphylaxis (*var. of* antianaphylaxis)
anangioplasia
anangioplastic
ANAP
  anionic neutrophil activating
  peptide
anaphase lag
anaphoresis
anaphylactic
  a. antibody
  a. intoxication
  a. shock
  a. transfusion reaction
anaphylactica
  enteritis a.
anaphylactogen
anaphylactogenesis
anaphylactogenic
anaphylactoid
  a. crisis
  a. purpura
  a. reaction
  a. shock
anaphylatoxin, anaphylotoxin
  C3a a.
  C4a a.
  C5a a.
  a. inactivator
anaphylaxis
  active a.
  aggregate a.
  antiserum a.
  chronic a.
  eosinophil chemotactic factor of a.
    (ECF-A)
  generalized a.
  inverse a.
  local a.
  reversed passive a.
  slow reacting factor of a. (SRF-A)
  slow reacting substance of a.
    (SRS-A)
  systemic a.
anaphylotoxin (*var. of* anaphylatoxin)

anaplasia
Anaplasma
  A. bovis
  A. phagocytophilum
  A. platys
Anaplasmataceae
anaplasmosis
anaplastic
  a. adenocarcinoma
  a. astrocytoma
  a. carcinoma
  a. cell
  a. large cell lymphoma
    (ALCL)
  a. lymphoma kinase (ALK)
  a. lymphoma kinase gene (ALK
    gene)
  a. malignant teratoma
  a. meningioma
  a. oligodendroglioma
  a. seminoma
anaplerotic
anapophysis
anarchic phenomenon
Ana-Sal HIV home test kit
anasarca
  fetoplacental a.
anasarcous
anastomoses (*pl. of* anastomosis)
anastomosing fiber
anastomosis, *pl.* **anastomoses**
  arteriovenous a. (AVA)
  artery-to-artery a.
  artery-to-vein a.
  vein-to-vein a.
anastomoticus
  varix a.
anatina
  Coenonia a.
anatipester
anatipestifer
  Moraxella a.
anatis
  Cochlosoma a.
  Gallibacterium a.
anatolicum
  Hyalomma a.
anatomic, anatomical
  a. change
  a. pathology
  a. tubercle
  a. tubercle
  a. wart
anatomical (*var. of* anatomic)
  a. element
  a. pathology
  a. wart
anatomicopathologic
anatomicopathological

anatomy
    cross-section a.
    general a.
    microscopic a.
    ultrastructural a.
anatoxic
anatoxin
Anatrichosoma
anaxon, anaxone
anaxone (*var. of* anaxon)
anazoturia
ANC
    absolute neutrophil count
ANCA
    antineutrophil cytoplasmic antibody
    antineutrophil cytoplasmic
      autoantibody
anchorage
    cell a.
    a. dependence
    a. independence
anchoring fibril
anchovy sauce pus
anchusin
ancient schwannoma
anconitis
ancoratus
ancrod
Ancylidae
Ancylobacter rudongensis
Ancylostoma, Ankylostoma
    A. braziliense
    A. caninum
    A. ceylanicum
    A. duodenale
    A. tubaeforme
ancylostomatic
ancylostomiasis
Andernach ossicle
Andersch ganglion
Anders disease
Andersen
    A. syndrome
    A. triad
Anderson
    A. and Goldberger test
    A. phenomenon
Anderson-Collip test
andersoni
    Dermacentor a.
Andes disease
Andrade
    A. indicator
    A. syndrome
André Thomas sign
Andrews
    A. lymphocyte curve
    A. nomogram
androblastoma

androgen
    a. independent prostate cancer
      (AIPC)
    a. insensitivity syndrome (AIS)
    a. receptor
    a. receptor gene
    a. unit (international)
androgen-binding protein (ABP)
androgenesis
androgenic
    a. anabolic agent (AAA)
    a. arrhenoblastoma
    a. hormone
    a. zone
androgenization
androgen-normal epithelium
androgen-secreting adrenal
andropathy
androstanediol
androstene
androstenediol
androstenedione test
androsterone
anectasis
Anellaria
anemia
    acanthocyte-associated hemolytic a.
    achlorhydric a.
    achrestic a.
    acquired hemolytic a. (AHA)
    acquired sideroblastic a.
    acute posthemorrhagic a.
    acute self-limited hemolytic a.
    Addison a.
    addisonian a.
    alloimmune hemolytic a.
    angiopathic hemolytic a.
    aplastic a.
    aregenerative a.
    asiderotic a.
    a. associated with chronic renal
      failure
    autoallergic hemolytic a.
    autoimmune hemolytic a. (AHA,
      AIHA)
    Belgian Congo a.
    Biermer a.
    blood loss a.
    brickmaker's a.
    cameloid a.
    chlorotic a.
    chronic autoimmune hemolytic a.
    chronic hemolytic a.
    cold autoimmune hemolytic a.
    cold-type autoimmune hemolytic a.
    congenital aplastic a.
    congenital aregenerative a.
    congenital dyserythropoietic a.
      (CDA)

congenital hypoplastic a. (CHA)
congenital nonregenerative a.
congenital nonspherocytic
  hemolytic a.
Cooley a.
cow's milk a.
crescent cell a.
Czerny a.
deficiency a.
Diamond-Blackfan a.
dilution a.
dimorphic a.
Diphyllobothrium a.
Dresbach a.
drug-induced autoimmune
  hemolytic a.
drug-induced immune hemolytic a.
dyserythropoietic congenital a.
dyshemopoietic a.
Ehrlich a.
elliptocytic a.
enzyme deficiency a.
enzyme-deficient a.
equine infectious a.
erythroblastic a.
Estren-Dameshek a.
Faber a.
factor deficiency a.
false a.
familial erythroblastic a.
familial hemolytic a.
familial hypoplastic a.
familial microcytic a.
familial pyridoxine-responsive a.
familial splenic a.
Fanconi a.
fish tapeworm a.
folate deficiency a.
folic acid deficiency a.
frank megaloblastic a.
genetic a.
globe cell a.
glucose-6-phosphate dehydrogenase
  deficiency a.
goat's milk a.
a. gravis
ground itch a.
Ham test for a.
Hayem-Widal a.
Heinz body hemolytic a.
hemolytic a.
hemorrhagic a.
hemotoxic a.
hereditary hemolytic a. (HHA)
hereditary nonspherocytic hemolytic
  a. (HNSHA)
hereditary sideroblastic a.
hookworm a.
hyperchromatic a.

hyperchromic a.
a. hypochromica sideroachrestica
  hereditaria
hypochromic microcytic a.
hypoferric a.
hypoplastic a.
hyporegenerative a.
iatrogenic a.
icterohemolytic a.
idiopathic refractory sideroblastic a.
  (IRSA)
idiopathic warm autoimmune
  hemolytic a.
immunohemolytic a.
a. infantum pseudoleukemica
infectious a.
intertropical a.
iron deficiency a. (IDA)
isochromic a.
isoimmune hemolytic a.
juvenile pernicious a.
lead a.
Lederer a.
leukoerythroblastic a.
local a.
a. lymphatica
macrocytic achylic a.
malignant a.
march a.
Marchiafava-Micheli a.
Mediterranean a.
megaloblastic a.
megalocytic a.
metaplastic a.
microangiopathic hemolytic a.
  (MAHA, MHA)
microcytic hypochromic a.
microdrepanocytic a.
milk a.
mixed a.
molecular a.
myelofibrosis a.
myelopathic a.
myelophthisic a.
neonatal a.
a. neonatorum
nonimmune hemolytic a.
nonmegaloblastic a.
normochromic a.
normocytic a.
nosocomial a.
nutritional a.
osteosclerotic a.
ovalocytic a.
oxidase-induced acute hemolytic a.
polar a.
posthemorrhagic a.
primaquine-sensitive a.
primary erythroblastic a.

anemia (*continued*)
    primary refractory a.
    production-defect a.
    protein deficiency a.
    pure red cell a.
    pyridoxine-responsive a.
    radiation a.
    a. refractoria sideroblastica
    refractory sideroblastic a.
    secondary refractory a.
    severe hemolytic a.
    sickle cell a.
    sideroachrestic a.
    sideroblastic a.
    sideropenic a.
    slaty a.
    spastic a.
    spherocytic a.
    splenic a.
    spur cell a.
    target cell a.
    thrombopenic a.
    toxic a.
    traumatic a.
    tropical a.
    unstable hemoglobin hemolytic a.
    variant sickling hemoglobin a.
    vitamin deficiency a.
    warm-and-cold-type autoimmune
      hemolytic a.
    warm autoimmune hemolytic a.
      (WAIHA)
AnemiaPro self-screening test
anemic
    a. anoxia
    a. halo
    a. hypoxia
    a. infarct
anemicus, anaemicus
    nevus a.
anemotrophy
anencephalia (*var. of* anencephaly)
anencephalic, anencephalous
anencephalous (*var. of* anencephalic)
anencephaly, anencephalia
anenterous
anenzymia catalasia
anephric
anergic leishmaniasis
anergy
    cachectic a.
    negative a.
    nonspecific a.
    positive a.
    a. skin test battery
    specific a.
anerythrogenesis
anerythroplasia
anerythroplastic

anerythroregenerative
anesthesia
    a. adjunct
    thalamic hyperesthetic a.
anesthetic leprosy
anetoderma
    a. erythematosum
    Schweninger-Buzzi a.
aneuploid
    a. cell
    a. tumor
aneuploidy
    DNA a.
    tumor a.
Aneurinibacillus danicus
aneurolemmic
aneurysm
    abdominal aortic a. (AAA)
    ampullary a.
    aortic arch a.
    arteriosclerotic aortic a.
    arteriosclerotic thrombosed a.
    arteriovenous a.
    atherosclerotic a.
    axial a.
    bacterial a.
    benign bone a.
    Bérard a.
    berry a.
    cardiac a.
    cirsoid a.
    compound a.
    congenital ruptured a.
    consecutive a.
    cylindroid a.
    cystogenic a.
    diffuse a.
    dissecting a.
    ectatic a.
    embolic a.
    embolomycotic a.
    endogenous a.
    erosive a.
    exogenous a.
    false a. (FA)
    fusiform a.
    hernial a.
    intracavernous a.
    intracranial a. (ICA)
    luetic a.
    miliary a.
    mural a.
    mycotic a.
    nondissecting aortic a.
    popliteal a.
    postoperative clipped a.
    Pott a.
    racemose a.
    Rasmussen a.

Richet a.
Rodrigues a.
ruptured a.
saccular a.
sacculated a.
serpentine a.
sinus of Valsalva a.
syphilitic a.
thoracic a.
thrombosed arteriosclerotic a.
traction a.
traumatic a.
true a.
tubular a.
varicose a.
ventricular a.
aneurysmal, aneurysmatic
a. bone cyst (ABC)
a. dilation
a. sac
a. varix
aneurysmatic (*var. of*
aneurysmal)
aneusomatic
aneusomy
AneuVysion prenatal test
ANF
antinuclear factor
Angelman syndrome
angel of death mushroom
Angelucci syndrome
Anger camera
angiectasia, angiectasis
congenital dysplastic a.
angiectasis (*var. of* angiectasia)
angiectatic
angiectopia
angiitic granulomatosis
angiitis, angitis
allergic granulomatous a.
Churg-Strauss a.
consecutive a.
cutaneous systemic a.
hypersensitivity a.
leukocytoclastic a.
a. livedo reticularis
necrotizing a.
angina
agranulocytic a.
Ludwig a.
lymphatic a.
a. lymphomatosa
monocytic a.
neutropenic a.
a. pectoris (AP)
Prinzmetal a.
Vincent a.
anginae
Saccharomyces a.

anginosa
scarlatina a.
anginose
a. scarlatina
anginosus
Streptococcus a.
anginosus-constellatus
Streptococcus a.-c.
angioblast
angioblastic cell
angioblastoma
angiocentric
a. immunoproliferative lesion (AIL)
a. lymphoproliferative lesion
a. pattern
a. T-cell lymphoma
angiocentricity
angiocholecystitis
angiocholitis
angiodermatitis
angiodestruction
angiodestructive pattern
angiodysgenetic myelomalacia
angiodystrophia
angioedema
angioelephantiasis
angioendothelioma
malignant endovascular papillary a.
angioendotheliomatosis
proliferating systematized a.
angiofibrolipoma
angiofibroma
juvenile a.
nasopharyngeal a. (NA)
angiofibrosis
angiogenesis
aberrant a.
a. factor
tumor a.
angiogenic switch
angioglioma
angiogliomatosis
angiogliosis
angiography
postmortem a.
angiohemophilia
angiohyalinosis
angiohypertonia
angiohypotonia
angioid streak
angioimmunoblastic
a. lymphadenopathy (AIL)
a. lymphadenopathy with dysproteinemia (AILD)
a. lymphoma (AIL)
a. T-cell lymphoma (AIL)
angioimmunoproliferative lesion (AIL)
angioinvasion
angioinvasive adenoma

angiokeratoma
    a. corporis diffusum
    diffuse a.
    Fordyce a.
    Mibelli a.
angiokeratosis
angioleiomyoma
angioleucitis
angiolipofibroma
angiolipoma
angiolith
angiolithic
    a. degeneration
    a. sarcoma
angiolymphatic invasion
**angiolymphoid hyperplasia with
  eosinophilia**
angioma, *pl.* **angiomata, angiomas**
    acquired tufted a
    cavernous a.
    cherry a.
    littoral cell a.
    a. lymphaticum
    a. serpiginosum
    spider a.
    telangiectatic a.
    a. venosum racemosum
angiomas (*pl. of* angioma)
angiomata (*pl. of* angioma)
angiomatodes
    nevus a.
angiomatoid tumor
angiomatosa
    elephantiasis congenita a.
angiomatosis
    bacillary a. (BA)
    cephalotrigeminal a.
    congenital dysplastic a.
    cutaneomeningospinal a.
    encephalotrigeminal a.
    oculoencephalic a.
    telangiectatic a.
angiomatous meningioma
angiomegaly
angiomyofibroblastoma
angiomyofibroma
angiomyolipoma (AML)
    pulmonary a.
    renal a.
angiomyoma
angiomyoneuroma
angiomyopathy
angiomyosarcoma
angiomyxoma
    aggressive a.
angioneuromyoma
angioneurotica
    purpura a.
angioneurotic edema

angioosteohypertrophy syndrome
angioparalysis
angioparesis
angiopathic hemolytic anemia
angiopathy
    amyloid a.
    British type amyloid a.
    cerebral amyloid a.
    congenital dysplastic a.
    congophilic a.
    diabetic a.
    prion protein cerebral amyloid a.
angiophacomatosis, angiophakomatosis
angiophakomatosis (*var. of*
  angiophacomatosis)
angioplany
angiopoietin
angioreninoma
angiorrhexis
angiosarcoma
    adrenal epithelioid a.
    low-grade a.
    salivary gland a.
    verrucous a.
angiosis
angiospasm
angiospastic
angiostaxis
angiostenosis
angiostrongylosis
Angiostrongylus
    A. cantonensis
    A. costaricensis
    A. malaysiensis
angiotelectasia (*var. of* angiotelectasis)
angiotelectasis, angiotelectasia
angiotensin
    a. 1 (A1)
    a. 2 (A2)
    a. 3 (A3)
    a. I
    a. I-converting enzyme
    a. I, II test
angiotensin-converting enzyme
angiotensinogen
angiotrophic lymphoma
angiotropic melanoma
angiotumoral complex
angiovascular
angitis (*var. of* angiitis)
angle
    Alsberg a.
    central collodiaphyseal a. (CCD)
    a. closure glaucoma
    critical a.
    a. head
    a. of incidence
    a. of reflection
    a. of refraction

solid a.
space of iridocorneal a.
angled soot pattern
angstrom (Å)
Ångstrom law
Anguillula
angular
a. acceleration
a. aperture
a. conjunctivitis
a. frequency
a. stomatitis
angularis
incisura a.
angulate cell
angulated lysosome
anguli (*pl. of* angulus)
Angulomicrobium amanitiforme
angulus, *pl.* **anguli**
ligamentum pectinatum anguli
ANH
acute normovolemic hemodilution
anhemolytic streptococcus
anhidrosis, anidrosis
anhidrotic ectodermal dysplasia
anhistic, anhistous
anhistous (*var. of* anhistic)
anhydrase
carbonic a.
anhydration
anhydride
acetic a.
basic a.
cyclic lysine a. (CLA)
heptafluorobutyric a. (HFBA)
resorcinol phthalic a.
trifluoroacetic a. (TFAA)
anhydrous
a. alcohol
a. sodium sulfite
ani (*pl. of* anus)
Anichkov (*var. of* Anitschkow)
anidrosis (*var. of* anhidrosis)
aniline
a. blue
a. blue modified trichrome stain
a. dye
a. fuchsin
a. gentian violet (AGV)
aniline, sulfur, formaldehyde (ASF)
anilinism
anilinophil, anilinophile
anilinophile (*var. of* anilinophil)
anilinophilous
animal
anthrax-infected a.
a. cell culture
conventional a.
Houssay a.

molluscous a.
normal a.
a. protein factor (APF)
sentinel a.
a. toxin
a. virus
animalcule
animatum
contagium a.
virus a.
anion
cyanide a.
a. exchanger 1 (AE1)
a. gap
a. gap test
a. interference
superoxide a.
anion-exchange
a.-e. chromatography
a.-e. resin
anionic
a. detergent
a. dye
a. neutrophil activating peptide
(ANAP)
anionotropy
aniridia
anisakiasis
anisakid
Anisakidae
Anisakis marina
anise oil
anisochromasia
anisochromia
anisocytosis
anisohypercytosis
anisohypocytosis
anisokaryosis
anisoleukocytosis
anisonucleosis
anisopoikilocytosis
anisotropic
a. disc
a. lipid
anisotropy
anitrata
Lingelsheimia a.
anitratus
Acinetobacter calcoaceticus a.
Anitschkow, Anichkov
A. cell
A. myocyte
Anixiella
Anixiopsis
ankle-type fibrous histiocytoma
ankyloblepharon
ankylocolpos
ankyloglossia
ankyloproctia

ankylosing spondylitis
ankylosis
    bony a.
    extracapsular a.
    fibrous a.
    intracapsular a.
    osseous a.
ankylostoma
ankylostomiasis
ankyrin
anlage, *pl.* anlagen
anlagen (*pl. of* anlage)
ANLL
    acute nonlymphocytic leukemia
Ann
    A. Arbor staging classification
    A. Arbor staging system
    A. Arbor tumor classification
annatto, annotto
anneal
annealing temperature
annelid
Annelida
annelloconidium
annexin
    a. A1 marker
    a. V
annexitis
annihilation
    positron a.
annotto (*var. of* annatto)
annua
    Artemisia a.
annulare
    granuloma a.
annularis
    Anopheles a.
    lichen a.
    lipoatrophia a.
    purpura a.
    rachitis fetalis a.
annulate lamellae
annulatus
    Boophilus a.
    Streptomyces a.
annulipes
    Anopheles a.
annulospiral
    a. ending
    a. organ
annuli (*pl. of* annulus)
annulus (*var. of* anulus), *pl.*
 annuli
annum
    Capsicum a.
ano
    fissure in a.
    fistula in a.
anochromasia

anodal
anode voltage
anodontia
anogenital wart
anomalad
anomalies (*pl. of* anomaly)
anomalous
    a. muscle band
    a. origin
    a. vascular distribution
    a. venous connection
    a. venous drainage
anomalus
    Hoplopsyllus a.
anomaly, *pl.* anomalies
    Alder a.
    Alder-Reilly a.
    Alius-Grignaschi a.
    cerebrovascular a.
    Chédiak-Steinbrinck-Higashi a.
    coloboma, heart disease, atresia
     choanae, retarded growth and
     development and ear anomalies
     (CHARGE)
    congenital a.
    developmental sequence a.
    dysraphic a.
    Ebstein a.
    Freund a.
    Hegglin a.
    Hüet-Pelger nuclear a.
    Jordan a.
    May-Hegglin a.
    Shone a.
    Uhl a.
    Undritz a.
    vascular a.
    vertebral defects, anal atresia,
     tracheoesophageal fistula with
     esophageal atresia, and radial and
     renal anomalies (VATER)
anomer
anomeric
Anopheles
    A. aconitus
    A. albimanus
    A. albitarsus
    A. annularis
    A. annulipes
    A. aquasalis
    A. arabiensis
    A. aztecus
    A. balabacensis
    A. barbirostris
    A. bellator
    A. brunnipes
    A. campestris
    A. crucians
    A. cruzi

A. *culicifacies*
A. *darlingi*
A. *flavirostris*
A. *fluviatilis*
A. *freeborni*
A. *funestus*
A. *gambiae*
A. *jeyporiensis*
A. *karwari*
A. *kweiyangensis*
A. *labranchiae*
A. *lesteri*
A. *leucosphyrus*
A. *maculatus*
A. *maculipennis*
A. *messeae*
A. *minimus*
A. *pseudopunctipennis*
A. *quadrimaculatus*
A. *stephensi*
A. *sundaicus*
A. *superpictus*
anophelicide
anophelifuge
Anophelinae
anopheline
Anophelini
anophelism
anophthalmia, anophthalmos
anophthalmos (*var. of* anophthalmia)
Anoplocephala perfoliata
Anoplocephalidae
Anoplura
anorchia
anorectal melanoma
anorectic, anoretic, anorexic
anoretic (*var. of* anorectic)
anorexia nervosa
anorexic (*var. of* anorectic)
anorexigenic neuropeptide
anosmia
anosteoplasia
anostosis
ANOVA
analysis of variance
anovular ovarian follicle
anovulation
anovulatory
anoxemia
anoxemic
anoxia
altitude a.
anemic a.
anoxic a.
fulminating a.
histotoxic a.
hypoxic a.
myocardial a.
a. neonatorum

oxygen affinity a.
a. reaction
stagnant a.
anoxic
a. anoxia
a. encephalopathy
Anoxybacillus
A. *ayderensis*
A. *contaminans*
A. *flavithermus*
A. *gonensis*
A. *kestanbolensis*
A. *pushchinoensis*
A. *voinovskiensis*
Anoxynatronum sibiricum
Anoxyphotobacteria
Anoxyphotobacteriae
ANP
atrial natriuretic peptide
ANS
antineutrophilic serum
arteriolonephrosclerosis
ansa, *pl.* **ansae**
Henle a.
ansae (*pl. of* ansa)
anserina
Borrelia a.
cutis a.
anserine
anseris
Amidostomum a.
ANSI
American National Standards
Institute
antagonism
bacterial a.
metabolic a.
microbial a.
salt a.
antagonist
beta-adrenergic a.
cholinergic a.
competitive a.
endothelin-1 receptor a.
enzyme a.
insulin a.
metabolic a.
narcotic a.
NMDA receptor a.
protein induced by vitamin K a.
(PIVKA)
sulfonamide a.
antarctica
Aequorivita a.
Oleispira a.
Pseudonocardia a.
Psychromonas a.
antarcticum
Exiguobacterium a.

antarcticus
>*Paenibacillus a.*
>*Planococcus a.*
>*Rhodoferax a.*

antecedent
>plasma thromboplastin a. (PTA)

antegrade

antemortem
>a. clot
>a. thrombus

antenatal

antepartum hemorrhage (APH)

anterior
>a. acute poliomyelitis
>a. centriole
>a. complete dislocation
>a. displacement
>a. elastic layer
>a. ethmoidal air cell
>glandula lingualis a.
>a. horn cell
>a. incisural space
>lamina elastica a.
>a. lateral myocardial infarct (ALMI)
>a. limiting layer of cornea
>a. lobe of hypophysis
>a. median fissure
>a. pituitary extract (APE)
>a. pituitary hormone (APH)
>a. pituitary hyperfunction
>a. pituitary-like (APL)
>a. semicircular canal
>a. wall
>a. wall infarction (AWI)
>a. wall myocardial infarction (AWMI)

anterioris
>cellulae ethmoidales anteriores
>endothelium camerae a.

anterochoanal

anterofacial dysplasia

anterograde

anteroposterior
>a. facial dysplasia
>a. dysplasia

anteroseptal myocardial infarct (ASMI)

anteverted/anteflexed

anthelminthic, anthelmintic

anthelmintic (*var. of* anthelminthic)

anthelmycin

antheridium

anthina
>*Burkholderia a.*

anthocyanidin

anthocyanin

Anthomyia
>*A. canicularis*
>*A. incisura*

Anthomyiidae

Anthopsis deltoidea

anthracemia

anthracene blue

anthracic

anthracin

anthracis
>*Bacillus a.*
>encapsulated *Bacillus a.*
>veterinary vaccine Stern strain *Bacillus a.*

Anthracobia

anthracoid

anthracometer

anthracosilicosis

anthracosis linguae

anthracotic
>a. pigment
>a. tuberculosis

anthracycline cardiotoxicity

anthramucin

anthranilic acid

anthrapurpurin

anthraquinone dye

anthrax
>abdominal a.
>a. as biological weapon
>a. bacillus
>a. belt
>a. capsule
>cutaneous a.
>a. epizootic
>gastrointestinal a.
>inhalational a.
>a. malignant pustule
>a. meningitis
>oropharyngeal a.
>a. pneumonia
>pulmonary a.
>a. septicemia
>septicemic a.
>a. spore
>a. toxin
>a. vaccine absorbed

anthrax-containing chocolate

anthrax-contaminated animal product

anthrax-infected
>a.-i. animal
>a.-i. body fluid

anthrone

anthropoid

anthropology
>forensic a.
>hematological a.

anthropometric

anthropometry
>forensic a.

anthropomorphic table

anthroponoses (*pl. of* anthroponosis)
anthroponosis, *pl.* **anthroponoses**
anthropophaga
    Cordylobia a.
    Ochromyia a.
anthropophilic
anthropozoonosis
anthurii
    Acidovorax a.
anti-A
    a.-A agglutinin
    a.-A antibody
antiadrenal antibody
antiagglutinin
antiaggregant
    platelet a.
antialexin
antialkaline phosphatase method
antiallergic
antiallotype
antialopecia factor
antianaphylaxis, ananaphylaxis
antiandrogen
    pure a.
antianemic
    a. factor
    a. principle
antiantibody
antiantitoxin
antiapoptotic protein
antiarachnolysin
antiasialoglycoprotein receptor
antiatherogenic activity
antiautolysin
anti-B
    a.-B agglutinin
    a.-B antibody
antibacterial
    a. agent
    a. agent susceptibility testing
antibasement
    a. membrane antibody (ABMA)
    a. membrane glomerulonephritis
    a. membrane nephritis
antibiogram
antibiont
antibiosis
antibiotic
    a. antitumor drug
    bactericidal a.
    bacteriostatic a.
    broad-spectrum a.
    a. enterocolitis
    a. level
    macrolide a.
    polyene a.
    a. sensitivity
    a. sensitivity test
    tetrin macrolide a.

antibiotica
    Kribbella a.
antibiotic-associated
    a.-a. colitis (AAC)
    a.-a. diarrhea (AAD)
antibiotic-resistant
antibody (Ab)
    A5B7 monoclonal a.
    ABO a.
    absorption of erythrocyte a.
    acetylcholine receptor a.
     (AChRAb)
    adrenal a.
    AE1 a.
    AE3 a.
    affinity a.
    a. affinity chromatography
    agglutinating a.
    albumin-agglutinating a.
    ALK1 a.
    allergen-specific IgE a.
    alloantin-D a.
    alpha globulin a.
    AMACR a.
    anaphylactic a.
    anti-A a.
    antiadrenal a.
    anti-B a.
    antibasement membrane a.
    anticardiolipin a. (ACA,
     ACLA)
    anti-CD11a humanized
     monoclonal a.
    anti-CD18 humanized a.
    anticentromere a.
    anti-Chido a.
    anticoilin a.
    anticytokeratin a.
    anticytoplasmic a. (ACPA)
    anti-DAK a.
    anti-DNA a.
    anti-EA a.
    anti-EGF-receptor a.
    antiendoglin a.
    anti fas/APO-1 a.
    antifibrin a.
    antifibrinogen a.
    anti-GBM a.
    anti-Goa a.
    antigranulocyte a.
    anti-hepatitis A a. (anti-HAV)
    anti-hepatitis C a. (anti-HCV)
    anti-hepatitis D a. (anti-HDV)
    antihistone a. (AHA)
    antiidiotype a.
    antiinsulin a.
    antiintrinsic factor a.
    anti-Js a.
    anti-kappa a.

antibody (*continued*)
    anti-Kell a.
    antikeratin AE1 a.
    antikeratin AE3 a.
    antikidney a.
    anti-LA a.
    antilambda a.
    antileukocyte a.
    antiliver-kidney microsomal a.
    anti-LKM-1 a.
    antilymphocytic a.
    anti-M a.
    antimetallothionein a. (MT)
    antimicrosomal a.
    antimitochondrial a. (AMA)
    antineutrophil cytoplasmic a.
     (ANCA)
    antinuclear a. (ANA)
    anti-P a.
    antiparietal cell a.
    Anti-PEP-1 a.
    Anti-Pep-8 a.
    antiphospholipid a. (APA)
    antiplatelet a.
    antireceptor a.
    anti-Rh a.
    anti-RNA a.
    anti-Ro a.
    anti-Rodgers a.
    anti-S a.
    anti-*Saccharomyces cerevisiae* a.
     (ASCA)
    antisera a.
    anti-Sm a.
    antismooth muscle a. (ASMA)
    anti-T-cell a.
    antithyroglobulin a.
    antithyroid peroxidase a.
    anti-*Toxoplasma* a. (ATA)
    antitubular basement membrane a.
    anti-VCA a.
    anti-VS a.
    APAAP a.
    ASCA a.
    autoantiidiotypic a.
    autoimmune a.
    autologous a.
    avidity a.
    B72.3 a.
    basal cell carcinoma specific a.
    basement membrane a.
    B-cell a.
    bcl-2 a.
    bcl-6 a.
    BE12 a.
    Ber-EP4 a.
    Ber-H2 a.
    BG8 monoclonal a.
    BH11 a.

    bivalent a.
    BLA 36 monoclonal a.
    blocking a. (BA)
    blood group a.
    BNH9 a.
    BrDu a.
    C219 a.
    C494 a.
    C8/144 a.
    CAM 5.2 a.
    cA2 monoclonal a.
    capture a.
    a. capture ligand assay
    a. catabolism
    cathepsin D a.
    CB11 a.
    CD a.
    CD14 a.
    CEJO65 monoclonal a.
    cell-bound a.
    centromere/kinetochore a.
    CF a.
    chimeric a.
    CH/RG a.
    chromogranin a.
    circulatory antigliadin a.
    Clonad monoclonal a.
    CM1 a.
    CMV a.
    coccidioidomycosis a.
    cold a.
    cold-reacting a.
    cold-reactive a.
    cold-type a.
    a. combining site
    complement-fixing a.
    complete a.
    coprecipitating a.
    Coulter CLONE monoclonal a.
    cross-reacting a.
    cryptosporidiosis a.
    cytokeratin CAM 5.2 a.
    cytomegalovirus a.
    cytophilic a.
    cytoplasmic antineutrophil
     cytoplasmic a. (cANCA)
    Cyto-Stat/Coulter CLONE
     monoclonal a.
    cytotoxic a.
    cytotropic a.
    D2-40 a.
    a. deficiency disease
    a. deficiency syndrome (ADS)
    desmin a.
    a. detection
    direct fluorescent a. (DFA)
    DL a.
    D2-40 monoclonal a.
    DO7 a.

Donath-Landsteiner a.
donor-specific HLA a.
Duffy a.
dystrophin a.
EMA a.
endomysial a.
enhancing a.
envoplakin a.
erythrocyte a. (EA)
a. excess
a. excess zone
extractable nuclear antigen a. (ENA)
ferritin-conjugated a. (FCA)
ferritin-coupled a.
fluorescein-labeled a.
fluorescent a. (FA)
fluorescent antinuclear a. (FANA)
fluorescent treponemal a. (FTA)
fluorochrome-conjugated
  monoclonal a.
Forssman a.
GB-7 a.
glomerular basement membrane a.
H a.
Ha-1A monoclonal a.
HAM 56 a.
HBME 1 a.
heat-labile a.
HECA-452 a.
hemagglutinating antipenicillin a.
  (HAPA)
hemagglutination-inhibition a. (HIA)
hepatitis a.
hepatitis A a.
hepatitis B core a. (HB$_c$Ab)
hepatitis Be a. (HB$_e$Ab)
hepatitis B surface a. (HB$_s$Ab)
HepPar1 a.
herpes simplex a.
heteroclitic a.
heterocytotropic a.
heterogenetic a.
heteroligating a.
heterophil a.
H1F1 a.
HHF 35 a.
HMB 45 a.
HMFG-2 a.
HMWK a.
homocytotropic a.
HTLV-I a.
human antichimeric a. (HACA)
human antimouse a. (HAMA)
human antimurine a. (HAMA)
humoral a.
hybrid a.
hybridoma a.
a. identification
idiotype a.

IgA-antigliadin a.
IgA endomysial a.
IgE a.
IgG desmoplakin a.
IgM a.
IgM-RF a.
immobilizing a.
immunosorbent a.
incomplete a.
indirect fluorescent a.
indirect fluorescent rabies a. (test)
inhibin a.
inhibiting a.
insulin a.
intrinsic factor a.
IOTest monoclonal a.
islet cell a. (ICA)
isoimmune a.
isophil a.
Ki-1 a.
Ki-67 a.
kidney-fixing a. (KFAb)
Ki-FDC1p a.
Ki-M4p a.
Ki-M1p a.
Ki-S5 a.
KO89-kit a.
KP1 a.
KP1/CD68 monoclonal a.
L26 a.
LCA a.
Legionnaire disease a.
LEMS a.
Leu 1–22 a.
LeuM1 a.
LeuM3 a.
LeuM5 a.
Lewis a.
LKM a.
LN1 a.
LN2 a.
LN3 monoclonal a.
lymphocytotoxic a.
lymphoid monoclonal a.
Mac387 a.
maternal a.
measles a.
Melan A/MART-1 a.
MIB1 a.
MIC2 a.
microsomal thyroid a.
mirror-image complementary a.
  (MICA)
mitochondrial a.
MOC31 monoclonal a.
monoclonal a. (MAb)
MSA a.
MTI a.
MUCI a.

antibody (*continued*)
    natural a.
    NCL-ARm monoclonal a.
    NCL-ARp polyclonal a.
    NCL-ER-LH2 monoclonal a.
    NCL-PCR monoclonal a.
    nephrotoxic a. (NTAB)
    neutralizing a. (NA)
    NK1-C3 a.
    no demonstrable antibodies
      (NDA)
    nonprecipitable a.
    nonprecipitating a.
    normal a.
    nuclear a.
    O a.
    OKT-9 a.
    OPD4 a.
    opsonizing a.
    OptiClone monoclonal a.
    Orthomune a.
    a. panning technique
    a. placental alkaline phosphatase
      (anti-PLAP)
    platelet a.
    p80NPM/ALK a.
    polyclonal antiplacental a.
    polyclonal prolactin a.
    Prausnitz-Kustner a.
    precipitating a.
    a. producing plasma cell
    reaginic a.
    Rh a.
    S-100 a.
    saline-agglutinating a.
    scleroderma a.
    a. screening
    a. screening test
    Sjogren a.
    skeletal muscle a.
    skin-sensitizing a. (SSA)
    smooth muscle a. (SMA)
    a. specificity prediction (ASP)
    sperm agglutinating a.
    a. stain
    synaptophysin a.
    T a.
    TAB 250 a.
    teichoic acid a.
    tetanus a.
    Thomsen a.
    thyroglobulin a.
    thyroid antimicrosomal a.
    thyroid antithyroglobulin a.
    thyroid microsomal a. (TMAb)
    thyrotropin-receptor a.
    TIA-1 a.
    a. titer
    TMH-1 a.

    a. to hepatitis B core antigen
      (HB$_c$Ab)
    a. to hepatitis B surface antigen
      (HB$_s$Ab)
    a. to SARS-CoV
    treponema-immobilizing a.
    treponemal a.
    tropomodulin-1 a. (TMOD1)
    TSH displacing a. (TDA)
    UCHL1 a.
    UCHL1^a a.
    UCL3D3 a.
    UJ127.11 a.
    UJ13A monoclonal a.
    ULCL4D12 a.
    univalent a.
    Vi a.
    vimentin a.
    warm reactive a.
    Wassermann a.
    white blood cell a.
    xenocytophilic a.
    Yersinia enterocolitica a.
    Yersinia pestis a.
    ZB4 a.
antibody-absorption
    fluorescent treponemal a.-a.
      (FTA-ABS)
antibody/antigen
    CD117 a.
    CD14 a.
**antibody-based lateral flow economical
  recognition ticket (ALERT)**
antibody-coated microprobe technique
antibody-conjugate
    antidigoxigenin alkaline phosphatase
      a.-c.
antibody-dependent
    a.-d. cell-mediated cytotoxicity
    a.-d. cell-mediated cytotoxicity
      reaction
    a.-d. immunity
antibody-forming cell
antibody-mediated
    a.-m. rejection
    a.-m. vascular damage
anti-BrdU
    anti-bromodeoxyuridine
anti-bromodeoxyuridine (anti-BrdU)
anticarcinoembryonic antigen
**anticardiolipin antibody
  (ACA, ACLA)**
anticariensis
    Halomonas a.
**anti-CD11a humanized monoclonal
  antibody**
anti-CD18 humanized antibody
anticentromere antibody
anti-c-*erb*B-2

anti-Chido antibody
anti-*Chlamydia* antibody test
anticholera serum
anticholinergic delirium
anticholinesterase
antichromogranin
antichymotrypsin
    alpha a. (ACT)
    alpha-1 a. (A1AC)
    a. test
anticoag
   anticoagulant
anticoagulant (AC)
    circulating a.
    a. heparin solution
    lupus a. (LA)
    a. protein
    a. therapy (ACT)
anticoagulant-citrate-dextrose
anticoagulant-citrate-phosphate-dextrose
anticoagulated blood
anticoagulative
anticoagulin
anticodon
anticoilin antibody
anticolibacillary serum
anticollagenase
anticommon leukocyte antigen
anticomplement
anticomplementary
    a. factor
    a. serum
anticontagious
anticytokeratin
    a. antibody
    a. immunohistochemistry
    a. stain
anticytoplasmic
    a. antibody (ACPA)
    a. autoantibody
anticytotoxin
anti-DAK antibody
antideoxyribonuclease
    a. B
    a. B titer test
antidesmin
antidigoxigenin
    a. alkaline phosphatase
      antibody-conjugate
    a. antibody peroxidase conjugate
anti-D immunoglobulin
antidiphtheric serum
antidiphtheritic globulin
antidiuretic
    a. hormone (ADH)
    a. hormone deficiency
    a. substance (ADS)
anti-DNA
    a.-D. antibody

    a.-D. antibody assay
    a.-D. topoisomerase
anti-DNase
anti-DNase B
antidote
    oxime a.
antidromic
anti-EA antibody
anti-EGF-receptor antibody
antiendoglin antibody
antiendomysial antibody test
antienzyme
antiepithelial serum
anti-Epstein-Barr nuclear antigen
antiestrogen receptor
antifactor I–IX disorder
anti-F1 antigen titer
anti-fas/APO-1 antibody
antifibrin antibody
antifibrinogen antibody
antifibrinolysin
antifibrinolytic
antifol
antifolic
antifungal agent
anti-GBM
    antiglomerular basement membrane
    a.-GBM antibody
    a.-GBM disease
antigen (Ag, AGN)
    A a.
    ABH a.
    ABO a.
    accessible a.
    acetone-insoluble a.
    A-like a.
    allogeneic a.
    alum-precipitated a.
    Am a.
    antibody to hepatitis B core a.
      (HB$_c$Ab)
    antibody to hepatitis B surface a.
      (HB$_s$Ab)
    anticarcinoembryonic a.
    anticommon leukocyte a.
    anti-Epstein-Barr nuclear a.
    Australia a. (AU Ag)
    autologous a.
    B a.
    B72.3 a.
    bacterial meningitis a.
    Be^a a.
    Becker a.
    Bi a.
    bile a.
    blood group a. (BGA)
    BR27.29 breast a.
    By a.
    C a.

antigen (*continued*)
 CA125 a.
 CA19-9 a.
 CA15-3 breast a.
 CAM 5.2 a.
 cancer a. (CA)
 cancer a. 125 (CA 125)
 capsular a.
 a. capture ligand assay
 carbohydrate a.
 carcinoembryonic a. (CEA)
 Cartwright a.
 C carbohydrate a.
 CD a.
 CD68 a.
 chick embryo a.
 Chlamydia a.
 cholesterinized a.
 ChrA a.
 CH/RG a.
 class histocompatibility a.
 clusterin a.
 cluster 1 small-cell lung cancer a.
 Colton a.
 common acute lymphoblastic
  leukemia a. (CALLA)
 common acute lymphocytic
  leukemia a.
 common enterobacterial a.
 complement-fixing a.
 complete a.
 complexed prostate-specific a. (cPSA)
 conjugated a.
 core a.
 cross-reacting a.
 cryptic T a.
 cryptococcal a. (CRY-AG)
 cyclin A a.
 cyclin E a.
 cytokeratin 1—20 a.
 cytokeratin CAM 5.2 a.
 D a.
 D10 a.
 delta a.
 DFA for capsular a.
 Dharmendra a.
 Di a.
 Diego a. (DiA)
 differentiation a. (DA)
 Dombrock a.
 Duffy a.
 DU-PAN-2 pancreatic
  cancer-associated a.
 E a.
 early a. (EA)
 endogenous a.
 envoplakin a.
 epidermal surface a.
 epithelial membrane a. (EMA)

 epsilon a.
 Epstein-Barr nuclear a. (EBNA)
 erythrocyte a.
 estrogen-receptor a.
 a. excess
 exogenous a.
 extractable nuclear a. (ENA)
 F a.
 1F6 a.
 fecal a.
 fetal a.
 fibrin-related a. (FRA)
 flagellar a.
 Forssman a.
 Frei a.
 Fy a.
 G a.
 a. gain
 gamma a.
 Ge a.
 Good a.
 Gr a.
 Gross virus a. (GSA)
 group a.'s
 group specific a.
 guinea pig a.
 H a. (HA)
 H-2 a.
 hapten X, Y a.
 HBA71 a.
 He a.
 heart a.
 heat-extracted a.
 hematopoietic progenitor cell a.
 hepatitis a.
 hepatitis-associated a. (HAA)
 hepatitis B core a. (HB$_c$Ag)
 hepatitis Be a. (HB$_e$Ag)
 hepatitis B surface a. (HB$_s$Ag)
 hepatitis D a.
 herpesvirus a.
 heterogeneic a.
 heterogenetic a.
 heterogenic enterobacterial a.
 heterophil a.
 hexon a.
 HHV 8 a.
 Hikojima a.
 histo-blood group a.
 histocompatibility a.
 HLA-A a.
 HLA-B a.
 HLA BW 54 a.
 HLA-D a.
 HLA-DR a.
 HMB 45 a.
 Ho a.
 homologous a.
 Hu a.

human leukemia-associated a.
human leukocyte a. (HLA)
human lymphocyte a.
human progenitor cell a.
H-Y a.
I a.
Ia a.
idiotypic a.
IGF-II a.
I/i a.
I(Ma) a.
Inaba a.
incomplete a.
inhalant a.
a. interferon
InV group a.
isophile a.
Ja a.
Jaa a.
Jaa-F11 a.
Jk a.
Jobbins a.
Js a.
K a.
K and k a.
KD a.
Kell a.
Ki-1 a.
Ki-67 a.
Kidd a.
Km a.
Kunin a.
Kveim a.
Kveim-Stilzbach a.
labeled a.
laminin a.
Lan a.
Le a.
Legionella urinary a. (LUA)
lens a.
Leu 1 a.
leukocyte common a. (LCA)
LeuM1 a.
Levay a.
Lewis a.
Lewis-X blood group a.
LP a.
Lu a.
Lw a.
Ly a.
Lyb a.
lymphocyte function associated a.
lymphogranuloma venereum a.
Lyt a.
M a.
M$_1$ a.
major histocompatibility a. (MHA)
Melan A/MART-1 a.
merozoite a.

Mi-2 a.
MIB1 a.
Miltenberger a.
minor histocompatibility a.
Mitsuda a.
monoclonal antibody-specific
   immobilization of platelet a.
   (MAIPA)
monoclonal antiepithelial
   membrane a.
mouse-specific lymphocyte a.
   (MSLA)
mu a.
mumps skin test a.
N a.
non-heat-extracted a.
nonspecific cross-reacting a. (NCA)
normal fecal a. (NFA-I)
NP a.
O a.
Ogawa a.
oncofetal a.
oncoprotein a.
organ-specific a.
Ot a.
Oz a.
P a.
p27 a.
P54 a.
p24 HIV a.
plasma cell a.
pollen a.
polyclonal anticarcinoembryonic a.
polyclonal carcinoembryonic a.
   (pCEA)
a. presentation
private a.
a. processing
proliferating cell nuclear a. (PCHA,
   PCNA)
Pronase a.
prostate-specific a. (PSA)
prostate-specific membrane a.
   (PSMA)
prostate stem cell a. (PSCA)
protective a. (PA)
Proteus OX2 a.
Proteus OX19 a.
Proteus OXK a.
public a.
Qa a.
R a.
a. receptor activation motif (ARAM)
a. recognition
recognition of a.
respiratory syncytial virus a.
a. retrieval
Rh a.
Rhus toxicodendron a.

antigen (*continued*)
    Rhus venenata a.
    rose bengal a. (RBA)
    S a.
    S and s a.
    SD a.
    a. sensitivity
    sensitized a.
    sequestered a.
    serologically defined a.
    shock a.
    Sialosyl-Tn a.
    single human leukocyte a.
    skin-specific histocompatibility a.
    Sm a.
    soluble human leukocyte a. (sHLA)
    soluble liver a. (SLA)
    somatic a.
    species-specific a.
    specific a.
    S-100 protein a.
    squamous-cell carcinoma a. (SCCA, SCC-Ag)
    SS-A/Ro a.
    SS-B/La a.
    Stobo a.
    Streptococcus M a.
    surface a.
    SV 40 T a.
    Sw^a a.
    Swann a.
    synthetic a.
    T a.
    Tac a.
    TAG-72 a.
    T-cell a.
    T-cell restricted intracellular a.
    T-dependent a.
    theta a.
    Thomas a.
    Thomsen-Friedenreich a.
    Thy-1 a.
    thymus-dependent a.
    thymus-independent a.
    thymus-leukemia a.
    tissue-specific a.
    TL a.
    Tn a.
    TRA a.
    TRA-1-60 human embryonal carcinoma marker a.
    transplantation a.
    tropomodulin-1 a.
    tumor a.
    tumor-associated rejection a. (TARA)
    tumor-associated transplantation a. (TATA)
    tumor-specific transplantation a. (TSTA)
    a. unit
    V a.
    Vel a.
    Ven a.
    Vi a.
    viral capsid a. (VCA)
    VLA a.
    von Willebrand factor a.
    Vw a.
    Wassermann a.
    Webb a.
    Wr^a a.
    Wr^b a.
    Wright a.
    Xg a.
    Yersinia pestis F1 capsular a.
    yolk sac a.
    Yta a.

antigen-antibody
    a.-a. complex
    a.-a. reaction

antigen-antiglobulin reaction

antigen-binding
    a.-b. capacity
    a.-b. region
    single-chain a.-b. (SCA)
    a.-b. site

antigen-combining site

antigenemia

antigenetic peptide

antigenic
    a. analysis
    a. assay
    a. competition
    a. complex
    a. deletion
    a. determinant
    a. difference
    a. distribution
    a. drift
    a. modulation
    a. shift
    a. similarity
    a. structural grouping

antigenicity

antigen-presenting cell (APC)

antigen-responsive cell

antigen-retrieval technique

antigen-sensitive cell

antigen-specific
    a.-s. helper factor
    a.-s. suppressor factor

antigen-transporting cell

antigen-triggered lymphocyte differentiation

antigenuria

anti-GFAP staining

antiglobulin test (AGT)
antiglomerular basement membrane
(anti-GBM)
anti-glomerular basement membrane
disease (anti-GBM d)
anti-glutamic acid decarboxylase
autoantibody
anti-Goa antibody
antigranulocyte antibody
anti-HBc
anti-HBe
    antibody to hepatitis B core antigen
anti-HBs
    antibody to hepatitis B surface
    antigen
antihemagglutinin
antihemolysin
antihemolytic
antihemophilic
    a. factor (AHF)
    a. factor A, B
    a. globulin (AHG)
    a. globulin A, B
    a. plasma
    a. plasma human
antihemorrhagic
antiheparin factor
antihepatic serum
anti-hepatitis
    a.-h. A antibody
    a.-h. C antibody
    a.-h. D antibody
antiheterolysin
antihistamine
antihistaminic
antihistone antibody
anti-HLA alloantibody
antihormone
antihuman
    a. globulin (AHG)
    a. globulin test
    a. lymphocyte serum (AHLS)
antihyaluronidase (AH)
    a. assay
    a. titer (AHT)
antihypercholesterolemic
antihypertensive
antiidiotype
    a. antibody
    a. autoantibody
antiinfective
antiinflammatory
    a. corticoid (AC)
    nonsteroidal a. (NSAID)
antiinsulin antibody
antiintrinsic factor antibody
antiisolysin
anti-Js antibody
anti-kappa antibody

anti-Kell antibody
antikeratin
    a. AE1
    a. AE3
    a. AE1 antibody
    a. AE3 antibody
antikidney
    a. antibody
    a. serum nephritis
anti-LA antibody
antilambda antibody
anti-LA/SS-B test
antileukocidin
antileukocyte antibody
antileukotoxin
antilewisite
    British a. (BAL)
antiliver-kidney microsomal antibody
anti-LKM-1 antibody
antilymphocyte
    a. globulin (ALG)
    a. plasma (ALP)
    a. serum (ALS)
antilymphocytic
    a. antibody
    a. globulin
antilysin
anti-M
    a.-M agglutinin
    a.-M antibody
antimacrophage
    a. globulin (AMG)
    a. serum (AMS)
antimalarial
antimediated cytotoxicity
antimeningococcus serum
antimetabolite drug
antimetallothionein antibody (MT)
antimicrobial
    a. spectrum
    a. therapy
antimicrosomal antibody
antimitochondrial
    a. antibody (AMA)
    a. antibody assay
antimode
antimony
    a. assay
    butter of a.
    a. chloride
    a. hydride
    a. pneumoconiosis
    a. poisoning
    a. stain
    a. trichloride
antimonyltartrate
    sodium a.
antimorph
antimorphic

antimouse
    a. lymphocyte serum (AMLS)
    a. thymocyte
antimüllerian hormone (AMH)
antimuscarinic effect
antimutagen
antimycotic
antimyoglobin
anti-N agglutinin
antineoplastic
antineurotoxin
antineutrophil
    a. cytoplasmic antibody (ANCA)
    a. cytoplasmic autoantibody (ANCA)
antineutrophilic serum (ANS)
antinsulin serum (AIS)
antinuclear
    a. antibody (ANA)
    a. antibody assay
    a. factor (ANF)
anti-oncogene
    DCC a.-o.
antioncogene
antioxidant
anti-P
    a.-P agglutinin
    a.-P antibody
    a.-P blood group specificity
anti-p53
antiparallel
antiparasitic
antiparietal
    a. cell antibody (APCA)
    a. cell antibody assay
antiparticle
antipedicular
antipediculotic
Anti-PEP-1 antibody
Anti-Pep-8 antibody
antiperiodic
antipernicious anemia factor (APA)
antipertussis serum
antiphagocytic polypeptide capsule
antiphospholipid
    a. antibody (APA, APAB)
    a. antibody syndrome
    a. syndrome (APS)
antiplague serum
antiplant pathogen
anti-PLAP
    antibody placental alkaline phosphatase
antiplasmin
    alpha 2 a.
antiplatelet
    a. antibody
    a. serum
antipneumococcic
antipneumococcus serum
antipodal cone

antiport
anti-Pr cold autoagglutinin
antiprecipitin
antiprogesterone receptor
antiprothrombin
anti-*Pseudomonas* human plasma
antipyogenic
antiqua
    Hylemya a.
antirabies serum (ARS)
antireceptor antibody
antireticular cytotoxic serum (ACS)
antiretroviral
    a. agent
    a. treatment (ART)
anti-Rh
    a.-R. agglutinin
    a.-R. antibody
    a.-R. titer
anti-Rho-D titer test
antiricin
anti-RNA antibody
anti-Ro antibody
anti-Rodgers antibody
anti-Ro/SS-A test
anti-S
    a.-S agglutinin
    a.-S antibody
anti-*Saccharomyces cerevisiae* antibody (ASCA)
antisarcomeric actin
antiscarlatinal serum
antisense probe
antisepsis
antiseptic
antiserum
    a. anaphylaxis
    antisera antibody
    blood group a.
    CALLA a.
    heterologous a.
    homologous a.
    human thymus a. (HUTHAS)
    monovalent a.
    nerve growth factor a. (NGF)
    NGF a.
    polyvalent a.
    specific a.
anti-Sm
    anti-Smith
    a.-S. antibody
    a.-S. test
anti-Smith (anti-Sm)
antismooth
    a. muscle actin
    a. muscle antibody (ASMA)
    a. muscle antibody assay
antisnake venom (ASV)
anti-S-100 protein

antistaphylococcic
antistaphylococcus serum
antistaphylolysin
antisteapsin
antistreptococcic
antistreptococcus serum
antistreptokinase
antistreptolysin (AS)
    a. O (ASO)
antistreptolysin-O titer
antisubstance
antisynthetase syndrome
anti-tac
anti-T-cell antibody
antitetanic serum (ATS)
antithoracic duct lymphocytic globulin
  (ATDLG)
antithrombin (AT, At)
    a. I
    a. III
    a. III test
    IL test liquid a.
    normal a.
antithromboplastin
antithymocyte
    a. globulin (ATG)
    a. serum (ATS)
antithyroglobulin (ATG)
    a. antibody
antithyroid peroxidase antibody
antitoxic serum
antitoxigen
antitoxin
    bivalent gas gangrene a.
    bothropic a.
    Bothrops a.
    botulinum a.
    botulism a.
    bovine a.
    Crotalus a.
    despeciated a.
    diphtheria a. (DAT)
    dysentery a.
    a. Einheit (AE)
    gas gangrene a.
    normal a.
    plant a.
    a. rash
    scarlet fever a.
    staphylococcus a.
    tetanus a. (TAT)
    tetanus-perfringens a.
    a. unit (AU)
antitoxinogen
anti-Toxoplasma antibody
  (ATA)
antitrypsin
    alpha a. (AAT)
    alpha₁ a. (A1AT)

    a. deficiency
    a. test
antitryptic index
antitubular basement membrane antibody
antitumor enzyme
antitumorigenesis
antityphoid serum
antiuvomorulin Fab fragment
anti-VCA antibody
antivenin
antivenomous serum
antivimentin
antiviral
    a. agent
    a. immunity
    a. protein
anti-VS antibody
anti-Xa assay
Anton
    A. syndrome
    A. test
Antoni type A, B neurilemmoma
Antopol-Goldman lesion
antral
    a. follicle
    a. gastritis
    a. G-cell hyperplasia
antralization
antranikianii
    Thermus a.
Antrodia
Antrodiella
antrum
    antra ethmoidalia
    follicular a.
anuclear
anucleated
anular pancreas
anuli (*pl. of* anulus)
anulus, annulus, *pl.* anuli
    a. fibrosus
    a. fibrosus disci intervertebralis
    a. fibrosus of aorta
anuresis
anuria
anus, *pl.* ani
    atresia ani
    Bartholin a.
    ectopic a.
    imperforate a. (IA)
    melanocarcinoma of a.
    a. vesicalis
    vestibular a.
    vulvovaginal a.
AO
    acridine orange
AOD
    arterial occlusive disease
Aonchotheca

Ao regurg
aortic regurgitation
aor regurg
aortic regurgitation
aorta, *pl.* **aortae**
anulus fibrosus of a.
coarctation of a.
cystic medial necrosis of ascending
a. (CMN-AA)
medial necrosis of a.
medionecrosis of the a.
postductal coarctation of a.
preductal coarctation of a.
aortae (*pl. of* aorta)
aortic
a. arch aneurysm
a. atresia
a. body
a. body tumor
a. dissection
a. explant assay
a. incompetence (AI)
a. knob
a. occlusion
a. regurgitation
a. septal defect
a. tunica adventitia
a. tunica intima
a. tunica media
a. valve replacement (AVR)
a. valvular insufficiency
a. valvular stenosis
aortica
glomera a.
aorticopulmonary
a. paraganglioma (APPG)
aorticosympathetic paraganglioma
aorticum
corpus a.
aortitis
bacterial a.
Döhle-Heller a.
giant cell a.
luetic a.
rheumatoid a.
syphilitic a.
aortocaval
aortoiliac
a. atherosclerosis
a. occlusive disease
aortosclerosis
AP
acid phosphatase
alkaline phosphatase
aminopeptidase
angina pectoris
antiplasmin
AP1
activator protein 1

APA
aldosterone-producing adenoma
aminopenicillanic acid
antipernicious anemia factor
antiphospholipid antibody
atypical polypoid adenomyofibroma
atypical polypoid adenomyoma
APAAP
alkaline phosphatase antialkaline
phosphatase
APAAP antibody
APAAP technique
APAAP test
APAB
antiphospholipid antibody
APACHE
Acute Physiology and Chronic Health
Evaluation
Apaf-1 adaptor protein
apallic syndrome
APA-LMP
atypical polypoid adenomyofibroma of
low malignant potential
apatite calculus
APC
activated protein C
adenoidal-pharyngeal-conjunctival
adenomatous polyposis coli
allophycocyanin
antigen-presenting cell
APC gene
APC gene stool test
APC resistance
APC virus
APC cofactor
APCA
antiparietal cell antibody
APCR
activated protein C
resistance
APE
anterior pituitary extract
Apec glucose analyzer
apeidosis
aperistalsis
esophageal a.
aperta
spina bifida a.
Apert-Crouzon disease
Apert disease
aperture
angular a.
numerical a.
APES
aminopropyltriethoxysilane
apeu virus
APF
anabolism-promoting factor
animal protein factor

A

APH
    antepartum hemorrhage
    anterior pituitary hormone
aphakia
Aphanoascus
Aphanocladium
aphasmid
Aphasmidia
apheresis platelet
aphrophilus
    Haemophilus a.
aphthosis
aphthous
        a. fever
        a. ileal ulcer
        a. stomatitis
        a. ulceration
Aphthovirus
aphylactic
aphylaxis
apical
        a. abscess
        a. dendrite
        a. gland
        a. granuloma
        a. process
        a. surface
apicitis
Apicomplexa
apiculate
apiculatus
    Saccharomyces a.
apiculus
apigenin
apii
    Cercospora a.
Apiocrea
Apiognomonia
Apiosordaria
apiospermum
    Monosporium a.
    Scedosporium a.
apiostomum
    Oesophagostomum a.
Apiotrichum
apista
API 20 Strep System
Apium
APL
    acute promyelocytic leukemia
    anterior pituitary-like
    antiphospholipid
aplanatic
        a. lens
        a. objective
aplasia
        bone marrow a.
        congenital thymic a.
        erythroid a.

        germ cell a.
        germinal cell a. (GCA)
        gonadal a.
        granulocytic a.
        hematopoietic a.
        lymphoid a.
        megakaryocytic a.
        nuclear a.
        pure red cell a. (PRCA)
        red cell a.
        retinal a.
        thymic-parathyroid a.
aplasia-thrombocytopenia
        radial a.-t.
aplasmic
aplastic
        a. anemia
        a. anemia syndrome
        a. bone marrow
        a. crisis
        a. lymph
Aplitest
apnea
        Bedbugg system for at-home
            diagnosis of sleep a.
        neonatal a.
        obstructive sleep a.
ApoA
    apolipoprotein A
ApoB
    apolipoprotein B
apobiosis
ApoC
    apolipoprotein C
apochromatic objective
apocrine
        a. adenoma
        a. adenosis
        a. carcinoma
        a. cyst
        a. ductal carcinoma in situ
        a. epithelium
        a. hidrocystoma
        a. hyperplasia
        a. lesion
        a. metaplasia
        a. miliaria
        a. nevus
        a. sweat gland
        a. tumor
apocynin
Apocynum
ApoD
    apolipoprotein D
ApoE
    apolipoprotein E
apoenzyme
apoferritin
apogamia, apogamy

apogamy (*var. of* apogamia)
apolar cell
apolipoprotein (Apo)
    a. A (ApoA)
    a. A1
    a. B (ApoB)
    a. C (ApoC)
    a. C2
    a. D (ApoD)
    a. E (ApoE)
apomixia
apomorphine-induced hypermobility
apomucin
aponeurosis
aponeurositis
aponeurotic fibroma
apophylaxis
apophysary (*var. of* apophysial)
apophyseal (*var. of* apophysial)
apophysial, apophyseal, apophysary
apophysis
apophysitis
    a. tibialis
    a. tibialis adolescentium
Apophysomyces elegans
apoplasmia
apoplectic
    a. coma
    a. cyst
apoplexy
apoprotein
ApopTag Plus kit
apoptosis
    cellular inhibitor of a. (cIAP)
    epithelial a.
    a. gene
    a. inhibitor
    lipoxygenase-induced a.
apoptotic
    a. body
    a. cell
    a. index
    a. keratinocyte
    a. process
aposome
Aposphaeria fuscidula
apothecium
apotransferrin
APP
    alum-precipitated pyridine
    amyloid precursor protein
    capsase mediated cleavage of APP
apparatus, *pl.* **apparatus**
    Abbe-Zeiss a.
    achromatic a.
    Barcroft a.
    Beckman Paragon SPE-II gel a.
    Benedict-Roth a.
    chromatic a.

    chromidial a.
    Golgi a.
    juxtaglomerular a.
    Langendorff a.
    nuclear mitotic a. (NuMA)
    Roughton-Scholander a.
    self-contained breathing a. (SCBA)
    subneural a.
    a. suspensorius lentis
    Van Slyke a.
apparent power
appearance
    amorphous eosinophilic a.
    batwing a.
    blush a.
    chicken fat a.
    cobblestone a.
    coffee ground a.
    cotton-wool a.
    currant jelly a.
    granular golden a.
    ground glass a.
    histologic a.
    immunoarchitectural a.
    jointed bamboo-rod cellular a.
    microscopic a.
    nutmeglike a.
    orange peel corneal a.
    owl-eye a.
    plucked-chicken a.
    pseudofollicular a.
    pseudoinvasive a.
    spike and dome a.
    starry-sky a.
    tram-track a.
    whorled a.
    window frame a.
    withering crypt a.
    wrinkled silk a.
appendage
    drumstick a.
appendiceal abscess
appendices (*pl. of* appendix)
appendicis (*gen. of* appendix)
appendicitis
    actinomycotic a.
    acute gangrenous a.
    acute suppurative a.
    catarrhal a.
    chronic a.
    focal a.
    gangrenous a.
    lumbar a.
    obstructive a.
    stercoral a.
    subperitoneal a.
    suppurative acute a.
appendicolithiasis, appendilothiasis,
appendilothiasis (*var. of* appendicolithiasis)

A

appendix *gen.* **appendicis,** *pl.* **appendices**
Corynebacterium appendicis
a. vermiformis
APPG
aorticopulmonary paraganglioma
apple-green birefringence
apple jelly nodule
applied
microiontophoretically a.
appliqué form
apposition
appositional growth
Appraise clinical densitometer
approach
clinicogenetic a.
appropriate for gestational age (AGA)
approximate lethal concentration (ALC)
APR
acute phase reactant
air-purifying respirator
amebic prevalence rate
apraxia
apri
Metastrongylus a.
apron
Hottentot a.
A68 protein
aprotic solvent
APS
antiphospholipid syndrome
APS1
autoimmune polyendocrine syndrome
type 1
Apscaviroid
APT
alum-precipitated toxoid
Apt
A. test
A. test for swallowed blood
Aptima Combo 2 assay
AP-TNAP
alkaline phosphatase, tissue-nonspecific
isozyme protein precursor
APTT, aPTT
activated partial thromboplastin time
activated partial thromboplastin time
APTT prolongation
APTT STA assay
APTT test
aptyalism
APUD
amine precursor uptake and
decarboxylation
apudoma
esophageal a.
apurinic acid
apyknomorphous
AQP1
aquaporin-1

Aquabacterium
A. citratiphilum
A. commune
A. parvum
Aquabirnavirus
aquagenic urticaria
Aquamicrobium defluvii
Aquamount
aquaporin (AQP)
aquaporin-1 (AQP1)
aquaregalis (*var. of* aqua
regia)
aqua regia, aquaregalis
Aquareovirus
aquasalis
Anopheles a.
Aquaspirillum
aquatica
Arcicella a.
Comamonas a.
Leifsonia a.
Tepidimonas a.
aquaticus
Gordius a.
Nocardioides a.
Thermus a.
aquatile
Flavobacterium a.
Fusobacterium a.
aquatilis
Sphingomonas a.
aqueduct
cochlear a.
Cotunnius a.
a. veil
aqueductus
a. cochleae
a. cotunnii
a. vestibuli
aqueous
a. humor
a. mounting medium
a. phase
a. solution
a. uranyl acetate
a. vaccine
aquibiodomus
Nitratireductor a.
Aquicella
A. lusitana
A. siphonis
Aquificaceae
Aquificae
Aquificales
aquilae
Corynebacterium a.
aquimarina
Kangiella a.
Sporosarcina a.

aquimarinus
  Algoriphagus a.
aquimaris
  Bacillus a.
aquiterrae
  Nocardioides a.
aquocobalamin
aquosa (*pl. of* aquosus)
aquosus, *pl.* aquosa
  humor a.
  polyemia aquosa
AR
  analytical reagent
  AR grade
arabiensis
  Anopheles a.
arabinomannan (Am)
arabinose operon
arabinoside
  adenine a.
  cytosine a. (CA)
arabinosuria
arabinotarda
  Shigella a.
arabitol test
Arabobacteria
arachidonate
arachidonic
  a. acid (AA)
  a. acid metabolite
  a. acidristocetin
  a. containing phosphatidyl
    ethanolamine
Arachis hypogaea
Arachnia propionica
Arachnida
arachnidism
Arachniotus
arachnodactyly
arachnoid
  a. cyst
  a. granulation
  a. trabecula
  a. trabeculae
  a. villus
arachnoideae
  granulationes a.
arachnoideus
  nevus a.
arachnoidism
arachnoiditis
  adhesive a.
  neoplastic a.
  obliterative a.
arachnolysin
Arachnomyces nodososetosus
araguata
  Stenella a.
Araldite

ARAM
  antigen receptor activation
  motif
Aran-Duchenne disease
araneism
araneosa
  Lentisphaera a.
araneus
  nevus a.
Arantius
  A. body
  A. canal
  A. duct
  A. ligament
  A. nodule
arborescence
arborescens
  lipoma a.
arborescent
arboris
  Ensifer a.
  Propionispira a.
arborization
arborize
arborizing pattern
arboroid
arborvirus (*var. of* arbovirus)
arboviral virus disease
arbovirus, arborvirus
  a. group A, B, C
  a. group unclassified
ARC
  AIDS-related complex
arcade
  Flint a.
Arcanobacterium
  A. haemolyticum
  A. hippocoleae
  A. pluranimalium
ARCD
  acquired renal cystic disease
arch
  Corti a.
Archaebacteria
Archaeobacteria
Archaeoglobaceae
Archaeoglobales
Archaeoglobea
Archaeoglobi
archamphiaster
Archangiaceae
archibaldi
  Leishmania donovani a.
archil
Architect
  A. Anti-HCV hepatitis assay
  A. AUSAB reagent kit
  A. HBsAg reagent immunoassay
architectonics

architectural
    a. pattern
    a. sheeting
architecture
    bone a.
    crypt a.
    loculated a.
archival brain tissue
arch-loop-whorl (ALW)
archnoid sheath
Arcicella aquatica
Arcobacter butzleri
arctation
arctica
    Desulfotalea a.
    Psychromonas a.
arcuata
    zona a.
arcuate
    a. nucleus
    a. zone
arcuatus uterus
arcus senilis
arc-welder's disease
ardor urinae
ARDS
    acute respiratory distress syndrome
    adult respiratory distress syndrome
area
    Betz cell a.
    body surface a.'s (BSA)
    Broca a.
    carcinoma with adenomatous a.'s
      (CWA)
    a. centralis
    clean a. (contamination-free)
    clinical laboratory maximum a.
    Cohnheim a.
    congested centrilobular a.
    a. cribrosa
    a. cribrosa papillae renalis
    dirty a. (contaminated)
    gray a.
    mean nuclear a. (MNA)
    a. postrema
    radiation emergency a. (REA)
    regulated a.
    skip areae
    a. striata
areata (*pl. of* areatus)
areatus *pl.* **areata**
    alopecia a.
arecoline
areflexia
areflexic quadriplegia
aregenerative anemia
arenacea
    corpora a.
    corpora arenaceacorpora a.

arenaceous
Arenaviridae
Arenavirus
Arenibacter
    A. certesii
    A. latericius
    A. troitsensis
arenosus
    Psychrobacter a.
areola, *pl.* **areolae**
    Chaussier a.
areolae (*pl. of* areola)
areolar
    a. connective tissue
    a. gland
areolares
    glandulae a.
ARF
    acute renal failure
    acute respiratory failure
    acute rheumatic fever
Argas
    A. persicus
    A. reflexus
argasid
Argasidae
argentaffin, argentaffine
    a. cell
    a. granule
    a. reaction
    a. stain
argentaffine (*var. of* argentaffin)
argentaffinity
argentaffinoma
argentation
Argentinean hemorrhagic fever
Argentine hemorrhagic fever virus
argentinense
    Clostridium a.
    rare clostridial strain of *Clostridium a.*
argentipes
argentophil, argentophile
argentophile (*var. of* argentophil)
argentum
arginase
arginine
    a. deiminase
    a. glutamate
    a. hydrochloride
    a. insulin tolerance test (AITT)
    a. monohydrochloride
    a. stimulation test
    suberyl a.
    a. tolerance test (ATT)
    a. vasopressin (AVP)
argininemia
argininosuccinate
    a. lyase
    a. lyase assay

argininosuccinate (*continued*)
    a. synthetase
    a. synthetase deficiency
argininosuccinic
    a. acid
    a. acidemia
argininosuccinicaciduria
arginyl
Argo cornstarch test
argon
Argonz-Del Castillo syndrome
Argyll
    A. Robertson pupil
    A. Robertson pupil sign
argyremia
argyria, argyrism, argyrosis
argyrism (*var. of* argyria)
argyrophil, argyrophile
    a. stain
argyrophile (*var. of* argyrophil)
argyrophilic
    a. ductal carcinoma in situ
    a. enterochromaffin-like cell
    a. fiber
    a. grain dementia
    a. nucleolar organizer region
    (AgNOR)
argyrosis (*var. of* argyria)
ariarii
    Trypanosoma a.
Arias-Stella
    A.-S. cell
    A.-S. effect
    A.-S. phenomenon
    A.-S. reaction (ASR)
Arias syndrome
ariboflavinosis
aristata
    Tetraploa a.
Arixtra
arizona
    A. hinshawii
    A. organism
arizonae
    Salmonella a.
    Salmonella choleraesuis subsp. *a.*
arizonensis
    Lactobacillus a.
ARM
    artificial rupture of membranes
arm
    dynein a.
armamentarium
Armanni-Ebstein
    A.-E. cell
    A.-E. change
    A.-E. disease
    A.-E. kidney
    A.-E. lesion

armata
    Taenia a.
armchair immunology
armed
    A. Forces Institute of Pathology
    (AFIP)
    a. macrophage
Armigeres obturbans
Armillaria
armillatus
    Armillifer a.
    Porocephalus a.
Armillifer
    A. armillatus
    A. moniliformis
armored heart
ARMS
    alveolar rhabdomyosarcoma
Armstrong disease
Arndt-Gottron syndrome
Arneth
    A. classification
    A. count
    A. formula
    A. index
    A. stage
Arnium leporinum
Arnold
    A. body
    A. bundle
    A. canal
    A. ganglion
    A. nerve reflex cough
    syndrome
    A. tract
Arnold-Chiari
    A.-C. deformity
    A.-C. malformation
    A.-C. syndrome
AROM
    active range of motion
    artificial rupture of
    membranes
aromatase
aromatic
    a. amine
    a. amino acid
    a. compound
    a. hydrocarbon
    a. l-amino acid decarboxylase
    (AADC)
    a. ring
aromaticity
aromaticivorans
    Novosphingobium a.
aromatization
AR-PKD
    autosomal recessive polycystic kidney
    disease

arrangement
    bcl-2 gene a.
    organoid a.
array
    Affymetrix GeneChip HU 95 a.
    A. 360, 360CE/CE-AL
      protein/drug/serology system
    oligonucleotide genomic a.
    whorl-like a.
array-based comparative genomic hybridization (aCGH)
arrector pili muscle
arrest
    cell cycle a.
    complete maturation a. (CMA)
    developmental a.
    epiphysial a.
    growth a.
    hematopoietic maturation a.
    maturation a.
    mitotic a.
    spermatogenic maturation a.
arrested tuberculosis
arrhaphia
Arrhenius
    A. doctrine
    A. equation
    A. formula
    A. theory
Arrhenius-Madsen theory
arrhenoblastoma
    androgenic a.
arrhinencephalia (*var. of* arrhinencephaly)
arrhinencephaly, arrhinencephalia
arrhizus
    Rhizopus a.
arrhythmogenicity
arrhythmogenic right ventricular dysplasia
arrival
    dead on a. (DOA)
Arroyo sign
ARS A
    acute radiation syndrome
    antirabies serum
ARS-A
    arylsulfatase A
arsenate
    sodium a.
arsenaticum
    Pyrobaculum a.
arsenazo III dye
arsenic
    a. assay
    a. hydride
    a. keratosis
    a. pigmentation
    a. poisoning

    a. stain
    a. trihydride
    a. trioxide (As_2O_3)
arsenical keratosis
arsenic-fast
Arsenicicoccus bolidensis
arseniciselenatis
    Bacillus a.
arsenide, arseniuret
    hydrogen a.
arsenious hydride
arseniuret (*var. of* arsenide)
arseniuretted hydrogen
arsenophilum
    Sulfurospirillum a.
arsenoxide
arsine
    a. gas
    NATO code for a. (SA)
ART
    absolute retention time
    Aerosol Resistant Tips
    antiretroviral treatment
    automated reagin test
artefact (*var. of* artifact)
Artemisia annua
arteria (*var. of* artery)
arteriae arcuatae renis
arterial
    a. blood collection
    a. blood gas (ABG)
    a. blood gas analysis
    a. blood oximetry
    a. cannulation
    a. capillary
    a. embolism
    a. hemangioma
    a. hypertension
    a. insufficiency
    a. line culture
    a. nephrosclerosis
    a. occlusive disease (AOD)
    a. oxygen saturation
    a. pCO_2
    a. pO_2
    a. pressure
    a. sclerosis
    a. spider
    a. thrombosis
arterialization of vein
arterialized blood
arterioatony
arteriocapillary sclerosis
arteriococcygeal gland
arteriolae rectae
arteriolar
    a. nephrosclerosis
    a. sclerosis
    a. thrombonecrosis

arteriole, arteriola
    hepatic a.
    tunica media of a.
arteriolith
arteriolitis
    necrotizing a.
arteriolization of venous blood
arteriolonecrosis
arteriolonephrosclerosis (ANS)
arteriolosclerosis
    hyaline a.
arteriolosclerotic kidney
arteriolovenular bridge
arteriomalacia
arteriomyomatosis
arterionephrosclerosis
arteriopathy
    hypertensive a.
    plexogenic pulmonary a.
arterioplania
arteriorrhexis
arteriosclerosis (AS, ATS)
    hyperplastic a.
    hypertensive a.
    medial a.
    Mönckeberg a.
    nodular a.
    a. obliterans
    senile a.
arteriosclerotic
    a. aortic aneurysm
    a. cardiovascular disease (ASCVD)
    a. gangrene
    a. heart disease (AHD)
    a. kidney
    a. thrombosed aneurysm
arteriostenosis
arteriosus
    double ductus a.
    patent ductus a. (PDA)
    pseudotruncus a.
    truncus a.
arteriovenous
    a. anastomosis (AVA)
    a. aneurysm
    a. carbon dioxide
    a. carbon dioxide difference
    a. fistula (AVF)
    a. malformation (AVM)
    a. oxygen difference (AVDO$_2$)
arteritica
    polymyalgia a.
arteritis
    cranial a.
    equine viral a.
    giant cell a.
    infectious a.
    a. nodosa
    a. obliterans

    obliterating a.
    rheumatic a.
    rheumatoid a.
    Takayasu a.
    temporal a.
Arterivirus
artery, arteria
    copper-wire a.
    distributing a.
    dolichoectatic a.
    end a.
    a. of pulp
    pipestem a.
    screw a.
    spiral a.
    supernumerary segmental a.
    transposition of great arteries (TGA)
artery-to-artery anastomosis
artery-to-vein anastomosis
Arthobotrys oligospora
arthragra
arthralgia
    rheumatic a.
    a. saturnina
Arthrinium
arthritic calculus
arthriticum
    tuberculum a.
arthritidis
    Actinobacillus a.
arthritis
    acute rheumatic a.
    atrophic a.
    chronic absorptive a.
    chronic proliferative a.
    chronic villous a.
    chylous a.
    crystal-induced a.
    a. deformans
    degenerative a.
    exudative a.
    filarial a.
    gonococcal a.
    gouty a.
    hypertrophic a.
    infectious a.
    inflammatory a.
    Jaccoud a.
    juvenile rheumatoid a. (JRA)
    a. mutilans
    navicular a.
    neuropathic a.
    a. nodosa
    ochronotic a.
    proliferative chronic a.
    psoriatic a.
    rheumatoid a. (RA)
    septic a.
    suppurative a.

a. uratica
vertebral a.
arthritis-dermatitis syndrome
Arthrobacter
    A. chlorophenolicus
    A. flavus
    A. gandavensis
    A. koreensis
    A. luteolus
    A. methylotrophus
    A. nasiphocae
    A. nitroguajacolicus
    A. roseus
    A. russicus
    A. sulfonivorans
Arthrobacteria
Arthrobotrys
arthrocentesis
arthrochondritis
arthroconidium
Arthroderma
arthrogram
Arthrographis langeroni
arthrography
    facet joint a.
arthrokatadysis
arthrolith
arthrolithiasis
arthroonychodysplasia
arthroophthalmopathy
    hereditary progressive a.
arthropathy
    Charcot a.
    hemophilic a.
    Jaccoud a.
    neurogenic a.
    osteopulmonary a.
arthrophyma
arthropica
    psoriasis a.
Arthropoda
arthropod-borne
    a.-b. viral disease
    a.-b. virus encephalitis
arthropodiasis
arthropodic, arthropodous
arthropod identification
arthropodous (*var. of*
 arthropodic)
Arthropsis hispanica
arthrosia
    exanthesis a.
arthrosis
arthrospore
arthrosynovitis
arthrotropic
Arthus
    A. phenomenon
    A. reaction

articular
    a. calculus
    a. capsule
    a. chondrocalcinosis
    a. corpuscle
    a. gout
    a. lamella
    a. leprosy
    a. rheumatism
articularia
    corpuscula a.
articularis
    capsula a.
    membrana fibrosa capsulae a.
    stratum fibrosum capsulae a.
articuli
    empyema a.
    hydrops a.
artifact, artefact
    bubble a.
    cautery a.
    crush a.
    electrical a.
    fixation a.
    iatrogenic a.
    movement a.
    retraction a.
    shock a.
    tissue a.
    xylene a.
artifactitious (*var. of* artifactual)
artifactual, artifactitious
artificial
    a. abortion
    a. active immunity
    a. insemination homologous
    (AIH)
    a. kidney
    a. leech
    a. melanin
    a. passive immunity
    a. rupture of membranes
Artyfechinostomum
arupensis
    Bartonella vinsonii
    subsp. *a.*
ARV
    AIDS-related virus
Arxiozyma
Arxula adeninivorans
arylaminopeptidase
arylesterase
aryl-ester hydrolase
aryl group
arylsulfatase (ARS)
    a. A (ARS A)
    a. test
arytenoid gland
arytenoiditis

AS
   Adams-Stokes
   antistreptolysin
   arteriosclerosis
   atherosclerosis
ASA
   acetylsalicylic acid
   Adams-Stokes attack
asaccharolytica
   Porphyromonas a.
asaccharolyticus
asahii
   Trichosporon a.
Asaia
   A. bogorensis
   A. krungthepensis
   A. siamensis
Asanoa
   A. ferruginea
   A. ishikariensis
ASAP biopsy system
asbestoid
ASBESTOS
   agent, state, body site, effects,
   severity, time course, other
   (diagnoses), synergism
asbestos
   a. body (AB)
   a. transformation
asbestosis
ASCA
   anti-*Saccharomyces cerevisiae* antibody
   ASCA antibody
**ascariasis, ascaridiasis, ascaridosis,
   ascariosis**
   a. serological test
ascaricidal
ascaricide
ascarid
Ascaridae
Ascaridata
Ascaridia
ascaridiasis (*var. of* ascariasis)
Ascaridida
Ascarididae
Ascaridoidea
Ascaridorida
ascaridosis (*var. of* ascariasis)
ascariosis (*var. of* ascariasis)
Ascaris
   A. alata
   A. canis
   A. equorum
   A. lumbricoides
   A. mystax
   A. pneumonitis
   A. suum
ascaron
Ascarops strongylina

ascending (asc)
   a. cholangitis
   a. chromatography
   a. degeneration
   a. myelitis
   a. pyelonephritis
Aschelminthes
Ascher syndrome
Aschheim-Zondek (AZ, A-Z)
   A.-Z. hormone
   A.-Z. pregnancy test
Aschoff
   A. body
   A. cell
   A. nodule
Aschoff-Rokitansky sinus
asci (*pl. of* ascus)
ascites
   abdominal a.
   a. adiposus
   cardiac a.
   chyliform a.
   a. chylosus
   chylous a.
   cirrhotic a.
   fatty a.
   gelatinous a.
   hemorrhagic a.
   malignancy-related a.
   milky a.
   nephrogenous a.
   pseudochylous a.
asciteschylosus (*var. of* chylous ascites)
ascitic
   a. agar
   a. fluid
ascitogenous
Ascobolus
ascocarp
Ascochyta
Ascocoryne
Ascodesmis
Ascodichaena
ascogenous
ascogonium
Ascoidea
Ascoli
   A. reaction
   A. test
ascomycete
Ascomycetes
ascomycetous
Ascomycota
Ascomycotina
ascorbate
   sodium a.
ascorbate-cyanide test
ascorbic
   a. acid

a. acid assay
a. acid test
Ascosphaera
Ascospora campanulae
ascospore
ascospore-forming fungus
Ascotricha novae-caledoniae
Ascovirus
ASCUS
  atypical squamous cells of
  undetermined significance
    ASM subset of ASCUS
ascus, *pl.* **asci**
ASCVD
  arteriosclerotic cardiovascular disease
  atherosclerotic cardiovascular disease
ASD
  aldosterone secretion defect
  atrial septal defect
asepsis
aseptate
aseptic
  a. meningitis
  a. necrosis
asexual reproduction
ASF
  aniline, sulfur, formaldehyde
Asfivirus
ASGPR
  asialoglycoprotein receptor
ASH
  asymmetric septal hypertrophy
Ashbya
Ashby differential agglutination method
Asherman syndrome
ashfordi
Ashkenazi screen
ash-leaf spot
asialoglycoprotein receptor (ASGPR)
asiatica
    Nocardia a.
Asiatic cholera
asiaticus
    Streptomyces a.
asiderosis
asiderotic anemia
asini
    Strongylus a.
asinigenitalis
    Taylorella a.
Askanazy cell
Askin tumor
Ask-Upmark kidney
ASM
  atypical squamous metaplasia
    ASM subset of ASCUS
ASMA
  alpha smooth muscle actin
  antismooth muscle antibody

ASMI
  anteroseptal myocardial infarct
ASN
  alkali-soluble nitrogen
Asn
  asparagine
ASO
  antistreptolysin O
    ASO probe
    ASO test
As$_2$O3
  arsenic trioxide
ASP
  antibody specificity prediction
Asp
  aspartic acid
asparaginase
asparagine (Asn, N)
asparaginic acid
asparaginyl
aspartate
  a. aminotransferase (AST)
  a. aminotransferase assay
  a. kinase
  potassium aspartate and magnesium
    a.
  a. transaminase
aspartic
  a. acid (Asp)
  a. proteinase
aspartokinase
aspartyl
aspartylglycosaminuria
asper
  aspergillosis
aspergilloma
aspergillosis
  allergic bronchopulmonary a.
    (ABPA)
  bronchopulmonary a.
  disseminated a.
  invasive a.
  pulmonary a.
  rhinocerebral a.
Aspergillus
  A. antibody test
  A. auricularis
  A. barbae
  A. bouffardi
  A. candidus
  A. clavatus
  A. concentricus
  A. fisherii
  A. flavus
  A. fumigatus
  A. fungus ball
  A. giganteus
  A. glaucus
  A. gliocladium

Aspergillus (*continued*)
  A. *mucoroides*
  A. *nidulans*
  A. *niger*
  A. *ochraceus*
  A. *parasiticus*
  A. *pictor*
  A. *repens*
  A. *serology*
  A. *terreus*
  A. *versicolor*
aspermatism
aspermatogenesis
  induced a.
aspermia
asperum
  Trichocladium a.
aspheric
asphyxia
  autoerotic a.
  intrauterine a.
  mechanical a.
  positional a.
asphyxial
asphyxiant
  chemical a.
  simple a.
asphyxiating
  a. thoracic chondrodystrophy
  a. thoracic dysplasia
  a. thoracic dystrophy
    (ATD)
asphyxiation
Aspiculuris tetraptera
aspidium oleoresin
aspirate
  bronchotracheal a.
  nasopharyngeal a.
aspiration
  a. biopsy
  a. biopsy cytology (ABC)
  bone marrow a.
  fine-needle a.
  foreign body a.
  lung a.
  meconium a.
  microsurgical epididymal sperm a.
    (MESA)
  mineral oil a.
  newborn a.
  a. of endometrium
  a. pneumonia
  a. pneumonitis
  suprapubic needle a.
  tracheal a. (trach asp)
  transbronchial needle a. (TBNA)
  uterine a. (UA)
  vacuum a. (VA)
  wound a.

aspirator
  water a.
aspirin
  long-term treatment with a.
  a. poisoning
  a. tolerance
  a. tolerance test
  a. toxicity
ASPIRINcheck urine test
AspirinWorks diagnostic urine test
asplenia
asplenic
ASPL-TFE3 fusion gene
asporogenic
asporogenous
asporous
asporulate
ASPS
  alveolar soft-part sarcoma
ASR
  aldosterone secretion rate
  aldosterone secretory rate
  analyte-specific reagent
  Arias-Stella reaction
assassin bug
assay
  Abbott AxSYM Prizm HCV a.
  Access testosterone a.
  acetaminophen a.
  acetylcholinesterase a.
  acid phosphatase a.
  adenosine deaminase a.
  ADH a.
  adhesion a.
  ADN-B a.
  adrenocorticotropic hormone a.
  agglutination inhibition a.
  AH a.
  air bleb a.
  alanine aminotransferase a.
  albumin a.
  alcohol a.
  aldolase a.
  aldosterone a.
  alkaline phosphatase a.
  alpha-2 antiplasmin functional a.
  alpha-1 fetoprotein a.
  Ames a.
  amino acid fractionation a.
  amitriptyline and nortriptyline a.'s
  ammonia a.
  amphetamine a.
  Amplicor Chlamydia a.
  amylase a.
  antibody capture ligand a.
  anti-DNA antibody a.
  anti-DNaseB a.
  antigen capture ligand a.
  antigenic a.

antihyaluronidase a.
antimitochondrial antibody a.
antimony a.
antinuclear antibody a.
antiparietal cell antibody a.
antismooth muscle antibody a.
anti-Xa a.
aortic explant a.
Aptima Combo 2 a.
APTT STA a.
Architect Anti-HCV hepatitis a.
argininosuccinate lyase a.
arsenic a.
ascorbic acid a.
aspartate aminotransferase a.
Auto Dimer a.
Aware Rapid HIV a.
bacterial inhibition a.
bacterial killing a.
barbiturate a.
Bayer Immuno 1 HER-2/neu a.
Bayer Versant HCV RNA 3.0 a.
Beckman a.
benzene a.
benzodiazepine a.
beta-hydroxybutyrate a.
bile acid a.
bilirubin a.
Bioclot protein S a.
biologic a.
biological a.
Bio-Rad protein a.
biotin a.
bismuth a.
blastogenesis a.
blood spot screening a.
B-lymphocyte a.
BoneTRAP A.
boron a.
branched DNA signal
  amplification a.
Breslow malignant melanoma a.
bromide a.
butanol-extractable iodine a.
CA125 a.
CA19-9 a.
cadmium a.
caffeine a.
calcitonin a.
calcium ionized a.
CALLA a.
camphor a.
capture a.
carbamazepine a.
carbaryl a.
carbon dioxide concentration a.
carbon disulfide a.
carbon monoxide a.
carbon tetrachloride a.

carboxyhemoglobin a.
Cardiac STATus rapid a.
Cardiac T rapid a.
carotene a.
catecholamine a.
^{13}C bicarbonate a.
CEA a.
CEDIA sirolimus a.
cell-mediated lympholysis a.
CellProbe HT caspase-3/7 whole
  cell a.
cerebrospinal fluid a.
ceruloplasmin a.
chemiluminescence a.
chemiluminescent a. (CLIA)
chemotaxis a.
Chlamydiazyme EIA a.
chloral hydrate a.
chloranil a.
chlorate a.
chlordiazepoxide a.
chlorinated hydrocarbon pesticide a.
chloroform a.
chlorohydrocarbon a.
chlorpromazine a.
cholesterol a.
cholinesterase a.
chorionic gonadotropin a.
chromatographic a.
chromium a.
chromogenic Xa inhibition a.
citric acid a.
clonogenic a.
Clostridium difficile toxin a.
coagulation factor a.
cobalt a.
cocaine metabolite a.
codeine a.
collagen gel invasion a.
4-color PCR a.
competitive binding a.
competitive protein-binding a.
complement binding a.
compressed spectral a. (CSA)
copper a.
coproporphyrin a.
cortisol a.
CPB a.
C-reactive protein a.
creatine kinase a.
creatinine a.
cresol a.
C-terminal a.
cyanide a.
cytochrome b5 reductase a.
cytolytic T-cell lysis a.
cytotoxicity a.
DCC a.
D-dimer a.

assay (*continued*)
  DDT a.
  DeBakey aortic a.
  delta aminolevulinic acid a.
  depramine a.
  desipramine a.
  DHPLC a.
  diazepam a.
  dihydroxycholecalciferol a.
  dimeric inhibin-A a.
  diquat a.
  direct fluorescence a. (DFA)
  direct fluorescent a. (DFA)
  disulfiram a.
  double antibody
    immunoenzymometric a.
  double antibody sandwich a.
  doxepin hydrochloride a.
  drug screening a.
  EAC rosette a.
  E erythrocyte rosette a.
  Elecsys Anti-HBe a.
  electrophoretic mobility shift a.
  ELISA titer a.
  ELISPOT enzymatic test a.
  endorphin a.
  endotoxin activity a. (EAA)
  enzyme a.
  enzyme-linked immunosorbent a.
    (ELISA)
  epinephrine and norepinephrine a.'s
  Epstein-Barr virus antibody a.
  Erlanger and Gasser peripheral
    nerve a.
  erythrocyte antibody complement
    rosette a.
  erythrocyte sedimentation rate a.
    (ESR assay)
  erythroid colony a.
  ESR a.
  estradiol a.
  estriol a.
  estrogen receptor a. (ERA)
  ethanol a.
  ethchlorvynol a.
  ethosuximide a.
  ethylene glycol a.
  factor III multimer a.
  fat a.
  fatty acid a.
  ferritin a.
  fibrin clot retraction a.
  fibrinogen a.
  FiF a.
  flow cytometric a.
  fluorescent cytoprint a.
  fluorescent protection a.
  fluoride a.
  fluoroacetate a.

  fluorocarbon a.
  folic acid a.
  follicle-stimulating hormone a.
    (FSH)
  fructose a.
  FSH a.
  FSH-RH a.
  galactose a.
  gastrin a.
  GeneSearch BLN a.
  GGT a.
  glucose a.
  glucosephosphate isomerase a.
  glucosylceramidase a.
  glutathione reductase a.
  glutethimide a.
  glycine a.
  glycosylated hemoglobin a.
  gold a.
  Groome a.
  guanine deaminase a.
  Guthrie bacterial inhibition a.
    (GBIA)
  halogenated hydrocarbon a.
  haloperidol a.
  halothane a.
  hamster egg penetration a.
  haptoglobin a.
  HDL cholesterol a.
  hemagglutination inhibition a.
  Hemochron Jr. Citrate PT a.
  hemoglobin F, H a.
  hemolytic plaque a.
  hemolytic tube a.
  heparin-induced platelet activation a.
    (HIPA)
  HercepTest breast cancer
    immunohistochemical a.
  heterogeneous a.
  hexachlorophene a.
  Hexaplex a.
  histocompatibility a.
  histoculture drug response a.
    (HDRA)
  Histoplasma antibody a.
  HitHunter cAMP enzyme fragment
    complementation a.
  homogeneous ligand a.
  hybridization protection a. (HPA)
  hydroxyapatite a.
  17-hydroxycorticosteroid a.
  5-hydroxyindoleacetic acid a.
  hydroxyproline a.
  25-hydroxyvitamin D a.
  iditol dehydrogenase a.
  ID-Tag RVP a.
  imipramine and desipramine a.'s
  ImmuKnow immune cell function a.
  Immulite free PSA a.

Immulite 2000 PSA a.
Immulite third-generation PSA a.
immune adherence hemagglutination
  a. (IAHA)
immune complex a.
immunochemical a.
immunoconcentration a.
immunocytochemical a. (ICA)
Immuno 1 DPD a.
immunoenzymometric a.
immunofluorescence a. (IFA)
immunofluorescent a.
immunoluminometric a.
immunometric a. (IMA)
immunoradiometric a. (IRMA)
indirect a.
inhibitor a.
in vitro invasion a.
iodide a.
ionized calcium a.
iron a.
isocitrate dehydrogenase a.
isoniazid a.
isopropanol a.
IVTT a.
Jaffe a.
Jerne plaque a.
17-ketogenic steroids a.
17-ketosteroid a.
lactate dehydrogenase a.
lactic acid a.
LATS a.
LDL cholesterol a.
lead a.
leukotactic a.
Liaison *Borrelia burgdorferi* a.
lidocaine a.
ligand a.
limulus amebocyte lysate a.
lipase a.
lipid a.
Lipi+Plus direct HDL a.
Lipi+Plus direct LDL a.
lipoprotein a.
liquid-phase hybridization
  protection a.
lithium a.
LMC a.
LOH a.
LRP a.
luteinizing hormone a.
lymphocyte marker a.
lymphocyte microcytotoxicity a.
lysergic acid diethylamide a.
lysozyme a.
macroglobulin a.
magnesium a.
manganese a.
MBP a.

meprobamate a.
mercury a.
mersalyl exchange a.
metanephrine a.
methadone a.
methanol a.
methaqualone a.
methemalbumin a.
3,4-methylenedioxyamphetamine a.
methyprylon a.
Metra BAP a.
Metra PYD a.
metronidazole a.
microalbumin immunoturbidimetric a.
microarray expression profiling a.
microbiologic a.
microbiological a. (MB)
microhemagglutination a. (MHA)
microlymphocytotoxicity a.
microtoxicity a.
mitogen a.
mixed lymphocyte culture a.
  (MLC)
MLC a.
molecular a.
morphine a.
MUC1 gene derived glycoprotein a.
mucoprotein a.
multiplex reverse transcription PCR
  enzyme hybridization a.
NAP modified LRP a.
NaSCN exchange a.
NBT reduction a.
nephelometric inhibition a. (NIA)
nitroblue tetrazolium dye
  reduction a.
noncompetitive a.
NucliSens CMV a.
NucliSens HIV-1 QT a.
one-stage factor a.
opiate a.
Opus cardiac troponin I a.
organothiophosphate compound a.
ornithine carbamoyltransferase a.
osteoblast proliferation
  fluorometric a.
osteoclastic factor a.
oxalic acid a.
plaque-forming cell a.
plasma clot solubility a.
plasminogen activator inhibitor a.
p-methoxyamphetamine a.
polychlorinated biphenyl a.
polyethylene glycol precipitation a.
porphobilinogen synthase a.
porphyrin a.
potassium a.
PP-CAP H. pylori IgA a.
^{32}P-postlabeling a.

assay (*continued*)
PRA-Stat enzyme linked immunosorbent a.
pregnanediol a.
PreVue *Borrelia burgdorferi* antibody detection a.
primidone a.
procainamide a.
Procleix HIV-1/HCV A.
progesterone receptor a. (PRA)
properdin a.
propoxyphene a.
propranolol a.
ProSpecT *Clostridium difficile* toxin A microplate a.
protamine sulfate a.
protein-bound iodine a.
protein-protein binding a.
protein truncation a.
protoporphyrin a.
protriptyline a.
PSFR a.
PTH a.
pyrimethamine a.
pyruvate kinase a.
pyruvic acid a.
quinidine a.
quinine a.
radioallergosorbent a.
radioenzymatic a. (REA)
radioimmunoprecipitation a. (RIPA)
radioligand a.
radioreceptor a. (RRA)
Raji cell radioimmune a.
rapid susceptibility a. (RSA)
receptor a.
recombinant immunoblot a. (RIBA)
renal venous renin a. (RVRA)
renin a.
Retic-Chex linearity a.
reverse hemolytic plaque a. (RHPA)
riboflavin a.
ribonuclease protection a. (RPA)
RID a.
saccharogenic a.
salicylate a.
sandwich nucleic acid hybridization a.
saturation and displacement a.
selenium a.
serial cardiac isoenzyme a.
serotonin a.
serotonin release a. (SRA)
Simplify D-dimer a.
single-agent kinetic enzyme a.
single-analyte immunologic a.
single-analyte molecular a.
slide immunoenzymatic a. (SIA)
sodium and potassium a.'s

spectrophotometric a.
sperm penetration a.
SPIFE acid hemoglobin a.
SPIFE alkaline hemoglobin a.
SSCP a.
Stamper-Woodruff a.
staphylococcal protein A binding a.
stem cell a.
stool toxin a.
strychnine a.
sucrose pad nuclear exchange a.
sugar assimilation a.
sugar fermentation a.
sulfonamide a.
sulfonylurea a.
superoxide a.
Syva EMIT-II a.
T and B lymphocyte subset a.
TBG a.
T/B lymphocyte a.
tellurium a.
telomeric repeat amplification protocol a.
thallium a.
theophylline a.
thiamine a.
thiamphenicol a.
thioridazine a.
thrombotic thrombocytopenic purpura a.
thyroid-stimulating hormone a.
thyroxine a.
thyroxine-binding globulin a.
tissue culture cytotoxin a. (TCCA)
total calcium a.
TPI a.
transferrin a.
transketolase a.
TRAP a.
Treponema pallidum hemagglutination a. (TPHA)
Treponema pallidum immobilization a.
triglyceride a.
triiodothyronine a.
triosephosphate isomerase a.
trypsin a.
TSH a.
TUNEL a.
two-site immunoenzymometric a.
tyrosine a.
UDP-glucose-hexose-1-phosphate uridylyltransferase a.
urea nitrogen a.
uric acid a.
urobilin a.
urobilinogen a.
uromucoid a.

uropepsinogen a.
uroporphyrin a.
vancomycin-resistant enterococcus a.
  (VRE)
Versant HCV RNA 3.0 a.
vitamin A and carotene a.'s
vitamin B_6 a.
vitamin B_{12} a.
vitamin D a.
vitamin E a.
vitamin K a.
Vitros anti-HBs a.
Vitros HBsAg a.
volatile organic substances a.
von Kossa calcium a.
von Willebrand factor a.
von Willebrand factor multimer a.
warfarin a.
Xpert EV a.
Xpert EV enterovirus a.
zinc a.

Asserachrom
A. APA immunoassay
A. D-Dimer kit

assessment
cancer risk a.
histocompatibility a.
purinergic receptor translocation a.

assignment statement
assimilation limit
assistant
Certified Laboratory A.
Assmann tuberculous infiltrate
associate
microbial a.
associated macrophage
association
American Clinical Laboratory A.
American Urological A. (AUA)
CHARGE a.
Clinical Laboratory
  Management A.
a. constant
independent practice a.
a. system
a. tract
associative reaction
assortative mating
assortment
independent a.
assurance
quality a. (QA)
AST
aspartate aminotransferase
AST test
astacoid rash
astasia
astatine
asteatosis

aster
asterixis
Asterococcus
asteroid body
asteroides
Nocardia a.
Trichophyton a.
Trichosporon a.
Asterophora
asthma
allergic a.
alveolar a.
atopic a.
bronchial a. (BA)
chronic bronchitis with a. (CBA)
cotton dust a.
a. crystal
emphysematous a.
essential a.
exercise-induced a.
extrinsic a.
grinder's a.
hay a.
intrinsic a.
miller's a.
miner's a.
potter's a.
steam-fitter's a.
stone-stripper's a.
summer a.
asthmatic bronchitis (AB)
asthmaticus
status a.
asthmogenic
astia
Xenopsylla a.
Astler-Coller modification of Dukes classification
astomatous
Astra blood chemistry profile
astral fiber
astringent
astroblastoma
astrocele
astrocyte
Alzheimer type I, II a.
atypical a.
fibrillar a.
fibrillary a.
fibrous a.
gemistocytic a.
protoplasmic a.
reactive a.
a. stain
a. staining
astrocytic
a. foot process
a. neoplasm
a. tumor

astrocytoma
 anaplastic a.
 cerebellar a.
 desmoplastic cerebral a.
 fibrillary a.
 fibrous a.
 gemistocytic a.
 grade I–IV a.
 juvenile cerebellar a.
 juvenile pilocytic a.
 low grade a.
 pilocytic a.
 piloid a.
 protoplasmic a.
 subependymal giant cell a.
astrocytosis cerebri
astroependymoma
astroglia cell
astrokinetic
astronyxis
 Acanthamoeba a.
astrosphere
Astrup method
Astwood test
ASV
 antisnake venom
 avian sarcoma virus
As/V
 ampere-second per volt
asymmetric, asymmetrical
 a. carbon atom
 a. chondrodystrophy
 a. septal hypertrophy (ASH)
 a. unit membrane
 a. uterus
asymmetrical (*var. of* asymmetric)
asymmetry
asymptomatic
 a. carrier
 a. coccidioidomycosis
 a. interval
 a. viremia
asymptote
asynapsis
asynchronism
asynchronous data transmission
asynchrony
asynechia
asystematic
AT
 adenosine triphosphate
ATA
 anti-*Toxoplasma* antibody
atabrine hydrochloride
Atadenovirus
atavistic phenomenon
ataxia, ataxy
 familial cerebellar a.
 Friedreich a.

 Friedrich a.
 a. telangiectasia
 a. telangiectasia syndrome
ataxia-telangiectasia
ataxin gene
ataxy (*var. of* ataxia)
ATC
 aggressive thyroid carcinoma
ATCC
 American Type Culture Collection
ATD
 asphyxiating thoracic dystrophy
ATDLG
 antithoracic duct lymphocytic
 globulin
atelectasis
 a. neonatorum
 obstructive a.
 primary a.
 round a.
 rounded a.
 secondary a.
atelia (*var. of* ateliosis)
ateliosis, atelia
ateliotic
Atelosaccharomyces
aterials
 secondary reference a.
ATG
 antithymocyte globulin
 antithyroglobulin
Athelia
atheroembolism
atherogenesis
atherogenic
atherogenicity
atheroma embolism
atheromatosis
atheromatous
 a. degeneration
 a. embolism
 a. embolus
 a. plaque
atherosclerosis (AS)
 aortoiliac a.
atherosclerotic
 a. aneurysm
 a. cardiovascular disease (ASCVD)
 a. heart disease (AHD)
atherosis
atherothromboembolism
atherothrombosis
atherothrombotic
athetoid
athetosis
athetotic
athlete's foot
athletic heart
athrepsia, athrepsy

athrepsy (*var. of* athrepsia)
athrocytosis
athrombia
ATL
    adult T-cell lymphoma
atlantica
    Ruegeria a.
atlanticus
    Aedes a.
    Croceibacter a.
    Thermococcus a.
atlantoaxial subluxation
ATLL
    adult T-cell leukemia/lymphoma
    adult T-cell lymphoma
    smoldering form of ATLL
atmosphere
    a. absolute
    explosive a.
atmospheric monitoring
ATN
    acute tubular necrosis
atom
    asymmetric carbon a.
atomic
    a. absorption
    a. absorption spectrophotometer
      (AAS)
    a. absorption spectrophotometry
      (AAS)
    a. absorption spectroscopy
    a. force microscopy (AFM)
    a. mass
    a. mass unit (amu)
    a. number
    a. spectrum
    a. weight
    a. weight unit (awu)
atomization
atomizer
atonia (*var. of* atony)
atony, atonia
atopen
atopic
    a. allergen
    a. allergy
    a. asthma
    a. dermatitis
    a. disease
    a. reagin
Atopobacter phocae
Atopobium
Atopostipes suicloacalis
atopy
ATP
    adenosine triphosphate
    extracellular ATP
    ATP pyrophosphohydrolase
    ATP synthesis

ATPase
    adenosine triphosphatase
    calcium-activated ATPase
    magnesium-activated ATPase
    Padykula-Herman stain for myosin
      ATPase
    ATPase stain
ATP7B gene
ATP-binding cassette (ABC)
ATPS
    ambient temperature and pressure,
    saturated
ATRA
    all-*trans*-retinoic acid
atrabiliaris
    glandula a.
atrabiliary capsule
atransferrinemia
    congenital a.
Atrax robustus
atrepsy
atresia
    anal a.
    a. ani
    aortic a.
    biliary a.
    choanal a.
    colon a.
    congenital a.
    duodenal a.
    esophageal a.
    extrahepatic biliary a. (EHBA)
    follicular a.
    intestinal a.
    mitral a.
    prepyloric a.
    pulmonary a.
    tricuspid a.
    ureteral a.
    vaginal a.
    valvular a.
atresic
atretic
    a. corpus luteum
    a. ovarian follicle
atreticum
    corpus a.
atretocystia
atretogastria
atria (*pl. of* atrium)
atrial
    a. infarction
    a. myxoma
    a. natriuretic factor
    a. natriuretic peptide (ANP)
    a. septal defect (ASD)
    a. septum
atrichous
atriodigital dysplasia

atriomegaly
atriopeptin
atrioventricular (AV)
    a. block
    a. bundle
    a. valve
atrioventricularis
    fasciculus a.
    truncus fascicularis a.
atrium
    accessory a.
Atropa
atrophedema
atrophia (*var. of* atrophy)
    acne a.
    a. blanche
    a. maculosa varioliformis cutis
atrophic
    a. arthritis
    a. chronic gastritis
    a. endometrium
    a. fenestration
    a. glossitis
    a. inflammation
    a. kidney
    a. lichen planus
    a. microcrypt
    a. pharyngitis
    a. rhinitis
    a. rhinitis of swine
    a. thrombosis
atrophica
    hyperkeratosis figurata centrifuga a.
    lineae atrophicae
    macula a.
    striae atrophicae
atrophicans
    acrodermatitis chronica a.
    dermatitis a.
atrophicus
    lichen sclerosus et a.
atrophied
atrophin gene
atrophoderma
    a. albidum
    a. maculatum
    a. neuriticum
    a. of Pasini and Pierini
    a. pigmentosum
    a. reticulatum
atrophy, atrophia
    acquired a.
    acute yellow a.
    brain a.
    brown a.
    cerebral a.
    Charcot-Marie-Tooth muscular a.
    circumscribed a.
    compensatory a.

    cyanotic a.
    cystic a.
    dentatorubral pallidoluysian a.
      (DRPLA)
    disuse a.
    endometrial a.
    essential a.
    exhaustion a.
    fatty a.
    focal a.
    gastric a.
    gelatinous a.
    granular a.
    Gudden a.
    gyrate a.
    hypertrophic polyneuritic-type
      muscular a.
    infantile muscular a.
    ischemic muscular a.
    Kienböck a.
    Leber optic a.
    lobar cerebral a.
    lobar pulmonary a.
    macular a.
    marantic a.
    mucinous a.
    multiple system a.
    muscular a.
    neuritic a.
    neurogenic muscular a. (NMA)
    neurotrophic a.
    olivocerebellar a.
    olivopontocerebellar a.
    optic a.
    polyneuritic-type hypertrophic
      muscular a.
    postmenopausal a.
    pressure a.
    progressive spinal muscular a.
    red a.
    senile a.
    serous a.
    simple a.
    subtotal villous a. (STVA)
    Sudeck a.
    traction a.
    traumatic a.
    villous a.
atropine
    a. autoinjector
    a. suppression test
atrosepticum
Atroxin solution
AT/RT
    atypical teratoid/rhabdoid tumor
ATS
    antitetanic serum
    antithymocyte serum
    arteriosclerosis

ATSDR
Agency for Toxic Substances &
Disease Registry
ATT
arginine tolerance test
atypical teratoid tumor
attached cranial section
attachment
epithelial a.
muscle-tendon a.
a. plaques
spindle a.
attack
Adams-Stokes a. (ASA)
agroterrorist a.
a. rate
transient ischemic a. (TIA)
vasovagal a.
attenuant
attenuate
attenuated
a. culture
a. familial adenomatous polyposis
rickettsia vaccine, a.
a. strain
a. tuberculosis
a. vaccine
a. viral form
a. virus
attenuation
ground glass a.
attenuator
AttoFluor RatioVision
attracted
chemotactically a.
attraction sphere
Attwood Stain
atypia
cellular a.
condylomatous a.
cytologic a.
cytonuclear a.
koilocytotic a.
atypica
Veillonella parvula subsp. a.
atypical
a. adenomatous hyperplasia (AAH)
a. apocrine hyperplasia
a. astrocyte
a. carcinoid
a. carcinoid tumor
a. cell
a. chronic myeloid leukemia
(aCML)
a. ductal hyperplasia (ADH)
a. endometrial hyperplasia
a. favor reactive
a. fibrous histiocytoma
a. fibroxanthoma (AFX)

a. glandular cell of undetermined
significance (AGUS)
a. glandular cell of unknown
significance (AGUS)
a. insulin
a. lipoma
a. lobular hyperplasia (ALH)
a. lymphocyte
a. measles
a. medullary carcinoma
a. melanocytic hyperplasia
a. melanocytic nevi of genital type
(AMNGT)
a. melanocytic nevus (AMN)
a. mycobacteria infection
a. polypoid adenomyofibroma (APA)
a. polypoid adenomyofibroma of
low malignant potential
(APA-LMP)
a. polypoid adenomyoma (APA)
a. primary pneumonia
a. regeneration
a. squamous cells of undetermined
significance (ASCUS)
a. squamous metaplasia (ASM)
a. teratoid/rhabdoid tumor (ATT/RhT)
a. teratoid/rhabdoid tumor of the
CNS
a. teratoid tumor (ATT)
a. verrucous endocarditis
atypicum
Corynebacterium a.
atypism
AUA
American Urological Association
AUA bladder cancer staging
classification
AU Ag
Australia antigen
Auchmeromyia luteola
audio amplifier
auditiva, *gen.* **auditivae**
cellulae pneumaticae tubae auditivae
lamina lateralis cartilaginis tubae
auditivae
lamina medialis cartilaginis tubae
auditivae
lamina membranacea cartilaginis
tubae auditivae
tuba a.
tunica mucosa tubae auditivae
auditivae (*gen. of* auditiva)
auditoria, *gen.* **auditoriae**
lamina lateralis cartilaginis tubae
auditoriae
lamina medialis cartilaginis tubae
auditoriae
tuba a.
auditoriae (*gen. of* auditoria)

auditory
- a. blast injury
- a. hair
- a. receptor cell
- a. string
- a. teeth
- a. tube

audouinii
- *Microsporum a.*

Audouin microsporon

Auer
- A. body
- A. rod

Auerbach
- A. ganglia
- A. nerve
- A. node
- A. plexus

Auger
- A. effect
- A. electron

augmented histamine test (AHT)

Aujeszky
- A. disease
- A. disease virus

AUL
- acute undifferentiated leukemia

Aulographina

AUO
- amyloid of unknown origin

aural polyp

auramine O fluorescent stain

auramine-rhodamine stain

auramine-stained buffy coat smear

aurantiaca
- *Actinocorallia a.*
- *Brevundimonas a.*
- *Gemmatimonas a.*
- *Pseudonocardia a.*
- *Sphingomonas a.*

aurantiacum
- *Cryptosporangium a.*
- *Virgisporangium a.*

aurantiacus
- *Agromyces a.*
- *Thermoascus a.*

aurantiasis

auranticolor
- *Actinokineospora a.*

Aurantimonas coralicida

Aurantiporus

aurati
- *Helicobacter a.*

aurea
- *Leifsonia a.*

Aureobasidium pullulans

aurescens
- *Escherichia a.*

aureus
- community-acquired methicillin-resistant *Staphylococcus a.* (CA-MRSA)
- glycopeptide-insensitive *Staphylococcus a.* (GISA)
- hospital-acquired methicillin-resistant *Staphylococcus a.* (HA-MRSA)
- lichen a.
- methicillin and aminoglycoside-resistant *Staphylococcus a.*
- methicillin-resistant *Staphylococcus a.* (MRSA)
- methicillin-susceptible *Staphylococcus a.*
- *Scopulariopsis a.*
- *Staphylococcus pyogenes a.*
- *Streptomyces a.*
- vancomycin-insensitive *Staphylococcus a.* (VISA)

Aureusvirus

auricular docimasia

Auricularia

auricularis
- *Aspergillus a.*

aurimucosum
- *Corynebacterium a.*

aurin tricarboxylic acid

auripigmenti
- *Desulfosporosinus a.*

auripigmentum
- *Desulfotomaculum a.*

auriscanis
- *Corynebacterium a.*

aurochromoderma

Aurococcus

aurothiomalate
- sodium a.

aurothiosuccinate
- sodium a.

aurothiosulfate
- sodium a.

auscultatory gap

Auspitz sign

austeni
- *Culicoides a.*

Australia (AU)
- A. antigen (AU Ag)

Australian
- A. X disease
- A. X disease virus
- A. X encephalitis
- A. X encephalitis virus

australiense
- *Propionibacterium a.*

australiensis
- *Bipolaris a.*

Quadricoccus a.
Tetrasphaera a.
australis
  Dermacentroxenus a.
  Leptospira a.
  Rickettsia a.
  Streptococcus a.
Austrobilharzia variglandis
autacoid (*var. of* autocoid)
autecic, autecious
autecious (*var. of* autecic)
Aution Max AX-4280 automated urine chemistry analyzer
autoabsorption
  cold a.
autoadhesive cellulose nitrate filter
autoadsorption
autoagglutination
autoagglutinin
  anti-Pr cold a.
  cold a.
autoallergic hemolytic anemia
autoallergization
autoallergy
autoanalyzer
  sequential multichannel a.
  (SMA)
autoanaphylaxis
autoantibody
  anticytoplasmic a.
  anti-glutamic acid decarboxylase a.
  (antiGAD-Ab)
  antiidiotype a.
  antineutrophil cytoplasmic a.
  (ANCA)
  cold a.
  cytoplasmic antineutrophil
  cytoplasmic a. (cANCA)
  Donath-Landsteiner cold a.
  hemagglutinating cold a.
  idiotype a.
  platelet a.
  specific a.
  thymocytotoxic a.
  warm a.
autoanticomplement
autoantigen
autoantiidiotypic antibody
autoanti-P
autoantitoxin
autoassay
autoblast
autocatalysis
autochthonous
autoclasia (*var. of* autoclasis)
autoclasis, autoclasia
autoclave (AC)
autocoid, autacoid
autocorrelation function

autocrine
  a. growth factor
  a. hypothesis
  a. motility factor (AMF)
  a. motility factor of the bladder
  a. motility factor receptor (AMFR)
autocrine-paracrine growth regulator
AutoCyte PREP system
autocytolysin
autocytolysis
autocytotoxin
autodigestion
Auto Dimer assay
autoerotic
  a. asphyxia
  a. death
autoerythrocyte
  a. sensitization
  a. sensitization syndrome
autoerythrophagocytosis
autofluorescence
autofluoroscope
autogamous
autogamy
autogeneic graft
autogenesis
autogenous vaccine
autograft
autografting
autohemagglutination
autohemagglutinin
autohemolysin
autohemolysis test
autohemotherapy
autoimmune
  a. antibody
  a. encephalomyelitis
  a. enteropathy
  a. gastritis
  a. hemolytic anemia (AHA, AIHA)
  a. hepatitis (AIH)
  a. leukopenia
  a. lymphoproliferative syndrome
  a. mechanism
  a. mucocutaneous disease
  a. neonatal thrombocytopenia
  a. orchitis
  a. pancytopenia
  a. polyendocrine syndrome type 1
  (APS1)
  a. reaction
  a. regulator (Aire)
  a. thrombocytopenic purpura
  a. thyroiditis
autoimmunity
autoimmunization
autoimmunocytopenia
autoimplant
autoinfection

autoinjector
    atropine a.
autoinoculable
autoinoculation
autoisolysin
Autolet blood glucose test
autologous
    a. antibody
    a. antigen
    a. blood and marrow transplantation (ABMT)
    a. bone marrow transplantation (ABMT)
    a. graft
    a. hemagglutinin
    a. leukapheresis, processing, and storage (ALPS)
    a. lymphokine activated killer cell
    a. peripheral blood stem cell (Auto-PBSC)
    a. peripheral blood stem cell bone marrow transplantation (Auto-PBSC BMT)
    a. transfusion
autolyse
autolysin
autolysis
    postmortem a.
autolysosome
autolytic enzyme
autolyze
automated
    a. activated partial thromboplastin
    a. assay optimization (AAO)
    a. bacteriology
    a. cell-counter technology
    a. cell image analysis
    a. cellular imaging system (ACIS)
    a. coagulation time
    a. differential leukocyte counter
    a. immunoprecipitation (AIP)
    a. motility factor
    a. multiphasic screening (AMS)
    a. reagin
    a. reagin test (ART)
    a. reticulocyte counting
    a. slide staining
automatic
    a. clinical analyzer
    a. fluorescent image analyzer
    a. hone
    a. tissue processing
automation
    blood cell count a.
    clinical chemistry a.
    differential leukocyte count a.
    a. initiative in laboratory management
    microbiology a.

    radioimmunoassay a.
    total laboratory a. (TLA)
Automeris io
autometallographic silver enhancement
autometallography (AMG)
automixis
autonomic
    a. dysfunction
    a. motor neuron
autonomous
    a. detection system (ADS)
    a. growth
autooxidation
autooxidative degradation
autoparenchymatous metaplasia
Autopath QC test
Auto-PBSC BMT
    autologous peripheral blood stem cell
autophagia, autophagy
autophagic
    a. granule
    a. vacuole
autophagocytosis
autophagolysosome
autophagosome
autophagy
autophosphorylation
autoplast
autoplastic graft
autoplasty
autoploidy
autopsy
    digital a.
    endoscopic a.
    forensic a.
    medicolegal a.
    psychological a.
    virtual a.
autoradiography
    storage phosphor a.
autoradiolysis
autoregulation
autoreinfection
autoreproduction
autosensitization
autosensitize
autosepticemia
autoserotherapy
autoserum therapy
autosomal
    a. dominant disorder
    a. dominant hemochromatosis
    a. dominant inheritance
    a. dominant osteopetrosis type 2 (ADO2)
    a. gene
    a. heredity
    a. recessive
    a. recessive disorder

a. recessive inheritance
a. recessive polycystic kidney disease (AR-PKD)
autosome translocation
Autostainer
Dako A.
Jung Autostainer XL
autotemnous
autotherapy
autotomy
autotoxemia
autotoxicus
horror a.
autotransformer
variable a.
autotransfusion
autotransplant
autotransplantation
autotroph
facultative a.
obligate a.
autotrophic
a. bacterium
a. fixation
autotrophica
Sulfurimonas a.
autotrophicum
Trichophyton equinum a.
autovaccination
autumnalis
Galerina a.
Leptospira a.
Neotrombicula a.
Trombicula a.
auxanography
Auxarthron
auxesis
auxetic growth
auxilytic
auxochrome
auxocyte
auxotroph
auxotrophic mutation
AV
atrioventricular
AV block
Av
avoirdupois
AVA
arteriovenous anastomosis
available
no data a. (NDA)
avalanche ionization
Avanti J-20XP, J-25, J-30I, J-HC, J-E centrifuge
avascular necrosis (AVN)
Avastrovirus
AVD O$_2$
arteriovenous oxygen difference

Avellis syndrome
Avenavirus
average
a. deviation
a. gradient
a. life
Walsh a.
weighted a.
averaging
signal a.
avermectinius
Streptomyces a.
avermitilis
Streptomyces a.
AVF
arteriovenous fistula
AVH
acute viral hepatitis
avian
a. diphtheria
a. encephalomyelitis virus
a. erythroblastosis virus
a. infectious encephalomyelitis
a. infectious laryngotracheitis
a. infectious laryngotracheitis virus
a. influenza
a. influenza virus
a. leukosis
a. leukosis-sarcoma complex
a. leukosis-sarcoma virus
a. lymphomatosis
a. lymphomatosis virus
a. monocytosis
a. myeloblastosis
a. myeloblastosis leukemia virus reverse transcriptase (AMLV-RT)
a. myeloblastosis virus
a. myelocytomatosis virus (AMV2)
a. neurolymphomatosis virus
a. pneumoencephalitis virus
a. reticuloendotheliosis
a. sarcoma
a. sarcoma virus (ASV)
a. tubercle bacillus
a. viral arthritis virus
Avibirnavirus
Avicenna gland
avidin
avidin-biotin
a.-b. based detection system
a.-b. complex
a.-b. complex immunodetection system
a.-b. immunoperoxidase technique
a.-b. peroxidase complex (ABC)
avidity
a. antibody
a. testing
avidum
Propionibacterium a.

Avihepadnavirus
avipoxvirus
    a.
avirulence
avirulent strain
avitaminosis
avium
    Mycobacterium a.
    Trypanosoma a.
avium-intracellulare
    Mycobacterium a.-i. (MAI)
AVM
    arteriovenous malformation
AVN
    avascular necrosis
Avogadro
    A. law
    A. number
avoirdupois (Av)
AvoSure INR test device
AVOXimeter 4000 CO oximeter
AVP
    arginine vasopressin
AVR
    aortic valve replacement
Avsunviroid
Avulavirus
avulsion
    a. fracture
    a. injury
A&W
    alive and well
aware
    A. HIV-1/2 oral fluid rapid
     test
    A. Rapid HIV assay
AWD
    alive with disease
AWI
    anterior wall infarction
AWMI
    anterior wall myocardial infarction
AWOD
    alive without disease
awu
    atomic weight unit
axanthum
    Acholeplasma a.
axei
    Trichostrongylus a.
Axenfeld syndrome
axenic
axes (*pl. of* axis)
axial
    a. aneurysm
    a. chordoma
    a. filament
axialensis
    Halomonas a.

axifugal
axile corpuscle
axillare
    hygroma a.
axillares
    nodi lymphoidei a.
axillaris
    trichomycosis a.
axillary sweat gland
axioplasm
axiopodium
axis, *pl.* axes
    brain-hair follicle a.
     (BHA)
    cell a.
    a. corpuscle
    a. cylinder
    hypothalamic-pituitary-testicular a.
    a. of rotation
    a. of symmetry
    renin-aldosterone a.
axoaxonic synapse
axodendritic synapse
axofugal
axolemma
axolysis
    terminal a.
axon
    bundle of a.
    cervix of the a.
    a. containing microtubule
    a. hillock
    motor a.
    a. of neuroglial cell
    a. of pyramidal cell
    a. staining method
    a. terminal
    unmyelinated a.
axonal
    a. degeneration
    a. demyelination
    a. process
    a. terminal bouton
axoneme
axonotmesis
axopetal
axoplasm
axoplasmic transport
axopodium
axosomatic synapse
axostyle
AxSYM
    AxSYM analyzer
    AxSYM CORE HBV antibody
     reagent kit
    AxSYM free PSA
     test
ayderensis
    Anoxybacillus a.

Ayerza
    A. disease
    A. syndrome
Ayoub-Shklar method
Ayre spatula
ayr phenotype
ayw phenotype
A-Z
    Aschheim-Zondek
azacytidine
azan stain
azar
    kala a.
azathioprine
azeotrope
azeotropic solution
azeotropy
azide
    sodium a.
azidothymidine
azin dye
azinphosmethyl
azo
    a. coupling reaction
    a. dye
Azoarcus
    A. buckelii
    A. toluvorans
azobenzene
azobilirubin
azocarmine
    a. B
    a. dye
    a. G
azoic dye
azolitmin paper
Azonexus fungiphilus
azoospermatism (*var. of* azoospermia)
azoospermia, azoospermatism
azophloxin
azoprotein
azoreducens
    Paenibacillus a.
azorense
    Sulfurihydrogenibium a.

azorensis
    Caloranaerobacter a.
Azospira oryzae
Azospirillum doebereinerae
azote
azotemia
    chloropenic a.
    extrarenal a.
    hypochloremic a.
    nonrenal a.
    postrenal a.
    prerenal a.
    renal a.
azotemic
Azotobacter
Azotobacteraceae
azotonutricium
    Treponema a.
azotorrhea
azoturia
azovan blue
Azovibrio restrictus
A-Z pregnancy test
aztecus
    Anopheles a.
azure
    a. A (aA)
    a. B (aB)
    a. C (aC)
    a. I, II
    a. II-methylene blue stain
    methylene a.
azure-eosin stain
azuresin
azurophil, azurophile
    a. granule
azurophile (*var. of* azurophil)
azurophilia
azurophilic granule
azymia
Azymoprocandida
Azzopardi
    A. criteria
    A. phenomenon
    A. sign

B
Baumé scale
Benoist scale
whole blood
B antigen
B cell
B cell activation
B cell lymphoma of MALT type
B cell lymphopoiesis
B lymphocyte
B lymphocyte stimulator (BLyS)
2b
Uvitex 2b
B₂
Sherman-Bourquin unit of vitamin B₂
4B
benzopurpurin 4B
B4
isolectin B4
B5
B5 fixative
B5 sodium acetate-sublimate formalin
B12a
vitamin B₁₂
BA
bacillary angiomatosis
bacterial agglutination
blocking antibody
bronchial asthma
Baastrup syndrome
Babcock tube
Babès
B. node
B. tubercle
Babès-Ernst
B.-E. body
B.-E. corpuscle
B.-E. granule
Babesia
B. divergens
B. microti
Babesiella
Babesiidae
babesiosis serological test
Babès nodule
Babinski-Fröhlich syndrome
Babinski-Nageotte syndrome
Babinski syndrome
Babinski-Vaquez syndrome
Babuvirus
baby
blue b.
collodion b.

BabyBIG
Babystart
B. fertility test kit
B. ovulation test
BAC
blood alcohol concentration
bronchioloalveolar carcinoma
BACA
bronchioalveolar carcinoma
BACE
beta site APP cleaving enzyme
Bachmann bundle
Bachman-Pettit test
Bachman test
Bacillaceae
Bacillales
bacillary
b. angiomatosis (BA)
b. body
b. dysentery
b. embolism
b. emulsion (tuberculin) (BE)
b. hemoglobinuria
b. layer
bacille bilíe de Calmette-Gúerin (BCG)
bacillemia
bacilli (*pl. of* bacillus)
bacilliform
bacilliformis
Bartonella b.
bacillisporus
Filobasidiella b.
bacillosis
bacilluria
Bacillus
B. aeolius
B. aerogenes capsulatus
B. aertrycke
B. algicola
B. alvei
B. ambiguus
B. anthracis
B. anthracis toxin
B. aquimaris
B. arseniciselenatis
B. barbaricus
B. bataviensis
B. botulinus
B. brevis
B. bronchisepticus
B. cereus
B. circulans
B. coli
B. decolorationis
B. diphtheriae

Bacillus (*continued*)
B. *drentensis*
B. *dysenteriae*
B. *endophyticus*
B. *enteritidis*
B. *faecalis alcaligenes*
B. *farraginis*
B. *fordii*
B. *fortis*
B. *fumarioli*
B. *funiculus*
B. *galactosidilyticus*
B. *gelatini*
B. *hemolyticus*
B. *histolyticus*
B. *hwajinpoensis*
B. *indicus*
B. *influenzae*
B. *jeotgali*
B. *krulwichiae*
B. *larvae*
B. *leprae*
B. *licheniformis*
B. *luciferensis*
B. *mallei*
B. *marisflavi*
B. *megaterium*
B. *nealsonii*
B. *necrophorus*
B. *neidei*
B. *novalis*
B. *odysseyi*
B. *oedematiens*
B. *oedematis maligni*
B. *okuhidensis*
B. *pertussis*
B. *pestis*
B. *pneumoniae*
B. *polymyxa*
B. *proteus*
B. *pseudomallei*
B. *psychrodurans*
B. *psychrotolerans*
B. *pumilus*
B. *pycnus*
B. *pyocyaneus*
B. *selenitireducens*
B. *shackletonii*
B. *siralis*
B. *soli*
B. *sonorensis*
B. *sphaericus*
B. *stearothermophilus*
B. *subterraneus*
B. *subtilis*
B. *suipestifer*
B. *tetani*
B. *thermantarcticus*
B. *thermodenitrificans*

B. *thuringiensis*
B. *tuberculosis*
B. *tularense*
B. *typhi*
B. *typhosus*
B. *vireti*
B. *vulcani*
B. *weihenstephanensis*
B. *welchii*
B. *whitmori*
bacillus, *pl.* **bacilli**
acid-fast b. (AFB)
anthrax b.
avian tubercle b.
Bang b.
Battey b.
Boas-Oppler b.
Bordet-Gengou b.
bovine tubercle b.
Calmette-Guérin b.
b. Calmette-Gúerin
cholera b.
coliform b.
colon b.
comma b.
diphtheria b.
diphtheroid bacilli
Döderlein b.
Ducrey b.
dysentery bacilli
enteric b.
Escherich b.
Fick b.
Flexner b.
Flexner-Strong b.
Friedländer b.
fusiform b.
Gärtner b.
Ghon-Sachs b.
glanders b.
gram-negative b.
gram-positive b.
Hansen b.
hay b.
Hofmann b.
human tubercle b.
Johne b.
Klebs-Löffler b.
Klein b.
Koch b.
Koch-Weeks b.
leprosy b.
Morax-Axenfeld b.
Morgan b.
Mott bacilli
Newcastle-Manchester b.
Nocard b.
nonfermentative b. (NFB)
plague b.

Preisz-Nocard b.
pseudotuberculosis b.
rhinoscleroma b.
Schmitz b.
Schmorl b.
Shiga b.
smegma b.
Sonne-Duval b.
Strong b.
swine rotlauf b.
tetanus b.
timothy b.
tubercle b. (TB)
typhoid b.
vegetative b.
vegetative anthrax bacilli
Vincent b.
vole b.
Weeks b.
Welch b.
Whitmore b.
bacitracin disc test
back
adolescent round b.
b. splatter
backbone
backcross
background
b. count
flame b.
b. interference
b. radiation
smear b.
backlash
backpropagation
backscatter
Backusia
backward failure
backwash ileitis
bacoti
Bdellonyssus b.
bact
bacterium
BacT/Alert automated microbial detection system
Bactec
B. blood culture system
B. 9000 MB system
B. MGIT 960
bacteremia, bacteriemia
clostridial b.
platelet-associated b.
bacteria (*pl. of* bacterium)
bacteria-free stage of bacterial endocarditis
bacterial
b. adherence
b. agar method
b. agglutination (BA)

b. allergy
b. aneurysm
b. antagonism
b. antigen detection method
b. aortitis
b. capsule
b. classification
b. culture
b. culturing
b. dissociation
b. encephalitis
b. endaortitis
b. endarteritis
b. endocarditis (BE)
b. enzyme
b. filter
b. genetics
b. hemolysin
b. infection
b. inhibition assay
b. interference
b. killing assay
b. lipochitooligosaccharide compound elicitor
b. meningitis
b. meningitis antigen
b. myocarditis
b. nephritis
b. opsonin
b. opsonization
b. overgrowth syndrome
b. pathogenicity
b. pericarditis
b. permeability-inducing (BPI)
b. plaque
b. prostatitis
b. serology
b. spore
b. stain
b. staining
b. susceptibility testing
b. toxin
b. transformation
b. transfusion reaction
b. urinary cast
b. vaginitis
b. vegetation
b. virus
b. zoonosis
bacterial-fungal interaction
bactericholia, bacteriocholia
bactericidal, bacteriocidal
b. antibiotic
b. concentration (BC)
bactericide (*var. of* bacteriocide)
bacterid
pustular b.
bacteriemia (*var. of* bacteremia)

bacteriform
bacterioagglutinin
bacteriocholia (*var. of* bactericholia)
bacteriocidal (*var. of* bactericidal)
bacteriocide, bactericide
 specific b.
bacteriocidin
bacteriocin factor
bacteriocinogen
bacteriocinogenic plasmid
bacterioclasis
bacteriogenic agglutination
bacterioid
bacteriological index (BI)
bacteriologic specimen
bacteriologist
bacteriology
 automated b.
 clinical diagnostic b.
 b. laboratory
 medical b.
 public health b.
 sanitary b.
 systematic b.
bacteriolysin
bacteriolysis
bacteriolytic
 b. amboceptor
 b. serum
bacteriolytica
 Algicola b.
bacteriolyze
bacterioopsonin
bacteriopexy
bacteriophage
 defective b.
 filamentous b.
 b. genetics
 b. immunity
 mature b.
 b. resistance
 temperate b.
 typhoid b.
 b. typing
 vegetative b.
 virulent b.
bacteriophagia
bacteriophagology
bacteriopsonic
bacteriopsonin
bacteriosis
bacteriostasis agar
bacteriostat
bacteriostatic
 b. agent
 b. antibiotic
bacteriotoxic
bacteriotropic substance
bacteriotropin

Bacteriovoracaceae
Bacteriovorax
 B. litoralis
 B. marinus
 B. starrii
 B. stolpii
bacteriovorus
 Bdellovibrio b.
bacterium (bact), *pl.* **bacteria**
 acid-fast b.
 aerobic b.
 anaerobic b.
 autotrophic b.
 beaded b.
 bifid b.
 Campylobacter b.
 chemoautotrophic b.
 chemoheterotrophic b.
 chromogenic b.
 commensal b.
 corkscrew-like bacteria
 denitrifying b.
 endogenous b.
 enterotoxigenic bacteria
 exogenous b.
 facultative b.
 fastidious b.
 gram-negative b.
 gram-positive b.
 heterotrophic b.
 higher bacteria
 hydrogen b.
 indigenous b.
 intermediate coliform bacteria
 lactic acid bacteria
 lysogenic b.
 mesophilic b.
 monocytogenes b.
 nitrifying b.
 nonlactose-fermenting b.
 nonmotile bacteria
 nonspore-forming b.
 organotropic b.
 ovoid b.
 psychrophilic b.
 pyogenic b.
 rod shaped b.
 rough b.
 smooth b.
 sulfur b.
 thermophilic b.
 toxigenic b.
 water b.
bacteriuria
 significant asymptomatic b.
 (SAB)
bacteroid
Bacteroidaceae
Bacteroideae

bacteroides
- *B. acidifaciens*
- *B. bivius*
- *Brevundimonas b.*
- *B. capillosus*
- *B. corrodens*
- *B. disiens*
- *B. distasonis*
- *B. fragilis*
- *B. funduliformis*
- *B. furcosus*
- *B. fusiformis*
- *B. melaninogenicus*
- *B. nodosus*
- *B. ochraceus*
- *B. oralis*
- *B. oris*
- *B. pneumonia*
- *B. pneumosintes*
- *B. praeacutus*
- *B. putredinis*
- *B. ruminicola*
- *B. serpens*
- *B. splanchnicus*
- *B. thetaiotamicron*
- *B. ureolyticus*

Bactigen

BactiSwab
- B. II
- B. NPG

Bacto
- B. Middlebrook
- B. Middlebrook 7H9 broth
- B. Middlebrook OADC Enrichment broth

Bactoderma

Bactometer

Bactrol Plus quality control culture

Bactron 1.5 anaerobic chamber

baculata
- *Heliorestis b.*

Baculoviridae

Badhamia utricularis

Badnavirus

Baehr-Lohlein lesion

Baelz disease

Baermann concentration

Baer vesicle

BAFF
- B-cell activating factor

Bäfverstedt syndrome

bag
- biohazard b.
- nuclear b.
- Speci-Gard specimen transport b.

bagassosis

Baggenstoss change in pancreas

bag-mask device

bag-valve-mask device, bag-mask device

baikonurensis
- *Rhodococcus b.*

Baillarger
- B. band
- B. line
- B. stria
- B. stripe

Bairnsdale ulcer

bajacaliforniensis
- *Spirochaeta b.*

Bakamjian deltopectoral flap

baker
- B. acid hematein
- B. acid hematein test
- B. cyst
- B. formol calcium
- B. pyridine extraction
- B. pyridine extraction test
- B. Sudan black method

baker's
- b. eczema
- b. yeast

BAL
- British antilewisite
- bronchoalveolar lavage
- BAL ointment

balabacensis
- *Anopheles b.*

balaenopterae
- *Granulicatella b.*

Balamuth
- B. aqueous egg yolk infusion medium
- B. buffer solution
- B. culture medium

Balamuthia mandrillaris

balance
- acid-base b.
- analytical b.
- calcium b.
- enzyme b.
- fluid b.
- genetic b.
- genic b.
- microchemical b.
- nitrogen b.
- b. translocation
- water b.

balanced
- b. polymorphism
- b. salt solution (BSS)

balanitis
- keratotic micaceous b.
- b. xerotica obliterans
- Zoon b.

balanoposthitis

balantidial
    b. colitis
    b. dysentery
balantidiasis, balantidosis
Balantidium
    B. coli
    B. suis
balantidosis (*var. of* balantidiasis)
Balbiani
    B. body
    B. chromosome
    B. nucleus
    B. ring
baldri
    Agrococcus b.
BALF
    bronchoalveolar lavage fluid
Balfour disease
balhimycina
    Amycolatopsis b.
baliensis
    Kozakia b.
Balint syndrome
Balkan
    B. grippe
    B. nephropathy
ball
    Aspergillus fungus b.
    chondrin b.
    food b.
    fungus b.
    hair b.
    pleural fibrin b.
    b. thrombus
B-ALL
    B-cell acute lymphoblastic leukemia
Baller-Gerold syndrome
Ballet disease
Ballingall disease
balloon
    b. cell
    b. cell nevus
    b. cytology
    b. dilation
    b. neuron
    b. scraping
ballooning
    b. colliquation
    b. degeneration
ball-valve
    b.-v. obstruction
    b.-v. thrombus
Balnearium lithotrophicum
balnei
    Mycobacterium b.
Balneimonas flocculans
Baló disease
BALT
    bronchus-associated lymphoid tissue

baltica
    Belliella b.
    Cellulophaga b.
    Idiomarina b.
    Rheinheimera b.
    Rhodopirellula b.
balticum
    Desulfotignum b.
Bamberger
    B. albuminuria
    B. disease
Bamberger-Marie
    B.-M. disease
    B.-M. syndrome
BamH1 enzyme
Bamle disease
banal cystitis
Bancroft
    B. filarial worm
    B. filariasis
bancrofti
    Filaria b.
    Wuchereria b.
bancroftian filariasis
bancroftiasis, bancroftosis
bancroftosis (*var. of* bancroftiasis)
band
    A b.
    alpha b.
    alpha-1 b.
    anomalous muscle b.
    Baillarger b.
    birefringent collagen b.
    b. cell
    centromeric b.
    chromosomal b.
    chromosome b.
    contraction b.
    creatine phosphokinase-myocardial b.
    (CPK-MB)
    b. form
    b. form granulocyte
    G b.
    giant b.
    H b.
    Hunter-Schreger b.
    I b.
    Kaes-Bekhterev b.
    b. keratopathy
    Ladd b.
    light b.
    M b.
    MB b.
    MM b.
    moderator b.
    monoclonal b.
    b. neutrophil
    nongermline b.
    oligoclonal b.

b. 3 protein
Q b.
Securline blood b.
Soret b.
b. spectrum
stromal collagen b.
subepithelial collagen b.
theta b.
thick fibrous b.
Z b.
banding
AgNOR b.
BrDu b.
C b.
chromosome b.
G b.
high-resolution b.
NOR b.
oligoclonal b.
prometaphase b.
Q b.
quinacrine b.
R b.
reverse b.
T b.
telomere b.
terminal b.
Bandl ring
bandpass
bands
cerebrospinal fluid oligoclonal b.
ghost b.
nondiscrete b.
band-shaped nucleus
bandwidth
bane
black b. (anthrax)
Banff renal allograft rejection classification
Bang
B. bacillus
B. disease
B. method
B. test
bank, banking
blood b. (BB)
gene b.
banking (*var. of* bank)
Bannayan-Riley-Ruvalcaba syndrome
Bannayan-Zonana syndrome
Bannister disease
Banti
B. disease
B. spleen
B. syndrome
bantianum
Cladosporium (Xylohypha) b.
Bantu siderosis

BAO
basal acid output
BAP
blood agar plate
bar
terminal bar
baragnosis, barognosis
Barany caloric test
baratii
Clostridium b.
rare clostridial strain of
Clostridium b.
Barbados leg
barbae
Aspergillus b.
folliculitis b.
tinea b.
trichophytosis b.
barbaricus
Bacillus b.
Barber psoriasis
barber's itch
barbiero
barbirostris
Anopheles b.
barbital
barbiturate
b. assay
b. level
b. spindle
Barclay-Baron disease
Barcoo
B. disease
B. rot
Barcroft apparatus
Bardet-Biedl syndrome
Bard needle
bare
b. lymphocyte syndrome type 1
b. lymphocyte syndrome
Bargen streptococcus
bariatric surgery
barium
b. granuloma
b. test
Barlow
B. disease
B. syndrome
Barnavirus
barnesae
Gallicola b.
Barnett-Bourne acetic alcohol-silver nitrate method
baroceptor (*var. of* baroreceptor)
barognosis (*var. of* baragnosis)
barometer
barometric
b. bomb
b. pressure (Pb)

barophilus
>   *Thermococcus b.*
baroreceptor, baroceptor
barosinusitis
barotrauma
Barr
>   B. body
>   B. body scoring
>   B. body test
>   B. chromatin body
Barraquer disease
Barré-Guillain syndrome
barrel chest
barreling distortion
Barrett
>   B. adenocarcinoma
>   (BCA)
>   B. epithelium (BE)
>   B. esophagus (BE)
>   B. metaplasia
>   B. syndrome
>   B. ulcer
Barrett-associated adenocarcinoma
barrier
>   blood-air b.
>   blood-aqueous b.
>   blood-brain b. (BBB)
>   blood-cerebral b.
>   blood-testis b.
>   blood-thymus b.
>   b. filter
>   glomerular b.
>   immune b.
>   b. isolation precaution
>   placental b.
>   protective osmatic b.
barrier-layer cell
barrier-sustained
>   cesarean-obtained b.-s. (COBS)
Barrnett-Seligman
>   B.-S. dihydroxydinaphthyl disulfide
>   method
>   B.-S. indoxyl esterase
>   method
Barroso-Moguel and Costero silver method
Bart
>   Hb B.
>   hemoglobin B.
>   B. syndrome
Bartholin
>   B. abscess
>   B. anus
>   B. cyst
>   B. duct
>   B., urethral, Skene (BUS)
bartholinitis
bartlettii
>   *Clostridium b.*

Bartonella
>   *B. bacilliformis*
>   *B. birtlesii*
>   *B. bovis*
>   *B. capreoli*
>   *B. chomelii*
>   *B. elizabethae*
>   *B. henselae*
>   *B. koehlerae*
>   *B. quintana*
>   *B. schoenbuchensis*
>   *B. vinsonii*
>   *B. vinsonii* subsp. *arupensis*
Bartonellaceae
bartonellosis
Bartter syndrome
baruria
basal
>   b. acid output (BAO)
>   b. apoptotic rate
>   b. body
>   b. cell
>   b. cell acanthoma
>   b. cell adenoma
>   b. cell ameloblastoma
>   b. cell carcinoma (BCC)
>   b. cell carcinoma specific antibody
>   b. cell epithelioma
>   b. cell hyperplasia
>   b. cell layer
>   b. cell nevus
>   b. cell nevus syndrome
>   b. cell papilloma
>   b. corpuscle
>   b. feet
>   b. gastric secretion test
>   b. granule
>   b. hemosiderosis
>   b. lamina
>   b. lamina of choroid
>   b. layer of choroid
>   b. metabolic rate (BMR)
>   b. metabolism
>   b. nucleus of Ganser
>   b. secretory flow rate (BSFR)
>   b. secretory flow rate test
>   b. squamous cell carcinoma
>   b. striation
>   b. tuberculosis
basale
>   stratum b.
basalis
>   decidua b.
>   stratum b.
basaloid
>   b. blastema
>   b. cell
>   b. growth pattern
>   b. hyperplasia

b. invasive squamous cell carcinoma (BISCC)
b. squamous cell carcinoma (BSCC)
b. tumor
basaloma
base
blood buffer b. (BB)
Brönsted-Lowry b.
buffer b. (BB)
complementary b.
conjugate b.
b. deficit (BD)
delta b.
b. excess (BE)
b. ionization constant
Lewis b.
b. lymphocyte syndrome (BLS)
National Cancer Data B. (NCDB)
b. pair (bp)
b. pairing
pressor b.
purine and pyrimidine b.'s
pyrimidine b.
b. ratio
Schiff b.
b. unit
Basedow disease
basement
b. lamina
b. membrane
b. membrane antibody
b. membrane component
b. membrane zone
basic
Acceava hCG B.
b. amino acid
b. anhydride
b. calcium phosphate (BCP)
b. calcium phosphate crystal
b. dye
b. fibroblast growth factor (bFGF)
b. fuchsin
b. fuchsin-methylene blue stain
b. helix-loop-helix transcription factor (bHLH)
b. magenta
b. metabolic panel (BMP)
basicaryoplastin
basichromatin
basichromiole
basicity
basicytoparaplastin
basidiobolae
entomophthoramycosis b.
basidiobolomycosis
Basidiobolus
B. haptosporus
B. ranarum

Basidiomycetes
Basidiomycota
basidiospore
basidium
basilar, basilaris
b. artery ischemia
b. cell
glandula basilaris
b. lamina
b. leptomeningitis
membrana basilaris
b. membrane of cochlear duct
b. meningitis
basilaris (*var. of* basilar)
basilemma
basilensis
Wautersia b.
basiparaplastin
basipetal
Basipetospora rubra
basis pontis
basisquamous (*var. of* basosquamous)
basket
b. cell
fibrillar b.
basket-weave pattern
baso
basophil
basophilic leukocyte
basocyte
basocytopenia
basocytosis
basoerythrocyte
basoerythrocytosis
basolateral membrane
basometachromophil, basometachromophile
basometachromophile (*var. of* basometachromophil)
basopenia
basophil (baso), basophile
b. adenoma
beta b.
b. cell
b. cell of anterior lobe of hypophysis
b. chemotactic factor (BCF)
b. degranulation test
b. granule
polymorphonuclear b. (PMB)
b. substance
tissue b.
basophile (*var. of* basophil)
basophilia
Grawitz b.
pituitary b.
punctate b.
substantia b.

basophilic, basophil
- b. cytoplasm
- b. deposit
- b. erythroblast
- b. granular degeneration
- b. granule
- b. hyperplasia
- b. leukemia
- b. leukocyte (baso)
- b. leukocytosis
- b. leukopenia
- b. marrow
- b. megakaryocyte
- b. megaloblast
- b. metamyelocyte
- b. mucin
- b. myelocyte
- b. normoblast
- b. promyelocyte
- b. stippling

basophilism
- Cushing b.
- pituitary b.

basophilocyte

basophilocytic
- b. leukemia

basoplasm

basosquamous, basisquamous
- b. carcinoma

Bassen-Kornzweig syndrome

bassiana
- Beauveria b.

bastinii
- Desulfovibrio b.

BAT
- biliary acid transporter

bataviensis
- Bacillus b.

batch analyzer

Bateman syndrome

bath
- flotation b.
- isopentane-dry ice b.
- water b.

bathochromic shift

bathophenanthroline

bathycardia

batsensis
- Oceanicola b.

Batson
- B. plexus
- B. system

Batten disease

Batten-Mayou syndrome

battered child

battery
- anergy skin test b.
- liver b.

Battey bacillus

Battey-type mycobacterium

battledore
- b. insertion
- b. placenta

batwing appearance

Bauer
- B. chromic acid leucofuchsin stain
- B. reaction

Bauer-Kirby test

Bauermeister scale

Bauhin gland

baumannii
- Acinetobacter b.
- Oceanimonas b.

Baumé
- B. law
- B. scale (B)

baumgartneri
- Caulochora b.

Baumgartner method

bauxite
- b. pneumoconiosis
- b. worker's disease

Bax
- B. apoptosis gene
- B. protein

Bayer
- B. AG II chemistry analyzer system
- B. Immuno 1 HER-2/neu assay
- B. Technicon H-2 analyzer
- B. Technicon H1 automated flow cytometer
- B. Versant HCV RNA 3.0 assay

Bayes theorem

Bayh-Dole Act

Bayle
- B. disease
- B. granulation

Baylisascaris procyonis

baylyi
- Acinetobacter b.

Bazex syndrome

Bazin disease

BB
- blood bank
- blood buffer base
- blue bloater
- breakthrough bleeding
- breast biopsy
- buffer base
  - creatine kinase BB (CK-BB)
  - glycogen phosphorylase isoenzyme BB (GPBB)
  - orseillin BB

BBB
- blood-brain barrier
- bundle-branch block

BC
    bactericidal concentration
    blood culture
BCA
    Barrett adenocarcinoma
    bicinchoninic acid method
BCAA
    branched-chain amino acid
BCB
    brilliant cresyl blue
BCC
    basal cell carcinoma
B-cell
    B-c. activating factor (BAFF)
    B-c. acute lymphoblastic leukemia
      (B-ALL)
    B-c. ALL
    B-c. antibody
    B-c. antigen receptor
    B-c. chronic lymphocytic leukemia
      (BCLL)
    B-c. chronic lymphocytic leukemia/
      small lymphocytic lymphoma
    B-c. chronic lymphoproliferative
      disorder (BCLPD)
    B-c. CLL/SLL
    B-c. count
    B-c. deficiency
    B-c. differentiating factor
    B-c. differentiation/growth factor
    B-c. growth factor I, II
    B-c. immunodeficiency
    B-c. lymphoma (BCL)
    B-c. lymphoproliferative disease
    B-c. lymphoproliferative disorder
      (BLPD)
    B-c. malignancy
    B-c. marker
    B-c. neoplasia
    B-c. neoplasm
    B-c. non-Hodgkin lymphoma
      (B-NHL)
    B-c. precursor lymphoblastic
      leukemia (BCP-LBL)
    B-c. prolymphocytic leukemia
      (B-PLL)
    B-c. stimulating factor
BCF
    basophil chemotactic factor
BCG
    bicolor guaiac test
    bronchocentric granulomatosis
    BCG vaccine
BChE
    butyrylcholinesterase
BCKA
    branched-chain keto acid
BCL
    B-cell lymphoma

bcl-**1 gene**
bcl-**2**
    b.-2 antibody
    b.-2 gene
    b.-2 gene arrangement
    b.-2 gene rearrangement
    b.-2 oncogene
    b.-2 protein
    b.-2 protooncogene
bcl-**6 antibody**
BCLL
    B-cell chronic lymphocytic leukemia
BCLPD
    B-cell chronic lymphoproliferative
    disorder
bcl-X_L **protein**
bCNU
    carmustine
BCP
    basic calcium phosphate
    BCP crystal
BCP-D
    bromocresol purple desoxycholate
BCP-LBL
    B-cell precursor lymphoblastic
    leukemia
BCR-ABL
    breakpoint cluster region-Abelson
    murine leukemia virus
    BCR-ABL hybrid protein
    BCR-ABL protein test
    BCR-ABL transcript
BD
    base deficit
    BD BBL CultureSwab Plus
      collection and transport system
    BD BeAware test
    BD Phoenix automated microbiology
      system
BD/BS
    bile duct-to-portal space ratio
BD-CHEK intestinal inflammation kit
Bdellomicrovirus
Bdellonyssus bacoti
Bdellovibrio bacteriovorus
BDG
    buffered desoxycholate glucose
b-DNA
    branched DNA
BDNF
    brain-derived neurotrophic factor
B-domain-deleted
    B-d.-d. factor VIII concentrate
    B-d.-d. rFVIII product
BDS
    biohazard detection system
BE
    bacillary emulsion (tuberculin)
    bacterial endocarditis

B

BE (*continued*)
    base excess
    bovine enteritis
Be^a antigen
bead
    agar b.
    controlled pore glass b.
    glutathione agarose b.'s
    IOBeads magnetic b.'s
beaded
    b. bacterium
    b. hair
beaked pelvis
beaker
    b. cell
    Griffin b.
Beale ganglion cell
beam
    electron b.
    b. splitting
bean
    castor b.
BE12 antibody
beard
    B. disease
    ringworm of b.
    B. test
beaten-egg-white-appearance colony
Beau
    B. disease
    B. line
    B. syndrome
Beauvais disease
Beauveria bassiana
Beaver direct smear method
Bechterew (*var. of* Bekhterev)
    B. disease
Beck
    B. disease
    B. triad
Becker
    B. antigen
    B. disease
    B. muscular dystrophy (BMD)
    B. nevus
    B. stain for spirochetes
Becker-type tardive muscular dystrophy
Beckman
    B. assay
    B. Paragon SPE-II gel apparatus
    B. Synchron CX-7 cholesterol analyzer
Beckmann thermometer
Beckwith syndrome
Beckwith-Wiedemann syndrome
becquerel

Becton-Dickinson needle
bed
    microcapillary b.
bedbug
Bedbugg system for at-home diagnosis of sleep apnea
Bednar tumor
Bedsonia
bedtime salivary cortisol test
beef tapeworm
beer
    b. drinker's cardiomyopathy
    b. drinker's potomania
    b. heart
    B. law
Beer-Boguer law
beeturia
bee venom toxin
Begbie disease
Beggiatoaceae
Beggiatoales
Begomovirus
Béguez César disease
behavior
    dementia pugilistica/autism with self-injury b.
    b. genetics
Behçet
    B. disease
    B. syndrome
behenic acid
Behnken unit (R)
Behr disease
Behring law
BEI
    butanol-extractable iodine
    BEI test
Beigel disease
beigelii
    Trichosporon b.
beijiangensis
    Streptomyces b.
beijingensis
    Nocardia b.
bejel
Bekhterev, Bechterew
    B. disease
    B. nucleus
bel
Belascaris
Belgian Congo anemia
beliardensis
    Legionella b.
belladonna
belladonnine
bellator
    Anopheles b.
bell-clapper abnormality
Bell disease

belli
    Isospora b.
Belliella baltica
Bellini
    B. duct
    B. duct carcinoma
    medullary ducts of B.
Bell-Magendie law
belly
    prune b.
belt
    anthrax b.
Belzer solution
Bence
    B. Jones (BJ)
    B. Jones albumin
    B. Jones albuminuria
    B. Jones albumosuria
    B. Jones body
    B. Jones cast nephropathy
    B. Jones cylinder
    B. Jones globulin
    B. Jones myeloma
    B. Jones protein
    B. Jones proteinemia
    B. Jones protein method
    B. Jones protein test
    B. Jones proteinuria
    B. Jones reaction
bench
    b. method
    B. needle biopsy
benchmark
Benditt hypothesis
benedeni
    Moniezia b.
Benedict
    B. method
    B. solution
    B. test
    B. test for glucose
Benedict-Hopkins-Cole reagent
Benedict-Roth apparatus
Benedikt syndrome
bengal
    rose b.
Bengston method
benign
    b. albuminuria
    b. bone aneurysm
    b. chronic bullous dermatosis of childhood
    b. cystic teratoma
    b. dry pleurisy
    b. dyskeratosis
    b. epithelial breast tumor
    b. epithelioma
    b. familial hematuria
    b. familial icterus

    b. familial pemphigus
    b. florid lymphoid hyperplasia
    b. giant lymph node hyperplasia
    b. glycosuria
    b. inoculation lymphoreticulosis
    b. inoculation reticulosis
    b. intracranial hypertension (BIH)
    b. juvenile melanoma
    b. lymphadenosis
    b. lymphocytic angiitis and granulomatosis
    b. lymphocytoma cutis
    b. lymphoepithelial lesion
    b. lymphoma of rectum
    b. mediastinal lymph node hyperplasia
    b. mesenchymoma
    b. mesothelioma
    b. mesothelioma of genital tract
    b. metastasizing leiomyoma
    b. monoclonal gammopathy (BMG)
    b. mucosal pemphigoid
    b. mucous membrane pemphigus
    b. myalgic encephalomyelitis
    b. neoplasm
    b. nephrosclerosis (BNS)
    b. paraganglioma (BPG)
    b. paroxysmal peritonitis
    b. pheochromocytoma (BPC)
    b. pheochromocytoma with histological invasion (BPCHI)
    b. proliferative lesion
    b. prostatic hyperplasia
    b. prostatic hypertrophy (BPH)
    b. tertian malaria
benigna
    variola b.
benignum
    empyema b.
    lymphogranuloma b.
Bennet corpuscle
Bennett
    B. disease
    B. sulfhydryl method
Bennhold
    B. Congo red method
    B. Congo red stain
Benoist scale (B)
Bensley
    B. aniline-acid fuchsin-methyl green method
    B. osmic dichromate fluid
    B. safranin acid violet
    B. specific granule
Benson disease
bentiromide test
bentonite flocculation test (BFT)
Benyvirus
benzalkonium chloride

B

benzanthracene
benzene
  b. assay
  b. derivative
  b. hexachloride (BHC)
  b. poisoning
benzeneamine
benzenivorans
  Pseudonocardia b.
benzenoid
benzidine
  b. method for myoglobin peroxidase
  b. test
benzilate
  3-quinuclidinyl b. (QNB)
benzimidazole
  budding uninhibited by b. (BUB)
benzin (*var. of* benzine)
benzine, benzin
benzoate
  caffeine sodium b.
  estradiol b. (EB)
  sodium b.
benzodiazepine assay
benzoic acid
benzol
benzopurpurin 4B
benzopyrene
benzoquinone
benzo sky blue method
benzosulfimide
  sodium b.
benzoxiquine
benzoylaminoacetic acid
benzoylation
benzoylecgonine
benzoylglycine
benzoyl phenylcarbinol
3,4-benzpyrene
benzyl alcohol
benzylamine
Beradinelli syndrome
Bérard aneurysm
berbera
  Borrelia b.
Ber-EP4
  B.-E. antibody
  B.-E. immunoperoxidase stain
Berg
  B. chelate removal method
  B. stain
bergamot oil
Berger
  B. cell
  B. disease
  B. focal glomerulonephritis

Bergeron
  B. chorea
  B. disease
Bergey classification
berghei
  Plasmodium b.
Bergmann
  B. cord
  B. fiber
  B. glia
Ber-H2 antibody
beriberi
  cardinal manifestation of wet b.
  dry b.
  b. heart
  wet b.
Berkefeld filter
berkelium
Berlin
  B. blue
  B. breakage syndrome
  B. disease
bermudensis
Bernard
  B. canal
  B. duct
  B. syndrome
Bernard-Horner syndrome
Bernard-Sergent syndrome
Bernard-Soulier syndrome (BSS)
Bernatz classification
Bernhardt disease
Bernhardt-Roth syndrome
Bernheim syndrome
Bernoulli
  B. law
  B. principle
  B. theorem
Bernstein test
Bernthsen methylene violet
berrensis
  Thermohalobacter b.
berry
  b. aneurysm
  b. cell
Berson test
Berthelot reaction
Bertiella studeri
bertiellosis
Bertin
  B. columns
  columns of B.
Bertolotti syndrome
berylliosis
beryllium granuloma
Besnier-Boeck disease
Besnier-Boeck-Schaumann
  B.-B.-S. disease
  B.-B.-S. syndrome

Besnier prurigo
Besnoitia
besnoitiasis (*var. of* besnoitiosis)
Besnoitiidae
besnoitiosis, besnoitiasis
Bessey-Lowry (BL)
    B.-L. unit (BLU)
Bessey, Lowry, Bock (BLB)
Bessman anemia classification
Best
    B. carmine stain
    B. disease
beta
    b. adrenergic blockade
    b. adrenergic receptor
    b. agglutination
    b. agglutinin
    b. amyloid precursor protein
      immunohistochemical stain
    b. antigen of adenovirus
    b. basophil
    b. burn
    b. catenin
    b. cell
    b. cell of hypophysis
    b. cell of pancreas
    b. corynebacteriophage
    b. decay
    b. emitter
    b. endorphin
    b. erythroidine
    estrogen receptor b.
    b. fetoprotein
    b. galactosidase
    b. galactosidase test
    b. globin gene
    b. globulin
    b. granule
    b. hCG
    b. hemolysin
    b. hemolysis
    b. hemolytic streptococcus (BHS)
    b. hydroxybutyrate (BHBA)
    interferon b.
    b. isoform
    b. lactoglobulin (BLG)
    b. lipoprotein
    b. lysin
    b. metachromasia
    b. monooxygenase
    b. myosin heavy chain
    b. naphthol
    NRG1 b.
    NRG2 b.
    b. oxidation
    b. particle
    b. phage
    b. quick strep test
    b. radiation

    b. ray
    b. ray microscope
    b. site APP cleaving enzyme
      (BACE)
    b. sitosterolemia
    b. staphylolysin
    b. streptococcus
    b. substance
    b. thalassemia major
    b. thalassemia minor
    b. thromboglobulin
    TNF b.
    transcription factor b.
    b. tubulin
    tumor necrosis factor b.
beta-adrenergic
    b.-a. antagonist
    b.-a. blocking agent
beta-1A globulin
beta-aminoisobutyric aciduria
beta-amyloid (Abeta)
    b.-a. compound
    b.-a. fibril
    b.-a. plaque
    b.-a. protein converting enzyme
beta-blocker
beta-catenin gene
beta-1C globulin
Betacryptovirus
betacyaninuria
beta-delta thalassemia
beta-d-glucuronidase deficiency
betae
    Bradyrhizobium b.
beta-1E globulin
beta-enolase
17 beta estradiol
beta-1F globulin
beta-galactosidase
    cerebroside b.-g.
betaglobulin
    steroid-binding b.
beta-glucosidase
    cerebroside b.-g.
beta-glucuronidase
beta-glycoprotein
    glycine-rich b.-g.
beta-hCG test
beta-hydroxybutyrate assay
beta-hydroxy-delta-5-steroid dehydrogenase
betaine
beta-lactamase
    b.-l. negative
    b.-l. positive
    b.-l. test
beta-lipoprotein
beta-methylcrotonylglycinuria
beta-2 microglobulin
beta-microglobulin

B

beta-N-acetylgalactosaminidase
beta-nicotyrine
Betanodavirus
beta-pleated sheet
Betaretrovirus
Betatetravirus
beta-tubulin
>neuron-associated class III b.-t.

betavasculorum
beta-VLDL
betel cancer
Bethesda
>B. Pap smear
>B. Pap smear rating scale
>B. system
>B. 2001 system diagnosis
>B. 2001 terminology for reporting results of cervical cytology
>B. unit (BU)

Bethesda-Ballerup group of *Citrobacter* (CBB)
Betke-Kleihauer
>B.-K. stain
>B.-K. test

Betke stain
Bettendorff test
Betula
betulina
>*Lenzites b.*

Betz
>B. cell
>B. cell area

beurmanni
>*Sporotrichum b.*

Beutler test
Bevan-Lewis cell
BeWo choriocarcinoma cell line
bezoar
Bezold
>B. abscess
>B. ganglion

bf
>bouillon filtrate

(b-f)-1:4-oxazepine (*var. of* NATO code for dibenz(b,f)-1:4-oxazepine)
B:F
>bound-free ratio

BF
>blastogenetic factor

bFGF
>basic fibroblast growth factor

BFP
>biologic false-positive

BFR
>biologic false-positive reactor
>bone formation rate

BFT
>bentonite flocculation test
>blunt force trauma

BFU-E
>burst-forming unit-erythroid

BG
>blood glucose
>bone graft
>Bordet-Gengou
>>BG test

BG8
>>BG8 immunostain
>>BG8 monoclonal antibody

BGA
>blood group antigen

BGG
>bovine gamma globulin

BGH
>bovine growth hormone

BGlu
>blood glucose

BGP
>biliary glycoprotein
>bone GLA-protein

BGSA
>blood granulocyte-specific activity

BGTT
>borderline glucose tolerance test

BHA
>brain-hair follicle axis

BH11 antibody
BHBA
>beta hydroxybutyrate

BHC
>benzene hexachloride

BHI
>brain-heart infusion

bHLH
>basic helix-loop-helix transcription factor

BHS
>beta hemolytic streptococcus

BHTU microscope
BH:VH
>body hematocrit to venous hematocrit ratio

BI
>bacteriological index
>burn index

Bial
>B. pentosetest
>B. reagent
>B. test

biallelic
Bianchi
>B. syndrome
>B. valve

Bi antigen
bias
>forward b.
>reverse b.

biased estimate

B

biatriatum
    cor pseudotriloculare b.
    cor triloculare b.
Biber-Haab-Dimmer corneal lattice dystrophy
bibulous
bicameral abscess
bicapsular
bicarb
    bicarbonate
    carbon dioxide
bicarbonate (bicarb, HCO₃)
    blood b.
    b. buffer
    b. buffer system
    b. ion
    plasma b.
    potassium b.
    serum b.
    sodium b.
    standard b.
    b. titration test
bicellular
Bichat
    B. canal
    B. fissure
    B. foramen
    B. membrane
    B. tunic
bichromate
    potassium b.
biciliate
bicinchoninic acid method (BCA)
biclonal
    b. gammopathy
    b. peak
    b. peakbiclonal peak
biclonality
bicolorata
    Agreia b.
bicolor guaiac test (BCG)
biconcave
biconvex
bicornis
    Ixodes b.
bicornuate uterus
bicytopenia
bidirectional information exchange
BIDLB
    block in posteroinferior division of left branch
Biebrich
    B. scarlet
    B. scarlet-picroaniline blue
    B. scarlet red
Biedl disease
Bielschowsky
    B. disease

    B. method
    B. stain
Bielschowsky-Jansky disease
Biemond syndrome
bieneusi
    Enterocytozoon b.
Biermer
    B. anemia
    B. disease
bifemoral
bifermentans
    Clostridium b.
bifid
    b. bacterium
    b. tongue
    b. ureter
    b. uterus
bifida
    spina b.
    Zimmermannella b.
Bifidobacteriaceae
Bifidobacteriales
Bifidobacterium
    B. bifidum
    B. dentium
    B. eriksonii
    B. infantis
    B. psychraerophilum
    B. scardovii
    B. thermacidophilum subsp. *porcinum*
    B. thermacidophilum subsp. *thermacidophilum*
bifidum
    Bifidobacterium b.
    cranium b.
bifidus
    Lactobacillus b.
biflexa
    Leptospira b.
biflorus
    Dolichos b.
biformata
    Robiginitalea b.
bifurcation
bifurcum
    Oesophagostomum b.
bigemina
    Isospora b.
bigeminal
bigeminy
    ventricular b.
biglycan
BIH
    benign intracranial hypertension
bilat
    bilateral
bilateral (bilat)
    b. left-sidedness

bilateral (*continued*)
  b. micronodular adrenal hyperplasia
  b. otitis media (BOM)
  bilateral, symmetrical, and equal
    (BSE)
  b. symmetry
bilayer
  protein-lipid b.
Bilderbeck disease
bile
  b. acid
  b. acid assay
  b. acid tolerance test
  b. antigen
  b. canaliculi
  b. capillary
  b. cast
  b. duct
  b. duct adenoma
  b. duct canaliculus
  b. duct carcinoma
  b. duct necrosis
  b. duct-to-portal space ratio
    (BD/BS)
  b. esculin agar
  b. esculin hydrolysis test
  b. extravasation
  b. fluid examination
  b. infarct
  b. lake
  b. nephrosis
  b. peritonitis
  b. pigment
  b. pigment hemoglobin
  b. pigment test
  b. salt agar
  b. salt breath test
  b. salt deficiency syndrome
  b. salts
  b. solubility test
  b. stasis
  b. thrombus
  white b.
Bilharzia
bilharzial
  b. deposition pigment
  b. dysentery
  b. granuloma
  b. pigment deposition
bilharziasis, bilharziosis
Bilharziella polonica
bilharziosis (*var. of* bilharziasis)
biliaris
  tunica mucosa vesicae b.
  tunica muscularis vesicae b.
  tunica serosa vesicae b.
biliary
  b. achalasia
  b. acid transporter (BAT)

  b. atresia
  b. calculus
  b. canaliculus
  b. cirrhosis
  b. colic
  b. disorder
  b. drainage
  b. duct
  b. ductule
  b. dyssynergia
  b. fistula
  b. glycoprotein
    (BGP)
  b. obstruction
  b. progenitor marker
  b. reflux
  b. scan
  b. stricture
  b. tract disease
  b. tract infection
  b. xanthomatosis
biliferi
  ductuli b.
  ductus b.
  tubuli b.
Bili-Labstix
bilineal acute leukemia
biliosae
  glandulae mucosae b.
biliousness
bilious remittent malaria
bilirubin
  amniotic fluid b.
  b. assay
  conjugated b.
  direct reacting b.
  b. encephalopathy
  b. glucuronide
  indirect reacting b.
  minimum concentration of b.
    (MCBR)
  neonatal b.
  b. scan
  serum b. (SB)
  b. tolerance test
  total serum b. (TSB)
  unconjugated b.
  volume of distribution of b.
    (VDBR)
bilirubinemia
  hereditary nonhemolytic b.
bilirubinometer
  Unistat b.
bilirubinuria
biliuria
biliverdin, biliverdine
biliverdine (*var. of* biliverdin)
biliverdinglobin
Billheimer method

Billroth
- B. cord
- B. disease
- B. venae cavernosae

bilobalide
bilobate placenta
biloculare
- cor b.

bilocular stomach
biloma
Bilopaque
Bilophila wadsworthia
bimetal thermometer
bimodal manner
bimolecular
bimorphic
bimucosa
- fistula b.

binary
- b. acid
- b. addition
- b. cytotoxin
- b. fission
- b. nomenclature
- b. variate

binasal hemianopsia
binax
- B. Now *Legionella* urine antigen test
- B. Now Malaria Test
- B. Now *Streptococcus pneumoniae* antigen test
- B. Now urinary antigen test

Bindazyme ANA Screening ELISA kit
binding
- albumin cobalt b. (ACB)
- b. constant
- cortisol b.
- b. energy
- protein b. (PB)
- b. protein protease (BPP)

Binet chronic lymphocytic leukemia classification
binocular microscope
binomial
- b. coefficient
- b. distribution
- b. nomenclature

Binswanger
- B. disease
- B. encephalopathy

binuclear, binucleate
- b. cell
- b. fiber

binucleate (*var. of* binuclear)
binucleated lymphocyte
binucleation disproportionate
binucleolate
Binz test

bioaccumulation
bioactive
bioanalysis
bioanalyst
bioassay
bioavailability
Biobarcode technology
biocenosis
biochem
- biochemical
- biochemistry

biochemical
- b. energetics
- b. fuel cell
- b. genetics
- b. metastasis
- b. profile
- b. sequestration
- b. testing

biochemically mediated effect
biochemistry
biochemorphic
biochemorphology
biocidal
bioclimatology
Bioclot protein S assay
bioconversion
biodefense
- Working Group on Civilian B.

biodegradability
biodegradable
bioelectronic sensor technology
bioenergetics
bioequivalence
bioethicist
biofidelic human surrogate
biogenesis
biogenetic
biogenic amine hypothesis
biographer
- GlucoWatch B.

biohazard
- b. bag
- b. detection system (BDS)

bioinjectable
biologic, biological
- b. assay
- b. false-positive (BFP)
- b. false-positive reactor (BFR)
- b. half-life
- b. WMD

biological (*var. of* biologic)
- b. alkylating agent
- b. assay
- b. clock
- b. half-life
- b. immunotherapy
- b. matrix reference materials
- b. safety cabinet (BSC)

B

biological (*continued*)
    B. Stain Commission
    b. standard unit
    b. terrorism
    b. vector
    b. warfare (BW)
    b. weapon
    B. Weapons and Toxins Convention
biologist
biology
    cellular b.
    molecular b.
    population b.
bioluminescence
bioluminescent method
biomarker
    ovarian cancer b.
biomass
biomechanical preparation
biomechanician
biomechanics
biomedical
    b. engineering
    b. scientist
Biomek 2000, 3000, FX, FX assay, NX laboratory automation workstation
biometrician
biometric identifier
biometry
biomicroscopy
biomonitor
Biomphalaria glabrata
Biondi-Heidenhain stain
Biondi ring
bionecrosis
bionics
biophage
biophagism, biophagy
biophagous
biophagy (*var. of* biophagism)
biophylactic
biophylaxis
biophysical profile
biophysics
bioplasm
bioplasmic
biopolitics
Biopore membrane device
Biopreparat
biopsy
    b. algorithm
    aspiration b.
    Bench needle b.
    blind punch b.
    bone b.
    bone marrow aspiration and b.
    breast b. (BB)
    bronchial brush b.
    cervical punch b.

    cone b.
    conventional core b. (CCB)
    core needle b. (CNB)
    CT-guided stereotactic b.
    deep wedge b.
    embryo b.
    endometrial b.
    endomyocardial b.
    excisional b.
    fine-needle aspiration b. (FNAB)
    formalin-fixed skin b.
    full-series b.
    image-guided breast b.
    image-guided core b.
    incisional b.
    jumbo b.
    kidney b.
    labial salivary gland b.
    large-needle aspiration b. (LNB)
    LSG b.
    lung b.
    lymph node b.
    minimally invasive breast b. (MIBB)
    muscle b.
    open lung b. (OLB)
    placental b.
    pleural b.
    prostate gland b.
    prostate needle core b.
    punch b.
    4 quadrant b.
    scalene node b. (SNB)
    sentinel lymph node b.
    sextant b.
    shave b.
    skin b.
    skin shave b.
    small-bowel b.
    b. specimen
    stereotactic brain b.
    stereotactic breast b.
    stereotactic core-needle b. (SCNB)
    suction-type b.
    synovial membrane b.
    thin-needle b.
    thyroid b.
    transbronchial lung b. (TBBx, TBLB)
    transition zone b.
    transrectal ultrasound-guided sextant b. (TRUS)
    trephine b.
    Tru-Cut b.
    urinary tract brush b.
    vacuum-assisted core b. (VACB)
biopterin
biopyoculture

Bio-Rad
>B.-R. H2500 microwave oven
>B.-R. protein assay

bioreagent

Biosafe TSH test

biosafety
>b. containment
>b. level (BSL)
>b. level 1 (BSL1)
>b. level 2 (BSL2)
>b. level 3 (BSL3)
>b. level 4 (BSL4)

biosampler
>Accelon Combi b.

biosciences
>Amersham B.

Bioshaf automated one-step fertility kit

biospectrometry

biospectroscopy

biospeleology

BioStar Strep A OIA MAX *Streptococcus* **A test**

biosynthesis

biosynthetic pathway

biotaxis

Bio-Tek EIx800 plate reader

bioterrorism
>food-based b.
>B. Preparedness and Response Program
>B. Readiness Plan

BioThrax

biotin
>b. assay
>labeled streptavidin b. (LSAB)

biotin-labeled probe

biotin-streptavidin-alkaline phosphatase method

biotin-streptavidin detection method

biotin-streptavidin-peroxidase method

biotinylated DNA probe

biotinylation

biotope

biotoxin

biotransformation

Biot respiration

biotype

biowarfare

BioWatch

BIP
>bismuth iodoform paraffin

biparasitism

biparental inheritance

biphasic
>b. blastoma
>b. helical CT
>b. hemolysis
>b. pattern

>b. response
>b. synovial sarcoma
>b. tumor

biphenotypic
>b. differentiation
>b. lymphoma

biphenotypy

biphenyl
>polychlorinated b. (PCB)

biphosphate
>sodium b.

bipolar
>b. cell
>b. depression disorder
>b. needle electrode
>b. neuron
>b. spindle
>b. stain
>b. staining
>b. uptake

Bipolaris
>B. *australiensis*
>B. *hawaiiensis*
>B. *spicifera*

bipotential cell

bipulmonary

bipunctata
>*Macromonas b.*

bipyramidal

bipyridyl

Birbeck granule

Birch-Hirschfeld stain

bird
>B. disease
>B. formula
>B. Nest filter
>b. unit

bird-breeder's
>b.-b. disease
>b.-b. lung

bird-fancier's
>b.-f. lung

birdseed agar

bird's nest lesion

birefringence
>apple-green b.
>crystalline b.
>flow b.
>form b.
>strain b.

birefringent
>b. collagen band
>b. crystal
>b. crystalline cleft

birgiae
>*Afipia b.*

Birnaviridae

Birnavirus

birth injury

birthmark (BMK)
    strawberry b.
    vascular b.
Birt-Hogg-Dube syndrome
birtlesii
    Bartonella b.
bis (b)
bisalbuminemia
BISCC
    basaloid invasive squamous cell
    carcinoma
bis(2-chloroethyl)sulfide
bischloromethyl ether
bisection
bishopi
    Latrodectus b.
Bismarck
    B. brown
    B. brown R, Y
bismuth
    b. assay
    B. cholangiocarcinoma classification
    b. iodide
    b. iodoform paraffin (BIP)
    b. pigmentation
    b. subnitrate
    b. triiodide
Bismuth-Corlette perihilar tumor
classification
bismuth-sulfite agar (BSA)
bisonis
    Cooperia b.
bisphosphate
    fructose b.
bisphosphatidylglycerol
2,3-bisphosphoglycerate
bisphosphoglycerate phosphatase
bisphosphoglyceromutase
bistratal
bistriata
    Trachybdella b.
bis-trimethylsilylacetamide
bis-trimethylsilyltrifluoroacetamide
(BSTFA)
bisulfate
bisulfide
    carbon b.
bisulfite
bit
    check b.
bitartrate
    potassium b.
bite
    b. cell
    insect b.
bitemporal hemianopsia
Bithynia
Bitot spot
bitropic

bitten colony
Bittner
    B. agent
    B. milk factor
    B. virus
biundulant
    b. meningoencephalitis
    b. milk fever virus
biurate
biuret
    b. reaction
    b. test
biuret-reactive material (BRM)
bivalent
    b. antibody
    b. gas gangrene antitoxin
    heteromorphic b.
    homomorphic b.
biventriculare
    cor triloculare b.
bivia
    Prevotella b.
bivius
    Bacteroides b.
bixin
bizarre
    b. leiomyoma
    b. megakaryocyte
    b. parosteal osteochondromatous
    proliferation (BPOP)
Bizzozero
    B. corpuscle
    B. platelet
    B. red cell
    Sudan black B.
BJ
    Bence Jones
    BJ protein
Bjerkandera
Bjork-Shiley mitral prosthesis
Björnstad syndrome
BK virus
black
    b. bane (anthrax)
    b. Bizzozero, Sudan
    b. currant rash
    b. death
    b. fly
    b. hairy tongue
    b. house rat
    b. jaundice
    b. lead
    b. light
    b. lung
    b. lung disease
    b. periodic acid method
    b. piedra
    b. plague
    b. powder

chlorazol b. E
Sudan b.
Sudan b. B (SBB)
b. thyroid adenoma
b. thyroid syndrome
b. urine
b. widow spider
black-dot ringworm
Blackfan-Diamond syndrome
blackhead
blackwater fever
bladder
    autocrine motility factor of the b.
    b. carcinoma
    b. disorder
    b. dysfunction
    exstrophy of the b.
    fasciculate b.
    low-compliance b.
    b. neck obstruction (BNO)
    neurogenic b.
    b. polyp
    poorly compliant b.
    b. spasm
    b. tumor (BT)
bladderworm
Blakeslea
BLA 36 monoclonal antibody
blanch
blanche
    atrophia b.
    tache b.
blanching
    tongue b.
bland
    b. embolism
    b. embolus
    b. infarct
    b. nucleus
Blandin gland
Blane
    amniotic infection syndrome of B.
Blaschko line
Blasius duct
blast
    b. cell
    b. cell leukemia
    b. chest
    b. crisis
    b. effect
    b. injury
    b. lung
    refractory anemia with excess of
      blasts (RAEB)
    rice b.
    b. wind
blastema
    basaloid b.
    b. cell

nodular b.
serpentine b.
blastemal cell
blastemic
blastic
    b. phase
    b. transformation
blast-induced
    b.-i. cognitive defect
    b.-i. memory defect
Blastobotrys
Blastococcus saxobsidens
Blastoconidium
Blastocystis hominis
blastocyte
blastocytoma
blastogenesis assay
blastogenetic, blastogenic
    b. factor (BF)
blastogenic (*var. of* blastogenetic)
blastoid
    b. variant
    b. variant of mantel cell lymphoma
      (BMCL)
blastoma
    biphasic b.
    epithelial predominant b.
    b. mantel cell lymphoma (BMCL)
    pleuropulmonary b.
    pluricentric b.
    pulmonary b.
    unicentric b.
blastomere
blastomogenic
Blastomonas ursincola
Blastomyces
    B. brasiliensis
    B. coccidioides
    B. dermatitidis
blastomycete
blastomycin
Blastomycoides
blastomycosis
    European b.
    North American b.
    pulmonary b.
    b. serology
    South American b.
blastophore
Blastopirellula marina
Blastoschizomyces capitatus
blastospore
blastula
blastulation
Blatin syndrome
Blatta
blattae
    Escherichia b.
Blattella

Blattidae
blauseare (Berlin blue acid)
BLB
    Bessey, Lowry, Bock
    Boothby, Lovelace, Bulbulian
      BLB mask
      BLB unit
bleb
    blunt b.
    cytoplasmic b.
    emphysematous b.
    plasma membrane b.
    subpleural b.
bleed
    acute b.
bleeder
bleeding (BL), bleed
    breakthrough b. (BB, BTB)
    dysfunctional uterine b.
    estrogen withdrawal b. (EWB)
    functional b.
    gastrointestinal b.
    implantation b.
    occult b.
    placentation b.
    b. polyp
    postmenopausal b.
    postmortem b.
    rectal b.
    b. time (BT)
    b. time test
blennadenitis
blennogenic
blennogenous
blennoid
blennorrhagia (*var. of* blennorrhea)
blennorrhagica
    keratoderma b.
    keratosis b.
blennorrhagic inflammation
blennorrhea, blennorrhagia
    b. adultorum
    b. inclusion
    inclusion b.
    b. neonatorum
blennorrheal conjunctivitis
blennuria
blepharitis ulcerosa
blepharoplast
blepharoptosia (*var. of* blepharoptosis)
blepharoptosis, blepharoptosia
Blessig
    B. groove
    B. space
BLG
    beta lactoglobulin
blighted ovum
blind
    b. fistula

    b. loop syndrome
    b. passage
    b. punch biopsy
    b. test
blindness
    hysterical b.
    river b.
B-lineage
blister
    b. agent
    blood b.
    b. cell
    cutaneous b.
    fever b.
    subepidermal b.
Blitz nevi
bloated cell
bloater
    blue b. (BB)
bloc
    en b.
Bloch
    B. method
    B. reaction
blochi
    Scopulariopsis b.
Bloch-Sulzberger
    B.-S. disease
    B.-S. syndrome
block
    atrioventricular b.
    AV b.
    bundle-branch b. (BBB)
    complete heart b. (CHB)
    complete left bundle-branch b.
      (CLBBB)
    complete right bundle-branch b.
      (CRBBB)
    b. diagram
    first-degree heart b.
    heart b.
    horse serum b.
    b. in anterosuperior division of left
      branch (BSDLB)
    incomplete right bundle-branch b.
    b. in posteroinferior division of left
      branch (BIDLB)
    left bundle-branch b.
    second-degree heart b.
    third-degree heart b.
blockade
    adrenergic neuron b.
    alpha adrenergic b.
    beta adrenergic b.
    cholinergic b.
    combined androgen b.
    narcotic b.
    renal b.
    virus b.

blocker
    histamine receptor b.
blocking
    b. agent
    b. antibody (BA)
    b. antibody reaction
    b. filter
    b. solution
block-like chromatin condensation
Blocq disease
blood (b)
    b. acylcarnitine analysis
    b. agar
    b. agar plate (BAP)
    b. agent
    b. albumin
    b. alcohol
    b. alcohol concentration (BAC)
    Almén test for b.
    anticoagulated b.
    Apt test for swallowed b.
    arterialized b.
    arteriolization of venous b.
    b. bank (BB)
    b. bicarbonate
    b. blister
    b. buffer base (BB)
    b. buffering capacity
    buffer value of the b.
    b. calcium level
    b. calculus
    b. capillary
    b. cast
    b. cell
    b. cell count
    b. cell count automation
    b. chemistry study
    chocolate b. (CB)
    b. cholesterol level
    citrated b.
    b. clot
    CMV-seronegative b.
    b. coagulation disorder
    b. coagulation factor
    b. component
    connective tissue supply b.
    cord b.
    b. corpuscle
    b. crisis
    b. crystal
    b. culture (BC)
    b. cyst
    b. cytolysate
    defibrinated b.
    b. disc
    b. dust
    b. dyscrasia
    b. extravasation
    b. film

    b. filter
    b. fluke
    fragility of the b.
    frozen b.
    b. gas
    b. gas analysis
    b. ghost
    b. glucose (BG, BGlu)
    b. granulocyte-specific activity
      (BGSA)
    b. group
    b. group agglutinin
    b. group agglutinogen
    b. group antibody
    b. group antigen (BGA)
    b. group antigen SLex
    b. group antiserum
    b. group chimera
    b. grouping
    b. grouping serum
    b. group-specific substances A, B
    b. group substance
    b. group systems (ABO)
    b. incompatibility
    b. indices
    intravascular coagulation of b.
    irradiated CPD b.
    b. island
    laky b.
    b. loss (BL)
    b. loss anemia
    b. lymph
    b. microvessel density
    mixed venous b.
    b. mole
    b. mote
    occult b.
    oxygen capacity of b.
    oxygen content of b.
    b. pH
    b. plasma
    b. plasma fraction
    b. plastid
    platelet-poor b. (PPB)
    b. poisoning
    b. pressure (BP)
    b. puzzles
    b. quotient
    red venous b. (RVB)
    b. salvage
    b. sinusoid
    sludged b.
    b. smear
    b. smear morphology
    b. spot
    b. spot screening assay
    stool occult b.
    strawberry-cream b.
    b. substitute

B

blood (*continued*)
  b. sugar (BS)
  b. trematode
  b. tumor
  b. type
  b. typing
  unspun peripheral b.
  b. urea clearance
  b. urea nitrogen (BUN)
  b. urea nitrogen test
  b. vessel
  b. vessel fibrosis
  b. volume (BV)
  b. volume measurement
  b. volume nomogram
  b. warming
  whole b. (B, WB)
blood-air barrier
blood-aqueous barrier
blood-brain barrier (BBB)
blood-cerebral barrier
blood-clot lysis time (BLT)
Bloodgood disease
bloodless glomeruli
bloodstain pattern analysis
blood-testis barrier
blood-thymus barrier
bloodworm
bloody
  b. feces
  b. stool
Bloom
  B. and Richardson classification
  B. syndrome
Bloom-Richardson scale
Bloor test
blot
  Southern b. (SB)
  b. test
  Western b.
blotting
Blount
  B. disease
  B. test
Blount-Barber disease
blowback
blowfly
blowout pipette
Bloxam test
BLPD
  B-cell lymphoproliferative disorder
BLS
  base lymphocyte syndrome
BLT
  blood-clot lysis time
BLU
  Bessey-Lowry unit
blue
  Alcian b. (AB)

alkaline toluidine b.O
aniline b.
anthracene b.
azovan b.
b. baby
Berlin b.
Biebrich scarlet-picroaniline b.
b. bloater (BB)
brilliant cresyl b. (BCB)
bromphenol b.
bromthymol b.
carbolic methylene b.
  (CMB)
celstine b. B
celestine b. B
b. cell pattern
b. cell tumor
cresyl b.
b. cytoplasm
dextran b. (DB)
Diagnex B.
b. diaper syndrome
b. dome cyst
b. edema
eosin-methylene b. (EMB)
Evans b.
b. formazan
indigo b.
insoluble Prussian b.
Isamine b.
isosulfan b.
Kühne methylene b.
leucomethylene b.
leuco patent b.
b. litmus paper
Löffler methylene b.
martius scarlet b. (MSB)
methyl b.
methylene b. (MB)
methylthymol b.
new methylene b.
Nile b.
Nile b. A
polychrome methylene b.
Prussian b.
b. pus
pyrrol b.
rhodanile b.
b. rubber bleb nevus
sky b.
b. spot
thymol b.
toluidine b. (TB)
toluidine b. O
trypan b.
Turnbull b.
Victoria b.
bluecomb virus
bluetongue virus

bluish
>eosin I b.

Blumenthal disease

Blum syndrome

blunt
>b. bleb
>b. duct adenosis
>b. end
>b. force trauma (BFT)
>b. head injury
>b. trauma

blush
>b. appearance
>tumor b.

BLV
>bovine leukemia virus

B-lymphocyte
>B-l. assay
>B-l. stimulatory factor (BSF)

BLyS
>B lymphocyte stimulator

BM
>body mass
>bone marrow

BMCL
>blastoid variant of mantel cell lymphoma
>blastoma mantel cell lymphoma

BMD
>Becker muscular dystrophy

BMG
>benign monoclonal gammopathy

BMI
>body mass index

B-mode

BMP
>basic metabolic panel

BMP4 gene

BMR
>basal metabolic rate

BMT
>bone marrow transplantation
>Auto-PBSC BMT

BN
>branchial neuritis
>BN ProSpec

BNH9 antibody

B-NHL
>B-cell non-Hodgkin lymphoma

BNO
>bladder neck obstruction

BNS
>benign nephrosclerosis

Boas
>B. point
>B. test

Boas-Oppler
>B.-O. bacillus
>B.-O. lactobacillus

boat clinger

boat-shaped heart

Bock
>Bessey, Lowry, B.

Bodansky unit (BU)

Bodian
>B. copper-protargol stain
>B. histochemical stain
>B. method

Bodo
>*B. caudatus*
>*B. saltans*
>*B. urinaria*
>*B. urinarius*

body
>acetone b.
>acidophil b.
>acidophilic b.
>adrenal b.
>alcoholic hyaline b.
>Alder b.
>Alder-Reilly b.
>alkapton b.
>Allison-Ghormley b.
>aortic b.
>apoptotic b.
>Arantius b.
>Arnold b.
>asbestos b. (AB)
>Aschoff b.
>asteroid b.
>Auer b.
>Babès-Ernst b.
>bacillary b.
>Balbiani b.
>Barr b.
>Barr chromatin b.
>basal b.
>Bence Jones b.
>Bollinger b.
>Borrel b.
>brassy b.
>bronchial obstruction by foreign b.
>Cabot ring b.
>Call-Exner b.
>cancer b.
>b. cavity
>cell b.
>central b.
>chromaffin b.
>chromatin b.
>chromatinic b.
>Civatte b.
>coccygeal b.
>colloid b.
>conchoidal b.
>Councilman hyaline b.
>Cowdry type A, B inclusion b.
>creola b.

body (*continued*)

curvilinear b.
cytoid b.
cytoplasmic inclusion b.
Deetjen b.
demilune b.
dense b. (DB)
Döhle inclusion b.
Donné b.
Donovan b.
Dutcher b.
Ehrlich inner b.
elementary b.
embryoid b.
eosinophilic viral inclusion b.
F b.
ferruginous b.
fibrin b.
fibrous b.
b. fluid
b. fluid analysis
foreign b. (FB)
fruiting b.
fuchsin b.
gall b.
Gamna-Favre b.
Gamna-Gandy b.
glass b.
glomus b.
Gordon b.
Guarnieri b.
Halberstaedter-Prowazek b.
Hassall b.
Heinz b.
Heinz-Ehrlich b.
b. hematocrit to venous hematocrit
  ratio (BH:VH)
hematoxylin b.
Herring b.
Hirano b.
HJ b.
Howell-Jolly b.
hyaline Civatte b.
hyaloid b.
immune b. (IB)
inclusion b. (IB)
intercarotid b.
intraocular foreign b. (IOFB)
intrauterine foreign b. (IUFB)
Jaworski b.
Joest b.
Jolly b.
juxtaglomerular b.
Kamino b.
ketone b. (KB)
Lafora b.
Lallemand b.
lamellar b.
lateral geniculate b.

LCL bodies
LE b.
Leishman-Donovan b.
Lewy b.
Lindner b.
Lipschütz b.
b. louse
Luse b.
Mallory b. (MB)
malpighian b.
Maragiliano b.
b. mass (BM)
b. mass index (BMI)
Masson b.
May-Hegglin b.
Medlar b.
melon seed b.
membranous cytoplasmic b.
  (MCB)
metachromatic b.
metallic foreign b. (MFB)
Michaelis-Gutmann b.
mineral oil foreign b.
Miyagawa b.
molluscum b.
multilamellar b.
multivesicular b.
myelin b.
Negri b.
nerve cell b.
neuroepithelial b.
Nissl b.
nodular b.
nuclear inclusion b.
Odland b.
b. of Luys syndrome
onion b.
oval fat b. (OFB)
oxyphil inclusion b.
pacchionian b.
pineal b.
Plimmer b.
polar b.
polyhedral b.
Prowazek-Greeff b.
psammoma b.
psittacosis inclusion b.
Renaut b. (RB)
residual b.
retained foreign b. (RFB)
reticulate b.
rice b.
ringworm of b.
Rushton b.
Russell b.
sand b.
Sandström b.
Schaumann b.
Schiller-Duval b.

Schmorl b.
sclerotic b.
selenoid b.
b. snatching
spiculated b.
striate b.
b. substance isolation (BSI)
suprarenal b.
b. surface areas (BSA)
b. surface burned (BSB)
tactoid b.
b. temperature
b. temperature, ambient pressure,
  saturated (BTPS)
thermostable b.
threshold b.
thyroid b.
tigroid b.
tingible b.
Todd b.
trachoma b.
Trousseau-Lallemand b.
tuffstone b.
tympanic b.
ultimobranchial b.
Verocay b.
Virchow-Hassall b.
vitreous b.
Weibel-Palade b.
Wesenberg-Hamazaki b.
Wolf-Orton b.
X chromatin b.
Y b.
yellow b.
zebra b.
Zuckerkandl b.
bodypacker syndrome
body-section radiography
Boeck
    B. disease
    B. sarcoid
Boeck-Drbohlav-Locke egg-serum medium
Boehmer hematoxylin
Boehringer
    B. in vitro transcription kit
    B. Mannheim DIG-Nucleic Detection
      kit
    B. Mannheim DIG-Oligonucleotide
      Tailing kit
    B. Mannheim Kermix cytokeratin
      cocktail
boenickei
    Mycobacterium b.
Boerhaave syndrome
Boettcher cell
Bogaert disease
bogorensis
    Asaia b.
Bogoriellaceae

bogoriensis
    Rhodobaca b.
bohemica
    Verpa b.
Bohr
    B. effect
    B. equation
boil
    Madura b.
boiling point (bp)
Bolande tumor
Boletus piperatus
bolidensis
    Arsenicicoccus b.
Boling burner
Bolivian hemorrhagic fever
boliviensis
    Halomonas b.
Boll cell
Bollinger
    B. body
    B. granule
bolteae
    Clostridium b.
Boltzmann constant
BOM
    bilateral otitis media
bomb
    ammonium nitrate b.
    barometric b.
    dirty b. (radiation dispersal device)
    fertilizer truck b.
    letter b.
    nail b.
    pipe b.
Bombardia
bombardment
Bombay
    B. blood group
    B. phenotype
bombesin
    b. peptide
    b. receptor
Bombidae
Bonanno test
bond
    chemical b.
    coordinate covalent b.
    covalent b.
    disulfide b.
    electron pair b.
    b. energy
    high-energy b.
    hydrogen b.
    intrachain disulphide b.
    ionic b.
    metallic b.
    sigma b.
    triple b.

bone

b. abscess
adamantinoma of long bones
b. age
b. architecture
b. aseptic necrosis
b. biopsy
brittle b.
bundle b.
b. canaliculus
cancellous b.
cartilage b.
b. chip
compact b.
b. corpuscle
cortical b.
b. cyst
decalcified b.
dermal b.
developing b.
b. disease
endochondral b.
epihyal b.
b. formation rate (BFR)
giant cell tumor of b. (GCTB)
b. GLA-protein (BGP)
b. graft (BG)
heterologous b.
b. infarct
lamellar b.
marble b.
b. marrow (BM)
b. marrow aplasia
b. marrow aspiration
b. marrow aspiration and biopsy
b. marrow carcinoma
b. marrow depression
b. marrow differential count
b. marrow disorder
b. marrow embolism
b. marrow embolus
b. marrow failure
b. marrow iron stores
b. marrow lesion
b. marrow macrophage
b. marrow particle
b. marrow precursor cell
b. marrow scan
b. marrow suppression
b. marrow transplant
b. marrow transplantation (BMT)
b. matrix
b. matrix alteration
membrane b.
b. morphogenetic protein 7 gene
nonlamellar b.
ping-pong b.
b. rarefaction
replacement b.

b. resorption
reticulated b.
b. sawing
b. sclerosis
septal b.
b. sialoprotein
sieve b.
spicule of b.
spongy b.
tibial cortical b.
b. tissue
trabecula of b.
trabecular b.
b. tumor
b. turnover
b. weapon
b. whorl
woven b.
bone-resorbing osteoclast
BoneTRAP Assay
bongori
   Salmonella b.
bonnei
Bonnet-Dechaume-Blanc syndrome
Bonnevie-Ullrich syndrome
Bonnier syndrome
bony
b. ankylosis
b. callus
b. heart
b. island
b. semicircular canal
bookeri
   Alcaligenes b.
Böök syndrome
Boolean function
BOOP
bronchiolitis obliterans organizing
   pneumonia
Boophilus annulatus
booster
b. dose
b. effect
b. response
Boothby, Lovelace, Bulbulian (BLB)
borate
sodium b.
Borchgrevink method
border
brush b.
b. cell
striated brush b.
vermilion b.
borderline
b. glucose tolerance test
  (BGTT)
b. leprosy
b. malignancy
b. ovarian tumor

Bordet amboceptor
Bordetella
    B. bronchiseptica
    B. hinzii
    B. holmesii
    B. parapertussis
    B. pertussis
    B. pertussis indirect fluorescent
    B. petrii
Bordet-Gengou
    B.-G. bacillus
    B.-G. culture medium
    B.-G. phenomenon
    B.-G. potato blood agar
    B.-G. reaction
    B.-G. test
borealis
    Paenibacillus b.
boreus
    Subtercola b.
boric
    b. acid
    b. acid broth
borism
Börjeson-Forssman-Lehmann syndrome
Börjeson syndrome
borkumensis
    Alcanivorax b.
Born
    B. method
    B. method of wax plate
      reconstruction
Borna
    B. disease
    B. disease virus
Bornavirus
Bornholm
    B. disease
    B. disease virus
boron
    b. assay
    b. trifluoride-methanol
borosilicate glassware
Borrel
    B. blue stain
    B. body
Borrelia
    B. afzelii
    B. anserina
    B. berbera
    B. burgdorferi
    B. burgdorferi sensu lato
    B. burgdorferi sensu stricto
    B. carteri
    B. caucasica
    B. crocidurae
    B. duttonii
    B. garinii
    B. hermsii

    B. hispanica
    B. kochii
    B. latyschewii
    B. mazzottii
    B. parkeri
    B. persica
    B. recurrentis
    B. refringens
    B. sinica
    B. turcica
    B. turicatae
    B. venezuelensis
    B. vincentii
borreliosis
    Lyme b.
Borrmann classification
Borst-Jadassohn type intraepidermal
  epithelioma
Bosea
    B. eneae
    B. massiliensis
    B. minatitlanensis
    B. vestrisii
bosselated
bosselation
Bostock disease
Boston exanthema
botfly
bothridium
bothriocephaliasis
Bothriocephalus
    B. cordatus
    B. latus
    B. mansoni
    B. mansonoides
bothrium
bothropic antitoxin
Bothrops
    B. antitoxin
    B. atrox serine proteinase
botniense
    Mycobacterium b.
Botox
    botulinum toxin
Botryoascus
Botryobasidium
Botryodiplodia theobromae
botryoid
    b. odontogenic cyst
    b. rhabdomyosarcoma
    b. sarcoma
    sarcoma b.
botryoides
    pseudosarcoma b.
Botryomyces caespitosus
botryomycosis
botryomycotic
botryosa
    Veronaea b.

Botryosphaeria rhodina
Botryotinia
Botryotrichum
Botrytis
bots
Böttcher
    B. cell
    B. crystal
bottle
    Nalgene PETG media b.
    Roux b.
botulin
botulinum
    b. antitoxin
    Clostridium b.
    b. toxin
botulinus
    Bacillus b.
    b. toxin
botulism
    b. antitoxin
    foodborne b.
    b. immune globulin intravenous (human)
    infant b.
    inhalational b.
    intestinal b.
    b. intoxication
    wound b.
Bouchard
    B. coefficient
    B. disease
    B. node
Bouchardat test
Boudierella
bouffardi
    Aspergillus b.
    B. black mycetoma
    B. white mycetoma
Bouguer law
Bouillaud
    B. disease
    B. syndrome
bouillon filtrate (bf)
Bouin
    B. fluid
    B. picroformol-acetic fixative
    B. solution
boulimia (*var. of* bulimia)
boundary lamina
bound-free ratio (B:F)
bound serum iron (BSI)
bouquet fever
Bourneville disease
Bourneville-Pringle disease
bouton
    axonal terminal b.
    b. en passage

    synaptic b.
    terminal b.
boutonneuse fever
Bouveret
    B. disease
    B. syndrome
bouvetii
    Acinetobacter b.
Bovicola
bovihominis
    Sarcocystis b.
bovine
    b. antitoxin
    b. colloid
    b. enteritis (BE)
    b. ephemeral fever
    b. gamma globulin (BGG)
    b. growth hormone (BGH)
    b. herpes mammillitis
    b. leukemia virus (BLV)
    b. leukosis virus
    b. malaria
    b. mastitis
    b. papular stomatitis
    b. papular stomatitis virus
    b. red blood cell (BRBC)
    b. rhinovirus
    b. serum albumin (BSA)
    b. smooth muscle cytosol
    b. spongiform encephalopathy (BSE)
    b. tubercle bacillus
    b. ulcerative mammillitis
    b. vaccinia mammillitis
    b. virus diarrhea
bovinum
    cor b.
bovis
    Actinomyces b.
    Anaplasma b.
    Bartonella b.
    Cysticercus b.
    Haemophilus b.
    Hypoderma b.
    Lachnobacterium b.
    Moraxella b.
    Mycobacterium b.
    Streptococcus b.
bowel
    b. bypass syndrome
    b. infarction
    b. perforation
Bowen
    B. disease
    B. precancerous dermatosis
bowenoid papulosis (BP)
Bowers-McComb unit
Bowie stain

Bowman
    B. capsule
    B. disc
    B. gland
    B. layer
    B. membrane
    B. space
bowmanii
    Clostridium b.
boxcar organism
Boyden
    B. chamber
    B. chamber assay device
boydii
    Allescheria b.
    Pseudallescheria b.
    Shigella b.
Boyle law
bozemanii
    Legionella b.
bp
    base pair
    boiling point
BP
    blood pressure
    bowenoid papulosis
    bypass
BPC
    benign pheochromocytoma
BPCHI
    benign pheochromocytoma with
      histological invasion
BPD
    bronchopulmonary dysplasia
BPG
    benign paraganglioma
BPH
    benign prostatic hypertrophy
BPI
    bacterial permeability-inducing
      BPI protein
180-bp ladder
B-PLL
    B-cell prolymphocytic leukemia
B-plus Fix
BPOP
    bizarre parosteal osteochondromatous
      proliferation
BPP
    binding protein protease
Bq
    becquerel
Braak neurofibrillary tangle staging
BRACAnalysis genetic susceptibility
  breast and ovarian cancer test
bracchium
    Agromyces b.
brachial
    b. dance

    b. gland
    b. plexitis
Brachiola
Brachmann-de Lange syndrome
Brachybacterium
    B. fresconis
    B. muris
    B. sacelli
brachycephalic, brachycephalous
brachycephalous (*var. of* brachycephalic)
Brachycladium
brachydactylia (*var. of* brachydactyly)
brachydactyly, brachydactylia
brachymesomelia-renal syndrome
Brachysporium
Brackiella oedipodis
Bracovirus
Bradford microassay procedure
Bradley disease
Bradshaw test
bradykinin
Bradyrhizobium
    B. betae
    B. yuanmingense
bradyzoite
BRAF
    BRAF mutation
    BRAF V600E mutation
Brailsford-Morquio disease
brain
    b. abscess
    b. atrophy
    b. cicatrix
    b. concussion
    b. congestion
    b. contusion
    b. death
    b. death syndrome
    b. edema
    b. lesion
    b. oxytocin
    primary Ki-1 lymphoma of b.
    respirator b.
    b. sand
    b. swelling
    b. tumor (BT)
brain-derived neurotrophic factor
  (BDNF)
Brainerd diarrhea
brain-hair follicle axis (BHA)
brain-heart
    b.-h. infusion (BHI)
    b.-h. infusion agar
    b.-h. infusion broth
    b.-h. infusion broth medium
brainstem, brain stem
    b. disease
    b. glioma
    b. tumor

B

braking radiation
branch
>block in anterosuperior division of
>left b. (BSDLB)
>block in posteroinferior division of
>left b. (BIDLB)

branched
>b. calculus
>b. chain
>b. chain ketoaciduria
>b. chain ketonuria
>b. DNA (b-DNA)
>b. DNA signal amplification
>assay

branched-chain
>b.-c. alpha keto acid decarboxylase
>b.-c. alpha keto acid dehydrogenase
>b.-c. amino acid (BCAA)
>b.-c. aminoaciduria
>b.-c. keto acid (BCKA)

brancher
>b. deficiency
>b. enzyme

branchial
>b. cleft cyst
>b. fistula
>b. neuritis (BN)

branching
>b. cardiac fiber
>b. decay
>b. enzyme
>b. fraction
>b. glycogen storage disease
>b. ratio

branchioma
Branhamaceae
Branhamella catarrhalis
brasilensis
>*Paenibacillus b.*

Brasil fixative
brasiliensis
>*Blastomyces b.*
>*Nocardia b.*
>*Vibrio b.*
>*Xenopsylla b.*

brassicacearum
>*Pseudomonas b.*

brassicae
>*Hylemya b.*

brassy
>b. body
>b. cough

BRAT diet
brauni
>*Digramma b.*
>*Diplogonoporus b.*

brawny edema
brazilein
Brazilian trypanosomiasis

brazilianum
>*Plasmodium b.*

braziliense
>*Ancylostoma b.*

braziliensis
>*Leishmania braziliensis b.*

brazilin
BRBC
>bovine red blood cell

BR27.29 breast antigen
BRCA1 gene
BRCA2 gene
bread-and-butter
>b.-a.-b. pericarditis
>b.-a.-b. pericardium

bread-loaf method
break
>DNA b.
>isochromatid b.

breakbone fever
breakdown
>protein b.
>starvation-induced protein b.

breaker
>circuit b.
>vacuum b.

breakpoint
>b. analysis
>b. cluster region-Abelson murine
>leukemia virus (BCR-ABL)
>b. cluster region rearrangement
>b. region

breakthrough bleeding (BTB)
breast
>b. biopsy (BB)
>b. cancer
>b. carcinoma
>b. cyst
>cystic hyperplasia of the b.
>b. duct
>fibrocystic disease of b.
>funnel b.
>medullary carcinoma of b.
>pleomorphic lobular carcinoma in
>situ of the b. (PLCIS)
>shotty b.
>b. specimen radiography
>b. tumor

breath
>b. analysis test
>b. hydrogen analysis

BreathTek UBT *H. pylori* test
Brecher-Cronkite method
Brecher new methylene blue technique
Breda disease
Breed smear
Breen and Tullis method
bregma
Breisky disease

bremensis
> Geobacter b.

bremneri
> Taenia b.

Bremsstrahlung radiation

Brennemann syndrome

brenneri
> Pseudomonas b.

Brenner tumor

Breslow
> B. malignant melanoma assay
> B. malignant melanoma classification
> B. thickness
> B. tumor index

Bretonneau disease

Brettanomyces

Breus mole

breve
> Flavobacterium b.
> Gymnodinium b.

Brevibacillus
> B. invocatus
> B. limnophilus

Brevibacteriaceae

Brevibacterieae

Brevibacterium
> B. luteolum
> B. paucivorans
> B. picturae
> B. sanguinis

brevicaeca
> Heterophyes b.

brevicaudum
> Oesophagostomum b.

brevicaulis
> Scopulariopsis b.

brevicollis
> dystrophia b.

Brevidensovirus

brevis
> Bacillus b.
> Janibacter b.
> Lactobacillus b.
> Sulfitobacter b.
> Thermomonas b.
> Trichostrongylus b.

Brevundimonas
> B. alba
> B. aurantiaca
> B. bacteroides
> B. diminuta
> B. intermedia
> B. nasdae
> B. subvibrioides
> B. variabilis
> B. vesicularis

Brewer infarct

brickdust deposit

brickmaker's anemia

brick-shaped virus

bridge
> alpha-methane b.
> arteriolovenular b.
> cell b.
> conjugation b.
> b. corpuscle
> cytoplasmic b.
> fibrinogen b.
> Gaskell b.
> intercellular b.
> myocardial b.
> b. rectifier
> salt b.
> Wheatstone b.

bridging
> b. fibrosis
> b. hepatic necrosis
> internuclear b. (INB)

bright
> b. contrast
> B. disease

bright-field microscopy

Brill disease

brilliant
> cresyl blue b.
> b. cresyl blue (BCB)
> b. crocein
> b. green
> b. green bile salt agar
> b. vital red
> b. yellow

Brill-Symmers disease

Brill-Zinsser disease

Brinton disease

Brion-Kayser disease

Briosia

Briquet syndrome

brisance

brisk infiltrate

Brissaud disease

Brissaud-Marie syndrome

Brissaud-Sicard syndrome

bristle cell

Bristowe syndrome

British
> B. antilewisite (BAL)
> B. Testicular Tumour Panel (BTTP)
> B. thermal unit (BTU)
> B. type amyloid angiopathy

brittle bone

BRM
> biuret-reactive material

broad
> b. fish tapeworm
> b. smear
> b. spectrum
> b. urinary cast

broad-beta disease

B

broad-betalipoproteinemia
broadening
broad-spectrum antibiotic
Broca area
Brock syndrome
Brocq disease
Broders
    B. classification
    B. tumor index
Brodie
    B. abscess
    B. disease
    B. knee
broegbernensis
    Pseudoxanthomonas b.
broken
    b. cell preparation
    b. compensation
bromate
bromcresol
    b. green
    b. purple
bromelain, bromelin
bromelin (*var. of* bromelain)
bromide
    aminoethylisothiouronium b. (AET)
    b. assay
    cetyltrimethylammonium b.
    ethidium b.
    formalin ammonium b.
    glycopyrronium b.
    hexamethonium b.
    methyl b.
    potassium b.
    sodium b.
bromination
bromine
brominism (*var. of* bromism)
bromism, brominism
bromobenzylcyanide
    NATO code for riot control agent
    b. (CA)
bromocresol purple desoxycholate
  (BCP-D)
bromocriptine suppression test
bromodeoxyuridine
5-bromodeoxyuridine (BrDu, BUdR)
bromoderma
bromodomain
bromoiodism
bromomethane
Bromovirus
bromphenol
    b. blue
    b. test
bromsulphalein
    b. test
bromthymol blue
bronchi (*pl. of* bronchus)

bronchial
    b. adenoma
    b. aspirate anaerobic culture
    b. asthma (BA)
    b. brush biopsy
    b. calculus
    b. carcinoid
    b. carcinoma
    b. challenge test
    b. cyst
    b. gland
    b. gland cell adenocarcinoma
    b. hyperreactivity
    b. lymphocyte
    b. obstruction by foreign body
    b. pneumonia
    b. polyp
    b. surface cell adenocarcinoma
    b. washing
    b. washing cytology
bronchialis
    Cyathostoma b.
    Gordonia b.
bronchic cell
bronchiectasia sicca
bronchiectasis
    cylindrical b.
    cystic b.
    dry b.
    fusiform b.
    saccular b.
bronchiectatic
bronchioalveolar carcinoma
  (BACA)
bronchiolar
    b. adenocarcinoma
    b. carcinoma
    b. exocrine cell
    b. lymphocyte
    b. metaplasia
bronchiole
    b. obstruction
    respiratory b.
    terminal b.
bronchiolectasia (*var. of* bronchiolectasis)
bronchiolectasis, bronchiolectasia
bronchioli respiratorii
bronchiolitis
    exudative b.
    b. fibrosa obliterans
    b. obliterans organizing pneumonia
    (BOOP)
    b. obliterans syndrome
    obliterative b.
    proliferative b.
    respiratory b.
bronchioloalveolar
    b. adenocarcinoma
    b. carcinoma (BAC)

bronchiorum
    tunica muscularis b.
bronchiostenosis
bronchiseptica
    Bordetella b.
    Brucella b.
bronchisepticus
    Alcaligenes b.
    Bacillus b.
    Haemophilus b.
bronchitic
bronchitis
    acute b.
    asthmatic b. (AB)
    chronic b. (CB)
    croupous b.
    fibrinous b.
    infectious avian b.
    b. obliterans
    obliterative b.
    plastic b.
    pseudomembranous b.
bronchitis/bronchiolitis
    acute b. (ABB)
bronchium (*var. of* bronchus)
bronchoalveolar
    b. lavage (BAL)
    b. lavage fluid (BALF)
bronchoaspergillosis
bronchoblastomycosis
bronchocandidiasis
bronchocavernous
bronchocentric granulomatosis (BCG)
bronchoconstriction
bronchoconstrictor
bronchodilatation
bronchodilator
bronchoedema
bronchoesophageal fistula
bronchofiberscopy
bronchogenic
    b. carcinoma
    b. cyst
    b. tumor
broncholith
broncholithiasis
bronchomalacia
bronchomycosis
bronchopathy
bronchopleural fistula
bronchopneumonia
    acute hemorrhagic b.
    confluent b.
    diffuse b.
    focal b.
    hemorrhagic b.
    necrotizing b.
    sequestration b.
    subacute b.

    tuberculous b.
    virus b.
bronchopneumopathy
bronchoprovocation
bronchopulmonary
    b. aspergillosis
    b. dysplasia (BPD)
    b. histoplasmosis
    b. lavage
    b. sequestration
bronchoscopic smear
bronchospasm
bronchostenosis
bronchotracheal aspirate
bronchovesicular
bronchus, bronchium, *pl.* **bronchi**
    mucous gland adenoma of b.
    (MGAB)
    tunica mucosa bronchi
bronchus-associated lymphoid tissue
(BALT)
Brönsted-Lowry
    B.-L. acid
    B.-L. base
bronzed disease
bronze diabetes, bronzed disease
bronzinum
    chloasma b.
brood cell
Brooke
    B. disease
    B. tumor
Brooker heterotopic ossification
    classification
broomstick extremity
broth
    Bacto Middlebrook 7H9 b.
    Bacto Middlebrook OADC
     Enrichment b.
    boric acid b.
    brain-heart infusion b.
    carbohydrate b.
    Casman b.
    chopped meat b.
    decarboxylase b.
    Eijkman lactose b.
    ethyl violet azide b.
    glucose-format b.
    glycerin b.
    glycerin-potato b.
    gram-negative b. (GN b)
    haricot b.
    hippurate b.
    Imago b.
    indole-nitrate b.
    inosite-free b.
    iron b.
    Kitasato b.
    Koser citrate b.

B

broth (*continued*)
    lactose-litmus b.
    lauryl sulfate b.
    lead b.
    MacConkey b.
    malachite green b.
    malt extract b.
    Martin b.
    methyl red, Voges-Proskauer b.
    Middlebrook b.
    MR-VP b.
    Mueller-Hinton b.
    nitrate b.
    nutrient b.
    Rosenow veal-brain b.
    selenite b.
    selenite-cystine b.
    serum b.
    sodium chloride b.
    Spirolate b.
    sterility test b.
    Stuart b.
    sugar b.
    tetrathionate enrichment b.
    thioglycolate b.
    Todd-Hewitt b.
    trypticase soy with agar b.
    urease test b.
    Voges-Proskauer b.
    wheat b.
    wort b.

brown
    b. adipose tissue
    b. atrophy
    Bismarck b.
    Bismarck b. R, Y
    b. bowel syndrome
    b. edema
    b. fat
    b. hemoglobin-derived pigment
    b. layer
    b. recluse spider
    b. striae
    Sudan b.
    b. tumor

Brown-Brenn
    B.-B. stain
    B.-B. technique

Brown-Hopp tissue Gram stain

brownian
    b. motion
    b. movement

Brown-Pearce tumor

Brown-Sequard
    B.-S. paralysis
    B.-S. syndrome

Brown-Symmers disease

brucei
    Trypanosoma brucei b.

Brucella
    B. abortus
    B. agar
    B. agglutination test
    B. bronchiseptica
    B. canis
    B. melitensis
    B. strain 19 vaccine
    B. suis

Brucellaceae
Brucelleae
brucellergin
brucellin
brucellosis agglutinin
Bruch
    B. gland
    B. membrane

Bruck disease
Brücke tunic
Brudzinski meningeal sign
Brugia
    B. malayi
    B. microfilariae

Brugsch
    B. syndrome
    B. syndrome

bruit
    flank b.

Brumimicrobium glaciale
brumpti
    Oesophagostomum b.

Brumpt white mycetoma
Brunchorstia
brunescens
    cataracta b.

Brunhilde virus
Brunn
    B. bud
    B. epithelial nest
    B. membrane

Brunner gland
brunneroma
brunnerosis
brunnipes
    Anopheles b.

Bruns
    B. glucose medium
    B. syndrome

Brunsting-Perry pemphigoid
Brunsting syndrome
brush
    b. bipolar cell
    b. border
    b. border enzyme
    endometrial b.
    protected catheter b.
    b. specimen

brush-border microvillus
Brushfield spot

brushings
    cytologic b.
    b. cytology
Bruton
    B. disease
    B. type agammaglobulinemia
    B. tyrosine kinase (BTK)
    B. X-linked agammaglobulinemia
    X-linked agammaglobulinemia of B.
Bryantella formatexigens
BS
    blood sugar
BSA
    bismuth-sulfite agar
    body surface areas
    bovine serum albumin
BSB
    body surface burned
BSC
    biological safety cabinet
BSCC
    basaloid squamous cell carcinoma
BSDLB
    block in anterosuperior division of left
    branch
BSE
    bilateral, symmetrical, and equal
    bovine spongiform encephalopathy
BSF
    B-lymphocyte stimulatory factor
BSFR
    basal secretory flow rate
      BSFR test
BSI
    body substance isolation
    bound serum iron
BSL
    biosafety level
BSL1
    biosafety level 1
BSL2
    biosafety level 2
BSL3
    biosafety level 3
BSL4
    biosafety level 4
BSP
    bromsulphalein
      BSP excretion test
BSS
    balanced salt solution
    Bernard-Soulier syndrome
    buffered saline solution
BSTFA
    bis-trimethylsilyltrifluoroacetamide
BT
    bladder tumor
    bleeding time
    brain tumor

BTB
    breakthrough bleeding
BTK
    Bruton tyrosine kinase
BTPS
    body temperature, ambient pressure,
    saturated
      BTPS conditions of gas
BTTP
    British Testicular Tumour
    Panel
BTU
    British thermal unit
BU
    Bethesda unit
    Bodansky unit
    busulfan
BUB
    budding uninhibited by benzimidazole
    cancer gene BUB
bubas
bubble
    b. artifact
    b. boy disease
    replication b.
bubo
    cervical b.
    climatic b.
    malignant b.
    primary b.
    tropical b.
bubonic plague
bubonulus
buccal
    b. gland
    b. psoriasis
    b. smear
buccale
    Mycoplasma b.
    Treponema b.
buccales
    glandulae b.
buccalis
    Amoeba b.
    Entamoeba b.
    Leptotrichia b.
    Tetratrichomonas b.
    Trichomonas b.
Buchner extract
buchneri
    Lactobacillus b.
Büchner tuberculin
buckelii
    Azoarcus b.
Buckley syndrome
Bucky grid
bud
    Brunn b.
    gustatory b.

B

bud (*continued*)
    taste b.
    vascular b.
Budd
    B. cirrhosis
    B. disease
    B. syndrome
Budd-Chiari syndrome
budding
    glandular b.
    b. uninhibited by benzimidazole
    (BUB)
Buerger disease
buetschlii
    Entamoeba b.
buffalo neck
buffalopox
buffer
    b. action
    b. amplifier
    b. base (BB)
    bicarbonate b.
    cacodylate b.
    b. capacity
    citrate b.
    diluent b.
    EDTA b.
    HEPES b.
    Holmes alkaline b.
    Joklik b.
    Krebs-Ringer bicarbonate b. (KRB)
    loading b.
    LST b.
    lysis b.
    Millonig phosphate b.
    protein b.
    proteinase K b.
    secondary b.
    Supre-Heme b.
    b. system
    Tris-HCl b.
    b. value
    b. value of the blood
    Vector Laboratories VectaShield
      antifading b.
    veronal b.
buffered
    b. desoxycholate glucose (BDG)
    b. formalin fixative
    b. implant
    b. neutral formalin
    b. saline solution (BSS)
buffy
    b. coat
    b. coat micromethod
    b. coat smear
    b. coat smear study
    b. coat smear test
    b. crust

buffy-coated cell
bug
    assassin b.
    cone-nose b.
    harvest b.
Bugula
Buhl disease
bulb
    end b.
    hair b.
    Krause end b.
    olfactory b.
    taste b.
bulbar
    b. conjunctiva
    b. myelitis
    b. palsy
bulbi (*pl. of* bulbus)
bulbitis
bulboid corpuscle
bulboidea
    corpuscula b.
bulbourethral gland
bulbourethralis
    glandula b.
bulbous pemphigoid
Bulbulian
    Boothby, Lovelace, B.
bulbus, *pl.* **bulbi**
    ligamentum anulare bulbi
    b. olfactorius
    b. pili
    stratum pigmenti bulbi
    tunica conjunctiva bulbi
    tunica fibrosa bulbi
    tunica vasculosa bulbi
bulgaricus
    Lactobacillus b.
bulimia, boulimia
bulla, *pl.* **bullae**
    intraepidermic b.
    pulmonary b.
    subcorneal b.
    subepidermic b.
    suprabasilar b.
bullae (*pl. of* bulla)
bullata
    Mycoplana b.
bulldog head
Bulleidia extructa
Bullera
Bulleromyces albus
bullet
    migrating b.
    b. wipe
    b. wound
bulliform cell
Bullis fever
bull neck

bullosa
      epidermolysis b. (EB)
      junctional epidermolysis b.
      keratitis b.
      Pseudostertagia b.
bullosis diabeticorum
bullosum
      erythema multiforme b.
bullous
      b. disease
      b. edema
      b. edema vesicae
      b. emphysema
      b. eruption
      b. granulomatous
        inflammation
      b. impetigo
      b. impetigo of newborn
      b. lichen planus
      b. myringitis
      b. pemphigoid
      b. syphilid
bull's
      b. eye
      b. eye granule
      b. eye lesion
bump
BUN
    blood urea nitrogen
BUN/creatinine ratio
bundle
      Arnold b.
      atrioventricular b.
      Bachmann b.
      b. bone
      b. branch block (BBB)
      Bürdach b.
      Clarke collateral b.
      collagen b.
      Helie b.
      His b. (HB)
      Keith b.
      Kent b.
      Kent-His b.
      Monakow b.
      muscle b.
      b. of axon
      b. of His
      Rathke b.
      tendon b.
      trunk of atrioventricular b.
bungpagga
bunion
Bunostomum
      B. phlebotomum
      B. trigonocephalum
Bunsen
      B. burner
      B. coefficient

bunyamwera
      B. fever
      B. virus
Bunyaviridae
Bunyavirus
buoyant density
buphthalmos
Burchard-Liebermann reaction
Bürdach
      B. bundle
      B. column
      B. cuneate fasciculus
      B. fissure
      B. tract
Burdach fiber
burden
      mutation b.
      radionuclide body b.
      tumor b.
buret, burette
burette (*var. of* buret)
burgdorferi
      Borrelia b.
Bürger-Grütz syndrome
Burkholderia
      B. ambifaria
      B. anthina
      B. caledonica
      B. cenocepacia
      B. cepacia
      B. dolosa
      B. fungorum
      B. hospita
      B. kururiensis
      B. mallei
      B. phymatum
      B. pseudomallei
      B. sacchari
      B. sordidicola
      B. stabilis
      B. terricola
      B. tuberum
      B. ubonensis
      B. unamae
      B. xenovorans
burkinensis
      Anaeroarcus b.
      Desulfovibrio b.
Burkitt
      B. lymphoma (BL)
      B. tumor
Burkitt-like lymphoma
burn
      beta b.
      b. culture
      first-degree b.
      flash b.
      fourth-degree b.
      full-thickness b.

B

burn (*continued*)
    b. index (BI)
    mustard-induced b.
    screen b.
    second-degree b.
    superficial b.
    third-degree b.
    ultraviolet b.
burned
    body surface b. (BSB)
burner
    Boling b.
    Bunsen b.
    Fischer b.
    laminar flow b.
burnetii
    Coxiella b.
Burnett
    B. disinfecting fluid
    B. syndrome
burn-in
burnt-out germ cell tumor
Burow solution
burr cell
burrow
burrowing pus
bursa-equivalent tissue
bursal
    b. abscess
    b. cyst
bursata
    exostosis b.
bursitis
    radiohumeral b.
    xanthogranulomatous b.
burst
    respiratory b.
    spider b.
burst-forming unit-erythroid (BFU-E)
Buruli ulcer
Bury disease
BUS
    Bartholin, urethral, Skene
    BUS glands
busanensis
    Legionella b.
Buschke
    B. disease
    B. scleredema
Buschke-Löwenstein
    giant condyloma of B.-L.
Buschke-Löwenstein
    B.-L. giant condyloma
    B.-L. tumor
Buschke-Ollendorf syndrome
buski
    Fasciolopsis b.
    Glyciphagus b.

Busquet disease
Buss disease
Busse-Buschke disease
Busse saccharomyces
busulfan (BSF, BU, BUS), busulphan
    b. lung
busulphan (*var. of* busulfan)
busy dermis
butabarbital
    sodium b.
butane
butanoic acid
butanol-extractable
    b.-e. iodine (BEI)
    b.-e. iodine assay
    b.-e. iodine test
butanone
Butchart tumor staging
bütschlii
    Iodamoeba b.
butter
    b. of antimony
    b. yellow
butterfly
    b. lung
    b. rash
button
    cell b.
    corneoscleral b.
buttonhole stenosis
butyl
    b. alcohol
    b. 2-cyanoacrylate
    b. methacrylate
butyraceous
butyrate esterase stain
butyric acid
butyricum
    Clostridium b.
    Mycobacterium b.
Butyrivibrio hungatei
butyrous colony
butyrylcholinesterase (BChE)
butzleri
    Arcobacter b.
buyo cheek cancer
BV
    blood volume
BW
    biological warfare
Bwamba
    B. fever
    B. fever virus
By antigen
Byetta
Byler
    B. disease
    B. syndrome

Bymovirus
bypass (BP)
    b. capacitor
    cardiopulmonary b.
byssina
    Dendrostilbella b.
byssinosis
Byssoascus

Byssochlamys
bystander
    b. hemolysis
    b. lysis
    b. suppression
Bywaters syndrome
BZ
    NATO code for QNB

B

C
calculus
carbon
Celsius temperature scale
centigrade
centigrade temperature
  scale
coulomb
large calorie
   C antigen
   C banding
   C carbohydrate antigen
   C cell
   C group virus
   C lactose test
   C peptide
   C region
   C virus

c
contact
small calorie

C1
   C1 complex
   C1 esterase
   C1 esterase inhibitor
   (C1EInh)

C2
   Clostridium botulinum cytotoxin type
   C2

C3
   C3 Nef factor
   C3 proactivator
   C3 proactivator convertase

CA
cancer
cancer antigen
carcinoma
chronological age
cold agglutinin
corpus amylaceum
croup-associated
cytosine arabinoside
NATO code for riot control agent
  bromobenzylcyanide
   CA virus

Ca
calcium
cancer

CA-125
cancer antigen 125
   CA-125 antigen
   CA-125 assay

CA15-3
   CA15-3 breast antigen
   CA15-3 RIA

CA19-9
   CA19-9 antigen
   CA19-9 assay
Ca2+
calcium ion
CA72-4
C3a anaphylatoxin
C4a anaphylatoxin
C5a anaphylatoxin
CABG
coronary artery bypass
  graft
cabinet
   biological safety c. (BSC)
c-abl oncogene
Cabot ring body
caccae
   Anaerostipes c.
Cacchi-Ricci syndrome
cache
   c. memory
   C. Valley virus
cachectic
   c. anergy
   c. endocarditis
   c. purpura
cachectin
cachexia
   cancerous c.
   c. exophthalmica
   malarial c.
   c. strumipriva
   thyroid c.
   uremic c.
CaCl2
calcium chloride
CaCN
calcium cyanide
cacocholia
cacodylate
   c. buffer
   sodium c.
cacodylic acid
cactinomycin
cacumen
CAD
compound absorption device
coronary artery disease
CaD
caldesmon
CADASIL
cerebral autosomal dominant
  arteriopathy with subcortical infarcts
  and leukoencephalopathy
cadaver donor

cadaveric
    c. ecchymosis
    c. spasm
cadaverine
cadaveris
    Clostridium c.
cadence
    counting c.
cadherin
    epithelial c. (E-cadherin)
    vascular endothelial c. (VE-cadherin)
cadherin/catenin complex
cadherin-6 gene
cadmium
    c. assay
    c. telluride detector
Ca-DTPA
    calcium diethylenetriaminepentaacetate
caduca
CAE
    chloroacetate esterase
caecum (*var. of* cecum)
caecutiens
    Chrysops c.
    Onchocerca c.
Ca-EDTA
    calcium ethylenediaminetetraacetic
CaEDTA
    calcium disodium edetate
Caenibacterium thermophilum
caerulea (*var. of* cerula)
    cataracta c.
caesar
    Lucilia c.
caespitosus
    Botryomyces c.
café au lait spot
caffeine
    c. assay
    c. sodium benzoate
Caffey
    C. disease
    C. syndrome
Caffey-Silverman syndrome
Ca2+-free perfusion
CAG
    chronic atrophic gastritis
    trinucleotide CAG
cagA toxin
CAH
    chronic active hepatitis
    congenital adrenal hyperplasia
CAHD
    coronary atherosclerotic heart disease
CAHM
    complex atypical hyperplasia/metaplasia
CAIS
    complete androgen insensitivity
    syndrome

caishijiensis
    Nocardia c.
caisson disease
Cajal
    C. astrocyte stain
    C. cell
    C. formol ammonium bromide
      solution
    C. gold sublimate method
    C. gold sublimate stain
    horizontal cell of C.
    C. interstitial nucleus
    C. uranium silver method
cajennense
    Amblyomma c.
cake kidney
cal
    small calorie
Cal
    large calorie
Calabar swelling
calbindin protein
calcanei (*pl. of* calcaneus)
calcaneonavicular
calcaneum (*var. of* calcaneus)
calcaneus, calcaneum, *pl.*
  calcanei
calcar
calcarea
    Nocardia c.
calcareous
    c. cystitis
    c. degeneration
    c. infiltration
    c. metastasis
calcarine
Calcarisporium
calcariuria
calcemia
calcergy
Cal-Chex for Cell-Dyn whole blood
  calibrator
calcicosis
calcific
    c. bicuspid aortic valve stenosis
    c. concretion
    c. nodular aortic stenosis
calcificans
    chondrodysplasia c.
calcification
    dystrophic c.
    egg-shell c.
    focal c.
    indeterminate c.
    c. line of Retzius
    medial c.
    metastatic c.
    mitral valve c.
    Mönckeberg medial c.

presenile dementia with tangles and c.'s

psammomatous c.

soft tissue c. (STC)

calcified
c. cartilage
c. gallbladder
c. granuloma
c. granulomatous inflammation

calcifying
c. ameloblastoma
c. epithelial odontogenic tumor (CEOT)
c. epithelioma of Malherbe
c. fibrous pseudotumor
c. pancreatitis

calcigerous

calcineurin (CN)

calcinosis
c. circumscripta
c. cutis
c. cutis, Raynaud phenomenon, sclerodactyly, and telangiectasia (CRST)
dystrophic c.
c. intervertebralis
calcinosis, Raynaud phenomenon, esophageal motility disorders, sclerodactyly, and telangiectasia (CREST)
reversible c.
tumoral c.
c. universalis

calciokinesis

calciokinetic

calciorrhachia

calciotropism

calcipenia

calcipexic

calcipexis, calcipexy

calciphilia

calciphylaxis (CPX)
systemic c.
topical c.

calcite

calcitonin
c. assay
c. gene-related peptide (CGRP)
plasma c.
c. receptor-like receptor
c. testing

calcitrans
Stomoxys c.

calcium (Ca)
c. acetate formalin
Baker formol c.
c. balance
c. channel agonist
c. chloride

c. cyanide (CaCN)
c. deposit demonstration
c. deposition
c. diethylenetriaminepentaacetate (Ca-DTPA)
c. disodium edetate
endogenous fecal c. (EFC)
c. ethylenediaminetetraacetic (Ca-EDTA)
c. gout
c. imbalance
c. ion (Ca2+)
ionized c.
c. ionized assay
leucovorin c.
c. oxalate (CO)
c. oxalate calculus
c. oxalate crystal
c. oxalate test
c. phosphate
c. phosphate calculus
c. pyrophosphate dehydrate
c. pyrophosphate deposition disease (CPPD)
c. pyrophosphate dihydrate (CPD)
c. red
c. time
urine c.

calcium-45

calcium-activated
c.-a. ATPase
c.-a. neutral protease

calcium-ATPase
sarcoendoplasmic reticulum c.-a. (SERCA)

calcium-magnesium-ATPase
Wachstein-Meissel stain for c.-m.-A.

calcium-sensing
c.-s. receptor
c.-s. receptor protein

calciuria

calcoaceticus
Acinetobacter c.

calcofluor white stain

calcospherite

calculated (calc)
c. mean organism (CMO)
c. serum osmolality

calculi (*pl. of* calculus)

calculosis

calculous pigment

calculus (C), *pl.* **calculi**
apatite c.
arthritic c.
articular c.
biliary c.
blood c.
branched c.
bronchial c.

calculus (*continued*)
    calcium oxalate c.
    calcium phosphate c.
    cardiac c.
    cerebral c.
    cholesterol c.
    combination c.
    coral c.
    cystine c.
    decubitus c.
    dendritic c.
    dental c.
    encysted c.
    fibrin c.
    fusible c.
    gastric c.
    hemic c.
    indigo c.
    intestinal c.
    joint c.
    lacrimal c.
    mammary c.
    matrix c.
    mixed c.
    mulberry c.
    nephritic c.
    oxalate c.
    pleural c.
    pocketed c.
    preputial c.
    primary renal c.
    prostatic c.
    renal c.
    salivary c.
    staghorn c.
    struvite c.
    urate c.
    ureteral c.
    uric acid c.
    urinary c.
    uterine c.
    vesical c.
    weddellite c.
    whewellite c.
Caldanaerobacter
    C. subterraneus
    C. subterraneus subsp. *acificus*
    C. subterraneus subsp. *subterraneus*
    C. subterraneus subsp. *tengcongensis*
    C. subterraneus subsp. *yonseiensis*
Caldariomyces
caldesmon (CaD)
    C. cell protein
Caldilinea aerophila
Caldimonas manganoxidans
Caldisphaera lagunensis
Caldithrix abyssi
Caldivirga maquilingensis

caldoxylosilyticus
    Geobacillus c.
caldus
    Acidithiobacillus c.
Caldwell-Moloy
    C.-M. classification
    C.-M. method
caledonica
    Burkholderia c.
calefacient
caliber (cal)
calibrate
calibration
    c. curve
    film density c.
    c. interval
    c. material
calibrator
    Advia Centaur anti-HBs c.
    Cal-Chex for Cell-Dyn whole blood c.
    dose c.
    Vitros Immunodiagnostic Products anti-HBc c.
calicectasis
caliciform, calyciform
    c. cell
    c. ending
Caliciviridae
calicivirus
    c.
calicoblast cell
calicoblastic epithelium
caliculus gustatorius
caliectasis
caliensis
California
    C. encephalitis (CE)
    C. encephalitis virus
    C. encephalitis virus titer
    C. myxoma virus
californiensis
    Anaerobranca c.
    Lentzea c.
    Thelazia c.
    Tindallia c.
californium (Cf)
caliper
    c. micrometer
    vernier dial c.
CALLA
    common acute lymphoblastic leukemia antigen
    C. antiserum
    C. assay
CALLA-positive ALL
Calleja
    islands of C.
    islets of C.

Call-Exner body
calligyrum
        Treponema c.
callipaeda
        Thelazia c.
Calliphora vomitoria
Calliphoridae
Callison fluid
Callitroga
callosity
callus
        bony c.
        central c.
        definitive c.
        ensheathing c.
        fracture c.
        myelogenous c.
        provisional c.
calmagite
calmative agent
Calmette-Gúerin
        bacille bilíe de C.-G.
        bacillus C.-G.
        C.-G. bacillus
        C.-G. vaccine
Calmette test
calmodulin
calnexin
Calocera
Calodium
calomel electrode
Calomys colossus
Calonectria
calor
        c. febrilis
        c. fervens
        c. innatus
Caloramator
        C. coolhaasii
        C. viterbiensis
Caloranaerobacter azorensis
caloric
        c. disease
        c. quotient
calorie, calory
        large c. (C, Cal)
        small c. (c, cal)
calorigenesis
calorigenic action
calorimeter
calorimetry
calory (*var. of* calorie)
Calospora
CALP
        calponin
calpain family of protease
calponin (CALP)
calretinin expression
calsequestrin

calvaria
Calvatia gigantea
Calvé-Perthes disease
Calvé-Perthes-Legg disease
calviensis
        Vibrio c.
calyciform (*var. of* caliciform)
Calymmatobacterium
        C. donovania
        C. granulomatis
CAM
        cell adhesion molecule
        chemical agent monitor
        AE1 plus CAM
        CAM 5.2 antibody
        CAM 5.2 antigen
cambium layer
Cambridge
        C. Biotech HIV-1 urine Western
          blot test
        factor V C.
cambriense
        Varibaculum c.
cameloid anemia
camelpox
camera
        Anger c.
        gamma c.
        Ikegami video c.
        Insight digital c.
        Nikon microprocessor-controlled c.
        scintillation c.
        Spot RT Monochrome Kodak
          KAI-2000 CCD digital c.
camera/microscope
        Coolscope digital c.
Cameron lesion
camerostome
camini
        Aeropyrum c.
Caminibacter
        C. hydrogeniphilus
        C. profundus
Caminicella sporogenes
caminithermale
        Clostridium c.
cA2 monoclonal antibody
cAMP
        adenosine 3′,5′-cyclic monophosphate
        adenosine 3′,5′-cyclic phosphate
        cyclic adenosine monophosphate
        cyclic AMP
camp
        c. fever
        c. response element binding
          activation transcription factor
          (CREB/ATF)
        c. response element binding protein
          (CREB)

C

CAMP
    Christie-Atkins-Munch-Petersen
      CAMP factor
      CAMP test
Campanacci
    osteofibrous dysplasia of C.
campanulae
    Ascospora c.
cAMP-dependent protein kinase
campestris
    Anopheles c.
Camp-Gianturco radiography method
camphor assay
camphorism
campinensis
    Ralstonia c.
    Wautersia c.
campisalis
    Halomonas c.
camptobactrum
    Leptodontium c.
camptocormia, camptocormy
camptocormy (*var. of* camptocormia)
camptothecin
Campylobacter
    C. bacterium
    C. cinaedi
    C. coli
    C. concisus
    C. curvus
    C. fennelliae
    C. fetus subsp. *fetus*
    C. fetus subsp. *venerealis*
    C. (Helicobacter) pylori
    C. hominis
    C. hyointestinalis
    C. jejuni
    C. lanienae
    C. lari
    C. rectus
    C. selective agar
    C. showae
    C. sputorum
Campylobacteraceae
Campylobacter-**like organism (CLO)**
Camurati-Engelmann disease
CANA
    convulsant antidote for nerve agent
Canada-Cronkhite syndrome
canadensis
    Chromohalobacter c.
    Helicobacter c.
    Onychocola c.
canal
    alimentary c.
    anterior semicircular c.
    Arantius c.
    Arnold c.
    Bernard c.

    Bichat c.
    bony semicircular c.
    central c.
    ciliary c.
    Cloquet c.
    Corti c.
    deferent c.
    dentinal c.
    Dorello c.
    haversian c.
    Hensen c.
    Holmgren-Golgi c.
    Hoyer c.
    hyaloid c.
    interfacial c.
    Kovalevsky c.
    Lambert c.
    lateral semicircular c.
    Leeuwenhoek c.
    Löwenberg c.
    lower anal c.
    nutrient c.
    obturator c.
    c. of Hering
    c. of Schlemm
    portal c.
    posterior semicircular c.
    Santorini c.
    semicircular c.
    Stilling c.
    Sucquet c.
    Sucquet-Hoyer c.
    uniting c.
    upper anal c.
    vestibular c.
    Volkmann c.
    Walther c.
    Wirsung c.
canalicular
    c. adenoma
    c. duct
    c. membrane
    c. organic anion
      transplant
    c. pattern
    c. space
canaliculization
canaliculum
canaliculus, *pl.* **canaliculi**
    bile canaliculi
    bile duct c.
    biliary c.
    bone c.
    canaliculi dentales
    intracellular c.
    pseudobile c.
    c. reuniens
    secretory c.
    Thiersch c.

canalis
   c. hyaloideus
   c. nutricius
   c. reuniens
   canales semicircularis ossei
canalization
canalized thrombus
canariasense
   Mycobacterium c.
canarypox virus
Canavalia
Canavan
   C. disease
   C. sclerosis
cANCA
   cytoplasmic antineutrophil cytoplasmic
     antibody
   cytoplasmic antineutrophil cytoplasmic
     autoantibody
cancellated
cancellous
   c. bone
   c. tissue
cancellus
cancer (CA, Ca)
   adrenal c.
   AJCC staging modification on
     prostate c.
   American Joint Committee on C.
     (AJCC)
   androgen independent prostate c.
     (AIPC)
   c. antigen (CA)
   c. antigen 125 (CA 125)
   betel c.
   c. body
   breast c.
   buyo cheek c.
   c. chemotherapy
   chimney-sweep's c.
   colloid c.
   colorectal c. (CRC)
   conjugal c.
   encephaloid c.
   c. en cuirasse
   endocervical c.
   epidermoid c.
   epithelial c.
   fallopian tube c.
   familial c.
   c. family
   foamy gland prostate c.
   gastrointestinal c.
   c. gene BUB
   glandular c.
   green c.
   hereditary diffuse gastric c. (HDGC)
   hereditary nonpolyposis colon c.
     (HNPCC)

   hereditary nonpolyposis colorectal c.
     (HNPCC)
   inherited c.
   c. juice
   kangri c.
   kidney c.
   laryngeal c.
   liver c.
   lung c.
   lymphatic c.
   lymph node c.
   lymphoreticular c.
   c. management therapy
   mule-spinner's c.
   mutated in colon c. (MCC)
   nonsmall cell c. (NSCC)
   nonsmall cell lung c. (NSCLC)
   ovarian c.
   pipe-smoker's c.
   pitch-worker's c.
   c. promoter
   prostate c.
   qualitative staging of breast c.
   c. risk assessment
   scar c.
   small cell c. (SCC)
   somatic mutation theory of c.
   spider c.
   c. staging
   stomach c.
   stump c.
   synchronous c.
   synovial c.
   telangiectatic c.
   testicular c.
   uterine c.
   vaginal c.
   vulvar c.
canceration
cancer-free white mouse (CFWM)
cancericidal, cancerocidal
cancerigenic
cancerization
   lobular c.
cancerocidal (*var. of* cancericidal)
cancerous cachexia
cancriform
cancroid
cancrum
   c. nasi
   c. oris
candela (cd)
CanDia5 candida rapid test
candicans
   corpus c.
Candida
   C. albicans
   C. dubliniensis
   C. endocarditis

Candida (*continued*)
    C. esophagitis
    C. glabrata
    C. guilliermondi
    C. krusei
    C. meningitis
    C. parapsilosis
    C. pneumonia
    C. precipitin test
    C. pseudotropicalis
    C. stellatoidea
    C. tropicalis
    C. vulvovaginitis
candidal
candidate
    c. tumor marker
    c. tumor suppressor gene
candidemia
candidiasis, candidosis
    chronic mucocutaneous c. (CMC)
    disseminated c.
    c. serologic test
    vulvovaginal c.
candidid
candidosis
candidum
    Geotrichum c.
candidus
    Aspergillus c.
    Thermoactinomyces c.
cangkringensis
    Streptomyces c.
canicola
    Leptospira c.
canicularis
    Anthomyia c.
    Fannia c.
canicular multispecific organic anion transporter (CMOAT)
canimorsus
    Capnocytophaga c.
canina
    Taenia c.
canine
    c. adenovirus 1 (CAV-1)
    c. carcinoma 1
    c. distemper virus
    c. herpesvirus
    c. herpetovirus
    c. oral papilloma
caninum
    Ancylostoma c.
    Dipylidium c.
    Episthmium c.
    Leishmania c.
    Neospora c.
canis
    Actinomyces c.
    Ascaris c.

    Brucella c.
    Ctenocephalides c.
    Ehrlichia c.
    Enterococcus c.
    hepatitis contagiosa c.
    Isospora c.
    Microsporum c.
    Streptococcus c.
    Toxocara c.
canities
canker sore
cannabina
    Pseudomonas c.
cannabinoid
cannabinol
Cannabis
cannabism
canning
    home c.
Cannizzaro reaction
cannulation, cannulization
    arterial c.
cannulization (*var. of* cannulation)
Cantharellula
cantharidin
C8/144 antibody
C219 antibody
C494 antibody
cantonensis
    Angiostrongylus c.
CAO
    chronic airway obstruction
caoutchouc pelvis
CAP
    College of American Pathologists
    CAP sweat analysis proficiency testing program
cap
    acrosomal c.
    c. cell
    cradle c.
    fibrin c.
    head c.
    TBG c.
capability
    morgue c.
capacitance
    membrane c.
capacitation
capacitive reactance
capacitor
    bypass c.
    ceramic c.
    coupling c.
    disc c.
    electrolytic c.
    filter c.
    junction c.
    Mylar c.

output c.
resistor c. (RC)
variable c.

capacity
antigen-binding c.
blood buffering c.
buffer c.
dye-binding c. (DBC)
forced vital c. (FVC)
functional reserve c. (FRC)
functional residual c. (FRC)
heat c.
inspiratory reserve c. (IRC)
iron-binding c. (IBC)
latent iron-binding c. (LIBC)
maximal sustained ventilatory c.
  (MSVC)
molar heat c.
proatherogenic c.
residual lung c. (RLC)
single breath carbon monoxide
  diffusing c.
slow vital c. (SVC)
specific heat c.
storage c.
total iron-binding c. (TIBC)
total lung c. (TLC)
trypsin-inhibitory c. (TIC)
unsaturated iron-binding c.
unsaturated vitamin B_{12}-binding c.
  (UBBC)
vitamin B_{12} unsaturated binding c.

Capdepont disease
Capella
tumor of C.
Capetown
hemoglobin J C.
Capgras syndrome
capillaceus
Actinoplanes c.
capillare
vas c.
capillarectasia
Capillaria
C. hepatica
C. philippinensis
capillariasis
capillarioscopy
capillaris
Muellerius c.
capillaritis
capillarity
capillaron
capillaropathy
capillaroscopy
capillary
c. action
arterial c.
bile c.

blood c.
c. blood sugar (CBS)
continuous c.
c. electrophoresis
c. electrophoresis electropherogram
c. embolism
erythrocyte in c.
fenestrated c.
c. flame
c. fragility
c. fragility test
c. hemangioma
c. loop
lymph c.
c. microscope
c. nevus
sinusoidal c.
c. tube
c. vein
venous c.
c. vessel
c. zone electrophoresis (CE)

capillary-like space
capillatus
Solenopotes c.
capillitii
Saccharomyces c.
capillosus
Bacteroides c.
Capillovirus
capillus
Capim virus
capistration
capita (*pl. of* caput)
capitation
capitatus
Blastoschizomyces c.
Dipodascus c.
capitis
pityriasis c.
tinea c.
trichophytosis c.
capitovis
Corynebacterium c.
capitular
capitulum
Caplan
C. nodule
C. syndrome
capneic
Capnocytophaga canimorsus
capnocytophagoides
Dysgonomonas c.
capnohepatography
capon-comb-growth test
capping
caprae
Mycobacterium c.
Mycobacterium bovis subsp. *c.*

caprate
  cellulose c.
capreoli
  Bartonella c.
capricola
  Trichostrongylus c.
caprine
  c. herpesvirus (CpHV)
  c. herpetovirus
caprinus
  Streptococcus c.
Capripoxvirus
Capronia pulcherrima
caprylate
  sodium c.
capsaicin
capsase mediated cleavage of APP
capsicum
  C.
  C. annum
  C. frutescens
  oleoresin c. (OC)
capsid
capsomer, capsomere
  c. capsular space
  c. capsule
capsomere (*var. of* capsomer)
capsula, *pl.* **capsulae**
  c. adiposa renis
  c. articularis
  c. cordis
  c. glomeruli
capsulae (*pl. of* capsula)
capsular
  c. antigen
  c. cell
  c. drop
  c. lipochondral degeneration
  c. precipitation reaction
  c. space
  c. synovial-like hyperplasia (CSH)
  c. tissue
capsulare
  lipoma c.
capsularis
  decidua c.
capsulata
  Emmonsiella c.
capsulatum
  Ajellomyces c.
  Histoplasma capsulatum c.
  Novosphingobium c.
capsulatus
  Bacillus aerogenes c.
  Endomyces c.
  Torula c.
capsule
  adipose c.

adrenal c.
anthrax c.
antiphagocytic polypeptide c.
articular c.
atrabiliary c.
bacterial c.
Bowman c.
capsomer c.
cartilage c.
c. cell
connective tissue c.
extreme c.
fibrous articular c.
fibrous membrane of joint c.
Friedländer stain for c.'s
Gerota c.
hyaline c.
joint c.
malpighian c.
Müller c.
Nicolle stain for c.'s
renal c.
sooty c.
suprarenal c.
tumor c.
capsulitis
  adhesive c.
  hepatic c.
capture
  c. antibody
  c. assay
  c. cross section
  electron c. (EC)
  Hybrid C. 2
  radiative c.
  viral hybrid c.
caput, *pl.* **capita**
  c. medusae
  c. quadratum
Caraparu virus
carateum
  Treponema c.
Caraway method
Carazzi hematoxylin
carb
  carbohydrate
carbamate
  hemoglobin c.
carbamazepine assay
carbamide
carbamino-carbon dioxide
carbamino compound
carbaminohemoglobin
carbamoyl
  c. phosphate synthetase
  (CPS)
  c. phosphate synthetase I
  deficiency

carbamoyltransferase
    ornithine c. (OCT)
carbamyl
    c. phosphate
    c. phosphate synthetase (CPS)
carbamylurea
carbanion
carbaprostacyclin
carbaryl assay
carbenicillin indanyl sodium
carbhemoglobin
carbinol
Carbitol
carbohemoglobin
carbohydrate (CHO)
    c. antigen
    c. broth
    fecal c.
    c. fermentation test
    c. identification test
    c. inversion
    c. metabolism index (CMI)
    stool c.
    c. tolerance test
    c. utilization test
carbohydrate-induced hyperlipidemia
carbohydraturia
carbolfuchsin (CF)
    c. stain
    Ziehl-Neelsen c.
carbolfuchsin-methylene blue staining method
carbolic
    c. acid
    c. methylene blue (CMB)
carbolism
carbol-thionin stain
carboluria
carbomycin
carbon
    c. bisulfide
    c. dioxide (bicarb, CO_2)
    c. dioxide absorbent
    c. dioxide acidosis
    c. dioxide challenge test
    c. dioxide combining power
    c. dioxide combining power measurement
    c. dioxide combining power test
    c. dioxide concentration
    c. dioxide concentration assay
    c. dioxide content
    c. dioxide dissociation curve
    c. dioxide electrode
    c. dioxide fixation
    c. dioxide myoglobin (MbCO)
    c. dioxide narcosis
    c. dioxide output (VI_{CO_2})
    c. dioxide production
    c. dioxide response curve
    c. dioxide tension
    c. disulfide
    c. disulfide assay
    c. disulfide poisoning
    c. gelatin mass
    c. inorganic compound
    c. 13-labeled ketoisocaproate breath test
    c. monoxide (CO)
    c. monoxide assay
    c. monoxide hemoglobin
    c. monoxide oximeter (CO-oximeter)
    c. monoxide poisoning
    c. monoxide test
    c. oxychloride
    c. resistor
    c. tetrachloride (CCl4)
    c. tetrachloride assay
    c. tetrachloride poisoning
carbon-11, -12, -13, -14
carbonaceous residue of combustion
carbonate
    c. dehydratase
    lithium c.
    potassium c.
    sodium c.
carbon-film resistor
carbon-hydrogen (C-H)
    c.-h. stretch
carbonic
    c. acid
    c. acid chloride
    c. anhydrase
    c. anhydrase inhibitor
    c. anhydrase-related protein (CA-RP)
carbonis
    Streptacidiphilus c.
carbonium ion
carbonized
carbonuria
    dysoxidative c.
carbonyl
    c. chloride
    c. cyanide p-(trifluoromethoxy)phenylhydrazone
carbonylhemoglobin
carbophenothion
Carborundum
Carbowax
Carboxydibrachium pacificum
Carboxydocella thermautotrophica
carboxyhemoglobin (CoHB, COHb, HbCO, HBCO)
    c. assay
carboxyhemoglobinemia
carboxyhemoglobinuria

C

carboxylase
    acetyl-CoA c.
    propionate c.
    propionyl-CoA c.
    pyruvate c.
carboxylate
    c. ion
    pyrrolidone c.
carboxylesterase
carboxylic acid
carboxyl terminal (Ct, C terminal)
carboxymethylcellulose (CM-cellulose)
carboxypeptidase
carbuncle
    kidney c.
    malignant c.
    renal c.
carbuncular
carbunculosis
carcinemia
carcinoembryonic
    c. antigen (CEA)
    c. antigen-related cell adhesion
      molecule 1 (CEACAM1)
    c. antigen test
carcinogen
    complete c.
    direct-reacting c.
    group 1 c.
carcinogenesis
    viral c.
carcinogenic hydrocarbon
carcinoid
    atypical c.
    bronchial c.
    foregut c.
    goblet cell c.
    c. heart disease
    intestinal tract c.
    lung c.
    mucous c.
    strumal c.
    c. syndrome
    c. tumor
carcinoides
carcinoid-like architectural pattern
carcinolytic
carcinoma (CA), *pl.* **carcinomas,**
  carcinomata
    acinar cell c. (ACC)
    acinic cell c.
    acinose c.
    acinous c.
    adenocystic c.
    adenoid cystic c. (ACC)
    adenoid squamous cell c.
    adenosquamous cell c. (ADSQC)
    adnexal c.
    adrenocortical c.

aggressive thyroid c. (ATC)
alveolar cell c.
ampullary c.
anal gland c.
anaplastic c.
apocrine c.
atypical medullary c.
basal cell c. (BCC)
basaloid invasive squamous cell c.
  (BISCC)
basaloid squamous cell c. (BSCC)
basal squamous cell c.
basosquamous c.
Bellini duct c.
bile duct c.
bladder c.
bone marrow c.
breast c.
bronchial c.
bronchioalveolar c. (BACA)
bronchiolar c.
bronchioloalveolar c. (BAC)
bronchogenic c.
canine c. 1
CD44v6 staining in prostate c.
cecal c.
ceruminous c.
cervical c.
chorionic c.
chromophobe c.
chromophobe renal cell c. (CRCC)
clear cell c. (CCC)
clear cell hepatocellular c.
  (HCC-CC)
clear cell myoepithelial c.
  (CCMEC)
clear cell odontogenic c.
clear cell renal cell c. (RCC-CC)
clinging c.
cloacogenic c.
collecting duct c. (CDC)
colloid c.
colon c.
colorectal c.
conventional papillary c. (CPC)
cribriform c.
cribriform-morular variant of
  papillary thyroid c.
crypt cell c.
cuboidal c.
c. cutaneum
cylindromatous c.
cystic c.
duct c.
ductal c.
duodenal c.
Ehrlich ascites c.
embryonal cell c.
endocervical c.

endometrial c.
endometrial intraepithelial c. (EIC)
endometrioid c.
endometrioid endometrial c. (EEC)
epidermoid c.
epimyoepithelial c.
epithelial-myoepithelial c. (EMEC)
esophageal c.
c. ex pleomorphic adenoma
fibrolamellar hepatocellular c.
fibrolamellar liver cell c.
follicular thyroid c. (FTC)
follicular variant of papillary thyroid
  c. (FVPTC)
gallbladder c.
gastric c.
gastrointestinal tract c.
gelatinous c.
giant cell c.
glandular c.
glassy cell c. (GCC)
grade 1, 2 neuroendocrine c.
granulosa cell c.
head and neck squamous cell c.
  (HNSCC)
hepatocellular c. (HCC)
hepatocellular bile duct c.
hereditary papillary renal cell c. (HPRC)
histiocytoid c.
Hürthle cell c.
hyalinizing clear cell c. (HCCC)
hypervascular hepatocellular c.
incidence of hepatocellular c.
infiltrating cribriform c.
infiltrating ductal c. (IDC)
infiltrating lobular c. (ILC)
infiltrating papillary c.
inflammatory c.
c. in situ (CIS)
c. in situ/intratubular germ cell
  neoplasia unclassified (CIS/ITGCNU)
insular c.
intermediate c.
intracystic papillary c.
intraductal papillary c. (IPC)
intraepidermal squamous cell c.
intraepithelial c.
invasive ductal c.
invasive lobular c.
invasive papillary c.
invasive squamous cell c. (ISCC)
ipsilateral intraductal c.
islet cell c.
Jewett bladder c.
juvenile c.
kangri burn c.
keratinizing invasive squamous cell c.
keratinizing squamous cell c.
  (KSCC)

Krompecher c.
large-cell neuroendocrine c.
  (LCNEC)
laryngeal c.
lateral aberrant thyroid c.
leptomeningeal c.
liver cell c.
lobular c.
Lucké c.
lung c.
lymphoepithelioma-like c. (LELC)
lymphoepithelioma-like thymic c.
  (LETC)
matrix-producing c.
medullary c. (MC)
medullary renal c. (MRC)
medullary thyroid c. (MTC)
melanotic c.
meningeal c.
mesometanephric c.
metachronous c.
metaplastic c.
metastatic c.
metastatic hepatocellular c. (HCC)
metatypical c.
microinvasive c.
micropapillary serous c. (MPSC)
minimally invasive follicular c.
  (MIFC)
mixed hepatocellular c.
mucin-depleted mucoepidermoid c.
mucinous bronchioloalveolar c.
mucinous tubular and spindle cell
  c. (MTSCC)
mucoepidermoid c. (MEC)
myoblastoid c.
myoblastomatoid c.
myoepithelial c.
c. myxomatodes
nasopharyngeal c. (NPC)
noncystic mucinous c.
noninfiltrating lobular c.
oat cell c.
occult c.
oncocytic c.
oncoplastic c.
ovarian c.
oxyphilic papillary c.
pilomatrix c.
piriform sinus c.
pleomorphic lobular c. (PLC)
poorly differentiated c.
primary thymic c. (PTC)
pseudoangiosarcomatous c.
pseudosarcomatous c.
pseudovascular adenoid squamous
  cell c. (PASCC)
recurrent c.
renal cell c. (RCC)

C

carcinoma (*continued*)
    renal clear cell c.
    reserve cell c.
    residual c.
    rhabdoid phenotype of large-cell c.
    Robson stage I, II renal c.
    Sakamoto poorly differentiated c.
    salivary gland c.
    sarcomatoid c.
    sarcomatoid thymic c. (STC)
    sarcomatoid urothelial c.
    scar c.
    schneiderian c.
    scirrhous c.
    sclerosing bronchioloalveolar c.
    sclerosing sarcomatoid transitional
      cell c.
    sebaceous c.
    secondary c.
    secretory c.
    serous c.
    serous epithelial ovarian c. (SEOC)
    sertoliform endometrioid c. (SEC)
    c. showing thymus-like
      differentiation (CASTLE)
    signet ring cell c.
    c. simplex
    sinonasal c.
    sinonasal undifferentiated c. (SNUC)
    skin c.
    small-cell lung c. (SCLC)
    small cell neuroendocrine c.
      (SCNC)
    small cell undifferentiated
      neuroendocrine c. (SCUNC)
    solid c.
    spindle cell c.
    sporadic papillary renal cell c.
    squamous cell c. (SCC)
    stomach c.
    stump c.
    superficial multicentric basal cell c.
    sweat gland c. (SGC)
    terminal duct c.
    testis c.
    thymic c.
    thyroid c.
    trabecular c.
    transitional cell c. (TCC)
    trichilemmal cystic squamous cell c.
    tubular c.
    tubulopapillary c.
    undifferentiated epidermoid c.
    undifferentiated squamous cell c.
    urachal c.
    ureteral c.
    urothelial c. (UcA)
    usual type papillary c. (UTPC)
    uterine endometrial c. (UEC)

    uterine serous c. (USC)
    uterine surface c.
    vaginal c.
    Vaterian c.
    verrucous c.
    villous c.
    Walker c.
    warty c.
    well-differentiated c. (WDCA)
    c. with adenomatous areas (CWA)
    Wolfe breast c.
    wolffian duct c.
    yolk sac c.
carcinomas (*pl. of* carcinoma)
carcinomata (*pl. of* carcinoma)
carcinomatoid
carcinomatosa
    lymphangitis c.
carcinomatosis
    leptomeningeal c.
    meningeal c.
carcinomatous
    c. component
    c. encephalomyelopathy
    c. epithelium
    c. implant
    c. meningoencephalopathy
    c. micrometastasis
    c. myelopathy
    c. myopathy
    c. neuromyopathy
    c. pericarditis
carcinosarcoma
    embryonal c.
    female genital tract c. (FGTCS)
    renal c.
    Walker c.
carcinosis
carcinostatic
carcoma
card
    CloneSaver c.
    ecarin clotting time test c.
    Guthrie c.
CARD
    catalyzed reporter deposition
card-amplified
    c.-a. nanogold-gold staining
    c.-a. nanogold-silver staining
cardiac
    c. albuminuria
    c. amyloidosis
    c. aneurysm
    c. ascites
    c. calculus
    c. catheterization
    c. cell necrosis
    c. cirrhosis
    c. concussion

c. decompensation
c. diet
c. dilation
c. disease
c. diuretic
c. edema
c. enlargement (CE)
c. enzymes/isoenzymes
c. failure (CF)
c. failure cell
c. gland
c. gland of esophagus
c. glycoside
c. hemoptysis
c. heterotaxia
c. histiocyte
c. index (CI)
c. muscle
c. muscle tissue
c. myocyte
c. myxoma (CM)
c. polyp
C. Reader
C. Reader D-Dimer test
C. Reader IQC test strip
C. Reader M myoglobin test
C. Reader T quantitative troponin-T test
c. sclerosis
c. shunt detection
c. silhouette
c. standstill
C. STATus CK-MB/myoglobin panel test
C. STATus CK-MB test
C. STATus controls for troponin I
C. STATus myoglobin/troponin I test
C. STATus rapid assay
C. STATus rapid format troponin I panel test
c. tamponade
c. thrombosis
C. T rapid assay
C. T rapid assay for troponin T
c. valve myxomatosis
c. valvular malformation
c. valvular regurgitation
cardiaca
adiposis c.
cardia intestinal metaplasia (CIM)
cardiasthenia
Cardiasure cardiac markers control
cardiectasis
cardiffensis
Actinomyces c.
cardinal manifestation of wet beriberi
cardioauditory
Cardiobacteriaceae
Cardiobacterium

C. hominis
C. valvarum
C. violaceum
cardiocentesis
cardiochalasia
cardiogenic shock
CardioGram
Cardio-Green (CG)
cardioid condenser
cardiolipin
c. antibody syndrome
c. test
cardiolith
cardiomalacia
cardiomegaly
cardiomyoliposis
cardiomyopathy (CMP)
alcoholic c.
beer drinker's c.
congestive c.
dilated c.
familial c.
hypertrophic obstructive c. (HOCM)
idiopathic c.
primary c.
restrictive c.
uremic c.
cardionecrosis
cardionector hypothesis
cardiopathy
cardioplegia
cardioptosia, cardioptosis
cardioptosis (*var. of* cardioptosia)
cardiopulmonary (CP)
c. bypass
c. exercise testing
c. function
c. sleep study
c. stress test
cardiotocography
cardiotoxicity
anthracycline c.
hydroxychloroquine c.
cardiotoxic myolysis
cardiovascular (CV)
c. disease (CVD)
c. malformation
c. renal disease (CVRD)
c. system and central nervous system (CVS/CNS)
Cardiovirus
carditis
rheumatic c.
streptococcal c.
verrucous c.
care
plan of c. (POC)
point of c. (POC)
Careside analyzer

C

caretaker gene
Carey Ranvier technique
carfentanil
Carica papaya
caricis
    Rathayibacter c.
caries
    dental c.
carinate
carinatum
carinii
    Pneumocystis c.
cariogenesis
carious
Carlavirus
carlsbadense
    Halosimplex c.
carlsbergensis
    Saccharomyces c.
carmalum
carminate
    Nonomuraea roseoviolacea
    subsp. *c.*
carmine
    alum c.
    chrome alum c.
    indigo c.
    lithium c.
    Schneider c.
carminic acid
carminophil, carminophile,
  carminophilous
carminophile (*var. of* carminophil)
carminophilous (*var. of* carminophil)
carmonensis
    Virgibacillus c.
Carmovirus
carmustine
carnaria
    Sarcophaga c.
carnea, *gen.* carneae
    columnae carneae
    trabeculae carneae
    tunica c.
carneae (*gen. of* carnea)
carneous
    c. degeneration
    c. mole
Carney
    C. complex
    C. syndrome
carnification
carniphilus
    Vagococcus c.
carnis
    Clostridium c.
carnitine
    c. palmitoyltransferase 2 (CPT2)
    c. palmitoyltransferase 2 deficiency

Carnobacterium
    C. inhibens
    C. maltaromaticum
    C. viridans
carnosa
    membrana c.
carnosinase
carnosine
carnosinemia
carnosinuria
carnosity
carnosus
Carnoy fixative
Caroli
    C. disease
carolinense
    Solanum c.
carotene assay
carotenemia
carotenoid
caroticum
    glomus c.
caroticus
    nodulus c.
carotid
    c. artery occlusion
    c. artery stenosis
    c. body tumor
    c. cavernous fistula
    c. disease
    c. endarterectomy
    c. sinus syndrome
carotovorum
CA-RP
    carbonic anhydrase-related protein
carpal
    c. tunnel decompression
    (CTD)
    c. tunnel syndrome
Carpenter syndrome
carpet tack follicular keratotic plug
Carpoglyphus passularum
carrageenin
    lambda c.
    c. solution
Carrell test
carrier
    asymptomatic c.
    c. cell
    convalescent c.
    female c.
    c. gas
    incubatory c.
    c. protein
    c. state
    c. strain
carrier-free (CF)
carrier-mediated transport
Carríon disease

carrionii
> *Cladosporium* c.
> *Hormodendrum* c.

Carr-Price
> C.-P. reaction
> C.-P. test

carry-over effect
Carson formalin
Carswell grape
cart
> Reach & Roll c.

Carter black mycetoma
carteri
> *Borrelia* c.

cartesian
> c. coordinates
> c. nomogram

cartilage
> c. and bone comparison
> c. bone
> calcified c.
> c. capsule
> c. cell
> cellular c.
> connecting c.
> elastic c.
> hyaline c.
> hypsiloid c.
> interosseous c.
> c. lacuna
> c. matrix
> c. matrix alteration
> precursory c.
> reticular c.
> c. space
> temporary c.
> uniting c.
> Y c.
> yellow c.

cartilage-hair hypoplasia (CHH)
cartilaginea
> exostosis c.

cartilaginoid
cartilaginous
> c. metaplasia
> c. rest
> c. tissue

cartilago
cartridge
> HDL direct test prefilled c.
> LDL direct test prefilled c.

Cartwright antigen
caruncle
> Santorini major c.
> Santorini minor c.
> urethral c.

Caryophanaceae
Caryophanales

caryothecae
> cisterna c.

Cary 100 UV-Vis spectrophotometer
CAS
> cold agglutinin syndrome
> CAS DNA staining kit
> CAS 200 Image Analysis system
> CAS 200 image cytometer

cascade
> chain-reaction c.
> coagulation c.
> c. filtration
> metastatic c.
> ras c.

case
> c. fatality rate
> c. history
> index c.
> sentinel c.

caseating
> c. granuloma
> c. granulomatous inflammation

caseation
> c. necrosis

case-control study
casei
> *Corynebacterium* c.
> *Lactobacillus* c.
> *Piophila* c.
> *Staphylococcus succinus*
> subsp. *c.*

casein
> c. agar
> c. hydrolysate

caseinate
> sodium c.

caseosa
> vernix c.

caseous
> c. abscess
> c. degeneration
> c. inflammation
> c. necrosis
> c. osteitis
> c. pneumonia
> c. tubercle

CaSki cell
Casman broth
Casoni intradermal test
caspase
> c. immunoreactivity
> c. protein

caspase-14
caspium
> *Corynebacterium* c.

cassette
> ATP-binding c. (ABC)

cassiicola
> *Corynespora* c.

C

cast
    bacterial urinary c.
    bile c.
    blood c.
    broad urinary c.
    coma c.
    corrosion c.
    crystal urinary c.
    decidual c.
    endometrial c.
    epithelial cell urinary c.
    false c.
    fatty urinary c.
    fibrinous c.
    fungal c.
    granular urinary c.
    hemoglobin c.
    hyaline urinary c.
    mucous c.
    muddy brown
     urinary c.
    OFB c.
    red blood cell c.
    renal c.
    RTE cell c.
    spurious c.
    tube c.
    urinary c.
    vascular corrosion c.
    waxy urinary c.
    WBC urinary c.
    white blood cell c.
Castellanella castellani
castellani
    Castellanella c.
    C. disease
    C. test
    Trypanosoma c.
castellanii
    Acanthamoeba c.
castenholzii
    Roseiflexus c.
casting
CASTLE
    carcinoma showing thymus-like
    differentiation
Castle factor
Castleman
    C. disease
    C. syndrome
castor bean
castration
    c. cell
    female c.
    male c.
casualty
    irradiated c.
cat
    c. distemper virus

    c. liver fluke
    c. unit
CAT
    chlormerodrin accumulation test
Cat
catabolic
    c. enzyme
    c. flow phase
catabolism
    antibody c.
    protein c.
catabolite
    c. activator protein
    c. repression
cataclysm
catagen
catagenesis
catalase
catalase-negative organism
catalase-positive organism
catalasia
    anenzymia c.
catalasitica
    Crocinitomix c.
Catalpa
catalysis
    contact c.
catalyst
    negative c.
catalytic
catalyze
catalyzed
    c. reporter deposition (CARD)
    c. signal amplification system
catalyzer
catanella
    Gonyaulax c.
cataphoresis
cataphoretic
cataphylaxis
cataplasia, cataplasis
cataplasis (*var. of* cataplasia)
catapulting
    pressure c.
cataract
    poikiloderma atrophicans and c.
    posterior subcapsular c. (PSC)
    progeria with c.
cataracta
    c. brunescens
    c. caerulea
    c. centralis pulverulenta
    c. complicata
    c. nigra
catarrh
    dry c.
catarrhal
    c. appendicitis
    c. conjunctivitis

c. dysentery
c. gastritis
c. inflammation
c. jaundice
catarrhalis
Branhamella c.
herpes c.
Moraxella c.
catastrophe
obstetric c.
catastrophic complication
catatorulin test
catatrichy
cat-bite fever
catechin
catechinic acid
catechol
catecholamine
adrenomedullary c.
c. assay
c. fraction
c. test
urinary c.
catechol-O-methyl transferase (COMT)
catechuic acid
categorical data
category
c. A, B, C agent
epizootic disease, c. A, B
catellatispora
Actinomadura c.
Catellatospora koreensis
Catellibacterium nectariphilum
Catenabacterium
catenaformis
Lactobacillus c.
catenating
catenatus
Catenibacterium mitsuokai
cateniformis
Coprobacillus c.
catenin
adherens junction-associated c.
alpha c.
beta c.
gamma c.
catenoid
catenulate
caterpillar
c. cell
urticating c.
Cathaemasia
cathartic colon
cathemoglobin
cathepsin
c. B, D, E, K, L, S
c. D antibody
c. D enzyme
c. K gene

cathepsin-mediated disease
catheptic enzyme
catheterization
cardiac c.
cathode
c. ray
c. ray tube
cati
Notoedres c.
Toxocara c.
cation
c. channel
c. exchange resin
c. interference
organic c.
cation-anion difference
cationic
c. charge
c. dye
c. trypsinogen gene
catoniae
Porphyromonas c.
cat's
c. cry syndrome
c. eye syndrome
cat-scratch disease (CSD)
cattle
c. plague
c. plague virus
c. wart
Cattoretti technique
catuli
Actinomyces c.
Catu virus
caucasica
Borrelia c.
caudal
c. dipygus duplication
c. sheath
caudalizing agent
caudate nucleus
caudati
corpus nuclei c.
caudatum
Uronema c.
caudatus
Bodo c.
caudorostral
cauliflower ear
Caulimovirus
Caulobacter
Caulobacteraceae
Caulobacterales
Caulobacterineae
Caulochora baumgartneri
causative
cause
constitutional c.
death of other c. (DOC)

cause (*continued*)
    c. of death (COD)
    predisposing c.
    proximate c.
cause-specific death rate
caustic
cauterant
cauterization
cautery artifact
CAV
    congenital absence of vagina
    congenital adrenal virilism
CAV-1
    canine adenovirus 1
Cavare disease
cave
    c. fever
    Meckel c.
Cavemovirus
caveola
caveolin
Cavernicola pilosa
cavernitis, cavernositis
    fibrous c.
cavernosae
    Billroth venae c.
cavernositis (*var. of* cavernitis)
cavernosorum
    trabeculae corporum c.
    tunica albuginea corporum c.
cavernosum
    lipoma c.
    lymphangioma c.
cavernosus
    nevus c.
cavernous
    c. angioma
    c. hemangioma
    c. lymphangiectasis
    c. malformation (CM)
    c. sinus
    c. sinus thrombosis
    c. space
    c. tissue
CAV1 gene
CAV2 gene
caviae
    Chlamydophila c.
    Neisseria c.
cavipalpus
    Ixodes c.
cavitary lesion
cavitating inflammation
cavitation
    temporary c.
cavity
    absorption c.
    body c.
    chorionic c.

    endometrial c.
    idiopathic bone c.
    inflammatory c.
    internal c.
    marrow c.
    maxillectomy c.
    oral c.
    synovial c.
    vitreous c.
cayenne
    mal de C.
    c. pepper spot
cayetanensis
    Cyclospora c.
Cazenave disease
CB
    centroblastic
    chocolate blood
    chronic bronchitis
        CB agar
CBA
    chronic bronchitis with asthma
C-banding stain
CB11 antibody
CBB
    Bethesda-Ballerup group of Citrobacter
C4b-binding protein (C4BP)
CBC
    complete blood count
CBCL
    cutaneous B-cell lymphoma
C5B-9 complex
CBF
    cerebral blood flow
    coronary blood flow
Cbfa1/Runx2 isoform
Cbfa1/Runx2
    transcription factor C.
CBG
    corticosteroid-binding globulin
    cortisol-binding globulin
^{13}C bicarbonate assay
CBN
    cellular blue nevus
CBP
    CREB binding protein
CBR
    chemical, biological, and radiological
CBRN
    chemical, biological, radiological or nuclear
        CBRN weapon
CBRNE
    chemical, biological, radiological, nuclear, explosive
CBS
    capillary blood sugar
    chronic brain syndrome
    citrate-buffered saline

CBV
    central blood volume
    circulating blood volume
    corrected blood volume
CBW
    chemical and biological warfare
CC
    cord compression
    creatinine clearance
CCA
    chick-cell agglutination
    chimpanzee coryza agent
CCAT
    conglutinating complement absorption
      test
CCB
    conventional core biopsy
CCC
    chronic calculous cholecystitis
    clear cell carcinoma
      primary salivary CCC
C$_3$, C$_4$ complement
CCD
    central collodiaphyseal angle
C-cell hyperplasia
CCF
    cephalin-cholesterol flocculation
    compound comminuted fracture
    congestive cardiac failure
CCFH
    cellular cutaneous fibrous histiocytoma
CCH
    circumscribed choroidal hemangioma
14C-cholylglycine breath excretion test
CCK
    cholecystokinin
CCl4
    carbon tetrachloride
CCl$_2$NOH
    dichloroformoxime C.
CC/MCL
    centrocytic/mantle-cell lymphoma
CCMEC
    clear cell myoepithelial carcinoma
C5 convertase
CCP
    ciliocytophthoria
    cyclic citrullinated peptide
CCSK
    clear cell sarcoma of the kidney
CCV
    columnar cell variant
    conductivity cell volume
CD
    cluster of differentiation
      CD antibody
      CD antigen
      CD+
      CD1a

CD1b
CD1c
CD2
CD3
CD5
CD6
CD7
CD9
CD11a
CD11b
CD11c
CDw12
CD13
CD14 antibody
CD14 antibody/antigen
CD16b
CDw17
CD18
CD19
CD20
CD23
CD24
CD25
CD26
CD27
CD28
CD29
CD30
CD31
CD32
CD33
CD35
CD36
CD37
CD38
CD39
CD40
CD41
CD42
CD42b
CD43
CD44
CD45
CD46
CD47
CD48
CD49
CD49a
CD49b
CD49c
CD49d
CD49e
CD49f
CD50
CD51
CD52
CD53
CD54
CD55

CD (*continued*)
    CD56
    CD57
    CD58
    CD59
    CDw60
    CD61
    CD63
    CD64
    CDw65
    CD66a
    CD66b
    CD66c
    CD66d
    CD66e
    CD68 antigen
    CD69
    CD70
    CD71
    CD72
    CD73
    CD74
    CDw75
    CDw76
    CD77
    CDw78
    CD79a
    CD79b
    CD80
    CD81
    CD82
    CD83
    CDw84
    CD85
    CD86
    CD87
    CD88
    CD89
    CDw90
    CD91
    CDw92
    CD93
    CD94
    CD95
    CD96
    CD97
    CD98
    CD100
    CDw101
    CD102
    CD103
    CD104
    CD105
    CD106
    CD107a
    CD107b
    CDw108
    CDw109
    CD115

    CD116
    CDw116
    CD117
    CD117 antibody/antigen
    CD120a
    CD120b
    CDw121a
    CDw121b
    CDw122
    CD123
    CDw124
    CD126
    CDw127
    CDw128
    CD129
    CDw130
    CD138
    CD molecule
    CD protease
    CD protein
    CD white blood
      cell
cd
    candela
CD$_{50}$
    median curative dose
2-CDA
    2-chlorodeoxyadenosine
CDA
    congenital dyserythropoietic anemia
      CDA type I–III
CD2AP
CDC
    cell-dependent cytotoxicity
    Centers for Disease Control
    chenodeoxycholic acid
    collecting duct carcinoma
      CDC Category A biological agents
        (the highest risk)
      CDC Category B biological agents
        (next highest risk)
      CDC Category C biological agents
        (third highest risk)
      CDC category of biological agent
      CDC test
CD4/CD8 count
CD11/CD18 deficiency
CD55/CD59
    Cellquant CD38/CD8-PE, C.
CD-Chex
    CD-C. C34 control for flow
      cytometry
    CD-C. Plus control for flow
      cytometry
CDH
    congenital dislocation of hip
CD44H
CDH1 gene
CD99 immunostain

CDK
cyclin-dependent kinase
CDK5
cyclin-dependent kinase 5
Cdk4/6-cyclin D complex
CDK4 gene
CDKI
cyclin-dependent kinase inhibitor
CD4 lymphopenia
CD15 marker
CD205 marker
cDNA
complementary DNA
cDNA clone
cDNA library
CDP
continuous distending pressure
cytidine diphosphate
CDP-diglyceride
CDP-ethanolamine
CDR
complementarity determining
region
CD10 stain
CD34 staining
CdTOX A OIA
CD44v6
CD44v6 score
CD44v6 staining in prostate
carcinoma
CD44v6-specific probe
CDX1 intestine-specific transcription factor
CDX2
CDX2 immunohistochemical marker
CDX2 intestine-specific transcription
factor
CE
California encephalitis
capillary zone electrophoresis
cardiac enlargement
CEA
carcinoembryonic antigen
crystalline egg albumin
CEA assay
CEA Gold-5 stain
CEA immunoperoxidase stain
CEA test
CEACAM1
carcinoembryonic antigen-related cell
adhesion molecule 1
CEACAM1 expression
ceanothus extract
CEAP
clinical manifestations, etiologic factors,
anatomic involvement,
pathophysiologic features
CEAP classification of venous
disorders

cebocephalus
cebocephaly
ceca (*pl. of* cecum)
cecal carcinoma
cecitis
cecum, caecum, *pl.* **ceca**
cedar oil
Cedecea
CEDIA
cloned enzyme donor immunoassay
CEDIA drug of abuse test
CEDIA sirolimus assay
cedrina
Pseudomonas c.
Ceelen-Gellerstedt syndrome
CEEV
Central European encephalitis virus
CEF
chick embryo fibroblast
cefaclor
cefamandole
cefoperazone
cefotaxime
cefoxitin
cefsulodin-Irgasan-novobiocin (CIN)
c.-I.-n. agar
C1EInh
C1 esterase inhibitor
CEJO65 monoclonal antibody
CEL
chronic eosinophilic leukemia
celebensis
Raillietina c.
Celebes vibrio
celestine blue B
celiac
c. crisis
c. disease
c. rickets
c. sprue
celiocentesis
celioma
celiomyositis
celioparacentesis
celiopathy
celitis
2-cell
cell
A c.
absorption c.
absorptive c.
acanthoid c.
accessory c.
acid c.
acidophil c.
acinar c.
acinous c.
acoustic c.
c. adhesion molecule (CAM)

cell (*continued*)
 adipose c.
 adrenal cortex c.
 adrenocorticotropic c.
 adult stem c.
 adventitial reticular c.
 c. aggregation
 agranular c.
 A549 human lung carcinoma c.
 air c.
 albuminous c.
 algoid c.
 alpha c.
 alveolar c.
 Alzheimer c.
 amacrine c.
 ameboid c.
 amniogenic c.
 amnion c.
 amphicrine c.
 amphophil c.
 anabiotic c.
 anaplastic c.
 c. anchorage
 aneuploid c.
 angioblastic c.
 angulate c.
 Anitschkow c.
 anterior ethmoidal air c.
 anterior horn c.
 antibody-forming c.
 antibody producing plasma c.
 antigen-presenting c. (APC)
 antigen-responsive c.
 antigen-sensitive c.
 antigen-transporting c.
 apolar c.
 apoptotic c.
 argentaffin c.
 argyrophilic enterochromaffin-like c.
 Arias-Stella c.
 Armanni-Ebstein c.
 Aschoff c.
 Askanazy c.
 astroglia c.
 atypical c.
 auditory receptor c.
 autologous lymphokine activated
  killer c.
 autologous peripheral blood stem c.
  (Auto-PBSC)
 c. axis
 axon of neuroglial c.
 axon of pyramidal c.
 B c.
 balloon c.
 band c.
 barrier-layer c.
 basal c.

 basaloid c.
 basilar c.
 basket c.
 basophil c.
 beaker c.
 Beale ganglion c.
 Berger c.
 berry c.
 beta c.
 Betz c.
 Bevan-Lewis c.
 binucleate c.
 biochemical fuel c.
 bipolar c.
 bipotential c.
 bite c.
 Bizzozero red c.
 blast c.
 blastema c.
 blastemal c.
 blister c.
 bloated c.
 c. block preparation
 blood c.
 c. body
 Boettcher c.
 Boll c.
 bone marrow precursor c.
 border c.
 Böttcher c.
 bovine red blood c. (BRBC)
 c. bridge
 bristle c.
 bronchic c.
 bronchiolar exocrine c.
 brood c.
 brush bipolar c.
 buffy-coated c.
 bulliform c.
 burr c.
 c. button
 C c.
 Cajal c.
 caliciform c.
 calicoblast c.
 cap c.
 capsular c.
 capsule c.
 cardiac failure c.
 carrier c.
 cartilage c.
 CaSki c.
 castration c.
 caterpillar c.
 CD white blood c.
 c. center
 centrifugal bipolar c.
 centroacinar c.
 centrocytelike c. (CLL)

centrofollicular c.
chalice c.
chief c.
chromaffin c.
chromophobe c.
chronic lymphosarcoma c.
ciliated c.
circulating reticuloendothelial c.
Clara c.
Claudius c.
clear c.
cleaved follicular center c.
clonal proliferated c.
clonogenic c.
clue c.
CMV-negative allogeneic c.
c. coat
cochlear hair c.
coelenterazine-treated c.
column c.
columnar absorptive c.
comet c.
commissural c.
committed c.
companion c.
compound granule c.
cone bipolar c.
conjunctival c.
connective tissue c.
contrasuppressor c.
control c.
Conway c.
cornified c.
Corti c.
c. count
c. counter
c. coupling
crenated c.
crescent c.
crystal c.
cuboidal c.
c. cycle
c. cycle arrest
c. cycle S phase
c. cycle time
cytomegalic c.
cytotoxic T c.
cytotrophoblastic c.
D c.
dark c.
daughter c.
Davidoff c.
c. death
c. death gene
decidual c.
decoy c.
deep c.
degenerating secretory c.
Deiters c.

delta c.
dendritic c. (DC)
dendritic clear c.
dendritic epidermal c.
deposit of amyloid in islet c.
dermal dendritic c.
destruction of pancreatic beta c.
c. differentiation
diffuse ganglion c.
diploid c.
displaced ganglion c.
dissociated islet c.
c. division
DNA-aneuploid tumor c.
Dogiel c.
dome c.
Dorothy Reed c.
Downey c.
ductular reactive c.
dust c.
early B c.
early myeloid progenitor c.
ectoblastic c.
ectodermal c.
effector c.
electrochemical c.
electrolytic c.
electromotive force c.
elongated c.
embryonic germ c.
embryonic stem c.
emigration of white cells
enamel c.
end c.
endocervical c.
endocrine c.
endodermal c.
endometrial c.
endothelial c.
c. engraftment
enterochromaffin c.
enteroendocrine c.
entodermal c.
c. envelope
ependymal c.
epidermic c.
epithelial reticular c.
epithelioid c.
epulis c.
E rosette-forming c.
erythrocytic blood c.
erythroid precursor c.
erythropoietin-responsive c. (ERC)
eta c.
ethmoidal c.
exocrine c.
exploding crypt c.
external pillar c.
exudation c.

C

cell (*continued*)
F+ c.
faggot c.
fasciculata c.
fat c.
fat-storing c.
FCL c.
Ferrata c.
Ficoll-Paque purified c.
fixed c.
flame c.
flat bipolar c.
flattened c.
floor c.
foam c.
folded c.
follicular cell lymphoma c. (FCL)
follicular center c. (FCC)
follicular dendritic c. (FDC)
follicular epithelial c.
follicular ovarian c.
foreign body giant c.
formative c.
free c.
frozen red blood c.
fuchsinophil c.
fusiform c.
c. fusion
G c.
galvanic c.
gamma c.
ganglion c.
gastric argentaffin c.
gastric parietal c.
gastric zymogenic c.
gastrointestinal mucosal c.
gastrointestinal pacemaker c.
Gaucher c.
Gegenbaur c.
gemistocytic c.
generative c.
genetically abnormal c.
Gerbich-negative red c.
germ c.
germinal c.
ghost c.
giant c.
Gierke c.
gitter c.
glandular c.
Gley c.
glia c.
glial c.
glitter c.
glomerulosa c.
glomus c.
goblet c.
Golgi c.
Goormaghtigh c.

granule c.
granulocytic blood c.
granulocytic precursor c.
granulosa lutein c.
grape c.
great alveolar c.
ground glass c.
guanine c.
guard c.
gustatory c.
gyrochrome c.
hair c. (HC)
hairy c.
hallmark of protein-secreting c.
hallmark of steroid-secreting c.
Hanseman c.
haploid c.
Hargraves c.
heart failure c.
HEK c.
HEL c.
HeLa c.
helmet c.
helper T c.
hematopoietic cord blood c.
hematopoietic progenitor c. (HPC)
hematopoietic stem c. (HSC)
HEMPAS c.
Hensen c.
hepatic progenitor c.
hepatic stellate c.
heteromeric c.
HGPRT-deficient c.
hilar c.
hilus c.
hobnail c.
Hodgkin and Reed-Sternberg c.
Hofbauer c.
homozygous typing c.
c. honeycombing
horny c.
horse red blood c. (HRBC)
Hortega c.
HOSE c.
hot c.
HPRT-deficient c.
HRS c.
human alpha-lactalbumin made lethal
  to tumor cells (HAMLET)
human dermal microvascular
  endothelial c. (HDMEC)
human umbilical vein endothelial c.
  (HUVEC)
Hürthle c.
hyaline c.
hybrid c.
c. hybridization
hyperchromatic c.
hyperdiploid c. (HDC)

hypertrophic amphophil c.
hypotetraploid c.
hypoxic c.
I c.
immunocompetent c. (ICC)
immunohistochemical stain for T c.
immunologically activated c.
immunologically competent c.
Immuno-trol c.
c. inclusion
inclusion c.
indifferent c.
inducer c.
infiltration of leukemic c.
inflammatory c.
c. injury
inner hair c.
inner phalangeal c.
innocent bystander c.
c. interaction (CI)
intercalary c.
intercapillary c.
intercellular canaliculus of
  parietal c.
interdigitating dendritic c. (IDC)
interdigitating reticulum c.
intermediate c.
internal pillar c.
internuncial c.
intestinal crypt c.
intimal c.
intracytoplasmic inclusion c.
intrasinusoidal cytokeratin-positive
  mesothelial c.
irreversibly sickled c. (ISC)
irritation c.
islet alpha c.
islet beta c.
islet delta c.
Ito c.
c. junction
juvenile c.
juxtaglomerular c.
K c.
karyochrome c.
keratinized c.
killer c. (K cell)
c. kinetics
Ki-67 positive c.
koilocytotic c.
Kulchitsky c.
Kupffer c.
L c.
C. Lab IC 100 image cytometer
labile c.
lacis c.
lactate dehydrogenase, aspartate
  aminotransferase, white blood c.'s
  (LAW)

lacunar c.
lacZ-tagged c.
Langhans giant c.
large c. (LC)
large unstained c. (LUC)
late cortical T c.
LE c.
Leclanché c.
Leishman chrome c.
lepra c.
leukocyte-poor packed red blood
  cells
leukocyte-reduced red blood cells
Leydig interstitial c.
L-H c.
light chain class-restricted B c.
c. line
c. lineage analysis
lining c.
lipid-rich neoplastic c.
Lipschtz c.
littoral c.
locomotive c.
Loevit c.
lupus erythematosus c.
luteal c.
lutein c.
luteum c.
lymph c.
lymphoblastic plasma c.
lymphocytic blood c.
lymphoid progenitor c.
lymphoid stem c.
lymphokine-activated killer c.
lymphoplasmacytoid c.
M c.
macroglia c.
malignant Hodgkin and
  Reed-Sternberg c.
malpighian c.
mammosomatotroph c.
Marchand wandering c.
marrow c.
Martinotti c.
mast c.
c. matrix
maturation B c.
mature B c.
mediator c.
medullary carcinoma c.
medullary interstitial c.
medullary T c.
medulloepithelial c.
megakaryocytic blood c.
melanotropic c.
c. membrane
c. membrane interdigitation
memory B, T c.
Merkel-Ranvier c.

C

cell (*continued*)

Merkel tactile c.
mesangial c.
mesenchymal c.
mesoderm c.
mesoglial c.
mesothelial c.
metallophil c.
metaphase c.
metaplastic c.
Mexican hat c.
Meynert c.
microfold c.
microglia c.
microglial c.
middle c.
midget bipolar c.
migratory c.
Mikulicz c.
mirror-image c.
mitral c.
modified red blood c.
monocytic blood c.
monocytic precursor c.
monocytoid c.
c. monolayer
mononuclear c.
monosomic c.
monosynaptic bipolar c.
mop bipolar c.
Mosher air c.
mossy c.
mother c.
motile c.
motor c.
Mott c.
MRC-5 human diploid fibroblast c.
^{99m}Tc labeled red blood c.
mucoalbuminous c.
mucoserous c.
mucous neck c.
Müller radial c.
multinucleated c.
multinucleated giant c. (MGC)
multipolar c.
mummified c.
mural c.
myeloid stem c.
myeloma c.
myocardial endocrine c.
myoepithelial c.
myogenic c.
myoid c.
Nageotte c.
naive c.
natural killer c.
navicular c.
neoplastic epidermal c.
nerve c.

c. nest
Neumann c.
neural crest c.
neurilemma c.
neuroectoderm-derived c.
neuroendocrine transducer c.
neuroepithelial c.
neuroglia c.
neuroglial c.
neurological c.
neuroprogenitor c.
neurosecretory c.
nevus c.
Niemann-Pick c.
no lymph nodes containing cancer
  c.'s (N0)
nonadherent c.
noncleaved follicular center c.
nonflagellated vegetative c.
nonfollicular center c. (non-FCC)
nonleukoreduced red c.
nonreplicating c.
normal complement of c.'s
nuclear wreath c.
nucleated red blood c.
null c.
nurse c.
oat c.
c. of Fañanás
olfactory receptor c.
oligodendrogenic c.
oligodendroglia c.
oligodendroglia-like c. (OLC)
oncocytic c.
Opalski c.
c. organelle
Ortho-Kung T c. (OKT)
osseous c.
osteochondrogenic c.
osteoclast-like giant c. (OLGC)
osteogenic c.
osteoprogenitor c.
outer hair c.
outer phalangeal c.
oval-shaped goblet c.
owl eye c.
oxyntic c.
oxyphil c.
oxyphilic c.
P c.
packed human blood c.'s
packed red blood c.'s (PRBC)
pagetoid foam c.
pillar c.
pineal c.
plaque-forming c. (PFC)
plasma c. (PC)
plasma blood c.
plasmacytic blood c.

pleomorphic binucleated giant c.
pleomorphic mononucleated giant c.
plump c.
pluripotent hematopoietic stem c.
pluripotential basal c.
pluripotential hemopoietic stem c.
pluripotential stem c. (PSC)
pluripotential stromal c.
pluripotent myeloid stem c.
pluripotent primitive mesodermal c.
polar c.
c. polarity
polychromatic c.
polychromatophil c.
polygonal c.
polyhedral c.
popcorn c.
Portland c.
positive c.
posterior c.
postmitotic c.
pre-B c.
preconfluent c.
precornified c.
precursor c.
predominant c.
pregnancy c.
pregranulosa c.
prickle c.
primary embryonic c.
primitive-looking c.
primitive neuroblastic c.
primitive reticular c.
primordial germ c.
primordial sex c.
principal c.
prismatic follicular c.
progenitor c.
prolactin c.
c. proliferation
prolymphocyte c.
pseudo-Gaucher c.
pseudosarcomatous c.
pseudounipolar c.
pseudoxanthoma c.
pulmonary neuroendocrine c. (PNEC)
pulpar c.
Purkinje c.
pus c.
pyknotic c.
pyramidal c.
pyroninophilic blast c.
pyrrol c.
RA c.
RACE c.
radiosensitivity of specialized c.
ragocyte c.
Raji c.
reactive c.

reagent red blood c.
red blood c. (RBC)
Reed c.
Reed-Sternberg c. (RS)
Reed-variant c.
regeneration c.
renal tubular epithelial c.
Renshaw c.
reproductive c.
reserve c.
resident c.
responder c.
resting B c.
resting wandering c.
restructured c.
reticular c.
reticularis c.
reticuloendothelial c.
reticulum c.
rhabdoid c.
rhagiocrine c.
Rieder c.
Rindfleisch c.
rod nuclear c.
rod photoreceptor c.
Rolando c.
rosette-forming c.
Rouget c.
round c.
rounded mononuclear c.
RTE c.
Russell-Crooke c.
S c.
Sala c.
c. salvage
c. sap
sarcogenic c.
satellite c.
scavenger c.
Schilling band c.
Schultze c.
Schwann c.
secretory c.
sedimented red c. (SRC)
c. seeding
segmented c.
self-renewing c.
sensitized c.
c. separation method
septal c.
seromucous c.
serous c.
Sertoli c.
sex c.
Sézary c.
shadow c.
sheep red blood c. (SRBC)
sickle c. (SC)
sickled c.

cell (*continued*)

signet ring c.
SiHa c.
silver c.
single-to-multiple layers of follicular c.
sinusoidal endothelial c.
skein c.
small cleaved c.
small noncleaved c. (SNCC)
smooth muscle c.
smudge c.
smudged c.
solid masses of epithelial c.
somatic c.
somatostatin-producing small c.
c. sorting analysis
sperm c.
spider c.
spindle c.
spindle-shaped neoplastic stromal c.
spindly squamoid c.
spine c.
splenic c.
spur c.
squamous alveolar c.
squamous epithelial c.
stab c.
stable c.
staff c.
static balance receptor c.
stellate c.
stem c.
Stem-Trol control c.
Sternberg giant c.
Sternberg-Reed c.
Sternheimer-Malbin positive c.
stichochrome c.
stimulator c.
stipple c.
c. strain
strap c.
stroma c.
subnuclear vacuolated c.
superficial c.
supporting c.
suppressor c.
surface absorptive c.
c. surface glycoprotein
c. surface immunophenotyping
c. surface marker
surface mucous c.
c. surface receptor
survival of cancer c.
suspicious c.
sustentacular c.
sympathetic formative c.
sympathicotropic c.
sympathochromaffin c.

sympathotropic c.
syncytiotrophoblastic c.
synovial c.
tactile c.
tadpole c.
tailed red c.
tanned red c. (TRC)
tapetal c.
target c.
tart c.
taste c.
T cytotoxic c.
TDTH c.
teardrop red c.
tendon c.
tennis racket c.
terphase c.
tetracarcinoma c.
Tg c.
theca interna c.
theca lutein c.
T helper c.
thryotroph c.
thymic epithelial c.
thymic reticulum c.
thymus-dependent c.
thymus-derived c.
thymus nurse c.
Tiselius electrophoresis c.
Tm c.
T-natural killer c. (TNK)
Toker clear c.
totipotent c.
totipotential stem c.
touch c.
Touton giant c.
c. traffic
transducer c.
c. transformation
transitional c.
transport of cancer c.
trisomic c.
trophoblast c.
T-suppressor c.
tube c.
tufted c.
tumor c.
tunnel c.
Türk c.
tympanic c.
type A intercalated c.
type B intercalated c.
type C nevus c.
type I c.
type II alveolar epithelial c.
typical smooth muscle c.
Tzanck c.
umbrella c.
undifferentiated c.

unipolar c.
unit c.
Unna c.
vacuolated c.
van Hansemann c.
vascular smooth muscle c. (VSMC)
vasoformative c.
vegetative c.
veil c.
veiled c.
Vero c.
vestibular hair c.
Vignal c.
Virchow c.
virgin B c.
virus-transformed c.
visual receptor c.
vitreous c.
c. volume (CV)
volume of packed c.'s (VPC)
volume of packed red c.'s
  (VPRC)
c. volume profile (CVP)
c. wall
c. wall defective bacteria culture
c. wall-deficient bacterial form
  (CWDF)
Walthard c.
wandering c.
Warthin-Finkeldey multinucleate
  giant c.
washed red c. (WRC)
washed red blood c.
wasserhelle c.
water-clear c.
c. web
white blood c. (WBC)
whorling c.
WI-38 c.
wing c.
xanthoma c.
yolk c.
Zeiss counting c.
zombie c.
zymogenic c.
CellaVision DM96 system
CellBIND cell culture surface
cell-bound antibody
cell-cell
  c.-c. adhesion molecule
  c.-c. contact region
  c.-c. interaction
Cell-Chex body fluid procedural control
cell-cycle
  c.-c. inhibitor
  c.-c. inhibitory protein
  c.-c. perturbation
  c.-c. regulator
cell-dependent cytotoxicity (CDC)

**Cell-Dyn 1200, 3200, 4000 automated
  cell counting instrument**
Cellfalcicula
cell-fat ratio
cell-free system
cellicolous
cell-mediated
  c.-m. immunity (CMI)
  c.-m. lympholysis assay
  c.-m. reaction
cellobiase
cellobiose
celloidin section
cellophane tape method
Cellosolve
CellPrep sample preparation system
CellProbe
  C. cytoenzymology reagent
  C. HT caspase-3/7 whole cell assay
Cellquant
  C. CD38/CD8-PE, CD55/CD59
  C. Kit
**CellQuest Pro 4.0 flow cytometry
  software**
cell-substrate adhesion molecule
cell-surface
  c.-s. carbohydrate chain
  c.-s. protein
cell-suspension flow cytometry
cell-to-cell adherent protein
cellula, *gen.* **and** *pl.* **cellulae**
  c. ethmoidales
  c. ethmoidales anteriores
  c. ethmoidales mediae
  c. ethmoidales posteriores
  c. pneumaticae tubae auditivae
  c. tympanicae
cellulae (*gen.* and *pl. of* cellula)
cellulans
  Cellulosimicrobium c.
cellular
  c. adaptation
  c. atypia
  c. biology
  c. blue nevus (CBN)
  c. cartilage
  c. cloning
  c. cutaneous fibrous histiocytoma
    (CCFH)
  c. debris
  c. debris centrifuge polarizing
    microscope
  c. degeneration
  c. dyscohesion
  c. embolism
  c. fibronectin
  c. hybridization
  c. immune theory
  c. immunity

C

cellular (*continued*)
  c. immunity deficiency syndrome (CIDS)
  c. infiltration
  c. inhibitor of apoptosis (cIAP)
  c. kinetics
  c. neurothekeoma
  c. pathology
  c. polyp
  c. respiration
  c. schwannoma
  c. senescence
  c. spill
  c. stroma
  c. swelling
  c. tenacity
  c. tumor
cellularity
  mixed c. (MC)
cellulase
cellulicidal
cellulifugal
cellulipetal
cellulite
cellulitic phlegmasia
cellulitis
  eosinophilic c.
  epizootic c.
  orbital c.
  streptococcal c.
cellulocutaneous plague
Cellulomonadaceae
Cellulomonas
  C. humilata
  C. iranensis
  C. persica
  C. xylanilytica
Cellulophaga
  C. algicola
  C. baltica
  C. fucicola
  C. lytica
  C. pacifica
  C. uliginosa
cellulosa
  vagina c.
cellulosae
  Cysticercus c.
cellulose
  c. acetate
  c. caprate
  DEAE c.
  diethylaminoethyl c. (DEAE)
  c. tape technique
cellulosilytica
  Xylanimonas c.
Cellulosimicrobium
  C. cellulans
  C. variabile

cellulosity
Cellvibrio
  C. fibrivorans
  C. fulvus
  C. gandavensis
  C. japonicus
  C. mixtus
  C. ostraviensis
  C. vulgaris
CELO
  chicken embryo lethal orphan CELO virus
celom (*var. of* coelom)
celomic metaplasia
celoschisis
celosomia
celozoic
Celsior solution
Celsius
  C. temperature scale (C)
  C. thermometer
Celsus kerion
cement
  c. corpuscle
  intercellular c.
  c. line
  polymethylmethacrylate c.
  c. substance
  tooth c.
cementification
cementifying fibroma
cementing substance
cementoblast
cementoblastoma
cementoclast
cementocyte
cementoma
  familial gigantiform c. (FGC)
cementosseous dysphasia (COD)
cementossifying fibroma (COF)
cementum
  afibrillar c.
  primary c.
  secondary c.
Cenangium
Cenarchaeales
cenobium
cenocepacia
  Burkholderia c.
Cenococcum
cenocyte, coenocyte
cenocytic
CenSlide 2000 urinalysis system
censored observation
census tract (CT)
center
  cell c.
  chiral c.
  chondrification c.

diaphysial c.
epiotic c.
follicular cell c.
Centers for Disease Control
(CDC)
germinal c. (GC)
ossific c.
Poison Control C.
primary ossification c.
progressive transformation of
germinal c. (PTGC)
proliferation c.
pseudofollicular growth c. (PFGC)
pseudofollicular proliferation c.
reaction c.
center-fire rifle wound
centigrade
c. temperature scale (C)
c. thermometer
centigram (cg)
centiliter (cL)
centimeter (cm)
cubic c. (cm³, cu cm)
centimeter-gram-second (CGS)
c.-g.-s. system
centimorgan (cM, cMO)
centipede
centipoise (cP)
centistoke (cSt)
central
c. achromia
c. blood volume (CBV)
c. body
c. callus
c. canal
c. chemoreceptor
c. chromatolysis
c. clonal deletion
c. collodiaphyseal angle (CCD)
c. core disease
c. diabetes insipidus
C. European encephalitis virus
(CEEV)
C. European tick-borne encephalitis
virus
C. European tick-borne fever
c. excitatory state (CES)
c. ganglioneuroma
c. hemorrhagic necrosis (CHN)
c. hyaline sclerosis
c. inhibitory state (CIS)
c. lacteal
c. lesion
c. limit theorem
c. necrosis
c. nervous system (CNS)
c. nervous system disorder
c. nervous system involvement
c. nervous system tuberculosis

c. nervous system tumor
c. neurocytoma
c. obesity
c. osteitis
c. osteocarcinoma
c. osteosarcoma
c. pit
c. pneumonia
c. pontine myelinolysis
c. pontine myelinosis
c. processing unit
c. radiolucency
c. Recklinghausen disease type II
c. spindle
c. spore
c. tendency
c. type neurofibromatosis
c. venous pressure (CVP)
centralis
area c.
fovea c.
substantia gelatinosa c.
substantia intermedia c.
central-patch infiltrate
centriacinar emphysema
centric fusion
Centriflo filter
centrifugal
c. bipolar cell
c. fast analyzer
c. flotation
c. force
centrifugalization
centrifugalize
centrifugation
cesium chloride gradient c.
density gradient c.
microhematocrit c.
zonal c.
centrifuge
Allegra 64R high-speed refrigerated
benchtop c.
Allegra 25R refrigerated benchtop c.
Allegra X-12, X-15R, X-22
benchtop c.
Avanti J-20XP, J-25, J-30I, J-HC,
J-E c.
CritSpin microhematocrit c.
CytoFuge 2 c.
Eppendorf 5702 c.
HemataSTAT Easy Read c.
J6-HC, J6-MC, J6-MI high capacity
c.
c. microscope
PK110 c.
Spinchron DLX, 15 series c.
Stat-60 c.
StatSpin Express 2 c.
StatSpin MP c.

C

centrifugum
  erythema annulare c.
  leukoderma acquisitum c.
centrilobar steatosis
centrilobular
  c. dilation
  c. emphysema
  c. fibrosis
  c. necrosis
  c. zone
centriole
  anterior c.
  distal c.
  posterior c.
  proximal c.
centripetal force
centroacinar cell
centroblast
centroblastic lymphoma
Centrocestus
centrocyte
centrocytelike cell (CLL)
centrocytic lymphoma
**centrocytic/mantle-cell lymphoma
  (CC/MCL)**
centrofollicular cell
centrolecithal
centromere (cen)
  c. banding stain
  c. enumeration probe (CEP)
  c. interference
centromere/kinetochore antibody
centromeric
  c. band
  c. region
centronuclear myopathy
centroplasm
centrosome
centrosphere
Centrospora acerina
Centruroides suffusus
cenuriasis (*var. of* cenurosis)
cenuris, coenuris
cenurosis, cenuriasis
CEOT
  calcifying epithelial odontogenic
  tumor
CEP
  centromere enumeration probe
  chronic eosinophilic pneumonia
  congenital erythropoietic porphyria
  counterelectrophoresis
    CEP 12 SpectrumOrange DNA
    probe kit
    CEP X, Y SpectrumOrange DNA
    probe kit
cepacia
  Burkholderia c.
  Pseudomonas c.

Cephaelis
cephalalgia, cephalgia
cephaledema
cephalemia
cephalgia (*var. of* cephalalgia)
cephalhematocele, cephalohematocele
cephalhematoma, cephalohematoma
cephalhydrocele
cephalic index
cephalin
  c. flocculation
  c. flocculation test
cephalin-cholesterol
  c.-c. flocculation (CCF)
  c.-c. flocculation test
cephaline
Cephaliophora irregularis
cephalitis
Cephaloascus
cephalocele
cephalocentesis
cephaloglycin
cephalohematocele (*var. of*
  cephalhematocele)
cephalohematoma (*var. of*
  cephalhematoma)
cephalohemometer
cephalomegaly
cephalomeningitis
Cephalomyia
cephalont
cephalooculocutaneous telangiectasia
cephalopathy
cephalopelvic disproportion (CPD)
Cephalopoda
cephaloridine
cephalosporin
Cephalosporium
  C. falciforme
  C. granulomatis
cephalothin
cephalothoracopagus
Cephalotrichum
cephalotrigeminal angiomatosis
cephamycin
**Ceprate SC stem cell concentration
  system**
CEQ 8000, 8800 genetic analysis system
cera
ceramic capacitor
ceramidase
ceramide
  c. dihexoside
  glycosyl c.
  c. lactoside
  lactosyl c.
  c. moiety
  c. trihexosidase
  c. trihexoside (CTH)

Cerasibacillus quisquiliarum
Ceratocystiopsis
Ceratocystis
Ceratophyllidae
Ceratophyllus punjatensis
Ceratopogonidae
c-erb-B2
    c-e.-B. oncoprotein
    c-e.-B. protooncogene
cercaria
cercaria-hullen reaction schistosomiasis
  test
cercarien-hullen-reaktion test
cerci (*pl. of* cercus)
cercocystis
cercomer
cercomonad
Cercomonas
Cercopithecus
Cercospora apii
cercus, *pl.* cerci
cerealis
    Oidiodendron c.
cerebellar
    c. agenesis
    c. amyloid plaque
    c. astrocytoma
    c. cortex
    c. cyst
    c. degeneration
    c. fissure
    c. pontine
    c. sarcoma
    c. tumor
cerebelli
    cortex c.
    fissurae c.
    stratum granulosum corticis c.
    stratum moleculare corticis c.
cerebellin
cerebellitis
cerebellomedullary malformation
  syndrome
cerebellopontine angle tumor
cerebellum
    molecular layer of c.
cerebral
    c. amyloid angiopathy
    c. atrophy
    c. autosomal dominant arteriopathy
      with subcortical infarcts and
      leukoencephalopathy (CADASIL)
    c. blood flow (CBF)
    c. calculus
    c. cladosporiosis
    c. compression
    c. cortex
    c. cortex perfusion rate (CPR)
    c. death

    c. dysplasia
    c. edema
    c. embolism
    c. epidural abscess
    c. glucose oxygen quotient (CG:OQ)
    c. hemorrhage
    c. hernia
    c. herniation
    c. infarct
    c. infarction (CI)
    c. layer of retina
    c. lupus
    c. metabolic rate (CMR)
    c. metabolic rate of glucose
      (CMRG)
    c. metabolic rate of oxygen (CMRO)
    c. palsy (CP)
    c. porosis
    c. salt-washing syndrome
    c. sphingolipidosis
    c. thrombosis (CT)
    c. tuberculosis
cerebralis
    adiposis c.
    Coenurus c.
    mycetism c.
cerebri
    astrocytosis c.
    commotio c.
    cortex c.
    epiphysis c.
    falx c.
    fungus c.
    gliomatosis c.
    hypophysis c.
    c. pseudotumor
cerebriform nucleus
cerebritis
    suppurative c.
cerebrocuprein
cerebrohepatorenal syndrome
cerebromalacia
cerebromeningitis
cerebronic acid
cerebropathia, cerebropathy
cerebropathy (*var. of* cerebropathia)
cerebrosclerosis
cerebroside
    c. beta-galactosidase
    c. beta-glucosidase
    c. lipidosis
    c. sulfatide
cerebrosidosis
cerebrospinal
    c. fever
    c. fluid (CSF)
    c. fluid albumin
    c. fluid albumin index
    c. fluid analysis

C

cerebrospinal (*continued*)
   c. fluid assay
   c. fluid culture
   c. fluid cytology
   c. fluid glucose
   c. fluid glutamine
   c. fluid IgG index
   c. fluid IgG synthesis rate
   c. fluid immunoglobulin
   c. fluid lactate
   c. fluid lactate dehydrogenase
     fractions
   c. fluid lactate dehydrogenase
     isoenzymes
   c. fluid leukocyte count
   c. fluid myelin basic protein
   c. fluid oligoclonal bands
   c. fluid pressure
   c. fluid protein electrophoresis
   c. fluid-to-serum albumin index
   c. fluid total protein
   c. meningitis (CSM)
cerebrospinalis
   liquor c.
cerebrospinant
cerebrosus
   Morococcus c.
cerebrotendinous
   c. cholesterolosis
   c. xanthomatosis
cerebrovascular
   c. accident (CVA)
   c. anomaly
   c. disease (CVD)
   c. malformation (CVM)
   c. obstructive disease (CVOD)
   c. resistance (CVR)
cereus
   Bacillus c.
cerevisiae
   Acetobacter c.
   Saccharomyces c.
Cerinosterus cyanescens
Cerithidea
cerium
ceroid
   c. lipofuscin
   c. pigment
   c. storage disease
ceroidosis
ceroplasty
cerradoensis
   Nocardia c.
cert
   certified
certesii
   Arenibacter c.
certification
   operator c.

certified (cert)
   C. Laboratory Assistant
   c. reference material
   c. stain
   c. standard
cerulea, caerulea
   macula c.
cerulein
ceruleus
   locus c.
ceruloplasmin
   c. assay
   c. level
   c. test
cerumen
ceruminal
ceruminoma
ceruminosae
   glandulae c.
ceruminous
   c. adenoma
   c. carcinoma
   c. gland
cervi
   Lipotena c.
   Setaria c.
cervical
   c. abortion
   c. adenitis
   c. bubo
   c. canal stenosis
   c. carcinoma
   c. culture
   c. disk syndrome
   c. diverticulum
   c. dysplasia
   c. fistula
   c. fracture
   c. gland
   c. gland of uterus
   c. Gram stain
   c. hygroma
   c. intraepithelial neoplasia
   (CIN)
   c. mucus sperm penetration
   test
   c. myalgia
   c. myelopathy
   c. polyp
   c. punch biopsy
   c. radiculitis
   c. rib syndrome
   c. scraper
   c. secretion
   c. smear
   c. somatosensory evoked potential
   c. spondylosis
cervicalis
   Onchocerca c.

cervical-vaginal
    c.-v. cytology
    c.-v. junction
cervices (*pl. of* cervix)
cervicitis
    cystic chronic c.
cervicovaginal
    c. lavage
    c. smear preparation
cervix, *pl.* **cervices**
    AIS of the c.
    epidermidization of c.
    GCC of the uterine c.
    incompetent c.
    c. of the axon
CES
    central excitatory state
cesarean-obtained barrier-sustained
(COBS)
cesium (Cs)
    c. chloride gradient centrifugation
Cestan-Chenais syndrome
Cestan-Raymond syndrome
Cestan syndrome
Cestoda
Cestodaria
cestode, cestoid
cestodiasis
cestoid (*var. of* cestode)
Cestoidea
Cetobacterium somerae
Cetraria
cetrimide agar
cetyl
cetylpyridium chloride test
cetyltrimethylammonium bromide
Ceuthospora
ceylanicum
        Ancylostoma c.
ceylonica
        Haemadipsa c.
Ceylon mouth sore
CF
    carbolfuchsin
    cardiac failure
    carrier-free
    chemotactic factor
    Christmas factor
    citrovorum factor
    complement fixation
    complement-fixing
    correction factor
    cystic fibrosis
        CF antibody
        CF antibody titer
        CF indicator system chloride patch
        CF test
Cf
    californium

cf
    centrifugal force
CFC
    chlorofluorocarbon
CFF
    critical flicker fusion
        CFF test
CFIDS
    chronic fatigue immune dysfunction
      syndrome
CFLP
    cleavase fragment length polymorphism
c-fos oncogene
CFP
    chronic false-positive
    cystic fibrosis of pancreas
CFS
    congenital fibrosarcoma
CFT
    complement-fixation test
CFTR
    cystic fibrosis transmembrane
      conductance regulator
        CFTR gene
CFU
    colony-forming unit
CFU-C
    colony-forming unit-culture
CFUC
    colony-forming unit-culture
CFU-E
    colony-forming unit-erythroid
CFU-GEMM
    colony-forming unit granulocyte,
      erythrocyte, monocyte, and
      megakaryocyte
CFU-GM
    colony-forming unit
      granulocyte-macrophage
CFU-Meg
    colony-forming unit-megakaryocyte
CFU/mL
    colony-forming units/mL
CFU-S
    colony-forming unit-spleen
CFWM
    cancer-free white mouse
CG
    Cardio-Green
    chorionic gonadotropin
    colloidal gold
cg
    centigram
CgA
    chromogranin A
CGD
    chronic granulomatous disease
CGG
    cytosine-guanine-guanine

C

CGH
    comparative genomic hybridization
CGL
    chronic granulocytic leukemia
C-glycocholic acid breath test
cGMP
    cyclic guanosine monophosphate
CGN
    chronic glomerulonephritis
7C gold urine protein test
CG:OQ
    cerebral glucose oxygen quotient
CGP
    chorionic growth hormone prolactin
    circulating granulocyte pool
CGRP
    calcitonin gene-related peptide
CGS
    centimeter-gram-second
CGT
    chorionic gonadotropin
CGTT
    cortisone-glucose tolerance test
CH
    cholesterol
    crown-heel
CHA
    congenital hypoplastic anemia
Chabert disease
Chabertia
chaeta
Chaetocladium
Chaetoconidium
Chaetomidium
Chaetomium
Chaetophoma dermo-unguis
Chaetosphaeronema
chaffeensis
    Ehrlichia c.
chagas
    C. disease
    C. disease serological test
Chagas-Cruz disease
chagasi
    Leishmania donovani c.
chagasii
    Vibrio c.
chagoma
Chagres virus
chahannaoensis
    Natrialba c.
chain
    alpha c.
    amyloid light c.
    beta myosin heavy c.
    branched c.
    cell-surface carbohydrate c.
    electron transport c.
    heavy c.

    hemolytic c.
    invariant c.
    c. isomerism
    J c.
    kappa light c.
    L c.
    lambda light c.
    laminin c.
    light c.
    monoclonal free light c.
    myosin heavy c. 9
    nuclear c.
    c. of custody
    c. reaction
    respiratory c.
    restricted light c.
    ricin A, B c.
    sympathetic c.
chaining
chain-reaction cascade
chains
    homology of c.
Chalara
chalasia, chalasis
chalasis (*var. of* chalasia)
chalaza (*var. of* chalazion)
chalazia (*pl. of* chalazion)
chalazion, chalaza, *pl.* **chalazia**
Chalciporus
chalcogen
chalcogenide
chalcone
chalcosis
chalice cell
chalicosis
challenge
    radioactive c.
    sulfite c.
chalone
chamaecephaly (*var. of* chamecephaly)
chamber
    Abbé-Zeiss counting c.
    anaerobic c.
    Bactron 1.5 anaerobic c.
    Boyden c.
    counting c.
    endothelium of anterior c.
    hyperbaric c.
    ionization c.
    multiwire proportional c.
    Sandison-Clark c.
    Shandon Cytospin c.
    Thoma counting c.
    Zappert counting c.
Chamberland filter
chamecephaly, chamaecephaly
Chameleon Cooler
Championnière disease
Champy fixative

chancre
  hard c.
  mixed c.
  monorecidive c.
  c. redux
  soft c.
  sporotrichositic c.
  tularemic c.
chancriform
  c. pyoderma
  c. syndrome
chancroid
chancroidal ulcer
chancrous
chandelier
  favic c.
Chang aniline-acid fuchsin method
change
  anatomic c.
  Armanni-Ebstein c.
  Crooke hyaline c.
  decidual c.
  degenerative c.
  desmoplastic c.
  DNA sequence copy number c.
  fatty c.
  harlequin color c.
  hyperplastic-like mucosal c. (HPC)
  myxoid c.
  onionskin c.
  polycystic c.
  polyneuropathy, organomegaly,
    endocrinopathy, monoclonal
    gammopathy, and skin changes
    (POEMS)
  postcurettage reparative c.
  progestagenic c.
  pseudobowenoid c.
  pseudocarcinomatous c.
  pseudoepitheliomatous c.
  pseudo-Pelger-Hüet c.
  reactive c.
  reversible c.
  single nucleotide c.
  Tenney c.
channel
  cation c.
  chloride c. 7
  epithelial sodium c. (ENaC)
  ion c.
  ligand-gated c.
  transmitter-gated ion c.
  transnexus c.
  voltage-gated c.
channel-forming integral protein
  (CHIP-1)
channelopathy
Chantemesse reaction
chaotic heart

Chapel Hill Consensus Conference
  classification
chapellei
  Geobacter c.
chaperone
  molecular c.
character
  acquired c.
  c. density
  dominant c.
  mendelian c.
  monogenic c.
  primary sex c.
  recessive c.
  secondary sex c.
  sex-conditioned c.
  sex-limited c.
  sex-linked c.
  X-linked c.
  Y-linked c.
characteristic
  c. curve
  organism c.
  c. pathologic
  receiver operating c. (ROC)
  ultrastructural c.
characterization
  definitive c.
  molecular c.
charcoal
  activated c.
  coelenterazine dextran-coated c.
  dextran-coated c. (DCC)
  c. yeast extract agar
Charcot
  C. arthropathy
  C. disease
  C. syndrome
  C. triad
Charcot-Böttcher crystalloid
Charcot-Bouchard microaneurysm
Charcot-Leyden
  C.-L. crystal
  C.-L. crystalloid
Charcot-Marie-Tooth
  C.-M.-T. disease
  C.-M.-T. muscular atrophy
Charcot-Neumann crystal
Charcot-Robin crystal
Charcot-Weiss-Baker syndrome
CHARGE
  coloboma, heart disease, atresia
    choanae, retarded growth and
    development and ear anomalies
charge
  C. association
  cationic c.
  elementary c.
  ionic c.

C

charge (*continued*)
    space c.
    C. syndrome
charged particle
charge-transfer complex
Charles law
Charlin syndrome
Charlouis disease
chart
    alignment c.
    flow c.
    Levey-Jennings c.
    quality control c.
chartarum
    Ulocladium c.
chattoni
    Entamoeba c.
Chauffard-Still syndrome
Chauffard syndrome
Chaussier areola
chauvoei
    Clostridium c.
CHB
    complete heart block
CHD
    congestive heart disease
ChE
    cholesterol ester
    cholinesterase
Cheadle disease
check
    alert c.
    c. bit
    delta c.
    c. digit
    limit c.
    linearity c.
    pacemaker c.
    previous value c.
checkerboard microdilution test
checkpoint
    mitotic spindle assembly c.
Chédiak-Higashi
    C.-H. disease
    C.-H. syndrome
Chédiak-Steinbrinck-Higashi
    C.-S.-H. anomaly
    C.-S.-H. syndrome
Chédiak test
cheek
    cleft c.
cheese
    c. washer's disease
    c. worker's lung
cheesy
    c. necrosis
    c. pus
cheilitis, chilitis
cheilosis, chilosis

Cheilospirura hamulosa
cheiragra
cheirarthritis
chejuensis
    Hahella c.
chelate
    Sequestrene iron c.
chelating agent
chelation therapy
chelerythrine
Chelex
    C. DNA amplification
    C. resin
chelicera
cheloid
chelonae
chem
    chemistry panel
    chemistry profile
chemical
    c. adsorption
    c. agent
    c. agent detector paper
    c. agent monitor (CAM)
    c. analysis
    c. and biological warfare (CBW)
    c. asphyxiant
    chemical, biological, and radiological (CBR)
    C. Biological Incident Response Force (of the U.S. Marine Corps)
    chemical, biological, radiological, nuclear, explosive (CBRNE)
    chemical, biological, radiological or nuclear (CBRN)
    c. bond
    c. environment
    c. equation
    c. equilibrium
    c. gastritis
    c. incompatibility
    incompatible c.
    c. inhibition isoamylase test
    c. interference
    c. mediator
    nuclear, biological, and c.
    nuclear, biological, c. (mass-casualty weapon)
    c. peritonitis
    c. pneumonia
    c. pneumonitis
    c. porphyria
    c. prophylaxis
    c. reaction
    c. shift
    c. spectrum
    c. splash suit
    c. styptic
    c. warfare (CW)

c. waste
c. WMD
chemically pure (CP)
chemical-resistant
c.-r. inner gloves
c.-r. outer gloves
chemiluminescence, chemoluminescence
c. assay
electrogenerated c. (ECL)
c. test
chemiluminescent
c. assay (CLIA)
c. immunoassay
c. probe
chemiosmotic hypothesis
chemiotaxis (*var. of* chemotaxis)
chemisorption
chemistry
analytical c.
clinical c.
histological c.
inorganic c.
International Federation of Clinical C.
International Union of Pure and
Applied C.
organic c.
c. panel (chem)
c. profile (chem)
ChemMate
C. capillary gap slide
C. multistep detection system
chemoattractant
chemoautotroph
chemoautotrophic bacterium
chemoceptor (*var. of* chemoreceptor)
chemocoagulation
chemodectoma
chemodectomatosis
chemodifferentiation
chemoheterotroph
chemoheterotrophic bacterium
chemoimmunology
chemoimmunotherapy (CI)
chemokine
Duffy antigen receptor for c.
(DARC)
chemokinesis
chemolithotroph
chemoluminescence (*var. of*
chemiluminescence)
chemoorganotroph
chemopreventive
chemoradioresistance
chemoreceptor, chemoceptor
central c.
medullary c.
c. tumor
chemoresistance
chemosensitive

chemostat
chemosterilant
chemosynthesis
chemotactic
c. activity
c. cytokine
c. factor (CF)
c. gradient
chemotactically attracted
chemotactin
chemotaxin
chemotaxis, chemiotaxis
c. assay
negative c.
positive c.
chemotherapeutic index (CI)
chemotherapy
ablative c.
adjuvant c.
c. and radiotherapy (chemrad)
cancer c.
cytotoxic c.
c. gastritis
high-dose c. (HDCT)
preoperative c. (preChx)
c. resistance
chemotransmitter
chemotroph
chemotropism
Chempack Project
chemrad
chemotherapy and radiotherapy
chemstrip
c.
C. BG test
C. dipstick
Micral c.
chemTRAK liquid chemistry control
CHEMXpress system
Cheney syndrome
chenodeoxycholate
chenodeoxycholic
c. acid (CDC)
c. acid test
chenopodium
C. ambroisiodes
c. oil
Chen test
cheopis
Pulex c.
Xenopsylla c.
Cherchevski disease
cherry
c. angioma
c. red spot
Cherry-Crandall
C.-C. procedure
C.-C. serum lipase test
cherubic facies

cherubism
Chesapeake
Hb C.
hemoglobin C.
chest
alar c.
barrel c.
blast c.
cobbler's c.
flail c.
foveated c.
funnel c.
pterygoid c.
c. radiography
tetrahedron c.
Chester disease
Cheyletiella parasitovorax
CHF
congestive heart failure
CHH
cartilage-hair hypoplasia
CHI
creatinine height index
Chiari
C. disease
C. II syndrome
C. net
Chiari-Arnold syndrome
Chiari-Budd syndrome
Chiari-Frommel syndrome
chiasm, chiasma, *pl.* **chiasmata**
glioma of optic c.
chiasma
chiasmal tumor
chiasmata (*pl. of* chiasm, chiasma)
chick
c. embryo antigen
c. embryo fibroblast (CEF)
chick-cell agglutination (CCA)
chicken
c. embryo lethal orphan
(CELO)
c. embryo lethal orphan virus
c. fat appearance
c. fat clot
c. louse
chickenpox
hemorrhagic c.
c. immune globulin (human)
c. immunoglobulin
c. virus
chicken-wire pattern
Chick-Martin test
chiclero ulcer
Chido/Rodgers
chief
c. agglutinin
c. cell
c. cell adenoma

c. cell of corpus pineale
c. cell of stomach
Chievitz
juxtaoral organ of C.
C. layer
C. organ
Chiffelle and Putt method
chigger
chigoe
chikungunya
c. fever virus
c. hemorrhagic fever
Chilaiditi syndrome
chilblain lupus
CHILD
congenital hemidysplasia with
ichthyosiform erythroderma and limb
defects
child, *pl.* **children**
acute lymphoblastic leukemia in
older children
battered c.
C. hepatic risk criteria
linear IgA bullous disease in
children
C. syndrome
childbed fever
childhood
benign chronic bullous dermatosis
of c.
chronic bullous dermatosis of c.
granulomatous disease of c.
c. hemolytic uremic syndrome
plexiform fibrohistiocytic tumor of c.
recurring digital fibroma of c.
transient erythroblastopenia of c.
(TEC)
children (*pl. of* child)
Child-Turcotte-Pugh score
chilensis
Sphingopyxis c.
chilitis (*var. of* cheilitis)
chill-fever reaction
chilomastigiasis
Chilomastix mesnili
chilomastosis
chilopod
Chilopoda
chilopodiasis
chilosis (*var. of* cheilosis)
chimaera
Mycobacterium c.
chimera
blood group c.
dispermic c.
heterologous c.
homologous c.
isologous c.
radiation c.

chimeric
    c. antibody
    c. gene
chimerism
    hematolymphoid c.
chimney-sweep's cancer
chimpanzee coryza agent (CCA)
chin
    galoche c.
chinensis
Chinese
    C. liver fluke
    C. restaurant syndrome
      (CRS)
chinjuensis
    Paenibacillus c.
chip
    Affymetrix human cancer c.
    bone c.
    DNA c.
    c. fracture
    TURP c.
CHIP-1
    channel-forming integral protein
chiral
    c. center
    c. crystal
chirality
Chiroptera
chi squared distribution
chitin
Chitinibacter tainanensis
Chitinimonas taiwanensis
chitinolyticus
    Paenibacillus c.
chix
    chickenpox
Chk1 kinase
Chk2 kinase
CHL
    classic Hodgkin lymphoma
chlamydia
    C. antigen
    C. culture
    C. group titer
    c. infection
    C. oculogenitalis
    C. OIA
    C. pneumoniae
    C. psittaci
    C. sepsis
    C. trachomatis
    C. trachomatis direct FA test
Chlamydiaceae
Chlamydiae
chlamydial
    c. disease
    c. pneumonia
Chlamydiales

Chlamydiamicrovirus
Chlamydiazyme
    C. EIA assay
    C. test
chlamydiosis
Chlamydoabsidia padenii
Chlamydobacteriaceae
Chlamydobacteriales
chlamydoconidium
Chlamydophila
    C. abortus
    C. caviae
    C. felis
    C. pecorum
    C. pneumoniae
    C. psittaci
Chlamydophrys
chlamydospore
Chlamydozoon
chloasma bronzinum
chloracetate
    c. esterase
    c. esterase histochemical stain
    naphthol AS-D c. (NASDCA)
chloracetic acid
chloracetophenone
    NATO code for c. (CS)
chloracne, chlorine acne
chloral
    c. hydrate
    c. hydrate assay
chlorambucil
chloramine-T
chloramphenicol
chloranil assay
chloranilate method
chloranilic acid
chlorate
    c. assay
    potassium c.
chlorazol
    c. black E
    c. black E stain
chlorbenside
chlordane
chlordiazepoxide assay
chloremia
chlorfenthion insecticide
chloride
    ammonium c.
    antimony c.
    benzalkonium c.
    calcium c.
    carbonic acid c.
    carbonyl c.
    c. channel 7
    cobaltous c.
    dansyl c.
    edrophonium c.

C

chloride (*continued*)
    fecal c.
    gold c.
    hydrogen c.
    c. imbalance
    indium 111 c.
    c. method
    methylene c.
    methylrosaniline c.
    NATO code for cyanogen c. ($CNCl_2$)
    Orion skin electrode for c.
    polyvinyl c. (PVC)
    potassium c. (KCl)
    pralidoxime c.
    Schales and Schales method for c.
    c. shield
    c. shift
    sodium c. (NaCl)
    stool c.
    urine c.
    vinyl c. (VC)
chloridimetry
Chloridium
chloridometer
    coulometric c.
chloriduria
chlorinated
    c. hydrocarbon pesticide
    c. hydrocarbon pesticide assay
chlorine (Cl)
Chloriridovirus
chloritidismutans
    Pseudomonas c.
chlormerodrin accumulation test (CAT)
chloroacetate
    c. esterase (CAE)
    c. esterase reaction
1-chloroacetophenone
    NATO code for 1-c. (CN)
chloroanemia
chloroarsine
    organic c.
Chlorobacteria
Chlorobacteriaceae
Chlorobacterium
Chlorobaculum
    C. limnaeum
    C. parvum
    C. tepidum
    C. thiosulfatiphilum
Chlorobea
chlorobenzilate
chlorobenzoica
    Thauera c.
chlorobenzylidene malonitrile
Chlorobiaceae

Chlorobiales
Chlorobium
    C. clathratiforme
    C. luteolum
Chlorochromatium
2-chlorodeoxyadenosine (2-CDA)
chloroethenivorans
    Pseudonocardia c.
Chloroflexi
chlorofluorocarbon (CFC)
chloroform
    c. assay
    methyl c.
    c. poisoning
chloroform-methanol
chloroguanide hydrochloride
chlorohydrin
    ethylene c.
chlorohydrocarbon assay
chloroleukemia
chlorolymphosarcoma
chloroma
chloromatous
chloromethanicum
    Hyphomicrobium c.
Chloromycetin
chloromyeloma
chloro-naphthol
chloropenia
chloropenic azotemia
chlorophenolicum
    Herbaspirillum c.
    Sphingobium c.
chlorophenolicus
    Arthrobacter c.
chlorophenol red
chlorophenoxy herbicide
Chlorophyllum molybdites
chlorophyll unit
chloropicrin
Chloropidae
chloroplast
chloropsia
chloroquine pump
chlororespirans
    Desulfitobacterium c.
chlorosis
Chlorothion
chlorotic anemia
chlorous acid reagent
Chlorovirus
chlorpromazine assay
chlortetracycline
chloruresis, chloruria
chloruria
CHN
    central hemorrhagic necrosis
CHO
    carbohydrate

choanal
  c. atresia
  c. polyp
Choanephora
choanoflagellate
choanomastigote
Choanotaenia infundibulum
chocolate
  anthrax-containing c.
  c. blood (CB)
  c. blood agar
  c. cyst
chocolatization
  medium c.
  c. of blood culture medium
choke
  ophthalmovascular c.
choking agent
cholagogic (*var. of* cholagogue)
cholagogue, cholagogic
cholaneresis
cholangeitis
cholangiectasis
cholangiocarcinoma (CCA)
cholangiocyte
cholangiofibrosis
cholangiogram
cholangiolar proliferation
cholangiole
cholangiolitic
  c. cirrhosis
  c. hepatitis
cholangiolitis
cholangioma
cholangiopancreatography
  endoscopic retrograde c. (ERCP)
cholangitic abscess
cholangitis, cholangeitis
  ascending c.
  primary sclerosing c. (PSC)
  pyogenic c.
  sclerosing c.
  suppurative c.
cholate
cholecalciferol
cholecyst
cholecystagogue
cholecystectasia
cholecystitis
  acalculous c.
  acute hemorrhagic c.
  chronic calculous c. (CCC)
  emphysematous c.
  follicular c.
  glandularis proliferans c.
  xanthogranulomatous c.
cholecystoduodenal fistula
cholecystogram
  oral c. (OCG)

cholecystokinin (CCK)
  c. test
cholecystokinin-pancreozymin
cholecystolithiasis
cholecystosis
  hyperplastic c.
choledochal cyst
choledoch duct
choledochitis
choledochocele
choledochoduodenal junction
choledocholith
choledocholithiasis
choledochus
  ductus c.
choleglobin
cholehemia
cholelith, chololith
cholelithiasis, chololithiasis
cholelithic, chololithic
cholemia
cholemic nephrosis
cholepathia
choleperitoneum
choleperitonitis
cholera
  Asiatic c.
  c. bacillus
  hog c.
  c. sicca
  c. toxin (CTX)
  typhoid c.
  c. vaccine
  c. vibrio
cholerae
  Vibrio c.
choleraesuis
choleragen
choleraic
choleraphage
cholera-red reaction
cholestasia, cholestasis
cholestasis (*var. of* cholestasia)
  chronic c.
cholestatic
  c. hepatitis
  c. jaundice
cholesteatoma
cholesteatomatous
**cholesteremia, cholesterolemia,
  cholesterinemia**
cholesterinemia (*var. of* cholesteremia)
cholesterinized antigen
cholesterinosis (*var. of* cholesterolosis)
cholesterinuria
cholesterol (CH, chol.)
  c. acyltransferase
  c. assay
  c. calculus

C

cholesterol (*continued*)
  c. cleft
  c. crystal
  c. deposition
  c. emboli
  c. embolism
  c. ester (ChE)
  c. esterase
  c. ester storage disease
  intracellular free c.
  C. Manager
  c. 1,2,3 noninvasive testing device
  c. polyp
  c. side-chain cleavage enzyme
    deficiency
  c. staining method
  c. test
  total c. (TC)
cholesterolemia (*var. of* cholesteremia)
cholesterol-free medium
cholesterol-lecithin flocculation test
cholesterolosis, cholesterinosis
  cerebrotendinous c.
  extracellular c.
cholesterol/phospholipid ratio
  (C:P)
cholesteroluria
CholesTrak
cholestyramine resin
cholic acid
cholicele
choliformis
  mycetism c.
choline
  c. acetyltransferase
  lysophosphatidyl c.
cholinergic
  c. antagonist
  c. blockade
  c. blocking agent
  c. crisis
  c. urticaria
cholinesterase (ChE, CHS)
  c. assay
  c. blood test
  c. enzyme
  c. inhibitor
  red blood cell c. (RBC-ChE)
chololith (*var. of* cholelith)
chololithiasis (*var. of* cholelithiasis)
chololithic (*var. of* cholelithic)
choloplania
cholothorax
choluria
cholylglycine
chomelii
  Bartonella c.
Chondodendron
chondral

chondralloplasia
chondrification center
chondrify
chondrin ball
chondritis
chondroblast
  differentiating c.
chondroblastic subtype
chondroblastoma
chondroblastoma-like osteosarcoma
chondrocalcinosis
  articular c. (ACC)
chondroclast
chondrocyte
  hypertrophied c.
  isogenous c.
  c. lacuna
  nuclei of c.
chondrodermatitis nodularis chronica
  helicis
chondrodysplasia
  c. calcificans
  c. punctata
chondrodystrophia (*var. of*
  chondrodystrophy)
    c. calcificans congenita
    c. congenita punctata
chondrodystrophic dwarfism
chondrodystrophy, chondrodystrophia
  asphyxiating thoracic c.
  asymmetric c.
chondroectodermal dysplasia
chondrofibroma
chondrogenic
chondrohypoplasia
chondroid
  c. chordoma
  c. lipoma
  c. metaplasia
  c. syringoma
  c. tissue
chondroitin
  c. sulfate
  c. sulfate proteoglycan
    (CSPG)
  c. sulfate stain
  c. sulfate staining
chondrology
chondroma
  extraskeletal c.
  juxtacortical c.
chondromalacia
  c. fetalis
  generalized c.
  c. of larynx
  c. patellae
  systemic c.
chondromatosis
  synovial c.

chondromatous
    c. exostosis
    c. giant cell tumor
chondrometaplasia
chondromucoprotein
chondromyxoid
    c. fibroma (CMF)
    c. metaplasia
chondromyxoma
chondronectin
chondroosseous
chondroosteodystrophy
chondropathy
chondrophila
    Waddlia c.
chondrophyte
chondroplast
chondroporosis
chondrosarcoma
    dedifferentiated c.
    extraskeletal myxoid c.
    (EMC)
    mesenchymal c.
    skeletal myxoid c. (SMC)
chondrosis
Chondrostereum
chondrotrophic hormone
chondrus
chopped
    c. meat broth
    c. meat medium
chorangiosis
chorda, *pl.* **chordae**
    Algoriphagus chordae
    chordae willisii
chordae (*pl. of* chorda)
chordalis
    endocarditis c.
chordee
chorditis
chordoblastoma
Chordodes morgani
chordoid features
chordoma
    axial c.
    chondroid c.
    familial clival c.
    sacrococcygeal c.
chorea
    Bergeron c.
    Huntington c. (HC)
    Sydenham c.
choreic
choreicus
    status c.
choreiform, choreoid
choreoathetosis
choreoid (*var. of* choreiform)
chorioadenoma destruens

chorioallantoic culture
chorioamnionic hemorrhage
chorioamnionitis
chorioangioma
chorioangiomatosis
chorioangiosis
choriocapillaris
    lamina c.
    membrana c.
choriocapillary layer
choriocarcinoma
    gestational c.
    monophasic c.
choriodecidual inflammatory response
  syndrome
choriodeciduitis
chorioepithelioma
chorioepitheliosis
chorioma
choriomeningitis
    lymphatic c. (LCM)
    lymphocytic c. (LCM)
chorion
    abnormal c.
    c. frondosum
    c. laeve
    mature abnormal c.
chorionic
    c. carcinoma
    c. cavity
    c. epithelioma
    c. gonadotropin (CG, CGT)
    c. gonadotropin-alpha subunit
    c. gonadotropin assay
    c. gonadotropin-beta subunit
    c. gonadotropin test
    c. gonadotropin unit (international)
    c. growth hormone prolactin
    (CGP)
    c. plate
    c. somatomammotropin (CS)
    c. villus
    c. villus embolism
    c. villus sampling (CVS)
Chorioptes
chorista
choristoblastoma
choristoma
    neuromuscular c.
    neuronal c.
choroid
    basal lamina of c.
    basal layer of c.
    c. plexus
    c. plexus papilloma
choroidal
    c. hemangioma
    c. neovascularization
    (CNV)

C

choroidea
    lamina basalis choroideae
    lamina vasculosa choroideae
    tela c.
choroideremia
choroiditis
choroidocapillaris
    lamina c.
Chotzen syndrome
CHR
  chromogranin
    CHR reaction
ChrA
  chromogranin A
    ChrA antigen
    ChrA immunoperoxidase stain
CH/RG
    CH/RG antibody
    CH/RG antigen
    CH/RG blood group
Christeller reaction
Christensen-Krabbe disease
Christensen urea agar
Christian
    C. disease
    C. syndrome
Christian-Hand-Schüller disease
Christian-Weber disease
Christie-Atkins-Munch-Petersen (CAMP)
Christison formula
Christmas
    C. disease
    C. factor (CF)
Christopherson nuclear grading system
Christopher spot
Christ-Siemens syndrome
Christ-Siemens-Touraine syndrome
chromaffin
    c. body
    c. cell
    Gomori method for c.
    c. hormone
    c. paraganglioma
    c. reaction
    c. reaction test
    c. system
    c. tissue
    c. tumor
chromaffinoma
    medullary c.
chromaffinopathy
chromaphil
chromate
    lead c.
    c. method
    sodium c.
    c. stain for lead
Chromatiaceae
Chromatibacteria

chromatic
    c. aberration
    c. apparatus
    c. fiber
    c. granule
chromatica
    trichomycosis c.
chromatid
    c. gap
    c. interference
    nonsister c.
    sister c.
chromatin
    c. body
    clock face c.
    c. dust
    heteropyknotic c.
    Klinger-Ludwig acid-thionin stain for
      sex c.
    marginated c.
    c. material
    c. network
    nucleolar-associated c.
    oxyphil c.
    c. particle
    c. reservoir
    sex c.
    c. spot
    X c.
    Y c.
chromatinic body
chromatin-negative
chromatinolysis
chromatinorrhexis
chromatin-positive
chromation
chromatism
chromatofocusing
    high-performance c. (HPCF)
chromatogram
chromatograph
    gas c.
chromatographic assay
chromatography
    adsorption c.
    affinity c.
    anion-exchange c.
    antibody affinity c.
    ascending c.
    DEAE anion exchange c.
    denaturing high-performance liquid
      c. (DHPLC)
    electric c.
    filter paper c.
    gas c. (GC)
    gas-liquid c. (GLC)
    gas-solid c. (GSC)
    gel-filtration c.
    gel-permeation c.

high-performance ion exchange c.
(HPIEC)
high-performance liquid c. (HPLC)
high-performance size exclusion c.
(HPSEC)
high-pressure liquid c. (HPLC)
immunoaffinity c.
instant thin-layer c. (ITLC)
ion-exchange c.
liquid c.
liquid-liquid c.
liquid-solid c.
microcolumn c.
molecular exclusion c.
molecular sieve c.
SDS gel filtration c.
serum thyroxine measured by
column c. ($T_4(C)$)
size-exclusion c.
thin-layer c. (TLC)
two-dimensional c.
vapor-phase c. (VPC)
chromatoid
chromatokinesis
chromatolysis, chromatinolysis
central c.
neuronal c.
retrograde c.
transsynaptic c.
chromatolytic
chromatometer
**chromatopectic, chromopectic,
chromopexic**
chromatopexis, chromopexis
chromatophil
chromatophilia
chromatophilic granule
chromatophilous
chromatophobia
chromatophore
chromatophorotropic hormone
chromatoplasm
chromatotaxis
chromatotropism
chromaturia
chrome
c. alum
c. alum carmine
c. alum hematoxylin-phloxine
method
c. alum hematoxylin-phloxine stain
c. hematoxylin
c. red
c. violet
c. violet CG
c. yellow
chromic
c. acid
c. acid fixative

chromidial
c. apparatus
c. net
c. substance
chromidiation
chromidiosis
chromidium
chromium (Cr)
c. assay
chromium-51 red cell survival
Chromobacterieae
Chromobacterium violaceum
chromoblastomycosis
chromocenter
chromocyte
chromodomain
chromogen
AEC c.
Porter-Silber c. (PSC)
tetramethylbenzidine c.
chromogenesis
chromogenic
c. bacterium
c. cephalosporin test
c. enzyme substrate test
c. Xa inhibition assay
chromogranin (CHR)
c. A (CgA, ChrA)
c. antibody
Chromohalobacter
C. canadensis
C. israelensis
C. marismortui
C. salexigens
chromolipid
chromolysis
chromolytic method
chromomere
chromometer
chromomycin A3
chromomycosis
chromonema
**chromopectic, chromatopectic,
chromopexic**
chromopexic (*var. of* chromatopectic,
chromopectic)
chromopexis (*var. of* chromatopexis)
chromophage
chromophil, chromophile
c. adenoma
c. granule
c. substance
chromophile (*var. of* chromophil)
chromophilia
chromophilic, chromophilous
chromophilous
chromophobe
c. adenoma
c. carcinoma

chromophobe (*continued*)
   c. cell
   c. cell of hypophysis
   c. granule
   c. renal cell carcinoma
    (CRCC)
   c. tumor
chromophobia
chromophobic adenoma
chromophore
chromophoric, chromophorous
chromophorous (*var. of* chromophoric)
chromoplastid
chromoprotein
chromoscopy
   gastric c.
chromosomal
   c. aberration
   c. abnormality
   c. band
   c. breakage syndrome
   c. deletion
   c. deletion syndrome
   c. derangement
   c. disorder
   c. endoreduplication
   c. instability (CIN)
   c. inversion
   c. linkage
   c. malformation syndrome
   c. marker
   c. mutagen
   nonhistone c. (NHC)
   c. RNA (cRNA)
chromosomally mediated resistant
 Neisseria gonorrhoeae
chromosome
   c. aberration
   accessory c.
   acrocentric c.
   c. alteration
   c. analysis
   Balbiani c.
   c. band
   c. banding
   c. breakage syndrome
   c. complement
   derivative c. (der)
   c. dicentric malformation
   double minute c.
   fragile X c.
   frontotemporal dementias with
    parkinsonism linked to c. 17
   gametic c.
   heteromorphic c.
   homologous c.
   i(12p) marker c.
   late replicating X c.
   long arm of c.

   c. map
   marker c.
   metaphase c.
   mitotic c.
   c. nomenclature
   c. painting
   polytene c.
   16q c.
   c. 14q tumor marker
   reduplication of meiotic c.
   ring c.
   sex c.
   somatic c.
   surnumerary c.
   c. translocation
   c. trisomy
   X c.
   Y c.
   yeast artificial c. (YAC)
Chromotorula
chromotoxic
chromotrope 2R
chromotropic acid
chronic
   c. abscess
   c. absorptive arthritis
   c. acholuric jaundice
   c. active hepatitis (CAH)
   c. active inflammation
   c. active liver disease
   c. adhesive pachymeningitis
   c. airway obstruction (CAO)
   c. allograft rejection
   c. anaphylaxis
   c. appendicitis
   c. atrophic gastritis (CAG)
   c. atrophic polychondritis
   c. atrophic thyroiditis
   c. atrophic vulvitis
   c. autoimmune hemolytic anemia
   c. brain syndrome (CBS)
   c. bronchitis (CB)
   c. bronchitis with asthma (CBA)
   c. bullous dermatosis of childhood
   c. calculus cholecystitis (CCC)
   c. carrier state
   c. cell leukemia
   c. cholestasis
   c. cicatrizing enteritis
   c. constrictive pericarditis
   c. cystic mastitis
   c. decubitus ulcer zone I, II
   c. discoid lupus
   c. discoid lupus erythematosus
   c. eczema
   c. eosinophilic leukemia (CEL)
   c. eosinophilic pneumonia (CEP)
   c. false-positive (CFP)
   c. familial icterus

c. familial jaundice
c. fatigue immune dysfunction syndrome (CFIDS)
c. fibrosing pancreatitis
c. follicular keratoconjunctivitis
c. glomerulonephritis (CGN)
c. granulocytic leukemia (CGL)
c. granulomatous disease (CGD)
c. hemolytic anemia
c. hypertrophic gastritis
c. hypertrophic vulvitis
c. idiopathic jaundice
c. idiopathic megacolon
c. idiopathic myelofibrosis (CIMF)
c. inflammatory demyelinating polyneuropathy (CIDP)
c. inflammatory disease
c. interstitial cystitis
c. interstitial hepatitis
c. interstitial nephritis (CIN)
c. interstitial salpingitis
c. intervillositis
c. intestinal pseudoobstructive syndrome (CIPS)
c. lobular hepatitis (CLH)
c. lymphatic leukemia (CLL)
c. lymphocytic leukemia (CLL)
c. lymphoproliferative disorder (CLPD)
c. lymphosarcoma cell
c. lymphosarcoma leukemia (CLSL)
c. membranous glomerulonephritis (CMGN)
c. monoblastic leukemia
c. monocytic leukemia
c. mucocutaneous candidiasis (CMC)
c. myelocytic leukemia (CML)
c. myelogenous leukemia (CML)
c. myeloid leukemia
c. myelomonocytic leukemia (CMML)
c. myeloproliferative disorder (CMPD)
c. neutrophilic leukemia
c. nonspecific inflammation
c. obstructive lung disease (COLD)
c. obstructive pulmonary disease (COPD)
c. passive congestion (CPC)
c. persistent hepatitis (CPH)
c. pneumonitis of infancy (CPI)
c. proliferative arthritis
c. prolymphocytic leukemia
c. pulmonary emphysema (CPE)
c. pulmonary vascular occlusive disease

c. pyelonephritis (CPN)
c. pyelonephritis/reflux nephropathy
c. renal disease (CRD)
c. renal failure (CRF)
c. respiratory failure
c. rheumatism
c. specific endometritis
c. subdural hematoma (CSH)
c. ulcer
c. ulcerative colitis (CUC)
c. ulcerative proctitis
c. villous arthritis
c. viral hepatitis
chronica
encephalitis subcorticalis c.
ileocolitis ulcerosa c.
mycosis cutis c.
pityriasis lichenoides c.
polyarthritis c.
chronicity index
chronicus
lichen simplex c.
chronological age (CA)
chronooncology
chronotropic
chronotropism
Chroobacteria
Chroococcales
chrotoplast
Chryseobacterium
   C. defluvii
   C. joostei
   C. meningosepticum
   C. miricola
chrysiasis
Chrysiogenaceae
Chrysiogenales
Chrysiogenetes
chrysocyanosis
chrysoidin
Chrysomyia
Chrysonilia sitophila
Chrysops
   C. caecutiens
   C. dimidiata
   C. discalis
   C. silacea
chrysorrhoea
   Euproctis c.
Chrysosporium parvum
chrysotile
Chrysovirus
CHS
   cholinesterase
CHUK
   conserved helix-loop-helix ubiquitous kinase
chungbukensis
   Sphingomonas c.

C

church spire papillomatosis
Churg-Strauss
    C.-S. angiitis
    C.-S. granuloma
    C.-S. syndrome
    C.-S. vasculitis
Churukian-Schenck stain
chutta
Chvostek sign
Chvostek-Weiss sign
chylangioma
chylaqueous
chyle
    c. corpuscle
    c. cyst
    c. peritonitis
    c. vessel
chylemia
chyli
    cisterna c.
chyliform ascites
chylocele
chyloderma
chylomediastinum
chylomicrograph
chylomicron
    c. composition
    lipoprotein c.
chylomicronemia
chylopericarditis
chylopericardium
chyloperitoneum
chylopleura
chylopneumothorax
chylorrhea
chylosus
    ascites c.
chylothorax
    congenital c.
    filarial c.
    nonfilarial c.
    traumatic c.
chylous
    c. arthritis
    c. ascites
    c. effusion
    c. hydrothorax
    c. urine
chyluria
chymase
    mast cell positive tryptase and c.
    (MCTC)
chyme, chymus
chymosin
chymotrypsin
    fecal c.
    c. stain
chymotrypsinogen enzyme
chymus (*var. of* chyme)

C.I.
    Colour Index
CI
    cell interaction
    cerebral infarction
    chemoimmunotherapy
    chemotherapeutic index
    confidence interval
    coronary insufficiency
    crystalline insulin
        CI molecule
        CI number
Ci
    curie
Ciaccio
    C. fluid
    C. gland
    C. method
    C. stain
Ciaccio-positive lipid
cIAP
    cellular inhibitor of apoptosis
Ciarrocchi disease
cibaria
    Weissella c.
cibinongensis
    Acetobacter c.
cicatrices (*pl. of* cicatrix)
cicatricial
    c. horn
    c. pemphigoid
cicatricosa
    Ambrosiozyma c.
cicatrix, *pl.* cicatrices
    brain c.
    meningocerebral c.
cicatrizant
cicatrization
cicatrizing enterocolitis
Cicuta
cicutoxin
CID
    cytomegalic inclusion disease
cidal level
CIDP
    chronic inflammatory demyelinating
     polyneuropathy
CIDS
    cellular immunity deficiency
     syndrome
    combined immunodeficiency syndrome
CIE
    countercurrent immunoelectrophoresis
CIEP
    countercurrent immunoelectrophoresis
    counterimmunoelectrophoresis
CIF
    clone-inhibiting factor
    congenital infantile fibrosarcoma

ciferii
 Stephanoascus c.
ciferrii
 Prototheca c.
cigarette-paper scar
cigar-shaped nucleus
ciguatera
ciguatoxin
Ci-hr
 curie-hour
ciliares (*gen. of* ciliaris)
ciliaris, *gen.* **ciliares**
 fibrae meridionales muscularis c.
 glandulae ciliares
 plicae ciliares
 stratum pigmenti corporis c.
 zona c.
 zonula c.
ciliary
 c. canal
 c. dysentery
 c. fold
 c. gland
 c. zone
 c. zonule
Ciliata
ciliated
 c. cell
 c. epithelium
 c. metaplasia
ciliate dysentery
ciliocytophthoria (CCP)
ciliogenesis
Ciliophora
ciliorum
 tinea c.
Cillobacterium
CIM
 cardia intestinal metaplasia
Cimex
 C. hemipterus
 C. lectularius
CIMF
 chronic idiopathic myelofibrosis
cimicosis
CIN
 cefsulodin-Irgasan-novobiocin
 cervical intraepithelial neoplasia
 chromosomal instability
 chronic interstitial nephritis
  CIN agar
cinaedi
 Campylobacter c.
 Helicobacter c.
cinchonism
cinemicrography
cinephotomicrography
cinerescens
 Volutella c.

cinereus
 Aedes c.
 Scopulariopsis c.
cinetoplasm, cinetoplasma
cinetoplasma (*var. of* cinetoplasm)
cingulate gyrus
cinnabarina
 Haemaphysalis c.
cinnamivorans
cinocentrum
CINtec
 CINtec cytology kit
 CINtec histology kit
cintus
CIP
 critical infrastructure protection
CipherGen Express software biomarker analysis system
CIPS
 chronic intestinal pseudoobstructive syndrome
circadian
 c. cycle
 c. quotient (CQ)
 c. rhythm
circinata
 tinea c.
circinate retinopathy
Circinella
circle of confusion
circling disease
Circovirus
circuit
 c. breaker
 delay c.
 open c.
 printed c.
 RC c.
 series c.
 short c.
circuitry
circulans
 Bacillus c.
circular
 c. dichroism
 c. fiber
 c. layer of muscular tunic
circulares
 fibrae c.
 plicae c.
circulating
 c. anticoagulant
 c. antithromboplastin disorder
 c. blood volume (CBV)
 c. granulocyte pool (CGP)
 c. pool
 c. reticuloendothelial cell

C

circulation
  c. rate
  c. time (CT)
circulatory
  c. antigliadin antibody
  c. collapse
  c. disease
  c. failure
  c. insufficiency
  c. overload
circumanales
  glandulae c.
circumanal gland
circumferential
  c. implantation
  c. lamella
circumgemmal
circummarginata
  placenta c.
circummarginate placenta
circumnevic vitiligo
circumnuclear
circumscribed
  c. atrophy
  c. choroidal hemangioma
    (CCH)
  c. craniomalacia
  c. edema
  c. inflammation
  c. mass
  c. peritonitis
  c. pyocephalus
circumscripta
  calcinosis c.
  lipoatrophia c.
  myositis ossificans c.
  osteitis fibrosa c.
  osteoporosis c.
circumscription
circumscriptum
  lymphangioma c.
circumscriptus
  keratoconus posticus c.
circumvallate
  c. papillae
  c. placenta
  c. placentation
circumvallation
cirrhogenic (*var. of* cirrhogenous)
cirrhogenous, cirrhogenic
cirrhonosus
cirrhosis
  alcoholic c.
  biliary c.
  Budd c.
  cardiac c.
  cholangiolitic c.
  congestive c.
  cryptogenic c.

diffuse septal c.
fatty c.
Glisson c.
Hanot c.
Indian childhood c. (ICC)
juvenile c.
Laënnec c.
necrotic c.
nutritional c.
obstructive c.
  c. pigment
pipestem c.
portal c.
posthepatitic c.
postnecrotic c.
primary biliary c. (PBC)
stasis c.
toxic c.
cirrhotic
  c. ascites
  c. glomerulosclerosis
cirrose, cirrous
cirrous (*var. of* cirrose)
cirrus
cirsocele
cirsoid
  c. aneurysm
  c. varix
cirsomphalos
CIS
  carcinoma in situ
  central inhibitory state
cis
  c. activation
  c. configuration
cis-acting locus
CIS/ITGCNU
  carcinoma in situ/intratubular germ cell
    neoplasia unclassified
CISM
  critical incident stress management
cisplatin
cistern
  c. of cytoplasmic reticulum
  c. of nuclear envelope
cisterna, *pl.* **cisternae**
  c. caryothecae
  c. chyli
  membranous cisternae
  sacroplasmic cisternae
  subsurface c.
  terminal c.
cisternae (*pl. of* cisterna)
cisternal
cisternogram
cis/trans test
cistron
CIT
  corneal impression test

Citelli syndrome
Citellus
Citeromyces matritensis
citrate
    c. agar
    c. agar gel electrophoresis
    c. buffer
    c. condensing enzyme
    gallium c.
    indole, methyl red, Voges-Proskauer, and c. (IMViC)
    c. intoxication
    lead c.
    c. phosphate dextrose (CPD)
    potassium c.
    Reynolds lead c.
    sodium acid c.
    standard saline c. (SSC)
    c. test
citrate-buffered saline (CBS)
citrated blood
citrate-phosphate-dextrose-adenine (CPD adenine)
citratiphilum
    Aquabacterium c.
citreus
    Erythrobacter c.
    Staphylococcus c.
citric
    c. acid
    c. acid assay
    c. acid cycle
Citricoccus muralis
Citrobacter
    C. amalonatica
    Bethesda-Ballerup group of *C.* (CBB)
    C. diversus
    C. freundii
    C. koseri
    C. murliniae
Citroclear
citrovorum factor (CF)
citrulline
    urine c.
citrullinemia
citrullinuria
Civatte
    C. body
    C. disease
    poikiloderma of C.
CJD
    Creutzfeldt-Jakob disease
CK
    creatine kinase
    cytokeratin
CK5 stain
CK7 marker
CK20 reactivity

CK-BB
    creatine kinase BB
c-Ki-ras gene
c-kit
    c-k. activity
    DayCytomation pharmDX c-k.
    c-k. oncogene
    c-k. protooncogene
    c-k. receptor
CK-MB tandem test
cL
    centiliter
Cl
    chloride
    chlorine
CLA
    cyclic lysine anhydride
Cladobotryum
Cladophialophora
Cladorchis watsoni
Cladorrhinum
cladosporioides
    Hormodendrum c.
cladosporiosis
    cerebral c.
    c. epidermica
Cladosporium
    C. carrionii
    C. mansonii
    C. trichoides
    C. werneckii
    C. (Xylohypha) bantianum
Cladothrix
clamp connection
clandestine aerosol release
Clara
    C. cell
    C. cell adenocarcinoma
    C. cell secretory protein gene
    C. hematoxylin
clarificant
Clark
    C. level
    C. malignant melanoma classification
    C. malignant melanoma staging
    C. nevus
    C. oxygen electrode
    C. rule
    C. test
Clark-Collip method
Clarke
    C. collateral bundle
    C. column
    C. dorsal nucleus
    C. fluid
Clarke-Hadfield syndrome
Clark-Elder malignant melanoma classification

C

CLAS
    congenital localized absence of skin
CLASH
    cryoglobulinemia, leukemia, arthritis,
      Sjögren syndrome, and hepatitis B
clasmatocyte
clasmatosis
class
    c. A, B, C, D pathogen
    Hallervorden-Spatz disease, tau
      pathology c.
    c. histocompatibility antigen
    immunoglobulin c.
    c. switch
    c. switching
classic
    c. hemophilia
    c. Hodgkin lymphoma (CHL)
    c. liver lobule
    c. RTA
classical
    c. complement pathway
    c. hemophilia
    c. swine fever
classification
    AJCC c.
    Ann Arbor staging c.
    Ann Arbor tumor c.
    Arneth c.
    Astler-Coller modification of
      Dukes c.
    AUA bladder cancer staging c.
    bacterial c.
    Banff renal allograft rejection c.
    Bergey c.
    Bernatz c.
    Bessman anemia c.
    Binet chronic lymphocytic
      leukemia c.
    Bismuth cholangiocarcinoma c.
    Bismuth-Corlette perihilar tumor c.
    Bloom and Richardson c.
    Borrmann c.
    Breslow malignant melanoma c.
    Broders c.
    Brooker heterotopic ossification c.
    Caldwell-Moloy c.
    Chapel Hill Consensus
      Conference c.
    Clark-Elder malignant melanoma c.
    Clark malignant melanoma c.
    Denver c.
    Dukes-Astler-Coller
      adenocarcinoma c.
    Dukes carcinoma c.
    Dutch c.
    Edmondson-Steiner hepatocellular
      carcinoma grading c.
    Eggel tumor c.

    Elder malignant melanoma c.
    Enzinger tumor c.
    FAB leukemia c.
    Fredrickson dyslipoproteinemia c.
    Gell and Coombs drug allergy c.
    Griffith c.
    Horie tumor c.
    Hyams esthesioneuroblastoma c.
    Isaacson gastric lymphoma c. (IC)
    Jansky human blood group c.
    Jensen trochanteric fracture c.
    Jewett bladder carcinoma c.
    Kauffman-White Salmonella
      serotype c.
    Keith-Wagener retinal changes c.
    Kiel non-Hodgkin lymphoma c.
    Klatskin tumor c.
    Lancefield c.
    Landsteiner c.
    Lauren c.
    Lennert c.
    Levine-Rosai tumor c.
    Ljubljana c.
    Lukes-Butler Hodgkin disease c.
    Lukes-Butler non-Hodgkin
      lymphoma c.
    Lukes-Collins non-Hodgkin
      lymphoma c.
    Masaoka c.
    McNeer gastric carcinoma c.
    MMH osteogenic c.
    Moss c.
    Portmann c.
    Rappaport c.
    REAL c.
    Revised European-American
      Lymphoma c. (REAL)
    Runyon c.
    Rye histopathologic Hodgkin
      disease c.
    Sakamoto c.
    c. scheme
    Schilling c.
    Seattle graft-versus-host disease c.
    Shimada c.
    Shimosato-Mukai c.
    Skinner partially edentulous c.
    Sydney c.
    Talerman c.
    WHO/ISUP c.
clastic
clastothrix
clathrate
clathratiforme
    Chlorobium c.
clathrin
clathrin-coated
    c.-c. pit
    c.-c. vesicle

Clathrochloris
Clathrocystis
Clauberg
    C. test
    C. unit
Claude Bernard-Horner syndrome
claudication
    intermittent c. (IC)
    venous c.
claudin 4 gene
Claudius cell
clause
    Delaney c.
claustrum
clausura
clavate papilla
clavatus
    Aspergillus c.
    Porocephalus c.
Claviceps purpurea
claviculus
Clavispora lusitaniae
clavus
claw
    griffin c.
clawfoot, claw foot
clawhand, claw hand
clay shoveler's fracture
CLBBB
    complete left bundle-branch block
ClCN7
    chloride channel 7
    ClCN7 gene
clean area (contamination-free)
clean-catch
    c.-c. collection method
    c.-c. urine culture
    c.-c. urine specimen
cleaning solution
cleanser
    AlcoSCRUB instant antiseptic
    hand c.
cleanup
    Wizard MagneSil PCR c.
    Wizard MagneSil sequencing c.
clean-voided specimen (CVS)
clear
    c. cell
    c. cell acanthoma
    c. cell adenocarcinoma
    c. cell adenoma
    c. cell borderline tumor
    c. cell carcinoma (CCC)
    c. cell cribriforming hyperplasia
    c. cell hepatocellular carcinoma
    (HCC-CC)
    c. cell hidradenoma
    c. cell leiomyoma
    c. cell meningioma

    c. cell morphology
    c. cell myoepithelial carcinoma
    (CCMEC)
    c. cell neoplasm
    c. cell odontogenic carcinoma
    c. cell pattern
    c. cell renal cell carcinoma
    (RCC-CC)
    c. cell sarcoma
    c. cell sarcoma of the kidney
    (CCSK)
    c. cell sugar tumor
    c. layer of epidermis
    c. plaque mutation
clearance
    albumin c.
    amylase c. (C_{am}, C_{Am})
    amylase/creatinine c.
    blood urea c.
    creatinine c. (CC)
    decreased creatine c.
    endogenous creatinine c.
    exogenous creatinine c.
    free water c.
    immune c.
    insulin c. (C_{in})
    interocclusal c.
    inulin c.
    iron plasma c.
    maximum urea c.
    osmolal c.
    osmolar c. (Cosm)
    osmotic c.
    p-aminohippurate c. (C_{pah})
    plasma c.
    serum creatinine c.
    sodium c.
    standard urea c.
    thyroidal c.
    total body c. (Q_B)
    urea c.
ClearCourse solution drug screening test
ClearCRIT microhematocrit tube
clearing
    c. factor
    c. factor lipase
    c. medium
ClearView C. Diff A test
Cleary
    method of C.
cleavage
    heterolytic c.
    homolytic c.
    c. line
    c. of ovum
    c. plane
    c. product
    progressive c.
    c. spindle

C

cleavase fragment length polymorphism (CFLP)
cleaved follicular center cell
cleft
    action potential synaptic c.
    birefringent crystalline c.
    c. cheek
    cholesterol c.
    c. face
    Larrey c.
    c. lip
    Maurer c.
    c. nose
    c. palate
    residual c.
    Schmidt-Lanterman c.
    c. spine
    synaptic c.
    c. tongue
clefting
    suprabasal c.
cleidocranial
    c. dysostosis
    c. dysplasia
cleistothecium
Cleland reagent
cleptoparasite
CLH
    chronic lobular hepatitis
    cutaneous lymphoid hyperplasia
CLIA
    chemiluminescent assay
    Clinical Laboratory Improvement Amendment
CLIA '88
    CLIA Laboratory Improvement Act of 1988
clidocranial
CLIF
    cloning inhibitory factor
cliftonensis
    Rubrimonas c.
c2-like viruses
Climacocystis
Climacodon
climacteric, climacterium
    delayed c.
climactericum
    keratoderma c.
climacterium (*var. of* climacteric)
climatic bubo
climbing fiber
clindamycin
cline
clinger
    boat c.
clinging
    c. carcinoma
    c. ductal carcinoma in situ

clinical
    c. chemistry
    c. chemistry automation
    c. chemistry quality control
    c. consideration
    c. cytogenetics
    c. diagnosis
    c. diagnostic bacteriology
    c. end point
    c. genetics
    c. indicator
    c. laboratory
    C. Laboratory Improvement Act of 1988 (CLIA '88)
    C. Laboratory Improvement Amendment (CLIA)
    C. Laboratory Management Association
    c. laboratory maximum area
    c. manifestations, etiologic factors, anatomic involvement, pathophysiologic features (CEAP)
    c. microbiology quality control
    c. microscopy
    c. pathology
    c. response
    c. sample
    c. sensitivity
    c. spectrometry
    c. spectroscopy
    c. spectrum
    c. toxicology
    c. trial
Clinician Outreach and Communication Activity (COCA)
clinicogenetic approach
clinicopathologic, clinicopathological
    c. analysis
    c. conference (CPC)
    c. study
clinicopathological (*var. of* clinicopathologic)
Clinistix
Clinitest stool test
clinodactyly
clinoscope
    exogenous creatinine c.
Clinostomum marginatum
clip
    Filschie c.
Clitocybe dealbata
Clitocybula
Clitopilus
clitoridauxe
clitoridis
    smegma c.
clivi (*pl. of* clivus)
clivus, *pl.* **clivi**

CLL
centrocytelike cell
chronic lymphatic leukemia
chronic lymphocytic leukemia
chronic myelogenous leukemia
Rai classification of CLL

CLL/SLL
B-cell CLL/SLL

CLO
Campylobacter-like organism
CLO test

cloaca, *pl.* **cloacae**
Aerobacter c.
ectopia c.
Enterobacter c.
Sphingomonas c.

cloacae (*pl. of* cloaca)

cloacal exstrophy

cloacogenic
c. carcinoma
c. polyp

clock
biological c.
c. face chromatin
real-time c.

clomiphene test

Clonad monoclonal antibody

clonal
c. deletion theory
c. disorder
c. eosinophilia
c. expansion
c. gene rearrangement
c. hematological nonmast cell
lineage disease
c. proliferated cell
c. seborrheic keratosis
c. selection theory
c. thrombocytosis

clonality study

clone
cDNA c.
complementary DNA c.
forbidden c.
genomic DNA c. (chromosomal)

cloned enzyme donor immunoassay
(CEDIA)

clone-inhibiting factor (CIF)

CloneSaver card

clonic

clonidine suppression test

cloning
cellular c.
gene c.
c. inhibitory factor
(CLIF)
molecular c.
therapeutic c.
c. vector

clonogenic
c. assay
c. cell

clonorchiasis, clonorchiosis

clonorchiosis (*var. of* clonorchiasis)

Clonorchis endemicus

Clontech gene expression profiling
procedure

clonus

Cloquet
C. canal
C. canal remnant
node of C.

closed
c. dislocation
c. fracture
c. loop obstruction

close range entrance wound

Closterovirus

Clostridiaceae

clostridial
c. bacteremia
c. collagenase
c. myonecrosis
c. myositis
c. strain

Clostridiales

clostridioforme
Clostridium c.

clostridiopeptidase A

Clostridium
C. acetobutylicum
C. acidisoli
C. akagii
C. algidixylanolyticum
C. amygdalinum
C. argentinense
C. baratii
C. bartlettii
C. bifermentans
C. bolteae
C. botulinum
C. botulinum cytotoxin type C2
C. botulinum neurotoxin type A, B,
C1, D, E, F, G
C. bowmanii
C. butyricum
C. cadaveris
C. caminithermale
C. carnis
C. chauvoei
C. clostridioforme
C. cochlearium
C. colicanis
C. difficile
C. difficile toxin
C. difficile toxin assay
C. diolis
C. estertheticum subsp. *laramiense*

C

Clostridium (*continued*)
  C. fallax
  C. frigoris
  C. gasigenes
  C. haemolyticum
  C. hathewayi
  C. hiranonis
  C. histolyticum
  C. histolyticum collagenase
  C. hungatei
  C. hylemonae
  C. innocuum
  C. jejuense
  C. kluyveri
  C. lactatifermentans
  C. lacusfryxellense
  C. novyi
  C. paraputrificum
  C. pasteurianum
  C. peptidivorans
  C. perfringens
  C. perfringens alpha toxin
  C. perfringens beta toxin
  C. perfringens enterotoxin
  C. perfringens enterotoxin iota
    (CPI)
  C. perfringens epsilon toxin
  C. perfringens iota toxin
  C. phytofermentans
  C. psychrophilum
  C. ramosum
  C. saccharobutylicum
  C. septicum
  C. sordellii
  C. sphenoides
  C. sporogenes
  C. stercorarium subsp.
    thermolacticum
  C. sticklandii
  C. tertium
  C. tetani
  C. tetanomorphum
  C. thermosaccharolyticum
  C. thiosulfatireducens
  C. uliginosum
  C. welchii
  C. xylanovorans
clostrisel agar
closure
  delayed primary c.
    (DPC)
clot
  antemortem c.
  blood c.
  chicken fat c.
  currant jelly c.
  c. lysis
  c. lysis time (CLT)
  postmortem c.

  c. reaction
  c. retraction
  c. retraction time
clothing
  disposable chemical-resistant c.
  hooded chemical-resistant c.
CLOT R
clottage
clotting
  c. factor
  c. factor deficiency
  c. time (CT)
Cloudman melanoma
cloudy
  c. swelling
  c. swelling degeneration
  c. urine
Clough-Richter syndrome
Clouston syndrome
clove oil
cloverleaf skull
CLPD
  chronic lymphoproliferative
    disorder
CLSL
  chronic lymphosarcoma leukemia
CLSM
  confocal laser scan microscopy
CLT
  clot lysis time
club hair
clubbed
  c. digit
  c. finger
  c. toe
clubbing
  digital c.
  hereditary c.
clubfoot, club foot
clubhand, club hand
clue cell
clump
clumping
  ex vivo platelet c.
cluster
  epithelioid cell c.
  glomerular-like c.
  metastatic c.
  c. of differentiation (CD)
  sinusoidal foam cell c.
  c. 1 small-cell lung cancer
    antigen
  temporal c.
clusterin
  c. antigen
  c. immunostaining
  c. marker
clustering
  hierarchical c.

Clutton joint
cM
  centimorgan
CM
  cardiac myxoma
  cavernous malformation
cm
  centimeter
cm3
  cubic centimeter
CMA
  complete maturation arrest
CM1 antibody
CMB
  carbolic methylene blue
CMC
  chronic mucocutaneous candidiasis
  critical micelle concentration
CM-cellulose
  carboxymethylcellulose
CMF
  chondromyxoid fibroma
CMGN
  chronic membranous glomerulonephritis
CMI
  carbohydrate metabolism index
  cell-mediated immunity
CMID
  cytomegalic inclusion disease
c/min
  cycle per minute
CML
  chronic myelocytic leukemia
  chronic myelogenous leukemia
CMM
  cutaneous malignant melanoma
cmm
  cubic millimeter
CMML
  chronic myelomonocytic leukemia
CMN
  congenital melanocytic nevi
  congenital mesoblastic nephroma
  cystic medial necrosis
CMN-AA
  cystic medial necrosis of ascending aorta
cMO
  centimorgan
CMO
  calculated mean organism
CMOAT
  canicular multispecific organic anion transporter
CMoL
  chronic monoblastic leukemia
  chronic monocytic leukemia
CMP
  cardiomyopathy

  colorimetric microtiter plate
  cytidine monophosphate
CMPD
  chronic myeloproliferative disorder
CMP-*N*-acetyl-d-neuraminate
c-mp1 receptor
CMR
  cerebral metabolic rate
  crude mortality ratio
CMRG
  cerebral metabolic rate of glucose
CMRO
  cerebral metabolic rate of oxygen
CMRR
  common mode rejection ratio
CMV
  cytomegalovirus
    CMV antibody
    CMV culture
    CMV isolation
CMV-negative allogeneic cell
CMV-seronegative blood
c-myc
    c-m. amplification
    c-m. gene
    c-m. marker
    c-m. cmyc oncogene
    c-m. oncoprotein
c-mycERTAM stem cell expansion technology
CN
  calcineurin
  NATO code for 1-chloroacetophenone
CN-
  cyanide radical
CNB
  core needle biopsy
Cnephia
CNHD
  congenital nonspherocytic hemolytic disease
Cnidospora
Cnidosporidia
CNS
  central nervous system
    atypical teratoid/rhabdoid tumor of the CNS
CNT
  cutaneous neural tumor
CNV
  choroidal neovascularization
  contingent negative variation
CNV
    interindividual CNV
CO
  calcium oxalate
  carbon monoxide
  corneal opacity

CO2
    carbon dioxide
        CO_2 output
        CO_2 production
CoA
    coenzyme A
coacervate
coacervation
coactivator
coactosinlike 1
Coag-a-mate prothrombin device
coagglutinin
coag
    coagulation
CoaguChek
        C. Pro/DM coagulometer
        C. Pro/DM system
coagulable
coagulant complex
coagulase test
coagulate
coagulated albumin
coagulating enzyme
coagulation (coag)
        c. cascade
        diffuse intravascular c. (DIC)
        disseminated intravascular c. (DIC)
        exogenous anticoagulant c.
        c. factor I
        c. factor assay
        c. factor inhibitor
        c. factor I–XIII
        c. factor transfusion
        fibrinolysin c.
        c. necrosis
        c. pathway
        plasmin c.
        spontaneous c.
        c. time (CT)
        c. time test
coagulative necrosis
coagulin-B
coagulogram
coagulometer
        CoaguChek Pro/DM c.
coagulopathy
        consumption c.
        dilutional c.
        intravascular consumption c. (IVCC)
        c. of liver disease
coagulum
        seminal c.
coal
        c. tar
        c. tar naphtha
        c. worker's pneumoconiosis (CWP)
coalescence
coalition
        tarsal c.

coarctate
coarctation
        infantile type c.
        c. of aorta
coarse
        c. gravel
        c. marking
        c. material
coarsening
coat
        buffy c.
        cell c.
        C. disease
        fuzzy c.
        sclerotic c.
        serous c.
coated electron-lucent vesicle
coating fixative
cobalamin
cobalt assay
cobalticyanide (CoCN6)
cobaltinitrite method
cobaltous chloride
Cobas
        C. Amplicor HIV-1 monitor test
        C. Fara H centrifugal analyzer
        C. Helios differential analyzer
        C. Integra Cyclosporine
            Immunoassay
cobbler's chest
cobblestone appearance
cobblestoning
Cobetia marina
Coblentz test method
cobra
        C. Amplicor analyzer
        c. hemotoxin
        c. venom
        c. venom cofactor
        c. venom factor
COBS
        cesarean-obtained barrier-sustained
COCA
        Clinician Outreach and Communication
            Activity
coca
        Erythroxylon c.
cocacinogen
Cocadviroid
cocaethylene
cocaine
        c. hydrochloride
        c. metabolite assay
        tetracaine, Adrenalin (epinephrine),
            and c.
cocarboxylase
cocarcinogen
cocarcinogenesis
cocarde reaction

coccal
cocci (*pl. of* coccus)
coccidia (*pl. of* coccidium)
coccidial
Coccidiasina
coccidioidal granuloma
coccidioides
    Blastomyces c.
    C. immitis
coccidioidin test
coccidioidoma
coccidioidomycosis
    c. antibody
    asymptomatic c.
    disseminate c.
    latent c.
    primary c.
    secondary c.
    subclinical c.
coccidiosis
coccidium, *pl.* **coccidia**
    C. hominis
coccinella
coccinellin
coccobacillus
    aerobic c.
    facultative c.
    intracellular c.
    obligate c.
coccobacteria
coccoid *Helicobacter pylori*
coccus, *pl.* **cocci**
    gram-negative cocci
    gram-positive cocci
coccygeal
    c. body
    c. fistula
    c. gland
coccygeum
    corpus c.
    glomus c.
Cochin China diarrhea
cochineal
cochlea, *pl.* **cochleae**
    aqueductus cochleae
    fenestra cochleae
    lamina basilaris cochleae
    ligamentum spirale
      cochleae
    membranous c.
cochleae (*pl. of* cochlea)
cochlear
    c. aqueduct
    c. duct
    c. hair cell
    c. hydrops
    c. otosclerosis
    c. window
cochleariform

cochlearis
    crista basilaris ductus c.
    ductus c.
    membrana tectoria ductus c.
    membrana vestibularis ductus c.
    stria vascularis ductus c.
cochlearium
    Clostridium c.
cochleate
Cochliobolus
Cochliomyia
    C. americana
    C. hominivorax
Cochlosoma anatis
$^{14}CO_2$**-cholyl-glycine breath test**
cockade reaction
Cockayne
    C. disease
    C. syndrome
Cockcroft-Gault equation
cockscomb
    c. polyp
    c. ulcer
cocktail
    Boehringer Mannheim Kermix
     cytokeratin c.
    DIG c.
    keratin c.
    Molotov c.
CoCN6
    cobalticyanide
coctoprecipitin
cocultivation
cocurrent
COD
    cause of death
    cementoosseous dysphasia
code
    degenerate c.
    gene c.
    genetic c.
    Hollerith c.
    mnemonic c.
    NATO c.
    object c.
    OP c.
    operation c.
    resistor color c.
    triplet c.
codeine assay
Code-On Immunoslide stainer
coding
    color c.
    polypeptide c.
    c. triplet
CODIS
    combined DNA index system
Codman tumor
codocyte

codominance
codominant
    c. gene
    c. inheritance
codon
    initiation c.
    start c.
    stop c.
    termination c.
coefficient
    absorption c.
    binomial c.
    Bouchard c.
    Bunsen c.
    conversion c.
    correlation c.
    creatinine c.
    decay c.
    diffusion c.
    dilution c.
    distribution c.
    extinction c.
    extraction c.
    hygienic laboratory c.
    inbreeding c.
    isotonic c.
    lethal c.
    linear attenuation c.
    Long c.
    mass attenuation c.
    c. of inbreeding
    c. of selection
    c. of variation (CV)
    osmotic c.
    oxygen utilization c.
    rank correlation c.
    regression c. (R)
    Rideal-Walker c.
    sedimentation c.
    solubility c.
    Spearman rank correlation c.
    Svedberg unit of sedimentation c. (S)
    temperature c. (Q_{10})
    urohemolytic c.
    urotoxic c.
    velocity c.
    volume c.
Coelenterata
coelenterate
coelenterazine dextran-coated charcoal
coelenterazine-treated cell
coeliaci
    nodi lymphoidei c.
coeloblastula
coelom, celom
coelomic
    c. epithelium
    c. granulocyte

Coemansia
coenocyte (*var. of* cenocyte)
coenocytic
Coenonia anatina
coenuris (*var. of* cenuris)
coenurosis
Coenurus
    C. cerebralis
    C. serialis
coenzyme
    c. A (CoA)
    acyl c. A (acyl-CoA)
    c. Q (CoQ)
    c. thiamine pyrophosphate
    d-3-hydroxyacyl c. A
    l-hydroxyacyl c. A
    malonyl c. A
coenzyme-labeled immunoassay
coeur en sabot
Coe virus
coexpression
COF
    cementoossifying fibroma
cofactor
    activated protein C c. (APC cofactor)
    cobra venom c.
    heparin c. (HC, HCF)
    c. of thromboplastin
    platelet c.
    ristocetin c. (RcoF)
coffee-bean groove
coffeegrounds appearance
coffin formation
Coffin-Lowry syndrome
Coffin-Siris syndrome
Cogan syndrome
COGTT
    cortisone-primed oral glucose tolerance test
COHb
    carboxyhemoglobin
coherent smallpox
cohesion
cohesiveness
Cohn fractionation
Cohnheim
    C. area
    C. field
    C. theory
cohort
    c. labeling
    c. study
coil
    c. gland
    Macroduct c.
    plectonemic c.
    primary c.

random c.
secondary c.
coincidence
c. correction
c. error
c. sum peak
coinfection
coin lesion
coinlike
cokeri
Septobasidium c.
Cokeromyces
COL4A5 gene
Colcemid
Colcher-Sussman x-ray pelvimetry method
colchicine
COLD
chronic obstructive lung disease
cold
c. abscess
c. agglutination
c. agglutinin (CA)
c. agglutinin disease
c. agglutinin screen
c. agglutinin syndrome (CAS)
c. agglutinin test
c. agglutinin titer
c. allergy
c. antibody
c. autoabsorption
c. autoagglutinin
c. autoantibody
c. autoimmune hemolytic anemia
c. gangrene
c. hemagglutinin
c. hemagglutinin disease
c. hemoglobinuria
c. hemolysin
c. hemolysin test
c. injury
c. intolerance
c. lesion
c. microtome
c. nodule
c. rigor point
c. room
rose c.
c. silver nitrate
c. sore
c. spot
c. stage
c. ulcer
c. urticaria
c. virus
cold-agglutination phenomenon
cold-knife conization

cold-reacting antibody
cold-reactive antibody
cold-sensitive mutation
cold-type
c.-t. antibody
c.-t. autoimmune hemolytic anemia
colectasia
Cole hematoxylin
Coleman Feulgen solution
Coleman-Schiff reagent
coleocanis
Actinomyces c.
coleohominis
Lactobacillus c.
Coleophoma
Coleoptera
coleoptosis
colestipol hydrochloride
Coleviroid
Coley toxin
coli
adenomatous polyposis c. (APC)
Amoeba c.
Bacillus c.
Balantidium c.
Campylobacter c.
diarrheagenic *E.* c.
Entamoeba c.
enteroaggregative *Escherichia* c. (EaggEC)
enterohemorrhagic *Escherichia* c.
enteroinvasive *Escherichia* c. (EIEC)
enteropathogenic *Escherichia* c. (EEC, EPEC)
enterotoxic *Escherichia* c. (ETEC)
enterotoxigenic *Escherichia* c. (ETEC)
Escherichia c.
extraintestinal pathogenic *Escherichia* c. (ExPEC)
familial adenomatous polyposis c.
familial polyposis c. (FPC)
Holophyra c.
juvenile polyposis c.
melanosis c.
polyposis c.
pseudomelanosis c.
stratum longitudinale tunicae muscularis c.
Streptococcus infantarius subsp. *c.*
teniae c.
tunica mucosa c.
tunica muscularis c.
tunica serosa c.
colibacillary
colibacillemia
colibacilluria
colibacillus

colic
- biliary c.
- endemic c.
- intestinal c.
- c. intussusception
- lead c.
- menstrual c.
- renal c.
- uterine c.
- verminous c.

colicanis
- *Clostridium c.*

colicin
colicinogeny
coliform bacillus
coliforme
colihominis
- *Anaerotruncus c.*

colinearity
colipase
coliphage
colistimethate sodium
colistin sulfate
colitides (*pl. of* colitis)
colitis, *pl.* colitides
- acute ulcerative c.
- amebic c.
- antibiotic-associated c. (AAC)
- balantidial c.
- chronic ulcerative c. (CUC)
- collagenous c.
- c. cystica profunda
- c. cystica superficialis
- diversion c.
- eosinophilic c.
- fulminant c.
- granulomatous c.
- c. gravis
- hemorrhagic c.
- indeterminate c.
- infectious c.
- ischemic c.
- lymphocytic c. (LC)
- metachronous collagenous c.
- microscopic c.
- mucous c.
- nonrelapsing c.
- nontyphoidal infectious c.
- pseudomembranous c. (PMC)
- radiation c.
- regional c.
- self-limited c.
- spastic c.
- toxic c.
- ulcerative c. (UC)
- uremic c.

colitose
colitoxicosis
colitoxin

coliuria
COLL
- collection
- colloidal

collacin
collagen
- c. bundle
- c. degeneration
- c. deposition
- c. disease
- c. disorder
- endomysial c.
- c. fiber
- c. fibril
- fibrous long-spacing c. (FLS)
- c. flower
- c. gel droplet-embedded drug sensitivity test
- c. gel invasion assay
- hyaluronidase c.
- lack of c.
- lamellar c.
- c. marker
- c. receptor deficiency
- ropey c.
- SLS c.
- c. staining method
- subepithelial c.
- c. type IX alpha 2 gene
- type I–XX c.
- wire-like c.
- c. X, XVIII
- Zyderm c.

collagenase
- clostridial c.
- *Clostridium histolyticum* c.
- c. synthesis

collagenation
collagenic
collagenization
collagenoblast
collagenocyte
collagenoma
- giant cell c. (GCC)

collagenosis
- reactive perforating c. (RPC)

collagenous
- c. colitis
- c. fiber
- c. fibroma
- c. spherulosis
- c. sprue
- c. stroma

collagen-vascular
- c.-v. disease

collapse
- circulatory c.
- hemodynamic c.
- c. induration

massive c.
structural c.
structure c.

collar
abrasion c.
c. button abscess
c. button lesion
false abrasion c.

collarette
collaring
collastin
collateral
collecting
c. duct
c. duct carcinoma (CDC)

collection
American Type Culture C. (ATCC)
arterial blood c.
GLOB c.
Macroduct system for sweat stimulation and c.
stool c.
UrAssist pum-assisted urine c.
urine specimen c.

collector
anaerobic specimen c.

College of American Pathologists
Colletotrichum
Collet-Sicard syndrome
Collet syndrome
colli
cystitis c.
fibromatosis c.
lipoma annulare c.

colliculi (*pl. of* colliculus)
colliculitis
colliculus, *pl.* **colliculi**
seminal c.

collidine
collier's lung
colligative
colligin
collimate
collimator
Collimonas fungivorans
Collinsella
C. aerofaciens
C. intestinalis
C. stercoris
collinsii
Trichococcus c.
colliquation
ballooning c.
reticulating c.

colliquative
c. albuminuria
c. degeneration
c. necrosis

collision tumor
collodion, collodium
c. baby
c. filter
collodium (*var. of* collodion)
colloid
c. adenocarcinoma
c. adenoma
c. body
bovine c.
c. cancer
c. carcinoma
c. corpuscle
c. cyst
c. degeneration
extrafollicular c.
c. goiter
c. milium
c. oncotic pressure (COP)
c. osmotic hemolysis
c. shift
c. shock
thyroid c.

colloidal
c. dispersion
c. electrolyte
c. gold (CG)
c. gold reaction
c. gold test
c. iron stain
c. osmotic pressure (COP)
c. silica gradient
c. silicon dioxide

colloides
struma c.

colloidin
colloidoclasia, colloidoclasis
colloidoclasis (*var. of* colloidoclasia)
colloid-osmotic lysis
collum folliculi pili
Collybia
Collyriclum
coloboma
c., heart disease, atresia choanae, retarded growth and development and ear anomalies (CHARGE)
c. syndrome

coloboma,
colocalization
colocutaneous fistula
coloenteric
coloileal fistula
colombiense
Aminobacterium c.
colon
c. atresia
c. bacillus
c. carcinoma
cathartic c.

colon (*continued*)
    giant c.
    c. glandular tissue
    irritable c. (IC)
    lead-pipe c.
    c. polyp
    sigmoid c.
    spastic c.
    c. tumor
colonic
    c. fistula
    c. hamartoma
    c. smear
    c. vomitus
colonization infection
colony
    beaten-egg-white-appearance c.
    bitten c.
    butyrous c.
    c. count
    curled hair c.
    D c.
    daughter c.
    dwarf c.
    effuse c.
    fried egg c.
    ground-glass appearance c.
    H c.
    hammered copper c.
    irregular border c.
    M c.
    c. morphology
    mucoid c.
    O c.
    opaque c.
    R c.
    raised c.
    rough c.
    S c.
    satellite c.
    shiny surface c.
    smooth c.
    c. stands up
    swirling comet tail c.
    wavy border c.
colony-forming
    c.-f. unit (CFU)
    c.-f. unit-culture (CFUC, CFU-C)
    c.-f. unit-erythroid (CFU-E)
    c.-f. unit granulocyte, erythrocyte, monocyte, and megakaryocyte (CFU-GEMM)
    c.-f. unit granulocyte-macrophage (CFU-GM)
    c.-f. unit-megakaryocyte (CFU-Meg)
    c.-f. units/mL (CFU/mL)
    c.-f. unit-spleen (CFU-S)

colony-stimulating
    c.-s. activity (CSA)
    c.-s. factor (CSF)
coloproctitis
    cryptal lymphocytic c.
coloptosia (*var. of* coloptosis)
coloptosis, coloptosia
color
    amniotic fluid c.
    c. coding
    complementary c.
    fecal c.
    primary c.
    spectral c.
    stool c.
Colorado
    C. tick fever
    C. tick fever virus
color-contrast microscope
colorectal
    c. cancer (CRC)
    c. carcinoma
    c. polyp
colorectitis
Colorfrost disposable microscope slide
colorimeter
colorimetric
    c. antibody detection
    c. method
    c. microtiter plate (CMP)
colorimetry
Colormark slide
Colormate Tlc.BiliTest system
ColorPAC toxin A test
4-color PCR assay
Coloscreen Self test
colossus
    Calomys c.
colostrum corpuscle
Colour Index (C.I.)
colovaginal fistula
colovesical fistula
colpatresia
colpectasia
colpitis
colpocystitis
colpocytology
colpohyperplasia
    c. cystica
    c. emphysematosa
Colpoma
Coltivirus
Colton antigen
colubriformis
    Trichostrongylus c.
Columbia
    C. blood agar
    C. medium
    C. SK virus

columbianum
 Oesophagostomum c.
columbium (Cb)
columella
column (COL)
 anal c.
 Bertin c.
 Bürdach c.
 c. cell
 Clarke c.
 DEAE-Sephacel ion exchange c.
 ion-exchange c.
 Morgagni c.
 c.'s of Bertin
 rectal c.
 renal c.
 Sertoli c.
columnae
 c. anales
 c. carneae
 c. renales
columnar
 c. absorptive cell
 c. cell hyperplasia
 c. cell variant (CCV)
 c. cuff
 c. epithelium
 c. layer
 c. metaplasia
Colwelliaceae
Colwellia piezophila
coma
 alcoholic c.
 apoplectic c.
 c. cast
 c. dépassé
 diabetic c.
 Harvard criteria of irreversible c.
 hepatic c.
 hyperosmolar diabetic c.
 irreversible c.
 metabolic c.
 uremic c.
Comamonadaceae
Comamonas
 C. aquatica
 C. denitrificans
 C. kerstersii
 C. koreensis
 C. nitrativorans
comatose
comb
combesi
 Eubacterium c.
comb-growth test
combination calculus
combinatorial immunity
combined
 c. androgen blockade

 c. DNA index system (CODIS)
 c. immunodeficiency
 c. immunodeficiency disease
 c. immunodeficiency syndrome
 (CIDS)
 c. pituitary function test
 c. sclerosis
 c. systems disease
 c. ventricular hypertrophy (CVH)
combining site
Combo
 Acceava hCG C.
 QuickVue+ One-Step hCG C.
combustible
 c. gas
 c. gas detector
 c. liquid
 c. vapor
combustion
 carbonaceous residue of c.
 heat of c.
comedo
 c. ductal carcinoma in situ
 c. necrosis
 c. nevus
comedocarcinoma
 infiltrating c.
comedomastitis
comedonecrosis
comedonicus
 nevus c.
comet cell
comma bacillus
commensal bacterium
commensalism
commercial insulin preparation
commingled remains
comminuted fracture
commission
 Biological Stain C.
commissura anterior grisea
commissural cell
commissure
 Ganser c.
 gray c.
committed cell
committee
 transfusion adult c.
common
 c. acute lymphoblastic leukemia
 antigen (CALLA)
 c. acute lymphocytic leukemia
 antigen
 c. bile duct
 c. bile duct obstruction
 c. cold virus
 c. enterobacterial antigen
 c. logarithm
 c. mode rejection ratio (CMRR)

C

215

common (*continued*)
    c. mode signal
    c. opsonin
    c. reference
    c. storage
    c. variable
    c. variable hypogammaglobulinemia (CVH)
    c. variable immunodeficiency (CVID)
    c. variable immunodeficiency syndrome
    c. viral etiology
    c. wart
commotio cerebri
commun dis
commune
    Aquabacterium c.
    integumentum c.
    Schizophyllum c.
communicable disease
communicans
    macula c.
communicate
    esophagus c.
communicating
    c. hydrocephalus
    c. junction
communication
    gap junction intercellular c.
communis
    macula c.
    Ricinus c.
    sacculus c.
    Sericopelma c.
community-acquired methicillin-resistant *Staphylococcus aureus*
commutator
Comovirus
compacta
    substantia c.
compact bone
compactum
    Fonsecaea c.
    Hormodendrum c.
    stratum c.
companion cell
comparascope
comparative
    c. genome hybridization
    c. genomic hybridization (CGH)
    c. pathology
comparator microscope
comparison
    cartilage and bone c.
    c. eyepiece
    c. microscope
    c. operation

compartment
    acidified prelysosomal c.
    c. syndrome
compartmental
    c. analysis
    c. syndrome
compatibility
    ABO c.
    c. test
compatible
compensated
    c. acidosis
    c. alkalosis
    c. eyepiece
compensating ocular
compensation
    broken c.
    dosage c.
    temperature c. (TC)
compensatory
    c. atrophy
    c. emphysema
    c. hypertrophy
    c. mechanism
    c. polycythemia
    c. regeneration
competence
    embryonic c.
    c. gene
    immunologic c.
    immunological c.
competition
    antigenic c.
    c. hybridization
competitive
    c. antagonist
    c. binding assay
    c. heterogeneous enzyme immunoassay
    c. inhibition
    c. protein-binding (CPB)
    c. protein-binding assay
    c. protein-binding test
    c. reverse transcription polymerase chain reaction (cRT-PCR)
competitor DNA
compiler
    optimizing c.
compile time
complement
    c. activation
    c. binding assay
    C_3, C_4 c.
    c. chemotactic factor
    chromosome c.
    c. component
    component of c.
    c. deficiency state
    c. direct Coombs test

dominant c.
endocellular c.
erythrocyte antibody c. (EAC)
c. fixation (CF)
c. inactivation
c. lysis sensitivity test
c. receptor (CR)
c. receptor 3 (CR3)
c. system
c. total
two's c.
c. unit
whole c. (WC)

complemental inheritance
complementarity
c. determining region (CDR)
dominant c.

complementary
c. base
c. color
c. DNA (cDNA)
c. DNA clone
c. gene
c. groove
c. hypertrophy
c. strand
c. symmetry amplifier

complementation
complement-fixation
c.-f. reaction
Reiter protein c.-f. (RPCF)
c.-f. test (CFT)

complement-fixing (CF)
c.-f. antibody
c.-f. antigen

complement-mediated cytotoxicity
complementophil
complete
c. abortion
c. androgen insensitivity syndrome (CAIS)
c. anterior dislocation
c. antibody
c. antigen
c. blood count (CBC)
c. carcinogen
c. fistula
c. heart block (CHB)
c. inferior dislocation
c. left bundle-branch block (CLBBB)
c. maturation arrest (CMA)
c. mole
c. obstruction
c. penetrance
c. posterior dislocation
c. reaction of degeneration (CRD)
c. right bundle-branch block (CRBBB)
c. superior dislocation

c. transduction
c. trisomy

complex
acrosomal c.
activated c.
c. adrenal endocrine disorder
AIDS-related c. (ARC)
angiotumoral c.
antigen-antibody c.
antigenic c.
c. atypical hyperplasia/metaplasia (CAHM)
avian leukosis-sarcoma c.
avidin-biotin c.
avidin-biotin peroxidase c. (ABC)
C1 c.
cadherin/catenin c.
Carney c.
C5B-9 c.
Cdk4/6-cyclin D c.
charge-transfer c.
coagulant c.
cytochrome bc1 c.
c. endometrial hyperplasia
electron transport chain c. I
feline leukemia-sarcoma virus c.
FN-MCD c.
gene c.
Ghon c.
Ghon-Sachs c.
glucocorticoid-glucocorticoid receptor c.
glucocorticoid-GR c.
Golgi c.
c. gonadal endocrine disorder
H-2 c.
healed Ghon c.
histocompatibility c.
HLA c.
homotetrameric c.
horseradish peroxidase conjugated streptavidin-biotin c.
immune c.
immune-stimulating c. (ISCOM)
junctional c.
juxtaglomerular c.
Kolliker-Fuse c.
major histocompatibility c. (MHC)
membrane attack c. (MAC)
Meyenburg c.
MHC I/calreticulin c.
minor histocompatibility c.
Mycobacterium avium-intracellulare c. (MAC)
Mycobacterium phlei cell wall DNA c. (MCC)
nuclear pore c.
c. number
c. odontoma

complex (*continued*)
   Ornithodoros moubata c.
   orthocresolphthalein c. (OPCP)
   ostiomeatal c.
   c. pituitary endocrine disorder
   platelet phospholipid c.
   primary c.
   prothrombin c.
   pyruvate dehydrogenase c. (PDC)
   renal dysplasia c.
   ribonucleoprotein c.
   ribosome-lamella c.
   RNP c.
   c. sclerosing lesion
   sicca c.
   steroid-receptor c.
   SWI/SNF c.
   synaptinemal c.
   synaptonemal c.
   T-cell receptor c.
   TCR c.
   tenase c.
   c. thyroid endocrine disorder
   triple symptom c.
   tuberous sclerosis c. (TSC)
   VATER c.
   vitamin B c.
   von Meyenburg c. (VMC)
complexed
   c. prostate-specific antigen (cPSA)
   c. PSA
complexity
   DNA c.
compliance
   dynamic pulmonary c.
   static pulmonary c.
complicata
   cataracta c.
complication
   catastrophic c.
   c. of silicosis
component
   amyloid P c.
   c. A of prothrombin
   basement membrane c.
   blood c.
   carcinomatous c.
   complement c.
   dense fibrillar c.
   epithelial c.
   epsilon c.
   extensive intraductal c. (EIC)
   Immunotech immunoassay c.
   inorganic c.
   late positive c. (LPC)
   M c.
   c. management
   micropapillary c. (MPC)
   no mineral c.

   c. of complement
   plasma thromboplastin c. (PTC)
   sarcomatous c.
   secretory c.
   sertoliform c.
   spindle cell c.
   stromal c.
   thromboplastic plasma c. (TPC)
composite lymphoma
composition
   chylomicron c.
   c. resistor
   three dimensional c.
composta
   Nocardiopsis c.
compound
   c. absorption device (CAD)
   acetone c.
   c. aneurysm
   aromatic c.
   beta-amyloid c.
   carbamino c.
   carbon inorganic c.
   c. comminuted fracture (CCF)
   condensation c.
   c. cyst
   c. dislocation
   gossypol c.
   c. granular corpuscle
   c. granule cell
   heterocyclic c.
   c. heterozygote
   c. leukemia
   meso c.
   c. microscope
   c. multiple fractures
   c. nevus
   OCT freezing c.
   c. odontoma
   organometallic c.
   organophosphate c.
   organosilicon c.
   polar c.
   c. presentation
   c. tumor
   volatile organic c. (VOC)
   c. X
compransoris
   Zavarzinia c.
compressed
   c. fracture
   c. gas storage
   c. spectral assay (CSA)
compression
   cerebral c.
   cord c. (CC)
   extrinsic c.
   c. fracture
   c. injury

c. of tissue
spinal cord c.
compressive myelopathy
compressus
fetus c.
computer
c. linkage analysis
sequential multiple analyzer c.
(SMAC)
computer-assisted image analysis
COMT
catechol-O-methyl transferase
ConA
concanavalin A
conarium
conc
concentrated
concentration
concameration
concanavalin
c. A (ConA)
c. A-horseradish peroxidase
concatenate
concatenation
Concato disease
concentrate
B-domain-deleted factor VIII c.
granulocyte c.
intrinsic factor c. (IFC)
malondialdehyde c.
marine protein c. (MPC)
metallothionein c.
platelet c.
random-donor platelet c.
Trizma buffer c.
concentrated (conc)
concentration (conc)
c. and dilution test
approximate lethal c. (ALC)
bactericidal c. (BC)
Baermann c.
blood alcohol c. (BAC)
carbon dioxide c.
cotinine urinary c.
critical micelle c. (CMC)
fecal c.
formalin-ether sedimentation c.
formalin-ethyl acetate sedimentation c.
gravity c.
hazardous c.
HCO_3 c.
hepatic iron c. (HIC)
high trough c.
hydrogen ion c. (pH)
hydroxyl c. (pOH)
ion c.
ionic c.
lethal c. (LC, LCt)
limiting isorrheic c. (LIC)

M c.
mass c.
maximum permissible c. (MPC)
maximum urinary c. (MUC)
mean cell hemoglobin c. (MCHC)
mean corpuscular hemoglobin c.
(MCHC)
microhematocrit c.
micromolar c.
minimal bactericidal c.
minimal inhibitory c. (MIC)
minimal isorrheic c.
minimal lethal c. (MLC)
minimum bactericidal c.
minimum complete-killing c. (MCC)
minimum detectable c. (MDC)
minimum inhibitory c. (MIC)
minimum lethal c. (MLC)
minimum mycoplasmacidal c. (MPC)
molar c. (c, molc)
c. of adenosine monophosphate
c. of creatinine in serum (Scr)
c. of creatinine in urine (Ucr)
c. of sodium in serum (SNa)
c. of sodium in urine (UNa)
c. of total oxygen
c. procedure
prothrombin complex c. (PCC)
radioactive c.
renal vein renin c. (RVRC)
serum p24 antigen c.
substance c.
time of maximum c. (T_{max})
total L-chain c. (TLC)
zinc sulfate flotation c.
concentration-dependent nanomolar response
concentration-time
c.-t. product (Ct)
c.-t. product for 50% of exposed group (Ct_{50})
concentrator
speed vacuum c.
concentric
c. fibroma
c. hypertrophy
c. intimal thickening
c. lamella
concentrica
encephalitis periaxialis c.
concentricum
Trichophyton c.
concentricus
Aspergillus c.
conception
retained products of c.
conchoidal body
concinna
Haemaphysalis c.

concisus
    Campylobacter c.
concomitant immunity
concordance
concrement
concrescence
concretio
    c. cordis
    c. pericardii
concretion
    calcific c.
concurrent infection
concussion
    brain c.
    cardiac c.
    c. myelitis
    spinal cord c.
condensans
    osteitis c.
    osteopathia c.
condensation
    block-like chromatin c.
    c. compound
    c. fibrosis
    c. polymer
condenser
    Abbé c.
    cardioid c.
    dark-field c.
condensing
    c. osteitis
    c. vacuole
condition
    RNase-free c.
    steady-state c.
    sufficient c.
conditional
    c. jump
    c. lethal mutation
    c. probability
conditional-lethal mutant
conditionally lethal mutant
conductance
conduction
    c. electron
    saltatory c.
    volume c.
conductive hearing loss
conductivity
    c. cell volume (CCV)
    thermal c. (TC)
    water c.
conductometry
conductor
conduit
conduplicate
condyloma, *pl.* **condylomas, condylomata**
    c. acuminatum
    Buschke-Löwenstein giant c.

    flat c.
    genital c.
    giant c.
    c. latum
    pointed c.
condylomas (*pl. of* condyloma)
condylomata (*pl. of* condyloma)
condylomatous atypia
cone
    antipodal c.
    c. biopsy
    c. bipolar cell
    c. cell of retina
    c. disc
    c. fiber
    c. granule
    Haller c.
    implantation c.
    retinal c.
    theca interna c.
    twin c.
    vascular c.
cone-nose bug
Conexibacter woesei
conexus
conference
    clinicopathologic c. (CPC)
confertus
confidence
    c. interval (CI)
    c. level
confidential unit exclusion (CUE)
configuration
    cis c.
    germline c.
    serpiginous c.
    signet-ring c.
    villiform c.
confined
    organ c. (OC)
    c. placental mosaicism (CPM)
confinement
    expected date of c. (EDC)
confirmatory
    c. test
    c. testing
confirmed diagnosis
confluent
    c. and reticulate papillomatosis
    c. bronchopneumonia
    c. hepatic necrosis
    c. inflammation
    c. pneumonia
    c. smallpox
confocal
    c. image
    c. laser scan microscopy (CLSM)
    c. microscopy

conformation
conformer
confusa
    Taenia c.
confusion
    circle of c.
congelans
    Pseudomonas c.
congelation urticaria
congener
congenita
    amyoplasia c.
    amyotonia c.
    chondrodystrophia calcificans c.
    dyskeratosis c.
    hyperkeratosis c.
    ichthyosis c.
    osteogenesis imperfecta c.
    osteosclerosis c.
    pachyonychia c.
congenital
    c. absence
    c. absence of vagina (CAV)
    c. achromia
    c. adrenal hyperplasia (CAH)
    c. adrenal virilism (CAV)
    c. afibrinogenemia
    c. agammaglobulinemia
    c. aganglionosis
    c. ahaptoglobinemia
    c. anomaly
    c. aplasia of thymus
    c. aplastic anemia
    c. aregenerative anemia
    c. atransferrinemia
    c. atresia
    c. biliary ectasia
    c. cardiovascular malformation
    c. chylothorax
    c. contracture
    c. cyst
    c. dislocation
    c. dislocation of hip (CDH)
    c. duplication
    c. dyserythropoietic anemia (CDA)
    c. dysphagocytosis
    c. dysplastic angiectasia
    c. dysplastic angiomatosis
    c. dysplastic angiopathy
    c. ectodermal defect
    c. ectodermal dysplasia
    c. elephantiasis
    c. erythropoietic porphyria (CEP)
    c. familial icterus
    c. familial nonhemolytic jaundice
    c. fibrosarcoma (CFS)
    c. generalized fibromatosis
    c. glaucoma
    c. goiter

    c. hemidysplasia with ichthyosiform erythroderma and limb defects (CHILD)
    c. hemolytic icterus
    c. hemolytic jaundice
    c. hepatic fibrosis
    c. hyperbilirubinemia
    c. hypophosphatasia
    c. hypoplastic anemia (CHA)
    c. infantile fibrosarcoma (CIF)
    c. lactase deficiency
    c. leukemia
    c. lobar emphysema
    c. localized absence of skin (CLAS)
    c. lymphedema
    c. megacolon
    c. melanocytic nevi (CMN)
    c. mesoblastic nephroma (CMN)
    c. methemoglobinemia
    c. muscular dystrophy
    c. musculoskeletal deformity
    c. myopathy
    c. nonregenerative anemia
    c. nonspherocytic hemolytic anemia
    c. nonspherocytic hemolytic disease (CNHD)
    c. pancytopenia
    c. pectus excavatum
    c. pterygium
    c. pulmonary lymphangiectasis (CPL)
    c. pyloric stenosis
    c. rest
    c. rubella syndrome
    c. ruptured aneurysm
    c. sebaceous hyperplasia
    c. spherocytosis
    c. sucrase-isomaltase deficiency (CSID)
    c. sutural alopecia
    c. thymic aplasia
    c. thymic dysplasia (CTD)
    c. torticollis
    c. total lipodystrophy
    c. toxoplasmosis
    c. valve
    c. valvular heart disease
    c. vascular weakness
congenitale
    hemangioma c.
    poikiloderma c.
congenitum
    megacolon c.
congested centrilobular area
congestion
    brain c.
    chronic passive c. (CPC)
    hypostatic c.

C

congestion (*continued*)
  postoperative c.
  pulmonary venous c. (PVC)
  venous c.
congestive
  c. cardiac failure (CCF)
  c. cardiomyopathy
  c. cirrhosis
  c. edema
  c. heart disease (CHD)
  c. heart failure (CHF)
  c. splenomegaly
conglobata
  acne c.
conglobate
conglobation
conglomerata
  elastosis colloidalis c.
conglomerate
conglomeratus
  Micrococcus c.
conglutinating complement absorption test (CCAT)
conglutination
conglutinin
conglutinogen-activating factor
Congo
  C. Corinth
  C. floor maggot
  C. red
  C. red paper
  C. red stain
  C. red test
  rubrum C.
congolense
  Trypanosoma c.
congolensis
  Actinomyces c.
  Dermatophilus c.
  Thysanotaenia c.
congophilic angiopathy
coni (*pl. of* conus)
conicae
conidial
conidiobolae
  entomophthoramycosis c.
Conidiobolus
  C. coronatus
  C. incongruus
conidiogenous
conidiophore
conidiospore
conidium
coniine
Coniochaeta
coniofibrosis
coniolymphstasis
coniophage
Coniophora

coniosis
Coniosporium
Coniothecium
Coniothyrium
Conium
conization
  cold-knife c.
conjoined twins
conjugal cancer
conjugant
conjugate
  c. acid
  c. acid-base pairs
  antidigoxigenin antibody peroxidase c.
  c. base
  c. division
  fluorochrome-avidin/streptavidin c.
  c. focus
  mercuric c.
  c. redox pair
conjugated
  c. antigen
  c. bilirubin
  c. estriol
  c. hapten
  c. hyperbilirubinemia I–III
  c. protein
conjugation bridge
conjugative plasmid
conjunctional
conjunctiva, *pl.* **conjunctivae**
  bulbar c.
  Dirofilaria conjunctivae
  Filaria conjunctivae
  lithiasis conjunctivae
  tela c.
  tunica c.
conjunctivae (*pl. of* conjunctiva)
conjunctival
  c. cell
  c. fungus culture
  c. gland
conjunctivales
  glandulae c.
conjunctive
conjunctivitis
  acute contagious c.
  acute epidemic c.
  acute follicular c.
  adult gonococcal c.
  allergic c.
  angular c.
  blennorrheal c.
  catarrhal c.
  follicular c.
  gonococcal c.
  granular c.
  inclusion c.

infantile purulent c.
lymphogranuloma venereum-trachoma
   inclusion c. (LGV-TRIC)
meningococcus c.
Moraxella c.
c. neonatorum
spring catarrhal c.
swimming pool c.
toxicogenic c.
trachoma-inclusion c. (TRIC)
tularemic c.
vernal c.
welder's c.
conjunctivoma
connectin
connecting
c. cartilage
c. ring
c. tubule
connection
anomalous venous c.
clamp c.
fetoscopic laser coagulation of
   vascular c.
connective
c. tissue
c. tissue capsule
c. tissue cell
c. tissue disease (CTD)
c. tissue disorder
c. tissue fiber
c. tissue group
c. tissue growth
   factor
c. tissue nevus
c. tissue septa
c. tissue stroma
c. tissue supply blood
c. tissue trabecula
c. tumor
connexin
connexus intertendinei musculi extensoris
   digitorum
conniventes
valvulae c.
Conn syndrome
Conocybe cyanopus
conoid
conoideum
   Hypoderaeum c.
conomyoidin
Conor and Bruch disease
conorii
   Rickettsia c.
conotruncal heart defect
Conradi disease
consanguineous
c. donor
c. mating

consanguinity
consecutive
c. aneurysm
c. angiitis
consent
informed c.
conservatrix
   Desulforegula c.
conserved helix-loop-helix ubiquitous
   kinase (CHUK)
consideration
clinical c.
differential diagnostic c.
consistency
fecal c.
stool c.
consistent estimate
consolidation
conspecific
conspicuum
   C. conspicuum
constant (k)
absorption c.
acid ionization c.
affinity c.
Ambard c.
association c.
base ionization c.
binding c.
Boltzmann c.
decay c.
dielectric c.
diffusion c.
disintegration c.
dissociation c.
equilibrium c.
Faraday c.
gas c.
ionization c.
Planck c. (h)
radioactive c.
rate c.
c. region
C. Spring mutation of
   hemoglobin
constellatus
   Diplococcus c.
   Streptococcus c.
constipation
functional c.
constituent
endocrine granule c.
   (EGC)
constitution
constitutional
c. cause
c. disease
c. dwarf
c. hepatic dysfunction

C

constitutional (*continued*)
    c. hyperbilirubinemia
    c. reaction
    c. thrombopathy
    c. ulcer
constitutive
    c. enzyme
    c. expression
    c. heterochromatin
    c. heterochromatin method
    c. mutation
    c. protein
constriction
    primary c.
    secondary c.
constrictive
    c. endocarditis
    c. pericarditis
constrictum
constrictus
    Porocephalus c.
constructible
construction
constructive
    c. interference
    c. proof
consultation
consumption
    alcohol c.
    c. coagulopathy
    oxygen c.
contact (c)
    c. activation product
    c. allergy
    c. catalysis
    c. dermatitis
    c. entrance wound
    hospital-acquired penetration c.
    c. hypersensitivity
    c. inhibition
    metal-to-metal c.
    c. sensitivity
contactant
contagion
    immediate c.
    mediate c.
contagiosa
    impetigo c.
contagiosum
    epithelioma c.
    molluscum c.
contagious
    c. bovine pleuropneumonia
    c. disease
    c. ecthyma
    c. ecthyma (pustular dermatitis)
     virus of sheep
    c. pustular dermatitis
    c. pustular stomatitis virus

contagiousness
contagium
    c. animatum
    c. vivum
contain
    to c. (TC)
contained criticality
container
    ALPS c.
    screw-cup c.
    c. size limitations
containment
    biosafety c.
contaminans
    Anoxybacillus c.
contaminant
contaminate
contaminated patient
contamination
    alpha c.
    c. irradiation
    primary c.
    secondary c.
contamination-free
content
    carbon dioxide c.
    dye c.
    gastrointestinal c.'s
    heat c.
    supranormal venous oxygen c.
    total carbon dioxide c.
contiguum
continence
continent
contingency table
**contingent negative variation
(CNV)**
continued fever
continuous
    c. capillary
    c. distending pressure (CDP)
    c. endothelium
    c. flow analyzer
    c. flow culture
    c. function
    c. phase
    c. spectrum
continua
    acrodermatitis c.
    epilepsia partialis c.
    Heterophyopsis c.
contorti
    tubuli c.
contortum
    Eubacterium c.
contortus
    Haemonchus c.
    tubulus renalis c.
contour line of Owen

contracted kidney
contractile
    c. ring
    c. vacuole
contraction
    c. band
    c. band necrosis
    isovolumic c. (IC)
    c. stress test
contracture
    congenital c.
    Dupuytren c.
    ischemic c.
    organic c.
    Volkmann c.
contrafissura
contraindication
contralat
    contralateral
contralateral (contralat)
    c. axillary metastasis
contrast
    bright c.
    c. media reaction
    c. medium
    c. stain
contrasuppressor cell
contrecoup
control
    Cardiasure cardiac markers c.
    c. cell
    Cell-Chex body fluid procedural c.
    Centers for Disease C. (CDC)
    chemTRAK liquid chemistry c.
    clinical chemistry quality c.
    clinical microbiology quality c.
    Elecsys PreciControl Anti-HBe c.
    ESR-Chex hematology c.
    c. experiment
    c. group
    healthy c.
    HemataCHEK hematology
      reference c.
    HepCheck whole blood c.
    ignition source c.
    infection c. (IC)
    Liquichek hematology-16 c.
    Liquichek hematology c. (A)
    Liquichek hematology c. (C)
    Liquichek immunology c.
    Liquichek qualitative urine
      toxicology c.
    Liquichek sedimentation rate c.
    Liquichek ToRCH Plus c.
    lupus anticoagulant positive c.
    Lyphochek anemia c.
    Lyphochek fertility c.
    Lyphochek hypertension markers c.
    Lyphochek maternal serum c.

    Lyphochek tumor marker c.
    Lyphochek whole blood c.
    c. material
    nicotinamide adenine dinucleotide
      diaphorase c. (NADH diaphorase
      control)
    process c.
    quality c. (QC)
    riot c.
    Sed-Chek 2 bilevel whole blood
      reference c.
    spill c.
    Sugar-Chex II glucose c.
    Virotrol syphilis total c.
controlled
    c. access laboratory
    c. pore glass bead
    c. substance
contusion
    brain c.
    incomplete muzzle c.
    muzzle c.
    scalp c.
    wind c.
conular
conus, *pl.* **coni**
    coni epididymidis
    coni vasculosi
convalescent
    c. carrier
    c. serum
convection
convention
    Biological Weapons and Toxins C.
conventional
    c. animal
    c. core biopsy (CCB)
    c. papillary carcinoma (CPC)
convergence
conversion
    c. coefficient
    c. electron
    internal c.
    Mantoux c.
    mediated c.
    c. of glucose
    c. ratio
    serum prothrombin c.
convertase
    C5 c.
    C3 proactivator c.
converter
    D/A c.
    digital-to-analog c. (DAC)
    voltage-to-frequency c.
convertin
converting enzyme
convexobasia
convoluted seminiferous tubule

C

225

convulsant antidote for nerve agent
  (CANA)
convulsion
Conway cell
COOH-terminal tagging
cookei
  Ixodes c.
cookii
  Paenibacillus c.
cooled-knife method
Cooler
  Chameleon C.
Cooley
  C. anemia
  C. disease
coolhaasii
  Caloramator c.
cooling
  Newton law of c.
Coolscope digital camera/microscope
Coomassie
  C. blue-stained gel
  C. brilliant blue R-250
Coombs
  C. serum
  C. test (CT)
Cooperative Human Tissue Network
Cooper disease
Cooperia
  C. bisonis
  C. curticei
  C. fieldingi
  C. oncophora
  C. pectinata
  C. punctata
  C. spatulata
Coopernail sign
coordinate covalent bond
coordinates
  cartesian c.
  polar c.
  spherical polar c.
  X-Y-Z beam scanning method c.
coossification
coossify
CO-oximeter
  carbon monoxide oximeter
COP
  colloidal osmotic pressure
  colloid oncotic pressure
  cryptogenic organizing pneumonia
COPD
  chronic obstructive pulmonary
    disease
Copelandia
copepod
Copepoda
Coplin jar
copolymer

copper (Cu)
  c. assay
  c. cyanide (CuCN)
  c. deposit demonstration
  c. grid
  c. metabolism
  c. reduction test
  c. storage protein
  c. sulfate
  c. sulfate method
  c. sulfate test
  urine c.
  c. wire effect
copper-binding protein test
copper-wire artery
coprecipitating antibody
coprecipitation
coprecipitin
copremesis
Coprinus
coproantibody
Coprobacillus cateniformis
coprogenus
  Saccharomyces c.
coprolith
coprology
coproma
Copromastix prowazeki
Copromonas subtilis
coprophagous
coprophagy
coprophil, coprophilic, coprophile
coprophile (*var. of* coprophil)
coprophilia
coprophilic (*var. of* coprophil)
coproporphyria (CP)
  erythropoietic c. (ECP)
  hereditary c. (HCP)
coproporphyrin (CP)
  c. assay
  free erythrocyte c. (FEC)
  c. test
  urinary c. (UCP)
  urine c.
coproporphyrinogen oxidase
coproporphyrinuria
coprostanol
coprostasis
coprosterol
coprozoa
coprozoic ameba
CoQ
  coenzyme Q
coracidium
coral calculus
coralicida
  Aurantimonas c.
coralliilyticus
  Vibrio c.

corallin
  yellow c.
Corallobothrium
Corbin rhinoplasty technique
Corbus disease
cord
  Bergmann c.
  Billroth c.
  c. blood
  c. blood screen
  c. compression (CC)
  dental c.
  c. factor
  hepatic c.
  lymph c.
  medullary c.
  psalterial c.
  red pulp c.
  rete c.
  sex c.
  splenic c.
  two-cell wide
    vertical c.
  velamentous c.
  Willis c.
Cordana
cordatum
  Diphyllobothrium c.
cordatus
  Bothriocephalus c.
cordis
  capsula c.
  concretio c.
  ectasia c.
  membrana c.
  mucro c.
  myofibrosis c.
  steatosis c.
  theca c.
cordocentesis
Cordyceps
Cordylobia anthropophaga
cordylobiasis
core
  air c.
  c. antigen
  hyaline c.
  hyalinized c.
  magnetic c.
  c. memory
  c. needle biopsy (CNB)
  c. pneumonia
  c. promoter mutant
corectasis
coremium
corepressor
Corex glassware
Cori
  C. cycle

C. disease
C. ester
coriaceus
  Ornithodoros c.
corii
  rete cutaneum c.
  sclerosis c.
  stratum papillare c.
  stratum reticulare c.
  tunica propria c.
Corinth
  Congo C.
Coriobacteriaceae
Coriobacteriales
Coriobacteridae
Coriolopsis
Coriolus
coriphosphine O
corium
  reticular layer of c.
corkscrew hair
corkscrew-like bacteria
cornea, *pl.* **cornea**
  anterior limiting layer of c.
  epithelium anterius corneae
  herpes corneae
  ichthyosis sebacea c.
  lamina limitans anterior corneae
  lamina limitans posterior corneae
  limbus corneae
  limiting layer of c.
  posterior limiting layer of c.
  substantia propria corneae
  substantia propria of c.
corneal
  c. corpuscle
  c. impression test (CIT)
  c. layer of epidermis
  c. margin
  c. opacity (CO)
  c. space
  c. ulcer
  c. vascularization
Cornelia de Lange syndrome
corneocyte envelope
corneoscleral
  c. button
  c. junction
  c. part of trabecular tissue of
    sclera
  c. tunic
corneous
Corner-Allen
  C.-A. test
  C.-A. unit
corn ergot
corneum
  Nosema c.
  stratum c.

C

cornification
    excessive c.
cornified
    c. cell
    c. layer of nail
cornifying form
cornmeal agar
cornoid lamella
cornu
    c. cutaneum
cornual pregnancy
corona, *pl.* **coronae**
    c. radiata
    c. veneris
coronae (*pl. of* corona)
coronal section
coronary
    c. artery bypass graft
      (CABG)
    c. artery disease (CAD)
    c. atherosclerotic heart disease
      (CAHD)
    c. blood flow (CBF)
    c. embolism
    c. insufficiency (CI)
    c. insufficiency syndrome
    c. occlusion
    c. ostial stenosis
    c. prognostic index (CPI)
    c. risk factor
    c. sinus
    c. tendon
    c. thrombosis (CT)
coronata
    Delacroixia c.
    Diploscapter c.
    Entomophthora c.
coronatum
    Cyathostomum c.
coronatus
    Conidiobolus c.
Coronaviridae
coronavirus (CoV)
    novel c.
    severe acute respiratory syndrome c.
      (SARS-CoV)
coroner
coronoidectomy
coronoid process fracture
corpora (*pl. of* corpus)
corps
    c. grains
    c. ronds
corpse temperature
corpulence, corpulency
corpulency (*var. of* corpulence)
corpus, *pl.* **corpora**
    c. albicans
    c. amylaceum (CA)

    c. aorticum
corpora arenacea
corpora arenaceacorpora arenacea
    c. atreticum
    c. candicans
    c. cavernosum urethrae
    c. coccygeum
    c. delicti
    c. glandulae sudoriferae
    c. hemorrhagicum
    c. hemorrhagicum cyst
corpora lutea cyst
corpora lutea twins
    c. luteum
    c. luteum cyst
    c. luteum hematoma
    c. luteum hormone
    c. luteum hormone unit
    c. luteum of pregnancy
    c. nuclei caudati
    c. papillare
corpora paraaortica
    c. pineale
    c. spongiosum
    c. spongiosum penis
    c. spongiosum urethrae muliebris
    c. striatum
tinea corporis
trichophytosis corporis
    c. vitreum
corpuscle
    amnionic c.
    amniotic c.
    amylaceous c.
    amyloid c.
    articular c.
    axis c.
    Babès-Ernst c.
    basal c.
    Bennet c.
    Bizzozero c.
    blood c.
    bone c.
    bridge c.
    bulboid c.
    cement c.
    chyle c.
    colloid c.
    colostrum c.
    compound granular c.
    corneal c.
    Dogiel c.
    Donné c.
    Drysdale c.
    dust c.
    Eichhorst c.
    exudation c.
    genital c.
    ghost c.

Gierke c.
Gluge c.
Golgi-Mazzoni c.
Grandry c.
Hassall concentric c.
Herbst c.
inflammatory c.
Jaworski c.
lamellated c.
lymph c.
lymphatic c.
lymphoid c.
malpighian c.
Mazzoni c.
Meissner c.
Merkel c.
Mexican hat c.
molluscum c.
Negri c.
Norris c.
oval c.
pacchionian c.
pacinian c.
plastic c.
Purkinje c.
pus c.
red c.
renal c.
reticulated c.
Ruffini c.
Russell c.
salivary c.
Schwalbe c.
shadow c.
splenic c.
tactile c.
taste c.
terminal nerve c.
third c.
thymic c.
touch c.
Toynbee c.
Traube c.
Tröltsch c.
Valentin c.
Vater c.
Vater-Pacini c.
Virchow c.
Wagner-Meissner c.
white c.
Zimmermann c.
corpuscula (*pl. of* corpusculum)
corpuscular
   c. lymph
   c. volume (CV)
corpusculum, *pl.* **corpuscula**
   corpuscula articularia
   corpuscula bulboidea
   corpuscula genitalia

corpuscula lamellosa
c. renis
corpuscula nervosa terminalia
c. tactus
corralin yellow
corrected
   c. blood volume (CBV)
   c. dextrocardia
   c. retention time
   c. sedimentation rate (CSR)
   c. transposition (CT)
correction
   Allen c.
   coincidence c.
   c. factor (CF)
correlation
   c. coefficient
   functional c.
   structural c.
corresponding ray
Corrigan disease
corrin ring
corrodens
   Bacteroides c.
   Eikenella c.
corrosion
   c. cast
   c. preparation
corrosive
   c. esophagitis
   c. gastric secretions
corrosivity
corrugata
   Acrocarpospora c.
cortex, *pl.* **cortices**
   adrenal c.
   agranular c.
   amorphous fraction of adrenal c.
   cerebellar c.
   c. cerebelli
   cerebral c.
   c. cerebri
   deep c.
   fetal adrenal c.
   ganglionic layer of cerebellar c.
   c. glandulae suprarenalis
   granular layer of cerebellar c.
   intercalated cell of the renal c.
   kidney c.
   layer of cerebellar c.
   layer of cerebral c.
   c. lentis
   molecular layer of cerebral c.
   multiform layer of cerebral c.
   c. nodi lymphatici
   c. of hair shaft
   c. of lens
   c. of lymph node
   c. of thymus

C

cortex (*continued*)
  c. ovarii
  provisional c.
  renal c.
  c. renalis
  stained c.
  suprarenal c.
  tertiary c.
  thymic c.
Corti
  C. arch
  C. auditory teeth
  C. canal
  C. cell
  C. ganglion
  C. membrane
  Mesocestoides c.
  C. organ
  C. pillar
  pillar cell of C.
  C. rod
  C. tunnel
cortical (cort)
  c. achromia
  c. bone
  c. defect
  c. dysplasia
  c. hormone
  c. necrosis
  c. osteitis
  c. stromal hyperplasia (CSH)
  c. substance
  c. thumb
  c. thymoma
  c. U-fiber
corticale
  Cryptostroma c.
corticalis
  substantia c.
corticalization
cortices (*pl. of* cortex)
Corticium
corticobasal degeneration
corticoid
  antiinflammatory c. (AC)
corticola
  Griphosphaeria c.
corticoliberin
corticomedullary junction
corticosteroid (CS)
  c. crystal
  inhalant c.
  c. myopathy
  rectal c.
  c. therapy
  topical c.
corticosteroid-binding
  c.-b. globulin (CBG)
  c.-b. protein

corticosterone
corticotrope adenoma
corticotroph cell hyperplasia
corticotropin
  hyperproduction of pituitary c.
corticotropin-releasing
  c.-r. factor (CRF)
  c.-r. hormone (CRH)
Corticoviridae
Corticovirus
Cortinarius orellanus
cortisol
  c. assay
  c. binding
  c. production rate
    (CPR)
  c. secretion rate (CSR)
  c. synthesis pathway
  urinary free c.
cortisol-binding globulin (CBG)
cortisone
cortisone-glucose tolerance test
  (CGTT)
cortisone-primed oral glucose tolerance
  test (COGTT)
cortol
cortolone
Cortrosyn
Corvac integrated serum separator
  tube
Corvisart disease
corymbifera
  Absidia c.
  Lechtheimia c.
corymbiform
Corynebacteriaceae
Corynebacterineae
corynebacteriophage
  beta c.
Corynebacterium
  C. amycolatum
  C. appendicis
  C. aquilae
  C. atypicum
  C. aurimucosum
  C. auriscanis
  C. capitovis
  C. casei
  C. caspium
  C. diphtheriae
  C. diphtheriae throat
    culture
  C. efficiens
  C. equi
  C. felinum
  C. freneyi
  C. glaucum
  C. glucuronolyticum
  C. halotolerans

C. hoagii
C. hofmanni
C. jeikeium
C. matruchotii
C. minutissimum
C. mooreparkense
C. mycetoides
C. nigricans
C. parvum
C. pseudodiphtheriticum
C. pseudotuberculosis
C. pyogenes
C. renale
C. simulans
C. sphenisci
C. spheniscorum
C. striatum
C. suicordis
C. testudinoris
C. tuberculostearicum
C. ulcerans
C. xerosis
coryneform group
Corynespora cassiicola
coryza
allergic c.
c. virus
coryzavirus
cosine
Cosm
osmolar clearance
cosmid
Cosmocephalus obvelatus
Cosmocerella
cosmopolitan
costa, *pl.* **costae**
costae (*pl. of* costa)
costal pleurisy
costantinii
Pseudomonas c.
costaricensis
Angiostrongylus c.
Morerastrongylus c.
Costello syndrome
Costen syndrome
costimulatory molecule
cosynthase
uroporphyrinogen III c.
cosyntropin test
Cotard syndrome
Cotasil silicone slide coating material
cothromboplastin
cotinine urinary concentration
Cotlove titrator
cotransport
cotton dust asthma
cotton-fiber embolism
cotton-wool appearance
Cotugno disease

cotunnii
aqueductus c.
liquor c.
Cotunnius
C. aqueduct
C. disease
C. liquid
cot value
Cotylaspis
cotyledon
fetal c.
maternal c.
Cotylogonimus
Cotylurus
cough
brassy c.
c. plate
whooping c.
coulomb (C)
C. law
coulometer
coulometric
c. chloridometer
c. titration
coulometry
Coulter
C. Clenz cleaning agent
C. CLONE monoclonal antibody
C. counter
C. Gen-S Cell hematology workstation
C. LH 500, 700, 750, 755, 1500 Series hematology analyzer
C. Manual CD4 Kit
C. MAXM hematology analyzer
C. reticONE system
C. STKS hematology analyzer
C. tetraONE system
C. TQ-Prep workstation
coumachlor
coumarin
Coumatrak prothrombin time device
Councilman
C. hyaline body
C. lesion
Councilmania
counseling
genetic c.
count
absolute eosinophil c.
absolute granulocyte c. (AGC)
absolute neutrophil c. (ANC)
Addis c.
agar plate c.
Arneth c.
background c.
B-cell c.
blood cell c.
bone marrow differential c.

C

count (*continued*)
    CD4/CD8 c.
    cell c.
    cerebrospinal fluid leukocyte c.
    colony c.
    complete blood c. (CBC)
    differential leukocyte c.
     (DLC)
    differential white blood c.
    egg c.
    eosinophil c.
    erythrocyte c.
    fecal leukocyte c.
    filament-nonfilament c.
    gastric aspirate cell c.
    c. information density
    leukocyte c.
    leukocyte differential c.
    microvessel c. (MVC)
    mitotic c.
    c. per minute (cpm)
    platelet c. (PC)
    proportional c.
    c. rate
    c. rate meter
    red blood cell c.
    red cell c.
    reticulocyte c.
    Schilling blood c.
    scintillation c.
    Sézary c.
    spinal fluid leukocyte c.
    stool leukocyte c.
    too numerous to c. (TNTC)
    total cell c.
    total ridge c. (TRC)
    viable cell c.
    white blood cell c.
    white cell c. (WCC)
counter
    automated differential
     leukocyte c.
    cell c.
    Coulter c.
    decade c.
    electronic cell c.
    frequency c.
    gamma well c.
    Geiger-Müller c.
    ion c.
    liquid scintillation c.
    Multisizer 3 Coulter c.
    proportional c.
    radiation c.
    ring c.
    ripple c.
    scintillation c.
    shift c.
    synchronous c.

    Sysmex R-1000 reticulocyte c.
    Z1, Z2 series Coulter c.
counterclockwise
countercurrent
    c. extraction
    c. immunoelectrophoresis (CIE,
     CIEP)
    c. mechanism
    c. multiplier system
counterelectrophoresis (CEP)
counterflow centrifugal elutriation
counterimmunoelectrophoresis (CIEP)
counterstain
counterstaining technique
counting
    automated reticulocyte c.
    c. cadence
    c. chamber
    liquid scintillation c.
    c. plate
couple
    redox c.
coupler
    acoustic c.
coupling
    c. capacitor
    cell c.
    c. defect
Courvoisier
    C. law
    C. sign
Courvoisier-Terrier syndrome
CoV
    coronavirus
covalent bond
**Covalink MicroElisa culture
  plate**
covariance
covariate
cover glass
coverglass
coverslip
Coverslipper
    Jung CV 5000 Robotic C.
cowanii
    Enterobacter c.
Cowden
    C. disease
    C. syndrome
Cowdria ruminantium
**Cowdry type A, B inclusion
  body**
cow kidney
Cowper
    C. cyst
    C. gland
cowperitis
cowpox virus
cow's milk anemia

Cox
- C. proportional hazards regression model
- C. regression analysis
- C. vaccine

COX-1
- cyclooxygenase-1

COX-2
- cyclooxygenase-2

coxa, *pl.* **coxae**
- c. magna
- c. plana

coxae (*pl. of* coxa)

Coxiella burnetii

coxitis

coxsackievirus encephalitis

cP
- centipoise

C:P
- cholesterol/phospholipid ratio

CP
- cardiopulmonary
- cerebral palsy
- chemically pure
- coproporphyrin
- cystosarcoma phyllodes

CPB
- competitive protein-binding
  - CPB assay

CPC
- chronic passive congestion
- clinicopathologic conference
- conventional papillary carcinoma

CPD adenine
- calcium pyrophosphate dihydrate
- cephalopelvic disproportion
- citrate phosphate dextrose
- contagious pustular dermatitis

CPDN
- cystic partially differentiated nephroblastoma

CPE
- chronic pulmonary emphysema

C-peptide test

CpG
- cytosine phosphate guanine
  - CpG island
  - CpG island methylator phenotype

CPH
- chronic persistent hepatitis

CpHV
- caprine herpesvirus

CPI
- chronic pneumonitis of infancy
- Clostridium perfringens enterotoxin iota
- coronary prognostic index

CPK
- creatine phosphokinase

CPK-MB
- creatine phosphokinase-myocardial band

CPL
- congenital pulmonary lymphangiectasis

cPLA2
- cytosol phospholipase A2

cpm
- count per minute

CPM
- confined placental mosaicism

CPN
- chronic pyelonephritis

CPPD
- calcium pyrophosphate deposition disease

CPR
- cerebral cortex perfusion rate
- cortisol production rate

CPS
- carbamoyl phosphate synthetase
- carbamyl phosphate synthetase
  - CPS deficiency

cPSA
- complexed prostate-specific antigen

CPT2
- carnitine palmitoyltransferase 2
  - CPT2 deficiency

CPX
- calciphylaxis

C1q
- C1q immune complex detection
- C1q nephropathy
- C1q radioassay

CQ
- circadian quotient

CR
- complement receptor
- crown rump
- NATO code for dibenz(b,f)-1:4-oxazepine

Cr
- chromium

CR3
- complement receptor 3

crab
- c. hand
- c. louse
- c. yaws

Crabtree effect

cracked heel

cradle cap

Craigia

Craigie
- C. tube
- C. tube method

Crandall syndrome

craniad

cranial
    c. arteritis
    c. gunshot wound
    c. insufflation
    c. monocephalus duplication
cranii
    osteoporosis circumscripta c.
craniocarpotarsal
    c. dysplasia
    c. dystrophy
craniocele
craniocleidodysostosis
craniodiaphysial dysplasia
craniofacial
    c. dysostosis
    c. fracture
craniomalacia
    circumscribed c.
craniomeningocele
craniometaphysial dysplasia
craniopagus
craniopathy
    metabolic c.
craniopharyngioma
    ameloblastomatous c.
    cystic papillomatous c.
craniorachischisis
cranioschisis
craniosclerosis
craniostenosis
craniosynostosis
craniotabes
craniotrypesis
cranium bifidum
Cranston hemoglobin
crapulent, crapulous
crapulous (*var. of* crapulent)
crassamentum
Crassicauda grampicola
crassicollis
    Taenia c.
crateriform ulceration
craw-craw, kra-kra
CRBBB
    complete right bundle-branch block
CRC
    colorectal cancer
CRCC
    chromophobe renal cell carcinoma
CrCl
    creatinine clearance
CRD
    chronic renal disease
    complete reaction of degeneration
CR3 deficiency
C-reactive
    C-r. protein (CRP)

    C-r. protein assay
    C-r. protein test
cream, creme
    leukocyte c.
    SoftGUARD hand c.
crease
    simian c.
creatine
    c. kinase (CK)
    c. kinase assay
    c. kinase BB (CK-BB)
    c. kinase isoenzyme
    c. kinase isoenzyme electrophoresis
    c. kinase test
    c. phosphate
    c. phosphokinase (CPK)
    c. phosphokinase-myocardial band (CPK-MB)
creatinemia
creatinine
    amniotic fluid c.
    c. assay
    c. clearance (CC)
    c. clearance test
    c. coefficient
    c. height index (CHI)
    urine c.
creatinuria
CREB
    cAMP response element binding protein
        CREB binding protein (CBP)
CREB/ATF
    cAMP response element binding activation transcription factor
Credé method
credentialing
creeping
    c. disease
    c. eruption
    c. ulcer
CREG
    cross-reactive group
        CREG matching
creme (*var. of* cream)
cremoricolorata
    Pseudomonas c.
cremoris
    Streptococcus c.
Crenarchaeota
crenate, crenated
crenated (*var. of* crenate)
    c. cell
crenation
crenocyte
crenocytosis
Crenosoma vulpis
Crenotrichaceae
crenulate

creola body
crepitans
  tenosynovitis c.
crescens
  Emmonsia parva c.
crescent
  c. cell
  c. cell anemia
  c. formation
  Giannuzzi c.
  glomerular c.
  Heidenhain c.
  c. sign
crescentic
  c. anti-GBM glomerulonephritis
  c. histiocyte
  c. nephritis
cresol
  c. assay
  c. red
cresol-ammonia spot test
crest
  acoustic c.
  ampullary c.
  embryonic neural c.
  neural c. (NC)
  neuroepithelium of
    ampullary c.
  obturator c.
  spiral c.
  C. syndrome
CREST
  calcinosis, Raynaud phenomenon,
  esophageal motility disorders,
  sclerodactyly, and telangiectasia
cresta
cresyl
  c. blue
  c. blue brilliant
  c. blue brilliant stain
  c. echt
  c. fast violet
  c. violet
  c. violet acetate
  c. violet stain
cresylecht violet
cretinism
Creutzfeldt-Jakob disease (CJD)
crevicular
  c. epithelium
  c. fluid
CRF
  chronic renal failure
  corticotropin-releasing factor
CRH
  corticotropin-releasing hormone
crib death
cribrate
cribration

cribriform
  c. carcinoma
  c. field of vision
  c. growth pattern
  c. nest
cribriform-morular
  c.-m. variant
  c.-m. variant of papillary thyroid
    carcinoma
cribrosa
  area c.
  macula c.
cribrosus
  status c.
cribrum
Crichton-Browne sign
cricothyroid
cri du chat syndrome
Crigler-Najjar
  C.-N. disease
  C.-N. syndrome
Crimean-Congo
  C.-C. hemorrhagic fever
  C.-C. hemorrhagic fever virus
Crimean hemorrhagic fever virus
crime scene investigation
criminal abortion
Crinipellis
Crinivirus
crinophagy
Cripavirus
Crippa lead tetraacetate method
crises (*pl. of* crisis)
crisis, *pl.* crises
  addisonian c.
  adrenal c.
  anaphylactoid c.
  aplastic c.
  blast c.
  blood c.
  celiac c.
  cholinergic c.
  hypercalcemic c.
  myasthenic c.
  myelocytic c.
  salt-losing c.
  scleroderma renal c.
  sequestration c.
  sickle cell c.
  thyroid c.
  c. value
  vasoocclusive c.
crispatum
  Eubacterium c.
crispatus
  Lactobacillus c.
crista, *pl.* cristae
  c. ampullaris
  c. basilaris ductus cochlearis

C

crista (*continued*)
    c. cutis
    c. of mitochondrion
    c. quarta
    c. spiralis
    swollen c.
    c. terminalis
    tubular cristae
cristae (*pl. of* crista)
criteria (*pl. of* criterion)
Crithidia **immunofluorescence**
  testing
critical
    c. angle
    c. flicker fusion (CFF)
    c. flicker fusion test
    c. illumination
    c. incident stress management
    (CISM)
    c. infrastructure protection (CIP)
    c. limit
    c. mass
    c. micelle concentration (CMC)
    c. path analysis
    c. pathway
    c. region
    c. staining level
    c. temperature
criticality
    contained c.
    c. incident
    c. locket dosimeter
    c. lockout
    uncontained c.
criticus
    status c.
Crit-Line
    C.-L. fluid monitor
    C.-L. III TQA fluid management
    and access device
    C.-L. III TQA system
CritSpin microhematocrit centrifuge
CRM
    cross-reacting material
cRNA
    chromosomal RNA
crocea
    Aequorivita c.
Croceibacter atlanticus
crocein
    brilliant c.
Crocicreas
crocidolite
crocidurae
    Borrelia c.
Crocinitomix catalasitica
Crocker silver impregnation
  technique
Crocq disease

Crohn
    C. disease
    C. ileitis
Cronkhite-Canada
    C.-C. polyp
    C.-C. syndrome
Crooke
    C. granule
    C. hyaline change
    C. hyaline degeneration
cross
    c. activation
    c. agglutination
    green c. (phosgene gas)
    hair c.
    c. hybridization
    c. infection
    Maltese c.
    c. product
    Ranvier c.
    c. reaction
    c. striation
    c. striation pattern
    three-point c.
    c. wall
cross-assembler
cross-bridge
    myosin c.-b.
cross-compiler
crossed
    c. grid
    c. immunoelectrophoresis
Crossiella
    C. cryophila
    C. equi
cross-link
    urine pyridinoline c.-l.
cross-linked N-telopeptide
cross-linking
crossmatch (XM)
    flow cytometric c.
    immediate-spin c.
    newborn c.
crossmatching
    donor-specific c.
crossover
    c. frequency
    c. hemoglobin
cross-protective immunity
cross-reacting
    c.-r. agglutinin
    c.-r. antibody
    c.-r. antigen
    c.-r. material (CRM)
cross-reactive group (CREG)
cross-reactivity
cross-sectional survey
cross-section anatomy
cross-striation

crossway
    sensory c.
crotalariae
crotalin
Crotalus **antitoxin**
crotonatoxidans
    Alkaliphilus c.
croton oil
croup
croup-associated (CA)
    c.-a. virus
crouposus
croupous
    c. bronchitis
    c. inflammation
    c. lymph
    c. membrane
    c. pharyngitis
Crouzon
    C. craniofacial
      dysostosis
    C. disease
    C. syndrome
crowded cell index
crowding
    c. effect
    gland c.
Crow-Fukase syndrome
crown
    C. needle
    radiate c.
    c. rump (CR)
crown-heel (CH)
CRP
    C-reactive protein
CRPH high-sensitivity C-reactive protein reagent
^{51}Cr red cell survival test
CRS
    Chinese restaurant syndrome
CRSFungal Profile diagnostic test
CRST
    calcinosis cutis, Raynaud phenomenon, sclerodactyly, and telangiectasia
    CRST syndrome
cRT-PCR
    competitive reverse transcription polymerase chain reaction
cruces pilorum
crucians
    Anopheles c.
cruciate ligament tear
Crucibulum
crude
    c. mortality ratio (CMR)
    c. rate
    c. urine
cruor

crura (*pl. of* crus)
crural diaphragm
crus, *pl.* **crura**
crush
    c. artifact
    c. injury
    c. kidney
    c. syndrome
crushing of tissue
crust
    buffy c.
    scale c.
crustae (*pl. of* crusta)
crusta, *pl.* **crustae**
    c. inflammatoria
    c. phlogistica
Crustacea
crusted ringworm
Cruveilhier
    C. disease
    C. paralysis
    C. ulcer
Cruveilhier-Baumgarten
    C.-B. disease
    C.-B. syndrome
Cruz-Chagas disease
cruzi
    Anopheles c.
    Schizotrypanum c.
    Trypanosoma c.
cryalgesia
crymophilic
crymophylactic
cryoablation
Cryobacterium psychrophilum
cryobank
cryobiology
cryocrit
CryoCults culture
cryoelectron microscopy
cryofibrinogen
cryofibrinogenemia
cryofracture
cryogammaglobulin
Cryo-Gel embedding medium
cryogenic spray
cryoglobulin
cryoglobulinemia
    crystal c.
    c., leukemia, arthritis, Sjögren syndrome, and hepatitis B (CLASH)
    mixed c.
cryoglobulinemic
    c. glomerulonephritis
    c. vasculitis
cryohydrocytosis
Cryokwik
cryolysis

C

CryoMed freezer
Cryomorphaceae
Cryomorpha ignava
cryopathic hemolytic syndrome
cryophila
    Crossiella c.
cryophile
cryophilic
cryophylactic
cryoprecipitated
    c. antihemophilic factor
    c. fibrinogen
cryoprecipitate-depleted plasma
cryoprecipitate transfusion
cryoprecipitation
cryopreservation
cryopreservative
    Microbank c.
cryoprobe
cryoprotectant
cryoprotein
Cryo rubber mold
    cryoablation
    cryoglobulin
cryoscope
cryoscopy
cryostat
    Ames Lab-Tek c.
    c. frozen sectioning aid
    c. section
CryoStor cell freezing solution
cryotolerant
Cryo-Vac-A cryostat vacuum
  system
Cryphonectria
crypt
    c. abscess
    adenomatous c.
    alveolar bony c.
    c. architecture
    c. cell carcinoma
    dental c.
    c. dilation
    c. disarray
    c. distortion
    enamel c.
    c. epithelium
    c. hypoplasia
    c. isolation technique
    lingual c.
    mutated c.
    regenerative c.
    synovial c.
    tonsillar c.
cryptal lymphocytic coloproctitis
crypta tonsillaris
cryptic
    c. enzyme
    c. T antigen

cryptitis
    acute c.
    neutrophilic c.
Cryptobacterium curtum
Cryptobia salmositica
Cryptococcaceae
cryptococcal
    c. antigen
    c. antigen titer
    c. meningitis
    c. polysaccharide
cryptococcemia
cryptococcoma
cryptococcosis
cryptococcus
    c.
    C. albidus
    C. antibody titer
    C. neoformans
cryptocrystalline
Cryptocystis trichodectis
Cryptodiaporthe
Cryptogamia
cryptogenic
    c. cirrhosis
    c. infection
    c. organizing pneumonia
    (COP)
    c. pyemia
    c. septicemia
cryptolith
cryptolytic lesion
cryptomenorrhea
cryptomere
Cryptomyces pleomorpha
cryptophthalmia (*var. of*
  cryptophthalmos)
cryptophthalmos, cryptophthalmia
cryptophthalmus syndrome
cryptoplasmic
cryptorchidism, cryptorchism
cryptorchid testis
cryptorchism (*var. of* cryptorchidism)
Cryptosporangium
    C. aurantiacum
    C. minutisporangium
cryptosporidia
cryptosporidiosis antibody
Cryptosporidium
    C. diagnostic procedure
    C. parvum
Cryptosporiopsis
Cryptostroma corticale
cryptostromosis
cryptoxanthin
cryptozoite
crypts of Lieberkuhn
cryptus
    Porphyrobacter c.

crystal
    ammonium biurate c.
    amorphous phosphate c.
    asthma c.
    basic calcium phosphate c.
    BCP c.
    birefringent c.
    blood c.
    Böttcher c.
    calcium oxalate c.
    c. cell
    Charcot-Leyden c.
    Charcot-Neumann c.
    Charcot-Robin c.
    chiral c.
    cholesterol c.
    corticosteroid c.
    c. cryoglobulinemia
    cystine c.
    c. deposition disease
    ear c.
    Florence c.
    hematoidin c.
    hippuric acid c.
    intracytoplasmic c.
    knife-rest c.
    leukocytic c.
    Leyden c.
    liquid c.
    Lubarsch c.
    mineral c.
    monosodium urate c. (MSU)
    MSU c.
    c. of Lubarsch
    Reinke c.
    scintillation c.
    sperm c.
    spermine c.
    talc c.
    thorn apple c.
    triple phosphate c.
    twin c.
    tyrosine c.
    urate c.
    uric acid c.
    c. urinary cast
    urine sediment c.
    c. violet
    c. violet stain
    c. violet vaccine
    Virchow c.
    whetstone c.
crystal-induced
    c.-i. arthritis
    c.-i. chemotactic factor
crystalline
    c. amylose
    c. birefringence
    c. egg albumin (CEA)

    c. insulin (CI)
    c. macromolecule alteration
    c. zinc insulin
crystallization
    intraglomerular c.
crystallography
    x-ray c.
crystalloid
    Charcot-Böttcher c.
    Charcot-Leyden c.
    Reinke c.
crystalluria
crystals
    urine c.
C&S
    culture and sensitivity
        C&S test
CS
    chorionic somatomammotropin
    corticosteroid
    NATO code for chloracetophenone
    NATO code for o-chlorobenzylidene
      malononitrile
        CS gas
Cs
    cesium
CSA
    colony-stimulating activity
    compressed spectral assay
CSD
    cat-scratch disease
CSF
    cerebrospinal fluid
    colony-stimulating factor
        CSF glutamine test
        CSF morphologic investigation
CSH
    capsular synovial-like hyperplasia
    chronic subdural hematoma
    cortical stromal hyperplasia
CSID
    congenital sucrase-isomaltase deficiency
Csillag disease
CSM
    cerebrospinal meningitis
CSPG
    chondroitin sulfate proteoglycan
CSR
    corrected sedimentation rate
    cortisol secretion rate
cSt
    centistoke
CT
    census tract
    cerebral thrombosis
    circulation time
    clotting time
    coagulation time
    Coombs test

C

CT (*continued*)
    coronary thrombosis
    corrected transposition
    cytotechnologist
        biphasic helical CT
        high-resolution CT (HRCT)
        CT number
Ct
    concentration-time product
Ct50, Ct_{50}
    concentration-time product for 50% of
    exposed group
        effective Ct_{50} (ECt_{50})
        incapacitating Ct_{50} (ICt_{50})
        lethal Ct_{50} (LCt_{50})
CTCL
    cutaneous T-cell lymphoma
CTD
    carpal tunnel decompression
    congenital thymic dysplasia
    connective tissue disease
Ctenocephalides canis
C-terminal
    carboxyl terminal
        C-t. assay
        C-t. fragment
C-terminus region
CT-guided stereotactic
biopsy
CTH
    ceramide trihexoside
CTL
    cytologic T lymphocyte
CTLA-4 interaction
CtO2
    concentration of total oxygen
CTP
    cytidine triphosphate
    cytosine triphosphate
CTX
    cholera toxin
cu
    cubic
Cu
    copper
Cuban itch
cubic (cu)
    c. centimeter (cm^3, cu cm)
    c. millimeter (cmm, cu mm, mm^3)
cuboidal
    c. carcinoma
    c. cell
    c. epithelium
    simple ciliated c.
cuboidalization
CUC
    chronic ulcerative colitis
CuCN
    copper cyanide

cucumerina
    Plectosphaerella c.
    Trichosanthes c.
cucumerinum
    Tracheophilus c.
    Typhlocoelum c.
Cucumovirus
cucurbitina
    Taenia c.
CUE
    confidential unit exclusion
cuff
    columnar c.
cuffing
    lymphocytic c.
    lymphoid c.
cuffitis
cuirasse
    cancer en c.
culbertsoni
    Acanthamoeba c.
cul-de-sac
    c.-d.-s. mass
    c.-d.-s. smear
Culex
    C. nigripalpus
    C. pipiens
    C. quinquefasciatus
    C. restuans
    C. salinarius
    C. tarsalis
culicicola
    Aeromonas c.
Culicidae
culicifacies
    Anopheles c.
culicis
    Agamomermis c.
Culicoides
    C. austeni
    C. furens
    C. milnei
culicosis
Culiseta
    C. inornata
    C. melanura
Cullen sign
cullin family protein
Cult-Dip Plus bacteriologic culture
-86C ULT freezer
cultivation
culture
    abscess aerobic c.
    acid-fast c. (AFC)
    Actinomyces c.
    adenovirus c.
    aerobic and anaerobic blood c.
    anaerobic bacteria c.
    c. and sensitivity (C&S)

animal cell c.
arterial line c.
attenuated c.
bacterial c.
Bactrol Plus quality control c.
blood c. (BC)
bronchial aspirate anaerobic c.
burn c.
cell wall defective bacteria c.
cerebrospinal fluid c.
cervical c.
Chlamydia c.
chorioallantoic c.
clean-catch urine c.
CMV c.
conjunctival fungus c.
continuous flow c.
Corynebacterium diphtheriae throat
  c.
CryoCults c.
Cult-Dip Plus bacteriologic c.
cytomegalovirus c.
direct c.
duodenal contents c.
ear c.
elective c.
endometrium anaerobic c.
enrichment c.
enterovirus c.
Epstein-Barr virus c.
fibroblast c.
flask c.
fluid c.
c. fluid supernatant
fungus c.
gastric c.
genital c.
gonorrhea c. (GC)
gravity-settling c. (GSC)
group A beta hemolytic streptococci
  throat c.
hanging-block c.
hanging-drop c.
Harada-Mori filter paper strip c.
Helicobacter pylori urease test and
  c.
herpes simplex virus c.
HSV c.
human immunodeficiency virus c.
  (HIV c)
influenza virus c.
Legionella pneumophila c.
Leptospira c.
c. medium
mixed leukocyte c. (MLC)
mixed lymphocyte c. (MLC)
mixed lymphocyte-tumor c. (MLTC)
monoxenic c.
mumps virus c.

mycobacteria c.
nasopharyngeal c.
needle c.
Neisseria gonorrhoeae c.
Nocardia c.
c. of vesicular fluid
organ c.
plate c.
polymicrobial c.
pouch c.
primary explant c.
print c.
pure c.
radioisotopic c.
RSV c.
rubella virus c.
secondary c.
semiquantitative viral c.
sensitized c.
shake c.
skin fungus c.
skin mycobacteria c.
slant c.
slope c.
smear c.
spinal fluid c.
sputum fungus c.
sputum mycobacteria c.
stab c.
Staphylococcus aureus
  nasopharyngeal c.
sterility c.
stock c.
stool fungus c.
stool mycobacteria c.
streak c.
synchronized c.
throat c.
thrust c.
tissue c. (TC)
tube c.
type c.
Ureaplasma urealyticum genital c.
urine fungus c.
urine mycobacteria c.
viral c.
VZV c.
wound c.
xenic c.
culturing
  bacterial c.
cummidelens
  Nocardia c.
cumulated activity ratio
cumulative
  c. action
  c. distribution
cumulative-frequency histogram
cumulative-summation technique (cusum)

C

cumulus
   c. oophorus
   c. ovaricus
cuneate
cuneiform
cuniculatum
   epithelioma c.
cuniculi (*pl. of* cuniculus)
cuniculus, *pl.* **cuniculi**
   Encephalitozoon cuniculi
   Gemella cuniculi
   Spilopsyllus cuniculi
   Treponema cuniculi
Cunninghamella elegans
cup
   cytospin c.
cupola (*var. of* cupula)
cupremia
cupric ion-inhibited acid phosphatase
cupriuresis
cuprizone model of chronic demyelination
cuprous
cupula, cupola, *pl.* **cupulae**
   c. ampullaris
   ampullary c.
cupulae (*pl. of* cupula)
curare
curariform paralysis
curative dose
curdy pus
curet, curette
curettage, curettement
   endocervical c. (ECC)
   endometrial c.
curette (*var. of* curet)
curettement (*var. of* curettage)
curetting
curie (Ci)
curie-hour (Ci-hr)
curiosum eroticum
curium
curled hair colony
Curling ulcer
currant
   c. jelly appearance
   c. jelly clot
currens
   larva c.
current
   alternating c.
   dark c.
   diffusion c.
   direct c.
   eddy c.
   c. gain
   c. regulator
   saturation c.
   three-phase c.

Curschmann
   C. disease
   C. spiral
curticei
   Cooperia c.
Curtis-Fitz-Hugh syndrome
Curtius syndrome
Curtobacterium herbarum
Curtovirus
curtum
   Cryptobacterium c.
curvata
   Syntrophomonas c.
curvatus
   Lactobacillus c.
curve
   Andrews lymphocyte c.
   calibration c.
   carbon dioxide dissociation c.
   carbon dioxide response c.
   characteristic c.
   distribution c.
   dye-dilution c.
   epidemic c.
   c. fitting
   indicator-dilution c.
   logarithmic c.
   multiple event c.
   oxygen-hemoglobin dissociation c.
   precipitin c.
   pressure-volume c.
   Price-Jones c.
   regression c.
   ROC c.
   sigmoid shape of the c.
   standard c.
   whole-body titration c.
curvilinear body
Curvularia
   C. geniculata
   C. lunata
   C. pallescens
   C. senagalensis
   C. verruculosa
curvus
   Campylobacter c.
Cushing
   C. basophilism
   C. disease
   C. syndrome
   C. ulcer
cushingoid facies
cushion
   muscular c.
custody
   chain of c.
customary temperature scale
cusum
   cumulative-summation technique

cutanea
    sclerosis c.
cutaneomandibular polyoncosis
cutaneomeningospinal angiomatosis
cutaneomucouveal syndrome
cutaneous
    c. amyloidosis
    c. anthrax
    c. anthrax infection
    c. B-cell lymphoma (CBCL)
    c. blister
    c. deciduosis
    c. dermal mucinosis
    c. emphysema
    c. extravascular necrotizing
      granuloma
    c. focal mucinosis
    c. fungus
    c. hemorrhoid
    c. horn
    c. larva migrans
    c. leishmaniasis (CL)
    c. leprosy
    c. lymphoid hyperplasia (CLH)
    c. lymphoma
    c. malformation
    c. malignant melanoma (CMM)
    c. meningioma
    c. myiasis
    c. necrotizing venulitis
    c. neural tumor (CNT)
    c. perifollicular
    c. pseudolymphoma
    c. reaction
    c. systemic angiitis
    c. systemic sclerosis
    c. T-cell lymphoma (CTCL)
    c. tissue
    c. tuberculin test
    c. tuberculosis
    c. vasculitis
cutaneum
    carcinoma c.
    cornu c.
    Trichosporon c.
cutdown
Cuterebra
cuticle of hair
cuticula vaginae folliculi pili
cutireaction test
cutis
    amyloidosis c.
    c. anserina
    atrophia maculosa varioliformis c.
    benign lymphocytoma c.
    calcinosis c.
    crista c.
    c. elastica
    glandulae c.

    c. hyperelastica
    hyperelastosis c.
    c. laxa
    leiomyoma c.
    leukemia c.
    neuroma c.
    osteoma c.
    osteosis c.
    stratum reticulare c.
    sulci c.
    tuberculosis c.
    c. vera
    c. verticis gyrata
cutization
cutoff frequency
cut surface
cutter
    agar c.
cutters
    rare base c.
cutting
    section c.
cuvet, cuvette, cuvette
cuvette (*var. of* cuvet)
CV
    cardiovascular
    cell volume
    coefficient of variation
    corpuscular volume
    cresyl violet
CVA
    cerebrovascular accident
      neonatal CVA
CVD
    cardiovascular disease
    cerebrovascular disease
CVH
    combined ventricular hypertrophy
    common variable
      hypogammaglobulinemia
CVID
    common variable immunodeficiency
      CVID syndrome
CVM
    cerebrovascular malformation
CVOD
    cerebrovascular obstructive disease
CVP
    cell volume profile
    central venous pressure
CVR
    cerebrovascular resistance
CVRD
    cardiovascular renal disease
CVS
    chorionic villus sampling
    clean-voided specimen
      transabdominal CVS
      transcervical CVS

C

CVS/CNS
  cardiovascular system and central
  nervous system
CW
  chemical warfare
CWA
  carcinoma with adenomatous areas
CWDF
  cell wall-deficient bacterial form
CWP
  coal worker's pneumoconiosis
CX
  NATO code for phosgene oxime
CX3, CX4, CX5 Delta clinical system
CX4
  CX4, CX5, CX9, CX500, CX1000
  PRO clinical system
  CX4, CX5, CX7 super clinical
  system
CX9 ALX clinical system
[14]C-xylose breath test
CyAn ADP analyzer
cyanemia
cyanescens
  Cerinosterus c.
cyanhemoglobin
cyanide
  c. anion
  c. antidote kit
  c. assay
  calcium c. (CaCN)
  carbonyl c.
    p-(trifluoromethoxy)phenylhydrazone
  copper c. (CuCN)
  diphenylarsine c. (DC)
  ethyl c.
  gold c. (AuCN)
  hydrogen c. (HCN)
  mercuric c.
  mercury c. (HgCN)
  c. poisoning
  potassium c. (KCN)
  c. radical (CN-)
  sodium c. (NaCN)
cyanide-ascorbate test
cyanide-nitroprusside test
cyanidol
cyanin
  alizarin c.
cyaniventris
  Dermatobia c.
cyanmethemoglobin
cyanoacrylate
  methyl c.
2-cyanoacrylate
  butyl 2-c.
Cyanobacteria
cyanochroic, cyanochrous
cyanochrous (*var. of* cyanochroic)

cyanocobalamin Co 57
cyanogen
cyanogriseus
  Actinoalloteichus c.
cyanohydrin metabolite
cyanophil, cyanophile
cyanophile (*var. of* cyanophil)
cyanophilia
  cytoplasmic c.
cyanophilous
cyanophoric glycoside
cyanopus
  Conocybe c.
cyanosed
cyanosis
  enterogenous c.
  false c.
  hereditary methemoglobinemic c.
  toxic c.
cyanotic
  c. atrophy
  c. induration
cyanuria
Cyathostoma bronchialis
Cyathostomum coronatum
Cyathus
cyberattack
cyberterrorism
cybrid
cyclamate
  sodium c.
cyclase
  adenyl c.
  adenylate c.
cycle
  cell c.
  circadian c.
  citric acid c.
  Cori c.
  eukaryotic cell c.
  futile c.
  glutamyl transfer c.
  hair c.
  Krebs c.
  Krebs-Henseleit c.
  menstrual c.
  mitotic c.
  operating c.
  c. per minute (c/min)
  c. per second (cps)
  pregnancy c.
  RANTES c.
  replication c.
  schizogonic c.
  suppression of cell c.
  tricarboxylic acid c.
    (TCA cycle)
  urea c.
cycler

cyclic, cyclical
    c. adenosine monophosphate (cAMP)
    c. albuminuria
    c. AMP (cAMP)
    c. AMP test
    c. citrullinated peptide (CCP)
    c. endoperoxide
    c. GMP
    c. guanosine monophosphate (cGMP)
    c. hydrocarbon
    c. lysine anhydride (CLA)
    c. neutropenia
    c. nucleotide
    c. tissue alteration
5′-cyclic
cyclical (*var. of* cyclic)
cyclicum
    Thialkalimicrobium c.
cyclin
    c. A antigen
    c. D1 gene
    c. D1 oncogene
    c. D1 protein
    c. D stain
    c. E antigen
cyclin-dependent
    c.-d. kinase (CDK)
    c.-d. kinase 5 (CDK5)
    c.-d. kinase inhibitor (CDKI)
    c.-d. protein
    c.-d. protein kinase 1
cycling probe
cyclitis
cyclitol
cyclitrophicus
    Vibrio c.
cyclization
cycloalkane
cycloalkene
cyclocreatine
cyclodiene hydrocarbon pesticide
cyclodimerization
Cyclodontostomum purvisi
cyclogeny
cyclohexane
cyclohexatriene
cycloheximide
cyclohexylamine
cyclohydrolase
    inosine c.
cyclonite
cyclooxygenase-1 (COX-1)
cyclooxygenase-2 (COX-2)
cyclooxygenase enzyme
cyclopea (*var. of* cyclopia)
cyclopentane
cyclopentanoperhydrophenanthrene
cyclophilin A (CypA)
Cyclophyllidea

cyclopia, cyclopea
Cyclops
cyclosarin
    NATO code for c. (GF)
cycloserine
    c. cefoxitin fructose agar
    c. mannitol agar
cyclosis
Cyclospora cayetanensis
cyclosporiasis
cyclosporin A
cyclosporine, cyclosporin A
cyclotron
cyclozoonosis
cylinder
    axis c.
    Bence Jones c.
    graduated c.
    Külz c.
cylinderization
cylindraxis
cylindrical
    c. bronchiectasis
    c. embryo
    c. epithelium
cylindricum
    stratum c.
cylindroadenoma
Cylindrocarpon
Cylindrocephalum
Cylindrocladium
cylindroid aneurysm
cylindroma
    dermal eccrine c.
cylindromatous carcinoma
cylindrosarcoma
cylindruria
Cymatoderma
Cymbal blood collection system
cynanche
    c. maligna
    c. tonsillaris
CYNAP
    cytotoxicity negative, absorption
    positive
cynarae
    Xanthomonas c.
cynodontis
    Leifsonia c.
    Leifsonia xyli subsp. *c.*
cynomolgi
    Plasmodium c.
CypA
    cyclophilin A
CYP2D6 drug screen test
Cyphellopsis
Cypovirus
cypricasei
    Lactobacillus c.

C

cyproheptadine hydrochloride
cyriacigeorgica
    Nocardia c.
Cyriax syndrome
cyrtometer
cyst
    adventitious c.
    allantoic c.
    alveolar hydatid c.
    aneurysmal bone c. (ABC)
    apocrine c.
    apoplectic c.
    arachnoid c.
    Baker c.
    Bartholin c.
    blood c.
    blue dome c.
    bone c.
    botryoid odontogenic c.
    branchial cleft c.
    breast c.
    bronchial c.
    bronchogenic c.
    bursal c.
    cerebellar c.
    chocolate c.
    choledochal c.
    chyle c.
    colloid c.
    compound c.
    congenital c.
    corpora lutea c.
    corpus hemorrhagicum c.
    corpus luteum c.
    Cowper c.
    Dandy-Walker c.
    daughter c.
    dental follicular c.
    dentigerous c.
    dermoid c.
    distention c.
    duplication c.
    echinococcus c.
    embryonal duct c.
    endometrial c.
    endothelial c.
    enterogenous c.
    ependymal c.
    epidermal inclusion c. (EIC)
    epidermoid inclusion c.
    epididymal c.
    epithelial inclusion c.
    extravasation c.
    exudation c.
    false c.
    fissural c.
    c. fluid cytology
    follicle c.
    follicular c.

    foregut c.
    ganglion c.
    Gartner c.
    gas c.
    germinal epithelial inclusion c.
    gingival c.
    glandular odontogenic c.
    globulomaxillary c.
    glomerular c.
    Gorlin c.
    granddaughter c.
    hemorrhagic c.
    hepatic c.
    hydatid c.
    implantation c.
    inclusion c.
    inflammatory odontogenic c.
    involution c.
    iodine c.
    junctional c.
    keratinous c.
    Kobelt c.
    lacteal c.
    leptomeningeal c.
    liver c.
    luteal c.
    luteinized follicular c.
    meibomian c.
    mesonephric c.
    mesothelial c.
    milium c.
    milk c.
    Morgagni c.
    mother c.
    mucinous c.
    mucous c.
    multilocular hydatid c.
    multiloculate hydatid c.
    myxoid c.
    nabothian c.
    nasolabial c.
    nasopalatine duct c.
    necrotic c.
    neural c.
    nonodontogenic c.
    odontogenic c.
    c. of Jadassohn
    oil c.
    oophoritic c.
    orbital c.
    orthokeratinized odontogenic c.
    (OOC)
    osseous hydatid c.
    ovarian c.
    pilar c.
    piliferous c.
    pilonidal c.
    pineal c.
    primordial c.

proliferation c.
proliferative c.
proliferous c.
pseudomucinous c.
radicular c.
ranular c.
Rathke cleft c.
renal c.
retention c.
sanguineous c.
sebaceous c.
secretory c.
seminal vesical c.
sequestration c.
serous c.
simple bone c.
simple renal c.
simple solitary c.
sinus c.
smooth-walled c.
solitary bone c.
sterile c.
sublingual c.
suprasellar c.
surgical ciliated c.
synovial c.
talgut c.
Tarlov c.
tarry c.
tarsal c.
tension c.
teratomatous c.
theca lutein c.
thyroglossal duct c.
thyroid c.
thyrolingual c.
traumatic bone c.
trichilemmal c.
tubular c.
umbilical c.
unicameral bone c.
unilocular hydatid c.
urachal c.
urinary c.
utricular c.
vellus hair c.
vitellointestinal c.
wolffian c.

cystacanth
cystadenocarcinoma
mucinous c.
pseudomucinous c.
serous c.
cystadenofibroma
serous c.
cystadenoma
hepatobiliary c.
c. lymphomatosum
mucinous c.

oncocytic papillary c.
pseudomucinous c.
serous c.
cystathionase
cystathionine
urine c.
cystathionine-beta-synthase
cystathionine-gamma-lyase
cystathioninuria
cystauchenitis
cystaugens
    Jannaschia c.
cysteamine
cystectasia, cystectasy
cystectasy (*var. of* cystectasia)
cysteic acid method
cysteine test
cysteinyl
cystic
c. acute inflammation
c. adenomatoid malformation
c. ameloblastoma
c. atrophy
c. bronchiectasis
c. carcinoma
c. chronic cervicitis
c. chronic inflammation
c. corpus hemorrhagicum
c. corpus luteum
c. degeneration
c. dermoid teratoma
c. diathesis
c. disease
c. duct
c. endometrial hyperplasia
c. fibrosis (CF)
c. fibrosis of pancreas (CFP)
c. fibrosis test
c. fibrosis transmembrane
  conductance regulator (CFTR)
c. fibrosis transmembrane
  conductance regulator gene
c. goiter
c. granulomatous inflammation
c. hamartoma
c. hygroma
c. hyperplasia of the breast
c. hypersecretory ductal carcinoma
  in situ
c. hypersecretory hyperplasia
c. kidney
c. lymphangiectasis
c. mastitis
c. mastopathy
c. medial necrosis (CMN)
c. medial necrosis of ascending
  aorta (CMN-AA)
c. medionecrosis
c. mole

C

247

cystic (*continued*)
    c. myxoma
    c. nephroma
    c. ovarian follicle
    c. papillomatous craniopharyngioma
    c. partially differentiated
      nephroblastoma (CPDN)
    c. polyp
    c. prostatic hyperplasia
    c. struma
cystica
    colpohyperplasia c.
    cystitis c.
    medionecrosis aortae
      idiopathica c.
    osteitis fibrosa c.
    osteitis tuberculosa
      multiplex c.
    pachyvaginitis c.
    pneumatosis intestinalis c.
    pyelitis c.
    spina bifida c.
    ureteritis c.
    vaginitis c.
cysticerci (*pl. of* cysticercus)
cysticercoid
cysticercosis
    mammary c.
    c. titer
cysticercus, *pl.* **cysticerci**
    C. bovis
    C. cellulosae
    C. fasciolaris
    C. ovis
    C. tenuicollis
cysticum
    acanthoma adenoides c.
    epithelioma adenoides c.
    hygroma colli c.
    lymphangioma c.
cysticus
    ductus c.
cystification
cystiform
cystigerous
cystine
    c. calculus
    c. crystal
    c. stone
    c. storage disease
    c. trypticase agar
    urine c.
cystinemia
cystinosin protein
cystinosis
cystinotic leukocyte
cystinuria
    familial c.
    c. test

cystiphorous
cystis
cystitis
    acute hemorrhagic c.
    banal c.
    calcareous c.
    chronic interstitial c.
    c. colli
    c. cystica
    eosinophilic c.
    erosive c.
    follicular c.
    c. follicularis
    c. glandularis
    hemorrhagic c.
    Hunner c.
    interstitial c. (IC)
    c. pneumatoides
    polypoid c.
    radiation c.
    schistosomal c.
    tuberculous c.
    ulcerative c.
cystoadenoma
cystocarcinoma
cystocele
Cystoderma
cystodiverticulum
cystoepithelioma
cystofibroma
Cystofilobasidium
cystogenic aneurysm
cystoid macular degeneration
cystolith
cystolithiasis
cystolithic
cystoma
    serous c.
cystomorphous
cystomyoma
cystomyxoadenoma
cystomyxoma
Cystoopsis scomber
cystopherous
cystoprostatectomy
cystoptosia, cystoptosis
cystoptosis (*var. of* cystoptosia)
cystopyelitis
cystopyelonephritis
cystosarcoma phyllode
cystoureteritis
cystourethritis
cystourethrocele
cystous
Cystoviridae
Cystovirus
cystyl
cytapheresis
    therapeutic c.

cytase
Cytauxzoon
cytauxzoonosis
cythemolytic icterus
cytidine
    c. diphosphate (CDP)
    c. monophosphate (CMP)
    c. triphosphate (CTP)
cytidine-5'-phosphate
cytidylic acid
cytidylyl
cytoadhesin
cytoanalyzer
cytoarchitectonics
cytoarchitectural
cytoarchitecture
cytobiology
cytobiotaxis
cytoblast
cytoblastema
cytoblock technique
cytocentrifugation
cytocentrifuge
    Aerospray c.
    CytoFuge 2 c.
    Cytopro c.
    Cyto-Tek c.
cytocentrum
cytochalasin B, D
cytochemical probe
cytochemistry
    leukocyte c.
cytochrome
    c. bc1 complex
    c. b5 reductase
    c. b5 reductase assay
    c. b5 reductase gene
    c. C protein
    c. oxidase (cyt ox)
    c. oxidase test
cytochylema
cytocidal
cytocide
cytoclasis
cytoclastic
cytoclesis
cytocrine secretion
cytocyst
cytode
cytodegenerative necrosis
cytodiagnosis
    exfoliative c.
cytodieresis
cytodifferentiation
cytofluorimetric analysis
cytofluorography
cytofluorometer
cytofluorometry
CytoFuge

C. 2 centrifuge
C. 2 cytocentrifuge
cytogene
cytogenetic
    c. analysis
    c. disorder
    c. map
    c. study
cytogenetics
    clinical c.
    population c.
cytogenous
cytoglucopenia
cytohyaloplasm
cytoid body
cytokeratin (CK)
    c. 1–20
    c. 1–20 antigen
    c. antigen-antibody reaction
    c. CAM 5.2 antibody
    c. CAM 5.2 antigen
    c. expression
    c. filament
    high molecular weight c. (HMW-CK)
    c. immunoreactivity
    c. neoepitope
    c. staining
cytokine
    chemotactic c.
    c. formation
    multiplexed fluorescent microsphere immunoassay for TH1, TH2 cytokines
    c. network
    proinflammatory c.
cytokinesis
cytolemma
cytolipin H
CytoLite luminescence assay system
cytologic
    c. abnormality
    c. alteration
    c. atypia
    c. brushings
    c. degeneration
    c. diagnosis
    c. engulfment
    c. examination
    c. filter preparation
    c. nuclear grading
    c. screening
    c. smear
    c. specimen
    c. T lymphocyte (CTL)
cytologist
cytology
    abrasive c.
    analytic c.

C

cytology (*continued*)
    aspiration biopsy c. (ABC)
    balloon c.
    Bethesda 2001 terminology for
      reporting results of cervical c.
    bronchial washing c.
    brushings c.
    cerebrospinal fluid c.
    cervical-vaginal c.
    cyst fluid c.
    cytomegalic inclusion disease c.
    effusion c.
    endometrial c.
    exfoliative c.
    fine-needle aspiration c.
      (FNAC)
    herpes c.
    image c.
    impression c.
    intraoperative c.
    nasal c.
    needle aspiration c.
    nipple discharge c.
    ocular c.
    oral cavity c.
    sputum c.
    thin-layer c.
    ThinPrep c.
    touch imprint c.
    urine c.
    washing c.
cytolymph
cytolysate
    blood c.
cytolysin
cytolysis
    immune c.
cytolysosome
CytoLyt fixative
cytolytic
    T (cell) c.
    c. T-cell lysis assay
cytoma
cytomatrix
cytomegalic
    c. cell
    c. inclusion disease
      (CID, CMID)
    c. inclusion disease cytology
    c. inclusion disease virus
cytomegalovirus (CMV)
    C. (CMV)
    c. antibody
    c. culture
    c. disease
    c. esophagitis
    c. infection
    c. isolation
    c. lymphadenitis

cytomegaly
cytomembrane
cytomere
cytometaplasia
cytometer
    Bayer Technicon H1 automated
      flow c.
    CAS 200 image c.
    Cell Lab IC 100 image c.
    Epics C flow c.
    Epics Profile flow c.
    FACScalibur flow c.
    FACScan flow c.
    FACSort flow c.
    FACStar Plus flow c.
    FACSVantage flow c.
    flow c.
    MAXM hematology flow c.
cytometric image analysis
cytometry
    CD-Chex C34 control for
      flow c.
    CD-Chex Plus control for flow c.
    cell-suspension flow c.
    DNA flow c.
    Feulgen c.
    flow c. (FC, FCM)
    gel and flow c.
    image c.
    multiparameter flow c.
cytomicrosome
Cytomics FC 500 series flow cytometry
  system
cytomorphology
cytomorphosis
cyton
cytonuclear
    c. atypia
    c. pleomorphism
cytopathic effect (CPE)
cytopathogenesis
cytopathogenic virus
cytopathologic, cytopathological
cytopathological (*var. of*
  cytopathologic)
cytopathologist
cytopathology
    nongynecologic c. (NGC)
cytopathy
cytopenia
Cytophagaceae
Cytophagales
cytophagic histiocytic panniculitis
cytophagous
cytophagy
cytophanere
cytopharynx
cytophil group
cytophilic antibody

cytophotometer
cytophotometry
    DNA c.
    flow c.
cytophylactic
cytophylaxis
cytophyletic
cytopipette
cytoplasm
    abundant c.
    amphophilic c.
    basophilic c.
    blue c.
    eosinophilic c.
    foamy c.
    glassy c.
    ground glass c.
    intensely basophilic c.
    lavender c.
    light-staining apical c.
    neurofibril in c.
    c. of neuron
    pale c.
    pink c.
    vacuolated c.
    water clear c.
cytoplasmic
    c. antineutrophil cytoplasmic antibody (cANCA)
    c. antineutrophil cytoplasmic autoantibody (cANCA)
    c. bleb
    c. bridge
    c. crystalline aggregate
    c. cyanophilia
    c. extension
    c. fiber alteration
    c. fibril alteration
    c. filament alteration
    c. glycogen
    c. granulation
    c. halo
    c. immunoreactivity
    c. inclusion
    c. inclusion body
    c. inheritance
    c. lipid aggregate
    c. lipid droplet alteration
    c. macromolecule aggregate
    c. matrix
    c. matrix alteration
    c. membrane
    c. organelle
    c. pattern
    c. peptidase
    c. process
    c. projection
    c. ratio
    c. snout

    c. staining
    c. striation
    c. tail
    c. vacuolation
    c. vacuole
cytoplast
cytopoiesis
cytopreparation
Cytopro cytocentrifuge
cytopuncture
    fine-needle c.
    c. smear
cytopyge
cytoreductive therapy
Cytorhabdovirus
CytoRich
    C. cervical cytology monolayer system
    C. Red fixative
cytorrhyctes (*var. of* cytoryctes)
cytoryctes, cytorrhyctes
cytoscopy
cytoscreener
cytosine
    c. arabinoside (CA)
    guanine c. (GC)
    c. phosphate guanine (CpG)
    c. triphosphate (CTP)
cytosine-guanine-guanine (CGG)
cytosis
cytoskeletal
    c. filament
    c. polymerization
    c. protein
    c. protein hyperphosphorylation disease
cytoskeleton
    actin c.
cytoskeleton-associated protein
cytosmear
cytosol
    aminopeptidase c.
    bovine smooth muscle c.
    c. phospholipase A2 (cPLA2)
cytosome
cytospin
    c. analysis
    c. cup
    c. slide centrifuge gram-stained smear
Cytospora
cytospray fixation
cytostasis
Cyto-Stat/Coulter CLONE monoclonal antibody
cytostatic
cytostome
cytotactic

C

cytotaxia (*var. of* cytotaxis)
cytotaxis, cytotaxia
    negative c.
    positive c.
cytotechnologist (CT)
Cyto-Tek cytocentrifuge
cytothesis
cytotoxic
    c. antibody
    c. chemotherapy
    c. edema
    c. hypersensitivity reaction
    c. necrosis
    c. protein
    T (cell) c. (Tc)
    c. T cell
cytotoxicity
    antibody-dependent cell-mediated c.
    antimediated c.
    c. assay
    cell-dependent c. (CDC)
    complement-mediated c.
    lymphocyte-mediated c. (LMC)
    c. negative, absorption positive
      (CYNAP)
cytotoxin

    binary c.
    vero c.
cytotrophic (*var. of* cytotropic)
cytotrophoblast
cytotrophoblastic cell
cytotropic, cytotrophic
    c. antibody
    c. antibody test
cytotropism
cytozoic
cytozoon
cytozyme
cyturia
Cytyc
    C. CytoLyt preservative solution
    C. PreservCyt preservative solution
Czapek-Dox
    C.-D. agar
    C.-D. medium
Czapek solution agar
Czermak
    globular space of C.
    C. space
Czerny
    C. anemia
    C. disease

D

D antigen
D cell
D colony
D line
D value

d

decigram

2D

two-dimensional
2D PAGE

D2-40

D2-40 antibody
D2-40 monoclonal
antibody

Daae disease
Daae-Finsen disease
DAB

diaminobenzidine
dimethylaminoazobenzene
DAB reaction

Dabska tumor
DAC

diazacholesterol
digital-to-analog converter

dacarbazine
Dacie method
D/A converter
DaCosta

D. disease
D. syndrome

dacrocyte
Dacron patch
Dacrymyces
dacryoadenitis
dacryoblennorrhea
dacryocyst
dacryocystitis
dacryocyte
dacryolith

Desmarres d.
Nocardia d.

dacryoma
dacryosolenitis
Dactylaria gallopava
dactylitis
Dactylium dendroides
Dactylogyrus
dactylolysis spontanea
DAD

diffuse alveolar damage

Daedalea
Daedaleopsis
daejeonensis

Paenibacillus d.

DAF

decay accelerating factor

Da Fano stain
DAG

diacylglycerol
diffuse antral gastritis

DAGT

direct antiglobulin test

DAH

disordered action of heart

DAI

diffuse axonal injury

Dakin solution
Dako

D. Artisan Staining System
D. Autostainer
D. Envision system peroxidase
D. Fast Red Substrate
System
D. hepatocyte immunostain
D. HercepTest
D. large volume LSAB2 alkaline
phosphatase kit
D. target retrieval solution

DakoCytomation EGFR pharmDx
colorectal cancer diagnostic kit
dalapon
Dale-Laidlaw clotting time method
Dalen-Fuchs nodule
Dale reaction
Dallas myocarditis criteria
DALM

dysplasia-associated lesion or
mass

Dalrymple disease
Dalton law
damage

antibody-mediated vascular d.
diffuse alveolar d.
(DAD)
end-organ d.
irradiation d.
irreversible d.
minimal brain d. (MBD)
myocardial d.
ossicular d.
radiation d.

damaged fibrotic valve
Damalinia
d-amino acid oxidase
dammar
dammini

Ixodes d.

damnosum

Simulium d.

D

253

dAMP
deoxyadenosine monophosphate
damping
Dam unit
decameter
danaparoid sodium
Danbolt-Closs syndrome
dance
brachial d.
hilar d.
hilus d.
St. Anthony d.
St. Guy d.
St. John d.
dandy fever
Dandy-Walker
D.-W. cyst
D.-W. malformation
D.-W. syndrome
Dane
D. and Herman keratin stain
D. method
D. particle
danicus
Aneurinibacillus d.
Danielssen-Boeck disease
Danielssen disease
dankaliense
Trichophyton d.
dankaliensis
Gymnoascus d.
Danlos syndrome
DANS
1-dimethylaminonaphthalene-5-sulfonic acid
dansyl chloride
D10 antigen
Danubian endemic familial nephropathy
Danysz phenomenon
DAP
death-associated protein
dihydroxyacetone phosphate
DAPI
4,6-diamidino-2-phenylindole-2-HCl
DAPI dye
DAPI stain
DAPT
direct agglutination pregnancy test
d-arabitol dehydrogenase
DARC
Duffy antigen receptor for chemokine
Darier disease
Darier-Roussy sarcoid
dark
d. cell
d. current
d. reaction
d. reactivation

dark-field
d.-f. condenser
d.-f. examination
fluorescent antibody d.-f. (FADF)
d.-f. microscope
d.-f. microscopy
dark-ground microscope
Darling disease
darlingi
Anopheles d.
Darlington amplifier
Darrow
D. red
D. red stain
d'Arsonval meter
dartoic tissue
dartos
d. muliebris
d. muscle
tunica d.
dashboard knee
dassonvillei
Nocardiopsis d.
Dasyprocta
DAT
differential agglutination titer
diphtheria antitoxin
direct agglutination test
direct antiglobulin test
database
GenBank d.
unigene d.
date fever
Datronia
Datura stramonium
daughter
d. cell
d. colony
d. cyst
daurensis
Heliorestis d.
Davainea
Davaineidae
Davenport graph
David disease
Davidoff cell
Davidsohn
D. differential absorption test
D. modification of Paul-Bunnell heterophile antibody test
Davies disease
davtiani
Teladorsagia d.
dawn phenomenon
Dawson encephalitis
DayCytomation pharmDX c-kit
16-day endometrium
Day test

DB
dextran blue
DBA
dibenzanthracene
DBC
dye-binding capacity
DBCL
dilute blood clot lysis
DBI
development-at-birth index
DC
dendritic cell
diphenylarsine cyanide
DCA
deoxycholate-citrate agar
DCC
dextran-coated charcoal
DCC anti-oncogene
DCC assay
DCF
direct centrifugal flotation
DCIS
ductal carcinoma in situ
DCO
diffusing capacity for carbon monoxide
DCOM
dilated cardiomyopathy
DCT
direct Coombs test
DCTMA
desoxycorticosterone trimethylacetate
DCTPA
desoxycorticosterone triphenylacetate
DDB2 gene
DDD
dense-deposit disease
dichlorodiphenyldichloroethane
digital differential display
dihydroxydinaphthyl disulfide
DDD analysis
DDGE
denaturing density gradient
electrophoresis
D-dimer
D-d. assay
D-d. test
DDR
discoidin domain receptor
DDS
dystrophy-dystocia syndrome
DDT
dichlorodiphenyltrichloroethane
DDT assay
DDVP
dimethyldichlorovinyl phosphate
de
d. Castro fluid
d. Clerambault syndrome
d. Galantha method for urates

d. Lange syndrome
d. Morgan spot
d. novo myelodysplastic syndrome
d. novo tissue formation
d. Quervain disease
d. Quervain tenosynovitis
d. Quervain thyroiditis
d. Ritis ratio
d. Sanctis-Cacchione syndrome
d. Toni-Fanconi syndrome
deacetylase
histone d. (HDAC)
deactivation
deacylase
acylsphingosine d.
deacylate
dead
d. fetus in utero (DFU)
d. finger
d. of disease
d. on arrival (DOA)
d. time
dead-end host
deadly agaric
dead-space hyponatremia
DEAE
diethylaminoethyl
diethylaminoethyl cellulose
DEAE anion exchange
chromatography
DEAE cellulose
DEAE-Sephacel ion exchange column
deafness
lentigines, electrocardiographic
abnormalities, ocular hypertelorism,
pulmonary stenosis, abnormalities
of genitalia, retardation of growth,
and d.
dealbata
Clitocybe d.
dealbation
dealcoholization
deallergization
deallergize
deaminase
adenine d.
adenosine d. (ADA)
adenylate d.
adenylic acid d.
AMP d.
guanine d.
histidine alpha d.
myoadenylate d.
porphobilinogen d.
deaquation
dearterialization
death
activation-induced cell d. (AICD)
autoerotic d.

D

death (*continued*)
    black d.
    brain d.
    cause of d. (COD)
    cell d.
    cerebral d.
    crib d.
    direct maternal d.
    early neonatal d.
    d. effector domain
    fetal d.
    d. fever
    functional d.
    indirect maternal d.
    infant d.
    infectious cause of d. (ICOD)
    intrauterine fetal d. (IUFD)
    d. investigation resources
    late neonatal d.
    local d.
    natural d.
    neonatal d. (ND, NND)
    nonrenal d. (NRD)
    d. notification
    d. of other cause (DOC)
    programmed cell d.
    somatic d.
    sports-related sudden d.
    sudden cardiac d. (SCD)
    sudden coronary d. (SCD)
    sudden intrauterine unexplained d.
        (SIUD)
    sudden unexpected d. (SUD)
    sudden unexpected, unexplained d.
        (SUUD)
    sudden unexplained d. (SUD)
    sudden unexplained infant d. (SUID)
    d. trance
    underlying cause of d.
death-associated protein (DAP)
DeBakey aortic assay
Debaromyces japonicus
Debaryomyces
    D. hansenii
    D. hominis
    D. neoformans
Debove membrane
debrancher deficiency limit dextrinosis
debranching enzyme
Debré phenomenon
Debré-Semelaigne syndrome
débridement
debris
    amorphous eosinophilic d.
    cellular d.
    inflammatory cell d.
    karyorrhectic nuclear d.
    lamellated collection of inspissated
        inflammatory d.

    purulent d.
    stonelike d.
debubbling
debug
debye
DEC1
    differentiated embryo-chondrocyte
    expressed gene 1
decade counter
decagram
decalcification
    AB d.
decalcified bone
Decalcifier
decalcify
decalcifying
decaliter
Decal Plus
decalvans
    folliculitis d.
decameter
decanoic acid
decanoyl-Arg-Val-Lys-Arg-
    chloromethylketone
    (dec-RVKR-cmk)
decant
decantation
decaplanina
    Amycolatopsis d.
decarboxylase
    aromatic l-amino acid d. (AADC)
    branched-chain alpha keto acid d.
    d. broth
    glutamate d.
    glutamic acid d. (GAD)
    histidine d. (HDC)
    hydroxytryptophan d.
    methylmalonyl-CoA d.
    ornithine d.
    orotidine-5′-phosphate d.
    orotidylate d.
    oxaloacetate d.
    uroporphyrinogen d. (UROD)
decarboxylation
    amine precursor uptake and d.
        (APUD)
decay (DK)
    d. accelerating factor (DAF)
    alpha d.
    d. antibody-accelerating factor
    beta d.
    branching d.
    d. coefficient
    d. constant
    exponential d.
    d. mode
    positron beta d.
    d. product
    radioactive d.

d. rate
d. scheme
deceleration of head
decentration
decerebrate rigidity
dechloracetivorans
    Desulfovibrio d.
Dechloromonas agitata
Dechlorosoma suillum
decibel
decidua
d. basalis
d. capsularis
ectopic d.
membrana d.
d. vera
decidual
d. alteration
d. cast
d. cell
d. change
d. endometritis
d. membrane
d. metaplasia
d. microvessel
d. plate
d. polyp
d. reaction
decidualis
decidualized endometrium
deciduitis
membranous d.
deciduoid
deciduoma
Loeb d.
deciduosis
cutaneous d.
deciduous
d. membrane
d. skin
decigram (d)
decile
deciliter (dL)
milligram per d. (mg/dL)
decimal reduction time
decimeter (dm)
decipiens
    Pseudoterranova d.
    Terranova d.
decision
d. table
warfarin dosing d.
DEC-205 marker
decoagulant
decode
decoder
decolorationis
    Bacillus d.
decolorize

decolorizer
decompensation
cardiac d.
d. injury
d. sickness
decomposition potential
decompression
carpal tunnel d. (CTD)
d. injury
d. sickness
decontaminating room
decontamination
dry d.
external d.
internal d.
d. wipe
d. zone
deconvolution fluorescence microscopy
decora
    Macrobdella d.
decorin
decorporate
decortication
decoy cell
decreased
d. cardiac output
d. creatine clearance
d. serum iron
decrease in bone mass
decrement
dec-RVKR-cmk
decanoyl-Arg-Val-Lys-Arg-
chloromethylketone
decubation
decubitus
d. calculus
d. ulcer
decurrent
decussate
decussatio
decussation
dedifferentiated
d. chondrosarcoma
d. liposarcoma
d. low-grade adenocarcinoma
dedifferentiation phenomenon
deefferentation
deep
d. agar
d. cell
d. cortex
d. fascia
d. penetrating nevus (DPN)
rapture of the d.
d. vein thrombosis (DVT)
d. wedge biopsy
deer
epizootic hemorrhagic disease of d.
hemorrhagic disease of d.

D

deerfly
    d. disease
    d. fever (tularemia)
Deetjen body
de-expression
def
    deficiency
defect
    acquired d.
    aldosterone secretion d. (ASD)
    aortic septal d.
    atrial septal d. (ASD)
    blast-induced cognitive d.
    blast-induced memory d.
    congenital ectodermal d.
    congenital hemidysplasia with
      ichthyosiform erythroderma and
      limb defects (CHILD)
    conotruncal heart d.
    cortical d.
    coupling d.
    diffusion d.
    dual hemostatic d.
    ectodermal d.
    endocardial cushion d.
    fibrous cortical d.
    filling d.
    focal bone marrow d.
    Gerbode d.
    hydrogen-detected ventricular septal
      d. (HVSD)
    interatrial septal d. (IASD)
    interventricular septal d. (IVSD)
    intraventricular conduction d.
      (IVCD)
    iodide transport d.
    iodotyrosine deiodinase d.
    labyrinthine d. (LD)
    mitotic spindle d.
    neural tube d.
    no significant d. (NSD)
    organification d.
    plasma d. (PD)
    platelet d. (PLD)
    protein d.
    red cell membrane protein d.
    septal d. (SD)
    serum d. (SD)
    solubilization d.
    surgical d.
    transport protein d.
    ventilation d.
    ventricular septal d. (VSD)
    zero defects (Z/D)
defective
    d. bacteriophage
    d. interfering (DI)
    d. phage
    d. probacteriophage

    d. prophage
    d. virus
defense
    host d.'s
    d. mechanism
defensin
deferens
    ductus d.
    vas d.
deferent
    d. canal
    d. duct
deferentis
    tunica mucosa ductus d.
    tunica muscularis ductus d.
deferentitis
deferoxamine
    d. challenge test
    d. mesylate
    d. mesylate infusion test
Deferribacter
    D. abyssi
    D. desulfuricans
    D. thermophilus
Deferribacteraceae
Deferribacterales
Deferribacteres
defervescent stage
defibrinated blood
defibrination syndrome
defibrinogenating effect
deficiency (def)
    A1AT d.
    acid maltase d.
    acquired C1EInh d.
    ADA d.
    adenosine deaminase d.
    adenylate kinase d.
    ADH d.
    alpha$_1$ antitrypsin d.
    alpha galactosidase A d.
    alphalipoprotein d.
    d. anemia
    antidiuretic hormone d.
    antitrypsin d.
    argininosuccinate synthetase d.
    B-cell d.
    beta-d-glucuronidase d.
    brancher d.
    carbamoyl phosphate synthetase I d.
    carnitine palmitoyltransferase 2 d.
    CD11/CD18 d.
    cholesterol side-chain cleavage
      enzyme d.
    clotting factor d.
    collagen receptor d.
    congenital lactase d.
    congenital sucrase-isomaltase d.
      (CSID)

CPS d.
CPT2 d.
CR3 d.
desmolase d.
dihydropteridine reductase d.
disaccharidase d.
d. disease
duplication d.
factor I, II, V, VII, VIII, IX, X,
 XI d.
ferrochelatase d.
fibrinogen d.
folate d.
folic acid d.
fructose 1,6-diphosphatase d.
galactokinase d.
GALT d.
glucose-6-phosphate dehydrogenase d.
glucosephosphate isomerase d.
GluR2 d.
glutathione reductase d.
glutathione synthetase d.
growth hormone d. (GHD)
heparin cofactor II d.
hepatic lipase d.
hereditary plasmathromboplastin
 component d.
hexosaminidase A d.
HLA class I d.
human growth hormone d.
IL-2 receptor alpha-chain d.
immune d.
immunological d.
iodine d.
lactase d.
LCAT d.
leukocyte adhesion d. (LAD)
lipoprotein lipase d.
medullary serotonergic network d.
mineralocorticoid d.
multiple carboxylase d. (MCD)
myeloperoxidase d.
myoadenylate deaminase d.
d. of gonadotropin
ornithine carbamoyltransferase d.
ornithine transcarbamoylase d.
PK d.
placental steroid sulfatase d.
plasma thromboplastin
 antecedent d.
plasminogen activator d.
PNP d.
porphobilinogen deaminase d.
porphobilinogen synthase d.
prothrombin d.
protoporphyrinogen oxidase d.
pseudocholinesterase d.
PTA d.
PTC d.

purine nucleoside phosphorylase d.
pyruvate kinase d.
red blood cell enzyme d.
secondary antibody d.
selective d.
SPCA d.
specific antibody d.
specific coagulation factor d.
stable factor d.
sulfite oxidase d.
systemic l-carnitine d.
tenascin-X d.
thiamine d.
thromboplastin antecedent d.
triosephosphate isomerase d.
tuftsin d.
tyrosinase d.
uroporphyrinogen decarboxylase d.
uroporphyrinogen III cosynthase d.
uroporphyrinogen synthase d.
vitamin B_{12} d.
vitamin K d.
ZAP-70 d.
zinc d.
ZPI d.

deficit
 base d. (BD)
defined
 d. culture medium
 serologically d. (SD)
 d. substrate (DS)
definition (df)
 recursive d.
definitive
 d. callus
 d. characterization
 d. erythroblast
 d. host
 d. lysosome
 d. method
 d. organism identification
deflagration
deflection signal
deflorescence
Defluvibacter lusatiensis
defluvii
 Aquamicrobium d.
 Chryseobacterium d.
 Pseudaminobacter d.
defoliant
deformability
deformans
 arthritis d.
 endarteritis d.
 hyperostosis corticalis d.
 osteitis d.
 osteochondrodystrophia d.
deformation
deforming

D

deformity
    acquired d.
    Arnold-Chiari d.
    congenital musculoskeletal d.
    Erlenmeyer flask d.
    gibbus d.
    J-sella d.
    Klippel-Feil d.
    lobster-claw d.
    Michel d.
    swan-neck d.
    valgus d.
    varus d.

degeneracy

degenerate
    d. code
    d. oligonucleotide-primed (DOP)
    d. oligonucleotide primed
      polymerase chain reaction
      (DOP-PCR)

degenerated
    d. intervertebral fibrocartilage
    d. meniscus

degenerating
    d. myelin demonstration
    d. secretory cell

degeneratio

degeneration
    adipose d.
    albuminoid d.
    albuminous d.
    Alzheimer fibrillary d.
    amyloid d.
    angiolithic d.
    ascending d.
    atheromatous d.
    axonal d.
    ballooning d.
    basophilic granular d.
    calcareous d.
    capsular lipochondral d.
    carneous d.
    caseous d.
    cellular d.
    cerebellar d.
    cloudy swelling d.
    collagen d.
    colliquative d.
    colloid d.
    complete reaction of d. (CRD)
    corticobasal d.
    Crooke hyaline d.
    cystic d.
    cystoid macular d.
    cytologic d.
    descending d.
    elastoid d.
    elastotic d.
    fatty d.

    feathery d.
    fibrinoid d.
    fibrinous d.
    fibrous d.
    floccular d.
    foamy d.
    granular d.
    granulovacuolar d.
    gray d.
    hepatolenticular d.
    hyaline d.
    hydatid d.
    hydropic d.
    lateral collateral ligament d.
    lenticular progressive d.
    lipid d.
    lipochondral d. (LCD)
    lipoid d.
    liquefaction d.
    liquefactive d.
    meniscal d.
    Mönckeberg d.
    mucinoid d.
    mucinous d.
    mucoid medial d.
    myelin d.
    myelinic d.
    myxohyaline d.
    myxoid d.
    myxomatous d.
    neurofibrillary d. (tau)
    Nissl d.
    pseudomucinous d.
    pseudotubular d.
    reaction of d. (DeR, DR)
    red d.
    reticular d.
    retrograde d.
    Schnabel cavernous d.
    secondary d.
    senile d.
    spongiform d.
    striatonigral d.
    subacute combined d. (SACD, SCD)
    transsynaptic d.
    Türck d.
    vacuolar d.
    wallerian d. (WD)
    waxy d.
    Zenker d.

degenerativa
    melanosis corii d.

degenerative
    d. arthritis
    d. change
    d. index
    d. inflammation
    d. joint disease (DJD)
    d. pannus

degenerativus
degerlachei
  Flavobacterium d.
deglycerolization
Degos
  D. disease
  D. syndrome
degradation
  autooxidative d.
  glycogen d.
  proteolytic d.
degranulation
degree
degrees of freedom (df)
Dehalobacter restrictus
dehalogenans
  Anaeromyxobacter d.
Dehalospirillum multivorans
dehiscence
dehydrase
  aminolevulinic acid d. (ALAD, ALA-D)
dehydratase
  carbonate d.
dehydrate
  calcium pyrophosphate d. (CPPD)
dehydrated alcohol
dehydration
dehydroascorbic acid
dehydrobilirubin
dehydroepiandrosterone (DHEA)
  d. sulfate (DHEAS)
dehydrogenase
  acyl-CoA d.
  alcohol d. (ADH)
  aldehyde d.
  alpha-keto acid d.
  beta-hydroxy-delta-5-steroid d.
  branched-chain alpha keto acid d.
  d-arabitol d.
  formaldehyde d.
  glucose-6-phosphate d. (G6PD)
  glutamate d.
  glyceraldehyde phosphate d. (GAPDH)
  heat-stable lactic d. (HLDH)
  hexosephosphate d.
  hydroxybutyrate d. (HBD, HBDH)
  hydroxybutyric d.
  iditol d.
  inosine d.
  inositol d.
  isocitrate d.
  isocitric d.
  isovaleryl-CoA d.
  lactate d. (LD)
  lactic d. (LD)
  l-arabinose d.

l-arabitol d.
l-xylulose d.
lysine d.
malate d.
malic d. (MDH)
mitochondrial pyruvate d.
NADH d.
oxoglutarate d.
oxoisovalerate d.
polyol d.
proline d.
pyrroline-5-carboxylate d.
saccharopine d.
sarcosine d.
serum hydroxybutyrate d. (SHBD)
serum isocitric d. (SICD)
serum lactate d. (SLD, SLDH)
Shikimate d.
sorbitol d.
succinate d.
tetrahydrofolate d.
triosephosphate d.
xylitol d.
dehydrogenate
dehydrogenation
dehydroisoandrosterone (DHIA)
DEIA
  DNA-enzyme immunoassay
deiminase
  arginine d.
Deinococcaceae
Deinococcales
Deinococci
Deinococcus indicus
deiodinase
deiodinate
deionization
deionized formamide
Deiters
  D. cell
  D. terminal frame
Dejerine
  D. disease
  D. syndrome
Dejerine-Klumpke
  D.-K. paralysis
  D.-K. syndrome
Dejerine-Roussy syndrome
Dejerine-Sottas
  D.-S. disease
  D.-S. syndrome
Dekkera
DEL1
  developmental endothelial locus 1
  DEL1 gene
Delacroixia coronata
Delafield
  D. fixative solution
  D. fluid

D

Delafield (*continued*)
    D. hematoxylin
    D. hematoxylin stain
Delaney clause
delay
    d. circuit
    d. line
delayed
    d. adrenarche
    d. allergy
    d. climacteric
    d. development
    d. graft function
    d. hemolytic transfusion
      reaction
    d. hypersensitivity
    d. hypersensitivity reaction
    d. menopause
    d. primary closure (DPC)
    d. puberty
    d. radiation toxicity
    d. traumatic intracerebral hematoma
      (DTICH)
    triage d.
delayed-phase skin response
delayed-type hypersensitivity
  (DTH)
delbrueckii
    Lactobacillus d.
deletion
    antigenic d.
    central clonal d.
    chromosomal d.
    gene d.
    gross d.
    hemizygous d.
    intercalary d.
    interstitial d.
    large d.
    d. mutation
    terminal d.
    d. theory
    X d.
DELFIA
    dissociation enhanced lanthanide
      fluoroimmunoassay
Delftia
    D. acidovorans
    D. tsuruhatensis
delicatus
    Sulfitobacter d.
delicti
    corpus d.
deliense
    Leptotrombidium d.
deliensis
    Trombicula d.
delipidated albumin
deliquescence

deliquescent
delirium
    anticholinergic d.
    excited d.
    d. tremens (DT)
delitescence
deliver
    to d. (TD)
delivery
    spontaneous d. (SD)
delle
delomorphous
delphian node
Delsa 440 SX Zeta potential
  analyzer
delta
    d. agent
    d. ALA acid
    d. aminolevulinic acid assay
    d. antigen
    d. base
    d. cell
    d. cell islet
    d. cell of anterior lobe of
      hypophysis
    d. cell of pancreas
    d. check
    d. fiber
    d. granule
    d. hepatitis
    d. ray
    d. staphylolysin
    d. storage pool disease
    d. thalassemia
    d. virus
Deltabacteria
delta-5 desaturase enzyme
delta^2-isopentenyl diphosphate
delta^3-isopentenyl diphosphate
deltalike 1 homolog (DLK1)
Deltaretrovirus
Deltavirus
deltoidea
    Anthopsis d.
demarcation
    line of d.
demargination
demarquayi
    Filaria d.
    Mansonella d.
Dematiaceae
dematiaceous fungus
dematioides
    Hormonema d.
Dematium
d'emblée
    mycosis fungoides d.
    tumeur d.
demeclocycline

dementia
  argyrophilic grain d.
  multiinfarct d.
  non-Alzheimer d.
  d. praecox
  d. pugilistica/autism with self-injury
    behavior
  tangle only d.
  transmissible d.
  vascular d.
demerariensis
  Raillietina d.
  Taenia d.
demethylchlortetracycline
demeton
  methyl d.
Demetria terragena
demilune
  d. body
  Giannuzzi d.
  Heidenhain d.
  serous d.
demineralization
deminutus
  Ternidens d.
demobilization
Demodex folliculorum
demonstration
  calcium deposit d.
  copper deposit d.
  degenerating myelin d.
  iron-positive pigment d.
  d. of organism
demyelinate
demyelinated myelitis
demyelinating
  d. disease
  d. encephalopathy
demyelination, demyelinization
  axonal d.
  cuprizone model of chronic d.
  spinal cord d.
demyelinization (*var. of* demyelination)
denaturation
  protein d.
denatured hemoglobin
denaturing
  d. density gradient electrophoresis
    (DDGE)
  d. gel
  d. gradient gel electrophoresis
    (DGGE)
  d. high-performance liquid
    chromatography (DHPLC)
dendraxon
dendriform
dendrite
  apical d.
dendritic

  d. calculus
  d. cell (DC)
  d. cell tumor
  d. clear cell
  d. cytoplasmic process
  d. epidermal cell
  d. spine
  d. synovitis
  d. thorn
dendriticum
  Diphyllobothrium d.
dendrocyte
  dermal d.
dendroid
dendroides
  Dactylium d.
dendron
Dendrosporobacter quercicolus
Dendrostilbella byssina
Dendryphion
dengue
  d. fever
  hemorrhagic d.
  d. hemorrhagic fever
  d. shock syndrome
  d. virus, types 1–4
denhamense
  Roseibium d.
Denhardt solution
denitrificans
  Achromobacter d.
  Alcaligenes d.
  Alicycliphilus d.
  Comamonas d.
  Kingella d.
  Listeria d.
  Shewanella d.
  Sterolibacterium d.
  Thialkalivibrio d.
denitrifying bacterium
Denitrobacterium detoxificans
Denitrovibrio acetiphilus
Dennie-Marfan syndrome
Dennis left atrium cannulation technique
Denonvilliers fascia
densa
  lamina d.
  macula d.
dense
  d. body
  d. deposit
  d. fibrillar component
  d. fibrous lamina (DFL)
  d. secondary granule
dense-core neurosecretory granule
dense-deposit disease (DDD)
densimeter
densitometer
  Appraise clinical d.

densitometry
density
    amniotic fluid bilirubin
      optical d.
    blood microvessel d.
    buoyant d.
    character d.
    count information d.
    extra electron d.
    fiber d.
    d. function
    d. gradient centrifugation
    intratumoral lymph vessel d.
    intratumor microvessel d.
    luminous flux d.
    macrophage d.
    microvessel d. (MVD)
    optical d. (OD)
    plating d.
    PSA d. (PSAD)
    scan information d.
    stellate d.
    subplasmalemmal d.
    total body d. (TBD)
    vascular d.
density-dependent repair
Densovirus
dental
    d. amalgam tattoo
    d. calculus
    d. caries
    d. cord
    d. crypt
    d. epithelium
    d. fluorosis
    d. follicle
    d. follicular cyst
    d. granuloma
    d. identification record
    d. lymph
    d. overexposure
    d. pathology
    d. plaque
    d. pulp
    d. sac
    d. tubule
dentales
    canaliculi d.
    tubuli d.
dentalis
    alveolus d.
    Amoeba d.
    alveoli pulmonis
dentata
    lamina d.
    Taenia d.
dentate
    d. line
    d. nucleus

**dentatorubral pallidoluysian atrophy
(DRPLA)**
dentatum
    Oesophagostomum d.
dentatus
    Stephanurus d.
dentes acustici
denticola
    Prevotella d.
    Treponema d.
denticolens
denticulate, denticulated
denticulated (*var. of*
  denticulate)
denticulatum
denticulatus
    Porocephalus d.
dentigerous
    d. cyst
    d. mixed tumor
dentin, dentine
    d. crystal alteration
    d. dysplasia
    d. globule
    d. tubule
dentinal
    d. canal
    d. fiber
    d. fluid
    d. pulp
    d. sheath
    d. tubule
dentine (*var. of* dentin)
dentinogenesis imperfecta
dentinoma
    fibroameloblastic d.
dentinum
dentis
    ebur d.
    pulpa d.
    substantia ossea d.
dentistry
    forensic d.
dentium
    Bifidobacterium d.
dentocariosa
    Rothia d.
dentrificans
    Jonesia d.
dentriticum
    Dicrocoelium d.
denucleated
denudation
    surface d.
Denver classification
Denys-Drash syndrome
Denys-Leclef phenomenon
deontology
deossification

deoxyadenosine
    d. monophosphate (dAMP)
    d. 5′-phosphate
deoxyadenylic acid
6-deoxy-beta-l-mannose
deoxycholate
deoxycholate-citrate agar (DCA)
deoxycholic acid
deoxycorticoid (DOC)
deoxycorticosterone (DOC)
    d. acetate (DOCA)
    d. test
deoxycortisol test
deoxycytidine
    d. monophosphate
    d. 5′-phosphate
deoxycytidylic acid
deoxygenated hemoglobin
deoxyguanosine
    d. monophosphate (dGMP)
    d. 5′-phosphate
    d. phosphate
2-deoxyguanosine 5′-triphosphate (dGTP)
deoxyguanylic acid
deoxyhemoglobin
6-deoxy-l-galactose
deoxynivalenol (DON)
deoxynucleotidyltransferase
    terminal d. (TdT)
deoxypyridinoline (DPD)
deoxyribonuclease (DNAse, DNase)
    d. agar
    d. digestion
    d. I, II
    d. test
deoxyribonucleic
    d. acid (DNA)
    d. acid stain
    d. acid staining
deoxyribonucleoprotein (DNP)
deoxyribonucleoside
deoxyribonucleotide
deoxyribose
deoxysugar
deoxythymidine triphosphate (dTTP)
deoxyuridine
    d. monophosphate (dUMP)
    d. 5′-phosphate
    d. phosphate
    d. suppression test
    d. triphosphate (DUTP)
deoxyuridylic acid
deoxyvirus
deparaffinization
department
    D. of Health and Human Services (DHHS)
    D. of Public Health (DPH)

dépassé
    coma d.
DEPC
    diethyl pyrocarbonate
DEPC-treated water
dependence, dependency
    anchorage d.
    drug d.
dependency (*var. of* dependence)
dependent
    d. edema
    d. variable
Dependovirus
depigmentation
deplasmolysis
depleted
    d. uranium (DU)
    d. uranium-containing explosion
depletion
    d. layer
    lipid d.
    mucin d.
    ovarian ascorbic acid d. (OAAD)
    plasma d.
    volume d.
depolarization
deposit
    basophilic d.
    brickdust d.
    dense d.
    endogenous pigments and deposits
    fingerprint d.
    hump d.
    iron d.
    lumpy-bumpy d.
    mesangial d.
    micrometastatic vascular d.
    d. of amyloid in islet cell
    posterior corneal d. (PCD)
    properdin d.
    washed out d.
deposition
    bilharzial pigment d.
    calcium d.
    catalyzed reporter d. (CARD)
    cholesterol d.
    collagen d.
    diffuse membrane hemosiderin d.
    diffuse perivillous fibrin d.
    fatty d.
    fibrin d.
    foreign material d.
    granular d.
    hemosiderin d.
    intestinal ceroid d.
    Kupffer cell iron d.
    linear d.
    malarial pigment d.

D

deposition (*continued*)
    subendothelial immune complex d.
    xanthomatous d.
depot
    fat d.
    d. reaction
depramine assay
depressant
depressed
    d. adenoma
    d. fracture
depression
    bone marrow d.
    myeloid d.
    respiratory d.
deprivation
    d. disease
    food d.
    severe protein d.
deproteinization
depth
    d. dose
    d. of field
    d. of focus
    relative sagittal d. (RSD)
depulization
depurination
der
    derivative chromosome
DER
    desmin ensheathment ratio
DeR
    reaction of degeneration
deradelphus
derangement
    chromosomal d.
Dercum disease
derepressed gene
derepression
    transient d.
derivation
derivative
    benzene d.
    d. chromosome
    purified protein d. (PPD)
derivative-standard
    purified protein d.-s. (PPD-S)
derived
    d. albumin
    d. protein
Dermabacteraceae
Dermacentor
    D. albopictus
    D. andersoni
    D. occidentalis
    D. reticulatus
    D. variabilis
Dermacentroxenus
    D. akari

    D. australis
    D. orientalis
    D. rickettsi
    D. sibericus
Dermacoccaceae
Dermacoccus nishinomiyaensis
dermal
    d. bone
    d. dendritic cell
    d. dendrocyte
    d. duct tumor
    d. eccrine cylindroma
    d. epidermal junction
    d. nevus
    d. papilla
    d. sinus
    d. tuberculosis
Dermanyssus avium et gallinae
dermatan sulfate
dermatica
    zona d.
dermatis
dermatitides (*pl. of* dermatitis)
dermatitidis
    Ajellomyces d.
    Blastomyces d.
    Fonsecaea d.
    Wangiella d.
dermatitis, *pl.* **dermatitides**
    actinic d.
    Ajellomyces d.
    allergic d.
    atopic d.
    d. atrophicans
    d. atrophicans diffusa
    d. atrophicans maculosa
    d. chronica atrophicans idiopathica
    contact d.
    contagious pustular d.
    eczematoid d.
    eczematous d.
    d. escharotica
    d. exfoliativa
    d. exfoliativa infantum
    d. exfoliativa neonatorum
    exfoliative d.
    factitious d.
    flaky paint d.
    follicular d.
    d. gangrenosa infantum
    d. herpetiformis
    infectious eczematoid d.
    lichenoid interface d.
    d. medicamentosa
    myositis sine dermatitides
    nickel d.
    nummular d.
    polymorphous d.
    psoriasiform d.

radiation d.
d. repens
Schamberg d.
seborrheic d.
spongiotic d.
stasis d.
subcorneal pustular d.
toxic d.
vacuolar interface d.
d. venenata
d. verrucosa
dermatoarthritis
lipoid d.
Dermatobia
D. cyaniventris
D. hominis
dermatobiasis
dermatocele
dermatocellulitis
dermatochalasis
dermatocyst
dermatofibroma (DF)
dermatofibrosarcoma protuberans (DFSP)
dermatofibrosis
d. lenticularis
d. lenticularis disseminata
dermatogen
dermatographism
dermatolysis
dermatoma
dermatome
trigeminal d.
dermatomegaly
dermatomycosis pedis
dermatomyoma
dermatomyositis
amyopathic d.
dermatopathia
d. pigmentosa
d. pigmentosa reticularis
dermatopathic
d. lymphadenitis
d. lymphadenopathy
dermatopathology
Dermatophagoides pteronyssinus
Dermatophilaceae
dermatophilosis
Dermatophilus
D. congolensis
D. penetrans
dermatophylaxis
dermatophyte test medium (DTM)
dermatophytid
dermatophytosis
dermatorrhagia
dermatorrhexis
dermatosclerosis
dermatoses (*pl. of* dermatosis)

dermatosis, *pl.* **dermatoses**
acantholytic d.
Bowen precancerous d.
dermolytic bullous d.
inflammatory d.
neutrophilic d.
d. papulosa nigra
progressive pigmentary d.
radiation d.
rheumatoid neutrophilic d.
subcorneal pustular d.
transient acantholytic d.
ulcerative d.
dermatozoiasis (*var. of* dermatozoonosis)
dermatozoon
dermatozoonosis, dermatozoiasis
dermatrophia, dermatrophy
dermatrophy (*var. of* dermatrophia)
Dermea
dermis
adventitial d.
busy d.
reticular d.
tombstone-like d.
Dermobacter
dermoepidermal interface
dermographia, dermographism
dermographism (*var. of* dermographia)
dermoid
d. cyst
d. cyst of ovary
implantation d.
inclusion d.
sequestration d.
d. tumor
dermolysis
dermolytic bullous dermatosis
dermonecrotic
dermopathy
diabetic d.
dermophlebitis
dermostenosis
dermostosis
dermosyphilopathy
dermotoxin
dermotuberculin reaction
dermo-unguis
Chaetophoma d.-u.
derodidymus
derotation
DES
diethylstilbestrol
des-Arg9-bradykinin
desaturase
acyl-CoA d.
desaturated phosphatidylcholine (DSPC)
desaturation
Descemet membrane
descemetocele

D

descending
    d. degeneration
    d. flaccid paralysis
descensus
    uterine d.
    d. ventriculi
description
    figure d.
    gross d.
desensitization
    drug d.
    heterologous d.
    homologous d.
    d. therapy
desensitize
desert fever
desetope
desferrioxamine
deshydremia
desiccant
desiccate
desiccation
desiccative
desiccator
designated blood donation
desipramine assay
Desmarres dacryolith
desmectasia
desmectasis
desmin
    d. antibody
    d. ensheathment ratio (DER)
desmitis
desmocollin
Desmodus
desmogenous
desmoglein
desmoglein-3
    IgG d.-3
desmoid
    extraabdominal d.
    d. fibromatosis
    d. tumor
desmoid-type fibromatosis (DTF)
desmolase
    17,20 d.
    20,22 d.
    d. deficiency
    mitochondrial enzyme d.
desmon
desmoplakin I
desmoplasia
    stromal d.
desmoplastic
    d. ameloblastoma
    d. cerebral astrocytoma
    d. change
    d. fibroblastoma
    d. fibroma

    d. infantile ganglioglioma
    d. medulloblastoma
    d. melanoma
    d. plaque
    d. small round cell tumor (DSRCT)
    d. stroma
    d. subtype
    d. trichoblastoma
    d. trichoepithelioma
desmosine
desmosomal protein
desmosome
desmosterol
desolvation
desoxycholate
    bromocresol purple d. (BCP-D)
desoxycorticosterone
    d. trimethylacetate (DCTMA)
    d. triphenylacetate (DCTPA)
11-desoxycorticosterone
despeciate
despeciated antitoxin
despeciation
despumation
desquamans
    herpes d.
desquamate
desquamation
    dry d.
    moist d.
desquamativa
    otitis d.
desquamative
    d. inflammatory vaginitis
    d. interstitial pneumonia (DIP)
    d. interstitial pneumonitis (DIP)
    d. interstitial poisoning
destruction
    immune-mediated d.
    d. of pancreatic beta cell
    red cell d.
    weapon of mass d. (WMD)
destructiva
    Ramularia d.
destructive
    d. distillation
    d. interference
destruens
    chorioadenoma d.
    Hyphomyces d.
Desulfacinum
    D. hydrothermale
    D. infernum
Desulfatibacillum
    D. aliphaticivorans
    D. alkenivorans
desulfhydrase
    homocysteine d.

Desulfitobacterium
　　D. chlororespirans
　　D. metallireducens
Desulfobacca acetoxidans
Desulfobacula
　　D. phenolica
　　D. toluolica
Desulfobulbus mediterraneus
Desulfocapsa sulfexigens
Desulfocella halophila
Desulfofaba
　　D. fastidiosa
　　D. gelida
　　D. hansenii
Desulfofrigus
　　D. fragile
　　D. oceanense
Desulfomicrobium
　　D. macestii
　　D. orale
Desulfomonile
　　D. limimaris
　　D. tiedjei
Desulfomusa hansenii
Desulfonatronum thiodismutans
Desulfonauticus submarinus
Desulfonispora thiosulfatigenes
Desulforegula conservatrix
Desulforhopalus
　　D. singaporensis
　　D. vacuolatus
Desulfosporosinus
　　D. auripigmenti
　　D. meridiei
　　D. orientis
Desulfotalea
　　D. arctica
　　D. psychrophila
Desulfotignum
　　D. balticum
　　D. phosphitoxidans
Desulfotomaculum
　　D. alkaliphilum
　　D. auripigmentum
　　D. gibsoniae
　　D. nigrificans
　　D. solfataricum
　　D. thermobenzoicum subsp.
　　　thermosyntrophicum
Desulfovibrio
　　D. alaskensis
　　D. alcoholivorans
　　D. aminophilus
　　D. bastinii
　　D. burkinensis
　　D. dechloracetivorans
　　D. gracilis
　　D. hydrothermalis
　　D. indonesiensis

　　D. magneticus
　　D. mexicanus
　　D. oxyclinae
　　D. piger
　　D. vietnamensis
　　D. zosterae
Desulfovirga adipica
desulfurans
　　Oceanithermus d.
desulfuricans
　　Deferribacter d.
　　Gordonia d.
Desulfurococcaceae
Desulfurococcales
Desulfurococcus amylolyticus
Desulfuromonas palmitatis
desynapsis
desynchronization
detached cranial section
detachment
　　retinal d.
detect, incident command, scene safety and security, assess hazard, support required, triage and treatment, evacuation, recovery (DISASTER)
detection
　　antibody d.
　　cardiac shunt d.
　　colorimetric antibody d.
　　C1q immune complex d.
　　digoxigenin-mediated d.
　　direct antigen d.
　　Filtracheck-UTI disposable
　　　colorimetric bacteriuria d.
　　nucleic acid d.
　　radiometric antibody d.
　　Vidiera NsD nucleic
　　　sample d.
detector
　　AD 340 absorbance d.
　　alpha particle d.
　　cadmium telluride d.
　　combustible gas d.
　　DTX series multimode d.
　　EC d.
　　electron capture d.
　　error d.
　　flame ionization d. (FID)
　　forward fluorescence d.
　　　(FED)
　　LD 400 luminescence d.
　　lithium-drifted d.
　　surface-barrier d.
　　TC d.
　　thermal conductivity d.
　　thermoluminescent d.
　　d. transfer function (DTF)
detergent
　　anionic d.

D

detergent (*continued*)
    nonionic d.
    oxidizing d.
determinant
    allotypic d.
    antigenic d.
    genetic d.
    d. group
    idiotypic antigenic d.
    immunogenic d.
    isoallotypic d.
    R d.
    resistance d. (RD)
    rough d.
determination
    activity d.
    fetal activity-acceleration d.
    lactate dehydrogenase isoenzyme d.
    sex d.
    Shimadzu hemoglobin d.
    shunt d.
deterministic
detersive
Dethiosulfovibrio
    D. acidaminovorans
    D. marinus
    D. russensis
detonation
detoxicate
detoxication
detoxificans
    Denitrobacterium d.
detoxification
    drug d.
    metabolic d.
detoxify
detrition
detritus
detrusor-external sphincter dyssynergia
detrusor-sphincter dyssynergia
detumescence
deuteranomaly
deuteranopia, deuteranopsia
deuteranopsia (*var. of* deuteranopia)
deuterium
deuterohemophilia
deuteromycetes
Deuteromycota
deuteron, deuton
deuteroplasm
deuterosome
deuterotocia, deuterotoky
deuterotoky (*var. of* deuterotocia)
deutomerite
deuton (*var. of* deuteron)
deutoplasm
deutoplasmic
deutoplasmigenon
deutoplasmolysis

Deutschländer disease
developing bone
development
    delayed d.
developmental
    d. arrest
    d. endothelial locus 1 (DEL1)
    d. mixoploid
    d. sequence anomaly
    d. synchronism
development-at-birth index (DBI)
Devergie disease
deviant
deviate
deviated septum
deviation
    average d.
    immune d.
    mean square d.
    no significant d. (NSD)
    relative standard d. (RSD)
    right axis d. (RAD)
    standard d. (SD)
    sum of square d.'s (SSD)
    d. to the right
Devic disease
device
    AvoSure INR test d.
    bag-valve-mask d.
    Biopore membrane d.
    Boyden chamber assay d.
    cholesterol 1,2,3 noninvasive testing d.
    Coag-a-mate prothrombin d.
    compound absorption d. (CAD)
    Coumatrak prothrombin time d.
    Crit-Line III TQA fluid management and access d.
    EMP d.
    HERF d.
    Hybrid Capture 2 (cervical cancer screening) d.
    improvised explosive d. (IED)
    intrauterine contraceptive d. (IUD)
    I/O d.
    IsoCode Stix d.
    OnTrak TestTcard drug testing d.
    OralScreen rapid oral fluid screening and test d.
    OraSure HIV-1 oral specimen collection d.
    Osteomark NTx point-of-care d.
    Ovabloc d.
    Profile-II ER drug screening d.
    ProTime INR test d.
    Qualitative Platform Immunoassay D. (QuPID)
    radiation dispersal d. (RDD)

Rheolog d.
Riechert-Mundiger stereotactic d.
semiconductor d.
Sepacell RZ-2000 d.
simple radiological d.
Status Cup Plus drug testing d.
Stratagene CastAway sequencing d.
stretch d.
Surgicutt d.
Tenderlett Plus finger-stick blood
  collection d.
thromboelastographic monitor d.
  (TEG)
TQA Sensor Pad blood-flow rate d.
venous access d. (VAD)
Verdict-II drug screening d.

devil's
  d. grip
  d. pinch

devolution

Devon polyposis syndrome

Devosia neptuniae

devriesei
  Streptococcus d.

Dewar flask

dexamethasone
  dexamethasone, insulin, and glucose
    (DIG)
  d. suppression test (DST)

**DexCom STS continuous glucose
monitoring system**

dexiocardia (*var. of* dextrocardia)

dextra

dextran
  d. blue (DB)
  low molecular weight d. (LMD,
    LMWD)

dextran-coated charcoal (DCC)

dextrin
  limit d.

dextrinase
  alpha d.

dextrinosis
  debrancher deficiency limit d.
  limit d.

dextrinosolvens
  Succinivibrio d.

dextrinuria

dextrocardia, dexiocardia
  corrected d.
  false d.
  isolated d.
  secondary d.
  type 1–4 d.
  d. with situs inversus

dextrogastria

dextrorotatory

dextrose
  d. agar

citrate phosphate d. (CPD)
d. in water (percent)
d. nitrogen ratio (DN)
d. solution mixture (DSM)
d. test
yeast peptone d.

dextrose-saline (DS)

dextrosuria

dextrothyroxine sodium

df
  degrees of freedom

DF
  dermatofibroma

DFA
  direct fluorescence assay
  direct fluorescent antibody
  direct fluorescent assay
    DFA for capsular antigen
    DFA test

DFA-TP
  direct fluorescent antibody *Treponema
    pallidum* test
    DFA-TP test

DFDT
  difluorodiphenyltrichloroethane

D-FISH
  double-fusion FISH

DFL
  dense fibrous lamina

DFS
  disease-free survival

DFSP
  dermatofibrosarcoma protuberans

DFU
  dead fetus in utero

DGGE
  denaturing gradient gel electrophoresis
    DGGE technique

DGLA
  dihomogammalinolenic acid

d-glucaric acid

dGMP
  deoxyguanosine monophosphate

dGTP
  2-deoxyguanosine 5′-triphosphate

DHA
  docosahexaenoic acid

dhakensis
  Aeromonas hydrophila subsp. *d.*

Dharmendra
  D. antigen
  D. antigenDharmendra antigen

DHE
  dihydroergotamine

DHEA
  dehydroepiandrosterone
    DHEA test

DHEAS
  dehydroepiandrosterone sulfate

D

d'Herelle phenomenon
DHFR
  dihydrofolate reductase
DHHS
  Department of Health and Human
  Services
DHIA
  dehydroisoandrosterone
DHL
  diffuse histocytic lymphoma
DHMA
  dihydroxymandelic acid
dhobie itch
DHPLC
  denaturing high-performance liquid
  chromatography
    DHPLC assay
DHT
  dihydrotachysterol
  dihydrotestosterone
    DHT test
d-3-hydroxyacyl coenzyme A
Di
  D. antigen
  D. Guglielmo disease
  D. Guglielmo syndrome
  D. particle
DI
  defective interfering
  ˙ DNA index
diabetes
  adult-onset d.
  alimentary d.
  bronze d.
  d. innocens
  d. insipidus
  insulin dependent d.
  juvenile-onset d.
  lipoatrophic d.
  maturity-onset d.
  d. mellitus
  Mosler d.
  renal d.
  Type 1 d.
  Type 2 d. (T2D)
diabetic
  d. acidosis
  d. amyotrophy
  d. angiopathy
  d. coma
  d. dermopathy
  d. diet
  d. gangrene
  d. glomerulosclerosis
  d. ketoacidosis (DKA)
  d. lipemia
  d. mastopathy
  d. microangiopathy
  d. myelopathy

  d. nephropathy
  d. neuropathy
  d. retinopathy (DR)
  d. ulcer
  d. urine
diabeticorum
  bullosis d.
  necrobiosis lipoidica d.
diabetogenic hormone
diacetemia
diacetic acid
diacetonuria
diaceturia
diacetyl monoxime
diaclasia (*var. of* diaclasis)
diaclasis, diaclasia
diacrinous
diacylglycerol (DAG)
diadenosine oligophosphate hydrolase
diag
  diagnosis
Diagnex
  D. Blue
  D. Blue test
diagnoses (*pl. of* diagnosis)
diagnosis (diag), *pl.* **diagnoses**
  Bethesda 2001 system d.
  clinical d.
  confirmed d.
  cytologic d.
  differential d.
  histologic d. (Histo-Dx)
  laboratory d.
  preimplantation genetic d.
    (PGD)
  prenatal d.
  presumptive d.
  provocative d.
  serum d.
  tumor stage at d.
diagnostic
  d. diphtheria toxin
  d. sensitivity
  d. serology
  d. specificity
  virtually d.
diagram
  acid-base d.
  block d.
  scatter d.
diakinesis
Dialister
  D. invisus
  D. pneumosintes
dial unit
dialysance
dialysate
dialysis dysequilibrium syndrome
diamagnetic

Diamanus montanus
diameter
    Mantoux d. (MD)
    mean cell d. (MCD)
    mean corpuscular d. (MCD)
    mean tubular d. (MTD)
    nuclear profile d.
    outside d. (OD)
diamide
4,6-diamidino-2-phenylindole-2-HCl (DAPI),
  6-diamidino-2-phenylindole-2-HCl
6-diamidino-2-phenylindole-2-HCl (*var. of* 4,6-diamidino-2-phenylindole-2-HCl)
diamine
    high iron d. (HID)
    low iron d. (LID)
diaminobenzidine (DAB)
    d. reaction
    d. stain
    d. tetrahydrochloride
diamniotic
diamond
    d. fuchsin
    D. TYM medium
Diamond-Blackfan
    D.-B. anemia
    D.-B. syndrome
Diamyl
Dianthovirus
diapause
diapedesis
Diaphane solution
diaphanometer
diaphanoscope
Diaphorobacter nitroreducens
diaphragm
    crural d.
    eventration of d.
    d. paralysis
diaphragmatic
    d. hernia
    d. peritonitis
    d. pleurisy
diaphyseal (*var. of* diaphysial)
diaphysial, diaphyseal
    d. aclasis
    d. center
    d. dysplasia
    d. juxtaepiphysial exostosis
diaphysitis
Diaporthe
Diaptomus
diarrhea
    antibiotic-associated d. (AAD)
    bovine virus d.
    Brainerd d.
    Cochin China d.
    hypokalemic d.

    medication-related d.
    opsoclonus-myoclonus d.
    traveler's d.
    tropical d.
diarrheagenic *E. coli*
diarrheogenic bacterial enterocolitis
diastase digestion
diastase-periodic
    d.-p. acid-Schiff (D-PAS)
    d.-p. acid-Schiff stain
diastase-resistant material
diastasic action
diastasis
diastasuria
diastatic
diastematocrania
diastematomyelia
diastereoisomer
diastereoisomerism
diastereomer
Diastix
diastolic hypertension
Diatest
    D. diabetes breath test
    D. diabetes breath test kit
diathermy
diatheses (*pl. of* diathesis)
diathesis, *pl.* **diatheses**
    cystic d.
    hemorrhagic d.
diathetic
diatom
diatomaceous earth
diauxic
diauxie
diazacholesterol (DAC)
diazepam
    d. assay
    d. breath test
diazinon
diazo
    d. reaction
    d. reagent
    d. stain for argentaffin granules
    d. staining method
diazomethane generator
diazonium salt
diazotize
dibasic
    d. acid
    d. aminoaciduria
    d. potassium phosphate (DKP)
dibenz[*a,h*]anthracene
dibenzanthracene (DBA)
dibenz(b,f)-1:4-oxazepine
dibenzopyridine
diborane
dibothriocephaliasis
Dibothriocephalus latus

dibrachius
  dicephalus dipus d.
  monocephalus tetrapus d.
  monocephalus tripus d.
1,2-dibromethane
dibromide
  ethylene d.
dibucaine number (DN)
DIC
  diffuse intravascular coagulation
  disseminated intravascular coagulation
dicarboxylic acid
dicelous
dicentric malformation
dicephalus
  d. dipus dibrachius
  d. dipus tetrabrachius
  d. dipus tribrachius
  d. dipygus
  d. tripus tribrachius
dicheirus
Dichelobacter nodosus
dichlobenil
dichloride
  ethylene d.
  ethylidene d.
  methylene d.
dichloroarisine
dichlorodiethyl sulfide
dichlorodiphenyldichloroethane (DDD)
dichlorodiphenyltrichloroethane (DDT)
1,1-dichloroethane
1,2-dichloroethane
dichloroformoxime CCl$_2$NOH
2,6-dichloroindophenol
dichloromethane
2,6-dichlorophenol-indophenol
dichlorophenoxy acetic acid
dichloropropene-dichloropropane mixture
dichlorvos
Dichomitus
dichorial (*var. of* dichorionic)
dichorionic, dichorial
  d. diamniotic placenta
  d. placenta twins
dichotic
Dichotomophthora portulacae
Dichotomophthoropsis nymphearum
dichotomous variable
dichotomy
dichroic filter system
dichroism
  circular d.
dichromate
  potassium d.
dichromatic erythrocyte
dichromophil, dichromophile
dichromophile (*var. of* dichromophil)

Dick
  D. method
  D. test
  D. test toxin
dicobalt edentate
dicofol
dicrocoeliosis
Dicrocoelium dentriticum
Dictyocaulus viviparus
Dictyonella
Dictyopanus
Dictyosporium
Dictyostelium
dictyotene
dicumarol
didelphis
  Streptococcus d.
dideoxy terminator
Didymella phacidiomorpha
didymitis
Diego
  D. antigen
  D. blood group system
diel
dieldrin
dielectric
  d. constant
  d. strength
diener
Dientamoeba fragilis
dieretic
diet
  BRAT d.
  cardiac d.
  diabetic d.
  elimination d.
  gluten-free d.
  low-fiber d.
dietary protein
Dieterle
  D. method
  D. stain
  D. stain
dietetic albuminuria
diethyl
  d. pyrocarbonate (DEPC)
  d. sulfate
diethylamide
  lysergic acid d. (LSD)
diethylamine
diethylaminoethyl (DEAE)
  d. cellulose
diethylcarbamazine
diethyldithiocarbamate
diethylene dioxide
diethylenetriaminepentaacetate
  calcium d. (Ca-DTPA)
diethylenetriaminepentaacetic acid
diethylstilbestrol (DES)

Dietzia
  D. *natronolimnaea*
  D. *psychralcaliphila*
Dietziaceae
dietziae
  Nonomuraea d.
Dieulafoy malformation
Difco ESP testing system
difference
  alveolar-arterial carbon dioxide d.
  alveolar-arterial oxygen d.
  d. amplifier
  antigenic d.
  arteriovenous carbon dioxide d.
  arteriovenous oxygen d.
  (AVDO$_2$)
  cation-anion d.
  electric potential d.
  fluorescence decay d.
  d. limen (DL)
  no significant d. (NSD)
  ultrastructural d.
differential
  d. agglutination titer (DAT)
  d. cell lysis
  d. diagnosis
  d. diagnostic consideration
  d. extraction
  d. leukocyte count (DLC)
  d. leukocyte count automation
  pressure d.
  d. renal function test
  d. stain
  d. thermometer
  d. ureteral catheterization test
  d. white blood count
differentiated
  d. embryo-chondrocyte expressed
    gene 1 (DEC1)
  moderately d. (MD)
  poorly d. (PD)
  teratoma d. (TD)
  d. teratoma
  well d.
differentiating chondroblast
differentiation
  acute monocytic leukemia with d.
    (M5b)
  acute monocytic leukemia without d.
    (M5a)
  acute myeloblastic leukemia without
    localized d. (M0)
  adipocyte d.
  amphicrine d.
  d. antigen
  antigen-triggered lymphocyte d.
  biphenotypic d.
  carcinoma showing thymus-like d.
    (CASTLE)

cell d.
cluster of d. (CD)
endothelial d.
epithelial d.
incomplete d.
invisible d.
leukotriene-dependent erythroid d.
meissnerian d.
mesenchymal d.
myofibroblastic d.
neuroendocrine d.
plasmacytoid d.
rhabdomyoblastic d.
sex d.
spindle cell epithelial tumor with
  thymus-like d. (SETTLE)
terminal d.
differentiator
difficile
  Clostridium d.
Diff-Quik
  D.-Q. histochemical stain
  D.-Q. smear
diffraction grating
DiffSpin slide spinner
diffusa
  dermatitis atrophicans d.
  leishmaniasis tegumentaria d.
diffusate
diffuse
  d. abscess
  d. acute inflammation
  d. acute peritonitis
  d. alveolar damage (DAD)
  d. amyloidosis
  d. aneurysm
  d. angiokeratoma
  d. antral gastritis (DAG)
  d. arterial ectasia
  d. axonal injury (DAI)
  d. bronchopneumonia
  d. chronic inflammation
  d. emphysema
  d. enlargement
  d. esophageal spasm
  d. extracapillary proliferative
    glomerulonephritis
  d. follicular variant
  d. ganglion
  d. ganglion cell
  d. histocytic lymphoma (DHL)
  d. hyperplasia
  d. hypertrophy
  d. idiopathic skeletal hyperostosis
  d. illumination
  d. infantile familial sclerosis
  d. infiltrative lung disease (DILD)
  d. interstitial fibrosis
  d. interstitial pneumonia

D

diffuse (*continued*)
    d. interstitial pulmonary disease
    d. intravascular coagulation (DIC)
    d. large B-cell lymphoma (DLBCL)
    d. large cell lymphoma (DLCL)
    d. lesion
    d. lymphatic tissue
    d. membrane hemosiderin deposition
    d. meningiomatosis
    d. mesangial hypercellularity (DMH)
    d. mesangial proliferation
    d. necrosis
    d. neuroendocrine system
    d. nontoxic goiter
    d. panbronchiolitis (DPB)
    d. pattern
    d. perivillous fibrin deposition
    d. phlegmon
    d. poorly differentiated lymphoma (DPDL)
    d. proliferative form
    d. proliferative lupus nephritis
    d. pyelonephritis
    d. reflection
    d. septal cirrhosis
    d. small cleaved cell lymphoma
    d. ulceration
    d. waxy spleen
diffusible
diffusing
    d. capacity for carbon monoxide (D_{CO}, DCO)
    d. capacity of lung for carbon monoxide (DLCO)
diffusion
    d. coefficient
    d. constant
    d. current
    d. defect
    double d.
    facilitated d.
    gel d.
    d. method
    Ouchterlony double d.
    d. potential
    radial d.
    d. shell
    single d.
diffusivity
diffusum
    angiokeratoma corporis d.
difluorodiphenyltrichloroethane (DFDT)
DIG
    dexamethasone, insulin, and glucose
    DIG cocktail
Digenea
Digene hc2 high-risk HPV DNA test
digenesis
digenetic

DiGeorge syndrome
digest
    TaqI restriction d.
digestion
    deoxyribonuclease d.
    diastase d.
    enzymatic d.
    glycogen d.
    hyaluronidase d.
    neuraminidase d.
    proteinase K d. (PKD)
    proteolytic d.
    sialidase d.
    d. vacuole
digestive
    d. albuminuria
    d. disorder
    d. glycosuria
    d. leukocytosis
    d. organ
    d. tract
    d. tube
digestorius
    tubus d.
digit
    check d.
    clubbed d.
    significant d.
digital
    d. autopsy
    d. clubbing
    d. differential display (DDD)
    d. fibrokeratoma
    d. infarct
    d. karyotyping
    d. macrophotography
    d. photomicrography
    d. rectal examination (DRE)
    d. voltmeter
digitalis
    d. glycoside
    herpes d.
    D. purpurea
    d. unit (international)
digital-to-analog converter (DAC)
digitata
    verruca d.
digitate wart
digitation
digiti hippocratici
digitize
digitizer
digitonin
    d. method
    d. reaction
digitopalmar
digitorum
    connexus intertendinei musculi extensoris d.

digitoxin
diglyceride
diglycosylated
digoxigenin-labeled riboprobe
digoxigenin-mediated detection
digoxigenin-UTP
digoxin
Digramma brauni
Di Guglielmo syndrome
Diheterospora
dihexoside
    ceramide d.
dihomogammalinolenic acid (DGLA)
dihydrate
    calcium pyrophosphate d. (CPD)
dihydric alcohol
dihydrobiopterin
dihydroergotamine (DHE)
dihydroethidine
dihydrofolate reductase (DHFR)
dihydrofolic acid
dihydrofolliculin
dihydropteridine
    d. reductase
    d. reductase deficiency
dihydropyridine receptor
dihydropyrimidinase
dihydropyrimidine
dihydropyrimidinuria
dihydrorhodamine
dihydrosphingosine
dihydrotachysterol (DHT)
dihydrotestosterone (DHT)
dihydroubiquinone
dihydrouridine
dihydroxyacetone phosphate (DAP)
dihydroxycholecalciferol assay
dihydroxydinaphthyl disulfide (DDD)
dihydroxymandelic acid (DHMA, DOMA)
dihydroxyphenylacetic acid
dihydroxyphenylalanine (DOPA)
diiodothyronine
diiodotyrosine (DIT)
diisocyanate
2,4-diisocyanate
    toluene 2.-d.
diisopropyl
    d. phosphate (DIP)
    d. phosphofluoridate
dikaryon
diktyoma
Dilantin
dilatation (*var. of* dilation)
    sinusoidal d.
    d. thrombosis
dilatator (*var. of* dilator)
dilate
dilated cardiomyopathy (DCOM)
dilation, dilatation

    aneurysmal d.
    balloon d.
    cardiac d.
    centrilobular d.
    crypt d.
    poststenotic d.
dilator, dilatator
    d. pupillae
    d. pupillae muscle
DILD
    diffuse infiltrative lung disease
diluent buffer
dilute
    d. blood clot lysis (DBCL)
    d. blood clot lysis method
    d. Russell viper venom time
      (DRVVT)
diluted
    d. whole blood clot lysis
    d. whole blood clot lysis test
dilution
    d. anemia
    d. coefficient
    doubling d.
    isotopic d.
    log d.
    maximum inhibiting d. (MID)
    nitrogen d.
    routine test d. (RTD)
    serial d.
    d. test
dilutional
    d. coagulopathy
    d. hypochloremia
    d. thrombocytopenia
dilution-filtration technique
DIM
    divalent ion metabolism
Dimastigamoeba
dimefox
dimension
    D. chemical analyzer
    double (gel) diffusion precipitin test
      in one d.
    double (gel) diffusion precipitin test
      in two d.'s
    gel diffusion precipitin test in one
      d.
    gel diffusion precipitin test in two
      d.'s
    single (gel) diffusion precipitin test
      in one d.
    single (gel) diffusion precipitin test
      in two d.'s
dimer
    thymine d.
dimercaprol
dimercaptopropanol
dimeric inhibin-A assay

D

dimerization
    ligand-dependent d.
    pyrimidine d.
dimerous
dimethoate
5-dimethoxyaniline
    N-ethyl-N-(2-hydroxy-3-sulfopropyl)-3,
    5-d.
dimethoxyphenylethylamine (DMPE)
dimethyl
    d. ether
    d. ketone
    d. sulfate
    d. sulfoxide
dimethyladenosine (DMA)
dimethylallyl diphosphate
dimethylaminoazobenzene (DAB)
dimethylaminobenzaldehyde (DMAB)
1-dimethylaminonaphthalene-5-sulfonic
  acid (DANS)
4-dimethylaminophenol (DMAP)
dimethylarsinic acid (DMA)
7,12-dimethylbenz[a]anthracene
dimethylbenzanthracene (DMBA)
dimethylbenzene
dimethyldichlorovinyl phosphate
  (DDVP)
dimethylguanosine
dimethylisopropylsilyl (DMIPS)
dimethylnitrosamine
5,5-dimethyl-2,4-oxazolidinedione
dimethylsulfoxide (DMSO)
dimidiata
    Chrysops d.
diminazene aceturate
diminuta
    Brevundimonas d.
    Hymenolepis d.
    Pseudomonas d.
    Taenia d.
diminutus
    Triodontophorus d.
dimorpha
    Mycoplana d.
dimorphic
    d. anemia
    d. pathogenic fungus
    d. structure
dimorphism
dimorphon
    Trypanosoma d.
dimorphous leprosy
dimple sign
DIN
    ductal intraepithelial
    neoplasia
dinitrate
    ethylene glycol d.
dinitrobenzene

4-dinitrobenzene (*var. of*
  fluoro-2,4-dinitrobenzene)
dinitrobenzoic acid
dinitrocarbanilide (DNC)
dinitrochlorobenzene (DNCB)
dinitrofluorobenzene (DNFB)
dinitrogen tetroxide
dinitroorthocresol (DNOC)
dinitrophenol
dinitrophenylhydrazine (DNPH)
    d. test
Dinobdella ferox
dinoflagellate toxin
dinormocytosis
dinucleotide
    flavin adenine d. (FAD, FADN)
    nicotinamide adenine d. (NAD,
      NADH)
    reduced nicotinamide-adenine d.
    d. repeat
Dioctophyma renale
dioctophymiasis
diolis
    Clostridium d.
diolivorans
    Lactobacillus d.
1,4-dioxane
    dioxane 1,4-d.
dioxane 1,4-dioxane
dioxathion
dioxide
    arteriovenous carbon d.
    carbamino-carbon d.
    carbon d. (bicarb, CO_2)
    colloidal silicon d.
    diethylene d.
    silicone d. (SiO_2)
    solid carbon d.
    sulfur d.
    thorium d.
dioxin
dioxygenase
    homogentisate d.
    p-hydroxyphenylpyruvate d.
    proline-2-oxoglutarate d.
1,2-dioxygenase
    homogentisate 1,2-d.
DIP
    desquamative interstitial pneumonia
    desquamative interstitial pneumonitis
    diisopropyl phosphate
    diploid
dipalmitoylphosphatidylcholine
dipeptidase
    aminoacyl-histidine d.
    glycyl-glycine d.
    glycyl-leucine d.
dipeptidyl peptidase IV protein
  (DPPIV)

Dipetalonema
  D. *perstans*
  D. *reconditum*
  D. *streptocerca*
dipetalonemiasis
diphacinone
diphasic
  d. meningoencephalitis virus
  d. milk fever
  d. milk fever virus
  d. wave
diphenadione
diphenhydramine (DPH)
  d. hydrochloride
diphenyl
diphenylaminearsine
  NATO code for d. (adamsite)
diphenylaminochloroarsine
  NATO code for d. (adamsite)
diphenylarsine cyanide (DC)
diphenyleneiodonium (DPI)
diphenylhexatriene (DPH)
diphenylhydantoin (DPH)
  d. gingivitis
  sodium d. (SDPH)
diphenylmethane dye
diphosphate
  adenosine d. (ADP)
  cytidine d. (CDP)
  delta^2-isopentenyl d.
  delta^3-isopentenyl d.
  dimethylallyl d.
  fructose d.
  geranylgeranyl d.
  guanosine d.
  hexose d.
  inosine d.
  thiamine d. (TDP)
  thymidine d. (dTDP)
  uridine d. (UDP)
5′-diphosphate
  adenosine 5.-d. (ADP)
  guanosine 5.-d. (GDP)
diphosphatidylglycerol
diphosphoglycerate
  d. mutase
  d. phosphatase
2,3-diphosphoglycerate mutase
diphosphoinositide
diphosphonate
diphosphopyridine nucleotide (DPN, DPNH)
diphosphosulfate
diphtheria
  d. antitoxin (DAT)
  d. antitoxin unit
  avian d.
  d. bacillus
  false d.

fowl d.
d. test
diphtheria, tetanus, and pertussis
  vaccine (DTP)
d. toxin
d. toxin immunization reaction
d. toxin normal (DTN)
d. toxoid, tetanus toxoid, and
  pertussis vaccine
diphtheriae
  Bacillus d.
  Corynebacterium d.
diphtheritic
  d. enteritis
  d. membrane
  d. ulcer
diphtheritica
  otitis d.
diphtheroid
  aerobic d.
  anaerobic d.
  d. bacilli
diphtherotoxin
diphyllobothriasis
Diphyllobothrium
  D. *anemia*
  D. *cordatum*
  D. *dendriticum*
  D. *hians*
  D. *houghtoni*
  D. *latum*
  D. *linguloides*
  D. *mansoni*
  D. *mansonoides*
  D. *nihonkaiense*
  D. *orcini*
  D. *pacificum*
  D. *parvum*
  D. *scoticum*
  D. *taenioides*
dipicolinic acid
diploalbuminuria
diplobacillus
diplobacterium
diploblastic
diplochromosome
diplococcemia
diplococcin
diplococci (*pl. of* diplococcus)
diplococcus, *pl.* **diplococci**
  D.
  D. *constellatus*
  gram-negative intracellular diplococci
    (GNID)
  D. *magnus*
  Morax-Axenfeld d.
  D. *morbillorum*
  D. *mucosus*
  d. of Morax-Axenfeld

D

diplococcus (*continued*)
    d. of Neisser
    D. paleopneumoniae
    D. plagarumbelli
    D. pneumoniae
    Weichselbaum d.
Diplodia
diploë
Diplogaster
Diplogonoporus
    D. brauni
    D. grandis
diploic
diploid
    d. adenoma
    d. cell
    d. merogony
    d. mosaicism
    d. nucleus
    d. number
    d. tumor
diploidea
    Sappinea d.
diploidy
diplokaryon
Diplomate of the National Board of Medical Examiners
diplomelituria
diplomyelia
diplonema
diplont
diplopia, dysphagia, dysarthria, dysphonia (4Ds)
diplopod
Diplopoda
Diploscapter coronata
diplosome
Diplosporium
diplotene
Dipodascus capitatus
dipodomis
    Pterygodermatites d.
dipolar
    d. ion
    d. structure
dipole moment
dipsosauri
    Gracilibacillus d.
dipstick
    Chemstrip d.
    Rapid One single drug screen d.
    screening d.
Diptera
dipteran
dipterous
Dipus sagitta
dipygus
    dicephalus d.
    d. parasiticus

dipylidiasis
Dipylidium caninum
diquat assay
direct
    d. agglutination
    d. agglutination pregnancy test (DAPT)
    d. agglutination test (DAT)
    d. antigen detection
    d. antiglobulin test (DAGT, DAT)
    d. bilirubin test
    d. centrifugal flotation (DCF)
    d. Coombs test (DCT)
    d. culture
    d. current
    d. fluorescence assay (DFA)
    d. fluorescent antibody (DFA)
    d. fluorescent antibody stain
    d. fluorescent antibody technique
    d. fluorescent antibody test
    d. fluorescent antibody-*Treponema pallidum* test (DFA-TP)
    d. fluorescent assay (DFA)
    d. hernia
    d. immunofluorescence
    d. immunofluorescence testing
    d. maternal death
    d. probe
    d. quenching fluorescent immunoassay
    d. reacting bilirubin
    d. sequencing
    d. transport
    d. vision spectroscope
    d. wet mount examination
direct-coupled amplifier
directed donor transfusion
Directigen Flu A + B test kit
directional selection
direct-reacting carcinogen
direct-reading potentiometer
Dirofilaria
    D. conjunctivae
    D. immitis
    D. repens
    D. tenuis
dirofilariasis
    pulmonary d.
dirty
    d. area (contaminated)
    d. bomb (radiation dispersal device)
    d. necrosis
disaccharidase deficiency
disaccharide tolerance test
disaggregated ribosome
disaggregation of membrane-bound polyribosomes
disappearance
    plasma iron d. (PID)
disappearing bone disease

disarray
    crypt d.
    lobular d.
    myocyte d.
disassociation (*var. of* dissociation)
disaster
    D. Medical Assistance Team
    (DMAT)
    D. Mortuary Team (DMORT)
DISASTER
  detect, incident command, scene safety
  and security, assess hazard, support
  required, triage and treatment,
  evacuation, recovery
disc, disk
    A d.
    Amici d.
    anisotropic d.
    d. approximation synergy test
    blood d.
    Bowman d.
    d. capacitor
    cone d.
    d. diffusion test
    d. electrophoresis
    H d.
    hair d.
    Hensen d.
    I d.
    intercalated d.
    intermediate d.
    isotropic d.
    d. kidney
    Merkel tactile d.
    Miller ocular d.
    proligerous d.
    Q d.
    Ranvier d.
    rod d.
    d. sensitivity method
    tactile d.
    transverse d.
    Z d.
discalis
    Chrysops d.
Discella
discharge
    double d.
    epileptiform d. (ED)
    exit d.
    d. frequency
    d. tube
    urethral d. (UD)
discharging tubule
disci (*pl. of* discus)
disciform, diskiform
disciformis
    keratitis d.
    Thiothrix d.

Disciotis
discitis, diskitis
disclosing
    d. agent
    d. solution
discocyte
discohesive
discoid
    d. lupus erythematosus (DLE)
    d. ulcer
discoidin domain receptor (DDR)
discontinuous
    d. endothelium
    d. epitope
    d. sterilization
discordance
discordant lymphoma
Discovery SE ultracentrifuge
discrete
    d. analyzer
    d. lesion
    d. nodule
    d. smallpox
    d. subaortic stenosis
discriminant
    d. function
    d. function analysis
discriminator
Discula
discus, *pl.* **disci**
    excavatio disci
    d. proligerus
discussive
discutient
disdiaclast
disease
    abortive viral d.
    accumulation d.
    Acosta d.
    acquired renal cystic d. (ARCD)
    acquired von Willebrand d.
    acute cardiovascular d. (ACVD)
    acute graft-versus-host d. (aGVHD)
    acute infectious d. (AID)
    acute respiratory d.
    Adams-Stokes d.
    Addison d.
    Addison-Biermer d.
    adrenal d.
    adult celiac d.
    adult polycystic kidney d.
    airway obstruction d.
    akamushi d.
    Akureyri d.
    Albarrán d.
    Albers-Schönberg d.
    Albert d.
    Albright d.
    Aleutian mink d.

D

disease (*continued*)
    Alexander d.
    alive with d. (AWD)
    alive without d. (AWOD)
    allergic airways d.
    Almeida d.
    Alpers d.
    alpha chain d.
    alpha heavy-chain d.
    alpha storage pool d.
    altitude d.
    alveolar hydatid d.
    Alzheimer d.
    Anders d.
    Andes d.
    antibody deficiency d.
    anti-GBM d.
    anti-glomerular basement membrane
      d. (anti-GBM d)
    aortoiliac occlusive d.
    Apert d.
    Apert-Crouzon d.
    Aran-Duchenne d.
    arboviral virus d.
    arc-welder's d.
    Armanni-Ebstein d.
    Armstrong d.
    arterial occlusive d. (AOD)
    arteriosclerotic cardiovascular d.
      (ASCVD)
    arteriosclerotic heart d. (AHD)
    arthropod-borne viral d.
    atherosclerotic cardiovascular d.
      (ASCVD)
    atherosclerotic heart d. (AHD)
    atopic d.
    Aujeszky d.
    Australian X d.
    autoimmune mucocutaneous d.
    autosomal recessive polycystic
      kidney d. (AR-PKD)
    Ayerza d.
    Baelz d.
    Balfour d.
    Ballet d.
    Ballingall d.
    Baló d.
    Bamberger d.
    Bamberger-Marie d.
    Bamle d.
    Bang d.
    Bannister d.
    Banti d.
    Barclay-Baron d.
    Barcoo d.
    Barlow d.
    Barraquer d.
    Basedow d.
    Batten d.

bauxite worker's d.
Bayle d.
Bazin d.
B-cell lymphoproliferative d.
Beard d.
Beau d.
Beauvais d.
Bechterew d.
Beck d.
Becker d.
Begbie d.
Béguez César d.
Behçet d.
Behr d.
Beigel d.
Bekhterev d.
Bell d.
Bennett d.
Benson d.
Berger d.
Bergeron d.
Berlin d.
Bernhardt d.
Besnier-Boeck d.
Besnier-Boeck-Schaumann d.
Best d.
Biedl d.
Bielschowsky d.
Bielschowsky-Jansky d.
Biermer d.
Bilderbeck d.
biliary tract d.
Billroth d.
Binswanger d.
Bird d.
bird-breeder's d.
black lung d.
Bloch-Sulzberger d.
Blocq d.
Bloodgood d.
Blount d.
Blount-Barber d.
Blumenthal d.
Boeck d.
Bogaert d.
bone d.
Borna d.
Bornholm d.
Bostock d.
Bouchard d.
Bouillaud d.
Bourneville d.
Bourneville-Pringle d.
Bouveret d.
Bowen d.
Bradley d.
Brailsford-Morquio d.
brainstem d.
branching glycogen storage d.

Breda d.
Breisky d.
Bretonneau d.
Bright d.
Brill d.
Brill-Symmers d.
Brill-Zinsser d.
Brinton d.
Brion-Kayser d.
Brissaud d.
broad-beta d.
Brocq d.
Brodie d.
bronzed d.
Brooke d.
Brown-Symmers d.
Bruck d.
Bruton d.
bubble boy d.
Budd d.
Buerger d.
Buhl d.
bullous d.
Bury d.
Buschke d.
Busquet d.
Buss d.
Busse-Buschke d.
Byler d.
Caffey d.
caisson d.
calcium pyrophosphate deposition d.
  (CPPD)
caloric d.
Calvé-Perthes d.
Calvé-Perthes-Legg d.
Camurati-Engelmann d.
Canavan d.
Capdepont d.
carcinoid heart d.
cardiac d.
cardiovascular d. (CVD)
cardiovascular renal d. (CVRD)
Caroli d.
carotid d.
Carríon d.
Castellani d.
Castleman d.
cathepsin-mediated d.
cat-scratch d. (CSD)
Cavare d.
Cazenave d.
celiac d.
central core d.
cerebrovascular d. (CVD)
cerebrovascular obstructive d.
  (CVOD)
ceroid storage d.
Chabert d.

Chagas d.
Chagas-Cruz d.
Championnière d.
Charcot d.
Charcot-Marie-Tooth d.
Charlouis d.
Cheadle d.
Chédiak-Higashi d.
cheese washer's d.
Cherchevski d.
Chester d.
Chiari d.
chlamydial d.
cholesterol ester storage d.
Christensen-Krabbe d.
Christian d.
Christian-Hand-Schüller d.
Christian-Weber d.
Christmas d.
chronic active liver d.
chronic granulomatous d. (CGD)
chronic inflammatory d.
chronic obstructive lung d. (COLD)
chronic obstructive pulmonary d.
  (COPD)
chronic pulmonary vascular
  occlusive d.
chronic renal d. (CRD)
Ciarrocchi d.
circling d.
circulatory d.
Civatte d.
clonal hematological nonmast cell
  lineage d.
coagulopathy of liver d.
Coat d.
Cockayne d.
cold agglutinin d.
cold hemagglutinin d.
collagen d.
collagen-vascular d.
combined immunodeficiency d.
combined systems d.
communicable d.
Concato d.
congenital nonspherocytic hemolytic
  d. (CNHD)
congenital valvular heart d.
congestive heart d. (CHD)
connective tissue d. (CTD)
Conor and Bruch d.
Conradi d.
constitutional d.
contagious d.
Cooley d.
Cooper d.
Corbus d.
Cori d.
coronary artery d. (CAD)

D

disease (*continued*)

coronary atherosclerotic heart d. (CAHD)
Corrigan d.
Corvisart d.
Cotugno d.
Cotunnius d.
Cowden d.
creeping d.
Creutzfeldt-Jakob d. (CJD)
Crigler-Najjar d.
Crocq d.
Crohn d.
Crouzon d.
Cruveilhier d.
Cruveilhier-Baumgarten d.
Cruz-Chagas d.
crystal deposition d.
Csillag d.
Curschmann d.
Cushing d.
cystic d.
cystine storage d.
cytomegalic inclusion d. (CID, CMID)
cytomegalovirus d.
cytoskeletal protein hyperphosphorylation d.
Czerny d.
Daae d.
Daae-Finsen d.
DaCosta d.
Dalrymple d.
Danielssen d.
Danielssen-Boeck d.
Darier d. (DD)
Darling d.
David d.
Davies d.
dead of d. (DOD)
deerfly d.
deficiency d.
degenerative joint d. (DJD)
Degos d.
Dejerine d.
Dejerine-Sottas d.
delta storage pool d.
demyelinating d.
dense-deposit d. (DDD)
deprivation d.
de Quervain d.
Dercum d.
Deutschländer d.
Devergie d.
Devic d.
diffuse infiltrative lung d. (DILD)
diffuse interstitial pulmonary d.
Di Guglielmo d.
disappearing bone d.

diverticular d.
dog d.
Döhle d.
dominantly inherited Lévi d.
Dubini d.
Dubois d.
Duchenne d.
Duchenne-Aran d.
Duchenne-Griesinger d.
Duhring d.
Dukes d.
Duncan d.
Durand d.
Durand-Nicolas-Favre d.
Durante d.
Duroziez d.
Dutton d.
Eales d.
Ebola virus d.
Ebstein d.
echinococcus d.
Economo d.
Edsall d.
endemic d.
endocrine d.
Engelmann d.
Engel-von Recklinghausen d.
English d.
Engman d.
eosinophilic endomyocardial d.
epidemic d.
epithelial cell d.
Epstein d.
Erb d.
Erb-Charcot d.
Erb-Goldflam d.
Erdheim d.
Erdheim-Chester d. (ECD)
Eulenburg d.
exanthematous d.
extramammary Paget d. (EPD)
extrapyramidal d.
Fabry d.
Fahr d.
familial nephronophthisis-medullary cystic d. (FN-MCD)
Farber d.
farmer's lung d.
fatal granulomatous d. (FGD)
fat-deficiency d.
Fauchard d.
Favre-Racouchot d.
Fede d.
Feer d.
femoropopliteal occlusive d.
Fenwick d.
fibrocontractive d.
fibrocystic d.
Fiedler d.

fifth d.
Filatov d.
fish-slime d.
Flajani d.
Flatau-Schilder d.
Flegel d.
flint d.
floating beta d.
focal d.
Folling d.
foot-and-mouth d. (FMD)
Forbes d.
Fordyce d.
Forestier d.
Förster d.
Fothergill d.
Fournier d.
Fox-Fordyce d.
Francis d.
Frankl-Hochwart d.
Franklin d.
Frei d.
Freiberg d.
Friedländer d.
Friedmann d.
Friedreich d.
Friend d.
Frommel d.
functional d.
Furstner d.
Gairdner d.
Gaisböck d.
gametic d.
gamma chain d.
gamma heavy-chain d.
Gamna d.
Gandy-Nanta d.
gannister's d.
Garré d.
gasping d.
gastroesophageal reflux d. (GERD)
gastrointestinal d.
Gaucher d.
gay-related immunodeficiency d.
Gee d.
Gee-Herter d.
Gee-Herter-Heubner d.
Gee-Thaysen d.
Gensoul d.
Gerhardt d.
Gerlier d.
gestational trophoblastic d. (GTD)
giant platelet d.
Gibney d.
Gierke d.
Gilbert d.
Gilchrist d.
Glanzmann d.
Glénard d.

Glisson d.
glomerular basement membrane d.
glomerulocystic kidney d. (GCKD)
glycogen storage d. (GSD)
Goldflam d.
Goldflam-Erb d.
Goldscheider d.
Goldstein d.
Gorham d.
Gougerot-Blum d.
Gougerot-Ruiter d.
Gougerot-Sjögren d.
Graefe d.
graft versus host d. (GVHD)
granulomatous d.
Graves d.
Greenfield d.
Greenhow d.
Griesinger d.
Gross d.
Grover d.
Guinon d.
Gull d.
Günther d.
Habermann d.
Haff d.
Haglund d.
Hagner d.
Hailey-Hailey d.
Hall d.
Hallervorden-Spatz d.
Hallopeau d.
Hamman d.
Hamman-Rich d.
Hammond d.
Hand d.
hand-foot-and-mouth d.
Hand-Schüller-Christian d.
Hanot d.
Hansen d.
hard pad d.
Harley d.
Hartnup d.
Hashimoto d.
heart d. (HD)
heavy chain d.
Heberden d.
Hebra d.
Heckathorn d.
Heerfordt d.
Heine-Medin d.
Heller-Döhle d.
helminthic d.
hemoglobin C d.
hemoglobin E-thalassemia d.
hemoglobin H d.
hemoglobin SO Arab sickle cell d.
Henderson-Jones d.
hepatic venoocclusive d.

D

disease (*continued*)

hepatolenticular d.
hepatorenal glycogen storage d.
hereditary d.
heredodegenerative d.
herpetic viral d.
herring-worm d.
Hers d.
Herter d.
Herter-Heubner d.
Heubner d.
hidebound d.
Hildenbrand d.
Hippel d.
Hippel-Lindau d.
Hirschfeld d.
Hirschsprung d. (HD)
His d.
His-Werner d.
Hjärre d.
hock d.
Hodara d.
Hodgkin d. (HD)
Hodgson d.
Hoffa d.
holoendemic d.
hoof-and-mouth d.
hookworm d.
Hoppe-Goldflam d.
Horton d.
Huchard d.
human lymphoproliferative d.
Hunt d.
Huntington d. (HD)
Hurler d.
Hutchinson d.
Hutchinson-Boeck d.
Hutchinson-Gilford d.
Hutinel d.
hyaline membrane d. (HMD)
hydatid d. (HD)
Hyde d.
hydrocephaloid d.
hyperendemic d.
hypertensive arteriosclerotic heart d.
  (HASHD)
hypertensive cardiovascular d.
  (HCVD)
hypertensive heart d.
hypertensive pulmonary vascular d.
  (HPVD)
hypopigmentation-
  immunodeficiency d.
iatrogenic d.
I-cell d.
idiopathic Bamberger-Marie d.
idiopathic Parkinson d.
IgE-mediated d.
immune complex d.

immune-deposit d.
immunodeficiency d.
immunoproliferative small intestinal
  d. (IPSID)
inborn lysosomal d.
inclusion body d.
inclusion cell d.
incompatible hemolytic blood
  transfusion d. (IHBTD)
infantile celiac d.
infantile polycystic kidney d.
infectious d.
infiltrative d.
inflammatory bowel d. (IBD)
inflammatory pelvic d. (IPD)
inherited d.
intercurrent d.
International Classification of
  Diseases (ICD)
interstitial lung d.
intestinal chronic graft-versus-host d.
iron-storage d.
Isambert d.
ischemic bowel d.
ischemic heart d. (IHD)
ischemic leg d. (ILD)
ischemic limb d. (ILD)
island d.
itai-itai d.
Jaffe-Lichtenstein d.
Jakob d.
Jakob-Creutzfeldt d.
Jaksch d.
Janet d.
Jansen d.
Jansky-Bielschowsky d.
Jensen d.
Johne d.
Johnson-Steven d.
joint d.
Jourdain d.
jumping d.
Jüngling d.
juvenile Paget d.
Kahlbaum d.
Kahler d.
Kalischer d.
Kashin-Bek d.
Kawasaki d.
Kayser d.
kedani d.
Keshan d.
Kienböck d.
Kikuchi d.
Kikuchi-Fujimoto d. (KFD)
Kimmelstiel-Wilson d.
Kimura d.
kinky hair d.
Kinnier Wilson d.

Kirkland d.
kissing d.
Klebs d.
Klemperer d.
Klippel d.
knight d.
Köhler d.
Köhlmeier-Degos d.
Koshevnikoff d.
Krabbe d.
Krishaber d.
Kufs d.
Kugelberg-Welander d.
Kuhnt-Junius d.
Kümmell d.
Kümmell-Verneuil d.
Kussmaul d.
Kussmaul-Maier d.
Kyasanur Forest d.
Kyrle d.
Läennec d.
Lafora d.
Lancereaux-Mathieu d.
Landouzy d.
Landry d.
Lane d.
Langdon-Down d.
Larrey-Weil d.
Larsen d.
Larsen-Johansson d.
Lasègue d.
Lauber d.
L-chain d.
Leber d.
Ledderhose d.
Legal d.
Legg d.
Legg-Calvé-Perthes d.
Legg-Perthes d.
Legionnaire's d. (LD)
Leigh d.
Leiner d.
Leloir d.
Lenègre d.
Leri-Weill d.
Leroy d.
Letterer-Siwe d.
Lev d.
Lévi d.
Lewandowski-Lutz d.
Leyden d.
Lhermitte-Duclos d.
Libman-Sacks d.
Lichtheim d.
light chain deposition d.
Lignac d.
Lindau d.
Lindau-von Hippel d.
lipid storage d.

Lipschütz d.
Little d.
Lobo d.
Lobstein d.
Löffler d.
long-segment Hirschsprung d.
Lorain d.
Lou Gehrig d.
Lowe d.
Lucas-Championnière d.
Luft d.
lumpy skin d.
lunger d.
Lutz-Splendore-Almeida d.
Lyell d.
Lyme d.
lymphocyte-depleted Hodgkin d.
  (LDHD)
lymphocyte-predominant Hodgkin d.
  (LPHD)
lymphoproliferative d. (LPD)
lymphoreticular d.
lysosomal storage d.
Madelung d.
Maffucci d.
Magitot d.
Maher d.
Majocchi d.
malabsorption d.
Malassez d.
mal de San Lazaro d.
maldigestive d.
Malherbe d.
Malibu d.
mammary Paget d.
Manson d.
maple bark stripper's d.
maple syrup urine d. (MSUD)
marble bone d.
Marburg virus d.
March d.
Marchiafava-Bignami d.
Marek d.
Marek herpesvirus d. (MDHV)
Marfan d.
Marie d.
Marie-Bamberger d.
Marie-Strümpell d.
Marie-Tooth d.
Marion d.
Marsh d.
Martin d.
mast cell d.
Mathieu d.
Maunier-Kuhn d.
Maxcy d.
McArdle d.
McArdle-Schmid-Pearson d.
McLean-Maxwell d.

D

disease (*continued*)
    Medin d.
    Mediterranean hemoglobin E d.
    medullary cystic d. (MCD)
    Meige d.
    Meleda d.
    Ménétrier d.
    Ménière d.
    Merzbacher-Pelizaeus d.
    metabolic bone d.
    metabolic stone d.
    metabolic storage d.
    Meyenburg d.
    Meyer d.
    Mibelli d.
    microdrepanocytic d.
    micrometastatic d.
    microvillus inclusion d.
    Mikulicz d.
    Mills d.
    Milroy d.
    Milton d.
    Minamata d.
    minimal-change d.
    minimal residual d. (MRD)
    Minor d.
    Mitchell d.
    mixed cellularity Hodgkin d. (MCHD)
    mixed connective tissue d. (MCTD)
    Miyasato d.
    Möbius d.
    molecular d.
    Möller-Barlow d.
    Molten d.
    Mondor d.
    Monge d.
    Morel-Kraepelin d.
    Morgagni d.
    Morquio d.
    Morquio-Ullrich d.
    Morton d.
    Morvan d.
    Moschcowitz d.
    motor neuron d.
    moyamoya d.
    Mucha d.
    Mucha-Habermann d.
    mucopolysaccharide storage d.
    mucosal d.
    mu heavy chain d.
    multicore d.
    multifactorial inherited d.
    Munchmeyer d.
    Myá d.
    myeloproliferative d.
    myocardial d.
    Nairobi sheep d.
    Neftel d.

neoautoimmune d.
neoplastic d.
Neumann d.
neuromuscular system d.
neuronal intermediate filament inclusion d. (NIFID)
neutral lipid storage d.
newborn hemolytic d.
newborn hemorrhagic d.
Newcastle d.
Newcastle virus d. (NVD)
Nicolas-Favre d.
Nidoko d.
Nieden d.
Niemann d.
Niemann-Pick d. (NPD)
nil d.
nodular lymphocyte-rich Hodgkin d.
nodular sclerosing Hodgkin d. (NSHD)
no evidence of d. (NED)
nonalcoholic fatty liver d. (NAFLD)
Nonne-Milroy d.
nonrelapsing d.
Nordau d.
Norwalk d.
no significant d. (NSD)
Notch3 gene polymorphism in ischemic cerebrovascular d.
Novy rat d.
oasthouse urine d.
obstructive airway d. (OAD)
obstructive lung d.
occupational lung d.
ocular inflammatory d. (OID)
d. of Hapsburg
Ofuji d.
Oguchi d.
Ohara d.
oid-oid d.
Ollier d.
Olmer d.
Opitz d.
Oppenheim d.
Oppenheim-Urbach d.
optic nerve d.
organic d.
Oriental lung fluke d.
Ormond d.
Osgood-Schlatter d.
Osler d.
Osler-Vaquez d.
Osler-Weber-Rendu d.
Otto d.
Owren d.
ox-warble d.
Paas d.
Pinkus d.
platelet-type von Willebrand d.

Plummer d.
polycystic kidney d. (PKD)
polycystic liver d.
polycystic ovary d.
polycystic renal d.
polyendocrine autoimmune d.
polyglutamine d.
Pompe d.
Poncet d.
Posada d.
Posada-Wernicke d.
posttransplant lymphoproliferative d. (PTLD)
Pott d.
Potter d.
Poulet d.
poultry handler's d.
Preiser d.
primary cold agglutinin d.
primary myocardial d. (PMD)
primary ovarian gestational trophoblastic d. (POGTD)
primary pigmented nodular adrenocortical d. (PPNAD)
Pringle d.
prion d.
prion-transmitted d.
Profichet d.
proliferative breast d. (PBD)
pseudo-von Willebrand d.
pulmonary heart d.
pulmonary thromboembolic d. (PTED)
pulmonary vascular d.
pulmonary veno-occlusive d. (PVOD)
pulseless d.
Purtscher d.
Pyle d.
pyramidal d.
quiet hip d.
Quincke d.
Quinquaud d.
Rangoon beggar's d.
Ranikhet d.
rat-bite d.
Rayer d.
Raynaud d. (RD)
Recklinghausen d.
Reclus d.
redwater d.
Reed-Hodgkin d.
Refsum d.
Reichmann d.
Reiter d.
relapsing d.
renal atheroembolic d.
renal cystic d.
Rendu-Osler-Weber d.

respiratory viral d.
restrictive lung d.
rheumatic heart d. (RHD)
rheumatic lung d.
rheumatoid heart d.
rhinocerebral d.
Rh$_{null}$ d.
Ribas-Torres d.
Riedel d.
Riga-Fede d.
Rigg d.
Ritter d.
Robinson d.
Roble d.
Roger d.
Rokitansky d.
Romberg d.
Rosai-Dorfman d. (RDD)
Rosenbach d.
Rossbach d.
Roth d.
Roth-Bernhardt d.
Rougnon-Heberden d.
Roussy-Lévy d.
Rubarth d.
Rummo d.
runt d.
Rust d.
Ruysch d.
Rye classification of Hodgkin d.
Sachs d.
salivary gland virus d.
Sanders d.
Sandhoff d.
Saunders d.
Savill d.
Schamberg d.
Schanz d.
Schaumann d.
Schenck d.
Scheuermann d.
Schilder d.
Schimmelbusch d.
Schlatter d.
Schlatter-Osgood d.
Schmorl d.
Scholz d.
Schönlein d.
Schottmuller d.
Schroeder d.
Schüller d.
Schüller-Christian d.
Schultz d.
Schweninger-Buzzi d.
sea-blue histiocyte d.
secondary cold agglutinin d.
Seitelberger d.
self-limited d.
Selter d.

D

disease *(continued)*
    Senear-Usher d.
    senile hip d.
    septic d.
    serum d.
    sexually transmitted d. (STD)
    Shaver d.
    Shichito d.
    shimamushi d.
    sickle cell hemoglobin C, D d.
    sickle cell thalassemia d.
    silo-filler's d.
    Simmonds d.
    Simons d.
    Siwe-Letterer d.
    sixth venereal d.
    Sjögren d.
    skeletal d.
    Skevas-Zerfus d.
    skinbound d.
    skip-segment Hirschsprung d.
    slow virus d.
    Sly d.
    Smith d.
    Smith-Strang d.
    Sneddon-Wilkinson d.
    specific d.
    Spencer d.
    sphingolipid storage d.
    Spielmeyer-Stock d.
    Spielmeyer-Vogt d.
    spinal cord d.
    sponge d.
    stable d. (SD)
    Stanton d.
    Stargardt d.
    Steinert d.
    Sternberg d.
    Sticker d.
    Stieda d.
    Still d.
    Stokes-Adams d.
    storage pool d.
    Strümpell d.
    Strümpell-Leichtenstern d.
    Strümpell-Lorrain d.
    Strümpell-Marie d.
    Strümpell-Westphal d.
    Sudeck d.
    d. susceptibility
    Sutton d.
    Swediaur d.
    Sweet d.
    Swift d.
    Swift-Feer d.
    swine vesicular d.
    Sydenham d.
    Sylvest d.
    Symmers d.

systemic autoimmune d.
systemic febrile d.
systemic mast cell d.
Takahara d.
Takayasu d.
Talfan d.
Talma d.
Tangier d.
Tarui d.
Taussig-Bing d.
Tay d.
Taylor d.
Tay-Sachs d. (TSD)
T-cell mediated d.
Teschen d.
thalassemia-sickle cell d.
Thaysen d.
Theiler d.
Thiemann d.
thin basement membrane d.
third d.
Thomsen d.
thromboembolic d. (TED)
Thygeson d.
thyrocardiac d.
thyrotoxic heart d.
Tillaux d.
Tommaselli d.
Tooth d.
Tornwaldt d.
Tourette d.
transfusion-associated graft-versus-host d. (TAGVHD)
transmissible d.
transplant vascular d.
transport d.
Trevor d.
trophoblastic d.
tropical d.
tsutsugamushi d.
tuberculosis-respiratory d. (TB-RD)
Tyzzer d.
ultrashort-segment Hirschsprung d.
Underwood d.
United States Army Medical Research Institute of Infectious D. (USAMRIID)
Unna d.
unstable hemoglobin d.
Unverricht d.
upper respiratory d. (URD)
Urbach-Oppenheim d.
Urbach-Wiethe d.
urinary tract d.
vagabond's d.
van Bogaert d.
van Buren d.
Vaquez d.
Vaquez-Osler d.

velogenic Newcastle d.
venereal d. (VD)
Verneuil d.
Verse d.
Vidal d.
Vincent d.
vinyl chloride d.
viral hematodepressive d. (VHD)
Virchow d.
virus X d.
vocal cord d.
Vogt-Spielmeyer d.
Volkmann d.
Voltolini d.
von Bechterew d.
von Economo d.
von Gierke d.
von Hippel d.
von Hippel-Lindau d.
von Jaksch d.
von Meyenburg d.
von Recklinghausen d.
von Willebrand d. (VW)
Voorhoeve d.
Vrolik d.
Wagner d.
Waldenström d.
Wardrop d.
Wartenberg d.
Wassilieff d.
wasting d.
Weber-Christian d.
Weber-Rendu-Osler d.
Wegner d.
Weil d.
Weir Mitchell d.
Wenckebach d.
Werdnig-Hoffmann d.
Werlhof d.
Werner-His d.
Werner-Schultz d.
Wesselsbron d.
Westphal d.
Westphal-Strümpell d.
Whipple d.
White d.
white muscle d.
white spot d.
Whitmore d.
Whytt d.
Wilkie d.
Willis d.
Wilson d. (WD)
Winckel d.
Windscheid d.
Winiwarter-Buerger d.
Winkler d.
Winton d.
Witkop d.

Wohlfart-Kugelberg-Welander d.
Wolman d.
woolsorter's d.
Woringer-Kolopp d.
X-linked lymphoproliferative d.
Zahorsky d.
Ziehen-Oppenheim d.
Zinsser-Brill d.
zoonotic d.
disease-associated bacterial toxin
disease-free survival (DFS)
disease-specific survival
disease-syphilis
venereal d.-s. (VDS)
disequilibrium
linkage d.
disfigurative
disgerminoma
dish
Stender d.
disiens
Bacteroides d.
Prevotella d.
disinfect
disinfectant
nonoemulsion d.
disinfection
disinsection, disinsectization
disinsectization (*var. of* disinsection)
disintegration constant
disintegrin protein
disjunction
disjunctive absorption
disjunctum
stratum d.
disk (*var. of* disc)
diskiform (*var. of* disciform)
diskitis (*var. of* discitis)
dislocation
anterior complete d.
closed d.
complete anterior d.
complete inferior d.
complete posterior d.
complete superior d.
compound d.
congenital d.
fracture d.
incomplete d.
inferior d.
inferior complete closed d.
inferior complete compound d.
lens d.
dismutase
extracellular superoxide d. (EC-SOD)
superoxide d.
disomic population
disomy
uniparental d. (UPD)

D

291

disopyramide
disorder
    absorptive d.
    acid-base d.
    amino acid d.
    antifactor I–IX d.
    autosomal dominant d.
    autosomal recessive d.
    B-cell chronic lymphoproliferative d.
      (BCLPD)
    B-cell lymphoproliferative d. (BLPD)
    biliary d.
    bipolar depression d.
    bladder d.
    blood coagulation d.
    bone marrow d.
    CEAP classification of venous d.'s
    central nervous system d.
    chromosomal d.
    chronic lymphoproliferative d.
      (CLPD)
    chronic myeloproliferative d.
      (CMPD)
    circulating antithromboplastin d.
    clonal d.
    collagen d.
    complex adrenal endocrine d.
    complex gonadal endocrine d.
    complex pituitary endocrine d.
    complex thyroid endocrine d.
    connective tissue d.
    cytogenetic d.
    digestive d.
    element d.
    fatty acid oxidation d. (FOD)
    fibrinolytic d.
    functional d.
    genital d.
    glomerular d.
    glycogen storage d. (GSD)
    gonadal endocrine d.
    growth d.
    hemolytic d.
    hemorrhagic d.
    heterozygous-type hemoglobin d.
    homozygous-type hemoglobin d.
    immune complex d.
    immunoglobulin d.
    immunoproliferative d.
    infectious d.
    inflammatory d.
    inherited giant platelet d. (IGPD)
    intestinal flow d.
    ion d.
    lipid transport d.
    lymphoproliferative d.
    lymphoreticular d.
    malabsorption d.
    metabolic d.

    mitochondrial d.
    myeloproliferative d.
    nasal allergic d.
    neurodegenerative d.
    neurovisceral storage d.
    neutrophil functional d.
    pituitary endocrine d.
    plasma iodoprotein d.
    polyglutamine expansion d.
    posttransplant lymphoproliferative d.
      (PTLD)
    proliferative d.
    Quebec platelet d.
    respiratory acid-base d.
    retinal d.
    sickling d.
    single gene d. (SGD)
    sleep d.
    T-cell d.
    thyroid endocrine d.
    tic d.
    transient myeloproliferative d.
    trinucleotide repeat d.
    uncommon developmental d.
    ureteral peristalsis d.
    urogenital d.
    vascular d.
    X-linked recessive d.
    XXX d.
    XXXX d.
    XXXXY d.
    XXXY d.
    XXYY d.
disordered
    d. action of heart (DAH)
    d. epithelial growth
    d. immunoregulation
    d. proliferative endometrium
disorganization
dispar
    Entamoeba d.
    Veillonella alcalescens subsp. *d.*
disparate
disparity
dispermia (*var. of* dispermy)
dispermic chimera
dispermy, dispermia
disperse phase
dispersion
    colloidal d.
    d. medium
    molecular d.
    optical rotary d. (ORD)
    population d.
dispersive medium
Dispira
displaceability
    tissue d.
displaced ganglion cell

displacement
  d. analysis
  anterior d.
  epithelial d.
  inferior d.
  mechanical d.
  tissue d.
display
  digital differential d. (DDD)
  seven-segment d.
Disporotrichum
disposable chemical-resistant clothing
disproportion
  cephalopelvic d. (CPD)
disproportionate
  binucleation d.
disrupter
  ultrasonic cell d.
disruption
  ossicular chain d.
dissecans
  endometritis d.
  osteochondritis d.
  pneumonia d.
dissect
dissecting
  d. aneurysm
  d. microscope
  d. osteitis
dissection
  aortic d.
  d. resorption
  retroperitoneal lymph node d.
    (RPLND)
  spontaneous coronary artery d.
    (SCAD)
  d. tubercle
  vascular d.
disseminata
  dermatofibrosis lenticularis d.
  leiomyomatosis peritonealis d.
  osteitis fibrosa d.
disseminate coccidioidomycosis
disseminated
  d. acute lupus erythematosus
  d. aspergillosis
  d. candidiasis
  d. condensing osteopathy
  d. foci (DF)
  d. inflammation
  d. intravascular coagulation
    (DIC)
  d. lipogranulomatosis
  d. sclerosis
  d. superficial actinic porokeratosis
    (DSAP)
  d. tuberculosis
dissemination
  hematogenous d.

disseminatum
  keratoma d.
  xanthoma d. (XD)
disseminatus
  lupus erythematosus d.
    (LED)
Disse space
dissociated islet cell
dissociation, disassociation
  albuminocytologic d.
  bacterial d.
  d. constant
  d. enhanced lanthanide
    fluoroimmunoassay (DELFIA)
  microbic d.
dissolution
Dissolve-A-Way tape
dissymmetry
distal
  d. centriole
  d. ileitis
  d. latency
  d. metastasis
  d. muscular dystrophy
  d. myopathy
  d. RTA
distal-type progressive muscular dystrophy
distance
  focal d.
  interelectrode d.
  d. learning
  skin-to-tumor d. (STD)
  working d.
distant
  d. organ metastasis
  d. range entrance wound
distantly vaccinated
distasonis
  Bacteroides d.
distemper
  feline d.
  d. virus
distensae
  striae cutis d.
distension (*var. of* distention)
distention, distension
  d. cyst
  d. ulcer
distill
distillate
distillation
  destructive d.
  fractional d.
  molecular d.
  vacuum d.
distilled oil
distincta
  Pseudoalteromonas d.

D

distinctive
>d. epithelium
>d. form

Distoma

distomatosis (*var. of* distomiasis)

distome

distomiasis, distomatosis
>pulmonary d.

Distomum

distortion
>barreling d.
>crypt d.

distortum
>*Microsporum canis* d.

distress
>fetal d.

distributa
>*Vulcanisaeta* d.

distributing artery

distribution
>actin d.
>anomalous vascular d.
>antigenic d.
>binomial d.
>chi squared d.
>d. coefficient
>cumulative d.
>d. curve
>dose d.
>extracellular in d.
>F d.
>fetal-maternal
> erythrocyte d.
>focal segmental d.
>frequency d.
>d. function
>gaussian d.
>intron-exon d.
>d. leukocytosis
>lognormal d.
>nitrogen d.
>Poisson d.
>probability d.
>reference d.
>sample d.
>skewed d.
>symmetric d.
>*t* d.

disulfide
>d. bond
>carbon d.
>dihydroxydinaphthyl d.
> (DDD)
>glutathione d. (GSSG)

disulfiram assay

disulfonate
>sodium indigotin d.

disulfoton

disuse atrophy

DIT
>diiodotyrosine
>drug-induced thrombocytopenia

dithionate
>sodium d.

dithionite test

dithiothreitol (DTT)

Dittrich
>D. plug
>D. stenosis

diuresis
>postobstructive d.

diuretic
>cardiac d.
>hemopoiesic d.
>loop d.
>mechanical d.
>osmotic d.
>potassium-sparing d.
>thiazide d.

diurna
>microfilaria d.

diurnal

diuron

diutinum
>erythema elevatum d.

divalent ion metabolism (DIM)

divarication

divergence

divergens
>*Babesia* d.

divergent

diversion
>d. colitis
>d. pouchitis
>d. proctocolitis

diversity
>methylation pattern d.
>NK clonal d.
>viral genomic d.

diversum
>*Mogibacterium* d.

diversus
>*Citrobacter* d.
>*Levinea* d.

diverticula (*pl. of* diverticulum)

diverticular disease

diverticulitis
>hemorrhagic d.
>obstructive d.

diverticuloma

diverticulosis
>segmental colitis associated with d.
> (SCAD)

diverticulum, *pl.* **diverticula**
>cervical d.
>duodenal d.
>epiphrenic d.
>false d.

hypopharyngeal d.
Meckel d.
pulsion d.
traction d.
true d.
urethral d.
ventricular d.
vesical d.
Zenker d.
divided dose
divider
voltage d.
diving goiter
divisio
division
cell d.
conjugate d.
equational d.
maturation d.
reduction d.
Dixon test
dizygotic twins
DJD
degenerative joint disease
DK
decay
DKA
diabetic ketoacidosis
DKC1 gene
dL
deciliter
DL
difference limen
Donath-Landsteiner
DL antibody
DL biphasic hemolysis
DL hemolysin
D-L Ab
D-lactic acidosis
DLBCL
diffuse large B-cell lymphoma
DLC
differential leukocyte count
DLCL
diffuse large cell lymphoma
DLCO
diffusing capacity of lung for carbon monoxide
DL2000 data management system
DLE
discoid lupus erythematosus
DLK1
deltalike 1 homolog
DLK1 gene
D-loop region
dm
decimeter
DM
myotonic dystrophy

DMA
dimethyladenosine
dimethylarsinic acid
DMAB
dimethylaminobenzaldehyde
DMAP
4-dimethylaminophenol
DMAT
Disaster Medical Assistance Team
DMBA
dimethylbenzanthracene
DMD
Duchenne muscular dystrophy
DME
drug metabolizing enzyme
DMH
diffuse mesangial hypercellularity
DMIPS
dimethylisopropylsilyl
DMORT
Disaster Mortuary Team
DMPE
dimethoxyphenylethylamine
DMPH
dysgenetic male pseudohermaphroditism
DMSO
dimethylsulfoxide
DN
dextrose nitrogen ratio
dibucaine number
DNA
deoxyribonucleic acid
DNA adduct level
amplifiable DNA
DNA aneuploidy
DNA array analysis
branched DNA (bDNA, b-DNA)
DNA break
DNA chip
competitor DNA
complementary DNA (cDNA)
DNA complexity
DNA copy number
DNA cytophotometry
double-stranded DNA (DS-DNA)
DNA fingerprint
DNA fingerprinting
DNA flow cytometry
fluorochrome-conjugated DNA
DNA gel electrophoresis
genomic DNA
hairpin DNA
DNA homology
DNA hybridization
DNA index (DI)
DNA ligase
DNA marker
DNA melting analysis
DNA methylation

D

DNA (*continued*)
    DNA microarray
    DNA microarray technology
    DNA multiploidy
    DNA nucleotidylexotransferase
    DNA nucleotidyltransferase
    plasma DNA
    DNA ploidy
    DNA polymerase
    DNA probe
    DNA reassociation
    recombinant DNA (rDNA)
    DNA renaturation
    DNA repair
    ribosomal DNA (rDNA)
    self-complementary DNA
    DNA sequence copy number change
    DNA sequencing
    single-stranded DNA (SS-DNA)
    DNA slot blot technique
    DNA synthesis
    DNA synthesis reagent
    DNA template
    DNA transfer
    DNA virus
DNA-aneuploid tumor cell
DNA-DNA hybridization
DNA-enzyme immunoassay (DEIA)
DNA-FluHunter test
DNA-Prep workstation & reagent system
DNA-RNA hybridization
DNA/RNA Protect
DNase
    deoxyribonuclease
    DNase agar
    DNase test
DNAzole cell suspension
DNC
    dinitrocarbanilide
DNCB
    dinitrochlorobenzene
DNET
    dysplastic neuroepithelial tumor
DNFB
    dinitrofluorobenzene
DNOC
    dinitroorthocresol
DNP
    deoxyribonucleoprotein
DNPH
    dinitrophenylhydrazine
    DNPH test
DOA
    dead on arrival
    drugs of abuse
DO7 antibody
DOC
    death of other cause
    deoxycorticoid

    deoxycorticosterone
    desoxycorticosterone
DOCA
    deoxycorticosterone acetate
docimasia
    auricular d.
    hepatic d.
    pulmonary d.
docosahexaenoic acid (DHA)
doctrine
    Arrhenius d.
documentation
    forensic d.
Döderlein bacillus
doebereinerae
    Azospirillum d.
dog
    d. disease
    d. distemper virus
    d. flea
    d. fly
    d. hookworm
    d. louse
    d. nose
    d. unit
Dogiel
    D. cell
    D. corpuscle
Döhle
    D. disease
    D. inclusion
    D. inclusion body
Döhle-Heller aortitis
Dold
    D. reaction
    D. test
dolens
    leukophlegmasia d.
dolichocolon
dolichoectatic artery
dolichol phosphate
Dolichos biflorus
dolipore
doll's
    d. eye movement
    d. kidney
dolor
doloresi
    Gnathostoma d.
dolorosa
    adiposis d.
    tubercula d.
dolosa
    Burkholderia d.
Dolosicoccus paucivorans
DOMA
    dihydroxymandelic acid
domain
    adhesive extracellular d.

a disintegrin and metalloproteinase
with thrombospondin d. 13
(ADAMTS 13)
amino-terminal d.
death effector d.
immunoglobulin d.
Dombrock antigen
dombrowskii
Halococcus d.
dome cell
dome-shaped
domestica
Musca d.
domesticus
Glyciphagus d.
Glycyphagus d.
domiciliated
dominance
incomplete d.
dominant
d. character
d. complement
d. complementarity
d. gene
d. inheritance
d. negative mutation
dominantly inherited Lévi
disease
DON
deoxynivalenol
Donath-Landsteiner (DL)
D.-L. antibody
D.-L. biphasic hemolysin
D.-L. cold autoantibody
D.-L. phenomenon
D.-L. syndrome
D.-L. test
donation
designated blood d.
NAT for HCV and HIV-1 in
blood d.
donensis
Superstitionia d.
Donkioporia
Donnan potential
Donné
D. body
D. corpuscle
D. test
Donohue syndrome
donor
cadaver d.
consanguineous d.
F d.
living d. (LD)
d. neocyte
proton d.
d. tissue
universal d.

donor-specific
d.-s. crossmatching
d.-s. HLA antibody
Donovan body
donovani
Herpetomonas d.
Leishmania donovani d.
donovania
Calymmatobacterium d.
D. granulomatis
DOP
degenerate oligonucleotide-primed
DOP PCR
DOPA
dihydroxyphenylalanine
DOPA stain
dopamine
d. hydroxylase
d. monooxygenase
urine d.
dopaminergic neuron
dopaquinone
DOP-PCR
degenerate oligonucleotide primed
polymerase chain reaction
doppel protein
Doppler effect
Dora
hemoglobin Koya D.
d'orange
peau d.
Doratomyces stemonitis
Dorea
D. formicigenerans
D. longicatena
Dorello canal
doricum
Mycobacterium d.
Doriden
dormancy
dormant
Dorner stain
Dorothy Reed cell
dorsal
dorsalis
Aedes d.
tabes d.
dorsi
elastofibroma d.
osteochondritis deformans juvenilis d.
dorsopancreaticus
ductus d.
dosage (*var. of* dose)
d. compensation
gene d.
high d. (HD)
dose, dosage
absorbed d.
d. account

dose (*continued*)
air d.
booster d.
d. calibrator
curative d.
depth d.
d. distribution
divided d.
effective d. (ED)
epilating d.
erythema d.
d. estimate
exit d.
fatal d. (FD)
genetically significant d.
guinea pig intraperitoneal infectious
d. (GPIPID)
incapacitating d.
infecting d. (ID)
infective d. (ID)
integral d.
L d.
L$^+$ d.
L$_0$ d.
lethal d. (LD)
Lf d.
loading d.
Lr d.
maximal permissible d. (MPD)
mean hemolytic d. (MHD)
median curative d. (CD$_{50}$)
median effective d. (ED$_{50}$)
median fatal d. (FD$_{50}$)
median infectious d. (ID$_{50}$)
median lethal d.
median tissue culture d. (TCD$_{50}$)
median tissue culture infective d.
(TCID$_{50}$)
medical internal radiation d.
(MIRD)
minimal erythema d. (MED)
minimal infecting d. (MID)
minimal lethal d.
minimal morbidostatic d.
(MMD)
minimal reacting d. (MRD)
minimum hemolytic d. (MHD)
minimum infective d. (MID)
minimum lethal d. (MLD)
normal single d. (NSD)
organ tolerance d. (OTD)
radiation absorbed d. (rad)
d. rate
sensitizing d.
shocking d.
skin test d. (STD)
threshold erythema d. (TED)
tissue culture d. (TCD)
tissue culture infective d. (TCID)

tissue tolerance d. (TTD)
titrated initial d. (TID)
tumor lethal d. (TLD)
dose-rate/meter
dose-reduction factor (DRF)
dosimeter
criticality locket d.
neutron personnel d.
pocket d.
quartz fiber d. (QFD)
thermoluminescent d. (TLD)
ultraviolet fluorescent d.
dosimetry
dot
d. blot test
Maurer d.
Mittendorf d.
d. product
d. scan
Schüffner d.
Ziemann d.
dot-blot
forward d.-b.
reverse d.-b.
Dothichiza
Dothiorella mangiferae
double
d. albuminemia
d. antibody immunoassay
d. antibody immunoenzymometric
assay
d. antibody method
d. antibody precipitation
d. antibody sandwich assay
d. antibody technique
d. blood supply
d. diffusion
d. diffusion test
d. discharge
d. ductus arteriosus
d. fluorescence labeling
d. (gel) diffusion precipitin test in
one dimension
d. (gel) diffusion precipitin test in
two dimensions
d. helix
d. immunodiffusion
d. immunolabeling
d. intussusception
d. minute chromosome
d. oxalate
d. phenotypic pattern
d. pneumonia
d. refraction
d. stain
d. staining technique
d. tertian malaria
d. trisomy
double-beam photometer

double-blind
    d.-b. experiment
    d.-b. study
double-contrast
    d.-c. examination
    d.-c. study
doublecortin
double-crossed immunoelectrophoresis
double-fluorescence
  microlymphocytotoxicity
double-fusion FISH (D-FISH)
double-layer fluorescent antibody
  technique
double-masked experiment
double-pole
    d.-p. double-throw switch
    d.-p. single-throw switch
double-precision variable
double-stranded
    d.-s. DNA (DS-DNA)
    d.-s. DNA virus
double-voided urine specimen
doubling
    d. dilution
    d. time
Doucas
    purpura of D.
doudoroffii
    Oceanimonas d.
Douglas
    D. abscess
    pouch of D.
dourine
Dowex
Down
    D. syndrome (DS)
    D. syndrome tau pathology
Downey cell
Downey-type lymphocyte
down-regulation
downstream
doxepin
    d. hydrochloride
    d. hydrochloride assay
Doyère eminence
D-PAS
    diastase-periodic acid-Schiff
      D-PAS stain
DPB
    diffuse panbronchiolitis
DPC
    delayed primary closure
DPC4 gene
Dpc4 immunohistochemical pancreatic
  cancer analysis
DPD
    deoxypyridinoline
DPDL
    diffuse poorly differentiated lymphoma

DPH
    Department of Public Health
    diphenhydramine
    diphenylhexatriene
    diphenylhydantoin
DPI
    diphenyleneiodonium
DPN
    deep penetrating nevus
    diphosphopyridine nucleotide
DPNH
    diphosphopyridine nucleotide
DPPIV
    dipeptidyl peptidase IV protein
DPX
    ER-Tracker blue-white DPX
DR
    diabetic retinopathy
    reaction of degeneration
Drabkin reagent
dracontiasis
dracunculiasis, dracunculosis
dracunculosis (*var. of*
  dracunculiasis)
Dracunculus
    D. lova
    D. medinensis
    D. oculi
    D. persarum
Dragendorff
    D. solution
    D. test
dragon
    d. worm
    d. worm infection
drainage
    anomalous venous d.
    biliary d.
drain-trap stomach
dramatic response
drancourtii
    Legionella d.
DRE
    digital rectal examination
Drechslera hawaiiensis
drench hose
drentensis
    Bacillus d.
drepanidium
Drepanidotaenia lanceolata
drepanocyte
drepanocythemia
drepanocytic
drepanocytosis
Drepanopeziza
Dresbach
    D. anemia
    D. syndrome
Dressler syndrome

D

DRF
  dose-reduction factor
dried
  d. blood spot
  d. human serum
  d. smear
  d. sodium phosphate
  d. yeast
drift
  antigenic d.
  genetic d.
  nosologic d.
  random genetic d.
drip-arm hyponatremia
dronabinol
drop
  capsular d.
  d. heart
  voltage d.
droplet
  electron-dense d.
  fat d.
  d. infection
  macrovesicular fat d.
  d. nuclei
  d. precautions
droplet-borne agent
dropsical
dropsy
  abdominal d.
Drosophila
  wingless signaling pathway in *D.*
drozanskii
  Legionella d.
drozdowiczii
  Streptomyces d.
DRPLA
  dentatorubral pallidoluysian atrophy
DR-70 tumor marker test
drug
  d. abuse screen
  afterload-reducing d.
  d. allergy
  antibiotic antitumor d.
  antimetabolite d.
  d. dependence
  d. desensitization
  d. detoxification
  d. interaction
  d. interference
  d. metabolism
  d. metabolizing enzyme (DME)
  drugs of abuse (DOA)
  ototoxic d.
  radioactive d.
  d. screening assay
  sulfa d.
  d. tolerance
  d. utilization review

drug-fast
drug-induced
  d.-i. autoimmune hemolytic anemia
  d.-i. hepatitis
  d.-i. immune hemolytic anemia
  d.-i. myocarditis
  d.-i. neutropenia
  d.-i. thrombocytopenia (DIT)
drug-resistant
drum membrane
drumstick
  d. appendage
  d. finger
  d. spore
drusen
DRVVT
  dilute Russell viper venom time
DRx quantitative hCG patient monitor test
dry
  d. abscess
  d. beriberi
  d. bronchiectasis
  d. catarrh
  d. decontamination
  d. desquamation
  d. gangrene
  d. leprosy
  d. objective
  d. pleurisy
  standard temperature and pressure, d.
  d. tap
drying agent
Drysdale corpuscle
4Ds
  diplopia, dysphagia, dysarthria, dysphonia
DS
  defined substrate
  dextrose-saline
  Down syndrome
DSAP
  disseminated superficial actinic porokeratosis
DS-DNA
  double-stranded DNA
DSM
  dextrose solution mixture
DSPC
  desaturated phosphatidylcholine
DSRCT
  desmoplastic small round cell tumor
DST
  dexamethasone suppression test
D-Stoff (phosgene gas)
DSX automated ELISA system
DT
  delirium tremens

dTDP
   thymidine diphosphate
DTF
   desmoid-type fibromatosis
   detector transfer function
DTH
   delayed-type hypersensitivity
DTICH
   delayed traumatic intracerebral
      hematoma
DTM
   dermatophyte test medium
DTN
   diphtheria toxin normal
DTP
   diphtheria, tetanus, and pertussis
      vaccine
**DTPA-Lys(40)-Exendin 4 radio-labeled
 imaging medium**
DTT
   dithiothreitol
dTTP
   deoxythymidine triphosphate
DTX series multimode detector
DU
   depleted uranium
dual hemostatic defect
dual-color
      d.-c. fluorescence
      d.-c. probe
dual-contrast study
dual-in-line package
dualism
Duane-Hunt relation
Duane syndrome
Dubini disease
Dubin-Johnson syndrome
Dubin-Sprinz syndrome
dubius
   Sulfitobacter d.
dubliniensis
   Candida d.
Dubois
      D. abscess
      D. disease
Duboisia myoporoides
duboisii
   Histoplasma capsulatum d.
Dubreuil-Chambardel syndrome
Dubreuilh
   precancerous melanosis of D.
Duchenne
      D. disease
      D. muscular dystrophy
       (DMD)
      D. syndrome
Duchenne-Aran disease
Duchenne-Erb syndrome
Duchenne-Griesinger disease

duck
   d. embryo origin vaccine
   d. hepatitis virus
   d. influenza virus
   d. plague
   d. plague virus
Ducrey
   D. bacillus
   D. test
ducreyi
   Haemophilus d.
duct
   aberrant d.
   accessory pancreatic d.
   alveolar d.
   anal d.
   Arantius d.
   Bartholin d.
   basilar membrane of cochlear d.
   Bellini d.
   Bernard d.
   bile d.
   biliary d.
   Blasius d.
   breast d.
   canalicular d.
   d. carcinoma
   choledoch d.
   cochlear d.
   collecting d.
   common bile d.
   cystic d.
   deferent d.
   efferent d.
   ejaculatory d.
   endolymphatic d.
   excretory d.
   galactophorous d.
   gall d.
   guttural d.
   hemithoracic d.
   Hensen d.
   Hoffmann d.
   intercalated d.
   interlobar d.
   interlobular d.
   intralobular d.
   lactiferous d.
   Luschka d.
   lymphatic d.
   mamillary d.
   mammary d.
   milk d.
   Müllerian d.
   d. of epididymis
   d. papilloma
   paramesonephric d.
   persistent vitelline d.
   prostatic d.

D

duct (*continued*)
    Rivinus d.
    salivary d.
    Santorini d.
    Schüller d.
    secretory d.
    semicircular d.
    spermatic d.
    Stensen d.
    striated d.
    submandibular d.
    submaxillary d.
    sudoriferous d.
    sweat d.
    testicular d.
    uniting d.
    utriculosaccular d.
    Walther d.
    Wharton d.
    Wirsung d.
    wolffian d.
ductal
    d. adenoma
    d. carcinoma
    d. carcinoma in situ (DCIS)
    d. hyperplasia (DH)
    d. intraepithelial neoplasia (DIN)
    d. lavage
    d. papilloma
    d. plate
ductectatic-type mucinous cystic tumor
ductibus
    glandulae sine d.
ductless gland
ductography
ductopenia
ductoscopy
ductular
    d. piecemeal necrosis
    d. reactive cell
ductule
    aberrant d.
    biliary d.
    efferent d.
    interlobular d.
    intralobular d.
    proliferating bile ductules (PBD)
    prostatic d.
ductuli (*pl. of* ductulus)
ductulus, *pl.* **ductuli**
    d. aberrans inferior
    d. aberrans superior
    ductuli aberrantes
    d. alveolaris
    ductuli biliferi
    ductuli efferentes testis
    ductuli excretorii glandula
    ductuli interlobulares
    ductuli paroophori
    ductuli prostatici
ductus, *pl.* **ductus**
    d. aberrantes
    d. biliferi
    d. choledochus
    d. cochlearis
    d. cysticus
    d. deferens
    d. deferens tumor
    d. dorsopancreaticus
    d. ejaculatorius
    d. endolymphaticus
    d. epididymidis
    d. excretorius
    d. excretorius vesiculae seminalis
    d. hemithoracicus
    d. lactiferi
    d. pancreaticus
    d. pancreaticus accessorius
    d. paraurethrales
    d. parotideus
    d. perilymphaticus
    d. prostatici
    d. reuniens
    d. semicirculares
    d. sublinguales minores
    d. sublingualis major
    d. submandibularis
    d. submaxillaris
    d. sudoriferus
    d. utriculosaccularis
Duddell membrane
Duffy
    D. antibody
    D. antibody Fya
    D. antibody Fyb
    D. antigen
    D. antigen receptor for chemokine (DARC)
    D. blood antibody type
    D. blood group system
Duganella violaceinigra
Duhamel technique
Duhring disease
Duke
    D. bleeding time test
    D. method
    D. method of bleeding time
Dukes
    D. A, B, C tumor stage
    D. carcinoma classification
    D. disease
    D. staging
Dukes-Astler-Coller adenocarcinoma classification
dullness, dulness
    Gerhardt d.
    relative hepatic d. (RHD)

dulness (*var. of* dullness)
dumbbell ganglioneuroma
Dumdum fever
dummy variable
dumoffii
    Legionella d.
dUMP
    deoxyuridine monophosphate
dumping syndrome
Duncan
    D. disease
    D. multiple-range test
    D. syndrome
Dunnett multiple component test
duodenal
    d. atresia
    d. carcinoma
    d. contents culture
    d. contents examination
    d. diverticulum
    d. fistula
    d. gland
    d. parasite
    d. smear
    d. ulcer
    d. ulcer perforation
    (DUP)
duodenale
    Ancylostoma d.
duodenales
    glandulae d.
duodenalis
    Uncinaria d.
duodeni
    pseudomelanosis d.
duodenitis
duodenocholangitis
duovirus
DUP
    duodenal ulcer perforation
DU-PAN-2 pancreatic cancer-associated antigen
Duplay syndrome
duplex
    Haemophilus d.
    d. ileum
    ileum d.
    d. kidney
    d. placenta
    d. scan
duplication
    caudal dipygus d.
    congenital d.
    cranial monocephalus d.
    d. cyst
    d. deficiency
    facial diprosopus d.
    fetal d.
    trunk d.

Dupré syndrome
Dupuytren
    D. contracture
    D. fibromatosis
dural sheath
dura mater
Durand disease
Durand-Nicolas-Favre disease
Duran-Reynals permeability factor
durans
    Streptococcus d.
Durante disease
Dura-Temp specimen transporter
Dürck node
Durella
Duret hemorrhage
Durham tube
durianis
    Lactobacillus d.
Durie and Salmon multiple myeloma clinical staging
Duroziez disease
durum
    papilloma d.
dusky erythema
dust
    blood d.
    d. cell
    chromatin d.
    d. corpuscle
    nuclear d.
Dutch classification
Dutcher body
DUTP
    deoxyuridine triphosphate
Dutton
    D. disease
    D. relapsing fever
    D. spirochete
Duttonella
duttonii
    Borrelia d.
Duverney gland
dux
    Sarcophaga d.
DVT
    deep vein thrombosis
D5W
    5 percent dextrose in water
D$_5$W
    5 percent dextrose in water
dwarf
    achondroplastic d.
    d. colony
    constitutional d.
    d. kidney
    pituitary d.
    primordial d.
    d. tapeworm

D

dwarfism
- achondroplastic d.
- acromelic d.
- chondrodystrophic d.
- Fröhlich d.
- Laron d.
- lethal d.
- Lorain d.
- mesomelic d.
- micromelic d.
- pituitary d.
- polydystrophic d.
- senile d.
- Silver-Russell d.
- snub-nose d.
- thanatophoric d.

DX
- dextran
- diagnosis

Dx
- diagnosis

DxI 800 immunoassay system

d-xylose
- d-x. absorption
- d-x. absorption test
- d-x. tolerance test

dyad

Dyadobacter fermentans

dydrogesterone

dye
- acid d.
- acidic d.
- acidophilic d.
- acridine d.
- aminoanthraquinone d.
- aminoketone d.
- amphoteric d.
- aniline d.
- anionic d.
- anthraquinone d.
- arsenazo III d.
- azin d.
- azo d.
- azocarmine d.
- azoic d.
- basic d.
- cationic d.
- d. content
- DAPI d.
- diphenylmethane d.
- endolymphatic d.
- d. exclusion test
- d. excretion test
- fluorescent d.
- Hoechst d.
- hydroxyketone d.
- indamine d.
- indigoid d.
- indophenol d.

- ketonimine d.
- lactone d.
- lipophilic d.
- metachromatic d.
- methine d.
- methylene blue d. (MBD)
- natural d.
- NBT d.
- nitro d.
- nitroblue tetrazolium d. (NTD)
- nitroso d.
- oxazin d.
- polycationic d.
- polymethine d.
- quinoline d.
- quinolinium d.
- rosanilin d.
- salt d.
- stilbene d.
- sulfur d.
- synthetic d.
- thiazin d.
- thiazole d.
- triarylmethane d.
- triphenylmethane d.
- vital d.
- xanthene d.

dye-binding capacity (DBC)

dye-dilution curve

dyed starch method

Dyggve-Melchior-Clausen syndrome

Dyke-Davidoff-Masson syndrome

dyn
- dyne

DyNA block 1000 microtiter plate

dynamic
- d. equilibrium
- d. ileus
- d. isomerism
- d. pulmonary compliance
- d. real-time telepathology
- d. storage allocation
- d. viscosity

dynamite heart

dyne (dyn)

dynein arm

Dynex Immulon 1B microtiter plate

dyphylline

Dyrenium

dysarthria

dysautonomia
- familial d.

dysbarism

dysbetalipoproteinemia
- familial d.

dysbolism

dyscephalia mandibulooculofacialis

dyschondrogenesis

dyschondroplasia with hemangiomas

dyschondrosteosis
dyscinesia (*var. of* dyskinesia)
dyscohesion
    cellular d.
dyscrasia
    blood d.
    lymphatic d.
    plasma cell d.
dyscrasic, dyscratic
dyscratic (*var. of* dyscrasic)
dysembryoma
dysembryoplastic neuroepithelial tumor
dysemia
dysencephalia splanchnocystica
dysenteriae
    Amoeba d.
    Bacillus d.
    Shigella d.
dysentery
    amebic d.
    d. antitoxin
    bacillary d.
    d. bacilli
    balantidial d.
    bilharzial d.
    catarrhal d.
    ciliary d.
    ciliate d.
    epidemic d.
    flagellate d.
    Flexner d.
    fulminant d.
    giardiasis d.
    malarial d.
    protozoal d.
    scorbutic d.
    Sonne d.
    spirillar d.
    sporadic d.
    viral d.
dyserythropoiesis
dyserythropoietic congenital anemia
dysferlin protein
dysfibrinogenemia
dysfunction
    autonomic d.
    bladder d.
    constitutional hepatic d.
    enterostomy d.
    infarctive placental d.
    minimal brain d. (MBD)
    multiorgan d.
    ovarian d.
    pituitary d.
    placental d.
    ventricular d.
dysfunctional uterine bleeding
dysgammaglobulinemia
    type I, II d.

dysgenesia (*var. of* dysgenesis)
dysgenesis, dysgenesia
    familial gonadal d.
    gonadal d.
    pure gonadal d. (PGD)
    renal tubular d. (RTD)
    reticular d. (RD)
    seminiferous tubule d.
    testicular d.
    XO gonadal d.
    XX gonadal d.
    XY gonadal d.
dysgenetic
    d. male pseudohermaphroditism
    (DMPH)
    d. testes
dysgerminoma
dysglobulinemia
dysgonic
Dysgonomonas
    D. capnocytophagoides
    D. gadei
    D. mossii
dysgranulopoiesis
dyshematopoiesis, dyshemopoiesis
dyshematopoietic, dyshemopoietic
    d. anemia
dyshemopoiesis (*var. of* dyshematopoiesis)
dyshemopoietic (*var. of* dyshematopoietic)
dyshesion
dyshesive
dyshidrosis, dyshidrotic eczema,
  dysidrosis, dyshydrosis
dyshidrotic eczema
dyshormonogenesis
dyshormonogenic goiter
dyshydrosis (*var. of* dyshidrosis)
dysidrosis (*var. of* dyshidrosis)
dyskaryosis
dyskaryotic
dyskeratoma
    warty d.
dyskeratosis
    benign d.
    d. congenita
    hereditary benign
     intraepithelial d.
    intraepithelial d.
    malignant d.
dyskeratotic
dyskinesia, dyskinesis, dyscinesia
    tracheobronchial d.
dyskinesis (*var. of* dyskinesia)
dyslipoproteinemia
dysmaturity
    placental d.
dysmegakaryocytopoiesis
dysmenorrhea
dysmetabolic iron overload

D

305

dysmorphia (*var. of* dysmorphism)
dysmorphic erythrocyte
dysmorphism, dysmorphia
    mandibulooculofacial d.
dysmorphogenesis
dysmorphologist
dysmorphology
dysmotility
    esophageal d.
dysmyelinisatus
    status d.
dysmyelopoietic syndrome
dysosteogenesis
dysostosis
    acrofacial d.
    cleidocranial d.
    craniofacial d.
    Crouzon craniofacial d.
    mandibuloacral d.
    mandibulofacial d.
    metaphysial d.
    d. multiplex
    orodigitofacial d.
    otomandibular d.
dysoxidative carbonuria
dyspallia
dyspepsia
    nonulcer d.
dysphagia, dysphagy
    d. lusoria
    sideropenic d.
dysphagocytosis
    congenital d.
dysphagy (*var. of* dysphagia)
dysphasia
    cementoosseous d. (COD)
    local cementoosseous d.
    (LOCD)
dysphonia
    diplopia, dysphagia, dysarthria, d.
    (4Ds)
dyspigmentation
dysplasia
    acquired d.
    anhidrotic ectodermal d.
    anterofacial d.
    anteroposterior facial d.
    arrhythmogenic right ventricular d.
    asphyxiating thoracic d.
    atriodigital d.
    bronchopulmonary d. (BPD)
    cerebral d.
    cervical d.
    chondroectodermal d.
    cleidocranial d.
    congenital ectodermal d.
    congenital thymic d. (CTD)
    cortical d.
    craniocarpotarsal d.

craniodiaphysial d.
craniometaphysial d.
dentin d.
diaphysial d.
ectodermal hereditary d.
endocervical glandular d.
  (EGD)
d. epiphysialis hemimelia
d. epiphysialis multiplex
d. epiphysialis punctata
epithelial d.
faciodigitogenital d.
fibromuscular d.
fibrous familial d.
fibrous monostotic d.
florid cementoosseous d.
florid local cementoosseous d.
  (FLCOD)
glandular d.
hereditary renal-retinal d.
hidrotic ectodermal d.
high grade d.
hypohidrotic ectodermal d.
intestinal neuronal d. (IND)
low-grade d. (LGD)
lymphopenic thymic d.
mammary d.
mandibulofacial d.
metaphysial d.
monostotic fibrous d.
mucoepithelial d.
multiple epiphysial d.
neuronal intestinal d.
nonsyndromal d.
oculoauriculovertebral d.
oculodentodigital d.
oculovertebral d.
ophthalmomandibulomelic d.
polyostotic fibrous d.
postradiation d. (PRDX)
precancerous d.
pseudoachondroplastic
  spondyloepiphysial d.
renal-retinal d.
right ventricular d.
septooptic d.
spondyloepiphysial d. (SED)
squamous d.
syndromal d.
thymic d.
trilineage d.
T-zone d.
ventriculoradial d.
vesical d.
Zenker d.
dysplasia-associated
    d.-a. lesion
    d.-a. lesion or mass (DALM)
    d.-a. mass

dysplastic
    d. cerebellar gangliocytoma
    d. epithelium
    d. focus
    d. neuroepithelial tumor (DNET)
    d. nevus
    d. nevus syndrome
    d. nodule
dyspoiesis
dyspoietic syndrome
dysprosium
dysproteinemia
    angioimmunoblastic lymphadenopathy
      with d. (AILD)
dysproteinemic neuropathy
dysprothrombinemia
dysraphic anomaly
dysraphicus
    status d.
dysregulation
    gene d.
dysrhythmia
dyssebacea (*var. of* dyssebacia)
dyssebacia, dyssebacea
dysspondylism
dyssynchronous
dyssynergia, dyssynergy
    biliary d.
    d. cerebellaris myoclonica
    d. cerebellaris progressive
    detrusor-external sphincter d.
    detrusor-sphincter d.
    progressive cerebellar d.
    vesico-sphincter d.
dyssynergy (*var. of* dyssynergia)
dystonia
dystonic
dystopia
dystopic
dystroglycan
    alpha d.
dystrophia (*var. of* dystrophy)
    d. brevicollis
    d. unguium

dystrophic
    d. calcification
    d. calcinosis
    d. neurite
dystrophica
    epidermolysis bullosa d.
dystrophin
    d. antibody
    d. gene
dystrophy, dystrophia
    adiposogenital d.
    asphyxiating thoracic d. (ATD)
    Becker muscular d. (BMD)
    Biber-Haab-Dimmer corneal lattice
     d.
    congenital muscular d.
    craniocarpotarsal d.
    distal muscular d.
    distal-type progressive muscular d.
    Duchenne muscular d. (DMD)
    facioscapulohumeral-type progressive
     muscular d.
    infantile neuroaxonal d. (INAD)
    infantile progressive spinal
     muscular d.
    Landouzy-Dejerine progressive
     muscular d.
    limb-girdle muscular d.
    lipoid d.
    muscular d. (MD)
    myotonic d. (DM)
    ocular muscle d. (OMD)
    ophthalmoplegic-type progressive
     muscular d.
    progressive muscular d. (PMD)
    reflex sympathetic d.
    Reis-Bücklers corneal lattice d.
    Thiel-Behnke corneal lattice d.
    thoracic asphyxiant d. (TAD)
    thoracic-pelvic-phalangeal d.
    vulvar d.
**dystrophy-dystocia syndrome
(DDS)**
dysuria-pyuria syndrome

D

E
erythrocyte
extraction fraction
glutamic acid
E antigen
E erythrocyte rosette assay
E rosette-forming cell
E test

E1
estrone

E2
estradiol

E3
estriol

E4
estetrol

EA
early antigen
erythrocyte antibody

EAA
endotoxin activity assay
extrinsic allergic alveolitis

EABA
endogenous avidin-binding activity

EAC
erythrocyte antibody complement
EAC rosette assay

Eadie-Hofstee equation
EAE
experimental allergic
encephalomyelitis

EAF
eosinophilic angiocentric fibrosis

EAG
experimental autoimmune
glomerulonephritis

EaggEC
enteroaggregative *Escherichia coli*

Eagle
E. basal medium
E. essential medium
E. minimum essential medium
(EMEM)
E. syndrome

EAHF
eczema, asthma, hay fever

EAHLG
equine antihuman lymphoblast globulin

EAHLS
equine antihuman lymphoblast serum

Eales disease
EAN
experimental allergic neuritis

EAP
epiallopregnanolone

ear
cauliflower e.
e. crystal
e. culture
e. lobule
scroll e.

eardrum
Earle
E. L fibrosarcoma
E. solution

early
E. Aberration Reporting System
(EARS)
e. antigen (EA)
e. B cell
e. invasion
e. myeloid progenitor cell
e. neonatal death
e. reaction
E. Surveillance Project (ESP)

early-phase response
EARS
Early Aberration Reporting System

earth
diatomaceous e.

earwax
eAST
erythrocyte aspartate aminotransferase
activity

East African (Rhodesian) trypanosomiasis
Eastern
E. equine encephalitis virus titer
E. equine encephalomyelitis (EEE)
E. equine encephalomyelitis virus
E. subtype Russian spring-summer
encephalitis

Eaton
E. agent
E. agent pneumonia

Eaton-Lambert syndrome
EB
epidermolysis bullosa
estradiol benzoate
EB virus

ebb phase
EBER
Epstein-Barr encoded RNA
EBER ISH

EBER1 riboprobe
Eberth
E. line
E. perithelium

Eberthella typhi
EBL
estimated blood loss

E

eBL
    endemic Burkitt lymphoma
EBNA
    Epstein-Barr nuclear antigen
Ebner
    E. gland
    imbrication line of von E.
    incremental line of von E.
    E. reticulum
Ebola
    E. hemorrhagic fever
    E. virus
    E. virus disease
Ebola-like viruses
Ebstein
    E. anomaly
    E. disease
    E. lesion
    E. malformation
ebur dentis
eburnation
eburnea
    substantia e.
eburneous
EBV
    Epstein-Barr virus
EC
    electron capture
    enteric-coated
    enterochromaffin cell hyperplasia
    extracellular
        EC detector
ECA
    ethacrynic acid
E-cad
    E-cadherin
E-cadherin
    epithelial cadherin
E-cadherin (E-cad)
    E-c. calcium-dependent
        molecule
    E-c. gene
    E-c. immunohistochemistry
    E-c. immunostain
    E-c. stain
    E-c. stain
ecarin clotting time test card
ECBO
    enteric cytopathogenic bovine
        orphan
        ECBO virus
ECBV
    effective circulating blood
        volume
ECC
    endocervical curettage
eccentric
    e. hypertrophy
    e. nucleus

eccentrica
    hyperkeratosis e.
    keratoderma e.
eccentrochondroplasia
ecchondroma, ecchondrosis
ecchondrosis (*var. of* ecchondroma)
ecchordosis physalifora
ecchymoma
ecchymosed
ecchymoses (*pl. of* ecchymosis)
ecchymosis, *pl.* **ecchymoses**
    cadaveric e.
    Tardieu ecchymoses
ecchymotic
eccrine
    e. acrospiroma
    e. gland
    e. poroma
    e. spiradenoma
    e. sweat gland secretion
    e. tumor
eccrinology
eccyesis
ECD
    Erdheim-Chester disease
ECDO
    enteric cytopathogenic dog orphan
        ECDO virus
ECE1
    endothelin-converting
        enzyme
ECF
    extracellular fluid
ECF-A
    eosinophil chemotactic factor of
        anaphylaxis
ECFV
    extracellular fluid volume
ecgonine
echidninus
    Laelaps e.
Echidnophaga gallinacea
echinata
    Memnoniella e.
echinate
Echinobotryum
Echinochasmus
echinococciasis (*var. of* echinococcosis)
echinococcosis, echinococciasis
    polyvisceral e.
    e. serological test
    unilocular e.
echinococcus
    e. cyst
    e. disease
    E. granulosus
    E. multilocularis
    Taenia e.
    E. vogeli

echinocyte
echinocytosis
Echinoparyphium recurvatum
Echinorhynchus gadi
echinosis
Echinostoma
    E. ilocanum
    E. lindoensis
    E. malayanum
    E. perfoliatum
    E. revolutum
echinostomiasis
echinulate
ECHO
    enteric cytopathogenic human orphan
      ECHO virus
echovirus, ECHO virus
echt
    cresyl e.
ECIS
    endometrial carcinoma in situ
Ecker plug
ECL
    electrogenerated chemiluminescence
    extracapillary lesion
eclampsia
    puerperal e.
    uremic e.
ECLIA
    electrochemiluminescence immunoassay
eclipse
    e. period
    e. phase
ECLT
    euglobulin clot lysis time
ECM
    erythema chronicum migrans
    extracellular material
    extracellular matrix
ECMO
    enteric cytopathogenic monkey orphan
    extracorporeal membrane oxygenation
      ECMO virus
ecogenetics
ecoid
E. coli
    Escherichia coli
ecologic niche
ecology
Economo disease
economy class syndrome
Eco RI enzyme
ecospecies
ecosystem
ecotaxis
ecotropic virus
ECP
    eosinophilic cationic protein
    erythropoietic coproporphyria

ecphyma
ECSO
    enteric cytopathogenic swine orphan
      ECSO virus
EC-SOD
    extracellular superoxide dismutase
ecstrophe
ECT
    ectomesenchymal chondromyxoid tumor
    euglobulin clot test
ECt50, ECt$_{50}$
    effective Ct$_{50}$
ectacolia
ectasia, ectasis
    congenital biliary e.
    e. cordis
    diffuse arterial e.
    gastric antral vascular e.
    (GAVE)
    hypostatic e.
    mammary duct e.
    mucinous ductal e.
    senile e.
    vascular e.
    e. ventriculi paradoxa
ectasis (*var. of* ectasia)
ectatic aneurysm
ecthyma
    contagious e.
    e. gangrenosum
    e. infectiosum
    e. infectiosum virus
ecthymatiform
ecthymiform
ectoantigen
ectoblastic cell
ectocervical smear
ectocornea
ectocyst
ectoderm
    stomodeal e.
ectodermal
    e. cell
    e. defect
    e. hereditary dysplasia
ectodermatosis
ectodermosis erosiva pluriorificialis
ectoenzyme
ectogenous
ectoglobular
ectomerogony
ectomesenchymal chondromyxoid tumor
  (ECT)
ectomesenchyme
ectomesenchymoma
ectonucleotide pyrophosphohydrolase
ectoparasite
ectoparasiticide
ectoparasitism

E

ectoperitonitis
ectophyte
ectopia, ectopy
    e. cloacae
    e. renis
    e. testis
    e. vesicae
ectopic (ect)
    e. ACTH syndrome
    e. anus
    e. decidua
    e. focus (EF)
    e. hormone
    e. hormone production
    e. pancreatic tissue
    e. pinealoma
    e. pregnancy (EP)
    e. testis
    e. thyroid tissue
ectoplasm
ectoplasmatic, ektoplasmic, ektoplastic
ectopy (*var. of* ectopia)
ectoretina
ectosarc
ectosteal
ectostosis
ectothrix infection
ectotoxin
Ectotrichophyton
ectozoic
ectozoon
ectromelia virus
ectromelus
ectrometacarpia
ectropion, ectropium
ectropium (*var. of* ectropion)
ECV
    effective circulating volume
    extracellular volume
ECW
    extracellular water
eczema
    allergic e.
    e., asthma, hay fever
      (EAHF)
    baker's e.
    chronic e.
    e. erythematosum
    facial e.
    e. herpeticum
    e. hypertrophicum
    lichenoid e.
    e. marginatum
    nummular e.
    e. vaccinatum
    e. verrucosum
    e. vesiculosum
eczematoid dermatitis
eczematous dermatitis

ED
    effective dose
    epileptiform discharge
ED50
    median effective dose
EDC
    expected date of confinement
E-DCIS
    endocrine ductal carcinoma in situ
Eddowes syndrome
eddy
    e. current
    squamous e.
eddy-current loss
edema
    allergic pulmonary e.
    alveolar e.
    angioneurotic e.
    blue e.
    brain e.
    brawny e.
    brown e.
    bullous e.
    cardiac e.
    cerebral e.
    circumscribed e.
    congestive e.
    cytotoxic e.
    dependent e.
    e. factor (EF)
    heat e.
    hereditary angioneurotic e. (HANE)
    inflammatory e.
    laryngeal e.
    lymphatic e.
    malignant e.
    e. neonatorum
    noncardiogenic pulmonary e.
    noninflammatory e.
    pitting e.
    pulmonary e. (PE)
    Quincke e.
    solid e.
    stromal e.
edematization
edematous
edentate
    dicobalt e.
edentatus
    Strongylus e.
edetate
    calcium disodium e.
    sodium calcium e.
edetic acid
edge
    e. effect
    spiculated e.
Edinger-Westphal nucleus
Edlefsen reagent

Edman reaction
Edmondson-Steiner hepatocellular
  carcinoma grading classification
Edmondson tumor grading system
edrophonium
    e. chloride
    e. chloride test
EDS
    Ehlers-Danlos syndrome
    energy dispersive spectrometer
    energy dispersive x-ray spectroscopy
Edsall disease
EDTA
    ethylenediaminetetraacetic acid
        EDTA buffer
        EDTA contamination of specimen
        potassium EDTA (K3 EDTA)
EDTA-associated leukoagglutination
EDTA-dependent pseudothrombocytopenia
Edwardsiella tarda
Edwardsielleae
Edwards-Patau syndrome
Edwards syndrome
EEC
    endometrioid endometrial carcinoma
    enteropathogenic *Escherichia coli*
EEE
    Eastern equine encephalomyelitis
        EEE virus
EEO
    electroendosmosis
E-EPE
    established extraprostatic extension
EF
    ectopic focus
    edema factor
    encephalitogenic factor
        EF protein
EFA
    essential fatty acid
EFC
    endogenous fecal calcium
EFE
    endocardial fibroelastosis
Effapoxy resin
effect
    antimuscarinic e.
    Arias-Stella e.
    Auger e.
    biochemically mediated e.
    blast e.
    Bohr e.
    booster e.
    carry-over e.
    copper wire e.
    Crabtree e.
    crowding e.
    cytopathic e.
    defibrinogenating e.

    Doppler e.
    edge e.
    end-organ e.
    excitatory e.
    Faraday e.
    founder e.
    Haldane e.
    intracellular signal transduction e.
    matrix e.
    monotypic e.
    muscarinic e.
    e. of fertilization
    oxygen e.
    polytopic e.
    radiation e.
    side e. (SE)
    Somogyi e.
    Soret e.
    Staub-Traugott e.
    Tyndall e.
    Whitten e.
    Wolff-Chaikoff e.
    zonation e.
effective
    e. circulating blood volume (ECBV)
    e. circulating volume (ECV)
    e. Ct_{50} (ECt_{50})
    e. dose (ED)
    e. half-life
    e. oxygen transport (EOT)
    e. refractory period (ERP)
    e. renal blood flow (ERBF)
    e. renal plasma flow (ERPF)
    e. temperature (ET)
effectiveness
    relative biological e. (RBE)
effector
    allosteric e.
    e. cell
    frangible anchor-linker e. (FRALE)
effemination
efferens
    vas e.
efferent
    e. duct
    e. ductule
    gamma e.
    e. lymphatic vessel
effervescent sodium
  phosphate
efficacy
efficiency
    geometric e.
efficiens
    Corynebacterium e.
efflorescence
efflux
effusa
    Hydrocarboniphaga e.

E

effuse colony
effusion
> chylous e.
> e. cytology
> exudative e.
> exudative pleural e.
> joint e.
> lymphoid-rich e.
> malignant pleural e. (MPE)
> pleural e.
> serofibrinous e.
> serosanguineous e.
> serous e.
> transudative pleural e.

EFV
> extracellular fluid volume

EGC
> endocrine granule constituent

EGD
> endocervical glandular dysplasia

EGE
> eosinophilic gastroenteritis

EGF
> epidermal growth factor

EGFP
> enhanced green fluorescent
> protein

EGFR
> epidermal growth factor receptor

egg
> e. count
> e. passage

Eggel tumor classification
Eggerthella lenta
egg-shell calcification
egg-white lysozyme (EWL)
egg-yolk agar
eglandulous
Eglis gland
EGOT
> erythrocyte glutamic oxaloacetic
> transaminase

EGP-2
> epithelial glycoprotein-2

EGTA
> ethylene glycol tetraacetic acid

Egyptian splenomegaly
EH
> epithelioid hemangioendothelioma
> essential hypertension

EHBA
> extrahepatic biliary atresia

EHBF
> estimated hepatic blood flow
> exercise hyperemia blood flow

EHE
> epithelioid hemangioendothelioma

EHEC
> enterohemorrhagic *Escherichia coli*

EHF
> exophthalmos-hyperthyroid factor

ehimensis
> *Paenibacillus e.*

EHL
> endogenous hyperlipidemia

Ehlers-Danlos syndrome (EDS)
EHLL
> epithelial hyperplastic laryngeal lesion

EHO
> extrahepatic obstruction

EHP
> excessive heat production

Ehrenreich and Churg membranous
nephropathy staging system
Ehrlich
> E. acid hematoxylin stain
> E. anemia
> E. aniline crystal violet stain
> E. ascites carcinoma
> E. benzaldehyde reaction
> E. diazo reaction
> E. diazo reagent
> E. hematoxylin
> E. inner body
> E. phenomenon
> E. postulate
> E. side-chain theory
> E. test
> E. triacid stain
> E. triple stain
> E. tumor
> E. unit (EU)

Ehrlichia
> *E. canis*
> *E. chaffeensis*
> *E. equi*
> *E. phagocytophila*
> *E. risticii*
> *E. sennetsu*

Ehrlichiaceae
Ehrlichieae
ehrlichiosis
> human granulocytic e. (HGE)
> human monocytic e. (HME)

EI
> enzyme inhibitor
> eosinophilic index

EIA
> enzyme-multiplied immunoassay
> EIA interface

EIC
> endometrial intraepithelial carcinoma
> enzyme immunochromatography
> epidermal inclusion cyst
> extensive intraductal component

Eichhorst corpuscle
eicosanoid synthesis
eicosapentaenoic acid (EPA)

EID
electroimmunodiffusion
EIEC
enteroinvasive *Escherichia coli*
eighth nerve tumor
Eijkman lactose broth
Eikenella corrodens
eiloid
Eimeria sardinae
Eimeriidae
Einarson
E. gallocyanin-chrome alum
E. gallocyanin-chrome alum stain
Einheit
antitoxin E. (AE)
einsteinium
Einthoven law
Eisenlohr syndrome
Eisenmenger
E. syndrome
tetralogy of E.
eisodic
ejaculate
ejaculatorius
ductus e.
ejaculatory duct
ejection murmur (EM)
EK
erythrokinase
Ekbom syndrome
EKC
epidemic keratoconjunctivitis
ekiri
Ektachem
ektoplasmic (*var. of* ectoplasmatic)
ektoplastic (*var. of* ectoplasmatic)
EL
electroluminescence
eLabNotebook
Eladia
Elaeophora schneideri
elaidic acid
E-LAM
endothelial-leukocyte adhesion
molecule
elastance
elastase
elastic
e. cartilage
e. fiber
e. fiber stain
e. lamellae
e. membrane
e. scattering
e. skin
e. tissue
elastica
cutis e.
Helvella e.

tela e.
tunica e.
e. van Gieson (EVG)
e. van Gieson stain
elasticity
wound e.
elasticum
pseudoxanthoma e. (PXE)
elastin
e. stain
Weigert stain for e.
elastin-binding protein
elastofibrolipoma
elastofibroma
e. dorsi
mediastinal e.
elastoid degeneration
elastoma
juvenile e.
Miescher e.
elastomer envelope
elastorrhexis
elastosis
e. colloidalis conglomerata
e. perforans serpiginosa
senile e.
solar e.
elastotic
e. degeneration
e. nodule
ELAT
enzyme-linked antiglobulin test
elaunin
Elavil
elbow
pitcher's e.
tennis e.
Elder malignant melanoma classification
Elecsys
E. Anti-HBe assay
E. free PSA immunoassay
E. 2010 modular immunoassay
analyzer
E. PreciControl Anti-HBe control
E. proBNP immunoassay
E. RBC folate hemolyzing reagent
E. total PSA immunoassay
E. total PSA test
E. troponin T immunoassay system
elective culture
Electra 1400C, 1800C coagulation system
electric
e. chromatography
e. field vector
e. potential
e. potential difference
e. susceptibility
electrical artifact
electroblot analysis

E

electrochemical cell
electrochemiluminescence immunoassay
  (ECLIA)
electrochemistry
electrode
      active e.
      bipolar needle e.
      calomel e.
      carbon dioxide e.
      Clark oxygen e.
      glass e.
      hydrogen e.
      e. impedance
      indicator e.
      indifferent e.
      inert e.
      ion-selective e. (ISE)
      e. of first kind
      e. of second kind
      Orion e.
      e. potential
      quinhydrone e.
      recording e.
      reference e.
      e. response time
      e. sensitivity
      Severinghaus e.
      silver/silver chloride e.
      standard hydrogen e.
      VaporTrode Vaporization E.
electroendosmosis (EEO)
electrogenerated chemiluminescence
  (ECL)
electroimmunoassay
electroimmunodiffusion (EID)
electroluminescence (EL)
electrolysis
      Faraday law of e.
electrolyte, *pl.* electrolytes
      amphoteric e.
      colloidal e.
      fecal electrolytes
      e. imbalance
      inorganic e.
      protein e.
      serum e.
      stool electrolytes
electrolytes (*pl. of* electrolyte)
electrolytic
      e. capacitor
      e. cell
      e. stripping
electromagnet
electromagnetic
      e. flowmeter (EMF)
      e. pulse (EMP)
      e. radiation
      e. unit (emu)
electrometer amplifier

electromotance
electromotive
      e. force (EMF)
      e. force cell
electron
      Auger e.
      e. beam
      e. capture (EC)
      e. capture detector
      conduction e.
      conversion e.
      free e.
      e. K-capture
      e. lens
      e. lucent granule
      e. micrograph
      e. microprobe
      e. microscope (EM)
      e. microscopy (EM)
      e. multiplier tube
      e. pair
      e. pair bond
      e. paramagnetic resonance
      e. spin resonance (ESR)
      e. transport chain
      e. transport chain complex I–IV
      e. transport inhibitor
      valence e.
      e. volt (eV)
electron-dense
      e.-d. droplet
      e.-d. hump
electronegative
electronegativity
electronic
      e. cell counter
      e. focal spot
      E. Surveillance System for the
      Early Notification of
      Community-based Epidemics
      (ESSENCE)
electron-lucent
      e.-l. fluff
      e.-l. vesicle
electronograph
electronystagmography
electroosmosis
electroosmotic flow
electroparacentesis
electropathology
electropherogram
      capillary electrophoresis e.
electrophile
electrophoresis (EP)
      acid e.
      acrylamide gel e.
      agar gel e.
      agarose gel e.
      alkaline phosphatase isoenzyme e.

capillary e.
capillary zone e. (CE)
cerebrospinal fluid protein e.
citrate agar gel e.
creatine kinase isoenzyme e.
denaturing density gradient e.
  (DDGE)
denaturing gradient gel e.
  (DGGE)
disc e.
DNA gel e.
gel e.
globin-chain e.
gradient gel e.
hemoglobin e.
high-resolution protein e. (HRE)
high-voltage e. (HVE)
IEF gel e.
immunofixation e. (IFE)
isoelectric focusing e.
isoenzyme e.
lipoprotein e. (LPE)
moving-boundary e.
polyacrylamide gel e. (PAGE)
protein e.
pulsed field gel e.
pulsed field gradient gel e.
  (PFGE)
SDS gel e.
serum immunofixation e.
serum protein and immunofixation
  e. (SPIFE)
serum protein e. (SPE, SPEP)
sodium dodecyl
  sulfate-polyacrylamide gel e.
  (SDS-PAGE)
temperature-gradient gel e.
  (TGGE)
temporal temperature gradient gel e.
  (TTGE)
e. test
thin-layer e. (TLE)
thyroxine-binding protein e.
two-dimensional gel e.
two-dimensional polyacrylamide
  gel e.
urine protein e. (UPEP)
zonal e.
zone e.
ElectrophoresisTUTOR
electrophoretic
  e. mobility
  e. mobility shift assay
electrophysiology study
electropositive
electroscope
electrospray (ES)
electrostatic unit (ESU)
electrosynthesis

electrotonic
  e. junction
  e. synapse
electrotransfer test
elegans
  Apophysomyces e.
  Cunninghamella e.
  Granulicatella e.
  Prosthenorchis e.
eleidin
Elek test
element
  anatomical e.
  e. disorder
  extrachromosomal e.
  labile e.
  morphologic e.
  neoplastic e.
  putative peroxisome proliferator
    response e. (PPRE)
  rare earth e.
  sacculotubular e.
  secretory acinar e.
  symmetry e.
  trace e.
  transposable e.
  ultra-trace e.
elementary
  e. body
  e. charge
  e. granule
  e. particle
eleoma
elephantiac, elephantiasic
elephantiasic (*var. of* elephantiac)
elephantiasis
  e. congenita angiomatosa
  congenital e.
  e. neuromatosa
  nevoid e.
  e. nostras
  e. scroti
  e. telangiectodes
  e. verrucosa nostrum
  e. vulva
elephantis
  Mycobacterium e.
elephant leg
Eleutherascus
elfin facies
elicitor
  bacterial lipochitooligosaccharide
    compound e.
elimination
  e. diet
  first-order e.
  immune e.
  e. reaction
  single-breath nitrogen e.

E

elinin
ELISA
  enzyme-linked immunosorbent
    assay
      N-MID osteocalcin ELISA
      ELISA titer assay
ELISPOT enzymatic test
  assay
elite
      Hemoccult Sensa e.
elizabethae
      Bartonella e.
ellipse
ellipsoid
ellipsoidal
elliptical
elliptocyte
elliptocytic anemia
elliptocytosis
      hereditary e. (HE)
      spherocytic hereditary e.
      stomatocytic hereditary e.
Ellis
      E. type 1 glomerulonephritis
      E. types 1, 2 nephritis
Ellis-van Creveld syndrome
Ellsworth-Howard test
ELMS
      epithelioid leiomyosarcoma
elongata
      Tetrasphaera e.
elongated cell
elongation factor
elongatus
      Metastrongylus e.
elongin
elongisporus
      Lodderomyces e.
ELT
      euglobulin lysis time
eluate
Elucigene CF29 analyte-specific reagent
  kit
eluent
elute
elution
      Kleihauer acid e.
      Kleihauer-Betke acid e.
elutriate
elutriation
      counterflow centrifugal e.
elyakovii
      Pseudoalteromonas e.
EM
      ejection murmur
      electron microscope
      electron microscopy
      erythema migrans
      erythrocyte mass

EMA
      epithelial membrane antigen
      EMA antibody
emaciation
emarginate
emargination
EMB
      eosin-methylene blue
      EMB Levine agar
Embadomonas
Embden-Meyerhof pathway
embed
embedding
      e. agent
      e. wax
Embellisia
embolemia
emboli (*pl. of* embolus)
embolic
      e. abscess
      e. aneurysm
      e. gangrene
      e. glomerulonephritis
      e. infarct
embolism
      air e.
      amniotic fluid e.
      arterial e.
      atheroma e.
      atheromatous e.
      bacillary e.
      bland e.
      bone marrow e.
      capillary e.
      cellular e.
      cerebral e.
      cholesterol e.
      chorionic villus e.
      coronary e.
      cotton-fiber e.
      fat e.
      gas e.
      infective e.
      lipid e.
      lymph e.
      lymphogenous e.
      miliary e.
      obturating e.
      oil e.
      plasmodium e.
      pulmonary e. (PE)
      pyemic e.
      retinal e.
      retrograde e.
      riding e.
      saddle e.
      spinal e.
      straddling e.
      systemic air e.

trichinous e.
tumor e.
venous e.
embolization
trophoblastic e.
embolomycotic aneurysm
embolus, *pl.* **emboli**
air e.
amniotic fluid e.
atheromatous e.
bland e.
bone marrow e.
cholesterol emboli
fat e.
foreign body e.
massive e.
recent e.
septic e.
tumor e.
valvular tissue e.
embryo
e. biopsy
cylindrical e.
nodular e.
stunted e.
embryocardia
embryogenesis
embryoid body
embryonal
e. adenoma
e. carcinosarcoma
e. cell carcinoma
e. duct cyst
e. leukemia
e. metaplasia
e. nephroma
e. rest
e. rhabdomyosarcoma (ERMS)
e. teratoma
e. tumor
embryonate
embryonic
e. competence
e. germ cell
e. hemoglobin
e. neural crest
e. sphere
e. spot
e. stem cell
e. tumor
embryoniform
embryonization
embryonum
smegma e.
embryophore
embryotoxicity
EMBT
endocervical mucinous borderline
tumor

EMC
encephalomyocarditis
extraskeletal myxoid chondrosarcoma
EMC virus
EMEC
epithelial-myoepithelial carcinoma
emeiocytosis (*var. of* emiocytosis)
EMEM
Eagle minimum essential medium
emergency
E. Medical Treatment and Labor
Act (EMTALA)
e. response planning guideline
(ERPG)
e. response to terrorism (ERT)
emerging virus
Emericella nidulans
Emericellopsis
emetica
Russula e.
emetine
EMF
electromagnetic flowmeter
electromotive force
endomyocardial fibrosis
erythrocyte maturation factor
EMG
exomphalos, macroglossia, and
gigantism
EMG syndrome
EMH
extramedullary hemopoiesis
emigration
e. of white cells
e. theory
eminence
Doyère e.
median e.
olivary e.
emiocytosis, emeiocytosis
emission
e. line
e. spectroscopy
e. spectrum
thermionic e.
EMIT
enzyme-multiplied immunoassay
technique
emitter
beta e.
Emmens S/L test
EMMM
epidermotropic metastatic malignant
melanoma
**Emmon modification of Sabouraud
dextrose agar**
Emmonsia
E. parva crescens
E. parva parva

E

Emmonsiella capsulata
emmprin
emotional leukocytosis
EMP
  electromagnetic pulse
  extramedullary solitary plasmacytoma
  EMP device
emperipolesis
  megakaryocytic e.
  thymic cell e.
emphraxis
emphysema
  bullous e.
  centriacinar e.
  centrilobular e.
  chronic pulmonary e. (CPE)
  compensatory e.
  congenital lobar e.
  cutaneous e.
  diffuse e.
  endolymphatic e.
  familial e.
  gangrenous e.
  generalized e.
  interstitial e.
  intestinal e.
  obstructive e.
  pink puffer e.
  pulmonary interstitial e. (PIE)
  subcutaneous e.
  surgical e.
  vesicular e.
emphysematosa
  colpohyperplasia e.
  vaginitis e.
emphysematous
  e. asthma
  e. bleb
  e. cholecystitis
  e. gangrene
  e. phlegmon
  e. vaginitis
empirical
emprosthotonos, emprosthotonus
emprosthotonus (*var. of* emprosthotonos)
empty
  e. marrow
  e. sella
  e. sella syndrome
empyema
  e. articuli
  e. benignum
  latent e.
  loculated e.
  e. necessitatis
  e. of pericardium
  pulsating e.
  subdural e.
empyemic

empyocele
EMS
  eosinophilia-myalgia syndrome
EMTALA
  Emergency Medical Treatment and
    Labor Act
emu
  electromagnetic unit
emulsify fat
emulsion
  bacillary e. (tuberculin) (BE)
EN
  erythema nodosum
en
  e. bloc
  e. face section
  e. grappe
  e. thyrse
ENA
  extractable nuclear antigen
  extractable nuclear antigen antibody
ENaC
  epithelial sodium channel
enamel
  e. cell
  e. crypt
  e. epithelium
  e. fiber
  e. hypoplasia
  interrod e.
  e. layer
  e. membrane
  mottled e.
  e. niche
  e. organ
  e. prism
  e. rod
  e. rod sheath
  e. tuft
enamelin
enamelogenesis imperfecta
enameloid
enamelum
Enamovirus
enanthem, enanthema
enanthema (*var. of* enanthem)
enantiobiosis
enantiomer
enantiomerism
enantiomorph
enantiomorphism
en-bloc stain
encainide
encapsulans
encapsulated
  e. *Bacillus anthracis*
  e. hemoglobin
encapsulation
encapsulatum

encapsuled
enceliitis (*var. of* encelitis)
encelitis, enceliitis
encephalemia
encephalitis
    acute hemorrhagic e.
    acute necrotizing e.
    allergic e.
    arthropod-borne virus e.
    Australian X e.
    bacterial e.
    California e. (CE)
    coxsackievirus e.
    Dawson e.
    Eastern subtype Russian
      spring-summer e.
    epidemic e.
    equine e.
    experimental allergic e.
    Far East Russian e.
    e. hemorrhagica
    herpes simplex virus e. (HSVE)
    hyperergic e.
    Ilhéus e.
    inclusion body e.
    Japanese B e. (JBE)
    e. japonica
    lead e.
    lethargic e.
    e. lethargica
    limbic e.
    Mengo e.
    Murray Valley e. (MVE)
    necrotizing e.
    e. neonatorum
    e. periaxialis concentrica
    postinfectious allergic e.
    postvaccinal e.
    postvaccination allergic e.
    Powassan e.
    purulent e.
    e. pyogenica
    Russian autumn e.
    Russian tick-borne e.
    secondary e.
    St. Louis e. (SLE)
    subacute inclusion body e.
    e. subcorticalis chronica
    suppurative e.
    tick-borne e. (Central European
      subtype)
    tick-borne e. (Eastern subtype)
    varicella e.
    Venezuelan equine e.
    vernal e.
    e. virus
    von Economo e.
    Western e. (WE)
    Western equine e.

    Western subtype Russian
      spring-summer e.
    woodcutter's e.
encephalitogen
encephalitogenic factor (EF)
Encephalitozoon
    E. cuniculi
    E. hellem
    E. intestinale
encephalocele
encephaloclastic microcephaly
encephalocraniocutaneous lipomatosis
encephalocystocele
encephalodysplasia
encephaloid cancer
encephaloma
encephalomalacia
encephalomeningitis
encephalomeningocele
encephalomeningopathy
encephalomyelitis
    acute disseminated e. (ADEM)
    acute necrotizing hemorrhagic e.
    allergic e.
    autoimmune e.
    avian infectious e.
    benign myalgic e.
    Eastern equine e. (EEE)
    enzootic e.
    epidemic myalgic e.
    equine e.
    experimental allergic e. (EAE)
    granulomatous e.
    herpes B e.
    induced allergic e.
    infectious porcine e.
    postinfectious e.
    postvaccination e. (PVEM)
    Venezuelan equine e. (VEE)
    viral e.
    Western e. (WE)
    Western equine e. (WEE)
    zoster e.
encephalomyelocele
encephalomyeloneuropathy
encephalomyelopathy
    carcinomatous e.
    epidemic myalgic e.
    infantile necrotizing e. (INE)
    necrotizing e.
encephalomyeloradiculitis
encephalomyeloradiculopathy
encephalomyocarditis (EMC)
    e. virus
encephalopathia (*var. of* encephalopathy)
    e. addisonia
encephalopathy, encephalopathia
    anoxic e.
    bilirubin e.

E

encephalopathy (*continued*)
Binswanger e.
bovine spongiform e. (BSE)
demyelinating e.
hepatic e.
HIV e.
hypercapnic e.
hypernatremic e.
hypertensive e.
hypoglycemic e.
hypoxic e.
ischemic e.
lead e.
metabolic e.
portal-systemic e. (PSE)
progressive subcortical e.
recurrent e.
saturnine e.
spongiform e.
subacute necrotizing e.
subacute spongiform e.
subcortical arteriosclerotic e.
thyrotoxic e.
transmissible mink e.
transmissible spongiform e. (TSE)
traumatic progressive e.
uremic e.
Wernicke e.
Wernicke-Korsakoff e.
encephalotrigeminal angiomatosis
enchondral
enchondroma
enchondromatosis
enchondromatosum
myxoma e.
enchondromatous
enchondrosarcoma
enclave
encode
encoder
encoding
encopresis
encrustation hypothesis
encysted
e. calculus
e. papillary lesion
e. pleurisy
encystment
end
e. artery
blunt e.
e. bulb
e. cell
e. organ
e. piece
e. plate
e. point
e. product
e. stage

endadelphos
Endamoeba
endangeitis (*var. of* endangiitis)
endangiitis, endangeitis
e. obliterans
endaortitis, endoaortitis
bacterial e.
endarterectomy
carotid e.
endarteritis, endoarteritis
bacterial e.
e. deformans
e. obliterans
obliterating e.
obliterative e.
e. proliferans
proliferating e.
end-brush
end-bulb
endemia
endemic
e. Burkitt lymphoma (eBL)
e. colic
e. disease
e. fluorosis
e. funiculitis
e. goiter
e. hemoptysis
e. hypertrophy
e. index
e. murine typhus
e. nonbacterial infantile
gastroenteritis
e. syphilis
e. typhus
endemicum
granuloma e.
endemicus
Clonorchis e.
endemoepidemic
endergonic reaction
endermosis
end-feet
ending
annulospiral e.
caliciform e.
epilemmal e.
flower-spray e.
free nerve e.
grape e.
hederiform e.
intraneural nerve e.
nerve e. (NE)
sole-plate e.
synaptic e.
Endo agar
endoamylase
endoaortitis (*var. of* endaortitis)
endoappendicitis

endoarteritis (*var. of* endarteritis)
Endobacteria
endobiotic
endobioticum
    Synchytrium e.
endobody
endobronchial
    e. tuberculosis
    e. tumor
endocardiac (*var. of* endocardial)
endocardial, endocardiac
    e. cushion defect
    e. fibroelastosis (EFE)
    e. plaque
    e. sclerosis
endocarditic
endocarditis
    abacterial thrombotic e.
    acute bacterial e.
    acute infective e.
    atypical verrucous e.
    bacteria-free stage of bacterial e.
    bacterial e. (BE)
    cachectic e.
    Candida e.
    e. chordalis
    constrictive e.
    Eubacterium e.
    infectious e.
    infective e.
    isolated parietal e.
    Libman-Sacks e.
    Löffler e.
    malignant e.
    marantic e.
    mural e.
    nonbacterial thrombotic e. (NBTE)
    nonbacterial verrucous e.
    polypous e.
    Q fever e.
    rheumatic e.
    septic e.
    Streptococcus e.
    subacute bacterial e. (SBE)
    subacute infective e.
    terminal e.
    thrombotic nonbacterial e.
    valvular e.
    vegetative e.
    verrucal atypical e.
    verrucal nonbacterial e.
    verrucous e.
endocardium
endocellular complement
endocervical
    e. cancer
    e. carcinoma
    e. cell
    e. curettage (ECC)

    e. glandular dysplasia (EGD)
    e. mucinous borderline tumor (EMBT)
    e. smear
endocervicitis
endocervicosis
endocervix
    vagina, ectocervix, e. (VCE)
endochondral
    e. bone
    e. ossification
endochondromatosis
    multiple e.
endochondromatous myxoma
Endoconidiophora
endocrinae
    glandulae e.
endocrine
    e. adenomatosis
    e. cell
    e. disease
    e. ductal carcinoma in situ
     (E-DCIS)
    familial multiple e.
    e. gland
    e. granule
    e. granule constituent (EGC)
    e. marker
    e. myopathy
    e. phenotype
    e. polyglandular syndrome
endocrinoma
    multiple e.
endocrinopathy
    multiple e.
endocyst
endocystitis
endocytosis
    receptor-mediated e.
endocytotically active
endodeoxyribonuclease
endodermal, endodermic
    e. cell
    e. pharyngeal pouch
    e. sinus tumor
endodermic (*var. of* endodermal)
Endodermophyton
endodyocyte
endodyogeny
endoenteritis
endoenzyme
endoesophagitis
endogamous
endogamy
endogastritis
endogenic (*var. of* endogenous)
endogenote
endogenous, endogenic
    e. aneurysm
    e. antigen

E

endogenous (*continued*)
    e. antigen cell-bound antibody reaction
    e. antigen-circulating antibody reaction
    e. antigen-transferred cell-bound antibody reaction
    e. antioxidant enzyme
    e. avidin-binding activity (EABA)
    e. bacterium
    e. creatinine clearance
    e. fecal calcium (EFC)
    e. hemosiderosis
    e. hyperglyceridemia
    e. hyperlipidemia (EHL)
    e. infection
    e. peroxidase
    e. pigments and deposits
    e. pneumoconiosis
    e. synthesis
    e. variable
endoglobular
endointoxication
Endolimax nana
endolymph
endolympha
endolymphatic
    e. duct
    e. dye
    e. emphysema
    e. hydrops
    e. stromal myosis
endolymphaticus
    ductus e.
endolymphic
endomerogony
endometrial
    e. adenocarcinoma
    e. atrophy
    e. biopsy
    e. blood supply
    e. brush
    e. carcinoma
    e. carcinoma in situ (ECIS)
    e. cast
    e. cavity
    e. cell
    e. curettage
    e. cyst
    e. cytology
    e. functionalis
    e. gestational alteration
    e. hyperplasia
    e. intraepithelial carcinoma (EIC)
    e. polyp
    e. smear
    e. stromal nodule (ESN)
    e. stromal sarcoma (ESS)
    e. stromatosis

endometrioid
    e. carcinoma
    e. endometrial carcinoma (EEC)
    e. tumor
endometrioma
endometriosis
    hematogenous theory of e.
    lymphatic dissemination theory of e.
    micronodular stromal e.
    stromal e.
    uterine e.
    vesical e.
endometritis
    chronic specific e.
    decidual e.
    e. dissecans
    granulomatous e.
    syncytial e.
endometrium
    e. anaerobic culture
    aspiration of e.
    atrophic e.
    16-day e.
    decidualized e.
    disordered proliferative e.
    FIGO adenocarcinoma of e.
    proliferative e.
    regenerative e.
    secretory e.
    Swiss cheese e.
endomitosis
Endomyces
    E. albicans
    E. capsulatus
    E. epidermidis
    E. geotrichum
Endomycetales
Endomycopsis
endomyocardial
    e. biopsy
    e. fibroelastosis
    e. fibrosis (EMF)
    e. sclerosis
endomyocarditis
endomyometritis
endomysial
    e. antibody
    e. collagen
endomysium
    fibrocyte in e.
endoneurial fibroblast
endoneurium
endonuclease
    restriction e.
endonucleolus
endoparasite
endoparasitism
endopeptidase
    zinc-containing e.

endoperiarteritis
endopericarditis
endoperimyocarditis
endoperitonitis
endoperoxide
    cyclic e.
    prostaglandin e.
endophlebitis
endophthalmitis
endophyte
endophytic
endophyticus
    Bacillus e.
endoplasm
endoplasmic reticulum (ER)
endoplast
endoplastic
endopolygeny
endopolyploidy
endoreduplication
    chromosomal e.
endoreplication
end-organ
    e.-o. damage
    e.-o. effect
endoribonuclease
endorphin
    e. assay
    beta e.
endosalpingiosis
endosalpingitis
endosalpinx
endosarc
endoscopic
    e. autopsy
    e. retrograde
     cholangiopancreatography
    e. ultrasonography
endosmosis
endosome
endosperm
endospore
endostatin
endosteal scalloping
endosteitis, endostitis
endosteoma
endosteum
endostitis (*var. of* endosteitis)
endostoma
endosulfan
endotendineum
endothelia (*pl. of* endothelium)
endothelial
    e. cell
    e. cyst
    e. differentiation
    high e.
    e. immunoglobin family adhesion
     protein

    e. leukocyte
    e. lining of vessel
    e. marker
    e. metaplasia
    e. myeloma
    e. phagocyte
    e. relaxing factor
    e. sarcoma
    e. thromboresistance
    e. tubuloreticular inclusion
endothelial-leukocyte adhesion molecule
  (E-LAM)
endothelin-2
endothelin-3 (ET3)
endothelin-A
    endothelin-A, -B receptor
endothelin-converting enzyme
  (ECE1)
endothelin-1 receptor antagonist
endothelin-receptor-B (ENDRB)
endotheliocyte
endothelioid habit
endotheliolytic serum
endothelioma
endotheliosis
endothelitis
endothelium, *pl.* endothelia
    e. camerae anterioris
    continuous e.
    discontinuous e.
    fenestrated e.
    e. of anterior chamber
endothelium-derived relaxing factor
endothermic
Endothia
endothrix
endotoxemia
    gram-negative e.
endotoxicosis
endotoxic shock
endotoxin
    e. activity assay (EAA)
    e. shock
endotracheal
    e. insufflation
endotrachelitis
endovasculitis
    hemorrhagic e. (HEV)
endovasculopathy
    hemorrhagic e.
endovenitis
end-piece
end-plate (*var. of* endplate)
endplate, end-plate
    motor e.
end-point measurement
end-product repression
ENDRB
    endothelin-receptor-B

E

endrin
endstage (*var. of* end stage)
end-systolic pressure (ESP)
end-tidal CO_2 tension
endyma
eneae
    Bosea e.
energetics
    biochemical e.
energy
    activation e.
    binding e.
    bond e.
    e. dispersed x-ray analysis
    e. dispersive spectrometer (EDS)
    e. dispersive x-ray microanalysis
    e. dispersive x-ray spectroscopy
      (EDS)
    free e.
    kinetic e. (KE)
    oxidative e.
    potential e.
    radiant e.
    e. resolution
    standard free e.
enflagellation
Engelmann disease
Engel-von Recklinghausen disease
engineering
    biomedical e.
    genetic e.
    human e.
English disease
englobe
englobement
Engman disease
engraftment
    cell e.
engulfment
    cytologic e.
Engyodontium album
enhanced green fluorescent protein
  (EGFP)
enhancement
    autometallographic silver e.
    immunologic e.
    immunological e.
enhancer
enhancing antibody
enhematospore
Enhygromyxa salina
enkephalin
ENL
    erythema nodosum leprosum
enlargement
    cardiac e. (CE)
    diffuse e.
    left atrial e. (LAE)
    left ventricular e. (LVE)

    right atrial e. (RAE)
    right ventricular e. (RVE)
enoeca
    Prevotella e.
enol
enolase
    neuron-specific e.
      (NSA, NSE)
enostosis
enoyl-coenzyme A hydratase
enrichment
    e. culture
    e. medium
ENS
    enteric nervous system
ensheathing callus
Ensifer
    E. arboris
    E. fredii
    E. kostiensis
    E. kummerowiae
    E. medicae
    E. meliloti
    E. saheli
    E. terangae
    E. xinjiangensis
entactin
entamebiasis
Entamoeba
    E. buccalis
    E. buetschlii
    E. chattoni
    E. coli
    E. dispar
    E. gingivalis
    E. hartmanni
    E. histolytica (Eh)
    E. histolytica serological test
    E. kartulisi
    E. moshkovskii
    E. nana
    E. nipponica
    E. polecki
    E. tetragena
    E. tropicalis
    E. undulans
entanii
    Gluconacetobacter e.
enteramine
enterectasis
enterelcosis
enteric
    e. bacillus
    e. cytopathogenic bovine orphan
      (ECBO)
    e. cytopathogenic dog orphan
      (ECDO)
    e. cytopathogenic human orphan
      (ECHO)

e. cytopathogenic monkey orphan (ECMO)
e. cytopathogenic swine orphan (ECSO)
e. helminthic zoonosis
human e. (virus)
e. nervous system (ENS)
e. orphan virus
e. tularemia
enteric-coated (EC)
enteric-type adenocarcinoma
entericus
    Streptococcus e.
enteritidis
    Bacillus e.
    E. salmonella
    Salmonella e.
enteritis
    e. anaphylactica
    bovine e. (BE)
    chronic cicatrizing e.
    diphtheritic e.
    eosinophilic e.
    feline infectious e.
    granulomatous e.
    e. necroticans
    e. of mink
    e. polyposa
    radiation e.
    regional e. (RE)
    staphylococcal e.
    transmissible e.
    typhoid e.
enteroaggregative *Escherichia coli* (EaggEC)
enterobacter
    E. aerogenes
    E. agglomerans
    E. alvei
    E. cloacae
    E. cowanii
    E. gergoviae
    E. hafniae
    E. liquefaciens
    E. pneumonia
    E. sakazakii
    E. subgroup C.
    e. urinary tract infection
Enterobacteriaceae
enterobiasis
Enterobius vermicularis
enterobrosia (*var. of* enterobrosis)
enterobrosis, enterobrosia
enterocele
enterocholecystostomy
enterochromaffin
    e. cell
    e. cell hyperplasia (EC)
    e. staining

enterochromaffin-like cell hyperplasia
enteroclysis
enterococci (*pl. of* enterococcus)
enterococcus, *pl.* **enterococci**
    E.
    E. canis
    E. faecalis
    E. faecium
    E. gilvus
    E. haemoperoxidus
    E. hermanniensis
    E. italicus
    E. moraviensis
    E. pallens
    E. phoeniculicola
    E. porcinus
    E. ratti
    e. urinary tract infection
    vancomycin-resistant *E.*
    E. villorum
enterocolitica
    Yersinia e.
enterocolitis
    acute necrotizing e.
    antibiotic e.
    cicatrizing e.
    diarrheogenic bacterial e.
    Hirschsprung-associated e. (HAEC)
    infectious enterocolitides
    lymphocytic e.
    necrotizing e.
    neonatal necrotizing e.
    pseudomembranous e.
    radiation e.
    regional e.
    Yersinia-related e.
enterocutaneous fistula
enterocyst, enterocystoma
enterocystoma
enterocyte
    rapid antigen uptake into the cytosol enterocytes (RACE)
Enterocytozoon bieneusi
enteroendocrine cell
enteroenteric fistula
enterogastritis
enterogastrone
enterogenous
    e. cyanosis
    e. cyst
    e. methemoglobinemia
enteroglucagon
enterohemorrhagic *Escherichia coli* (EHEC)
enterohepatitis
enteroinvasive *Escherichia coli* (EIEC)
enterokinase
enterolith
enterolithiasis

E

enteromegalia (*var. of* enteromegaly)
enteromegaly, enteromegalia
Enteromonas hominis
enteromycosis
enteronitis
enteropathica
    acrodermatitis e.
enteropathogen
enteropathogenic *Escherichia coli* (EEC, EPEC)
enteropathy
    acrodermatitis e.
    autoimmune e.
    familial e.
    gluten-induced e.
    gluten-sensitive e. (GSE)
    protein-losing e.
    tufting e.
enteropathy-associated T-cell lymphoma
enteropeptidase
enterophila
    Oerskovia e.
enteroptosia (*var. of* enteroptosis)
enteroptosis, enteroptosia
enteroptotic
EnteroScreen 4 single-tube pathogen test
enterosepsis
enterostenosis
enterostomy dysfunction
enterotoxic *Escherichia coli* (ETEC)
enterotoxigenic
    e. bacteria
    e. *Escherichia coli* (ETEC)
enterotoxin
    Clostridium perfringens e.
    Escherichia coli e.
    staphylococcal e.
    staphylococcal e. B (SEB)
enterovaginal fistula
enterovesical fistula
Enterovibrio norvegicus
enteroviral meningitis
enterovirus (EV)
    e. culture
    e. type 71 (EV 71)
enterozoic
enterozoon
enthalpy of reaction
enthesitis
enthesopathic
enthesopathy
enthetic
Entner-Doudoroff pathway
entochoroidea
entocornea
entodermal cell
Entoloma sinuatum
Entomobirnavirus

entomology
Entomophthora coronata
Entomophthorales
entomophthoramycosis, entomophthoromycosis
    e. basidiobolae
    e. conidiobolae
entomophthoromycosis (*var. of* entomophthoramycosis)
Entomoplasmataceae
Entomoplasmatales
entomopox virus
Entomopoxvirus A, B, C
entopic
entoplasm
entoretina
entosarc
entozoal
entozoic
entozoon
entrance wound
entrapment
    e. neuropathy
    tendon e.
    ulnar nerve e.
entropion, entropium
entropium (*var. of* entropion)
entropy
entry
    e. wound
    e. zone
enucleate
enucleation
enumeration
    lymphocyte subset e.
envelope
    cell e.
    cistern of nuclear e.
    corneocyte e.
    elastomer e.
    nuclear e.
    viral e.
envenomation
environment
    a hypotonic e.
    chemical e.
environmental
    e. illness
    E. Protection Agency (EPA)
    e. sample
    e. stress
    e. toxicology
EnVision non-avidin-biotin detection system
envoplakin
    e. antibody
    e. antigen
Enzact
    Pro-PredictRx E.

enzanensis
    Actinokineospora e.
Enzinger tumor classification
enzootic
    e. bovine leukosis
    e. encephalomyelitis
    e. encephalomyelitis virus
    e. infection
enzymatic, enzymic
    e. adaptation
    e. antigen unmasking
    e. digestion
    e. digestion method
    e. fat necrosis
    e. liquidation
    e. poisoning
enzyme
    activating e.
    acyl e.
    adaptive e.
    allosteric e.
    alpha glucan-branching e.
    amino acid-activating e.
    amylolytic e.
    e. analyzer
    angiotensin-converting e. (ACE)
    angiotensin I-converting e.
    e. antagonist
    antitumor e.
    e. assay
    autolytic e.
    bacterial e.
    e. balance
    BamH1 e.
    beta-amyloid protein converting e.
      (BACE)
    beta site APP cleaving e. (BACE)
    brancher e.
    branching e.
    brush border e.
    catabolic e.
    cathepsin D e.
    catheptic e.
    cholinesterase e.
    chymotrypsinogen e.
    citrate condensing e.
    coagulating e.
    constitutive e.
    converting e.
    cryptic e.
    cyclooxygenase e.
    debranching e.
    e. deficiency anemia
    delta-5 desaturase e.
    e. demonstration method
    drug metabolizing e. (DME)
    Eco RI e.
    endogenous antioxidant e.
    endothelin-converting e. (ECE1)

    extracellular matrix-degrading e.
    FADD-like interleukin-1 beta
      converting e. (FLICE)
    fatty acid beta oxidation e.
    fibrinolytic e.
    flippase e.
    glucan-branching e.
    glycogen branching e.
    glycolytic e.
    hydrolytic e.
    immobilized e.
    e. immunochromatography (EIC)
    inducible e.
    e. induction
    e. inhibition
    e. inhibitor (EI)
    inhibitory e.
    inverting e.
    key e.
    lipocortin e.
    lipolytic e.
    lipoxygenase e.
    e. marker
    microsomal e.
    Nagao e.
    poly-ADP-ribose-polymerase e.
    proteolytic e.
    receptor-destroying e. (RDE)
    e. repression
    restriction e.
    SERCA e.
    serum e.
    steatolytic e.
    e. study
    telomerase e.
    terminal addition e.
    topoisomerase II e.
    e. unit (EU)
    urease e.
enzyme-assisted immunoassay technique
enzyme-deficient anemia
enzyme-dependent colorimetric
  technique
enzyme-enhancement immunoassay
enzyme-labeled oligonucleotide
enzyme-linked
    e.-l. antibody test
    e.-l. antiglobulin test (ELAT)
    e.-l. immunosorbent assay (ELISA)
enzyme-multiplied
    e.-m. immunoassay (EIA)
    e.-m. immunoassay technique
      (EMIT)
enzymes/isoenzymes
    cardiac e.
enzymic (*var. of* enzymatic)
    e. fat necrosis
enzymolysis
enzymopathy

Eobacteria
E6-oncoprotein
E7-oncoprotein
eos
eosinophil
eosinophilic leukocyte
eosin
alcohol-soluble e.
e. B, Y
ethyl e.
hematoxylin and e. (H&E)
e. I bluish
e. Y derivative of fluorescein stain
e. yellowish
e. Ys
eosin-methylene blue (EMB)
eosinocyte
Eosinofix reagent
eosinopenia
eosinophil, eosinophile
e. adenoma
e. chemotactic factor
e. chemotactic factor of anaphylaxis
(ECF-A)
e. count
e. granule
e. leukocytic infiltrate
polymorphonuclear e. (PME)
e. protein X (EPX)
e. smear
e. stimulation promoter (ESP)
eosinophile (*var. of* eosinophil)
eosinophilia
angiolymphoid hyperplasia with e.
clonal e.
granulomatous angiitis with e.
nonallergic rhinitis with e.
(NARES)
pulmonary e.
pulmonary infiltration and e. (PIE)
sclerosing mucoepidermoid carcinoma
with e. (SMECE)
simple pulmonary e.
tropical e.
eosinophilia-myalgia syndrome (EMS)
eosinophilic
e. abscess
e. angiocentric fibrosis (EAF)
e. cationic protein (ECP)
e. cell metaplasia
e. cellulitis
e. colitis
e. cystitis
e. cytoplasm
e. endomyocardial disease
e. enteritis
e. esophagitis
e. fasciitis
e. gastritis

e. gastroenteritis (EGE)
e. granularity
e. granule
e. granuloma
e. granuloma of lung
e. granulomatosis
e. hyperplasia
e. index (EI)
e. leukemia
e. leukocyte (eos)
e. leukocytosis
e. leukopenia
e. lung
e. macronucleus
e. marrow
e. meningoencephalitis
e. metamyelocyte
e. myelocyte
e. pneumonia
e. pneumonitis
e. promyelocyte
e. proteinaceous granular material
e. pustular folliculitis
e. viral inclusion body
eosinophilocytic leukemia
eosinophiluria
eosinotactic
eosin-stained microscopic section
EOT
effective oxygen transport
EP
ectopic pregnancy
electrophoresis
EP test
EP toxicity
EPA
eicosapentaenoic acid
Environmental Protection Agency
EPC
epilepsia partialis continua
EPCA-2 prostate cancer test
EPD
extramammary Paget disease
EPE
extraprostatic extension
EPEC
enteropathogenic *Escherichia coli*
ependyma
ependymal
e. cell
e. cyst
e. layer
e. zone
ependymitis
ependymoblastoma
ependymocyte
ependymoma
epithelial e.
grade I-IV e.

malignant e.
myxopapillary e.
Eperythrozoon
EPF
exophthalmos-producing factor
exposed protruding form
ephapse
ephedrine
ephelis
nevi, atrial myxoma, myxoid
neurofibroma, and ephelides
ephemeral fever virus
Ephemerovirus
epi
epiglottis
epinephrine
epiallopregnanolone (EAP)
epiblast
epibole (*var. of* epiboly)
epiboly, epibole
epibulbar
epicanthal fold
epicardial
epicatechin gallate
epichlorohydrin
Epicoccum purpurascens
epicondylitis
lateral e.
medial e.
Epics
E. Altra cell sorting system
E. C flow cytometer
E. Profile flow cytometer
E. XL, XLMCL flow cytometer
system
epicutaneous testing
epicystitis
epicyte
epidemic
e. benign dry pleurisy
e. curve
e. disease
e. dysentery
Electronic Surveillance System for
the Early Notification of
Community-based E.'s (ESSENCE)
e. encephalitis
e. exanthema
e. gastroenteritis virus
e. hemoglobinuria
hemorrhagic fever e.
e. hemorrhagic fever
e. hepatitis
E. Information Exchange (Epi-X)
e. keratoconjunctivitis (EKC)
e. keratoconjunctivitis virus
e. louse-borne typhus
e. myalgia
e. myalgia virus

e. myalgic encephalomyelitis
e. myalgic encephalomyelopathy
e. myositis
e. nausea
e. nonbacterial gastroenteritis
e. parotitides
e. parotitis virus
e. pleurodynia
e. pleurodynia virus
e. polyarthritis
e. roseola
e. tremor
typhus e.
e. vomiting
epidemica
nephropathia e.
epidemicity
epidemiography
epidemiology
hospital e.
molecular e.
E. Program Office (EPO)
epiderm, epiderma
epiderma (*var. of* epiderm)
epidermal, epidermatic
e. dermal nevus
e. growth factor (EGF)
e. growth factor receptor (EGFR)
e. inclusion cyst (EIC)
e. ridge
e. surface antigen
epidermalization, epidermization
epidermal-melanin unit
epidermatic (*var. of* epidermal)
epidermic
e. cell
e. pearl
epidermica
cladosporiosis e.
Saccharomyces e.
epidermic-dermic nevus
epidermides (*pl. of* epidermis)
epidermidis
Endomyces e.
nonpenicillinase-producing
Staphylococcus e.
Staphylococcus e.
stratum basale e.
stratum corneum e.
stratum granulosum e.
stratum spinosum e.
epidermidization of cervix
epidermidosis
epidermis, *pl.* **epidermides**
clear layer of e.
corneal layer of e.
granular layer of e.
horny layer of e.
keratohyalin granule of e.

E

epidermitis
epidermization (*var. of* epidermalization)
epidermodysplasia verruciformis
epidermoid
    e. cancer
    e. carcinoma
    e. carcinoma in situ
    e. inclusion cyst
    e. metaplasia
epidermolysin
epidermolysis
    e. bullosa (EB)
    e. bullosa acquisita
    e. bullosa dystrophica
    e. bullosa lethalis
    e. bullosa simplex
epidermolytic hyperkeratosis
epidermophytid
Epidermophyton
    E. floccosum
    E. inguinale
    E. rubrum
epidermophytosis
epidermosis
epidermotropic metastatic malignant
  melanoma (EMMM)
epidermotropism
epididymal cyst
epididymides (*pl. of* epididymis)
epididymidis (*gen. of* epididymis)
epididymis, *gen.* epididymidis, *pl.*
  epididymides
    coni epididymidis
    duct of e.
    ductus epididymidis
    lobule of e.
    lobuli epididymidis
epididymitis
epididymoorchitis
epidural
    e. abscess
    e. hematoma
    e. meningitis
epifluorescence microscopy
epigastric hernia
epigastrius parasiticus
epigenesis
epigenetics
epigenetic silencing
epigenotype
epiglottiditis, epiglottitis
epiglottis (epi)
epiglottitis (*var. of* epiglottiditis)
epignathus
epihyal bone
epiillumination
epilamellar
epilans
    Trichophyton e.

epilating dose
epilation
epilemma
epilemmal ending
epilepidoma
epilepsia (*var. of* epilepsy)
    e. partialis continua (EPC)
epilepsy, epilepsia
    familial myoclonic e.
    focal cortical e.
    grand mal e.
    jacksonian e.
    minor e.
    myoclonic e.
    posttraumatic e.
    psychomotor e.
    rolandic e.
    sudden unexplained death in e.
      (SUDEP)
    temporal lobe e.
    uncinate e.
epilepticus
    status e.
epileptiform discharge (ED)
epileptogenic, epileptogenous
    e. focus
    e. zone
epileptogenous (*var. of*
  epileptogenic)
epiloia
epimastical fever
epimastigote
epimembranous glomerulonephritis
epimer
epimerase
epimerite
epimerization
epimicroscope
epimorphic regeneration
epimyoepithelial carcinoma
epimysium
epinephrine (epi)
    e. and norepinephrine assays
    ferric chloride reaction of e.
    iodate reaction of e.
    iodine reaction of e.
    urine e.
epinephros
epineurial
epineurium
epionychium
epiotic center
epiphenomenon
epiphenotype
epiphrenic diverticulum
epiphyseal (*var. of* epiphysial)
epiphysial, epiphyseal
    e. arrest
    e. aseptic necrosis

e. giant cell tumor
e. plate
epiphysis
e. cerebri
stippled e.
epiphysitis
epiphyte
epiploic
epiploica
episcleralis
lamina e.
episcleral lamina
episcleritis, episclerotitis
rheumatoid e.
episclerotitis (*var. of* episcleritis)
episialin
episode
mitochondrial encephalopathy, lactic
acidosis, and strokelike e.'s
(MELAS)
transient cerebral ischemic e. (TCIE)
transient ischemic e. (TIE)
episomal
episome
resistance transferring e.
episplenitis
epistasis
epistasy
epistatic
epistaxis
Episthmium caninum
epitaxy
epitendineum
epitenon
epitestosterone
epithalaxia
epithelia (*pl. of* epithelium)
epithelial
e. apoptosis
e. attachment
e. attachment of Gottlieb
e. basement membrane
e. cadherin (E-cadherin)
e. cancer
e. cell disease
e. cell urinary cast
e. choroid layer
e. component
e. differentiation
e. displacement
e. dysplasia
e. ependymoma
e. foot process
e. glycoprotein-2 (EGP-2)
human ovarian surface e. (HOSE)
e. hyperchromasia
e. hyperplasia
e. hyperplastic laryngeal lesion
(EHLL)

e. inclusion cyst
e. lamina
e. marker immunohistochemistry
e. membrane antigen (EMA)
e. neoplasm
e. nest
e. pearl
e. pigment
e. predominant blastoma
renal tubular e. (RTE)
e. rest
e. reticular cell
e. sodium channel (ENaC)
e. thymoma
e. tissue
e. tumor
epithelialis
lamina choroidea e.
epithelialization, epithelization
epithelial-myoepithelial carcinoma
(EMEC)
epithelial-stromal tumor
epitheliitis
epitheliocyte
thymic e.
tumor of thymic e.
epitheliofibril
epithelioglandular
epithelioid
e. cell
e. cell cluster
e. cell melanoma
e. cell nevus
e. hemangioendothelioma (EH, EHE)
e. histiocyte
e. leiomyoma
e. leiomyosarcoma (ELMS)
e. morphology
e. phenotype
e. sarcoma (ES)
e. soft-tissue neoplasm (ESTN)
epitheliolysis
epitheliolytic
epithelioma
e. adenoides cysticum
basal cell e.
benign e.
Borst-Jadassohn type intraepidermal e.
chorionic e.
e. contagiosum
e. cuniculatum
Malherbe calcifying e.
multiple self-healing squamous e.
sebaceous e.
epitheliomatous
epitheliopathy
epithelioserosa
zona e.
epitheliosis

E

epitheliotropism
epithelium, *pl.* **epithelia**
  adenomatous e.
  androgen-normal e.
  e. anterius corneae
  apocrine e.
  Barrett e.
  calicoblastic e.
  carcinomatous e.
  ciliated e.
  coelomic e.
  columnar e.
  crevicular e.
  crypt e.
  cuboidal e.
  cylindrical e.
  dental e.
  distinctive e.
  e. ductus semicircularis
  dysplastic e.
  enamel e.
  foveolar e.
  germinal e.
  gingival e.
  glandular e.
  inner dental e.
  junctional e.
  laminated e.
  e. lentis
  mesenchymal e.
  metaplastic columnar e.
  muscle e.
  neoplastic e.
  odontogenic e.
  e. of lens
  olfactory e.
  oncocytic e.
  pseudostratified columnar e.
  reduced enamel e.
  respiratory e.
  seminiferous e.
  specialized e.
  squamous e.
  sulcular e.
  surface e.
  transitional e.
  vaginal e.
  e. with mitotic figure
epithelization
epitope
  discontinuous e.
  e. mapping
  e. masking
  e. retrieval
  e. unmasking
epitoxoid
epitrichium
epituberculous infiltration
epitype

Epi-X
  Epidemic Information Exchange
epizoic
epizoon
epizootic
  anthrax e.
  e. cellulitis
  e. disease, category A, B
  e. hemorrhagic disease of deer
  e. lymphangitis
epizootica
  lymphangitis e.
EPM
  extraosseous plasmacytoma of the
    mediastinum
EPO
  Epidemiology Program Office
Epon-Araldite resin
Epon tissue-embedding medium
eponychium
epoophori
  tubuli e.
epoophoron
  transverse ductules of e.
e-positive RBCs
epoxide
  heptachlor e.
  e. leukotriene LTA4
  e. reductase
epoxyeicosatrienoic acid
epoxy resin
EPP
  erythropoietic protoporphyria
Eppendorf
  E. 5702 centrifuge
  E. filtertip
  E. MicroChisel
  E. MicroDissector
  E. Repeater Pro pipette
  E. tube
EPS
  exophthalmos-producing substance
Epsilobacteria
epsilon
  e. acid
  e. antigen
  e. clostridial toxin
  e. component
  e. isoform
  e. staphylolysin
Epsilonretrovirus
Epstein
  E. disease
  E. syndrome
Epstein-Barr (EB)
  E.-B. encoded RNA (EBER)
  E.-B. nuclear antigen (EBNA)
  E.-B. virus (EBV)
  E.-B. virus antibody assay

E.-B. virus culture
E.-B. virus-encoded RNA in situ
 hybridization
E.-B. virus serology
epulis cell
EPX
 eosinophil protein X
eq
 equivalent
equal
 bilateral, symmetrical, and e.
 (BSE)
equation
 alveolar air e.
 Arrhenius e.
 Bohr e.
 chemical e.
 Cockcroft-Gault e.
 Eadie-Hofstee e.
 Friedewald e.
 Hanes e.
 Hasselbalch e.
 Henderson-Hasselbalch e.
 Hill e.
 Hüfner e.
 Lineweaver-Burk e.
 Michaelis-Menten e.
 Nernst e.
 Scatchard e.
 Svedberg e.
 van der Waals e.
equational division
equi
 Corynebacterium e.
 Crossiella e.
 Ehrlichia e.
 Lactobacillus e.
 Rhodococcus e.
 Streptococcus e.
equilibration
equilibrium
 chemical e.
 e. constant
 dynamic e.
 radioactive e.
 secular e.
 sedimentation e.
 thermal e.
 thermodynamic e.
 transient e.
equina
 Setaria e.
 Taenia e.
equine
 e. abortion virus
 e. antihuman lymphoblast globulin
 (EAHLG)
 e. antihuman lymphoblast serum
 (EAHLS)

e. arteritis virus
e. coital exanthema virus
e. encephalitis
e. encephalomyelitis
e. encephalomyelitis virus
e. gonadotropin unit (international)
e. infectious anemia
e. infectious anemia virus
e. influenza
e. influenza virus
e. morbillivirus (Hendra virus)
e. rhinopneumonitis (ERP)
e. rhinopneumonitis virus
e. rhinovirus
e. serum hepatitis
e. viral arteritis
equinum
 Fusobacterium e.
 Trichophyton e.
 Trypanosoma e.
equinus
 Rhizopus e.
 Strongylus e.
equiperdum
 Trypanosoma e.
equipment
 eyewash e.
 individual protective e. (IPE)
equipotential line
equivalence, equivalency
 e. point
 e. relation
 e. zone
 zone of e.
equivalency (*var. of* equivalence)
equivalent (eq)
 age e. (AEq)
 lethal e.
 metabolic e. (MET)
 nitrogen e.
 tissue e.
 toxic e.
equorum
 Ascaris e.
equuli
 Actinobacillus e.
ER
 endoplasmic reticulum
 estrogen receptor
Er
 erbium
ERA
 estrogen receptor assay
eradication therapy
Eranko fluorescence stain
erb
 e. A oncogene
 e. B, B-2 oncogene
 e. B protooncogene

E

erb (*continued*)
  E. disease
  E. syndrome
Erb-Charcot disease
ERBF
  effective renal blood flow
Erb-Goldflam disease
erbium (Er)
ERC
  erythropoietin-responsive cell
ERCC2 gene
ERCC3 gene
ERCC4 gene
ERCC5 gene
Erdheim
  E. disease
  E. rest
  E. tumor
Erdheim-Chester disease (ECD)
erectile
  e. myxoma
  e. tissue
Eremascus
Eremomyces langeronii
Eremothecium
ergastoplasm
ERGIC-53 gene product
ergocalciferol
ergoloid mesylate
ergometer
ergonovine provocation test
ergoreceptor activation
ergosterol
ergot
  corn e.
ergothioneine
ergotism
ergotoxine
eriksonii
  Actinomyces e.
  Bifidobacterium e.
erinacei
  Trichophyton e.
  Trichophyton mentagrophytes e.
Erlanger and Gasser peripheral nerve assay
Erlenmeyer
  E. flask
  E. flask deformity
  E. flask-like
ERMS
  embryonal rhabdomyosarcoma
erode
E-rosette test
erosion
erosive
  e. adenomatosis of nipple
  e. aneurysm

  e. cystitis
  e. esophagitis
  e. gastritis
  e. inflammation
eroticum
  curiosum e.
ERP
  effective refractory period
  equine rhinopneumonitis
  estrogen receptor protein
ERPF
  effective renal plasma flow
ERPG
  emergency response planning guideline
Errantivirus
erraticus
  Ornithodoros e.
error
  coincidence e.
  e. detector
  machine e.
  preanalytic e.
  probable e.
  random e.
  e. rate
  standard e. (SE)
  systematic e.
  type I, II e.
ERRT
  extrarenal rhabdoid tumor
ERT
  emergency response to terrorism
ER-Tracker blue-white DPX
eruption
  bullous e.
  creeping e.
  Kaposi varicelliform e.
  macular e.
  maculopapular e.
  polymorphic light e.
  polymorphous e.
  varicelliform e.
eruptione
  variola sine e.
eruptive fever
Erwinia
  E. amylovora
  E. herbicola
  E. papayae
Erwinieae
erysipelas
erysipeloid
Erysipelothrix
  E. inopinata
  E. insidiosa
  E. rhusiopathiae
Erysipelotrichaceae
Erysiphe graminis

erythema
  e. ab igne
  e. annulare centrifugum
  e. chronicum migrans (ECM)
  e. dose
  dusky e.
  e. dyschromicum perstans
  e. elevatum diutinum
  e. exfoliativa
  figurate e.
  e. figuratum
  gyrate e.
  e. gyratum repens
  e. induratum
  e. infectiosum
  e. iris
  e. keratodes
  macular e.
  e. marginatum
  e. marginatum rheumaticum
  e. migrans (EM)
  mottled e.
  e. multiforme
  e. multiforme bullosum
  e. multiforme exudativum
  necrolytic migratory e.
  e. neonatorum
  e. nodosum (EN)
  e. nodosum leprosum (ENL)
  Osler e.
  e. pernio
  e. perstans
  e. polymorphe
  toxic e.
  e. toxicum
erythematosum
  anetoderma e.
  eczema e.
erythematosus
  acute disseminated lupus e.
  chronic discoid lupus e.
  discoid lupus e. (DLE)
  disseminated acute lupus e.
  lupus e. (LE)
  systemic lupus e. (SLE)
erythrasma
erythremia
erythremic myelosis
erythrinae
  Samsonia e.
erythritol
Erythrobacillus
Erythrobacter
  E. citreus
  E. flavus
  E. longus
Erythrobasidium
erythroblast
  basophilic e.

  definitive e.
  polychromatophilic e.
  primitive e.
erythroblastemia
erythroblastic
  e. anemia
  e. island
erythroblastoma
erythroblastomatosis
erythroblastopenia
erythroblastosis
  fetal e.
  e. fetalis
  e. neonatorum
erythroblastotic
erythrocatalysis
erythrochromia
erythroclasis
erythroclast
erythroclastic
erythrocuprein
erythrocytapheresis
erythrocyte (E)
  e. adherence phenomenon
  e. adherence test
  e. antibody (EA)
  e. antibody complement (EAC)
  e. antibody complement rosette
   assay
  e. antigen
  e. aspartate aminotransferase activity
   (eAST)
  e. count
  dichromatic e.
  dysmorphic e.
  e. fragility
  e. fragility test
  e. glutamic oxaloacetic transaminase
   (EGOT)
  hypochromic microcytic e.
  e. in capillary
  e. indices
  e. mass (EM)
  e. maturation factor (EMF)
  e. membrane
  microcytic e.
  normocytic e.
  e. protoporphyrin test
  reticulated e.
  e. rosette
  e. sedimentation
  e. sedimentation rate (ESR)
  e. sedimentation rate assay
  sickled e.
  e. transketolase
  e. zinc protoporphyrin
erythrocyte-sensitizing substance
(ESS)
erythrocythemia

E

erythrocytic
  e. blood cell
  e. marrow
  e. series
erythrocytoblast
erythrocytolysin
erythrocytolysis
erythrocytometer
erythrocytometry
erythrocytopenia
erythrocytophagy
erythrocytopoiesis
erythrocytorrhexis
erythrocytoschisis
erythrocytosis
  absolute e.
  leukemic e.
  e. megalosplenica
  relative e.
  stress e.
erythrocyturia
erythrodegenerative
erythroderma, erythrodermia
  e. exfoliativa
  Sézary e.
erythrodermia (*var. of* erythroderma)
erythrodextrin
erythrodysesthesia syndrome
erythrogenesis imperfecta
erythrogenic toxin
erythroglutinin
erythrogonium
erythrohepatic porphyria
erythroid
  e. aplasia
  e. colony assay
  e. hyperplasia
  e. hypoplasia
  e. leukemia
  e. precursor
  e. precursor cell
erythroidine
  beta e.
erythrokeratodermia variabilis
erythrokinase (EK)
erythrokinetics
erythrokinetic study
erythroleukemia
  acute e. (M6)
erythroleukosis
erythrolysin
erythrolysis
erythromelalgia
erythromelia
erythromyeloblastic leukemia
erythron
erythroneocytosis
erythropenia
erythrophage

erythrophagia
erythrophagocytosis
erythrophil
erythrophilic
erythrophobic
erythrophore
erythroplakia
erythroplasia of Queyrat
erythropoiesis
  extramedullary e.
  increased e.
  ineffective e.
  megaloblastic e.
erythropoietic
  e. coproporphyria (ECP)
  e. hormone
  e. porphyria
  e. porphyrin
  e. protoporphyria (EPP)
erythropoietic-stimulating factor
  (ESF)
erythropoietin (Epo)
  inappropriate production of e.
  recombinant e.
  e. test
erythropoietin-responsive cell (ERC)
erythropyknosis
erythrorrhexis
erythrose
erythrosin B
Erythrovirus
Erythroxylon coca
erythruria
ES
  electrospray
  epithelioid sarcoma
  Ewing sarcoma
Esbach reagent
escape
  e. mask
  e. mutant
ES300-Cardiac T ELISA troponin T
  immunoassay system
eschar
  localized black e.
escharotica
  dermatitis e.
Escherich bacillus
Escherichia
  E. adecarboxylata
  E. albertii
  E. aurescens
  E. blattae
  E. coli
  E. coli enterotoxin
  E. coli 0157:h7
  E. coli pneumonia
  E. coli urinary tract infection
  E. fergusonii

E. hermanii
E. vulneris
Escherichieae
escomelis
    Trypanosoma e.
esculenta
    Gyromitra e.
    Helvella e.
esculin hydrolysis test
E-selectin
ESF
    erythropoietic-stimulating factor
ES-FISH
    extra signal FISH
ESFT
    Ewing sarcoma family of tumors
ESN
    endometrial stromal nodule
esodic
esoethmoiditis
esogastritis
esophageae
    glandulae e.
esophageal
    e. achalasia
    e. acid infusion test
    e. aperistalsis
    e. apudoma
    e. atresia
    e. carcinoma
    e. dysmotility
    e. gland
    e. gland proper
    e. hernia
    e. hypomotility
    e. motility study
    e. perforation
    e. reflux
    e. ring
    e. rupture
    e. smear
    e. spasm
    e. stricture
    e. tumor
    e. varices
    e. web
esophagectasia, esophagectasis
esophagectasis (*var. of* esophagectasia)
esophagi (*pl. of* esophagus)
esophagitis
    Candida e.
    corrosive e.
    cytomegalovirus e.
    eosinophilic e.
    erosive e.
    fungal e.
    herpes e.
    infectious e.
    irradiation e.

monilial e.
pill e.
pill-induced e.
reflux e.
esophagogastric junction
esophagogastritis
esophagomalacia
esophagomycosis
esophagoptosia (*var. of* esophagoptosis)
esophagoptosis, esophagoptosia
esophagosalivary reflex
esophagostenosis
esophagostomiasis
esophagus, *pl.* **esophagi**
    Barrett e.
    cardiac gland of e.
    e. communicate
    tunica mucosa esophagi
    tunica muscularis esophagi
esosphenoiditis
ESP
    Early Surveillance Project
    end-systolic pressure
    eosinophil stimulation promoter
    ESP II system
espundia
ESRA-10 erythrocyte sedimentation rate analyzer
ESR
    electron spin resonance
    erythrocyte sedimentation rate
    ESR assay
ESR-Auto Plus sedimentation rate analyzer
ESR-Chex hematology control
ESS
    endometrial stromal sarcoma
    erythrocyte-sensitizing substance
ESSENCE
    Electronic Surveillance System for the Early Notification of Community-based Epidemics
essential
    e. albuminuria
    e. asthma
    e. atrophy
    e. fatty acid (EFA)
    e. fever
    e. fructosuria
    e. hematuria
    e. hypercholesterolemia
    e. hyperlipidemia
    e. hypertension (EH)
    e. macroglobulinemia
    e. monoclonal gammopathy
    e. oil
    e. pentosuria
    e. telangiectasia
    e. thrombocythemia (ET)

E

essential (*continued*)
   e. thrombocytopenia
   e. thrombocytosis
established
   e. cell line
   e. extraprostatic extension
   (E-EPE)
ester
   acridinium e.
   cholesterol e. (ChE)
   Cori e.
   fatty acid methyl e. (FAME)
   hexosephosphoric e.'s
   nonfluorescent acetoxymethyl e.
   tetra-methylrhodamine ethyl e.
esterase
   alpha-naphthyl acetate e.
   (ANAE)
   Cl e.
   chloracetate e.
   chloroacetate e. (CAE)
   cholesterol e.
   leukocyte e.
   naphthol-AS-D-chloracetate e.
   (NASDCE)
   neuron-specific e. (NSE)
   neuropathy target e. (NTE)
   nonspecific e. (NSE)
   e. staining method
   e. test
   urine leukocyte e.
esterification
estetrol (E$_4$)
esthesioneuroblastoma
   olfactory e.
esthesioneurocytoma
esthiomene
esthiomenous
estimate
   biased e.
   consistent e.
   dose e.
   interval e.
   median unbiased e.
   point e.
   pooled e.
   standard error of e. (SEE)
   unbiased e.
estimated
   e. blood loss (EBL)
   e. hepatic blood flow (EHBF)
Estlander flap
ESTN
   epithelioid soft-tissue neoplasm
estradiol (E$_2$)
   e. assay
   e. benzoate (EB)
   e. benzoate unit (international)
   17 beta e.

   e. receptor
   e. test
Estren-Dameshek anemia
estriol (E$_3$)
   e. assay
   conjugated e.
   free e.
   maternal urine e.
   serum e.
   total e.
   unconjugated e.
   urinary e.
   urine placental e.
estrogen
   plant e.
   e. receptor (ER)
   e. receptor alpha
   e. receptor assay (ERA)
   e. receptor beta
   e. receptor MRNA
   e. receptor protein (ERP)
   e. stimulation test
   total e. (excretion)
   total urine e.
   urine total e.
   e. withdrawal bleeding (EWB)
estrogenic hormone
estrogen-receptor antigen
estrone (E$_1$)
   e. unit (international)
estunensis
   Acetobacter e.
ESU
   electrostatic unit
ET
   effective temperature
   endotoxin
   essential thrombocythemia
   etiology
   exchange transfusion
ET3
   endothelin-3
eta
   e. cell
   e. isoform
état mamelonné
ETEC
   enterotoxic *Escherichia coli*
   enterotoxigenic *Escherichia coli*
ethacrynic acid (ECA)
ethambutol
ethane
ethanedial
ethanedinitrile
ethanoic acid
ethanol
   e. assay
   e. gelation test
   e. level

ethanolamine
    arachidonic containing
      phosphatidyl e.
ethchlorvynol assay
ethene
ether
    bischloromethyl e.
    dimethyl e.
    ethyl e.
    e. storage
ethidium
    e. bromide
    e. bromide stain
ethiodized oil
ethion
ethionamide
ethionine
ethmoid
ethmoidal
    e. cell
    e. sinus
ethmoidalia
    antra e.
ethmoidalis
    cellulae ethmoidales
    fovea e.
    lamina cribrosa ossis e.
    sinus ethmoidales
ethmoiditis
ethosuximide assay
ethoxazene hydrochloride
ethyl
    e. acetate
    e. alcohol (EtOH,
      ETOH)
    e. alcohol poisoning
    e. cyanide
    e. eosin
    e. ether
    e. green
    e. orange
    e. violet azide broth
ethylbromoacetate grenade
ethylcarbazole
    e. amino 9
ethylcocaine
ethyldichloroarsine
ethylene
    e. chlorohydrin
    e. dibromide
    e. dichloride
    e. glycol
    e. glycol assay
    e. glycol dinitrate
    e. glycol intoxication
    e. glycol poisoning
    e. glycol tetraacetic acid (EGTA)
    e. oxide
    e. tetraacetic acid

ethylenediaminetetraacetate
ethylenediaminetetraacetic
    e. acid (EDTA)
    calcium e. (Ca-EDTA)
ethylidene dichloride
ethylphosphonofluoridate
    NATO code for nerve agent
      isopropyl e. (GE)
ethylphosphonothioate
    NATO code for nerve agent O-ethyl
      S-[2-(diethylamino)ethyl] e. (VE)
ethyne
etiocholanolone
etiol
    etiology
etiologic, etiological
    e. agent
    e. factor
etiological (*var. of* etiologic)
etiology (ET, etiol)
    common viral e.
    genetic e.
    idiopathic e.
    pyrexia of unknown e.
      (PUE)
    unknown e.
    villitis of unknown e. (VUE)
etiopathogenic factor
ETOH, EtOH
    ethyl alcohol
etorphine
EU
    Ehrlich unit
    enzyme unit
eubacteria
Eubacteriales
Eubacterieae
Eubacteriineae
Eubacterium
    E. aerofaciens
    E. aggregans
    E. alactolyticum
    E. combesi
    E. contortum
    E. crispatum
    E. endocarditis
    E. filamentosum
    E. lentum
    E. limosum
    E. minutum
    E. moniliforme
    E. parvum
    E. poeciloides
    E. pseudotortuosum
    E. pyruvativorans
    E. quartum
    E. quintum
    E. rectale
    E. tenue

E

Eubacterium (*continued*)
    E. *tortuosum*
    E. *ventriosum*
eucalyptus oil
eucapnia
Eucaryotae (*var. of* Eukaryotae)
eucaryote (*var. of* eukaryote)
eucaryotic (*var. of* eukaryotic)
Eucestoda
eucholia
euchromatic
Eucoleus
Euflagellata
Euglena
    E. *gracilis*
    E. *viridis*
Euglenidae
euglenoid movement
euglobin lysis time
euglobulin
    e. clot lysis
    e. clot lysis time
      (ECLT)
    e. clot test (ECT)
    e. lysis test
    e. lysis time (ELT)
euglycemia
euglycemic
eugnosia
eugonic
Eugregarinida
eukaryon
eukaryosis
eukaryotae, eucaryotae
eukaryote, eucaryote
eukaryotic, eucaryotic
    e. cell cycle
eukeratin
Eulenburg disease
eumelanin
eumelanosome
eumetria
eumorphism
eumycetes
Eumycetozoea
eumycotic mycetoma
eunuchoid
eunuchoidism
    hypogonadotropic e.
euosmia
euparal
Euparyphium
Eupenicillium
euplasia
euplastic lymph
euploid
euploid-polyploid pattern
euploidy
eupraxia

Euproctis chrysorrhoea
Eurasina
europaeiscabiei
    Streptomyces e.
europaeus
    Ulex e. (UE)
European
    E. blastomycosis
    E. hookworm
    E. rat flea
europium
Eurotium malignum
Euryarchaeota
eurystrepta
    Spirochaeta e.
eurytherma
    Amycolatopsis e.
eurythermal
Eurythermea
Eurytrema pancreaticum
euscope
Eusimulium
eustachian
    e. tonsil
    e. tube
eustachiana, eustachii
    tuba e.
eustachii (*var. of* eustachiana)
Eustoma rotundatum **parasitic worm**
Eustrongylides
Eustrongylus
eutectic temperature
euthyroidism
euthyroid sick state
eutonic
Eutriatoma
Eutrombicula alfreddugesi
eutropha
    Nitrosomonas e.
    Wautersia e.
eutrophic
euvolemic
    e. hypotonic hyponatremia
    e. volume
eV
    electron volt
EV
    extravascular
EVAC
    evacuation
evacuation (EVAC)
evagination
evaluation
    Acute Physiology and
      Chronic Health E.
      (APACHE)
    forensic e.
    hormonal e.

pneumonectomy e.
tilt table e.

Evans
E. blue
E. syndrome

evansi
Trypanosoma e.

evaporation

event
agroterrorist e.
late e.
low probability, high consequence e.
(LPHC)
sentinel e.

eventration of diaphragm

eversion

EVG
elastica van Gieson

evidence
e. gathering process
short-lived e.

evil
king's e.

evisceration

evisceroneurotomy

evocative testing

evolutus
Streptococcus e.

EWB
estrogen withdrawal bleeding

Ewing
E. sarcoma (ES)
E. sarcoma family of tumors
(ESFT)
E. sarcoma gene
E. sarcoma/peripheral
neuroectodermal tumor
E. sarcoma/primitive neuroectodermal
tumor

Ewingella

EWL
egg-white lysozyme

EWS-WT1 chimeric transcript

EX
exophthalmos
extract
extraction

ex
exophthalmos
e. vivo
e. vivo platelet clumping

**ExacTech blood glucose meter
test**

exam (*var. of* examination)

examination, exam
bile fluid e.
cytologic e.
dark-field e.
digital rectal e. (DRE)

direct wet mount e.
double-contrast e.
duodenal contents e.
fecal e.
full blood e. (FBE)
gastric residue e.
national e.
ova and parasite e.
pleural fluid e.
postmortem e.
semen e.
sputum e.
stool e.
synovial fluid e.

examiner
Diplomate of the National Board of
Medical E.'s
medical e.

exanthem (*var. of* exanthema)

exanthema, exanthem
Boston e.
epidemic e.
e. subitum
vesicular e.

exanthematous
e. disease
e. fever
e. inflammation

exanthesis arthrosia

excavatio
e. disci
e. papilla
e. papillae

excavation

excavatum
congenital pectus e.

excess (XS)
antibody e.
antigen e.
base e. (BE)
negative base e.

excessive
e. cornification
e. fatigue
e. heat production (EHP)
e. weakness
e. weight gain

exchange
bidirectional information e.
Epidemic Information E. (Epi-X)
fetomaternal molecular e.
gas e.
e. pairing
plasma e.
therapeutic plasma e.
e. transfusion (ET)

exchangeable
e. mass
e. sodium

E

exchanger
    anion e. 1 (AE1)
    organic
      anion-dicarboxylate/tricarboxylate e.
    organic anion-X e.
excipient
excision
    marginal e. (ME)
excisional biopsy
excitation spectrum
excitatory effect
excited
    e. delirium
    e. skin syndrome
    e. state
exciter filter
excitomotor
excitotoxin protein
exclusion
    allelic e.
    confidential unit e. (CUE)
    steric e.
exconjugant
excoriation
excrescence
    Lambl e.
    mesothelial/monocytic incidental
      cardiac e. (MICE)
    polypoid e.
excretion
    pseudouridine e.
excretorius
    ductus e.
excretory
    e. duct
    e. duct of seminal vesicle
    e. duct of sweat
    e. gland
    e. portion
    e. urogram (XU)
excurrent duct system
excystation
execute
execution time
exencephalia (*var. of* exencephaly)
exencephalic, exencephalous
exencephalocele
exencephalous (*var. of* exencephalic)
exencephaly, exencephalia
exenteration
exenteritis
exercise
    e. hyperemia blood flow
    (EHBF)
    e. intolerance
exercise-induced
    e.-i. asthma
exergonic reaction
exflagellation

exfoliatin
exfoliation
exfoliativa
    dermatitis e.
    erythema e.
    erythroderma e.
    keratolysis e.
exfoliative
    e. cytodiagnosis
    e. cytologic alteration
    e. cytology
    e. dermatitis
    e. gastritis
    e. psoriasis
exhalans
    Nocardiopsis e.
exhaust
    slot e.
exhaustion
    e. atrophy
    secretory e.
exhumation
Exidia
exigua
    Slackia e.
Exiguobacterium
    E. antarcticum
    E. undae
existence proof
exit
    e. access
    e. discharge
    e. dose
    e. wound
exiting projectile
exoantigen test
Exobasidium
exocellular
exocervix
exochorial pregnancy
exocrine
    e. cell
    e. gland
    e. pancreas
    e. phenotype
exocytosis
exodus
exoenzyme
exoerythrocytic plasmodium
Exoflagellata
exogamy
exogenetic
exogenote
exogenous
    e. aneurysm
    e. anticoagulant coagulation
    e. antigen
    e. antigen cell-bound antibody
      reaction

e. antigen-circulating antibody
reaction
e. bacterium
e. creatinine clearance
e. creatinine clinoscope
e. growth factor
e. hemochromatosis
e. hemosiderosis
e. hyperglyceridemia
e. infection
e. lipid pneumonia
e. obesity
e. pigmentation
e. variable
exomphalos, macroglossia, and gigantism (EMG)
exon
exonuclease
exopeptidase
Exophiala
E. jeanselmei
E. mycetoma
E. pisciphila
E. werneckii
exophthalmica
cachexia e.
exophthalmic goiter
exophthalmos (ex), exophthalmus
exophthalmos-hyperthyroid factor (EHF)
exophthalmos-producing
e.-p. factor (EPF)
e.-p. substance (EPS)
exophthalmus (*var. of* exophthalmos)
exophyte
exophytic
e. growth
e. papilla
exoplasm
exoribonuclease
exoskeleton
exosmosis
exosome
exospore
Exosporina
exosporium
exostoses (*pl. of* exostosis)
exostosis, *pl.* **exostoses**
e. bursata
e. cartilaginea
chondromatous e.
diaphysial juxtaepiphysial e.
hereditary multiple exostoses
ivory e.
multiple e.
osteocartilaginous e.
exotaxin/CCL11 gene
exothermic
exotoxic

exotropia
expander
plasma volume e.
expansa
Moniezia e.
expansion
clonal e.
volume e.
ExPEC
extraintestinal pathogenic *Escherichia coli*
expected date of confinement (EDC)
expectoration
prune juice e.
experiment
control e.
double-blind e.
double-masked e.
experimental
e. allergic encephalitis
e. allergic encephalomyelitis (EAE)
e. allergic neuritis (EAN)
e. autoimmune glomerulonephritis (EAG)
e. pathology
explant
explantation
explode
exploding crypt cell
explosion
depleted uranium-containing e.
explosion-proof
explosive
e. atmosphere
chemical, biological, radiological, nuclear, e. (CBRNE)
high e.
e. limit
low e.
e. material
Expo 32 flow cytometry software
exponent
hydrogen e.
exponential
e. decay
e. function
e. phase
exposed protruding form (EPF)
exposure
neutron e.
ExpressDetect technology
expressed RNA
expression
active protein e.
calretinin e.
CEACAM1 e.
constitutive e.
cytokeratin e.
FMC7 e.

E

expression (*continued*)
    gene e.
    hNIS gene e.
    inhibin e.
    latent membrane protein-1 e.
    MUC4 e.
    myoid marker e.
    oncogene e.
    p57 KIP^2 e.
    podoplanin e.
    profile of gene e.
    reduced Fhit protein e.
    serial analysis of gene e. (SAGE)
    serological expression of cDNA e.
     (SEREX)
    surface e.
    survivin e.
    total protein e.
    TRK-A gene e.
    underphosphorylated protein e.
    e. vector
expressivity
exsanguinate
exsanguination
exsanguine
Exserohilum longirostratum
exsiccant
exsiccate
exsiccated sodium sulfite
exsiccation
exsiccosis
exstrophy
    cloacal e.
    e. of the bladder
    e. of the cloaca
extended insulin zinc suspension
extension
    cytoplasmic e.
    established extraprostatic e.
     (E-EPE)
    extraprostatic e. (EPE)
    focal extraprostatic e. (F-EPE)
extensive
    e. accumulation
    e. intraductal component (EIC)
    e. regression
extensum
    hemangioma planum e.
externa
    hematorrhachis e.
    hepatitis e.
    muscularis e.
    otitis e.
    pachymeningitis e.
    theca e.
    tunica e.
external
    e. decontamination
    e. elastic lamellae

    e. elastic lamina
    e. fistula
    e. hemorrhoid
    e. irradiation
    e. meningitis
    e. pillar cell
    e. pudendal vein
    e. pyocephalus
    e. pyramidal layer
    e. root sheath
    e. spiral sulcus
    e. storage
externum
externus
    sulcus spiralis e.
exteroceptor
extima
    tunica e.
extinction coefficient
extinguishing
extra
    e. electron density
    e. signal FISH (ES-FISH)
extraabdominal
    e. desmoid
    e. fibromatosis
extracapillary lesion (ECL)
extracapsular
    e. ankylosis
    e. tumor
extracellular (EC)
    e. aggregate alteration lipid
    e. ATP
    e. cholesterolosis
    e. fibril alteration
    e. fluid (ECF)
    e. fluid volume (ECFV, EFV)
    e. granule
    e. ground substance
    e. in distribution
    e. lipid aggregate
    e. macromolecule aggregate
    e. material (ECM)
    e. matrix (ECM)
    e. matrix alteration
    e. matrix-degrading enzyme
    e. matrix glycoprotein
    e. matrix protein
    e. parasite
    e. plasma
    e. structural alteration
    e. superoxide dismutase
     (EC-SOD)
    e. tachyzoite
    e. toxin
    e. vacuole
    e. volume (ECV)
    e. water (ECW)
extrachorial placentation

extrachromosomal
    e. element
    e. inheritance
extracorporeal
    e. membrane oxygenation (ECMO)
    e. photophoresis
    e. photophoresis technique
extracorpuscular
extract
    adipose tissue e.
    adrenocortical e. (ACE)
    allergenic e.
    allergic e.
    anterior pituitary e. (APE)
    Buchner e.
    ceanothus e.
    lipopolysaccharide e.
    pollen e.
    streptomycin assay agar with yeast
    e.
    whole ragweed e. (WRE)
extractable
    e. nuclear antigen (ENA)
    e. nuclear antigen antibody (ENA)
extraction
    Baker pyridine e.
    e. coefficient
    countercurrent e.
    differential e.
    e. fraction (E)
    Gibco-BRL TriZol DNA e.
    guanidinium e.
    solvent e.
    testicular sperm e. (TESE)
Extract-N-Amp Blood PCR kit
extractor
    RNAzol Reagent E.
extracystic
extradural hematorrhachis
extraembryonic mesoblast
extrafollicular colloid
extrafusal muscle fiber
extraglomerular mesangium
extragonadal germ cell tumor
extrahepatic
    e. biliary atresia (EHBA)
    e. obstruction (EHO)
extraintestinal
    e. manifestation
    e. pathogenic *Escherichia coli*
    (ExPEC)
extralobar sequestration
extramammary Paget disease (EPD)
extramedullary
    e. erythropoiesis
    e. hemopoiesis (EMH)
    e. myelogenous leukemia
    e. myelopoiesis
    e. solitary plasmacytoma (EMP)

extramembranous glomerulonephritis
extramural
extraneural
extranodal
    e. marginal zone
    e. marginal zone lymphoma
extranuchal nuchal fibroma
extranuclear
extraosseous
    e. ameloblastoma
    e. plasmacytoma
    e. plasmacytoma of the mediastinum
    (EPM)
extraparenchymal
extrapineal pinealoma
extraplacental
extrapleural
extrapolation
extraprostatic extension (EPE)
extraprostatitis
extrapulmonary tuberculosis
extrapyramidal disease
extrarenal
    e. azotemia
    e. rhabdoid tumor (ERRT)
extraserous
extraskeletal
    e. chondroma
    e. myxoid chondrosarcoma
    (EMC)
    e. osteosarcoma
extratarsal
extrathymic tissue
extrauterine-extraovarian endometrioid
  stromal tumor
extrauterine pregnancy
extravasate
extravasation
    bile e.
    blood e.
    e. cyst
    e. feces
    e. gas
    mucus e.
extravascular (EV)
    e. hemolysis
    e. migratory metastasis
    mechanism
    e. site
    e. space
extreme
    e. capsule
    e. gastric hypersecretion
extremitas (*var. of* extremity)
extremity, extremitas
    broomstick e.
extremorientalis
    Pseudomonas e.
extrication

E

347

extrinsic
  e. allergic alveolitis
    (EAA)
  e. asthma
  e. compression
  e. factor
  e. hemolysis
  e. pathway
  e. semiconductor
  e. system
extructa
  Bulleidia e.
extrude
extrusion
exuberant
  e. infection
  e. tumor
exudate
  fibrinonecrotic e.
  inflammatory e.
  mucopurulent e.
exudation
  e. cell
  e. corpuscle
  e. cyst
  fibrinous e.
exudative
  e. arthritis
  e. bronchiolitis
  e. effusion
  e. glomerulonephritis
  e. granulomatous inflammation
  e. pleural effusion
exudativum
  erythema multiforme e.
exude
exulcerans
exuvia, *pl.* **exuviae**
exuviae (*pl. of* exuvia)
eye
  bull's e.
  fibrous tunic of e.
  owl e.
  raccoon e.'s
  e. spot
  e. tumor
  white of e.
eyelid
  heliotrope e.
eyepiece
  comparison e.
  compensated e.
  high eyepoint e.
  huygenian e.
  Ramsden e.
  widefield e.
eyepoint
eyespot
eyewash equipment
eyeworm
EZ-HP *Helicobacter pylori* **test**
ezrin

F

Fahrenheit
farad
feces
female
force
gilbert (unit of magnetomotive force)
  F agent
  F antigen
  F body
  F distribution
  F donor
  F factor
  F genote
  F pili
  F plasmid
  F thalassemia

F1

first filial generation

F2

second filial generation

FA

fluorescent antibody
  FA technique

FA-A gene
FAA protein
FAB

French-American-British
  FAB leukemia classification
  FAB tumor staging

Fab

  F. fragment
  F. piece

Fabavirus
Faber

  F. anemia
  F. syndrome

Fabry disease
face

  adenoid f.
  cleft f.
  hippocratic f.
  f. of polyhedron (P)
  f. shield
  trans f.

facet, facette

  f. joint arthrography
  f. joint injection
  f. syndrome

facette (*var. of* facet)
facial

  f. diprosopus duplication
  f. eczema
  f. hemiatrophy

  f. myiasis
  f. palsy
  f. trophoneurosis

faciale

  granuloma f.
  tinea f.

facialis

  herpes f.
  zona f.

facies

  adenoid f.
  cherubic f.
  cushingoid f.
  elfin f.
  f. hepatica
  hippocratic f.
  hound-dog f.
  hurloid f.
  Hutchinson f.
  leonine f.
  leprechaun f.
  Marshall Hall f.
  Potter f.
  scaphoid f.

facilitated diffusion
facility

  high-containment BSL4 f.
  medical treatment f. (MTF)

faciodigitogenital dysplasia
facioscapulohumeral-type progressive muscular dystrophy
Facklam classification scheme
Facklamia

  F. miroungae
  F. sourekii
  F. tabacinasalis

FAC protein
FACS

fluorescence-activated cell sorter

FACScalibur flow cytometer
FACScan flow cytometer
FACSort flow cytometer
FACStar Plus flow cytometer
FACSVantage flow cytometer
F-actin

  F-a. binding protein
  F-a. ring

factitia

  thyrotoxicosis f.

factitial panniculitis
factitious

  f. dermatitis
  f. melanin
  f. urticaria

F

factor

f. A
ABO f.
accelerator f.
acquired genetic f.
activated clotting f.
adipocyte determination and
 differentiation f. 1 (ADD1)
adrenocorticotropic hormone-releasing
 f. (ACTH-RF)
AHG f.
f. alpha
amplification f.
anabolism-promoting f. (APF)
angiogenesis f.
animal protein f. (APF)
antialopecia f.
antianemic f.
anticomplementary f.
antigen-specific helper f.
antigen-specific suppressor f.
antihemophilic f. A, B (AHF)
antiheparin f.
antinuclear f. (ANF)
antipernicious anemia f. (APA)
atrial natriuretic f.
autocrine growth f.
autocrine motility f. (AMF)
automated motility f.
f. B
bacteriocin f.
basic fibroblast growth f. (bFGF)
basic helix-loop-helix transcription f.
 (bHLH)
basophil chemotactic f. (BCF)
B-cell activating f. (BAFF)
B-cell differentiating f.
B-cell differentiation/growth f.
B-cell stimulating f.
Bittner milk f.
blastogenetic f. (BF)
blood coagulation f.
B-lymphocyte stimulatory f. (BSF)
brain-derived neurotrophic f. (BDNF)
CAMP f.
cAMP response element binding
 activation transcription f.
 (CREB/ATF)
Castle f.
CDX2 intestine-specific transcription
 f.
CDX1 intestine-specific
 transcription f.
chemotactic f. (CF)
Christmas f. (CF)
citrovorum f. (CF)
clearing f.
clone-inhibiting f. (CIF)
cloning inhibitory f.

clotting f.
C3 Nef f.
cobra venom f.
colony-stimulating f. (CSF)
complement chemotactic f.
conglutinogen-activating f.
connective tissue growth f.
cord f.
coronary risk f.
correction f.
corticotropin-releasing f. (CRF)
cryoprecipitated antihemophilic f.
crystal-induced chemotactic f.
f. D
decay accelerating f. (DAF)
decay antibody-accelerating f.
f. deficiency anemia
dose-reduction f. (DRF)
Duran-Reynals permeability f.
f. E
edema f. (EF)
elongation f.
encephalitogenic f. (EF)
endothelial relaxing f.
endothelium-derived relaxing f.
 (EDRF)
eosinophil chemotactic f.
epidermal growth f. (EGF)
erythrocyte maturation f. (EMF)
erythropoietic-stimulating f. (ESF)
etiologic f.
etiopathogenic f.
exogenous growth f.
exophthalmos-hyperthyroid f.
 (EHF)
exophthalmos-producing f. (EPF)
extrinsic f.
F f.
Fc f.
fertility f.
fibrin stabilizing f. (FSF)
fibroblast growth f. (FGF)
Fitzgerald f.
Fitzgerald-Williams-Flaujeac f.
Flaujeac f.
Fletcher f.
G f.
glass f.
glial cell line-derived neurotropic f.
 (GDNF)
glucose tolerance f. (GTF)
gonadotropin-releasing f. (GRF)
granulocyte colony-stimulating f.
 (G-CSF)
granulocyte-macrophage
 colony-stimulating f. (GM-CSF)
growth hormone-releasing f. (GH-RF,
 GRF)
growth inhibitory f.

Hageman f. (HF)
heat shock f. 1
hemophilic f. A
hepatocyte growth f. (HGF)
hepatocyte growth factor/scatter f. (HGF/SF)
histamine-releasing f. (HRF)
homeodomain transcription f.
human antihemophilic f.
humoral thymic f. (THF)
hydrazine-sensitive f.
hyperglycemic-glycogenolytic f. (HGF)
hypoxia inducible f. (HIF)
hypoxia inducible f. 1 (HIF-1)
f. II gene
f. I, II, III, IV, V, VII, VIII, VIII:C, VIII:R, IX, X, Xa, XI, XII, XIII, XIIIa
f. III multimer assay
f. I, II, V, VII, VIII, IX, X, XI deficiency
immunoglobulin-binding f. (IBF)
immunoglobulin M-rheumatoid f. (IgM-RF)
inherited genetic f.
inhibiting f.
inhibition f.
f. inhibitor
initiation f.
insulinlike growth f.
interferon regulatory f. 1
intrinsic f. (IF)
keratinocyte growth f. 2
labile f.
Lactobacillus bulgaricus f. (LBF)
Laki-Lorand f.
LE f.
Leiden f.
lethal f. (LF)
leukemia inhibitory f. (LIF)
leukocyte inhibitory f.
leukocytosis-promoting f. (LPF)
leukopenic f.
ligand-activated transcription f.
L-L f.
load f.
luteinizing hormone-releasing f. (LH-RF)
lymph node permeability f. (LNPF)
lymphocyte-activating f.
lymphocyte blastogenic f.
lymphocyte mitogenic f.
lymphocyte-transforming f.
lymphocytosis-promoting f. (LPF)
macrophage activation f. (MAF)
macrophage agglutination f. (MAggF)
macrophage chemotactic f. (MCF)

macrophage chemotactic and activating f. (MCAF)
macrophage colony stimulating f. (M-CSF)
macrophage-derived growth f.
macrophage growth f.
macrophage inhibiting f. (MIF)
macrophage migration inhibition f.
megakaryocyte growth and development f. (MGDF)
melanocyte-stimulating hormone inhibiting f. (MIF)
melanocyte-stimulating hormone releasing f. (MRF)
microphthalmia-associated transcription f. (MITF)
migration inhibition f. (MIF)
migration-inhibitory f.
milk f.
mitogenic f.
monocyte-derived neutrophil chemotactic f. (MDNCF)
myeloid progenitor inhibitory f. 1
myocardial depressant f. (MDF)
natural killer cell-stimulating f. (NKSF)
necrotizing f.
nephritic f.
nerve growth f. (NGF)
neurohumoral f.
neurotrophic f.
neutrophil activating f. (NAF)
neutrophil chemotactant f.
neutrophil chemotactic f. (NCF)
neutrophilic chemotactic f.
Nod f.
obligate osteogenic transcription f.
octamer-binding transcription f. 4
orexigenic f.
osteoclast activating f.
Ovenstone f. (OF)
pivotal transcription f.
plasma atrial natriuretic f.
plasma clotting f.
plasma labile f.
plasma thromboplastin f. B (PTF)
plasmin prothrombin conversion f. (PPCF)
platelet f. 1–4
platelet-activating f. (PAF)
platelet-aggregating f. (PAF)
platelet-derived growth f. (PDGF)
platelet tissue f.
polymorphonuclear neutrophil chemotactic f.
postulated pathogenetic f.
preadipocyte f. (Pref-1)
predisposing f.
prognostic f.

F

factor (*continued*)

prolactin-inhibiting f. (PIF)
prolactin-releasing f. (PRF)
proliferation inhibitory f. (PIF)
properdin f. A, B, D, E
prothrombokinase f.
Prower f.
Prower-Stuart f.
quality f. (QF)
R f.
RB1 protein transcription f.
recognition f.
recombinant human insulin-like
  growth f. (rhIGF)
recombinant platelet-derived growth
  f. (rPDGF)
releasing f. (RF)
renal erythropoietic f. (REF)
resistance f.
resistance inducing f. (RIF)
resistance transfer f. (RTF)
Rh f.
rheumatoid f. (RF)
rheumatoid arthritis f. (RAF)
rho f.
ripple f.
risk f.
rough f.
secretor f.
serum prothrombin conversion
  accelerator f.
plasma f. X
Simon septic f.
skin-reactive f. (SRF)
somatotroph release inhibiting f.
somatotropin-releasing f.
  (SRF)
SPCA f.
specific macrophage-arming f.
  (SMAF)
spreading f.
stable f.
stem cell f. (SCF)
stem cell renewal f.
Stuart f.
Stuart-Prower f.
sulfation f.
T f.
T-cell growth f. (TGF)
T-cell replacing f. (TRF)
termination f.
testis-determining f. (TDF)
thymic humoral f.
thymic lymphopoietic f.
thymic replacing f.
thyroid-stimulating hormone-releasing
  f. (TSH-RF)
thyrotoxic complement-fixation f.
thyrotropin-releasing f. (TRF)

tissue f.
tissue-coding f. (TCF, TSF)
tissue-damaging f. (TF)
tissue plasminogen f.
transcription f.
transfer f. (TF)
transforming growth f. X
translocation f.
trefoil family f. (TFF)
tumor angiogenic f. (TAF)
tumor-cell migration-inhibition f.
  (TMIF)
tumor necrosis f. (TNF)
tumor receptor-associated f.
  (TRAF)
undegraded insulin f. (UIF)
upstream binding f.
uterine-relaxing f. (URF)
vascular endothelial growth f.
  (VEGF)
vascular permeability f.
f. V Cambridge
f. VIII-crossed immunoelectrophoresis
virulence f.
f. V Leiden mutation test
von Willebrand f.
W f.
Williams f.
Wnt inhibitory f. (WIF)
f. X for *Haemophilus*
f. XIIIa

factor-1

insulinlike growth f.-1
T-cell growth f.-1
thyroid transcription f.-1 (TTF-1)

factor-2

fibroblast growth f.-2
T-cell growth f.-2

factorial

facultative

f. anaerobe
f. autotroph
f. bacterium
f. coccobacillus
f. heterochromatin
f. histiocyte
f. organism
f. parasite

FAD

flavin adenine dinucleotide

FADD

FAS-associated death domain protein

**FADD-like interleukin-1 beta converting
enzyme (FLICE)**

FADF

fluorescent antibody dark-field

faecale

Trichosporon f.

Faecalibacterium prausnitzii

faecalis
>   *Alcaligenes f.*
>   *Enterococcus f.*
>   *Psychrobacter f.*
>   *Rhodopseudomonas f.*
>   *Streptococcus f.*
>   *Zimmermannella f.*

faecium
>   *Enterococcus f.*
>   *Streptococcus f.*

faeni
>   *Frigoribacterium f.*
>   *Micropolyspora f.*
>   *Sphingomonas f.*

faggot cell
Fahey and McKelvey method
Fahr disease
Fahrenheit (F)
>   F. thermometer

failure
>   acute renal f. (ARF)
>   acute respiratory f. (ARF)
>   adrenal f.
>   anemia associated with chronic renal f.
>   backward f.
>   bone marrow f.
>   cardiac f. (CF)
>   chronic renal f. (CRF)
>   chronic respiratory f.
>   circulatory f.
>   congestive cardiac f. (CCF)
>   congestive heart f. (CHF)
>   forward f.
>   fulminant hepatic f. (FHF)
>   heart f. (HF)
>   hepatic f.
>   high-output cardiac f.
>   left ventricular f. (LVF)
>   liver f.
>   mean time between f.'s
>   multiple-organ system f. (MOSF)
>   myonecrosis, myoglobinuria, renal f.
>   f. of all vital forces (FOAVF)
>   ovarian f.
>   pituitary gonadotropic f.
>   f. rate
>   renal f.
>   respiratory f.
>   right ventricular f.
>   testicular f.
>   f. to thrive
>   ventilatory f.

Fajersztajn crossed sciatic sign
FAK
>   focal adhesion kinase

falcate
falcatus
>   *Stellantchasmus f.*

falciform
falciforme
>   *Cephalosporium f.*

falciparum
>   f. fever
>   f. malaria
>   *Plasmodium f.*

falcular
FA-L gene
fallax
>   *Clostridium f.*

falling drop procedure
fallonii
>   *Legionella f.*

fallopian
>   f. tube cancer
>   f. tube tumor

Fallot
>   F. syndrome
>   tetralogy of F. (tet, TF)

false
>   f. abrasion collar
>   f. agglutination
>   f. albuminuria
>   f. anemia
>   f. aneurysm
>   f. cast
>   f. cyanosis
>   f. cyst
>   f. dextrocardia
>   f. diphtheria
>   f. diverticulum
>   f. hematuria
>   f. hypertrophy
>   f. knot (umbilical cord)
>   f. labor
>   f. membrane
>   f. mole
>   f. negative
>   f. neuroma
>   f. positive

false-negative (FN)
>   f.-n. reaction

false-positive (FP)
>   biologic f.-p. (BFP)
>   chronic f.-p. (CFP)
>   f.-p. reaction

false-resistant
false-susceptible
falx cerebri
FAME
>   fatty acid methyl ester

familial
>   f. adenomatous polyposis (FAP)
>   f. adenomatous polyposis coli
>   f. benign pemphigus
>   f. cancer
>   f. cardiomyopathy
>   f. cerebellar ataxia

F

familial (*continued*)
    f. clival chordoma
    f. cyclic neutropenia
    f. cystinuria
    f. dysautonomia
    f. dysbetalipoproteinemia
    f. emphysema
    f. enteropathy
    f. erythroblastic anemia
    f. erythrophagocytic
      lymphohistiocytosis (FEL)
    f. gigantiform cementoma (FGC)
    f. goiter
    f. gonadal dysgenesis
    f. hemiplegic migraine (FMH)
    f. hemolytic anemia
    f. hemophagocytic
      lymphohistiocytosis (FMLH)
    f. hypercholesterolemia (FH)
    f. hyperlipoproteinemia I, II, IIa,
      IIb, III–V
    f. hypertriglyceridemia
    f. hypocalciuric hypercalcemia
    f. hypoceruloplasminemia
    f. hypoplastic anemia
    f. intestinal polyposis
    f. juvenile nephrophthisis
      (FJN)
    f. juvenile polyp (FJP)
    f. Mediterranean fever (FMF)
    f. mental retardation (FMR)
    f. microcytic anemia
    f. multiple endocrine
    f. multiple endocrine adenomatosis,
      type 1, 2
    f. myoclonic epilepsy
    f. nephritis
    f. nephronophthisis-medullary cystic
      disease (FN-MCD)
    f. nephrophthisis
    f. nephrosis
    f. nonhemolytic jaundice
    f. paroxysmal polyserositis
    f. paroxysmal rhabdomyolysis
    f. periodic paralysis
    f. polycythemia
    f. polyposis
    f. polyposis coli
    f. primary systemic amyloidosis
    f. pyridoxine-responsive anemia
    f. recurrent polyserositis
    f. splenic anemia
family
    cancer f.
    human ABC transporter f.
    melanoma antigen-encoding gene f.
    MyoD gene f.
    14-3-3 protein f.
    ras gene f.

    septin gene f.
    Trefoil Factor F.
FAN
    fuchsin, amido black, and naphthol
      yellow
fan
    macular f.
FANA
    fluorescent antinuclear antibody
      FANA test
Fañanás
    cell of F.
Fanconi
    F. anemia
    F. pancytopenia
    F. syndrome
Fanconi-Zinsser syndrome
fan-in
Fannia
    F. canicularis
    F. scalaris
fan-out
1F6 antigen
FAP
    familial adenomatous polyposis
farad (F)
Faraday
    F. constant
    F. effect
    F. law of electrolysis
faradic shock
Farber
    F. disease
    F. lipogranulomatosis
    F. syndrome
    F. test
Farber-Uzman syndrome
farciminosus
    Histoplasma f.
farcinica
    Nocardia f.
farcy
Far East Russian encephalitis
farmer's
    f. lung disease
    f. skin
Farr
    F. law
    F. test
farraginis
    Bacillus f.
Farrant
    F. medium
    F. mounting fluid
**Farrzyme human high avidity
anti-dsNA enzyme immunoassay
kit**
FAS
    fatty acid synthase

Fas
> F. ligand
> F. receptor

FAS-associated death domain protein (FADD)

fascia
> f. adherens
> deep f.
> Denonvilliers f.
> Gerota f.
> Monakow f.
> renal f.
> f. renalis

fascial fibrosarcoma

fasciatus
> *Nosopsyllus f.*
> *Pulex f.*

fascicle
> herringbone f.
> muscle f.
> nerve f.

fascicular
> f. pattern
> f. sarcoma

fasciculata
> f. cell
> zona f.

fasciculate bladder

fasciculation

fasciculi (*pl. of* fasciculus)

fasciculus, ** *pl.* **fasciculi
> f. atrioventricularis
> Bürdach cuneate f.
> f. gracilis

fasciitis, fascitis
> eosinophilic f.
> infiltrative f.
> necrotizing f.
> nodular f.
> proliferative f.
> pseudosarcomatous f.

fascin

Fasciola
> *F. gigantica*
> *F. hepatica*

fasciolaris
> *Cysticercus f.*

fascioliasis

fasciolid

Fascioloides magna

fasciolopsiasis

Fasciolopsis
> *F. buski*
> *F. rathouisi*

fascitis (*var. of* fasciitis)

Fas-Fas ligand protein

FAST
> fluorescent allergosorbent
> test

fast
> f. action potential
> f. green (FG)
> f. green FCF stain
> f. hemoglobin
> low-voltage f. (LVF)
> f. smear
> f. turnaround time
> f. x-scanning
> f. yellow

fasted state

fastFISH amnio test

fastidiosa
> *Amycolatopsis f.*
> *Desulfofaba f.*

fastidious bacterium

fastigium

fasting
> f. blood sugar (FBS)
> f. plasma glucose (FPG)

fastness

fastosum
> *Platynosomum f.*

FastPack blood analyzer system

FAT
> fluorescent antibody
> test

fat
> f. absorption
> f. absorption study
> f. absorption test
> f. assay
> brown f.
> f. cell
> f. depot
> f. droplet
> f. embolism
> f. embolism syndrome
> f. embolus
> emulsify f.
> fecal f.
> f. free
> f. in stool
> multilocular f.
> f. necrosis
> f. staining
> subcutaneous f.
> f. tide
> total body f. (TBF)
> unilocular f.
> white f.
> yellow f.

fatal
> f. dose (FD)
> f. granulomatous disease

fat-deficiency disease

fat-free
> f.-f. dry weight (FFDW)

F

fat-free (*continued*)
    f.-f. mass (FFM)
    f.-f. wet weight (FFWW)
FAT1 gene
fatigue
    excessive f.
fat-induced hyperlipidemia
fat-mobilizing
    f.-m. hormone
    f.-m. substance (FMS)
fat-pad, fat pad
    Imlach f.-p.
fat-storing cell
fatty
    f. acid
    f. acid assay
    f. acid beta oxidation enzyme
    f. acid-binding protein
    f. acid methyl ester
      (FAME)
    f. acid oxidation
    f. acid oxidation disorder
      (FOD)
    f. acid profile
    f. acid synthase (FAS)
    f. acid synthesis
    f. ascites
    f. atrophy
    f. change
    f. cirrhosis
    f. degeneration
    f. deposition
    f. heart
    f. infiltration
    f. intraosseous tissue
    f. kidney
    f. liver
    f. metamorphosis
    f. oil
    f. phanerosis
    f. urinary cast
fauces, *gen.* **faucium**
    Mycoplasma faucium
Fauchard disease
faucial tonsil
faucitis
faulty union
faun tail nevus
FAV
    feline ataxia virus
faveolate
faveolus
favic chandelier
favid
favism
favisporus
    Paenibacillus f.
favosa
    porrigo f.

    tinea f.
    trichomycosis f.
Favre-Racouchot disease
favus
FB
    foreign body
FBE
    full blood examination
F-box protein
FBP
    fibrinogen breakdown product
FBS
    fasting blood sugar
    fetal bovine serum
FC
    flow cytometry
Fc
    Fc factor
    Fc fragment
    Fc piece
    Fc receptor
FCA
    ferritin-conjugated antibody
FCC
    follicular center cell
FCCP
    trifluorocarbonylcyanide phenylhydrazone
      protonophore FCCP
F^+ **cell**
FCL
    follicle center lymphoma
    follicular cell lymphoma cell
      FCL cell
FCM
    flow cytometry
FCS
    fluorescence correlation spectroscopy
FD
    fatal dose
FD50, FD$_{50}$
    median fatal dose
FDC
    follicular dendritic cell
FDNB
    fluoro-2,4-dinitrobenzene
FDP
    fibrin degradation product
    fibrin/fibrinogen degradation product
    fibrinogen degradation product
F-duction
Fe
    iron
feathery degeneration
feature
    chordoid f.'s
    clinical manifestations, etiologic
      factors, anatomic involvement,
      pathophysiologic f.'s (CEAP)
    fibroblastic-myofibroblastic f.

general f.
morphologic f.
organotypic f.
febricitans
febrile
f. agglutination
f. agglutination test
f. agglutinin
f. albuminuria
hydroa f.
f. nonhemolytic transfusion reaction
f. urine
febrilis
calor f.
herpes f.
FEC
free erythrocyte coproporphyrin
fecal
f. abscess
f. antigen
f. carbohydrate
f. chloride
f. chymotrypsin
f. color
f. concentration
f. consistency
f. electrolytes
f. examination
f. fat
f. fat stain
f. fat test
f. fistula
f. impaction
f. incontinence
f. leukocyte
f. leukocyte count
f. lipids
f. marker
f. mucus
f. muscle fiber
f. nitrogen
f. occult blood test (FOBT)
f. osmolality
f. pH
f. porphyrin
f. porphyrin analysis
f. potassium
f. reducing substances test
f. sodium
f. trypsin
f. tumor
f. urobilinogen (FU)
f. vomitus
fecalith
fecaloma, scatoma
fecal-oral transmission
feces (F)
bloody f.

extravasation f.
impacted f.
Fechner tumor
Fechtner syndrome
FED
forward fluorescence detector
Fede disease
feedback
f. inhibition mutation
f. loop
feed forward loop
feeleii
Legionella f.
Feer disease
FEF
forced expiratory flow
Fehleisen streptococcus
Fehling
F. solution
F. test
FEL
familial erythrophagocytic lymphohistiocytosis
Felicola subrostratus
feline
f. agranulocytosis
f. ataxia virus (FAV)
f. distemper
f. infectious enteritis
f. infectious peritonitis
f. leukemia
f. leukemia-sarcoma virus complex
f. leukemia virus (FeLV)
f. panleukopenia virus
f. rhinotracheitis virus
f. viral rhinotracheitis
felineum
Microsporum f.
felineus
Opisthorchis f.
felinum
Corynebacterium f.
felis
Afipia f.
Chlamydophila f.
Haemophilus f.
Isospora f.
Rickettsia f.
Felix-Weil reaction (FWR)
felleae
tunica mucosa vesicae f.
tunica muscularis vesicae f.
tunica serosa vesicae f.
Fellomyces
Felton phenomenon
feltwork
Kaes f.
Felty syndrome

F

FeLV
    feline leukemia virus
female (F)
    f. carrier
    f. castration
    f. genital tract (FGT)
    f. genital tract carcinosarcoma
      (FGTCS)
    f. hormone
    f. pseudohermaphrodite
    f. pseudohermaphroditism
    f. sex chromatin pattern
    XY f.
femininae
    glandulae urethrales f.
    tunica mucosa urethrae f.
    tunica muscularis urethrae f.
feminization
    f. syndrome, adrenal
    testicular f.
feminizing tumor
femoral
    f. hernia
    f. puncture
femorocele
femoropopliteal occlusive disease
femtoliter (fL)
femtometer (fm)
femtomole (fmol)
femur
    proximal f.
FENa
    fractional excretion of sodium
fenac
fenestra, *pl.* **fenestrae**
    alveolar f.
    f. cochleae
    hepatic f.
    f. of the vestibule
    f. ovalis
    f. rotunda
    f. vestibuli
fenestrae (*pl. of* fenestra)
fenestrata
    placenta f.
fenestrated
    f. capillary
    f. capillary showing
    f. endothelium
    f. membrane
    f. placenta
fenestration
    atrophic f.
Fennellia
fennelliae
    Campylobacter f.
    Helicobacter f.
Fennellomyces
fenofibrate

fentanyl
fenthion insecticide
Fenton reaction
Fenwick disease
Fenwick-Hunner ulcer
FEP
    free erythrocyte protoporphyrin
F-EPE
    focal extraprostatic extension
FEPP
    free erythrocyte protoporphyrin
fergusonii
    Escherichia f.
ferintoshensis
    Lactobacillus f.
ferment
fermentans
    Acidaminococcus f.
    Dyadobacter f.
    Geothrix f.
    Halanaerobium f.
    Mycoplasma f.
fermentation
    mannitol f.
    mixed acid f.
    salicin f.
    f. test
    f. tube
Fermentotrichon
fermentum
    Amphibacillus f.
    Lactobacillus f.
fermium (Fm)
Fernandez reaction
Fernbach flask
ferning
fern test
ferox
    Dinobdella f.
    prurigo f.
Ferrata cell
ferredoxin
Ferrein
    F. pyramid
    F. tube
    F. vasa aberrantia
ferreini
    processus f.
Ferribacterium limneticum
ferric
    f. ammonium sulfate stain
    f. chloride, perchloric acid, nitric
      acid (FPN)
    f. chloride reaction of epinephrine
    f. chloride test
    f. ferricyanide reduction test
    f. ferrocyanide
    f. iron
    f. oxide

ferricyanide
>ferrous f.
>potassium f.

ferrihemoglobin

ferrimagnetic

Ferrimonadaceae

ferriorganovorum
>*Thermovenabulum f.*

ferriphilum
>*Leptospirillum f.*

ferriprotoporphyrin (FPP)

ferrireducens
>*Geovibrio f.*
>*Rhodoferax f.*

ferrite

ferritin assay

ferritin-conjugated antibody (FCA)

ferritin-coupled antibody

Ferrobacteria

ferrocalcinosis

ferrochelatase deficiency

ferrocyanide
>ferric f.

ferroflocculation

ferrokinetic

ferrokinetics study

ferrooxidans
>*Acidithiobacillus f.*
>*Leptospirillum f.*

ferrophilus

Ferroplasma acidiphilum

Ferroplasmaceae

ferrous
>f. citrate Fe 59
>f. ferricyanide
>f. iron

ferroxidase

ferrugination

ferruginea
>*Asanoa f.*

ferrugineum
>*Microsporum f.*
>*Trichophyton f.*

ferrugineus
>*Pseudorhodobacter f.*

ferruginosa
>*Tubifera f.*

ferruginous
>f. body
>f. micelles

fertile eunuch syndrome

fertility
>f. agent
>f. factor
>f. inhibition

fertilization
>effect of f.

fertilizer truck bomb

FertilMARQ
>F. fertility screening test
>F. male fertility screening test kit

fervens
>calor f.

Fervidobacterium pennivorans

FES
>flame emission spectroscopy
>forced expiratory spirogram

fester

festoon

festooning

festucae
>*Rathayibacter f.*

FET
>forced expiratory time

fetal
>f. abnormality
>f. activity-acceleration determination
>f. adenocarcinoma
>f. adenoma
>f. adrenal cortex
>f. alcohol syndrome
>f. antigen
>f. antigen test
>f. biophysical profile
>f. bovine serum (FBS)
>f. cotyledon
>f. death
>f. distress
>f. duplication
>f. erythroblastosis
>f. face syndrome
>f. fat cell lipoma
>f. fibronectin (FFN)
>f. hemoglobin (HbF)
>f. hemoglobin test
>f. hydantoin syndrome
>f. karyotyping in mid-trimester IUFD
>f. life
>f. lobulation
>f. lung maturity (FLM)
>f. neuron
>f. nuchal translucency
>f. oxygen saturation monitoring
>f. prematurity
>f. repertoire gradient
>f. reticularis
>f. stem artery thrombosis
>f. trimethadione syndrome
>f. vaccinia
>f. zone

fetalis
>*Alishewanella f.*
>chondromalacia f.
>erythroblastosis f.
>Hb Bart hydrops f.
>hydrops f.

F

fetalis (*continued*)
    ichthyosis f.
    keratosis diffusa f.
    rachitis f.
fetalization
fetal-maternal erythrocyte distribution
FETI
    fluorescence excitation transfer
    immunoassay
fetid rhinitis
fetoglobulin
    alpha-1 f.
fetomaternal
    f. hemorrhage
    f. incompatibility
    f. molecular exchange
fetoplacental anasarca
fetoprotein
    alpha f. (AFP)
    alpha-1 f.
    beta f.
    gamma f.
fetoscopic laser coagulation of vascular
  connection
fetoscopy
fetotoxicity
FETS
    forced expiratory time in seconds
fetu
    fetus in f.
fetus
    f. acardiacus
    f. amorphus
    Campylobacter fetus subsp. *f.*
    f. compressus
    harlequin f.
    hydropic f.
    f. in fetu
    macerated f.
    minimum dose causing death or
      malformation of 100% of fetuses
      (T/LD_{100})
    f. papyraceus
    f. sanguinolentis
    stunted f.
Feuerstein-Mims syndrome
Feulgen
    F. cytometry
    F. reaction
    F. stain
    F. test
FEV-1, FEV1
    forced expiratory volume at
    1 second
fever
    abortus f.
    acute rheumatic f. (ARF)
    Aden f.
    aestivoautumnal f.

African hemorrhagic f.
African swine f.
African tick-borne f.
aphthous f.
Argentinean hemorrhagic f.
blackwater f.
f. blister
Bolivian hemorrhagic f.
bouquet f.
boutonneuse f.
bovine ephemeral f.
breakbone f.
Bullis f.
Bunyamwera f.
Bwamba f.
camp f.
cat-bite f.
f. caused by infection (FI)
cave f.
Central European tick-borne f.
cerebrospinal f.
chikungunya hemorrhagic f.
childbed f.
classical swine f.
Colorado tick f.
continued f.
Crimean-Congo hemorrhagic f.
dandy f.
date f.
death f.
deerfly f. (tularemia)
dengue hemorrhagic f.
desert f.
diphasic milk f.
Dumdum f.
Dutton relapsing f.
Ebola hemorrhagic f.
eczema, asthma, hay f. (EAHF)
epidemic hemorrhagic f.
epimastical f.
eruptive f.
essential f.
exanthematous f.
falciparum f.
familial Mediterranean f. (FMF)
Flinders Island spotted f.
flood f.
food f.
Fort Bragg f.
glandular f.
Haverhill f.
hay f.
hematuric bilious f.
hemoglobinuric f.
hemorrhagic f.
herpetic f.
hospital f.
Ilhéus f.
intermittent malarial f.

inundation f.
island f.
jail f.
Japanese river f.
jungle yellow f.
Katayama f.
kedani f.
Kenya tick f.
Korean hemorrhagic f.
Lassa hemorrhagic f.
laurel f.
louse-borne relapsing f.
malarial f.
malignant tertian f.
Malta f.
Manchurian hemorrhagic f.
Marseilles f.
marsh f.
Mediterranean f.
metal fume f. (MFF)
miliary f.
miniature scarlet f.
monoleptic f.
mud f.
f. of undetermined origin (FUO)
f. of unknown origin (FUO)
Omsk hemorrhagic f.
O'nyong-nyong f.
Oroya f.
polka f.
polyleptic f.
Pontiac f.
protein f.
puerperal f.
Pym f.
pyogenic f.
Q f.
quartan f.
Queensland tick f.
quotidian f.
rabbit f. (tularemia)
rat-bite f.
recrudescent typhus f.
relapsing f.
remittent malarial f.
rheumatic f. (RF)
Rift Valley f.
Rocky Mountain spotted f.
 (RMSF)
Ross River f.
sandfly f.
San Joaquin Valley f.
scarlet f. (SF)
septic f.
ship f.
Siberian tick f.
Sindbis f.
slow f.
solar f.

spotted f.
steroid f.
swamp f.
swine f.
symptomatic f.
syphilitic f.
tertian f.
three-day f.
tick f.
traumatic f.
trench f.
tsutsugamushi f.
typhoid f.
undifferentiated type f.
undulant f.
uveoparotid f.
valley f.
viral hemorrhagic f. (VHF)
vivax f.
Wesselsbron f.
West African f.
West Nile f.
Whitmore f.
Wolhynia f.
wound f.
yellow f.
Zika f.

feverish urine

F-18, ^{18}F
  fluorine 18

FFA
  free fatty acid

FFDW
  fat-free dry weight

FFF
  Fuzzy Functional Form
    FFF technology

FFL
  floral variant of follicular lymphoma

FFM
  fat-free mass

FFN
  fetal fibronectin
    FFN test

FFP
  fresh frozen plasma

FFPE
  formalin-fixed paraffin-embedded

FFWW
  fat-free wet weight

FGC
  familial gigantiform cementoma

FGF
  fibroblast growth factor

FGT
  female genital tract
    FGT cytologic smear

FGTCS
  female genital tract carcinosarcoma

F

FH
  familial hypercholesterolemia
  follicular hyperplasia
FH4
    N_5-formyl FH$_4$
FHF
  fulminant hepatic failure
FHIT
  fragile histidine triad
    FHIT gene
    FHIT protein
FI
  fever caused by infection
FIA
  fluorescent immunoassay
fiber, fibra, fibre
    A f.
    amianthoid collagen f.'s
    anastomosing f.
    argyrophilic f.
    astral f.
    Bergmann f.
    binucleate f.
    branching cardiac f.
    Burdach f.
    chromatic f.
    circular f.
    climbing f.
    collagen f.
    collagenous f.
    cone f.
    connective tissue f.
    delta f.
    f. density
    dentinal f.
    elastic f.
    enamel f.
    extrafusal muscle f.
    fecal muscle f.
    f. FISH analysis
    gamma f.
    gray f.
    intrafusal f.
    Korff f.
    Mahaim f.
    meat f.
    medullated nerve f.
    mossy f. (MF)
    Müller f.
    myelinated nerve f.
    nerve f.
    nonmedullated f.
    nuclear bag f.
    nuclear chain f.
    osteocollagenous f.
    osteogenetic f.
    oxytalan f.
    pilomotor f.
    precollagenous f.

    Prussak f.
    Purkinje f. (PF)
    red f.
    Remak f.
    reticular f.
    reticulin f.
    Retzius f.
    rod f.
    Rosenthal f.
    Rosenthal f.
    Sharpey f.
    skeinoid f.
    skeletal muscle f.
    sling f.
    f. spectrum
    spindle f.
    stool muscle f.
    stress f.
    striatonigral f.
    sudomotor f.
    target f.
    tautomeric f.
    thin elastic f.
    Tomes f.
    transseptal f.
    U f.
    unmyelinated f.
    wavy f.
    white f.
    yellow f.
    zonular f.
fiber-FISH
fiberoptic
fibra (*var. of* fiber), *pl.* fibrae
    fibrae circulares
    fibrae lentis
    fibrae meridionales muscularis
      ciliaris
    fibrae obliquae tunicae muscularis
    fibrae zonulares
fibrae (*pl. of* fibra)
fibre (*var. of* fiber)
fibremia
Fibricola seoulensis
fibril
    Alzheimer f.
    amyloid f.
    anchoring f.
    beta-amyloid f.
    collagen f.
    fibronectin f.
    muscular f.
fibrilla
fibrillar, fibrillary
    f. astrocyte
    f. basket
fibrillary (*var. of* fibrillar)
    f. astrocyte
    f. astrocytoma

f. gliosis
f. glomerulonephritis
f. neuroma
fibrillate
fibrillated
Fibrillenstruktur
fibrillin gene
fibrillogenesis
fibrin
f. body
f. breakdown product
f. calculus
f. cap
f. clot retraction assay
f. degradation product (FDP)
f. degradation product method
f. deposition
f. foam
Fraser-Lendrum stain for f.
f. glue
f. histochemical stain
intervillous f.
lighter layer of f.
f. matrix
f. monomer
Nitabuch f.
f. plate lysis
reptilase f.
f. stabilizing factor (FSF)
f. stabilizing factor test
f. staining
subchorionic f.
fibrin, subchorionic
f. thrombus
f. titer
f. titer test
Weigert stain for f.
fibrinase
fibrin/fibrinogen degradation product (FDP)
fibrin-like proteinaceous material
fibrin-linked platelet plug
fibrinocellular
fibrinogen
f. assay
f. breakdown product (FBP)
f. bridge
cryoprecipitated f.
f. deficiency
f. degradation product (FDP)
functional intact f. (FiF)
f. I-125
f. method
plasma f.
f. split product (FSP)
f. titer test
fibrinogenase
fibrinogenemia

fibrinogen-fibrin conversion syndrome
fibrinogenic, fibrinogenous
fibrinogenolysis
fibrinogenopenia
fibrinogenous (*var. of* fibrogenic)
fibrinohemorrhagic peritonitis
fibrinoid
f. degeneration
f. necrosis
f. necrotizing inflammation
fibrinokinase
fibrinolysin
f. coagulation
seminal f.
streptococcal f.
fibrinolysis
primary f.
fibrinolysokinase
fibrinolytic
f. disorder
f. enzyme
f. protein
f. purpura
f. split product (FSP)
f. system
f. therapy
fibrinonecrotic exudate
fibrinopenia
fibrinopeptide
f. A, B
f. test
fibrinopurulent inflammation
fibrinous
f. acute lobar pneumonia
f. acute pleuritis
f. adhesion
f. bronchitis
f. cast
f. degeneration
f. exudation
f. inflammation
f. lymph
f. pericarditis
f. peritonitis
f. pleurisy
f. polyp
f. pseudomembrane
fibrin-related antigen (FRA)
fibrin-split product
fibrinuria
fibrivorans
Cellvibrio f.
fibroadenoma
giant f.
giant intracanalicular f.
intracanalicular f.
juvenile f.
fibroadenosis
fibroadipose tissue

F

fibroameloblastic
    f. dentinoma
    f. odontoma
fibroareolar
fibroblast
    f. and fibrocyte
    chick embryo f. (CEF)
    f. culture
    endoneurial f.
    f. growth factor (FGF)
    f. growth factor-2
    f. growth factor receptor
    f. interferon
    proliferation of f.
    radiation f.
fibroblastic
    f. lesion
    f. meningioma
    f. meningoblastoma
    f. tumor
fibroblastic-myofibroblastic feature
fibroblastoma
    desmoplastic f.
    giant cell f. (GCF)
fibrocalcific nodule
fibrocarcinoma
fibrocartilage
    degenerated intervertebral f.
    f. matrix alteration
fibrocartilaginous
fibrocartilago
fibrocaseous
    f. inflammation
    f. peritonitis
fibrocellular
fibrochondritis
fibrochondroma
fibrocollagenous stroma
fibrocongestive
    f. hypertrophy
    f. splenomegaly
fibrocontractive disease
fibrocyst
fibrocystic
    f. disease
    f. disease of breast
    f. mastitis
    f. mastopathy
fibrocystoma
fibrocyte
    fibroblast and f.
    f. in endomysium
fibrodysplasia ossificans progressiva
fibroelastic
fibroelastogenesis
fibroelastosis
    endocardial f. (EFE)
    endomyocardial f.
    intimal f.

fibroenchondroma
fibroepithelial
    f. lesion
    f. papilloma
    f. polyp
    f. tumor
fibroepithelioma
fibrofatty plaque
fibrofolliculoma
fibrogenesis imperfecta ossium
fibrogenic proliferation
fibrogliosis
fibrohistiocytic
    f. lesion
    f. marker
fibrohistiocytoma
fibrohyaline tissue
fibrohyalinosis
fibroid
    f. adenoma
    f. inflammation
    f. tumor
    f. uterus
fibroin
fibroinflammatory lesion
fibrointimal thickening
fibrokeratoma
    acquired f.
    digital f.
fibrolamellar
    f. hepatocellular carcinoma
    f. liver cell carcinoma
fibroleiomyoma
fibrolipoma
fibroliposarcoma
fibroma
    ameloblastic f.
    aponeurotic f.
    cementifying f.
    cementoossifying f. (COF)
    chondromyxoid f. (CMF)
    collagenous f.
    concentric f.
    desmoplastic f.
    extranuchal nuchal f.
    garlic-clove f.
    giant cell f.
    irritation f.
    juvenile ossifying f.
    localized f.
    f. molle
    f. molle gravidarum
    myxoid f.
    f. myxomatodes
    nonossifying f.
    nuchal f.
    odontogenic f.
    ossifying f.
    pleomorphic f.

pleural f.
rabbit f.
senile f.
Shope f.
telangiectatic f.
fibromatoid
fibromatosis
abdominal f.
aggressive infantile f.
f. colli
congenital generalized f.
desmoid f.
desmoid-type f. (DTF)
Dupuytren f.
extraabdominal f.
inclusion body f.
infantile digital f.
juvenile hyalin f.
juvenile palmoplantar f.
mesenteric f.
musculoaponeurotic f.
nodular palmar f.
plantar fascia f.
retroperitoneal f.
somatic f.
fibromatous
fibromembranous
fibrometer
fibromuscular
f. dysplasia
f. hyperplasia
fibromyalgia (FM)
fibromyoma
fibromyositis
fibromyxoid
f. sarcoma
f. tumor
fibromyxolipoma
fibromyxoma
fibromyxosarcoma
fibronectin
cellular f.
fetal f. (FFN, fFN)
f. fibril
plasma f.
tissue f.
fibroneuroma
fibronexus junction
fibroodontoma
ameloblastic f.
fibroosseous lesion
fibroosteoma
fibropapilloma
fibroplasia
retrolental f. (RLF)
fibroplastic
fibroplastica
gastritis f.
fibroplate

fibropolypus
fibroreticularis
lamina f.
fibroreticulate
fibrosa, *pl.* **fibrosae** (*var. of* fibrous)
localized osteitis f.
multifocal osteitis f.
myositis f.
osteitis f.
tunica f.
fibrosae (*pl. of* fibrosa)
fibrosarcoma (FS)
ameloblastic f.
congenital f. (CFS)
congenital infantile f. (CIF)
Earle L f.
fascial f.
infantile f.
inflammatory f.
medullary f.
odontogenic f.
sclerosing epithelioid f.
fibrosarcomatous variant of dermatofibrosarcoma protuberans (FS-DFSP)
fibrosclerosing lesion
fibrose
fibroserous
fibrosiderotic nodule
fibrosing
f. adenomatosis
f. adenosis
f. alveolitis
fibrosis
blood vessel f.
bridging f.
centrilobular f.
condensation f.
congenital hepatic f.
cystic f. (CF)
diffuse interstitial f.
endomyocardial f. (EMF)
eosinophilic angiocentric f. (EAF)
focal f.
hepatic f.
honeycomb f.
idiopathic endomyocardial f.
idiopathic pulmonary f. (IPF)
idiopathic retroperitoneal f. (IRF)
interstitial pulmonary f. (IPF)
islet cell focal f.
leptomeningeal f.
marrow f.
mediastinal f.
multifocal f.
nodular subepidermal f.
pipestem f.
pleural f.
portal f.

F

fibrosis (*continued*)
    postinflammatory pulmonary f.
    progressive massive f. (PMF)
    pulmonary f.
    replacement f.
    retroperitoneal f.
    striped form of interstitial f.
    subadventitial f.
    subepidermal f.
    subsinusoidal f.
    Symmers clay pipestem f.
fibrositis
FIBROSpec test
fibrosum
    adenoma f.
    lipoma f.
    molluscum f.
    myxoma f.
fibrosus
    anulus f.
fibrothecoma
fibrothorax
fibrotic focus
fibrous, fibrosa
    f. adhesion
    f. ankylosis
    f. articular capsule
    f. astrocyte
    f. astrocytoma
    f. bacterial virus
    f. body
    f. cavernitis
    f. cortical defect
    f. degeneration
    f. dysplasia of jaw
    f. dysplasia protuberans
    f. familial dysplasia
    f. goiter
    f. histiocytoma
    f. hypertrophic pachymeningitis
    f. layer
    f. long-spacing collagen (FLS)
    f. membrane of joint capsule
    f. mesothelioma
    f. monostotic dysplasia
    f. nodule
    f. obliteration
    f. osteoma
    f. plug
    f. polyp
    f. protein
    f. pseudotumor
    f. repair
    f. replacement
    f. spindle cell lipoma
    f. streak
    f. tendon sheath
    f. thyroiditis
    f. tissue (FT)

    f. tubercle
    f. tunic of eye
    f. union
    f. xanthoma
fibrovascular
    f. septum
    f. stroma
fibroxanthoma
    atypical f. (AFX)
ficain (*var. of* ficin)
ficin, ficain
Fick
    F. bacillus
    F. law
    F. principle
Ficoll-Hypaque technique
Ficoll-Paque purified cell
ficulneum
    Leuconostoc f.
FID
    flame ionization detector
fidelis
    Shewanella f.
Fiedler
    F. disease
    F. myocarditis
field
    Cohnheim f.
    depth of f.
    f. effect transistor
    high-power f. (HPF)
    low-power f. (LPF)
    magnetic f.
    f. method
    microscopic f.
    f. of microscope
    f. of view
    oil immersion f. (OIF)
    F. rapid stain
    red blood cells per high-power f.
      (RBC/hpf)
    spiral visual f.
    tubular visual f.
    f. vole
    white blood cells per high-power f.
      (WBC/hpf)
fieldingi
    Cooperia f.
Fielding membrane
Fiessinger-Leroy-Reiter syndrome
FIF
    forced inspiratory flow
FiF
    functional intact fibrinogen
    FiF assay
    FiF test
fifth
    f. disease
    f. disease virus

FIGLU
> formiminoglutamic acid
>> FIGLU excretion test

FIGO
> International Federation of Gynecology
> and Obstetrics
>> FIGO adenocarcinoma of endometrium
>> FIGO classification of tumor staging

Figueira syndrome

figurata
> keratosis rubra f.

figurate erythema

figuratum
> erythema f.

figure
> f. description
> epithelium with mitotic f.
> flame f.
> mitotic f.
> myelin f. (MF)

fig wart

Fijivirus

filaceous

filaggrin

filaggrin-like immunoreactivity

filamen, filamin

filament
> actin f.
> algal f.
> Ammon f.
> axial f.
> cytokeratin f.
> cytoskeletal f.
> filopodia-like f.
> glial f.
> intermediate f. (IF)
> keratin f.
> myosin f.
> f. polymorphonuclear
> f. polymorphonuclear leukocyte
> spermatic f.
> Z f.

filamenta (*pl. of* filamentum)

filamented neutrophil

filament-nonfilament count

filamentosum
> *Eubacterium f.*

filamentous
> f. bacterial virus
> f. bacteriophage

filamentum, *pl.* **filamenta**
> *Prototheca filamenta*

filamin (*var. of* filamen)

filar
> f. mass
> f. micrometer
> f. substance

filaria
> *F. bancrofti*

F. conjunctivae
F. demarquayi
F. hominis oris
F. juncea
F. labialis
F. lentis
F. loa
F. lymphatica
F. medinensis
Ozzard f.
F. ozzardi
F. palpebralis
F. philippinensis
F. sanguinis
F. tucumana
F. volvulus

filarial
> f. arthritis
> f. chylothorax
> f. dance sign
> f. funiculitis

filariasis
> Bancroft f.
> bancroftian f.
> lymphatic f.
> Malayan f.
> onchocerciasis-type f.
> f. serological test

filaricidal

filaricide

filariform

Filarioidea

Filaroides hirthi

Filatov, Filatow
> F. disease

Filatow (*var. of*
> Filatov)

file
> Indian f.
> master f.
> Rare Donor F.

filensin

Filifactor alocis

filiform
> f. growth pattern
> f. hyperkeratosis
> hyperkeratosis f.
> f. papilla
> f. papillae
> f. process
> f. wart

filiformis
> verruca f.

filigree pattern

filipin fluorometry

filling defect

film
> blood f.
> f. density calibration

F

film (*continued*)
    fixed blood f.
    gelatin f.
    spot f.
    sulfa f.
    X-Omat AR f.
Filobacillus milosensis
Filobasidiella
    F. bacillisporus
    F. neoformans
Filobasidium
Filomicrobium fusiforme
filopodia-like filament
filopodium
filovaricosis
Filoviridae
filovirus
    f.
Filschie clip
filter
    autoadhesive cellulose
     nitrate f.
    bacterial f.
    barrier f.
    Berkefeld f.
    Bird Nest f.
    f. bleeding time
    blocking f.
    blood f.
    f. capacitor
    Centriflo f.
    Chamberland f.
    collodion f.
    exciter f.
    gelatin f.
    Gelman f.
    glass fiber f.
    HEPA f.
    high-pass f.
    Hybond N f.
    f. hybridization
    inherent f.
    interference f.
    line f.
    low-pass f.
    membrane f.
    microaggregate f.
    Millex-GS plasma f.
    Millipore f.
    Nalgene capsule f.
    Nuclepore f.
    f. paper
    f. paper chromatography
    f. paper microscopic (FPM)
    f. paper microscopic test
    f. photometer
    polyether sulfone f.'s
    Seitz f.
    Selas f.

    Tetko nylon mesh f.
    Wratten f.
filterable virus
filtering
filtertip
    Eppendorf f.
Filtracheck-Uti
    F.-U. colorimetric filtration system
    F.-U. disposable colorimetric
     bacteriuria detection system
    F.-U. disposable colormetric
     bacteriuria detection
    F.-U. test
filtrate
    bouillon f.
    glomerular f.
    tuberculin f. (TF)
filtration
    cascade f.
    gel f.
    glomerular f.
    lymph f.
    Millipore f.
    f. slit
    f. space
filum terminale
fimbria, *pl.* **fimbriae**
    fimbriae of uterine tube
    fimbriae tubae uterinae
fimbriae (*pl. of* fimbria)
fimbriate, fimbriated
fimbriated (*var. of* fimbriate)
finding
    in situ f.
FineFix
Finegoldia magna
finegoldii
    Alistipes f.
finely stippled chromatin pattern
fine-needle
    f.-n. aspiration (FNA)
    f.-n. aspiration biopsy (FNAB)
    f.-n. aspiration cytology
     (FNAC)
    f.-n. cytopuncture
fine structure
finger
    clubbed f.
    dead f.
    drumstick f.
    hippocratic f.
    mallet f.
    promyelocytic leukemia zinc f.
     (PLZF)
    rudimentary f.
    sausage f.
    spade f.
    waxy f.
    webbed f.

fingerprint
> f. deposit
> DNA f.
> genetic f.
> high-resolution f. (HRF)
> f. pattern

fingerprinting
> DNA f.
> plasmid f.

finite element modeling
Fink-Heimer stain
Finn chamber patch test
FiO2
> fractional concentration of inspired
> oxygen

fire
> Saint Anthony's f.

Firmicutes
firmware
first
> f. arch syndrome
> F. Check 12 Drug test
> F. Check Ecstasy test kit
> F. Check home-screening
> test
> f. filial generation (F_1)
> f. morning urine specimen
> f. responder
> F. Warning System

first-degree
> f.-d. burn
> f.-d. frostbite
> f.-d. heart block
> f.-d. radiation injury

first-order
> f.-o. elimination
> f.-o. kinetics
> f.-o. reaction

first-pass metabolism
first-set graft rejection
Fischer
> F. burner
> F. exact test
> F. projection

fischeri
> *Neosartorya f.*
> *Trichophyton f.*

FISH
> fluorescence in situ hybridization
> double-fusion FISH(D-FISH)
> extra signal FISH
> (ES-FISH)
> multicolored FISH

fish
> f. gelatin
> f. skin
> f. tapeworm
> f. tapeworm anemia

Fishberg concentration test

Fisher
> F. exact test
> F. Scientific Histo-freeze 2000
> freezing spray
> F. syndrome

fisherii
> *Aspergillus f.*

Fisher-Race nomenclature
Fishman-Lerner unit
fish-slime disease
fission
> binary f.
> f. fungus
> f. product
> uncontrolled f.

fissiparity
fissiparous
fissurae cerebelli
fissural cyst
fissure
> Ammon f.
> anal f.
> anterior median f.
> Bichat f.
> Bürdach f.
> cerebellar f.
> Henle f.
> f. in ano
> Rolando f.
> Santorini f.

fissured nucleus
fistula (fist.), *pl.* **fistulae, fistulas**
> abdominal f.
> amphibolic f.
> anal f.
> arteriovenous f. (AVF)
> biliary f.
> f. bimucosa
> blind f.
> branchial f.
> bronchoesophageal f.
> bronchopleural f.
> carotid cavernous f.
> cervical f.
> cholecystoduodenal f.
> coccygeal f.
> colocutaneous f.
> coloileal f.
> colonic f.
> colovaginal f.
> colovesical f.
> complete f.
> duodenal f.
> enterocutaneous f.
> enteroenteric f.
> enterovaginal f.
> enterovesical f.
> external f.
> fecal f.

F

fistula (*continued*)
    gastric f.
    gastrocolic f.
    gastrocutaneous f.
    gastroduodenal f.
    gastrointestinal f.
    genitourinary f.
    hepatic f.
    hepatopleural f.
    horseshoe f.
    f. in ano
    incomplete f.
    inflammatory f.
    internal f.
    intestinal f.
    lacteal f.
    mammary f.
    metroperitoneal f.
    mouth f.
    nuisance f.
    pilonidal f.
    pulmonary arteriovenous f. (PAF)
    rectolabial f.
    rectourethral f.
    rectovaginal f.
    rectovesical f.
    rectovestibular f.
    rectovulvar f.
    salivary f.
    sigmoidovesical f.
    spermatic f.
    stercoral f.
    thoracic duct f. (TDF)
    thyroglossal f.
    tracheobiliary f.
    tracheoesophageal f. (TEF)
    umbilical f.
    urachal f.
    ureterocutaneous f.
    ureterovaginal f.
    urethrovaginal f.
    urinary bladder f.
    urogenital f.
    uteroperitoneal f.
    vesical f.
    vesicocolic f.
    vesicocutaneous f.
    vesicointestinal f.
    vesicouterine f.
    vesicovaginal f.
    vesicovaginorectal f.
fistulae (*pl. of* fistula)
fistulas (*pl. of* fistula)
fistulation, fistulization
Fistulina
fistulization (*var. of* fistulation)
fistulous
FITC
    fluorescein isothiocyanate

Fite
    F. method
    F. stain
Fite-Faraco stain
fitter cell theory
fitting
    curve f.
Fitzgerald factor
Fitzgerald-Williams-Flaujeac factor
Fitz-Hugh and Curtis syndrome
Fitz syndrome
fix
    F. and Perm Cell Permeabilization Kit
    B-plus F.
fixation
    alcohol f.
    AMeX f.
    f. artifact
    autotrophic f.
    carbon dioxide f.
    complement f. (CF)
    cytospray f.
    microwave f.
    f. reaction
    secondary f.
    f. test
    Treponema pallidum complement f. (TPCF)
fixative
    acetone f.
    AFA f.
    alcohol-glycerin f.
    aldehyde f.
    Altmann f.
    B5 f.
    Bouin picroformol-acetic f.
    Brasil f.
    buffered formalin f.
    Carnoy f.
    Champy f.
    chromic acid f.
    coating f.
    CytoLyt f.
    CytoRich Red f.
    Flemming f.
    formaldehyde f.
    formalin f.
    formol-calcium f.
    formol-Müller f.
    formol-saline f.
    formol-Zenker f.
    Gendre f.
    glacial acetic acid f.
    glutaraldehyde f.
    Golgi osmiobichromate f.
    Helly f.
    Hermann f.
    Hollande f.

Jores f.
Kaiserling f.
Karnovsky f.
lead f.
Luft potassium permanganate f.
Marchi f.
mercuric f.
methanol f.
Millonig phosphate-buffered formalin f.
Müller f.
neutral buffered formalin f.
Newcomer f.
Orth f.
osmic acid f.
PreservCyt f.
PVA f.
Regaud f.
Saccomanno f.
SAF f.
Schaudinn f.
Shandon f.
single vial f.
Spray-Cyte slide f.
Supermount slide f.
Thoma f.
Trump f.
wick f.
Zenker f.
fixative/solution
Hollande f.
isopentane f.
methylbutane f.
fixed
f. blood film
f. cell
f. macrophage
f. oil
f. sediment method
f. virus
fixed-point variable
fixed-time method
FJN
familial juvenile nephrophthisis
FJP
familial juvenile polyp
FL
follicular lymphoma
Fl
fluid
fluor
fluorescence
follicle lysis
fL
femtoliter
fl
follicle lysis
flaccid
flaccidity

flagella (*pl. of* flagellum)
flagellar
f. agglutination
f. agglutinin
f. antigen
Flagellata
flagellated
flagellate dysentery
flagellin
flagellosis
flagellum, *pl.* **flagella**
flail
f. chest
f. scallop
Flajani disease
flaky paint dermatitis
flame
f. background
capillary f.
f. cell
f. emission spectrophotometry
f. emission spectroscopy (FES)
f. figure
f. intensity zone
f. ionization detector (FID)
manometric f.
f. nevus
f. photometer
f. photometry
flame-shaped retinal hemorrhage
flammability
flammable
flammeus
nevus f.
Flammulina
flank bruit
flap
Bakamjian deltopectoral f.
Estlander f.
Gillies f.
Karapandzic lip reconstruction f.
Wookey skin f.
flash burn
flash-point temperature
flask
f. culture
Dewar f.
Erlenmeyer f.
Fernbach f.
Florence f.
hatching f.
vacuum f.
volumetric f.
flask-like
Erlenmeyer f.-l.
flask-shaped heart
flat
f. bipolar cell
f. condyloma

F

flat (*continued*)
　f. smallpox
　f. substrate method
　f. urothelial hyperplasia
　f. wart
Flatau-Schilder disease
flat-field objective
flattened
　f. cell
　f. shape
flatworm
Flaujeac factor
flava (*pl. of* flavum)
flavescens
　Aedes f.
　Mycobacterium f.
　Neisseria f.
　Trichophyton f.
flavianic acid
flavida
　Kribbella f.
flavin, flavine
　f. adenine dinucleotide (FAD)
　f. mononucleotide (FMN)
flavine (*var. of* flavin)
flavirostris
　Anopheles f.
flaviscutellata
　Lutzomyia f.
flaviscutellatus
flavithermus
　Anoxybacillus f.
flaviverrucosa
　Lentzea f.
Flaviviridae
flavivirus
Flavobacteria
Flavobacteriaceae
Flavobacterium
　F. aquatile
　F. breve
　F. degerlachei
　F. frigidarium
　F. frigoris
　F. gelidilacus
　F. gillisiae
　F. limicola
　F. meningosepticum
　F. micromati
　F. omnivorum
　F. xanthum
　F. xinjiangense
flavoenzyme
flavogenita
　Stemonitis f.
flavoprotein
flavum, *pl.* **flava**
　macula flava
　medulla ossium flava

　Neisseria flava
　Oxalicibacterium f.
　Saccharopolyspora flava
flavus
　Arthrobacter f.
　Aspergillus f.
　Erythrobacter f.
　Plantibacter f.
flaxseed oil
FLCOD
　florid local cementoosseous dysplasia
flea
　American rat f.
　dog f.
　European rat f.
　human f.
　Indian rat f.
flea-bitten kidney
Flegel disease
Fleischer ring
Fleischner syndrome
Fleitmann test
Flemming
　F. fixative
　germinal center of F.
　intermediate body of F.
　F. triple stain
flesh
　proud f.
fleshfly
fleshy
　f. mole
　f. polyp
Fletcher factor
fleurettii
　Staphylococcus f.
flexilis
　Thiothrix f.
Flexistipes sinusarabici
Flexner
　F. bacillus
　F. dysentery
　F. serum
flexneri
　Shigella f.
Flexner-Strong bacillus
Flexner-Wintersteiner rosette
FlexSure
　F. HP
　F. OBT
flexure
　splenic f.
FL11 gene
FLICE
　FADD-like interleukin-1 beta
　converting enzyme
FLICE-like inhibitory protein (FLIP)
flight
　time of f.

Flinders Island spotted fever
flint
>F. arcade
>f. disease
>f. glass

FLIP
>FLICE-like inhibitory protein

flippase enzyme
FLM
>fetal lung maturity
>fluorescence lifetime imaging
>>FLM imaging
>>FLM microscopy

floater
floating
>f. beta disease
>f. organ

floating-point variable
floc
>flocculation

floccose
floccosum
>*Acrothesium f.*
>*Epidermophyton f.*
>*Trichophyton f.*

flocculable
flocculans
>*Balneimonas f.*
>*Rubritepida f.*

floccular degeneration
flocculate
flocculation (floc)
>cephalin f.
>cephalin-cholesterol f. (CCF)
>limes f. (Lf)
>limit of f. (LF)
>f. reaction (FR)
>f. test
>thymol f. (TF)

floccule
>toxoid-antitoxoid f. (TAF)

flocculence
flocculent
flocculus
flood
>f. fever
>f. plate
>f. source

floor cell
flora
>intestinal f.
>oral f.

floral
>f. variant
>f. variant of follicular lymphoma (FFL)

Florence
>F. crystal
>F. flask

Florescent Amplification Catalyzed by T7-polymerase Technique
Florey unit
florid
>f. adenosis
>f. cementoosseous dysplasia
>f. local cementoosseous dysplasia (FLCOD)
>f. oral papillomatosis

Florisil
flotation
>f. bath
>centrifugal f.
>direct centrifugal f. (DCF)
>f. rate
>f. technique
>f. test
>f. unit

flow
>abnormal f.
>f. birefringence
>cerebral blood f. (CBF)
>f. chart
>coronary blood f. (CBF)
>f. cytometer
>f. cytometric assay
>f. cytometric crossmatch
>f. cytometric immunophenotyping
>f. cytometric platelet counting procedure
>f. cytometric reticulocyte analysis
>f. cytometry (FC, FCM)
>f. cytophotometry
>effective renal blood f. (ERBF)
>effective renal plasma f. (ERPF)
>electroosmotic f.
>estimated hepatic blood f. (EHBF)
>exercise hyperemia blood f. (EHBF, EXBF)
>forced expiratory f. (FEF)
>forced inspiratory f. (FIF)
>gene f.
>hepatic blood f. (HBF)
>high f. (HF)
>increased f.
>inspiratory f.
>maximal midexpiratory f. (MMEF)
>maximum expiratory f. (MEF)
>maximum inspiratory f. (MIF)
>pseudopod f.
>pulmonary blood f.
>f. rate (FR)
>reactive hyperemia blood f. (RHBF)
>renal plasma f. (RPF)
>splanchnic blood f. (SBF)
>uterine blood f. (UBF)
>f. volume loop

flower
    collagen f.
flower-spray
    f.-s. ending
    f.-s. organ of Ruffini
flowing hyperostosis
flowmeter (FM)
    electromagnetic f. (EMF)
flow-sorted aneuploid fraction
FLS
    fibrous long-spacing collagen
FLSA
    follicular lymphosarcoma
flu (*var. of* influenza)
    influenza
        FLU OIA A/B rapid test
fluctuation
    IP3 dependent calcium f.
flucytosine
fludrocortisone
fluff
    electron-lucent f.
Fluhmann lumen
fluid (fl)
    Altmann f.
    amniotic f.
    anthrax-infected body f.
    ascitic f.
    f. balance
    Bensley osmic dichromate f.
    body f.
    Bouin f.
    bronchoalveolar lavage f.
      (BALF)
    Burnett disinfecting f.
    Callison f.
    cerebrospinal f. (CSF)
    Ciaccio f.
    Clarke f.
    crevicular f.
    f. culture
    culture of vesicular f.
    de Castro f.
    Delafield f.
    dentinal f.
    extracellular f. (ECF)
    Farrant mounting f.
    gastric f. (GF)
    Gendre f.
    gingival f.
    Helly f.
    interstitial f.
    intracellular f. (ICF, IF)
    intraocular f.
    looped f.
    f. mosaic model
    Orth f.
    pleural f.
    prostatic f.

    proteinaceous f.
    Rees-Ecker f.
    respiratory tract f. (RTF)
    f. retention
    Saccomanno collection f.
    seminal f.
    serous f.
    f. shear stress
    spinal f.
    subretinal f. (SRF)
    sulcular f.
    synovial f.
    tissue f.
    transcellular f.
    tubular f. (TF)
    f. volume (FV)
    Zamboni f.
    Zenker f.
fluid-borne agent
fluke
    blood f.
    cat liver f.
    Chinese liver f.
    giant intestinal f.
    giant liver f.
    lancet f.
    liver f.
    lung f.
    Manson blood f.
    Oriental blood f.
    Oriental lung f.
    sheep liver f.
    vesical blood f.
    Yokogawa f.
fluminea
    Nocardia f.
fluor
fluorescein
    f. isothiocyanate (FITC)
    f. mercuric acetate
    f. sodium
fluorescein-labeled antibody
fluorescein-to-protein ratio (F:P)
fluorescence
    f. correlation spectroscopy (FCS)
    f. decay difference
    dual-color f.
    f. excitation transfer immunoassay
      (FETI)
    f. in situ hybridization (FISH)
    laser-activated f.
    f. lifetime imaging (FLM)
    f. microscope
    f. microscopy
    f. plus Giemsa stain
    f. polarization immunoassay
      (FPIA)
    f. quenching
    relative f. (RF)

resonance f.
f. resonance energy transfer (FRET)
f. spectrum
time-resolved f. (TRF)
fluorescence-activated cell sorter (FACS)
fluorescens
    Pseudomonas f.
fluorescent
f. allergosorbent test (FAST)
f. antibody (FA)
f. antibody dark-field (FADF)
f. antibody technique
f. antibody test (FAT)
f. antinuclear antibody (FANA)
f. antinuclear antibody test
Bordetella pertussis indirect f.
f. cytoprint assay
f. dye
f. immunoassay (FIA)
f. in situ hybridization
f. material
f. microscope
f. microscopy
f. probe
f. protection assay
f. resonance energy transfer
  (FRET)
f. staining
f. treponemal antibody (FTA)
f. treponemal antibody-absorption
  (FTA-ABS)
f. treponemal antibody-absorption
  test
fluoride
f. assay
hydrogen f.
f. number
sodium f.
fluorine (F)
f. 18
fluorite objective
fluoroacetamide
fluoroacetate
f. assay
sodium f.
fluorocarbon assay
fluorochrome
molecule of equivalent soluble f.
  (MESF)
fluorochrome-avidin/streptavidin conjugate
fluorochrome-conjugated
f.-c. DNA
f.-c. monoclonal antibody
fluorochroming
fluorocyte
5-fluorocytosine
fluorodeoxyuridine (FUDR)
fluoro-2,4-dinitrobenzene (FDNB),
  4-dinitrobenzene

Fluorognost HIV-1 IFA assay kit
fluoroimmunoassay
dissociation enhanced lanthanide f.
  (DELFIA)
polarization f.
fluoro jade staining
fluorometry
filipin f.
time-resolved f. (TRF)
fluorophosphonate
methylarachidonyl f. (MAFP)
fluoroscopic diaphragmatic paralysis sniff
  test
fluorosilicate
sodium f.
fluorosis
dental f.
endemic f.
skeletal f.
Fluorospheres
Immuno-Brite F.
fluosol-DA
Flury
F. strain rabies virus
F. strain vaccine
fluvialis
  Vibrio f.
fluviatilis
  Anopheles f.
flux
luminous f.
magnetic f.
FLx/TDx immunoassay analyzer
fly
f. agaric
black f.
dog f.
fruit f.
larva f.
f. larva
stable f.
tsetse f.
warble f.
flying spot microscope
Flynn-Aird syndrome
FM
flowmeter
Fm
fermium
fm
femtometer
FMC7 expression
FMD
foot-and-mouth disease
FMD virus
FMF
familial Mediterranean fever
FMH
familial hemiplegic migraine

F

FMLH
familial hemophagocytic lymphohistiocytosis
fMLP
formyl methionyl leucyl phenylalanine
fMLP receptor
FMN
flavin mononucleotide
fmol
femtomole
FMR
familial mental retardation
FMR-I gene
FMS
fat-mobilizing substance
fms oncogene
FN
false-negative
FNA
fine-needle aspiration
FNAB
fine-needle aspiration biopsy
FNAC
fine-needle aspiration cytology
FNH
focal nodular hyperplasia
FN-MCD
familial nephronophthisis-medullary cystic disease
FN-MCD complex
foam
f. cell
fibrin f.
f. stability index (FSI)
f. stability test (FST)
foam/shake test
foamy
f. agent
f. cytoplasm
f. degeneration
f. gland prostate cancer
f. histiocyte
f. macrophage
f. virus
FOAVF
failure of all vital forces
FOBT
fecal occult blood test
focal
f. adhesion kinase (FAK)
f. amyloidosis
f. appendicitis
f. atrophy
f. axonal injury
f. bone marrow defect
f. bronchopneumonia
f. calcification
f. cortical epilepsy
f. dermal hypoplasia

f. dermal hypoplasia syndrome
f. disease
f. distance
f. embolic glomerulonephritis
f. epithelial hyperplasia
f. extraprostatic extension (F-EPE)
f. fibrosis
f. hypertrophy
f. infarct
f. infection
f. involvement
f. length
f. lymphocytic thyroiditis
f. necrosis
f. necrotizing glomerulonephritis
f. nesidioblastosis
f. nodular hyperplasia (FNH)
f. plane
f. plaque rupture
f. pneumonia
f. proliferative lupus nephritis
f. reaction
f. regression
f. sclerosing glomerulopathy
f. segmental distribution
f. segmental glomerular sclerosis
f. segmental glomerular sclerosis and hyalinosis (FSGSH)
f. segmental glomerulosclerosis (FSGS)
f. ulcer
f. zone
FocalCheck microsphere
foci (*pl. of* focus)
focus, *pl.* foci
aberrant crypt f.
conjugate f.
depth of f.
disseminated foci (DF)
dysplastic f.
ectopic f. (EF)
epileptogenic f.
fibrotic f.
Ghon f.
Ghon-Sachs f.
low-voltage f. (LVF)
metastatic f.
necrotic f.
principal f.
proliferating f.
focused grid
focusing
isoelectric f. (IEF)
FOD
fatty acid oxidation disorder
foenisicii
foetidus
foetus
Trichomonas f.

fog oil (SGF2)
foil
    air f.
Foix-Alajouanine myelitis
Foix syndrome
folate
    f. deficiency
    f. deficiency anemia
    red cell f. (RCF)
    f. reductase
    sodium f.
    whole-blood f. (WBF)
fold
    ciliary f.
    epicanthal f.
    giant gastric f.
    Kerckring f.
    longitudinal f.
    mucobuccal f.
    numerous mucosal f.'s
folded
    f. cell
    f. nucleus
folded-cell index
folded-lung syndrome
folding
    sarcolemmal f.
foliacée
    lame f.
foliaceous
folia linguae
foliar
foliatae
foliate
    f. papilla
    f. papillae
folic
    f. acid
    f. acid assay
    f. acid deficiency
    f. acid deficiency anemia
    f. acid receptor
Folin
    F. and Wu (FW)
    F. and Wu method
    F. test
Folin-Ciocalteu
    F.-C. reagent
    F.-C. test
folinic acid
Folin-Looney test
foliose
follicle
    anovular ovarian f.
    antral f.
    atretic ovarian f.
    f. center lymphoma (FCL)
    f. cyst

    cystic ovarian f.
    dental f.
    gastric f.
    graafian f.
    growing ovarian f.
    hair f.
    intestinal f.
    Lieberkühn f.'s
    lingual f.
    lymphatic f.
    lymphoid f.
    f. lysis (Fl)
    mature ovarian f.
    Montgomery f.
    multilaminar primary f.
    nabothian f.
    ovarian f.
    polyovular ovarian f.
    primary lymphoid f.
    primary ovarian f.
    primordial ovarian f.
    sebaceous f.
    secondary lymphoid f.
    secondary ovarian f.
    solitary f.
    splenic lymph f.
    thyroid f.
    unilaminar primary f.
    vellus anagen f.
    vellus telogen f.
    vesicular ovarian f.
follicle-cell lymphoma
follicle-stimulating
    f.-s. hormone (FSH)
    f.-s. hormone assay
    f.-s. hormone releasing hormone (FSH-RH)
    f.-s. principle
follicular
    f. abscess
    f. adenoma
    f. ameloblastoma
    f. and papillary adenocarcinoma
    f. antrum
    f. atresia
    f. cell center
    f. cell lymphoma cell (FCL)
    f. center cell (FCC)
    f. cholecystitis
    f. conjunctivitis
    f. cyst
    f. cystitis
    f. dendritic cell (FDC)
    f. dendritic cell sarcoma
    f. dermatitis
    f. epithelial cell
    f. gland
    f. goiter
    f. hyperplasia (FH)

F

follicular (*continued*)
  f. inflammation
  f. infundibula
  f. inverted keratosis
  f. lymphoma (FL)
  f. lymphosarcoma (FLSA)
  f. mucinosis
  f. ovarian cell
  f. pattern
  f. pharyngitis
  f. salpingitis
  f. stigma
  f. thyroid carcinoma
  f. urethritis
  f. variant of papillary thyroid
    carcinoma
    (FVPTC)
follicularis
  cystitis f.
  isolated dyskeratosis f.
  keratosis f.
  f. keratosis
folliculi (*pl. of* folliculus)
folliculitis
  f. abscedens et suffodiens
  f. barbae
  f. decalvans
  eosinophilic pustular f.
  f. keloidalis
  pseudolymphomatous f.
  f. ulerythematosa reticulata
folliculocentricity
folliculogenesis
folliculoma
folliculorum
  Acarus f.
  Demodex f.
  Simonea f.
folliculosis
folliculotropic mycosis fungoides
folliculus, *pl.* **folliculi**
  folliculi glandulae thyroideae
  hydrops folliculi
  folliculi linguales
  folliculi lymphatici aggregati
  folliculi lymphatici aggregati
    appendicis vermiformis
  folliculi lymphatici gastrici
  folliculi lymphatici laryngei
  folliculi lymphatici lienales
  folliculi lymphatici recti
  folliculi lymphatici solitarii
  f. lymphaticus
  f. ovaricus primarius
  f. ovaricus vesiculosus
  f. pili
  theca folliculi
  tunica externa thecae folliculi
  tunica interna thecae folliculi

Folling disease
follow-up (*var. of* followup)
followup, follow-up
  lost to f. (LTF)
fomes
Fomitopsis
fondaparinux
Fonio solution
Fonsecaea
  F. compactum
  F. dermatitidis
  F. jeanselmei
  F. pedrosoi
Fontana
  F. methenamine silver stain
  F. space
Fontana-Masson
  F.-M. silver stain
  F.-M. staining method
fontislapidosi
  Idiomarina f.
food
  f. allergy
  f. ball
  f. deprivation
  f. fever
  f. intolerance
  Inuit traditional f.
  medical f.
  f. poisoning
food-based bioterrorism
foodborne
  f. botulism
  f. infection
  f. pathogen
**foodSCAN food allergy
  test**
foot
  athlete's f.
  basal feet
  fungous f.
  Hong Kong f.
  immersion f.
  Madura f.
  Morand f.
  mossy f.
  f. plate
  f. process
  F. reticulin impregnation
    stain
  F. reticulin method
  sandal f.
  trench f.
foot-and-mouth
  f.-a.-m. disease (FMD)
  f.-a.-m. disease virus
  f.-a.-m. disease virus vaccine
foot-plate (*var. of* footplate)
footplate, foot-plate, foot plate

foramen, *pl.* **foramina**
 Bichat f.
 foramina nervosa
 f. nutricium
 nutrient f.
 obturator f.
 f. of Luschka
 f. ovale
 foramina papillaria renis
foramina (*pl. of* foramen)
Foraminifera
foraminiferous
foraminosus
 tractus spiralis f.
foraminulum
Forbes-Albright syndrome
Forbes disease
forbidden clone
force (F)
 centrifugal f.
 centripetal f.
 Chemical Biological Incident
  Response F. (of the U.S. Marine
  Corps)
 electromotive f. (EMF)
 failure of all vital f.'s (FOAVF)
 London f.
 relative centrifugal f. (RCF)
 van der Waals f.'s
forced
 f. expiratory flow (FEF)
 f. expiratory spirogram (FES)
 f. expiratory time (FET)
 f. expiratory time in seconds
  (FETS)
 f. expiratory volume at 1 second
  (FEV-1, FEV1)
 f. inspiratory flow (FIF)
 f. inspiratory oxygen
 f. vital capacity (FVC)
forceps
 air powered f.
 large-cup f.
 Spencer-Wells f.
Forcipomyia glauca
fordii
 Bacillus f.
Fordyce
 F. angiokeratoma
 F. disease
 F. granule
 F. spot
foregut
 f. carcinoid
 f. cyst
forehead
 olympian f.
foreign (for.)
 f. body (FB)

 f. body aspiration
 f. body embolus
 f. body giant cell
 f. body granuloma
 f. body odditis
 f. body reaction
 f. body salpingitis
 f. body tumorigenesis
 f. material deposition
 f. protein
 f. protein therapy
 f. serum
forensic
 f. anthropology
 f. anthropometry
 f. autopsy
 f. dentistry
 f. documentation
 f. evaluation
 f. evaluation of handgun wound
 f. odontology
 f. photograph
 f. radiology
 f. toxicology
 f. urine drug testing (FUDT)
forespore
Forestier disease
forest yaws
fork
 replication f.
forkhead box J1 gene
form
 accolé f.
 appliqué f.
 attenuated viral f.
 band f.
 f. birefringence
 cell wall-deficient bacterial f. (CWDF)
 cornifying f.
 diffuse proliferative f.
 distinctive f.
 exposed protruding f. (EPF)
 Fuzzy Functional F. (FFF)
 ghost f.'s
 intramural protruding f. (IPF)
 involution f.
 myocardial infarction in dumbbell f.
 noncornifying f.
 replicative f.
 ring f.
 spore f.
 sunburst f.
 ulcerating f. (UF)
Formad kidney
formaldehyde
 aniline, sulfur, f. (ASF)
 f. dehydrogenase
 f. fixative
 f. solution

F

formaldehyde-induced fluorescence method
formalin
    alcoholic f.
    f. ammonium bromide
    B5 sodium acetate-sublimate f.
    buffered neutral f.
    calcium acetate f.
    Carson f.
    f. fixative
    f. pigment
    f. solution
    zinc f.
formalin-ether
    f.-e. sedimentation concentration
    f.-e. sedimentation method
formalin-ethyl acetate sedimentation concentration
formalin-fixed
    f.-f. paraffin-embedded (FFPE)
    f.-f. paraffin-embedded sample
    f.-f. skin biopsy
    f.-f. tissue
    f.-f. tissue section
formalinize
formamide
    deionized f.
format
    low-volume air thermal cycle f.
formatexigens
    Bryantella f.
formation
    coffin f.
    crescent f.
    cytokine f.
    de novo tissue f.
    formazan f.
    heat of f.
    ketone body f.
    localized plaque f. (LPF)
    mesencephalic reticular f. (MRF)
    morule f.
    reticular f.
    Roman bridge f.
    rouleau f.
    standard enthalpy of f.
    tubule f.
formatio reticularis
formative cell
formazan
    blue f.
    f. formation
forme
    f. fruste
    f. tardive
formic
    f. acid
    f. aldehyde

formication
formicigenerans
    Dorea f.
formicigenes
    Tepidibacter f.
formicophilia
formiminoglutamic acid (FIGLU)
formin
formol-calcium fixative
formol-gel test
formol-Müller fixative
formol-saline fixative
formol-Zenker fixative
formonitrile
Formosa algae
formula
    Arneth f.
    Arrhenius f.
    Bird f.
    Christison f.
    Häser f.
    Haworth f.
    Long f.
    Poisson-Pearson f.
    Ranke f.
    Reuss f.
    Runeberg f.
    Trapp f.
    Trapp-Häser f.
    Van Slyke f.
formulary
formyl methionyl leucyl phenylalanine (fMLP)
Forney syndrome
fornicalis
    Lactobacillus f.
fornices (*pl. of* fornix)
fornix, *pl.* **fornices**
forskolin-stimulated intracellular cAMP accumulation
Forssman
    F. antibody
    F. antigen
    F. antigen-antibody reaction
    F. lipoid
    F. shock
Förster disease
Forsure One Step Dip Read drug screen test
forsythensis
    Tannerella f.
Fort Bragg fever
fortis
    Bacillus f.
    Vibrio f.
fortuitum
    Mycobacterium f.
fortuitum-chelonae
    Mycobacterium f.-c.

forward
  f. bias
  f. blood typing
  f. dot-blot
  f. failure
  f. fluorescence detector (FED)
  f. mutation
  f. scatter (FSC)
Foshay test
fosphenytoin
fossa, *pl.* **fossae**
  adipose f.
  infratemporal f.
  f. navicularis
fossae (*pl. of* fossa)
fossula, *pl.* **fossulae**
fossulae (*pl. of* fossula)
Foster Kennedy syndrome
Fothergill disease
Fouchet
  F. reagent
  F. stain
  F. test
founder effect
four
  f. locus
  f. subunit
Fourier
  F. analysis
  F. transform infrared
    microspectroscopy (FTIR)
Fournier
  F. disease
  F. gangrene
  syphiloma of F.
fourth-degree
  f.-d. burn
  f.-d. frostbite
  f.-d. radiation injury
fovea
  f. centralis
  f. centralis maculae luteae
  f. ethmoidalis
foveate, foveated
foveated (*var. of* foveate)
  f. chest
Foveavirus
foveola, *pl.* **foveolae**
  f. gastrica
  f. papillaris
foveolae (*pl. of* foveola)
foveolar
  f. epithelium
  f. hyperplasia
foveolate
foveolin
Foville syndrome
fowl
  f. diphtheria

  f. erythroblastosis virus
  f. leukosis
  f. lymphomatosis
  f. lymphomatosis virus
  f. myeloblastosis virus
  f. neurolymphomatosis virus
  f. paralysis
  f. pest
  f. plague
  f. plague virus
fowleri
  Naegleria f.
Fowler solution
fowlpox virus
fox encephalitis virus
Fox-Fordyce disease
fozii
  Psychrobacter f.
F:P
  fluorescein-to-protein ratio
FP
  false-positive
  freezing point
  frozen plasma
FPG
  fasting plasma glucose
FPIA
  fluorescence polarization
    immunoassay
FPM
  filter paper microscopic
FPN
  ferric chloride, perchloric acid,
    nitric acid
    FPN reagent
FPP
  ferriprotoporphyrin
FR
  flocculation reaction
  flow rate
Fr
  francium
FRA
  fibrin-related antigen
fract
  fracture
fractal texture
fraction
  blood plasma f.
  branching f.
  catecholamine f.
  cerebrospinal fluid lactate
    dehydrogenase f.'s
  extraction f. (E)
  flow-sorted aneuploid f.
  growth f.
  heparin-precipitable f. (HPF)
  mole f. (molfr, x)
  f. of inspired oxygen

F

fraction (*continued*)
    O_2Hb f.
    plasma protein f. (PPF)
    saponifiable f.
    S-phase f.
    urine estradiol f.
    urine estriol f.
fractional
    f. allelic loss
    f. concentration of inspired oxygen (FiO_2)
    f. distillation
    f. excretion of sodium (FENa)
    f. sterilization
    f. urinalysis
fractionated
    f. alkaline phosphatase
    f. erythrocyte porphyrin
fractionation
    Cohn f.
    free catecholamine f.
    17-ketosteroid f.
    lipoprotein-cholesterol f.
    nucleocytoplasmic f.
    protein f.
fracture (fract)
    avulsion f.
    f. callus
    cervical f.
    chip f.
    clay shoveler's f.
    closed f.
    comminuted f.
    compound comminuted f. (CCF)
    compound multiple f.'s
    compressed f.
    compression f.
    coronoid process f.
    craniofacial f.
    depressed f.
    f. dislocation
    Frykman hand f.
    greenstick f.
    healed f.
    Hunt and Hess hand f.
    impacted f.
    incomplete compound f.
    Judet epiphysial f.
    linear f.
    Neer shoulder f. I
    nonunion f.
    oblique f.
    orbital f.
    result of severe f.
    Salter-Harris 1 — 5 f.
    scaphoid f.
    simple f.
    spiral f.
    stellate f.

    stress f.
    transverse f.
    ununited f.
fragi
    Pseudomonas f.
fragile
    Desulfofrigus f.
    f. histidine triad (FHIT)
    f. histidine triad gene
    f. X chromosome
    f. X syndrome
fragilis
    Bacteroides f.
    Dientamoeba f.
fragilitas
    f. ossium
    f. sanguinis
fragility
    capillary f.
    erythrocyte f.
    increased capillary f.
    mechanical f.
    f. of the blood
    osmotic f.
    red cell f.
    f. test
fragilocyte
fragilocytosis
fragment
    antiuvomorulin Fab f.
    C-terminal f.
    Fab f.
    Fc f.
    Klenow f.
    f. length
    N-terminal f.
    N-terminal mid f. (NMID)
    P-radiolabeled DNA probe f.
    retained placental f.
    telomeric restriction f. (TRF)
    f. Y
fragmentation myocarditis
fragmenting projectile
fragmentography
    mass f.
FRALE
    frangible anchor-linker effector
Fraley syndrome
frambesia
frame
    Deiters terminal f.
    open reading f. (ORF)
    reading f.
frame-scanning segment
frameshift mutation
framework
Franceschetti-Jadassohn syndrome
Franceschetti syndrome
Francis

F. disease
F. skin test
Francisella
F. philomiragia
F. tularensis
F. tularensis biovar Jellison type A, B
francium (Fr)
François syndrome
frangible anchor-linker effector (FRALE)
Frankiaceae
Frankineae
Frankl-Hochwart disease
Franklin disease
frank megaloblastic anemia
Frank-Starling mechanism
Fraser-Lendrum stain for fibrin
Fraser syndrome
Fras1 gene
frataxin gene
fraterna
Hymenolepis nana f.
fraternal twins
FRC
functional reserve capacity
functional residual capacity
freckle
Hutchinson melanotic f.
melanotic f.
frederiksbergense
Mycobacterium f.
frederiksbergensis
Pseudomonas f.
frederiksenii
Yersinia f.
fredii
Ensifer f.
Fredrickson dyslipoproteinemia classification
free
f. beta test
f. catecholamine fractionation
f. cell
f. electron
f. energy
f. erythrocyte coproporphyrin (FEC)
f. erythrocyte protoporphyrin (FEP, FEPP)
f. estriol
fat f.
f. fatty acid (FFA)
germ f.
gluten f. (GF)
f. macrophage
f. nerve ending
f. protein S test
f. radical
f. ribosome
f. T_4

f. thyroxine index (FTI, FT_4I)
f. toxicology
f. T_4 ratio
f. triiodothyronine (FT_3)
f. triiodothyronine index (FT_3I)
f. (unbound) thyroxine (FT_4)
f. urinary cortisol test
f. water clearance
freeborni
Anopheles f.
freedom
degrees of f. (df)
Freeman-Sheldon syndrome
FreeStyle blood glucose monitoring system
free/total
f. PSA index
f. PSA ratio test
freeze-clamp
freeze-cleave method
freeze-drying
freeze-etch method
freeze-fracture
f.-f. replica
f.-f. technique
freeze-fracture-etch method
freezer
CryoMed f.
-86C ULT f.
Gentle Jane Snap F.
freeze-substitution
freezing
f. injury
f. microtome
f. point (FP)
f. point depression osmometer
Frei
F. antigen
F. disease
F. test
Freiberg disease
Frei-Hoffmann reaction
French-American-British (FAB)
French proof agar
freneyi
Corynebacterium f.
Frenkel anterior ocular traumatic syndrome
frenulum linguae
frequence-time histogram
frequency
angular f.
f. counter
crossover f.
cutoff f.
discharge f.
f. distribution
gene f.
high f. (HF)

F

frequency (*continued*)
    mean dominant f. (MDF)
    medium f. (MF)
    f. polygon
    recombination f.
    urinary f.
    very-high f.
frequens
    Ixodes f.
Frerichs theory
fresconis
    Brachybacterium f.
fresh frozen plasma (FFP)
Fresnel fringe
FRET
    fluorescence resonance energy transfer
    fluorescent resonance energy transfer
freudenreichii
    Propionibacterium f.
Freund
    F. anomaly
    F. complete adjuvant
    F. incomplete adjuvant
freundii
    Citrobacter f.
Frey syndrome
friable
Friderichsen-Waterhouse syndrome
fried egg colony
Friedewald equation
Friedländer
    F. bacillus
    F. bacillus pneumonia
    F. disease
    F. pneumobacillus
    F. stain for capsules
Friedmann
    F. disease
    F. vasomotor syndrome
Friedmanniella
    F. lacustris
    F. spumicola
Friedman test
Friedreich
    F. ataxia
    F. disease
Friedrich ataxia
Friend
    F. disease
    F. leukemia virus
frigidarium
    Flavobacterium f.
frigidity
frigoramans
    Subtercola f.
Frigoribacterium faeni
frigoris
    Clostridium f.
    Flavobacterium f.

frigorism
frill
    iris f.
fringe
    Fresnel f.
    synovial f.
frisingense
    Herbaspirillum f.
fritillariae
    Okibacterium f.
friuliensis
    Actinoplanes f.
Froehlich (*var. of* Fröhlich)
frog test
Fröhlich, Froehlich
    F. dwarfism
    F. syndrome
Frohn reagent
Froin syndrome
Froment paper sign
Frommel-Chiari syndrome
Frommel disease
frond
frondosum
    chorion f.
frontotemporal dementias with parkinsonism linked to chromosome 17 (FTDP-17)
Froriep induration
frostbite
    first-degree f.
    fourth-degree f.
    second-degree f.
    third-degree f.
frosted
    f. heart
    f. liver
frotteurism
frozen
    f. blood
    f. pelvis
    f. plasma (FP)
    f. red blood cell
    f. section (FS, FZ)
    f. section method
fructofuranose
fructokinase
fructopyranose
fructosamine
    AccuMeter f.
fructose
    f. assay
    f. bisphosphate
    f. 1,6-diphosphatase deficiency
    f. diphosphate
    f. intolerance
    f. test
fructose-bisphosphate aldolase
fructosemia

fructosum
> *Leuconostoc f.*

fructosuria
> essential f.

fructosyl

fruit fly

fruiting body

frumenti
> *Lactobacillus f.*

fruste
> forme f.

frustrated phagocytosis

frutescens
> *Capsicum f.*

Frykman hand fracture

Fryn syndrome

fryxellensis
> *Loktanella f.*

FS
> fibrosarcoma
> frozen section

FSC
> forward scatter

FS-DFSP
> fibrosarcomatous variant of dermatofibrosarcoma protuberans

FSF
> fibrin stabilizing factor

FSGS
> focal segmental glomerular sclerosis

FSGSH
> focal segmental glomerular sclerosis and hyalinosis

FSH
> follicle-stimulating hormone
> follicle-stimulating hormone assay
> FSH assay

FSH-RH
> follicle-stimulating hormone releasing hormone
> FSH-RH assay

FSI
> foam stability index

FSP
> fibrinogen split product
> fibrinolytic split product

FSR
> fusiform skin revision

FST
> foam stability test

FT
> fibrous tissue

FT3
> free triiodothyronine

FT4
> free (unbound) thyroxine

FTA
> fluorescent treponemal antibody

FTA-ABS
> fluorescent treponemal antibody-absorption
> FTA-ABS test

FTDP-17
> frontotemporal dementias with parkinsonism linked to chromosome 17

FT$_3$I
> free triiodothyronine index

FT$_4$I
> free thyroxine index

FTI
> free thyroxine index

FTIR
> Fourier transform infrared microspectroscopy

FU
> fecal urobilinogen

Fuchs
> F. adenoma
> F. syndrome

fuchsianus

fuchsin
> acid f.
> aldehyde f. (AF)
> fuchsin, amido black, and naphthol yellow (FAN)
> aniline f.
> basic f.
> f. body
> diamond f.
> new f.
> f. stain

fuchsinophil
> f. cell
> f. granule
> f. reaction

fuchsinophilia

fuchsinophilic

fuchuensis
> *Lactobacillus f.*

fucicola
> *Cellulophaga f.*

fucosidosis

fucosyl moiety

FUDR
> fluorodeoxyuridine

FUDT
> forensic urine drug testing

fuelleborni
> *Strongyloides f.*

fugacity

fugax
> amaurosis f.

fugitive swelling

Fuhrman
> F. grade tumor

F

Fuhrman (*continued*)
    F. nuclear grade
    F. system
fujisawaense
    Methylobacterium f.
Fujiwara reaction
full
    f. blood examination (FBE)
    f. house pattern
    f. scale
full-body x-ray
fuller's earth pneumoconiosis
full-mutation allele
full-series biopsy
full-thickness burn
full-wave rectifier
full-width half-maximum
fulminans
    purpura f.
fulminant
    f. colitis
    f. dysentery
    f. hepatic failure (FHF)
    f. hepatitis
    f. myocarditis
fulminating
    f. anoxia
    f. smallpox
Fulvimarina pelagi
Fulvimonas soli
fulvum
    Microsporum f.
fulvus
    Cellvibrio f.
fumagillin
fumarase
fumarate hydratase
fumaric acid
fumarioli
    Bacillus f.
fume hood
fumigation
fumigatus
    Aspergillus f.
Funalia
functio laesa
function
    abnormal beta cell f.
    autocorrelation f.
    Boolean f.
    cardiopulmonary f.
    continuous f.
    delayed graft f.
    density f.
    detector transfer f. (DTF)
    discriminant f.
    distribution f.
    exponential f.
    line-spread f.

    liver f.
    Maddrey discriminant f.
    modulation transfer f.
    monocular f.
    neonatal biliary f.
    progressive impairment of renal f.
    quadratic f.
    respiratory f.
    split renal f. (SRF)
    step f.
    telomerase f.
    transfer f.
functional
    f. aerobic impairment
    f. affinity
    f. albuminuria
    f. bleeding
    f. constipation
    f. correlation
    f. death
    f. disease
    f. disorder
    f. group
    f. group isomerism
    f. hypertrophy
    f. intact fibrinogen (FiF)
    f. pathology
    f. reserve capacity (FRC)
    f. residual capacity (FRC)
    f. terminal innervation ratio
    f. tumor
functionale
    stratum f.
functionalis
    endometrial f.
fundamentalis
    substantia f.
Fundibacter jadensis
fundic
    f. gland
    f. mucosa
funduliformis
    Bacteroides f.
funestus
    Anopheles f.
fungal
    f. antibody screen
    f. cast
    f. esophagitis
    f. hyphae
    f. pericarditis
    f. pneumonia
    F. Prions
    f. serology
    f. skin testing
    f. spore
    f. stain
Fungalase-F stain
fungate

fungating
  f. adenocarcinoma
  f. sore
fungemia
fungi (*pl. of* fungus)
fungicidal
fungicide
fungiform
  f. papilla
  f. papillae
fungiformes
fungilliform
fungiphilus
  Azonexus f.
fungistatic
fungitoxic
fungitoxicity
fungivorans
  Collimonas f.
Fungizone
fungoid
fungoides
  folliculotropic mycosis f.
  mycosis f. (MF)
fungoma
fungorum
  Burkholderia f.
fungosa
  gastrosia f.
fungosity
fungous foot
fungus, *pl.* **fungi**
  ascospore-forming f.
  f. ball
  f. cerebri
  f. culture
  cutaneous f.
  dematiaceous f.
  dimorphic pathogenic f.
  fission f.
  Fusarium f.
  Gridley stain for fungi
  imperfect f.
  Fungi Imperfecti
  mosaic f.
  mycelial f.
  f. smear
  f. staining
  thrush f.
  yeast f.
funicular
  f. myelitis
  f. myelosis
funiculi (*pl. of* funiculus)
funiculitis
  endemic f.
  filarial f.
funiculus, *pl.* **funiculi**
  Bacillus f.

funis
funisitis
  necrotizing f.
funkei
  Actinomyces f.
funnel
  f. breast
  f. chest
  separatory f.
FUO
  fever of undetermined origin
  fever of unknown origin
furan
furanose
furanoside
furazolidone
furcal
furcate
furcosus
  Bacteroides f.
furens
  Culicoides f.
furfur
  Malassezia f.
  Microsporum f.
  Pityrosporum f.
furfural
  f. reaction
  f. reagent
furfurans
  porrigo f.
furnissii
  Vibrio f.
Furovirus
furrow
  Liebermeister f.
Furstner disease
Furst-Ostrum syndrome
furuncle
furunculoid
furunculosa
  Herpetomonas f.
  Leishmania f.
furunculosis
fusariomycosis
Fusarium
  F. fungus
  F. moniliforme
  F. oxysporum
  F. solanae
fusca
  membrana f.
  Mollisia f.
  Thermomonas f.
fuscans
  Trichosporon f.
fuscicauda
  Sarcophaga f.

F

fuscidula
  Aposphaeria f.
fuseau
fused
  f. glandular pattern
  f. kidney
  f. novel gene
Fusellovirus
Fusibacter paucivorans
fusible calculus
Fusicoccum
fusidate
  sodium f.
Fusidium
fusiform
  f. aneurysm
  f. bacillus
  f. bronchiectasis
  f. cell
  f. layer
  f. skin revision (FSR)
fusiforme
  Filomicrobium f.
  Fusobacterium f.
fusiformis
  Bacteroides f.
  F. necrophorus
  Sarcocystis f.
fusimotor
fusion
  Alpha-TFEB gene f.
  cell f.
  centric f.
  critical flicker f. (CFF)
  gene f.
  f. gene
  heat of f.
  f. protein
  protoplast f.
  splenogonadal f.
  testicular-splenic f.
  TMPRSS2-ERG gene f.
  whole-arm f.
fusispora
  Acrophialophora f.
Fusobacterium
  F. aquatile
  F. equinum

F. fusiforme
F. glutinosum
F. gonidiaformans
F. mortiferum
F. naviforme
F. necrophorum
F. nucleatum
F. plauti-vincentii
F. prausnitzii
F. russii
F. symbiosum
F. varium
fusocellular
fusospirillary
fusospirillosis
fusospirochetal infection
fusospirochetosis
fustic
futile cycle
FU-48 Zenker fixative solution
fuzzy
  f. coat
  F. Functional Form (FFF)
FV
  fluid volume
FVC
  forced vital capacity
FVPTC
  follicular variant of papillary thyroid
  carcinoma
FW
  Folin and Wu
  FW method
FWM
  Folin-Wu method
FWR
  Felix-Weil reaction
Fx
  Icon Fx
fx
  fractional
Fya
  Duffy antibody F.
Fy antigen
Fyb
  Duffy antibody F.
FZ
  frozen section

G
  gauss
  giga
  gonidial (colony)
    G agent
    G antigen
    azocarmine G
    G band
    G banding
    G cell
    G factor
    G protein
    G protein-coupled receptor
    G protein-linked receptor
    G syndrome
    G to A stage tumor transition
    G unit of streptomycin
g
  gram
GAA repeat in the frataxin gene
GABA
  gamma aminobutyric acid
    GABA receptor
GAD
  glutamic acid decarboxylase
Gadd153 gene
Gaddum and Schild test
gadei
    Dysgonomonas g.
gadfly
gadi
    Echinorhynchus g.
gadolinium
Gadus
gaetbuli
    Shewanella g.
Gaeumannomyces
Gaffky
    G. scale
    G. table
Gaffkya tetragena
GAG
  glycosaminoglycan
gag reflex
Gail index of breast cancer risk
gain
    antigen g.
    current g.
    excessive weight g.
gain-of-function abnormality
Gairdner disease
Gaisböck
    G. disease
    G. syndrome
galactan

galactanivorans
    Zobellia g.
galactic
galacticolus
    Saccharomyces g.
galactitol
galactoblast
galactocele
galactocerebroside beta galactosidase
galactography
galactokinase deficiency
galactolipid
galactolipin
galactometer
Galactomyces geotrichum
galactophore
galactophori
    tubuli g.
galactophoritis
galactophorous duct
galactopoietic hormone
galactorrhea
galactosamine
galactose
    g. assay
    g. breath test
    g. oxidase Schiff reaction
    g. phosphate uridyltransferase
      (GPUT)
    g. tolerance test
galactosemia
galactose-1-phosphate uridyltransferase
  (GALT)
galactosidase
    beta g.
    galactocerebroside beta g.
    o-nitrophenyl beta g.
galactoside
galactosidilyticus
    Bacillus g.
galactosuria
galactosylceramidase
galactosylhydrolase
galacturia
galacturonic acid
GA LAW
    glucose, age, lactate, dehydrogenase,
    aspartate aminotransferase, white
    blood cells
Galeati gland
galectin
Galerina autumnalis
gall
    g. body
    g. duct

G

gallate
:   epicatechin g.
gallbladder
:   calcified g.
:   g. carcinoma
:   hourglass g.
:   g. hydrops
:   g. polyp
:   porcelain g.
:   sandpaper g.
:   strawberry g. (SGB)
Gallego differentiating solution
gallein
Gallibacterium anatis
Gallicola barnesae
gallicus
:   *Vibrio* g.
gallinacea
:   *Echidnophaga* g.
gallinaceus
:   *Streptococcus* g.
gallinae
:   *Acarus* g.
:   *Dermanyssus avium* et g.
:   *Microsporum* g.
:   *Trichophyton* g.
gallinarum
:   neurolymphomatosis g.
:   osteopetrosis g.
:   *Trichomonas* g.
gallinatum
gallinifaecis
:   *Ochrobactrum* g.
Gallionellaceae
gallisepticum
:   *Mycoplasma* g.
gallium-67
gallium citrate
gallocyanin, gallocyanine
gallocyanine (*var. of* gallocyanin)
gallopava
:   *Dactylaria* g.
gallstone ileus
gallus adenolike virus
Gallyas
:   G. method
:   G. silver staining technique
galoche chin
GALT
:   galactose-1-phosphate uridyltransferase
:   gastrointestinal associated lymphoid tissue
:   gut-associated lymphoid tissue
:   GALT deficiency
GaLV
:   gibbon ape lymphosarcoma virus
galvanic
:   g. cell
:   g. skin response (GSR)

galvanism
galvanometer
GAL virus
gambiae
:   *Anopheles* g.
Gambian trypanosomiasis
gambiense
:   *Trypanosoma brucei* g.
gametangium
gamete
gametic
:   g. chromosome
:   g. disease
gametocide
gametocyst
gametocyte
gametocytemia
gametogenesis
gametogonia
gametogony
gametoid theory
gametokinetic
gametophagia
gamma
:   g. aminobutyric acid (GABA)
:   g. antigen
:   g. camera
:   g. catenin
:   g. cell
:   g. chain disease
:   g. efferent
:   g. fetoprotein
:   g. fiber
:   g. globulin (GG)
:   g. glutamyltransferase (GGT)
:   g. glutamyl transpeptidase (GGTP)
:   g. heavy-chain disease
:   g. hemolysis
:   IFN g.
:   interferon g.
:   g. loop
:   g. metachromasia
:   g. motor neuron
:   g. motor system
:   g. phage lysis
:   g. photo
:   g. ray
:   g. spectrometer
:   g. spectrometry
:   g. staphylolysin
:   g. streptococcus
:   g. thalassemia
:   g. well counter
gamma-aminobutyrate
gamma-carboxyglutamate
gammaglobulinopathy
gamma-ray spectrum
Gammaretrovirus

gammatolerans
    Thermococcus g.
gammopathy
    benign monoclonal g. (BMG)
    biclonal g.
    essential monoclonal g.
    monoclonal g.
    polyclonal g.
Gamna disease
Gamna-Favre body
Gamna-Gandy
    G.-G. body
    G.-G. nodule
gamogony
gamont
gamophagia
Gamsia
Gamstorp syndrome
gandavensis
    Arthrobacter g.
    Cellvibrio g.
Gandy-Gamna
    G.-G. nodule
    G.-G. spleen
Gandy-Nanta disease
ganghwensis
    Nocardioides g.
    Thalassomonas g.
    Zooshikella g.
ganglia (*pl. of* ganglion)
gangliitis
ganglioblast
gangliocyte
gangliocytoma
    dysplastic cerebellar g.
    hypothalamic g.
ganglioglioma
    desmoplastic infantile g.
gangliolysis
ganglioma
ganglion, *pl.* **ganglia, ganglions**
    aberrant g.
    Acrel g.
    Andersch g.
    Arnold g.
    Auerbach ganglia
    Bezold g.
    g. cell
    g. cell of retina
    Corti g.
    g. cyst
    diffuse g.
    Ganser g.
    Lobstein g.
    nerve g.
    nodose g.
    Soemmerring g.
    Troisier g.
ganglioneuroblastoma (GNB, GNBL)

ganglioneuroma
    central g.
    dumbbell g.
ganglioneuromatosis
ganglionic
    g. blocking agent (GBA)
    g. layer of cerebellar cortex
    g. motor neuron
ganglionitis
ganglionopathy
ganglions (*pl. of* ganglion)
ganglioside
    g. GD2 stain
    g. GM_1
    g. GM_2
gangliosidosis
    generalized g.
    GM_1 g.
    GM_2 g.
gangosa
gangrene
    arteriosclerotic g.
    cold g.
    diabetic g.
    dry g.
    embolic g.
    emphysematous g.
    Fournier g.
    gas g.
    hemorrhagic g.
    hot g.
    Meleney g.
    moist g.
    presenile spontaneous g.
    progressive bacterial synergistic g.
    static g.
    symmetrical g.
    thrombotic g.
    trophic g.
    venous g.
    wet g.
    white g.
gangrenescens
    granuloma g.
gangrenosa
    vaccinia g.
gangrenosum
    ecthyma g.
    pyoderma g. (PG)
gangrenosus
gangrenous
    g. appendicitis
    g. emphysema
    g. necrosis
    g. pharyngitis
    g. pneumonia
    g. stomatitis
ganmani
    Helicobacter g.

G

gannister's disease
Ganoderma
Ganser
>   basal nucleus of G.
>   G. commissure
>   G. ganglion
>   nucleus basalis of G.
>   G. syndrome

GANT
>   gastrointestinal autonomic nerve tumor

gap
>   anion g.
>   auscultatory g.
>   chromatid g.
>   isochromatid g.
>   g. junction
>   g. junction intercellular
>   communication
>   osmolal g.
>   osmolar g.

GAPDH
>   glyceraldehyde phosphate
>   dehydrogenase

gapes
gapeworm
gapped ligase chain reaction
gap$_0$period
gap$_1$period
gap$_2$period
Garciella nitratireducens
Gardner-Diamond syndrome
Gardnerella vaginalis
Gardner syndrome
gargantuan mastitis
gargoylism type of histiocyte
garinii
>   *Borrelia g.*
garlic-clove fibroma
garnhami
>   *Leishmania mexicana g.*
Garré
>   G. disease
>   G. sclerosing osteomyelitis
Gärtner bacillus
Gartner cyst
garvieae
>   *Streptococcus g.*
gas
>   g. abscess
>   g. amplification
>   arsine g.
>   arterial blood g. (ABG)
>   blood g.
>   BTPS conditions of g.
>   carrier g.
>   g. chromatograph
>   g. chromatography (GC)
>   g. chromatography-mass spectrometry
>   (GC-MS)

combustible g.
>   g. constant
>   CS g.
>   g. cyst
>   g. embolism
>   g. exchange
>   extravasation g.
>   g. gangrene
>   g. gangrene antitoxin
>   HCN g.
>   hemolytic g.
>   hepatic portal venous g. (HPVG)
>   ideal g.
>   g. law
>   mustard g.
>   nettle g.
>   oxidizing g.
>   P-50 blood g.
>   g. peritonitis
>   g. phlegmon
>   g. retention
>   sneeze g.
>   g. sterilizer
>   g. storage limit
>   STPD conditions of g.
>   tear g.
>   g. thermometer
>   tritiated g.
>   water g.
GASDirect test
gas-discharge lamp
gaseous spectrum
gasicomitatum
>   *Leuconostoc g.*
gasigenes
>   *Clostridium g.*
Gaskell bridge
gas-liquid chromatography (GLC)
gasometry
gasping disease
Gasser syndrome
gas-solid chromatography (GSC)
Gasteromycetes
Gasterophilidae
Gasterophilus
gastradenitis, gastroadenitis
gastrectasia
gastrectasis, gastrectasia
gastri
>   *Mycobacterium g.*
gastric, gastricus
>   g. acid
>   g. acid stimulation test
>   g. algid malaria
>   g. analysis
>   g. antral vascular ectasia (GAVE)
>   g. argentaffin cell
>   g. aspirate cell count
>   g. atrophy

g. calculus
g. carcinoma
g. chromoscopy
g. culture
g. emptying half time (GET1/2)
g. emptying time (GET)
g. fistula
g. fluid (GF)
g. follicle
g. function test
g. gland
g. incisura
g. inhibitory peptide (GIP)
g. inhibitory polypeptide (GIP)
g. lamina propria
g. lavage
g. lymphoid nodule
g. mucosa
g. myiasis
g. parietal cell (GPC)
g. parietography
g. phenotype lesion
g. pit
g. polyp
g. residua
g. residue examination
g. smear
g. tubular adenoma
g. tumor
g. ulcer (GU)
g. volvulus
g. zymogenic cell

gastrica
foveola g.
glandulae gastricae
tunica mucosa g.

gastrici
folliculi lymphatici g.

gastricus (*var. of* gastric)

gastrin
g. assay
g. releasing peptide (GRP)

gastrin-calcium infusion stimulation test
gastrinoma triangle
gastrin-protein stimulation test
gastrin-secretin stimulation test
gastritis
acute hemorrhagic erosive g.
antral g.
atrophic chronic g.
autoimmune g.
catarrhal g.
chemical g.
chemotherapy g.
chronic atrophic g. (CAG)
chronic hypertrophic g.
g. cystica polyposa
g. cystica profunda
diffuse antral g. (DAG)

eosinophilic g.
erosive g.
exfoliative g.
g. fibroplastica
giant hypertrophic g.
granulomatous g.
Helicobacter g.
hemorrhagic g.
hypertrophic g.
interstitial g.
lymphocytic g.
multifocal atrophic g. (MAG)
polypous g.
pseudomembranous g.
radiation g.
reflux g.
sclerotic g.
Sydney classification for g.
varioliform g.

gastroadenitis (*var. of* gastradenitis)
Gastroccult test
gastrocele
gastrocolic fistula
gastrocolitis
gastrocoloptosis
gastrocutaneous fistula
Gastrodiscoides hominis
Gastrodiscus hominis
gastroduodenal fistula
gastroduodenitis
gastroenteritis
acute infectious nonbacterial g.
endemic nonbacterial infantile g.
eosinophilic g. (EGE)
epidemic nonbacterial g.
infantile g.
porcine transmissible g.
transmissible g.
viral g.
g. virus type A, B

gastroenterocolitis
gastroenteroptosis
gastroesophageal
g. reflux
g. reflux disease (GERD)
gastroesophagitis
gastroileitis
gastrointestinal (GI)
g. adsorbent
g. anthrax
g. anthrax infection
g. associated lymphoid tissue (GALT)
g. autonomic nerve tumor (GANT)
g. blast injury
g. bleeding
g. bleed localization study
g. blood loss test
g. cancer

G

gastrointestinal (*continued*)
   g. contents
   g. disease
   g. fistula
   g. hemorrhage
   g. hormone
   g. ischemia
   g. mucosal cell
   g. pacemaker cell
   g. pacemaker cell tumor (GIPACT)
   g. protein loss test
   g. smooth muscle tumor
   g. stromal tumor (GIST)
   g. tract carcinoma
   g. tuberculosis
   upper g. (UGI)
gastrojejunal
gastrolienal
gastrolith
gastrolithiasis
gastromalacia
gastromegaly
gastropathy
   hypertrophic hypersecretory g.
gastropexy
Gastrophilidae
Gastrophilus
gastropod
Gastropoda
gastroptosia (*var. of* gastroptosis)
gastroptosis, gastroptosia
gastrorrhagia
gastrorrhexis
gastroschisis
gastrosia fungosa
Gastrospirillum hominis
gastrostaxis
gastrostenosis
gastrostom
   percutaneous endoscopic g. (PEG)
gastrotoxin
GATA3 gene mutation
gate
gating
Gaucher
   G. cell
   G. disease (GD)
   G. type of histiocyte
gauge
   vacuum g.
Gauma virus
gauss (G)
gaussian distribution
GAVE
   gastric antral vascular ectasia
gay
   G. gland
   g. lymph node syndrome
Gay-Lussac law

gay-related immunodeficiency disease
GB
   NATO code for sarin
GBA
   ganglionic blocking agent
G-banding stain
GB-7 antibody
GBIA
   Guthrie bacterial inhibition assay
GBM
   glioblastoma
   glomerular basement membrane
GBS
   group B streptococcus
   Guillain-Barré syndrome
GC
   gas chromatography
   germinal center
   gonococcus
   gonorrhea culture
   guanine cytosine
      GC agar
      GC OIA
      GC OID
      GC value
GCA
   germinal cell aplasia
g-cal
   gram-calorie
GCC
   giant cell collagenoma
   glassy cell carcinoma
      GCC of the uterine cervix
GCDFP
   gross cystic disease fluid protein
GCDFP-15 protein
G-cell tumor
GCF
   giant cell fibroblastoma
GCH
   giant cell hepatitis
GCIS
   isolated gland carcinoma in situ
GCKD
   glomerulocystic kidney disease
g-cm
   gram-centimeter
GC-MS
   gas chromatography-mass
   spectrometry
G-CSF
   granulocyte colony-stimulating factor
GCTB
   giant cell tumor of bone
GCT-LMP
   giant cell tumor of low malignant
   potential
GCTTS
   giant cell tumor of tendon sheath

GD
> NATO code for soman

gDNA
> genomic deoxyribonucleic acid

GDNF
> glial cell line-derived neurotropic factor

GDP
> guanosine 5′-diphosphate

GDP-d-mannose
GDP-l-fucose
G:E
> granulocyte/erythroid ratio

GE
> NATO code for nerve agent isopropyl ethylphosphonofluoridate

Ge antigen
Gedoelstia
gedoelstiosis
Gee disease
Gee-Herter disease
Gee-Herter-Heubner disease
Gee-Thaysen disease
Gegenbaur cell
Geiger-Müller counter
gel
> aluminum hydroxide g.
> g. and flow cytometry
> Coomassie blue-stained g.
> denaturing g.
> g. diffusion
> g. diffusion precipitin test
> g. diffusion precipitin test in one dimension
> g. diffusion precipitin test in two dimensions
> g. diffusion reaction
> g. electrophoresis
> g. electrophoresis pattern
> g. filtration
> hydrophilic g.
> hydrophobic g.
> NuPAGE Bis-Tris g.
> polyacrylamide g.
> silica g.

Gelasinospora
gelatin
> g. agar
> g. film
> g. filter
> fish g.
> g. hydrolysis
> g. slide adhesive
> g. sponge particle
> g. zymography

gelatinase
gelatini
> *Bacillus g.*

gelatinoid

gelatinolytic activity
gelatinosa
> substantia g.

gelatinous
> g. acute inflammation
> g. acute pneumonia
> g. adenocarcinoma
> g. ascites
> g. atrophy
> g. carcinoma
> g. infiltration
> g. polyp
> g. substance
> g. tissue

gelatinovorans
> *Ruegeria g.*

gelation
gel-embedded GA-fixed skeleton
gel-filtration chromatography
gelida
> *Desulfofaba g.*

Gelidibacter
> *G. algens*
> *G. mesophilus*

gelidilacus
> *Flavobacterium g.*

Gélineau syndrome
Gell
> G. and Coombs drug allergy classification
> G. and Coombs reaction

Gelman filter
gelosis
gel-permeation chromatography
Gelria glutamica
gem-diol
Gemella
> *G. cuniculi*
> *G. morbillorum*
> *G. palaticanis*
> *G. sanguinis*

geminate
geminatus
> *Anaeroglobus g.*

geminin gene
gemistocyte
gemistocytic
> g. astrocyte
> g. astrocytoma
> g. cell
> g. tumor

gemistocytoma
GEMM
> granulocyte, erythrocyte, monocyte, and megakaryocyte

gemma
Gemmatimonadaceae
Gemmatimonadales
Gemmatimonadetes

G

Gemmatimonas aurantiaca
gemmation
gemmule
 Hoboken g.'s
genal gland
genavense
 Mycobacterium g.
GenBank database
gender reassignment
Gendre
 G. fixative
 G. fluid
gene
 adducin g.
 Aire g.
 allelic g.
 alpha globin g.
 amino acid transporter E16 g.
 g. amplification
 anaplastic lymphoma kinase g.
 (ALK gene)
 androgen receptor g.
 APC g.
 apoptosis g.
 g. arrangement study
 ASPL-TFE3 fusion g.
 ataxin g.
 ATP7B g.
 atrophin g.
 autosomal g.
 g. bank
 Bax apoptosis g.
 bcl-1 g.
 bcl-2 g.
 beta-catenin g.
 beta globin g.
 BMP4 g.
 bone morphogenetic protein 7 g.
 BRCA1 g.
 BRCA2 g.
 cadherin-6 g.
 candidate tumor suppressor g.
 caretaker g.
 cathepsin K g.
 cationic trypsinogen g.
 CAV1 g.
 CAV2 g.
 CDH1 g.
 CDK4 g.
 cell death g.
 CFTR g.
 chimeric g.
 g. chip technology
 c-Ki-ras g.
 Clara cell secretory protein g.
 claudin 4 g.
 ClCN7 g.
 g. cloning
 c-myc g.

 g. code
 codominant g.
 COL4A5 g.
 collagen type IX alpha 2 g.
 competence g.
 complementary g.
 g. complex
 cyclin D1 g.
 cystic fibrosis transmembrane
  conductance regulator g.
 cytochrome b5 reductase g.
 DDB2 g.
 DEL1 g.
 g. deletion
 derepressed g.
 differentiated embryo-chondrocyte
  expressed g. 1
 DKC1 g.
 DLK1 g.
 dominant g.
 g. dosage
 DPC4 g.
 g. dysregulation
 dystrophin g.
 E-cadherin g.
 ERCC2 g.
 ERCC3 g.
 ERCC4 g.
 ERCC5 g.
 Ewing sarcoma g.
 exotaxin/CCL11 g.
 g. expression
 g. expression pattern
 g. expression profiling
 g. expression signature
 FA-A g.
 factor II g.
 FA-L g.
 FAT1 g.
 FHIT g.
 fibrillin g.
 FL11 g.
 g. flow
 FMR-I g.
 forkhead box J1 g.
 fragile histidine triad g.
 Fras1 g.
 frataxin g.
 g. frequency
 fused novel g.
 g. fusion
 fusion g.
 GAA repeat in the frataxin g.
 Gadd153 g.
 geminin g.
 GLEPP1 g.
 glucocerebrosidase g.
 Grb14 g.
 Grb7 g.

Grem1 g.
Grip1 g.
H g.
heme oxygenase-1 g.
heparan sulfate 2-sulfotransferase g.
HER-2 g.
HER-2/neu g.
hexon g.
hexosaminidase A g.
HFE g.
histocompatibility g.
HLA-DM g.
hMLH 1 g.
holandric g.
hologynic g.
homeobox g.
hPMS2 g.
hRAD30 g.
H-ras g.
HRPT2 g.
human androgen receptor g.
  (HUMARA)
human lamin A g. (LMNA)
huntingtin g.
IGH g.
immune response g.
Ir g.
Is g.
Jagged1 g.
jumping g.
Kibra g.
g. knockout
laminin β2 g.
laminin α3β1 g.
laminin α5 g.
lethal g.
g. library
LMX1B g.
LYP g.
major g.
g. mapping
marker g.
MCC g.
Melan-A (MART-1) g.
merlin g.
mismatch repair g.
MLH1 g.
MMR g.
mobile g.
modifying g.
Mrf4 g.
MSH2 g.
MSH6 g.
MTND2 g.
MTND5 g.
MTTA g.
mucin-4 g. (MUC4)
mutant g.
mutator g.

mutL g.
mutS g.
myf3 g.
myf4 g.
myf5 g.
MYH9 g.
MyoD family of g.'s
MyoD1 regulatory g.
myopodin g.
myotonin protein kinase g.
NEDD8 g.
neurofibromin g.
NF-1 g.
NF2 g.
NOD2 g.
nonfunctional factor VIII-related g.
nonstructural g.
N-ras g.
NuMA g.
operator g.
p15 g.
p16 g.
p53 g.
Pbxl g.
PDGF-B g.
PDGFR-β g.
PDGFR-A g.
p16INK4A g.
PMP22 g.
PMS1 g.
PMS-1, -2 g.
PMS2 g.
Pod1 g.
podocalyxin g.
pol g.
g. pool
ppENK g.
p22phox g.
PRAD1 g.
PRCC-TFE3 fusion g.
procollagen alpha1(I) g.
g. product (gp)
programmed cell death 4 g.
  (PDCD4)
prothrombin g.
PTEN tumor suppressor g.
ras g.
RB g.
R-cadherin g.
g. rearrangement
recessive g.
regulator g.
regulatory g.
repressor g.
retinoblastoma g. (RB1)
retinoic acid binding protein 1 g.
14-3-3s g.
S100A g.
S100 calcium binding protein A1 g.

G

gene (*continued*)
    secretor g.
    selenoprotein P g.
    SEPT9 g.
    sex-linked g.
    SHH g.
    g. silencing
    silent g.
    single copy g.
    SMN telomeric g.
    SMO g.
    specific g.
    g. splicing
    split g.
    steroid sulfatase g.
    structural g.
    STS g.
    suicide g.
    superoxide dismutase g.
    supplementary g.
    suppressor g.
    survival motor neuron
      telomeric g.
    synaptopodin g.
    tau g.
    tensin g.
    g. therapy
    thioredoxin reductase g.
    g. transcription
    transfer g.
    transforming g.
    TRPC6 g.
    TSC1 g.
    TSC2 g.
    TSLC1 g.
    tumor suppressor g.
    type I collagen g.
    UP1a uroplakin g.
    UP1b uroplakin g.
    UPII g.
    UPIII g.
    VEGF-A g.
    VHL g.
    VHL g.
    von Hippel-Lindau g.
    wild-type g.
    wingless g.
    Wnt11 g.
    Wnt9b g.
    WRN g.
    wt1 g.
    XAP101 g.
    XLA g.
    X-linked g.
    XLP g.
    XPC g.
    Y-linked g.
    zinc finger g.
    ZYF g.

GeneAmp PCR System 9600
  thermocycler
GeneChip
GenePhor
    G. DNA fragment analyzer
    G. DNA silver staining kit
general
    g. anatomy
    g. dissection technique
    g. feature
    g. gonadotropic activity (GGA)
    g. immunity
    g. paresis (GP)
    g. pathology
    g. peritonitis
    g. radiation
    g. transduction
    g. tuberculosis
generalisata
    hyperostosis corticalis g.
generalisatus
    herpes g.
generalized
    g. activation of thrombosis
    g. anaphylaxis
    g. chondromalacia
    g. cortical hyperostosis
    g. emphysema
    g. eruptive histiocytoma
    g. gangliosidosis
    g. linear mixed model (GLMM)
    g. panhypopituitarism
    g. pustular psoriasis of Zambusch
    g. Sanarelli-Shwartzman reaction
      (GSSR)
    g. Shwartzman phenomenon
    g. Shwartzman reaction (GSR)
    g. transduction
    g. transudation
    g. tuberculosis
    g. vaccinia
    g. xanthelasma
generation
    alternation of g.'s
    first filial g. (F_1)
    second filial g. (F_2)
    spontaneous g.
    g. time
generative cell
generator
    aerosol g.
    diazomethane g.
    random number g.
generic
    g. name
    g. substitution
GeneSearch BLN assay
genesistasis
genestatic

gene-targeting
genetic
- g. abnormality
- g. abnormality analysis
- g. adaptation
- g. algorithm (GA)
- g. anemia
- g. balance
- g. code
- g. counseling
- g. determinant
- g. drift
- g. engineering
- g. etiology
- g. fingerprint
- g. hits
- g. linkage analysis
- g. map
- g. mapping
- g. marker
- g. mutation
- g. recombination
- g. regulation
- g. screening
- g. susceptibility
- G. Systems HIV-1 Western blot test

genetically
- g. abnormal cell
- g. significant dose

genetics
- bacterial g.
- bacteriophage g.
- behavior g.
- biochemical g.
- clinical g.
- mathematical g.
- medical g.
- mendelian g.
- microbial g.
- molecular g.
- population g.
- reverse g.
- somatic cell g.

Gengou phenomenon
genic balance
geniculata
- *Curvularia g.*

geniculocalcarine tract
geniculotemporal tract
geniculum
genioglossus muscle
geniohyoid
genital
- g. condyloma
- g. corpuscle
- g. culture
- g. disorder
- g. gland
- g. herpes

- g. mycoplasma
- g. tract actinomycosis
- g. tubercle
- g. wart

genitalia
- ambiguous external g.
- corpuscula g.

genitalis
- herpes g.
- *Treponema g.*

genitalium
- *Mycoplasma g.*

genitourinary (GU)
- g. fistula
- g. malformation
- g. myiasis

genoblast
genocopy
genodermatosis
genome
- haploid g.
- human g.
- g. mutation
- g. sequencing
- g. stability
- viral g.

GenomeLab
- G. GeXP genetic analysis system
- G. SNPstream genotyping system

genomic
- g. deoxyribonucleic acid (gDNA)
- g. DNA
- g. DNA clone (chromosomal)
- g. imprinting
- g. integration
- g. probe

genophenotypic
genospecies
genote
- F g.

genotype
- PiMM g.
- PiMZ g.

genotypic blot hybridization
genotyping
- hereditary hemochromatosis g.

GenProbe
Gen-S
- G.-S automated cell counting instrument
- G.-S hematology analyzer

Gensoul disease
GenSpin gDNA purification kit
Genta
- G. slide
- G. stain

gentian, gentian root
- g. aniline water
- g. orange stain

G

gentian (*continued*)
    g. violet (GV)
    g. violet stain
gentianophil, gentianophile
gentianophile (*var. of* gentianophil)
gentianophilous
gentianophobic
gentiobiase
Gentle Jane Snap Freezer
Gentra Systems Puregene DNA isolation kit
genu
    g. recurvatum
    g. valgum
    g. varum
Geobacillus
    G. caldoxylosilyticus
    G. kaustophilus
    G. stearothermophilus
    G. subterraneus
    G. thermocatenulatus
    G. thermodenitrificans
    G. thermoglucosidasius
    G. thermoleovorans
    G. toebii
    G. uzenensis
Geobacter
    G. bremensis
    G. chapellei
    G. grbiciae
    G. hydrogenophilus
    G. pelophilus
    G. sulfurreducens
Geobacteraceae
Geobacteria
Geodermatophilaceae
Geodermatophilus
Geoglobus ahangari
geographic
    g. necrosis
    g. pathology
    g. tongue
geolei
    Thermosipho g.
geometric
    G. Data Miniprep slide maker
    g. efficiency
    g. isomerism
    g. optics
geometrical model
geometricus
    Latrodectus g.
Geomyces pannorus
geophagia, geophagism, geophagy
geophagism (*var. of* geophagia)
geophagy (*var. of* geophagia)
geophilic
Geophilus

geophylla
    Inocybe g.
Georgenia muralis
Georgetown
    hemoglobin C G.
georgianum
    Oesophagostomum g.
Geothrix fermentans
Geotrichoides
geotrichosis
geotrichum
    g.
    G. candidum
    Endomyces g.
    Galactomyces g.
    G. immite
geotropism
Geovibriales
Geovibrio
    G. ferrireducens
    G. thiophilus
Geraghty test
geranylgeranyl diphosphate
Gerbich blood group system
Gerbich-negative
    G.-n. phenotype
    G.-n. red cell
Gerbode defect
GERD
    gastroesophageal reflux disease
gergoviae
    Enterobacter g.
Gerhardt
    G. disease
    G. dullness
    G. ferric chloride test
    G. reaction
    G. syndrome
    G. test for acetoacetic acid
    G. test for urobilin in the urine
GERL
    Golgi endoplasmic reticulum lysosome
Gerlach
    G. tonsil
    G. valvula
Gerlier disease
germ
    aberrant g.
    g. cell
    g. cell aplasia
    g. cell deoxyribonucleic acid (germ cell DNA)
    g. cell neoplasm
    g. cell tumor
    g. free (GF)
    g. layer
    g. line
    g. theory

g. tube
g. tube test
German
  G. measles
  G. measles virus
germanium
germicidal
germicide
germinal
  g. cell
  g. cell aplasia (GCA)
  g. center (GC)
  g. center of Flemming
  g. center of lymphatic
   nodule
  g. center of lymph node
  g. epithelial inclusion cyst
  g. epithelium
  g. spot
  g. vesicle
germination tube test
germinativa
  macula g.
germinative
  g. layer
  g. layer of nail
germinativum
  stratum g.
germinoma
  hypophysial stalk g.
  pineal g.
Germiston virus
germline (GL)
  g. configuration
  g. mosaicism
  unrearranged g.
  g. variant
germ-time mutation
gerneri
  Acinetobacter g.
geroderma osteodysplastica
geromarasmus
gerontine
Gerota
  G. capsule
  G. fascia
  G. method
Gerronema
Gerstmann-Straussler-Scheinker disease
(Indiana kindred), tau pathology class I
Gerstmann syndrome
gestagen
gestational
  g. age (GA)
  g. alteration
  g. choriocarcinoma
  g. proteinuria
  g. trophoblastic disease (GTD)
  g. trophoblastic neoplasia

gestationis
  herpes g.
  prurigo g.
gestosis
GET
  gastric emptying time
GET1/2
  gastric emptying half time
geV
  giga electron volt
GF
  gastric fluid
  germ free
  gluten free
  NATO code for cyclosarin
  NATO code for nerve agent
   cyclohexyl methylphosphonofluoridate
GFAP
  glial fibrillary acidic protein
GFP
  green fluorescence protein
GFR
  glomerular filtration rate
GG
  gamma globulin
GGA
  general gonadotropic activity
GGE
  gradient gel electrophoresis
GGT
  gamma glutamyltransferase
   GGT assay
GGTP
  gamma glutamyl transpeptidase
GH
  growth hormone
GHD
  growth hormone deficiency
Ghent
  albumin G.
GH-IH
  growth hormone-inhibiting hormone
Ghon
  G. complex
  G. focus
  G. primary lesion
  G. tubercle
Ghon-Sachs
  G.-S. bacillus
  G.-S. complex
  G.-S. focus
  G.-S. primary lesion
  G.-S. tubercle
ghost
  g. bands
  blood g.
  g. cell
  g. corpuscle
  g. forms

G

ghoul hand
GH-RF
  growth hormone-releasing factor
GH-RH
  growth hormone-releasing hormone
GH-RIH
  growth hormone release inhibiting
    hormone
GHz
  gigahertz
Gi
  gilbert (unit of magnetomotive force)
GI
  gastrointestinal
Giannuzzi
  G. crescent
  G. demilune
Gianotti-Crosti syndrome
giant
  g. anorectal condyloma acuminatum
  g. band
  g. blue nevus
  g. cell
  g. cell aortitis
  g. cell arteritis
  g. cell carcinoma
  g. cell collagenoma (GCC)
  g. cell fibroblastoma (GCF)
  g. cell fibroma
  g. cell glioblastoma
  g. cell hepatitis (GCH)
  g. cell interstitial pneumonia (GIP)
  g. cell myeloma
  g. cell myocarditis
  g. cell reaction
  g. cell reparative granuloma
  g. cell thyroiditis
  g. cell tumor
  g. cell tumor of bone (GCTB)
  g. cell tumor of low malignant
    potential (GCT-LMP)
  g. cell tumor of tendon sheath
    (GCTTS)
  g. colon
  g. condyloma
  g. condyloma of
    Buschke-Lowenstein
  g. fibroadenoma
  g. follicle lymphoma
  g. follicular lymphoblastoma
  g. follicular lymphoma
  g. gastric fold
  g. hairy nevus
  g. hamartoma
  g. hives
  g. hypertrophic gastritis
  g. intestinal fluke
  g. intracanalicular fibroadenoma
  g. liver fluke

  g. melanosome
  g. mitochondrion
  g. neutrophil
  g. neutrophilia
  g. osteoid osteoma
  g. pigmented nevus
  g. platelet
  g. platelet disease
  g. platelet syndrome
  g. urticaria
giantism (*var. of* gigantism)
Giardia
  G. intestinalis
  G. lamblia
giardiasis dysentery
Giardiavirus
Gibberella
gibbon ape lymphosarcoma virus
  (GaLV)
gibbus deformity
Gibco-BRL TriZol DNA extraction
Gibney disease
Gibson-Cooke sweat test
gibsoniae
  Desulfotomaculum g.
gibsonii
  Streptomyces g.
Giemsa
  G. chromosome banding stain
  G. method
Gierke
  G. cell
  G. corpuscle
  G. disease
Gieson
  elastica van G. (EVG)
  Verhoeff-van G. (VVG)
giga (G)
  g. electron volt (geV)
gigahertz (GHz)
gigantea
  Calvatia g.
  urticaria g.
giganteum
  Trichosporon g.
giganteus
  Aspergillus g.
gigantica
  Fasciola g.
gigantism, giantism
  exomphalos, macroglossia, and g.
    (EMG)
  Sotos syndrome of cerebral g.
gigantocellular glioma
gigantomastia
Gigantorhynchus
gigohm
GIK
  glucose, insulin, and potassium

gilardii
    Roseomonas g.
    Wautersia g.
gilbert
    G. disease
    G. syndrome
    g. (unit of magnetomotive force) (F, Gi)
Gilchrist
    G. disease
    G. mycosis
gill-arch skeleton
Gilles de la Tourette syndrome
Gill #2 hematoxylin blue stain
Gillies flap
gillisiae
    Flavobacterium g.
Gillisia limnaea
Gilmaniella
gilvus
    Enterococcus g.
GIM
    gonadotropin-inhibitory material
Gimenez stain
gingival
    g. cyst
    g. epithelium
    g. fluid
    g. hyperplasia
    g. tissue
gingivalis
    Entamoeba g.
gingivitis
    acute necrotizing ulcerative g.
    diphenylhydantoin g.
    hypertrophic g.
    necrotizing ulcerative g. (NUG)
    scorbutic g.
gingivodental ligament
gingivosis
gingivostomatitis
    herpetic g.
    necrotizing ulcerative g.
ginkgetin
ginkgolide
GIP
    gastric inhibitory peptide
    gastric inhibitory polypeptide
    giant cell interstitial pneumonia
GIPACT
    gastrointestinal pacemaker cell tumor
Girard
    G. method
    G. reagent
GISA
    glycopeptide-insensitive *Staphylococcus aureus*
GIST
    gastrointestinal stromal tumor

gitalin
gitaloxin
Gitelman syndrome
gitoxin
GITT
    glucose insulin tolerance test
gitter cell, gitterzelle
gitterzelle (*var. of* gitter cell)
GKA
    glucokinase activator
GL
    germline
    greatest length
glabellar
glabra
    verruca g.
glabrata
    Biomphalaria g.
    Candida g.
    Torulopsis g.
glabrosa
    tinea g.
glabrous skin
glabrum
    Trichophyton g.
glacial
    g. acetic acid
    g. acetic acid fixative
glaciale
    Brumimicrobium g.
Glaciecola
    G. mesophila
    G. pallidula
    G. polaris
    G. punicea
gladiatorum
    herpes g.
gland
    accessory g.
    acid g.
    acinotubular g.
    acinous g.
    admaxillary g.
    adrenal g.
    aggregate g.
    agminate g.
    albuminous g.
    alveolar g.
    anal g.
    apical g.
    apocrine sweat g.
    areolar g.
    arteriococcygeal g.
    arytenoid g.
    Avicenna g.
    axillary sweat g.
    Bauhin g.
    Blandin g.
    Bowman g.

G

gland (*continued*)
brachial g.
bronchial g.
Bruch g.
Brunner g.
buccal g.
bulbourethral g.
BUS g.'s
cardiac g.
ceruminous g.
cervical g.
Ciaccio g.
ciliary g.
circumanal g.
coccygeal g.
coil g.
conjunctival g.
Cowper g.
g. crowding
ductless g.
duodenal g.
Duverney g.
Ebner g.
eccrine g.
Eglis g.
endocrine g.
esophageal g.
excretory g.
exocrine g.
follicular g.
fundic g.
Galeati g.
gastric g.
Gay g.
genal g.
genital g.
Gley g.
Guérin g.
hemal g.
hematopoietic g.
hemolymph g.
hibernating g.
holocrine g.
hyperplastic g.
interscapular g.
interstitial g.
intestinal g.
intraepithelial g.
jugular g.
Knoll g.
Krause g.
labial g.
labial salivary g. (LSG)
lacrimal g.
lactiferous g.
laryngeal g.
Lieberkühn glands
Littré g.
Luschka cystic g.

lymph g. (LG)
malpighian g.
mammary g.
marrow-lymph g.
master g.
maxillary g.
meibomian g.
merocrine g.
mesenteric g.
milk g.
Moll g.
mucilaginous g.
muciparous g.
mucus secreting cervical g.
nasal g.
Nuhn g.
odoriferous g.
g. of internal secretion
oil g.
olfactory g.
oxyntic g.
pacchionian g.
pileous g.
pineal g.
pituitary g.
Poirier g.
prehyoid g.
preputial g.
prostate g.
pyloric g.
racemose g.
Rivinus g.
Rosenmüller g.
saccular g.
salivary g.
sebaceous g.
secretory g.
sentinel g.
seromucous g.
serous g.
Serres g.
sexual g.
Sigmund g.
Skene g.
solitary g.
sublingual g.
submaxillary g.
sudoriferous g.
suprahyoid g.
suprarenal g.
Suzanne g.
sweat g.
target g.
tarsal g.
Terson g.
Theile g.
thymus g.
thyroid g.
Tiedemann g.

tracheal g.
trachoma g.
tubular g.
tubuloacinar g.
tubuloalveolar mucous g.
tympanic g.
Tyson g.
unicellular g.
uterine g.
vaginal g.
vascular g.
vesical g.
vestibular g.
vulvovaginal g.
Waldeyer g.
Wasmann g.
Weber g.
Wepfer g.
Wölfler g.
Wolfring g.
Zeis g.

glanders
g. bacillus
g. pneumonia
gland-forming malignancy
glandilemma
glandula, *pl.* **glandulae**
glandulae areolares
g. atrabiliaris
g. basilaris
glandulae buccales
g. bulbourethralis
glandulae ceruminosae
glandulae cervicales uteri
glandulae ciliares
glandulae circumanales
glandulae conjunctivales
glandulae cutis
ductuli excretorii g.
glandulae duodenales
glandulae endocrinae
glandulae esophageae
glandulae gastricae
glandulae lacrimales accessoriae
glandulae suprarenales accessoriae
glandulae glomiformes
glandulae intestinales
glandulae labiales
g. lacrimalis
glandulae laryngeae
g. lingualis anterior
g. mammaria
g. mucosa
glandulae mucosae biliosae
glandulae nasales
glandulae olfactoriae
glandulae oris
glandulae palatinae
g. parathyroidea

g. parotidea
g. parotidea accessoria
g. parotis
g. parotis accessoria
glandulae pharyngeales
g. pituitaria
glandulae preputiales
g. prostatica
glandulae pyloricae
g. salivaria
glandulae sebaceae
g. seromucosa
g. serosa
glandulae sine ductibus
g. sublingualis
g. submandibularis
glandulae sudoriferae
g. suprarenalis
glandulae tarsales
g. thyroidea
g. thyroidea accessoria
glandulae tracheales
glandulae tubariae
glandulae urethrales femininae
glandulae urethrales masculinae
glandulae uterinae
glandulae vestibulares minores
g. vestibularis major
glandulae (*pl. of* glandula)
glandular
g. budding
g. cancer
g. carcinoma
g. cell
g. dysplasia
g. epithelium
g. fever
g. hyperplasia
g. mastitis
g. metaplasia
g. odontogenic cyst
g. pharyngitis
g. proliferation
g. schwannoma
g. structure
g. system
glandularis
cystitis g.
g. proliferans cholecystitis
pyelitis g.
ureteritis g.
glandule
glandulous
glans
Glanzmann
G. disease
G. thrombasthenia
Glanzmann-Naegeli thrombasthenia
Glanzmann-Riniker syndrome

G

GLA-protein
    bone G.-p. (BGP)
glass
    g. body
    cover g.
    g. electrode
    g. factor
    g. fiber filter
    flint g.
    ground g.
    heat-resistant g.
    low-actinic g.
    object g.
    optical g.
    Wood g.
glass-bead retention method
glass-blower's mouth
glassware
    aluminosilicate g.
    borosilicate g.
    Corex g.
    Kimax g.
    Pyrex g.
    soda-lime g.
    Vycor g.
glassy
    g. cell carcinoma (GCC)
    g. cytoplasm
    g. membrane
glauca
    Forcipomyia g.
glauciflava
    Actinomadura g.
glaucoma
    angle closure g.
    congenital g.
    infantile g.
    open-angle g. (OAG)
    primary g.
    secondary g.
glaucomatous
    g. habit
    g. pannus
glaucosuria
glaucum
    Corynebacterium g.
glaucus
    Aspergillus g.
GLC
    gas-liquid chromatography
Gleason
    G. pattern
    G. prostate carcinoma
      score
    G. tumor grade
Glénard disease
Glenner-Lillie stain for pituitary
Glenospora graphii
GLEPP1 gene

Gley
    G. cell
    G. gland
glia
    Bergmann g.
    g. cell
gliacyte
gliadin
gliae
    membrana limitans g.
glial
    g. cell
    g. cell line-derived neurotropic
      factor (GDNF)
    g. fibrillary acidic protein (GFAP)
    g. filament
glicentin
glioblast
glioblastoma (GBM)
    g. cell line
    giant cell g.
    g. multiforme
gliocladium
    Aspergillus g.
gliofibrillary acidic protein
glioma
    brainstem g.
    gigantocellular g.
    lipidized g.
    malignant g.
    mixed g.
    nasal g.
    g. of optic chiasm
    optic nerve g.
    subependymal g.
    telangiectatic g.
Gliomastix murorum
gliomatosis
    g. cerebri
    g. peritonei
gliomatous
gliomyxoma
glioneuroma
gliosarcoma
gliosis
    fibrillary g.
    isomorphous g.
    g. of brain stem
    pulvinar g.
    g. uteri
gliotoxin
Glisson
    G. cirrhosis
    G. disease
glissonian sheath
glissonitis
glitter cell
GLMM
    generalized linear mixed model

GLOB collection
globe cell anemia
globi (*pl. of* globus)
Globicatella sulfidifaciens
Globidium
globin-chain
    g.-c. electrophoresis
    g.-c. synthesis
globin insulin
globispora
    Sporosarcina g.
Globocephalus
globoid
    g. cell leukodystrophy
    g. encapsulated tumor
globose specialization
globoside
globular
    g. leukocyte
    g. monomer
    g. protein
    g. space of Czermak
    g. sputum
    g. thrombus
    g. value
globular-fibrous transformation
globule
    acidophilic yolk g.
    dentin g.
    hyaline g.
    polar g.
globuliferous phagocyte
globulin
    accelerator g. (AcG)
    alpha g.
    alpha-1 g.
    alpha-2 g.
    antidiphtheritic g.
    antihemophilic g. A, B (AHG)
    antihuman g. (AHG)
    antilymphocyte g. (ALG)
    antilymphocytic g.
    antimacrophage g. (AMG)
    antithoracic duct lymphocytic g.
      (ATDLG)
    antithymocyte g. (ATG)
    Bence Jones g.
    beta g.
    beta-1A g.
    beta-1C g.
    beta-1E g.
    beta-1F g.
    bovine gamma g. (BGG)
    chickenpox immune g. (human)
    corticosteroid-binding g. (CBG)
    cortisol-binding g. (CBG)
    equine antihuman lymphoblast g.
      (EAHLG)
    gamma g. (GG)

    hepatitis B immune g. (HBIG)
    horse antihuman thymus g.
      (HAHTG)
    human-derived botulism immune g.
    human gamma g. (hGG)
    human milk factor g.
    human rabies immune g. (HRIG)
    immune serum g. (ISG)
    liver-derived sex steroid-binding g.
    measles immune g. (human)
    plasma accelerator g.
    poliomyelitis immune g. (human)
    rabies immune g.
    $Rh_o(D)$ immune g.
    serum accelerator g.
    sex hormone-binding g.
    specific immune g. (human)
    steroid hormone binding g. (SHBG)
    g. test
    testosterone-estradiol binding g.
      (TeBG)
    tetanus immune g.
    thyroid-binding g. (TBG)
    thyroxine-binding g. (TBG)
    unbound thyroxine-binding g.
      (UTBG)
    vaccinia immune g. (VIG)
    g. X
    zoster immune g. (ZIG)
globulinemia
    IgA g.
globulinuria
globulomaxillary cyst
globulus
globus, *pl.* **globi**
Gloeobacterales
Gloeobacteria
Gloeocystidiellum
Gloeophyllum
Gloeosporium
glomangioma
glomangiomatous osseous malformation
  syndrome
glomangiopericytoma
glomangiosis
    pulmonary g.
glome
glomerata
    Actinocorallia g.
Glomerella
glomerular, glomerulose
    g. barrier
    g. basal lamina
    g. basement membrane (GBM)
    g. basement membrane antibody
    g. basement membrane disease
    g. crescent
    g. cyst
    g. disorder

G

glomerular (*continued*)
   g. filtrate
   g. filtration
   g. filtration rate (GFR)
   g. nephritis
   g. sclerosis
   g. tuft
glomerular-like cluster
glomerule
glomeruli (*pl. of* glomerulus)
glomerulitis
glomerulocystic kidney disease (GCKD)
glomeruloid hemangioma
glomerulonephritides (*pl. of*
  glomerulonephritis)
glomerulonephritis (GN), *pl.*
  glomerulonephritides
   acute g. (AGN)
   acute crescentic g.
   acute exudative g.
   acute hemorrhagic g.
   acute poststreptococcal g.
   acute proliferative g.
   antibasement membrane g.
   Berger focal g.
   chronic g. (CGN)
   chronic membranous g. (CMGN)
   crescentic anti-GBM g.
   cryoglobulinemic g.
   diffuse extracapillary proliferative g.
   Ellis type 1 g.
   embolic g.
   epimembranous g.
   experimental autoimmune g. (EAG)
   extramembranous g.
   exudative g.
   fibrillary g.
   focal embolic g.
   focal necrotizing g.
   healed g.
   hemorrhagic g.
   hypocomplementemic g.
   idiopathic pauciimmune necrotizing
    crescentic g.
   immune complex g.
   immunotactoid g.
   induced g.
   lobular g.
   local g.
   membranoproliferative g. (MPGN)
   membranous g. (MGN)
   mesangial proliferative g.
   mesangiocapillary g.
   mesangioproliferative g.
   necrotizing g.
   postinfectious g.
   poststreptococcal g. (PSGN)
   proliferative g.
   rapidly progressive g. (RPGN)

   segmental g.
   subacute g.
   type II membranoproliferative g.
glomerulopathy
   focal sclerosing g.
   immune complex g.
   immunotactoid g.
   nonmyloidotic fibrillary g.
   proliferative g.
glomerulosa
   g. cell
   zona g.
glomerulosclerosis
   cirrhotic g.
   diabetic g.
   focal segmental g.
   intercapillary g.
   nodular g.
glomerulose (*var. of* glomerular)
glomerulus, *pl.* **glomeruli**
   bloodless glomeruli
   capsula glomeruli
   malpighian g.
   obsolescent g.
   g. of pronephros
   olfactory g.
   Ruysch g.
glomiformes
   glandulae g.
glomus
   glomera aortica
   g. body
   g. caroticum
   g. cell
   g. coccygeum
   g. jugulare tumor
   g. pulmonale
   g. vagale
gloriae
   Trichophyton g.
Glossina
   G. morsitans
   G. pallidipes
   G. palpalis
glossinidius
   Sodalis g.
glossitis
   atrophic g.
   Hunter g.
   median rhomboid g.
glottis
glove juice technique
gloves
   chemical-resistant inner g.
   chemical-resistant outer g.
   Skinsense g.
glow modulator tube
Glu
   glutamic acid

glucagon (GL, Gln, GN)
gut g.
g. hypersecretion
immunoreactive g. (IRG)
plasma g.
g. response test
glucagonoma
glucaldrate
potassium g.
glucan-branching
g.-b. enzyme
g.-b. glycosyltransferase
Glucatell beta-glucagan blood test kit
glucitol
glucocerebrosidase gene
glucocerebroside
glucocorticoid
g. receptor (GR)
g. suppressible aldosteronism
g. therapy
glucocorticoid-glucocorticoid receptor complex
glucocorticoid-GR complex
glucocorticosteroid
glucofuranose
glucogenesis
glucogenic amino acid
glucohemia
glucokinase activator
Gluconacetobacter
G. entanii
G. intermedius
G. johannae
G. oboediens
gluconate
potassium g.
gluconeogenesis
gluconeogenetic
glucopenia
glucopyranose
glucosamine
glucose
glucose, age, lactate dehydrogenase, aspartate aminotransferase, white blood cells (GA LAW)
g. assay
Benedict test for g.
blood g. (BG)
buffered desoxycholate g.
cerebral metabolic rate of g. (CMRG)
cerebrospinal fluid g.
conversion of g.
dexamethasone, insulin, and g. (DIG)
fasting plasma g. (FPG)
g. fingerstick test
glucose, insulin, and potassium (GIK)

g. insulin tolerance test (GITT)
maximal tubular reabsorption of g. (T_{mg})
g. metabolism
mole of g.
g. oxidase
g. oxidase method
g. oxidase paper strip test
g. oxidase test
postprandial g.
premeal g.
g. suppression test
g. tolerance (GT)
g. tolerance factor (GTF)
g. tolerance test (GTT)
urine g.
glucose-format broth
glucose-nitrogen ratio (G:N)
glucose-6-phosphatase hepatorenal deficiency glycogenosis
glucose-1-phosphate
glucose-6-phosphate
g.-6-p. dehydrogenase (G6PD)
g.-6-p. dehydrogenase deficiency
g.-6-p. dehydrogenase deficiency anemia
g.-6-p. dehydrogenase screen
g.-6-p. dehydrogenase test
glucosephosphate
g. isomerase
g. isomerase assay
g. isomerase deficiency
1,4-glucosidase
alpha 1.-g.
glucosidase
alpha g.
glucoside
glucosuria
glucosyl
glucosylceramidase assay
GlucoWatch Biographer
glucuronate
glucuronic acid
glucuronide, glucuronoside
bilirubin g.
glucuronolyticum
Corynebacterium g.
glucuronoside (*var. of* glucuronide)
glucuronosyl transferase
glue
fibrin g.
Gluge corpuscle
glumarum
Puccinia g.
GluR2 deficiency

G

glutamate
    arginine g.
    g. decarboxylase
    g. dehydrogenase
    monosodium g. (MSG)
    g. semialdehyde
    sodium g.
glutamate-pyruvate transaminase
glutamatergic transmission
glutamic
    g. acid (E, Glu)
    g. acid decarboxylase (GAD)
    g. aciduria
glutamica
    Gelria g.
glutamic-oxaloacetic transaminase (GOT)
glutamic-pyruvic transaminase (GPT)
glutaminase
glutamine
    cerebrospinal fluid g.
    g. synthetase
glutaminyl
glutaminyl-peptide gamma glutamyltransferase
glutamyl
    g. transfer cycle
    g. transpeptidase (GT)
glutamyltransferase
    gamma g. (GGT)
    glutaminyl-peptide gamma g.
glutaral
glutaraldehyde fixative
glutaric
    g. acid
    g. acidemia
    g. aciduria type 2 syndrome
glutarica
glutathione (GSH)
    g. agarose beads
    g. disulfide (GSSG)
    g. instability test
    oxidized g. (GSSG)
    g. peroxidase
    reduced g.
    g. reductase (GR)
    g. reductase assay
    g. reductase deficiency
    g. stability test
    g. synthetase
    g. synthetase deficiency
glutathionemia
glutathionuria
gluten free (GF)
gluten-free diet
glutenin
gluten-induced enteropathy
gluten-sensitive enteropathy (GSE)
glutethimide assay

glutin
glutinis
    Saccharomyces g.
glutinosum
    Fusobacterium g.
glutinous
glutitis
GLUT-1 marker
GLUT5 transporter
Gly
    glycine
    glycyl
glycan
glycanilyticus
    Paenibacillus g.
glycemia
glyceraldehyde phosphate dehydrogenase (GAPDH)
Glycergel
    G. mounting medium
    Sigma G.
glyceride
glycerin
    g. broth
    g. method
glycerinated lymph
glycerin-potato broth
glycerol gelatin medium
glycerolization
glycerolize
glycerol-3-phosphate oxidase (GOI)
glycerophosphate
    potassium g.
glycerophosphatide
glyceryl triacetate
glycine (Gly)
    g. assay
    urine g.
glycine-arginine reaction
glycinemia
glycine-rich beta-glycoprotein
glycinuria
Glyciphagus
    G. buski
    G. domesticus
Glycobacteria
glycocalyx
glycochenodeoxycholate
glycochenodeoxycholic acid
glycocholate
glycocholic acid
glycoconjugate
    lipid-linked g.
glycodelin glycoprotein
glycodeoxycholic acid
glycogen
    g. acanthosis
    g. branching enzyme
    cytoplasmic g.

g. degradation
g. digestion
g. granule
hepatic g.
g. infiltration
intracytoplasmic g.
g. particle
g. phosphorylase
g. phosphorylase isoenzyme BB
(GPBB)
g. stain
g. staining
g. (starch) synthase
g. storage
g. storage disease (GSD)
g. storage disorder (GSD)
g. storage test
g. synthesis
tissue g.
glycogenesis
glycogenic acanthosis
glycogenolysis
glycogenolytic
glycogenosis
glucose-6-phosphatase hepatorenal
deficiency g.
hepatophosphorylase deficiency g.
hepatorenal g.
idiopathic generalized g.
myophosphorylase deficiency g.
type V g.
glycoglycinuria
glycohistochemistry
glycol
ethylene g.
g. methacrylate
polyethylene g.
propylene g.
glycolate
sodium g.
glycolic
g. acid
g. acid test
g. aciduria
glycolipid
g. layer
g. lipidosis
g. stain
g. staining
glycolithocholic acid
glycolysis
anaerobic g.
glycolytic enzyme
Glycomycetaceae
Glycomycineae
glycone
glyconeogenesis
glycopenia
glycopeptide

glycopeptide-insensitive *Staphylococcus*
aureus **(GISA)**
Glycophagus
glycophorin A staining
glycoprotein (GP)
acid g.
alpha-1 acid g.
alpha acid g.
biliary g. (BGP)
cell surface g.
extracellular matrix g.
glycodelin g.
g. hormone
nonlineage specific
transmembrane g.
platelet membrane g.
P-selectin g.
g. receptor
g. stain
g. staining
submaxillary g.
thrombomodulin g. (TM)
tumor-associated g. (TAG)
glycoprotein-1
glycoprotein-2
epithelial g.-2 (EGP-2)
glycoproteinase
glycoptyalism
glycopyrrolate
glycopyrronium bromide
glycorrhachia
glycorrhea
glycosaminoglycan (GAG)
glycosaminolipid
glycosialia
glycosidase
glycoside
cardiac g.
cyanophoric g.
digitalis g.
sterol g.
glycosphingolipid
glycosuria
alimentary g.
benign g.
digestive g.
normoglycemic g.
renal g.
toxic g.
glycosuric melituria
glycosylase
uracil DNA g. (UDG)
glycosylated
g. hemoglobin
g. hemoglobin assay
g. hemoglobin test
glycosylation
N-linked g.
glycosyl ceramide

G

glycosylphosphatidylinositol (GPI)
  g. specific phospholipase D
    (GPI-PLD)
glycosyltransferase
  alpha glucan-branching g.
  glucan-branching g.
glycuresis
glycuronuria
glycyl (Gly)
glycyl-glycine dipeptidase
glycyl-leucine dipeptidase
glycyltryptophan test
Glycyphagus domesticus
glyodin
glyoxylate reductase
glyoxylic acid test
g-m
  gram-meter
GM-CSF
  granulocyte-macrophage
    colony-stimulating factor
Gmelin test
GM instrument
3′,5′-GMP
  guanosine 3′,5′-cyclic phosphate
3′:5′-GMP
GMS
  Grocott-Gomori methenamine silver
    GMS stain
GMW
  gram molecular weight
G:N
  glucose-nitrogen ratio
gnat
Gnathostoma
  G. doloresi
  G. hispidum
  G. nipponicum
  G. siamense
  G. spinigerum
gnathostomiasis
GNB
  ganglioneuroblastoma
GNBL
  ganglioneuroblastoma
GNID
  gram-negative intracellular
    diplococci
Gnomonia
Gnomoniopsis
gnotobiology
gnotobiota
gnotobiote
gnotobiotic
gnotophoresis
GnRH
  gonadotropin-releasing
    hormone
goatpox

goat's milk anemia
goblet
  g. cell
  g. cell adenocarcinoma
  g. cell carcinoid
  g. cell metaplasia
Godwin tumor
Gofman test
GOG
  gynecologic oncology group
GOI
  glycerol-3-phosphate oxidase
goiter
  aberrant g.
  acute g.
  adenomatous g.
  colloid g.
  congenital g.
  cystic g.
  diffuse nontoxic g.
  diving g.
  dyshormonogenic g.
  endemic g.
  exophthalmic g.
  familial g.
  fibrous g.
  follicular g.
  hyperplastic nodular g.
  lingual g.
  lymphadenoid g.
  microfollicular g.
  multinodular g.
  multiple colloid adenomatous g.
    (MCAG)
  nodular colloid g.
  nodular hyperplastic g.
  nontoxic g. (NTG)
  simple g.
  sporadic diffuse g.
  sporadic nodular g.
  substernal g.
  suffocative g.
  thoracic g.
  toxic g. (TG)
  wandering g.
goitrous
gold
  g. assay
  g. chloride
  g. chloride reagent
  colloidal g. (CG)
  g. cyanide
  g. particle
  protein A g. (PAG)
  g. sol test
  g. standard
  g. therapy
  g. toning
gold-198

Goldberg-Maxwell syndrome
Goldblatt
    G. hypertension
    G. kidney
Goldenhar syndrome
Goldflam disease
Goldflam-Erb disease
Goldner trichrome stain
Goldscheider disease
Goldstein disease
Goldz-Gorlin syndrome
golf hole ureteral orifice
Golgi
    G. apparatus
    G. cavity alteration
    G. cell
    G. complex
    G. endoplasmic reticulum lysosome
    (GERL)
    G. internal reticulum
    G. membrane alteration
    G. osmiobichromate fixative
    G. stain
    G. tendon organ
    G. vacuole alteration
    G. vesicle alteration
    G. zone
Golgi-Mazzoni corpuscle
golgiokinesis
Goltz syndrome
GOM
    granular osmiophilic material
Gomori
    G. aldehyde fuchsin stain
    G. chrome alum
    hematoxylin-phloxine stain
    G. methenamine silver stain (GMS
    stain)
    G. method for chromaffin
    G. nonspecific acid phosphatase
    stain
    G. nonspecific alkaline phosphatase
    stain
    G. one-step trichrome stain
    G. silver impregnation stain
Gomori-Jones periodic acid-methenamine
silver stain
Gomori-Takamatsu
    G.-T. procedure
    G.-T. stain
gonad
    streak g.
gonadal
    g. agenesis
    g. aplasia
    g. dysgenesis
    g. endocrine disorder
    g. ridge
    g. shield

    g. streak
    g. stromal tumor
gonadoblastoma
gonadotrope adenoma
gonadotroph
gonadotrophin (*var. of* gonadotropin)
gonadotropic
    g. hormone (GTH)
gonadotropin, gonadotropic hormone,
    gonadotrophin
    chorionic g. (CG, CGT)
    deficiency of g.
    human chorionic g. (HCG, hCG)
    human menopausal g. (HMG)
    human pituitary g. (hPG)
    menopausal g.
    pituitary g.
    pregnant mare serum g. (PMSG)
    g. test
    total urinary g. (TUG)
    urinary chorionic g. (UCG)
gonadotropin-inhibitory material
    (GIM)
gonadotropin-producing adenoma
gonadotropin-releasing
    g.-r. agent
    g.-r. factor (GRF)
    g.-r. hormone (GnRH)
    g.-r. hormone stimulation test
gonarthritis
gonatagra
gonatocele
gondii
    Toxoplasma g.
gondwanensis
    Psychroflexus g.
gonecystolith
gonensis
    Anoxybacillus g.
Gongronella
Gongylonema pulchrum
gongylonemiasis
gonidiaformans
    Fusobacterium g.
gonidial (colony) (G)
gonioma
gonitis
gonocele
gonococcal
    g. arthritis
    g. arthritis-dermatitis syndrome
    g. conjunctivitis
    g. ophthalmia
    g. peritonitis
gonococcemia
gonococcus (GC)
gonocyte
gonohemia
gonophage

G

gonorrhea
g. culture (GC)
venereal disease g.
gonorrheal
g. ophthalmia
g. rheumatism
g. salpingitis
gonorrhoeae
chromosomally mediated resistant
Neisseria g.
Neisseria g.
gonorrhoica
macula g.
gonotoxemia
gonotoxin
gonotyl
Gonyaulax catanella
Good
G. antigen
G. syndrome
goodfellowii
Leptotrichia g.
Goodpasture
G. stain
G. syndrome
Goormaghtigh cell
Gopalan syndrome
Gordius
G. aquaticus
G. robustus
Gordon
G. agent
G. and Sweets stain
G. body
G. syndrome
G. test
gordonae
Mycobacterium g.
Gordonia
G. aichiensis
G. amarae
G. amicalis
G. bronchialis
G. desulfuricans
G. hirsuta
G. hydrophobica
G. namibiensis
G. nitida
G. paraffinivorans
G. polyisoprenivorans
G. rubropertincta
G. sihwensis
G. sinesedis
G. sputi
G. terrae
G. westfalica
Gordoniaceae
gordoniae
Rhodococcus g.

gordonii
Streptococcus g.
Gordon-Sweet staining
Gorham disease
Goriaew rule
Gorlin
G. cyst
G. syndrome
Gorlin-Chaudhry-Moss syndrome
Gorlin-Goltz syndrome
Gorlin-Psaume syndrome
gormanii
Legionella g.
Gorman syndrome
gorondou
gossypol compound
GOT
glutamic-oxaloacetic transaminase
Göthlin capillary fragility test
Gottlieb
epithelial attachment of G.
Gottron papule
gottschalkii
Anaerobranca g.
Gougerot-Blum
G.-B. disease
G.-B. syndrome
Gougerot-Carteaud syndrome
gougerotii
Sporotrichum g.
Gougerot-Ruiter disease
Gougerot-Sjögren disease
goundou
gourvilii
Trichophyton g.
gout
abarticular g.
articular g.
calcium g.
lead g.
g. nephropathy
saturnine g.
tophaceous g.
gouty
g. arthritis
g. nephropathy
g. tophus
g. urine
Gower 1, 2 hemoglobin
Gowers
G. solution
G. syndrome
GP
general paresis
glycoprotein
gram-positive
group
GPAIS
guinea pig antiinsulin serum

GPBB
glycogen phosphorylase isoenzyme BB
GPC
gastric parietal cell
GPC-R5b receptor
GPC-R5c receptor
GPC-R5d receptor
G6PD
glucose-6-phosphate dehydrogenase
A or B isozyme of G6PD
G$_0$ phase
G$_1$ phase
GPI
glycosylphosphatidylinositol
gram-positive identification
Vitek GPI
GPIIb
platelet fibrinogen receptor GPIIb I
platelet receptor GPIIb I
GPIIb/IIIa
platelet G.
GPIPID
guinea pig intraperitoneal infectious
dose
GPI-PLD
glycosylphosphatidylinositol specific
phospholipase D
GPK
guinea pig kidney
GPKA
guinea pig kidney absorption (test)
GPS
gray platelet syndrome
guinea pig serum
GPT
glutamic-pyruvic transaminase
GPUT
galactose phosphate uridyltransferase
GR
glucocorticoid receptor
glutathione reductase
graafian follicle
grab urine specimen
gracile
Trichosporon g.
Gracilibacillus
G. dipsosauri
G. halotolerans
Gracilicutes
gracilis
Desulfovibrio g.
Euglena g.
fasciculus g.
Hylemonella g.
Nitrospina g.
g. syndrome
grade
ACS g.
analytical reagent g.

AR g.
Fuhrman nuclear g.
Gleason tumor g.
high g. (HG)
histological tumor g.
g. I–IV astrocytoma
g. I-IV ependymoma
g. 1, 2 neuroendocrine carcinoma
Nottingham histologic g.
nuclear g.
prostatic intraepithelial neoplasia,
mild dysplasia or low g. (PIN 1)
prostatic intraepithelial neoplasia,
moderate dysplasia or high g.
(PIN 2)
prostatic intraepithelial neoplasia,
severe dysplasia or high g. (PIN
3)
reagent g.
weapon g.
Gradenigo syndrome
gradient
average g.
chemotactic g.
colloidal silica g.
fetal repertoire g.
g. gel electrophoresis (GGE)
serum ascites albumin g. (SAAG)
sucrose density g. (SDG)
transmural g.
grading
cytologic nuclear g.
histologic g.
Kernohan malignant astrocytoma g.
Nottingham modification of
Scarff-Bloom-Richardson g.
tumor g.
graduated
g. cylinder
g. pipette
Graefe disease
Graffi virus
graft
allogeneic g.
autogeneic g.
autologous g.
autoplastic g.
bone g. (BG)
coronary artery bypass g. (CABG)
heterologous g.
heteroplastic g.
heterospecific g.
homologous g.
homoplastic g.
interspecific g.
isogeneic g.
isologous g.
isoplastic g.
material g.

G

graft (*continued*)
    g. rejection
    serum chemistry g. (SCG)
    skin g. (SG)
    split-thickness skin g. (STSG)
    syngeneic g.
    g. versus host disease (GVHD)
    g. versus host reaction (GVHR)
    white g.
    xenogeneic g.
Graham
    G. law
    G. Little syndrome
Graham-Cole test
Grahamella
grain
    corps g.'s
    g. count halving time
    g. itch
    g. itch mite
gram (g)
    g. iodine
    g. ion
    g. method
    g. molecular weight (GMW)
    G. solution
    G. stain
gram-calorie (g-cal)
gram-centimeter (g-cm)
Gram-chromotrope stain
gramicidin
graminea
    Vicia g.
graminis
    Erysiphe g.
    Paenibacillus g.
    Puccinia g.
graminophila
    Heterodera g.
gram-meter (g-m)
gram-negative (GN)
    g.-n. bacillus
    g.-n. bacterium
    g.-n. broth
    g.-n. cocci
    g.-n. endotoxemia
    g.-n. intracellular diplococci (GNID)
grampicola
    Crassicauda g.
gram-positive (GP)
    g.-p. bacillus
    g.-p. bacterium
    g.-p. cocci
    g.-p. identification (GPI)
Gram-Sure reagent
Gram-Weigert stain
granddaughter cyst
grandis
    Diplogonoporus g.

grand mal epilepsy
Grandry corpuscle
Granger method
Granit loop
granivorans
    Paenibacillus g.
granular
    g. atrophy
    g. cell ameloblastoma
    g. cell myoblastoma
    g. cell schwannoma
    g. cell tumor
    g. conjunctivitis
    g. degeneration
    g. deposition
    g. endoplasmic reticulum
    g. golden appearance
    g. kidney
    g. layer of cerebellar cortex
    g. layer of epidermis
    g. leukoblast
    g. leukocyte
    g. osmiophilic material (GOM)
    g. pharyngitis
    g. pneumocyte
    g. pneumonocyte
    g. urethritis
    g. urinary cast
    g. vaginitis
granulare
    Trichophyton g.
granularity
    eosinophilic g.
granularum
    Acholeplasma g.
    Mycoplasma g.
granulation
    arachnoid g.
    Bayle g.
    cytoplasmic g.
    pacchionian g.
    g. tissue
    toxic g.
granulationes arachnoideae
granule
    acidophil g.
    acrosomal g.
    acrosome g.
    alpha g.
    Altmann g.
    amphophil g.
    argentaffin g.
    autophagic g.
    azurophil g.
    azurophilic g.
    Babès-Ernst g.
    basal g.
    basophil g.
    basophilic g.

Bensley specific g.
beta g.
Birbeck g.
Bollinger g.
bull's eye g.
g. cell
chromatic g.
chromatophilic g.
chromophil g.
chromophobe g.
cone g.
Crooke g.
delta g.
dense-core neurosecretory g.
dense secondary g.
diazo stain for argentaffin g.'s
electron lucent g.
elementary g.
endocrine g.
eosinophil g.
eosinophilic g.
extracellular g.
Fordyce g.
fuchsinophil g.
glycogen g.
Grawitz g.
haloed g.
Heinz g.
intranuclear perichromatin g.
iodophil g.
juxtaglomerular g.
kappa g.
keratohyalin g.
keratohyalin-like g.
lamellar g.
Langerhans g.
Langley g.
light-staining g.
lipofuscin g.
membrane-coating g.
metachromatic g.
mucigen g.
mucinogen g.
neurosecretory g.
Neusser g.
neutrophil g.
Nissl g.
oxyphil g.
primary g.
proacrosomal g.
prosecretion g.
rod g.
round secretory g.
sand g.
Schüffner g.
secondary g.
secretory g.
seminal g.
siderocytic g.

siderotic g.
smoker's g.
specific g.
sulfur g.
toxic g.
Zimmermann g.
zymogen g.
Granulicatella
  G. adiacens
  G. balaenopterae
  G. elegans
granuloblast
granulocyte
  band form g.
  coelomic g.
  g. colony-stimulating factor
    (G-CSF)
  g. concentrate
  granulocyte, erythrocyte, monocyte,
    and megakaryocyte (GEMM)
  hypersegmented g.
  hypogranular g.
  hyposegmented g.
  immature g.
  g. pheresis
  polymorphonuclear g.
  g. recovery
  segmented g.
  g. transfusion
  g. transfusion support
granulocyte/erythroid ratio (G:E)
granulocyte-macrophage
  colony-forming unit g.-m.
    (CFU-GM)
  g.-m. colony-stimulating factor
    (GM-CSF)
granulocytic
  g. aplasia
  g. blood cell
  g. hyperplasia
  g. hypoplasia
  g. leukemia
  g. precursor cell
  g. sarcoma (GS)
  g. series
granulocytopenia
granulocytopoiesis
granulocytopoietic
granulocytosis
granulogenesis
granuloma, *pl.* **granulomata**
  amebic g.
  g. annulare
  apical g.
  barium g.
  beryllium g.
  bilharzial g.
  calcified g.
  caseating g.

G

granuloma (*continued*)
   Churg-Strauss g.
   coccidioidal g.
   cutaneous extravascular necrotizing
      g.
   dental g.
   g. endemicum
   eosinophilic g.
   g. faciale
   foreign body g.
   g. gangrenescens
   giant cell reparative g.
   histiocytic g.
   Hodgkin g.
   infectious g.
   g. inguinale
   g. inguinale tropicum
   intramucosal loose g.
   Kaposi sarcoma-like g.
   laryngeal g.
   lethal midline g.
   lipoid g.
   lipophagic g.
   Majocchi g.
   malignant g.
   midline lethal g.
   midline malignant reticulosis g.
   mineral oil g.
   multifocal eosinophilic g.
   necrobiotic g.
   noncaseating g.
   nonnecrotizing g.
   oily g.
   plasma cell g. (PCG)
   pulmonary hyalinizing g. (PHG)
   pyogenic g.
   g. pyogenicum
   reparative giant cell g.
   reticulohistiocytic g.
   ring g.
   g. sarcoid
   sarcoid g.
   sarcoidal g.
   schistosome g.
   sea urchin g.
   silica g.
   silicone g.
   spermatocytic g.
   spermatogenic g.
   suture g.
   swimming pool g.
   g. telangiectaticum
   tuberculoid g.
   tuberculoid-type g.
   unifocal eosinophilic g.
   uterine g.
   Windelmann g.
   zirconium g.
granulomata (*pl. of* granuloma)

granulomatis
   Calymmatobacterium g.
   Cephalosporium g.
   Donovania g.
granulomatosis
   allergic g.
   angiitic g.
   benign lymphocytic angiitis and g.
   bronchocentric g. (BCG)
   g. disciformis chronica et
      progressiva
   eosinophilic g.
   Langerhans cell g. (LCG)
   lipophagia g.
   lipophagic intestinal g.
   lymphomatoid g. (LYG)
   Miescher g.
   necrotizing sarcoid g. (NSG)
   g. siderotica
   Wegener g.
granulomatous
   g. angiitis with eosinophilia
   g. colitis
   g. disease
   g. disease of childhood
   g. encephalomyelitis
   g. endometritis
   g. enteritis
   g. gastritis
   g. hepatitis
   g. inflammation
   g. lesion
   g. mastitis
   g. orchitis
   g. polyp
   g. process
   g. thyroiditis
granulomere
granulopenia
granuloplasm
granuloplastic
granulopoiesis
granulopoietic
granulopoietin
granulosa
   g. cell carcinoma
   g. cell tumor
   g. lutein cell
   membrana g.
   Oospora g.
granulosa-stromal cell tumor
granulosa-theca cell tumor
granulosis
   Noguchia g.
   g. rubra nasi
granulosity
granulosum
   Propionibacterium g.
   stratum g.

Trichophyton g.
Trichosporon g.
granulosus
    Echinococcus g.
    Noguchia g.
    Oceanicola g.
granulovacuolar degeneration
Granulovirus
granum
granzyme B
grape
    Carswell g.
    g. cell
    g. ending
    g. mole
graph
    Davenport g.
    g. tablet
graphanesthesia (*var. of* graphesthesia)
graphesthesia, graphanesthesia
graphic
    g. analysis
    g. terminal
graphii
    Glenospora g.
    Verticillium g.
graphite pneumoconiosis
Graphium
graphomotor
graphospasm
grappe
    en g.
grating
    diffraction g.
    replica g.
gravel
    coarse g.
Graves disease
grave wax
gravidarum
    fibroma molle g.
    hyperemesis g.
    molluscum fibrosum g.
    nephritis g.
    striae g.
gravimetric method of Sobel
Gravindex pregnancy test
gravis
    anemia g.
    colitis g.
    icterus g.
    myasthenia g.
gravitation abscess
gravity
    g. concentration
    increased specific g.
    specific g. (SG, sp gr)
gravity-settling culture (GSC)
Gravlee jet wash

Grawitz
    G. basophilia
    G. granule
    G. tumor
gray, grey
    g. area
    g. commissure
    g. degeneration
    g. fiber
    g. hepatization
    g. induration
    g. infiltration
    g. patch
    g. platelet syndrome (GPS)
    g. scale
    g. zone lymphoma
grayi
    Listeria g.
gray-patch ringworm
Grb7 gene
Grb14 gene
grbiciae
    Geobacter g.
great
    g. alveolar cell
    g. pestilence
    G. Smokies Diagnostic Laboratories
        intestinal permeability test kit
    g. vessel
greater omentum
greatest length (GL)
green
    brilliant g.
    bromcresol g.
    g. cancer
    g. cross (phosgene gas)
    ethyl g.
    fast g.
    g. fluorescence protein (GFP)
    guinea g. B
    g. hemoglobin
    indocyanine g. (ICG)
    Janus g. B
    malachite g.
    methyl g.
    g. monkey virus
    g. pus
    g. sickness
    g. sputum
Greenfield disease
Greenhow disease
greenstick fracture
gregaloid
Gregarina
gregarine
Gregarinia
gregarinosis
Greig syndrome
Greiner Vacuette coagulation plastic tube

G

Grem1 gene
Gremmeniella
grenade
    ethylbromoacetate g.
grenz
    g. ray
    g. zone
gresilensis
    Legionella g.
grey (*var. of* gray)
    G. Turner sign
GRF
    gonadotropin-releasing factor
    growth hormone-releasing factor
grid
    aligned g.
    Bucky g.
    copper g.
    crossed g.
    focused g.
    g. index
    Kova Glasstic Slide #10 with G.'s
    g. line
    nickel g.
    ocular g.
    Potter-Bucky g.
    g. ratio
    Westgard selection g.
Gridley
    G. stain
    G. stain for fungi
Griesinger disease
Griess reagent
griffe
    main en g.
griffin
    G. beaker
    g. claw
Griffith
    G. classification
    G. point
Grifola
grignonense
    Ochrobactrum g.
Grimelius
    G. argyrophil reaction
    G. argyrophil stain method
    G. stain
Grimontia hollisae
grimontii
    Acinetobacter g.
    Pseudomonas g.
grinder
    Potter-Elvehjem handheld tissue g.
grinder's asthma
grip
    devil's g.
Grip1 gene
Griphosphaeria corticola

grippe
    Balkan g.
grippotyphosa
    Leptospira g.
Griscelli syndrome
grisea
    commissura anterior g.
    Madurella g.
griseofulvin
Grisonella ratellina
gristle
Grocott-Gomori
    G.-G. methenamine silver method
    G.-G. methenamine silver stain
    (GMS)
Grocott methenamine silver (GMS)
groin ulcer
Grönblad-Strandberg syndrome
Groome assay
groove
    Blessig g.
    coffee-bean g.
    complementary g.
    Harrison g.
    Liebermeister g.
    liver g.'s
    nuclear g.
    g. of nail matrix
    g. sign
    skin g.
gross
    g. cystic disease fluid protein
    (GCDFP)
    g. deletion
    g. description
    G. disease
    g. hematuria
    g. lesion
    G. leukemia virus
    G. virus antigen
ground
    g. glass
    g. glass appearance
    g. glass attenuation
    g. glass cell
    g. glass cytoplasm
    g. glass hepatocyte
    g. glass opacity
    g. itch anemia
    g. lamella
    g. state
    g. substance
ground-glass appearance colony
group
    g. A beta hemolytic streptococci
    throat culture
    acetyl g.
    acyloxy g.
    g. agglutination

g. agglutinin
g. A hapten
alkyl g.
g. antigens
arbovirus g. A, B, C
aryl g.
g. A *Streptococcus*
g. B arbor virus
blood g.
Bombay blood g.
g. B *Streptococcus* (GBS)
g. 1 carcinogen
CH/RG blood g.
concentration-time product for 50% of exposed g. (Ct$_{50}$)
connective tissue g.
control g.
coryneform g.
cross-reactive g. (CREG)
cytophil g.
determinant g.
g. D *Streptococcus*
functional g.
guanidinium g.
gynecologic oncology g. (GOG)
high mobility g. (HMG)
hydroxyl g.
I blood g.
g. I-IV mycobacteria
g. immunity
isogenous g.
Kell blood g. (K)
Kell-Cellano blood g.
keto g.
Kidd blood g.
Lewis blood g.
linkage g.
Lutheran blood g.
MNSs blood g.
National Bladder Cancer Collaborative G. (NBCCG)
g. N *Streptococcus*
P blood g.
platinum g.
polycomb g.
P-related blood g.
prenyl g.
prosthetic g.
proteus g.
psittacosis-lymphogranuloma venereum-trachoma g.
g. reaction
Rh blood g.
salmonella g.
g. specific amplification
g. specific antigen
spotted fever g. (SFG)
sulfhydryl g.
symmetry g.

thiocarbonyl g.
g. transfer
ventral respiratory g.
Vibrio g. F (EF-6)
grouping
antigenic structural g.
blood g.
haptenic g.
Lancefield g.
reverse g.
Grover disease
grower
rapid g.
growing
g. ovarian follicle
g. point
growth
g. acceleration
accretionary g.
g. alteration
appositional g.
g. arrest
autonomous g.
auxetic g.
g. disorder
disordered epithelial g.
exophytic g.
g. fraction
g. fraction with Ki-67
g. hormone (GH)
g. hormone deficiency (GHD)
g. hormone-inhibiting hormone (GH-IH)
g. hormone-producing adenoma
g. hormone release inhibiting hormone (GH-RIH)
g. hormone-releasing factor (GH-RF, GRF)
g. hormone-releasing hormone (GH-RH)
g. hormone suppression test
g. inhibitory factor
interstitial g.
intussusceptive g.
multiplicative g.
new g.
g. pattern
g. plate
Regaud pattern of g.
g. retardation
Schmincke pattern of g.
turban g.
growth-stimulating hormone (GSH)
GRP
gastrin releasing peptide
Gruber-Frantz tumor
Gruber syndrome
Gruber-Widal reaction
Grubyella

G

gru.nous
gryochrome
GS
    granulocytic sarcoma
GSA
    group specific amplification
GSC
    gas-solid chromatography
    gravity-settling culture
GSD
    glycogen storage disease
    glycogen storage disorder
GSE
    gluten-sensitive enteropathy
GSH
    glutathione
    growth-stimulating hormone
GSR
    galvanic skin response
    generalized Shwartzman reaction
    gunshot residue
        GSR test
GSSG
    glutathione disulfide
    oxidized glutathione
GSSR
    generalized Sanarelli-Shwartzman
      reaction
GT
    glucose tolerance
    glutamyl transpeptidase
GTD
    gestational trophoblastic disease
GTF
    glucose tolerance factor
GTH
    gonadotropic hormone
GTP
    guanosine triphosphate
GTPase-activating protein
GTT
    glucose tolerance test
GU
    gastric ulcer
guaiac
    stool g.
    g. test
guaiac-based fecal occult blood test
guaiacin
guaiacolsulfonate
    potassium g.
Guam
    amyotrophic lateral
      sclerosis/parkinsonism±dementia
      complex of G.
Guama virus
Guanarito virus
guanase
guanidine isothiocyanate method

guanidinemia
guanidinium
    g. extraction
    g. group
guanidino-aminovaleric acid
guanine
    g. cell
    g. cytosine (GC)
    cytosine phosphate g. (CpG)
    g. deaminase
    g. deaminase assay
guanosine
    g. $3',5'$-cyclic phosphate ($3',5'$-GMP)
    g. $5'$-diphosphate (GDP)
    g. diphosphate
    g. monophosphate
    g. $5'$-phosphate
    g. triphosphate
guanylic acid
guanyl-nucleotide-binding protein
guanylyl
guard cell
Guarnieri body
Guaroa virus
guaymasensis
Gubler
    G. line
    G. paralysis
    G. syndrome
    G. tumor
Gudden atrophy
Guérin gland
guideline
    emergency response planning g.
    (ERPG)
Guignardia
Guillain-Barré syndrome (GBS)
Guilliermondella
guilliermondi
    Candida g.
guinea
    g. green B
    g. pig antigen
    g. pig antiinsulin serum (GPAIS)
    g. pig intraperitoneal infectious dose
    (GPIPID)
    g. pig kidney (GPK)
    g. pig kidney absorption (test)
    (GPKA)
    g. pig serum (GPS)
    g. worm infection
Guinon disease
Gulf War syndrome
Gull disease
Gull-Sutton syndrome
Gulosibacter molinativorax
gumma, *pl.* **gummata, gummas**
    syphilitic g.
    tuberculous g.

gummas (*pl. of* gumma)
gummata (*pl. of* gumma)
gummatous
    g. abscess
    g. syphilid
    g. ulcer
gummosa
    scrofuloderma g.
gummy
Gumprecht shadow
gums
    strawberry g.
Gun Hill hemoglobin
gun-needle probe
Gunning-Lieben test
Gunn syndrome
gunpowder
    g. mark lesion
    g. stippling
gunshot
    g. residue (GSR)
    g. wound
Günther disease
Günzberg
    G. reagent
    G. test
Gussenbauer artificial larynx
gustation
gustatorius
    caliculus g.
    porus g.
gustatory
    g. bud
    g. cell
    g. organ
    g. pore
    g. sweating syndrome
gustus
    organum g.
gut-associated lymphoid tissue (GALT)
gut glucagon
Guthrie
    G. bacterial inhibition assay (GBIA)
    G. card
    G. test
Gutman unit
guttata
    morphea g.
Guttavirus

gutter
guttiformis
    Staleya g.
guttural duct
gutturotetany
Gutzeit test
guyanensis
    Leishmania braziliensis g.
GV
    gentian violet
GVHD
    graft versus host disease
GVHR
    graft versus host reaction
gyiorum
    Kerstersia g.
Gymnamoebida
Gymnascella
Gymnoascaceae
Gymnoascus dankaliensis
Gymnodinium breve
Gymnophalloides seoi
Gymnopilus
gymnothecium
gynandrism
gynandroblastoma
gynandromorphism
gynecogen
gynecoid
gynecologic oncology group (GOG)
gynecomastia, gynecomasty
gynecomasty (*var. of* gynecomastia)
gypseum
    Microsporum g.
    Trichophyton g.
gyrata
    cutis verticis g.
gyrate
    g. atrophy
    g. erythema
gyrectomy
gyri (*pl. of* gyrus)
gyrochrome cell
Gyrodactylus
Gyromitra esculenta
GyroTwister
Gyrovirus
gyrus, *pl.* **gyri**
    cingulate g.

G

H
- Hauch
- Holzknecht unit
- Hounsfield unit
- NATO code for impure sulfur mustard
  - H agglutination
  - H agglutinin
  - H and E staining
  - H antibody
  - H antigen
  - H band
  - H colony
  - cytolipin H
  - H disc
  - H gene
  - h nucleus
  - H substance

h
- Planck constant

H+
- increased arterial H+

H-2
- H-2 antigen
- H-2 complex

H3
- tritium

HA
- hemagglutination
- hyaluronic acid

HAA
- hepatitis-associated antigen

Haagensen test
Ha-1A monoclonal antibody
habenulae perforatae
Habermann disease
Haber syndrome
Haber-Weiss reaction
habit
- endothelioid h.
- glaucomatous h.
- leukocytoid h.

habitual abortion
habituation
Habronema
- H. majus
- H. megastoma
- H. microstoma
- H. muscae

habronemiasis
HACA
- human antichimeric antibody

HACEK
- *Haemophilus, Actinobacillus, Cardiobacterium, Eikenella, Kingella*

Haddad syndrome
Hadfield-Clarke syndrome
Hadobacteria
Hadrurus
HAEC
- Hirschsprung-associated enterocolitis

Haemadipsa ceylonica
Haemagogus
Haemamoeba
Haemaphysalis
- H. cinnabarina
- H. concinna
- H. leachi
- H. leporis-palustris
- H. spinigera

haematobium
- Schistosoma h.

Haematopinus
Haematopota
Haemobartonella
haemocanis
- Mycoplasma h.

Haemococcidium
Haemodipsus ventricosus
haemofelis
- Mycoplasma h.

haemoglobin (*var. of* hemoglobin)
haemoglobinophilus
- Haemophilus h.

Haemogregarina
haemolytica
- Thermomonas h.

haemolyticum
- Arcanobacterium h.
- Clostridium h.

haemolyticus
- Haemophilus h.
- Staphylococcus h.

haemomuris
- Mycoplasma h.

Haemonchus
- H. contortus
- H. placei

haemoperoxidus
- Enterococcus h.

Haemophileae
haemophilum
- Mycobacterium h.

Haemophilus
- H., Actinobacillus, Cardiobacterium, Eikenella, Kingella (HACEK)
- H. actinomycetemcomitans
- H. aegyptius
- H. aphrophilus

H

Haemophilus (*continued*)
    H. bovis
    H. bronchisepticus
    H. ducreyi
    H. duplex
    factor X for *H.*
    H. felis
    H. haemoglobinophilus
    H. haemolyticus
    H. influenzae
    H. influenzae pneumonia
    Koch-Weeks *H.*
    H. parahaemolyticus
    H. parainfluenzae (HPI)
    H. parapertussis
    H. paraphrophilus
    H. paratropicalis
    H. pertussis vaccine (HPV)
    H. segnis
    H. suis
    H. vaginalis
Haemoproteus
haemorrhoidalis
    Sarcophaga h.
Haemosporida
Haemosporina
haemostasis (*var. of* hemostasis)
Haenszel test
haeundaensis
    Paracoccus h.
Haff disease
Haffkine vaccine
Hafnia alvei
hafniae
    Enterobacter h.
hafnium
Hagedorn
    neutral protamine H.
Hageman factor (HF)
hageni
    Otomyces h.
Haglund disease
Hagner disease
Hahella chejuensis
Hahn
    H. oxine reagent
    H. oxine reagentHahn oxine reagent
HAHTG
    horse antihuman thymus globulin
HAI
    hemagglutinin inhibition
    histologic activity index
    HAI titer
Hailey-Hailey disease
hair
    h. analysis
    auditory h.
    h. ball
    beaded h.

    h. bulb
    h. cell (HC)
    club h.
    corkscrew h.
    h. cross
    cuticle of h.
    h. cycle
    h. disc
    h. follicle
    ingrown h.
    lanugo h.
    h. papilla
    h. root
    Schridde cancer h.
    taste h.
    telogen h.
    vellus h.
hair-like filamentous projection
hairpin
    h. DNA
    h. loop
hairpin-mediated polymerase slippage model
HAIRscreen drug test
hairworm
hairy
    h. cell
    h. cell leukemia (HCL)
    h. heart
    h. mole
Hakim syndrome
Halanaerobacter salinarius
Halanaerobiaceae
Halanaerobiales
Halanaerobium
    H. fermentans
    H. kushneri
Halberstaedter-Prowazek body
Haldane
    H. effect
    H. hypothesis
Hale colloidal iron stain
half-bandwidth
half-cell
half-life
    biologic h.-l.
    biological h.-l.
    effective h.-l.
    terminal h.-l. (T 1/2)
half-maximum
    full-width h.-m.
half-moon
    red h.-m.
half-reaction
half time
half-value layer (HVL)
half-wave
    h.-w. potential
    h.-w. rectifier

Haliangium
    H. ochraceum
    H. tepidum
Halicephalobus
halichoeri
    Streptococcus h.
halide
halisteresis phenomenon
halisteretic
Hall
    H. disease
    H. pterygium method
Haller
    H. cone
    H. line
    H. tunica vasculosa
    H. vas aberrans
    H. vascular tissue
Hallermann-Streiff-François syndrome
Hallermann-Streiff syndrome
Hallervorden-Spatz
    H.-S. disease
    H.-S. disease, tau pathology
      class
    H.-S. syndrome
Hallervorden syndrome
Hallgren syndrome
hallmark
    h. of protein-secreting cell
    h. of steroid-secreting cell
Hallopeau disease
Hallopeau-Siemens syndrome
hallucination
    shared h.
hallucinogen
halo
    anemic h.
    cytoplasmic h.
    h. melanoma
    h. nevus
Haloarcula quadrata
Halobacillus
    H. karajensis
    H. locisalis
    H. salinus
Halobacteria
Halobacteriaceae
Halobacteriales
Halobacteroidaceae
Halobiforma
    H. haloterrestris
    H. nitratireducens
Halococcus dombrowskii
halocynthiae
    Halomonas h.
halodurans
    Alkalilimnicola h.
    Roseivivax h.
haloed granule

Haloferax
    H. alexandrinus
    H. lucentense
halogen
halogenated hydrocarbon assay
halogenation
halogenoderma
Halomebacteria
halometer
Halomicrobium mukohataei
Halomonadaceae
Halomonas
    H. alimentaria
    H. anticariensis
    H. axialensis
    H. boliviensis
    H. campisalis
    H. halocynthiae
    H. hydrothermalis
    H. magadiensis
    H. marisflavi
    H. maura
    H. muralis
    H. neptunia
    H. organivorans
    H. sulfidaeris
    H. ventosae
Halonatronum saccharophilum
Halon system
haloperidol assay
halophila
    Desulfocella h.
    Hongiella h.
    Nitrosomonas h.
    Prauserella h.
    Saccharomonospora h.
halophile
halophilus
    Aestuariibacter h.
    Algoriphagus h.
    Halothiobacillus h.
haloprogin
halorespirans
    Sulfurospirillum h.
Halorhabdus utahensis
Halorhodospira neutriphila
Halorubrum
    H. tebenquichense
    H. terrestre
    H. tibetense
    H. xinjiangense
Halosimplex carlsbadense
Halospirulina tapeticola
halosteresis
haloterrestris
    Halobiforma h.
Haloterrigena
    H. thermotolerans
    H. turkmenica

H

halothane
  h. assay
  h. hepatitis
Halothiobacillus
  H. halophilus
  H. hydrothermalis
  H. kellyi
  H. neapolitanus
halotolerans
  Corynebacterium h.
  Gracilibacillus h.
  Jeotgalicoccus h.
  Nesterenkonia h.
  Nocardiopsis h.
  Roseivivax h.
  Yania h.
Halsted
  H. law
  H. mastectomy
Halteridium
halzoun
HAM
  HTLV-1 associated myelopathy
  human alveolar macrophage
  HAM 56 antibody
ham
  H. paroxysmal nocturnal
    hemoglobinuria test
  H. test for anemia
HAMA
  human antimouse antibody
  human antimurine antibody
**Hamamatzu high-sensitivity
  photomultiplier tube**
hamartia
hamartin protein
hamartoblastoma
hamartochondromatosis
hamartoma
  colonic h.
  cystic h.
  giant h.
  leiomyomatous h.
  mesenchymal h.
  neurocristic h.
  neuronal lipofibromatous h.
  neurovascular h.
  pulmonary h.
  renal h.
  respiratory epithelial adenomatoid h.
  urothelial leiomyomatous h.
hamartomatous
  h. polyp
  h. tumor
hamburgensis
  Nitrobacter h.
Hamburger
  H. law
  H. phenomenon

hamelinense
  Roseibium h.
Hamel test
Hamigera
Hamilton
  H. pseudophlegmon
  H. Rating Scale (HRS)
Hamman
  H. disease
  H. syndrome
Hamman-Rich
  H.-R. disease
  H.-R. syndrome
Hammarsten
  H. reagent
  H. test
hammered copper colony
Hammerschlag method
Hammersmith hemoglobin
hammock ligament
Hammond disease
hamster
  h. egg penetration assay
  h. egg penetration test
hamulosa
  Cheilospirura h.
HAN
  Health Alert Network
hand
  crab h.
  H. disease
  ghoul h.
  mechanic's h.
  opera-glass h.
  skeleton h.
  spade h.
  trident h.
hand-foot-and-mouth
  h.-f.-a.-m. disease
  h.-f.-a.-m. disease virus
hand-foot syndrome
hand-foot-uterus syndrome
handgun
  semiautomatic h.
handling
  toxic chemical h.
Hand-Schüller-Christian
  H.-S.-C. disease
  H.-S.-C. type of histiocyte
HandyStep electronic repeating pipette
HANE
  hereditary angioneurotic edema
Hanes equation
Hanger test
hanging-block culture
hanging-drop culture
Hanhart syndrome
Hanker-Yates reagent
Hannebertia

Hanot
> H. cirrhosis
> H. disease

Hanot-Chauffard syndrome
Hansel stain
Hanseman cell
Hansemann macrophage
Hansen
> H. bacillus
> H. disease

Hanseniaspora
hansenii
> *Debaryomyces h.*
> *Desulfofaba h.*
> *Desulfomusa h.*

Hansenula
Hantaan virus
hantavirus pulmonary syndrome
HAP
> heredopathia atactia polyneuritiformis

HAP1
> huntingtin-associated protein 1

HAPA
> hemagglutinating antipenicillin
> antibody

hapalonychia
Haplographium
haploid
> h. cell
> h. genome
> h. number

haploidy
haploinsufficiency
haploinsufficient
Haplorchis
Haplosporangium parvum
Haplosporidia
haplotype association study
happy puppet syndrome
Hapsburg
> disease of H.

hapten
> conjugated h.
> group A h.
> h. inhibition of precipitation
> h. mechanism
> h. X, Y antigen

haptenic grouping
haptoglobin
> h. assay
> haptoglobin, Hp^1 and
> Hp^2
> h. test

haptosporus
> *Basidiobolus h.*

haptotaxis
Harada syndrome
**Harada-Mori filter paper strip
culture**

Ha-ras mutation
hard
> h. chancre
> h. pad disease
> h. pad virus
> h. papilloma
> h. sore
> h. tissue
> h. tubercle
> h. ulcer

hardened pelvis
harderoporphyria
Harding-Passey melanoma
Hardy-Weinberg law
Hare syndrome
Hargraves cell
haricot broth
Harleco synthetic resin
Harlem
> hemoglobin C H.

harlequin
> h. color change
> h. fetus

Harley disease
harmaline
harmine
harmonic
Harris
> H. alum hematoxylin
> H. and Ray test
> H. staining method
> H. syndrome

Harrison
> H. groove
> H. test

Hartmann
> H. pouch
> H. solution

Hartmannella
> *H. hyalina*
> *H. veriformis*

hartmannellae
> *Neochlamydia h.*

hartmanni
> *Entamoeba h.*

Hartnup
> H. disease
> H. syndrome

**Harvard criteria of irreversible
coma**
harvest
> h. bug
> h. mite

Harzia
Hasegawaea
Häser formula
HASH
> human achaete-scute homolog

Hasharon hemoglobin

H

HASHD
    hypertensive arteriosclerotic heart disease
Hashimoto
    H. disease
    H. struma
    H. thyroiditis
Hassall
    H. body
    H. concentric corpuscle
Hassall-Henle wart
Hasselbalch equation
hassiacum
    Novosphingobium h.
Hassin syndrome
HAT
    heparin-associated thrombocytopenia
    hypoxanthine-aminopterin-thymidine
hatchetti
    Acanthamoeba h.
hatching
    h. flask
    h. test
hathewayi
    Clostridium h.
Hauch (H)
    ohne H.
Haute
    hemoglobin Terre H.
HAV
    hepatitis A virus
Haverhill fever
Haverhillia
    H. moniliformis
    H. multiformis
haversian
    h. canal
    h. lamella
    h. space
    h. system
Hawaii agent
hawaiiensis
    Bipolaris h.
    Drechslera h.
hawkinsin
hawkinsinuria
Hawkins sign
Haworth formula
HAX protein
hay
    h. asthma
    h. bacillus
    h. fever
Hayem
    H. hematoblast
    H. solution
Hayem-Widal
    H.-W. anemia
    H.-W. syndrome

Hayflick limit
Haygarth node
hazard
    h. identification
    radiation h.
    h. ratio (HR)
    h. symbol
hazardous
    h. concentration
    h. material
    h. materials labeling
    H. Materials Response Unit (HMRU)
    h. substance
HB, Hb
    heart block
    hemoglobin
        Hb Bart
        Hb Bart hydrops fetalis
        Hb Chesapeake
        Hb CS
        Hb D
        Hb Kansas
        Hb Köln
HBA71 antigen
HbA1c
    glycosylated hemoglobin
HB$_c$Ab
    antibody to hepatitis B core antigen
    hepatitis B core antibody
HB$_c$Ag
    hepatitis B core antigen
HBc antigen immunodetection
HBCO
    carboxyhemoglobin
HbCO
    carboxyhemoglobin
HBD, HBDH
    hydroxybutyrate dehydrogenase
    hydroxybutyric dehydrogenase
HB$_e$Ab
    hepatitis Be antibody
HB$_e$Ag
    hepatitis Be antigen
HBF
    hepatic blood flow
HbF
    fetal hemoglobin
Hb1 - Hb4 protein
HBI
    high serum-bound iron
HBIG
    hepatitis B immune globulin
HBLV
    human B lymphotropic virus
HBME 1 antibody

HbO2
oxyhemoglobin
HbS
sickle cell hemoglobin
sulfhemoglobin
HB$_s$Ab
hepatitis B surface antibody
HB$_s$Ag
hepatitis B surface antigen
HbSS
homozygous hemoglobin S
HBV
hepatitis B virus
HBV DNA marker
HBW
high birth weight
HBx protein
HC
hair cell
Huntington chorea
hydroxycorticoid
hc2
Hybrid Capture 2
hc2 CMV DNA test
hc2 HPV DNA test
HCA
hepatocellular adenoma
h-caldesmon (HCD)
HCC
hepatocellular carcinoma
hydroxycholecalciferol
metastatic hepatocellular
carcinoma
HCCC
hyalinizing clear cell carcinoma
HCC-CC
clear cell hepatocellular carcinoma
HCD
h-caldesmon
H-CD marker
HCG, hCG
human chorionic gonadotropin
HCG alpha subunit
beta hCG
HCG beta subunit
Icon II HCG
HCL
hairy cell leukemia
HCN
hydrogen cyanide
HCN gas
NATO code for HCN (AC)
HCO3
bicarbonate
HCO$_3$ concentration
HCP
hereditary coproporphyria
HCR
hypocretin

hCSM
human chorionic somatomammotropin
HCT
homocytotrophic
hydrochlorothiazide
Hct
hematocrit
HCTZ
hydrochlorothiazide
HCU
homocystinuria
HCV
hepatitis C virus
HCVD
hypertensive cardiovascular disease
HD
heart disease
high dosage
Hirschsprung disease
Hodgkin disease
Huntington disease
hydatid disease
HDA
heteroduplex analysis
HDAC
histone deacetylase
HDAC inhibitor
HD allele version
HDC
histidine decarboxylase
hyperdiploid cell
HDCT
high-dose chemotherapy
HDCV
human diploid cell rabies vaccine
HDGC
hereditary diffuse gastric cancer
HDH
heart disease history
HDI
histologically detectable iron
HDJ1 protein
HDL
high-density lipoprotein
AccuMeter H.
H. cholesterol assay
H. direct test prefilled cartridge
HDL-C
high-density lipoprotein-cholesterol
HDMEC
human dermal microvascular
endothelial cell
HDN
hemolytic disease of newborn
hemorrhagic disease of newborn
alloimmune HDN
Kell HDN
HDRA
histoculture drug response assay

H

HDS
herniated disc syndrome
HDV
hepatitis delta virus
hepatitis D virus
HDW
hemoglobin distribution
width
H&E
hematoxylin and eosin
HE
hereditary elliptocytosis
human enteric (virus)
head
h. and neck squamous cell
carcinoma (HNSCC)
angle h.
bulldog h.
h. cap
deceleration of h.
hydrophilic h.
H. line
h. louse
Medusa h.
h. space analysis
headache
tension h.
healed
h. fracture
h. Ghon complex
h. glomerulonephritis
h. infarct
h. tuberculosis
h. ulcer
healing
scarless h.
wound h.
health
H. Alert Network (HAN)
Department of Public H.
immediately dangerous to life or h.
(IDLH)
H. Insurance Portability and
Accountability Act (HIPAA)
National Institute for Occupational
Safety and H. (NIOSH)
National Institutes of H. (NIH)
h. physics
H. Resources and Services
Administration (HRSA)
HealthCheck
H. HDL home-screening test
H. One-Step One Minute pregnancy
test
H. total cholesterol home-screening
test
HealthEssist urine-based test
healthy control
He antigen

heart
h. antigen
armored h.
athletic h.
beer h.
beriberi h.
h. block (HB)
boat-shaped h.
bony h.
chaotic h.
h. disease (HD)
h. disease history (HDH)
disordered action of h. (DAH)
drop h.
dynamite h.
h. failure (HF)
h. failure cell
fatty h.
h. fatty acid binding protein
(H-FABP)
flask-shaped h.
frosted h.
hairy h.
hypoplastic h.
icing h.
h. infusion agar
luxus h.
movable h.
muscle of h.
myxedema h.
ox h.
sabot h.
stone h.
tabby cat h.
thrush breast h.
tiger h.
tiger lily h.
trilocular h.
h. tumor
valvular disease of h. (VDH)
heart-hand syndrome
heart-lung preparation
heartwater
heartworm
HEAT
human erythrocyte agglutination test
heat
h. antigen retrieval protocol
h. capacity
h. coagulation test
h. content
h. edema
h. instability test
h. intolerance
h. killed (HK)
h. labile
h. labile test
latent h.
h. of combustion

h. of formation
h. of fusion
h. of reaction
h. of solution
h. of sublimation
h. of vaporization
h. precipitation test
h. shock factor 1 (HSF1)
h. shock protein (HSP)
h. shock response
h. sink
specific h.
h. stability test
h. unit (HU)
heater
SlidePro slide h.
heat-extracted antigen
heat-induced epitope retrieval (HIER)
heat-killed *Listeria monocytogenes* (HKLM)
heat-labile
h.-l. antibody
h.-l. protein
heat-mediated
h.-m. antigen retrieval
heat-resistant glass
heat-stable (HS)
h.-s. alkaline phosphatase
h.-s. lactic dehydrogenase (HLDH)
heavy
h. chain
h. chain disease
h. meromyosin
h. metal
h. metal poisoning
h. metal screen
h. metal screening test
h. water
hebdomidis
Leptospira h.
hebeiensis
Streptomyces h.
Hebeloma mesophaeum
Heberden
H. disease
H. node
Hebra
H. disease
prurigo of H.
hebraeum
Amblyomma h.
HECA-452 antibody
hecateromeric
hecatomeral, hecatomeric
hecatomeric (*var. of* hecatomeral)
Hecht pneumonia
Heckathorn disease

heckeshornense
Mycobacterium h.
hectogram
hectometer
hederiform ending
hedgehog
sonic h. (SHH)
heel
cracked h.
Heerfordt
H. disease
H. syndrome
Hegglin
H. anomaly
H. syndrome
heidelberg
Salmonella enteritidis serotype *h.*
Heidenhain
H. azan stain
H. crescent
H. demilune
H. iron hematoxylin
H. iron hematoxylin stain
H. syndrome
height (ht)
heilmannii
Helicobacter h.
Heine-Medin disease
Heinz
H. body
H. body hemolytic anemia
H. body stain
H. body test
H. granule
Heinz-Ehrlich body
HEK
human embryo kidney
human embryonic kidney
HEK cell
Hektoen
H. enteric agar
H. phenomenon
HEL
human embryo lung
HEL cell
HeLa cell
Helcococcus sueciensis
Heleidae
helenine
helgolandensis
Jannaschia h.
helianthine
helical
helicase
h. protein
ReQ h.
helicis
chondrodermatitis nodularis chronica h.

H

Helicobacter
  H. aurati
  H. canadensis
  H. cinaedi
  H. fennelliae
  H. ganmani
  H. gastritis
  H. heilmannii
  H. hepaticus
  H. mesocricetorum
  H. pylori
  H. pylori breath test
  H. pylori gII test
  H. pylori serology
  H. pylori urease
  H. pylori urease test and
    culture
  H. typhlonius
Helicostylum
helicotrema
Helicotylenchus
Helie bundle
heliencephalitis
Heliobacterium
  H. sulfidophilum
  H. undosum
Heliorestis
  H. baculata
  H. daurensis
heliotrinireducens
  Slackia h.
heliotrope eyelid
Heliozoea
Helisal rapid blood test
helium equilibration time (HET)
helix, *pl.* helices
  alpha h.
  double h.
  right-handed alpha h.
helix-loop-helix protein
hellem
  Encephalitozoon h.
hellenicus
  Staphylothermus h.
Heller-Döhle disease
helle zellen (pale cells)
HELLP
  hemolysis, elevated liver enzymes, and
    low platelets
  HELLP syndrome
Helly
  H. fixative
  H. fluid
helmet cell
helminthagogue
helmintheca
  Neorickettsia h.
helminthemesis
helminthiasis, helminthism

helminthic (*var. of* helmintic)
  h. disease
helminth identification procedure
helminthism (*var. of* helminthiasis)
helminthoid
helminthology
helminthoma
Helminthosporium oryzae
helmintic, helminthic
  h. infection
Heloderma
Helophilus
Helotium
helper
  h. T cell
  h. T lymphocyte
  h. virus
helper/suppressor cell ratio
Helvella
  H. elastica
  H. esculenta
helvola
  Zimmermannella h.
helvolus
  Pseudoclavibacter h.
Helweg-Larssen syndrome
hemachrome
hemachrosis
hemacytometer (*var. of* hemocytometer)
hemacytozoon
hemadsorption
  h. inhibition test
  mixed h. (MHA)
  h. virus test
  h. virus type 1, 2
hemafacient
hemagglutinating
  h. antipenicillin antibody (HAPA)
  h. cold autoantibody
  h. unit (HU)
hemagglutination
  indirect h. (IH, IHA)
  h. inhibition (HI)
  h. inhibition assay
  h. inhibition titer
  reverse passive h.
  h. test
  treponemal h. (TPH)
  h. treponemal test for syphilis
  Treponema pallidum h. (TPH)
  viral h.
hemagglutination-inhibition
  h.-i. antibody (HIA)
  h.-i. test (HIT)
hemagglutinin
  autologous h.
  cold h.
  heterologous h.
  homologous h.

h. inhibition (HAI)
warm h.
hemal
h. gland
h. node
hemalum
Mayer h.
hemamebiasis
hemanalysis
hemangiectatic hypertrophy
hemangioblast
hemangioblastoma
hemangioendothelial sarcoma
hemangioendothelioblastoma
hemangioendothelioma
epithelioid h. (EH, EHE)
infantile hepatic h.
retiform h.
h. tuberosum multiplex
hemangiofibroma
juvenile h.
hemangiolipoma
hemangioma, *pl.* **hemangiomas,**
hemangiomata
ameloblastic h.
arterial h.
capillary h.
cavernous h.
choroidal h.
circumscribed choroidal h. (CCH)
h. congenitale
dyschondroplasia with h.'s
glomeruloid h.
infantile h.
microvenular h.
nuchal h.
placental h.
h. planum extensum
racemose h.
renal h.
sclerosing h.
senile h.
h. simplex
targetoid hemosiderotic h.
hemangiomas (*pl. of* hemangioma)
hemangiomata (*pl. of* hemangioma)
hemangioma-thrombocytopenia syndrome
hemangiomatosis
pulmonary capillary h. (PCH)
hemangioperic-like
hemangiopericytic
hemangiopericytoma (HPC)
lipomatous h. (LHPC)
orbital h.
hemangiopericytomatous growth pattern
hemangiosarcoma
splenic h.
hemapheic
hemaphein

hemapheism
hemapheresis
hemarthrosis
Hemastainer
hemastrontium
hemat
hematology
HemataCHEK hematology reference
control
hematapostema
HemataSTAT Easy Read centrifuge
hematein
Baker acid h.
h. test
Hematek 2000 slide stainer
hematemesis
hematencephalon
Hematest reagent tablet test
hematherapy
hemathidrosis
hemathorax (*var. of* hemothorax)
hematic
hematid
hematidrosis
hematimeter
hematin
acid formaldehyde h.
h. albumin
h. pigmentation
reduced h.
hematinemia
hematinic principle
hematite pneumoconiosis
hematobilia (*var. of* hemobilia)
hematobium
Schistosoma h.
hematoblast
Hayem h.
hematocele
hematocelia
hematocephaly
hematochezia
hematochlorin
hematochyluria
hematocolpos
hematocrit
large vessel h. (LVH)
mean circulatory h.
total body h. (TBH)
venous h. (VH)
whole-blood h. (WBH)
hematocrystallin
hematocyst
hematocystis
hematocyte
hematocytoblast
hematocytolysis
hematocytometer
hematocytozoon

H

hematocyturia
hematodermic neoplasm
hematodyscrasia
hematodystrophy
hematogen
hematogenesis
hematogenic (*var. of* hematogenous)
hematogenous, hematogenic
    h. abscess
    h. dissemination
    h. hyalin
    h. jaundice
    h. metastasis
    h. osteitis
    h. pigment
    h. theory of endometriosis
hematogone
hematohistioblast
hematohyaloid
hematoid
hematoidin
    h. crystal
    h. pigmentation
hematological anthropology
hematologic malignant neoplasm
hematologist
hematology
    International Committee for
      Standardization in H.
hematolymphangioma
hematolymphoid
    h. chimerism
    h. malignancy
hematolysis
hematolytic
hematoma
    chronic subdural h. (CSH)
    corpus luteum h.
    delayed traumatic intracerebral h.
      (DTICH)
    epidural h.
    intracranial h.
    intramural h.
    organized h.
    puerperal h.
    retroplacental h.
    subdural h.
hematometra, hemometra
hematometry
hematomyelia
hematomyelopore
hematonic
hematopathology
hematopathy
hematopenia
hematophagia
hematophagous
hematophagus
hematophilia

hematoplastic
hematopneic index
hematopoiesis (*var. of* hemopoiesis)
    intrathoracic extramedullary h.
hematopoietic (*var. of* hemopoietic)
    h. aplasia
    h. cell cytoplasmic alteration
    h. cell origin
    h. cord blood cell
    h. gland
    h. hyperplasia
    h. hypoplasia
    h. malignancy
    h. maturation
    h. maturation alteration
    h. maturation arrest
    h. progenitor cell (HPC)
    h. progenitor cell antigen
    h. progenitor cell transplantation
    h. stem cell (HSC)
    h. system
    h. tissue
    h. tumor
hematopoietin
hematoporphyrinemia
hematoporphyrinuria
hematorrhachis, hemorrhachis
    h. externa
    extradural h.
    h. interna
    subdural h.
hematosalpinx, hemosalpinx
hematosepsis
hematoside
hematosis
hematospectroscope
hematospectroscopy
hematospermatocele
hematospermia
hematostatic
hematostaxis
hematotoxic
hematotoxin
hematotropic
hematoxic
hematoxin
hematoxylin
    alum h.
    h. and eosin (H&E)
    h. body
    Boehmer h.
    Carazzi h.
    chrome h.
    Clara h.
    Cole h.
    Delafield h.
    Ehrlich h.
    Harris alum h.
    Heidenhain iron h.

iron h.
Lillie h.
Mayer h.
silver nitrate with h.
h. stain
Weigert iron h.
hematoxylin-malachite green-basic fuchsin stain
hematoxylin-phloxine B stain
hematoxylin-phloxine-saffron (HPS)
hematozoon
hematuria
benign familial h.
essential h.
false h.
gross h.
initial h.
microscopic h.
nonglomerular h.
renal h.
terminal h.
total h.
urethral h.
vesical h.
hematuric bilious fever
heme
h. moiety
h. oxygenase (HO)
h. oxygenase-1 (HO 1)
h. oxygenase/carbon monoxide (HO/CO)
h. oxygenase-1 gene
h. synthetase (HS)
h. test
hemendothelioma
heme-porphyrin fecal occult blood test
hemerythrin
HemeSelect
hemiacardius
hemiacetal
hemianopia, hemianopsia, hemiopia
hemianopsia (*var. of* hemianopia)
binasal h.
bitemporal h.
hemiaplasia
hemiatrophy
facial h.
hemiballism (*var. of* hemiballismus)
hemiballismus, hemiballism
hemiblock
hemic calculus
Hemichorda (*var. of* Hemichordata)
Hemichordata, Hemichorda
hemicranicus
status h.
hemidesmosome
hemidrosis
hemiglobin
hemiglobincyanide

hemiglobinemia
hemiglobinuria
hemihidrosis
hemihyperhidrosis
hemilesion
hemimelia
dysplasia epiphysialis h.
hemimetabolous
hemin
hemiopia (*var. of* hemianopia)
Hemiptera
hemipterus
Cimex h.
hemipyonephrosis
Hemispora stellata
hemisyndrome
hemithoracic duct
hemithoracicus
ductus h.
Hemivirus
hemizygosity
hemizygous deletion
hemoagglutination
hemoagglutinin
hemoantitoxin
Hemobartonella
hemobilia, hematobilia
hemoblast
hemoblastosis
hemocatharsis
hemocatheresis
hemocatheretic
Hemoccult
H. fecal occult blood test
H. ICT
H. ICT immunoassay
H. II Sensa fecal occult blood test
H. Sensa
H. Sensa elite
hemocele
hemocholecyst
hemocholecystitis
hemochromatosis
autosomal dominant h.
exogenous h.
hereditary h. (HH, HHC)
juvenile h.
neonatal h.
non-HFE-related h.
secondary h.
hemochromogen
Hemochron
H. Jr. Citrate PT assay
H. P214 glass-activated ACT tube
hemoclasia (*var. of* hemoclasis)
hemoclasis, hemoclasia
hemoclastic
h. reaction
h. shock

H

hemoconcentration
hemoconia
hemoconiosis
hemocryoscopy
HemoCue
    H. B-Glucose analyzer
    H. hemoglobin test system
hemocyanin
    keyhole-limpet h. (KLH)
hemocystinuria
hemocyte
hemocytoblast
hemocytocatheresis
hemocytolysis
hemocytometer, hemacytometer
    Neubauer h.
hemocytometry
hemocytotripsis
hemocytozoon
hemodiagnosis
hemodialyzer
    ultrafiltration h.
hemodilution
    acute normovolemic h. (ANH)
    h. test
hemodynamic collapse
hemodyscrasia
hemodystrophy
hemofiltration
hemoflagellate
    mitochondrion of h.
hemofuchsin
    Mallory stain for h.
hemofuscin pigmentation
hemogenesis
hemogenic
hemoglobin (Hb, HB, Hbg, hemo, hg,
  HG, Hgb, hgb, HGB), haemoglobin
    h. A
    h. A_2
    aberrant h.
    h. A1c
    adult h.
    alkali-resistant h.
    h. Bart
    bile pigment h.
    h. carbamate
    carbon monoxide h.
    h. cast
    h. C disease
    h. C Georgetown
    h. C Harlem
    h. Chesapeake
    h. Constant Spring
    Constant Spring mutation of h.
    h. content of reticulocytes
    Cranston h.
    crossover h.
    h. D

denatured h.
deoxygenated h.
h. distribution width (HDW)
h. D Punjab
h. E
h. electrophoresis
embryonic h.
encapsulated h.
h. E-thalassemia disease
h. E trait
h. F
fast h.
fetal h. (HbF)
h. F, H assay
glycosylated h.
Gower 1, 2 h.
h. G Philadelphia trait
green h.
Gun Hill h.
h. H
Hammersmith h.
Hasharon h.
h. H disease
hereditary persistence of fetal h.
  (HPFH)
homozygous h. S (HbSS)
h. I
h. Icaria
h. identification
h. Indianapolis
h. J
h. J Capetown
h. Kansas
Köln h.
h. Koya Dora
h. Lepore
h. Lepore trait
lipid vesicle-encapsulated h.
h. M
mean cell h. (MCH)
mean corpuscular h. (MCH)
h. M Hyde Park
h. M-Saskatoon
muscle h.
oxygenated h.
oxygen half-saturation pressure of h.
h. pigmentation
h. Portland
h. Rainier
reduced h. (HHb)
h. S
h. SC-alpha thalassemia
Seal Rock h.
sickle cell h. (HbS)
sickling h.
slow h.
h. SO Arab sickle cell disease
solubilized h.
h. S test

stroma-free h.
h. Terre Haute
total h.
total circulating h. (TCH)
unionized h. (HHb)
unstable h.
variant h.
h. Yakima
h. Zurich
hemoglobinated
hemoglobinemia
hemoglobinocholia
hemoglobinolysis
hemoglobinometer
hemoglobinometry
hemoglobinopathy
　heterozygous h.
　homozygous h.
　mixed h.
hemoglobinopepsia
hemoglobinophilic
hemoglobin-polyoxyethylene
　pyridoxalated h.-p. (PHP)
hemoglobinuria
　bacillary h.
　cold h.
　epidemic h.
　intermittent h.
　malarial h.
　march h.
　toxic h.
hemoglobinuric
　h. fever
　h. nephropathy
　h. nephrosis
hemogram
hemohistioblast
hemokinesis
hemolamella
hemoleukocyte
hemolith
hemology
hemolymph
　h. gland
　h. heteroagglutinin
　h. node
hemolysate
hemolysin
　alpha h.
　bacterial h.
　beta h.
　cold h.
　DL h.
　Donath-Landsteiner biphasic h.
　heterophil h.
　immune h.
　natural h.
　h. saponin
　specific h.

h. unit
warm-cold h.
hemolysinogen
hemolysis
　alpha h.
　beta h.
　biphasic h.
　bystander h.
　colloid osmotic h.
　DL biphasic h.
　hemolysis, elevated liver enzymes,
　　and low platelets (HELLP)
　extravascular h.
　extrinsic h.
　gamma h.
　immune h.
　h. interference
　intramedullary h.
　intravascular h.
　macrovascular h.
　nonimmune h.
　osmotic h.
　traumatic h.
hemolytic
　h. amboceptor
　h. anemia
　h. anemia of newborn
　h. chain
　h. disease of newborn (HDN)
　h. disorder
　h. gas
　h. index
　h. jaundice
　h. malaria
　microangiopathic h.
　h. plaque assay
　h. reaction
　h. splenomegaly
　h. streptococcus
　h. substance
　h. transfusion reaction
　h. tube assay
　h. unit
hemolytic-uremic syndrome (HUS)
hemolyticus
　Bacillus h.
hemolyzable
hemolyzation
hemolyze
hemometra (*var. of* hematometra)
hemometry
hemonchosis
hemonephrosis
hemopathology
hemopathy
hemoperfusion
hemopericardium
hemoperitoneum
hemopexin

H

hemophagia
hemophagocytic
    h. lymphohistiocytosis
      (HLH)
    h. syndrome (HPS)
hemophagocytosis
hemophil, hemophile
hemophile (*var. of* hemophil)
hemophilia
    h. A, B, C
    h. B Leyden
    h. Bm
    classic h.
    classical h.
    vascular h.
hemophiliac
hemophilic
    h. arthropathy
    h. factor A
hemophilus of Koch-Weeks *(Haemophilus aegypticus)*
hemophoresis
hemophthalmia, hemophthalmus
hemophthalmus (*var. of* hemophthalmia)
hemophthisis
hemoplastic
hemoplasty
hemopneumopericardium
hemopneumothorax
hemopoiesic diuretic
hemopoiesis
    extramedullary h.
hemopoietic
hemopoietin
hemoprecipitin
hemoprotein
hemoptysis
    cardiac h.
    endemic h.
    Oriental h.
    vicarious h.
hemopyelectasia (*var. of* hemopyelectasis)
hemopyelectasis, hemopyelectasia
HemoQuant fecal blood test
hemorepellant
hemorrhachis (*var. of* hematorrhachis)
hemorrhage
    antepartum h. (APH)
    cerebral h.
    chorioamnionic h.
    Duret h.
    fetomaternal h.
    flame-shaped retinal h.
    gastrointestinal h.
    intracerebral h.
    intracranial h.
    intrapulmonary h.
    intraventricular h. (IVH)

    massive pulmonary h.
    maternal-fetal h.
    neonatal gastrointestinal h.
    pinpoint h.
    postpartum h. (PPH)
    punctate h.
    renal h.
    subarachnoid h. (SAH)
    transplacental h. (TPH)
    traumatic basal subarachnoid h. (TBSAH)
    traumatic subarachnoid h. (TSAH)
hemorrhagic
    h. anemia
    h. ascites
    h. bronchopneumonia
    h. chickenpox
    h. colitis
    h. colitis syndrome
    h. cyst
    h. cystitis
    h. dengue
    h. diathesis
    h. disease of deer
    h. disease of newborn
    h. disorder
    h. diverticulitis
    h. endovasculitis (HEV)
    h. endovasculopathy
    h. fever (HF)
    h. fever epidemic
    h. fever with renal syndrome
    h. gangrene
    h. gastritis
    h. glomerulonephritis
    h. infarct
    h. inflammation
    h. lobar pneumonia
    h. malaria
    h. mediastinitis
    h. meningitis
    h. nephritis
    h. pachymeningitis
    h. pancreatitis
    h. pericarditis
    h. plague
    h. pleurisy
    h. rickets
    h. shock
    h. smallpox
    h. thoracic lymphadenitis
    h. thrombocythemia
    h. ulcer
hemorrhagica
    encephalitis h.
    purpura h.
    scarlatina h.
    variola h.

hemorrhagicum
> corpus h.
> cystic corpus h.

hemorrhagin unit

hemorrhoid
> cutaneous h.
> external h.
> internal h.
> thrombosed h.

hemorrhoidal
> h. nerve
> h. vein
> h. zone

hemosalpinx (*var. of* hematosalpinx)

hemosiderin
> h. deposition
> local deposition of h.
> Puchtler-Sweat stain for hemoglobin and h.
> h. stain
> stainable h.
> h. staining
> h. test

hemosiderin-laden macrophages

hemosiderinuria test

hemosiderosis
> basal h.
> endogenous h.
> exogenous h.
> idiopathic h.
> idiopathic pulmonary h. (IPH)
> pulmonary h.
> secondary pulmonary h. (SPH)

hemosiderotic fibrohistiocytic lipomatous lesion (HFLL)

HemoSite hemoglobin meter

hemospermia
> h. spuria
> h. vera

Hemosporidium

hemosporines

hemostasia (*var. of* hemostasis)

hemostasis, hemostasia, haemostasis

hemostatic

hemosuccus pancreaticus

hemotherapeutics (*var. of* hemotherapy)

hemotherapy, hemotherapeutics

hemothorax, hemathorax

hemotoxic anemia

hemotoxin
> cobra h.

hemotropic

hemozoic

hemozoin

hemozoon

HEMPAS
> hereditary erythrocytic multinuclearity with positive acidified serum
> HEMPAS cell

hemuresis

henchirensis
> *Ramlibacter h.*

Hench-Rosenberg syndrome

Henderson-Hasselbalch equation

Hendersonia

Henderson-Jones disease

Hendersonula toruloidea

Henipavirus

Henle
> H. ansa
> H. fenestrated elastic membrane
> H. fiber layer
> H. fissure
> loop of H.
> H. nervous layer
> H. plexus
> H. reaction
> H. sheath
> H. tubule

Henoch purpura

Henoch-Schönlein
> H.-S. purpura (HSP)
> H.-S. syndrome

henpuye

Henry
> H. fructose test
> H. law

henselae
> *Bartonella h.*
> *Rochalimaea h.*

Hensen
> H. canal
> H. cell
> H. disc
> H. duct
> H. line
> H. node
> H. stripe

HEP
> hepatoerythropoietic porphyria

HEPA
> high-efficiency particulate air
> HEPA filter
> HEPA filter mask

Hepacivirus

Hepadnaviridae

heparan
> h. sulfate
> h. sulfate-antithrombin III system
> h. sulfate PG stain
> h. sulfate proteoglycan
> h. sulfate proteoglycan stain
> h. sulfate 2-sulfotransferase gene

heparanese

heparan-*N*-sulfatase

heparin
> h. cofactor
> h. cofactor II deficiency

H

441

heparin (*continued*)
    h. lithium
    h. unit
heparinase
heparin-associated thrombocytopenia
  (HAT)
heparinate
heparinemia
heparinic acid
heparin-induced
    h.-i. platelet activation assay
      (HIPA)
    h.-i. thrombocytopenia (HIT)
    h.-i. thrombocytopenia-thrombosis
      (HITT)
heparinize
heparinolytica
    Prevotella h.
heparin-precipitable fraction
  (HPF)
hepar lobatum
hepatarius
    Vibrio h.
hepatatrophia, hepatatrophy
hepatatrophy (*var. of* hepatatrophia)
hepatic
    h. abscess
    h. acinus
    h. adenoma
    h. arteriole
    h. blood flow (HBF)
    h. capsulitis
    h. coma
    h. cord
    h. cyst
    h. docimasia
    h. encephalopathy
    h. failure
    h. fenestra
    h. fibrosis
    h. fistula
    h. function test
    h. glycogen
    h. hydrothorax
    h. iron concentration (HIC)
    h. iron index (HII)
    h. laminae
    h. lipase deficiency
    h. lobule
    h. porphyria
    h. portal venous gas (HPVG)
    h. progenitor cell
    h. sinusoid
    h. steatosis
    h. stellate cell (HSC)
    h. transaminase
    h. tumor
    h. vein thrombosis
    h. venoocclusive disease

hepatica
    adiposis h.
    Capillaria h.
    facies h.
    Fasciola h.
Hepaticola
hepaticus
    Helicobacter h.
hepatis
    lobulus h.
    tunica fibrosa h.
    tunica serosa h.
    venae centrales h.
hepatitic
hepatitides (*pl. of* hepatitis)
hepatitis, *pl.* **hepatitides**
    h. A antibody
    h. A, B, C, D, E
    active chronic h.
    acute focal h.
    acute parenchymatous h.
    acute viral h. (AVH)
    alcoholic h.
    h. antibody
    h. antigen
    autoimmune h. (AIH)
    h. A virus (HAV)
    h. B core antibody (HB$_c$Ab)
    h. B core antigen (HB$_c$Ag)
    h. Be antibody (HB$_e$Ab)
    h. Be antigen (HB$_e$Ag)
    h. B immune globulin (HBIG)
    h. B surface antibody (HB$_s$Ab)
    h. B surface antigen (HB$_s$Ag)
    h. B surface antigen test
    h. B vaccine
    h. B virus (HBV)
    cholangiolitic h.
    cholestatic h.
    chronic active h. (CAH)
    chronic interstitial h.
    chronic lobular h. (CLH)
    chronic persistent h. (CPH)
    chronic viral h.
    h. contagiosa canis
    cryoglobulinemia, leukemia, arthritis,
      Sjögren syndrome, and h. B
      (CLASH)
    h. C serology
    h. C virus (HCV)
    h. D antigen
    delta h.
    h. delta virus (HDV)
    drug-induced h.
    h. D serology
    h. D virus (HDV)
    h. E-like viruses
    epidemic h.
    equine serum h.

h. E virus (HEV)
h. externa
fulminant h.
h. GB virus (HGBV)
giant cell h. (GCH)
granulomatous h.
h. G virus (HGV)
halothane h.
icteric serum h. (ISH)
infectious h. (IH)
infectious canine h.
ischemic h.
La Brea h.
long incubation h.
lupoid h.
MS-1 h.
MS-2 h.
murine h.
NANB h.
neonatal h.
non-A h.
non-A, non-B h.
non-B h.
nonviral h.
plasma cell h.
posttransfusion h. (PTH)
serum h. (SH)
short incubation h.
Simbu h.
subacute h.
suppurative h.
transfusion h.
transfusion-mediated viral h.
unresolved h.
h. virus
wilsonian fulminant h.
hepatitis-associated antigen (HAA)
hepatization
gray h.
red h.
yellow h.
hepatobiliary cystadenoma
hepatoblastoma
hepatocarcinoma
hepatocavopathy
obliterative h.
hepatocele
hepatocellular
h. adenoma (HCA)
h. bile duct carcinoma
h. carcinoma (HCC)
h. jaundice
h. necrosis
hepatocholangitis
hepatocuprein
Hepatocystis
hepatocyte
ground glass h.
h. growth factor (HGF)

h. growth factor/scatter factor
(HGF/SF)
h. nuclear factor 1 alpha
hepatoerythropoietic porphyria (HEP)
hepatogenic, hepatogenous
hepatogenous (*var. of* hepatogenic)
h. jaundice
h. pigment
hepatohemia
hepatoid
hepatojugular reflux
hepatolenticular
h. degeneration
h. disease
hepatolienomegaly
hepatolith
hepatolithiasis
hepatolysin
hepatoma
malignant h.
hepatomalacia
hepatomegalia (*var. of* hepatomegaly)
hepatomegaly, hepatomegalia
hepatomelanosis
hepatonecrosis
hepatonephoric syndrome
hepatonephric (*var. of* hepatorenal)
hepatonephromegaly
hepatoperitonitis
hepatophosphorylase deficiency
 glycogenosis
hepatophyma
hepatopleural fistula
hepatoptosis
hepatorenal, hepatonephric
h. glycogenosis
h. glycogen storage disease
h. syndrome
hepatorrhexis
hepatosplenitis
hepatosplenomegaly (HSM)
hepatotoxemia
hepatotoxic
hepatotoxicity type I, II
hepatotoxin
Hepatovirus
Hepatozoon
HepCheck whole blood control
hepcidin
h. peptide
h. peptide hormone
HEPES buffer
HEPES-buffered KSOM
Hepevirus
HepPar1 antibody
heptabarbital
heptacarboxyporphyrin
urine h.
heptachlor epoxide

H

heptafluorobutyric anhydride (HFBA)
heptane
Hepzyme
HER-2
    human epidermal growth receptor 2
    HER-2 gene
    HER-2 protein
herald patch
herbarius
    Alicyclobacillus h.
herbarum
    Curtobacterium h.
    Pleospora h.
Herbaspirillum
    H. chlorophenolicum
    H. frisingense
    H. lusitanum
    H. seropedicae
herbicide
    chlorophenoxy h.
herbicidovorans
    Sphingobium h.
herbicola
    Erwinia h.
Herbst corpuscle
HercepTest
    H. breast cancer
      immunohistochemical assay
    Dako H.
    H. IHC kit
    H. immunohistochemical test
Herceptin
Hercospora
herd immunity
hereditaria
    anemia hypochromica
      sideroachrestica h.
    porphyria cutanea tarda h.
    protocoproporphyria h.
hereditary
    h. acanthocytosis
    h. adynamia
    h. angioneurotic edema (HANE)
    h. benign intraepithelial dyskeratosis
    h. clubbing
    h. coproporphyria (HCP)
    h. diffuse gastric cancer (HDGC)
    h. disease
    h. elliptocytosis (HE)
    h. enzymatic-type
      methemoglobinemia
    h. erythroblastic multinuclearity
    h. erythrocytic multinuclearity with
      positive acidified serum
      (HEMPAS)
    h. flat adenoma syndrome (HFAS)
    h. fructose intolerance (HFI)
    h. hemochromatosis (HH, HHC)
    h. hemochromatosis genotyping

    h. hemolytic anemia (HHA)
    h. hemorrhagic telangiectasia
      (HHT)
    h. hemorrhagic thrombasthenia
    h. hypersegmentation
    h. lymphedema
    h. methemoglobinemic cyanosis
    h. mixed polyposis syndrome
    h. multiple exostoses
    h. multiple trichoepithelioma
    h. nephritis (HN)
    h. nonhemolytic bilirubinemia
    h. nonpolyposis colon cancer
      (HNPCC)
    h. nonpolyposis colorectal cancer
      (HNPCC)
    h. nonspherocytic hemolytic anemia
      (HNSHA)
    h. orotic aciduria
    h. osteoonychodysplasia (HOOD)
    h. papillary renal cell carcinoma
      (HPRC)
    h. persistence of fetal hemoglobin
      (HPFH)
    h. plasmathromboplastin component
      deficiency
    h. progressive arthroophthalmopathy
    h. pyropoikilocytosis (HPP)
    h. renal-retinal dysplasia
    h. sensory radicular neuropathy
    h. sideroblastic anemia
    h. spherocytosis (HS)
    h. stomatocytosis
    h. thrombophilia
    h. tyrosinemia
heredity
    autosomal h.
    sex-linked h.
    X-linked h.
heredodegenerative disease
heredopathia atactia polyneuritiformis
  (HAP)
HERF
    high-energy radiofrequency
    HERF device
Hericium
Hering
    canal of H.
Herlitz syndrome
hermanii
    Escherichia h.
Hermann fixative
hermanniensis
    Enterococcus h.
Hermansky-Pudlak syndrome
hermaphrodism (*var. of* hermaphroditism)
hermaphroditism, hermaphrodism
Hermetia illucens
hermetic seal

hermsi
> Ornithodoros *h.*

hermsii
> Borrelia *h.*

HER-2/neu
> HER-2/neu gene
> HER-2/neu oncogene
> HER-2/neu overexpression
> HER-2/neu protein
> serum HER-2/neu
> HER-2/neu serum test

hernia, *pl.* **herniae**
> cerebral h.
> diaphragmatic h.
> direct h.
> epigastric h.
> esophageal h.
> femoral h.
> hiatal h.
> hiatus h.
> incarcerated h.
> incomplete h.
> indirect h.
> inguinal h.
> irreducible h.
> Larrey h.
> meningeal h.
> Morgagni h.
> obturator h.
> retrocolic h.
> retrosternal h.
> Richter h.
> rolling h.
> strangulated h.
> umbilical h.
> urinary bladder h.
> h. uteri inguinale

herniae (*pl. of* hernia)
hernial aneurysm
herniated
> h. disc syndrome (HDS)
> h. nucleus pulposus (HNP)

herniation
> cerebral h.
> uncal h.

heroin-associated nephropathy
herophili
> torcular h.

herpangina virus
herpes
> h. B encephalomyelitis
> h. catarrhalis
> h. corneae
> h. cytology
> h. desquamans
> h. digitalis
> h. esophagitis
> h. facialis
> h. febrilis

> h. generalisatus
> genital h.
> h. genitalis
> h. gestationis
> h. gladiatorum
> h. iris
> h. labialis
> neonatal h.
> h. pneumonitis
> h. progenitalis
> h. simplex (HS)
> h. simplex antibody
> h. simplex lymphadenitis
> h. simplex virus (HSV)
> h. simplex virus culture
> h. simplex virus encephalitis (HSVE)
> h. simplex virus I (HSV-I)
> h. simplex virus II (HSV-II)
> h. simplex virus infection
> h. simplex virus isolation
> traumatic h.
> h. virus
> h. whitlow
> h. zoster
> h. zoster ophthalmicus
> h. zoster varicellosus
> h. zoster virus (HZV)

HerpeSelect type specific IgG antibody detection kit
herpeslike virus
herpes-type virus (HTV)
Herpesviridae
herpesvirus (HV), herpes virus
> h. antigen
> canine h.
> caprine h.
> H. hominis (HVH)
> human h. 1–8 (HHV)
> h. papio 2
> *H. simiae*
> suid h.

herpetic
> h. fever
> h. gingivostomatitis
> h. keratitis
> h. keratoconjunctivitis
> h. meningoencephalitis
> h. paronychia
> h. stomatitis
> h. ulcer
> h. viral disease
> h. whitlow

herpetica
herpeticum
> eczema h.

herpetiformis
> dermatitis h.
> morphea h.

H

Herpetomonas
  H. donovani
  H. furunculosa
  H. tropica
Herpetoviridae
herpetovirus
  canine h.
  caprine h.
Herpotrichia
Herring body
herringbone
  h. fascicle
  h. pattern
herring-worm disease
Herrmann syndrome
Hers disease
Herter
  H. disease
  H. test
Herter-Heubner disease
hertz (Hz)
Herxheimer
  H. reaction
  H. spiral
hesitation wound
Hespellia
  H. porcina
  H. stercorisuis
hesperidum
  Alicyclobacillus h.
H&E stain
HET
  helium equilibration
  time
hetastarch
heterakid
Heterakis
heterauxesis
heteraxial
heterecious
heterecism
heteroagglutination
heteroagglutinin
  hemolymph h.
heteroallele
heteroantibody
heteroantigen
heteroantiserum
heteroatom
Heterobasidion
Heterobilharzia
heteroblastic
heterobrachial inversion
heterocellular
heterocentric
heterochromatic
heterochromatin
  constitutive h.
  facultative h.

  nuclear h.
  satellite-rich h.
heterochromatinization
heterochromia
heterochromic iridocyclitis
heterochromous
heterochthonous
heteroclitic antibody
heterocycle
heterocyclic compound
heterocytotropic antibody
Heterodera
  H. graminophila
  H. marioni
  H. radicicola
heterodermic
heterodimer
  TAP1/TAP2 h.
Heterodoxus spiniger
heteroduplex analysis (HDA)
heterodyne
heterofermentation
heterogametic sex
heterogamy
heterogeneic antigen
heterogeneity, heterogenicity
heterogeneous
  h. assay
  h. nucleation
  h. pattern
heterogenetic
  h. antibody
  h. antigen
heterogenic enterobacterial antigen
heterogenicity (*var. of* heterogeneity)
heterogenote
heterogenous vaccine
heterogony
heterograft
heterokaryon
heterokaryotic twins
heterokeratoplasty
heterolactic
heteroligating antibody
heterologous
  h. antiserum
  h. bone
  h. chimera
  h. desensitization
  h. graft
  h. hemagglutinin
  h. metaplasia
  h. protein
  h. serotype
  h. serum
  h. tumor
heterology
heterolysin
heterolysis

heterolysosome
heterolytic cleavage
heteromastigote
heteromeric cell
heterometabolous
heterometaplasia
heteromorphic
    h. bivalent
    h. chromosome
heteroosteoplasty
heteropathy
heterophagic vacuole
heterophagosome
heterophagy
heterophil, heterophile
    h. agglutinin
    h. antibody
    h. antibody test
    h. antigen
    h. antigen reaction
    h. hemolysin
heterophile (*var. of* heterophil)
heterophilic leukocyte
Heterophyes
    H. brevicaeca
    H. katsuradai
heterophyiasis
heterophyid
Heterophyidae
Heterophyopsis continua
heteroplasia
heteroplasmy
heteroplastic graft
heteroplastid
heteroplasty
heteroploid
heteroploidy
heteropolymer
heteropolysaccharide
heteropyknotic chromatin
heteroscedasticity
heterosis
heterosomal aberration
heterosome
heterospecific graft
heterotaxia, heterotaxy
    cardiac h.
heterotaxic
heterotaxy (*var. of* heterotaxia)
heterothallic
heterothallism
heterotopia, heterotopy
    intestinal h.
    neuronal nodular h.
    occult nodular h.
heterotopic transplantation
heterotopous
heterotopy (*var. of* heterotopia)
heterotransplantation

heterotremus
heterotroph
heterotrophic bacterium
heterovaccine therapy
heteroxenous
heterozygosis (*var. of* heterozygosity)
heterozygosity, heterozygosis
    loss of h. (LOH)
heterozygote
    compound h.
    manifesting h.
    selection against h.'s
heterozygous
    h. alpha thalassemia 1
    h. hemoglobinopathy
    h. point mutation
    h. thalassemia
heterozygous-type hemoglobin disorder
Heublein method
Heubner disease
heuristic method
HEV
    hemorrhagic endovasculitis
    hepatitis E virus
    high-endothelial venule
hexacanth
hexacarboxyporphyrin
    urine h.
hexachloride
    benzene h. (BHC)
hexachlorobenzene
1,2,3,4,5,6-hexachlorocyclohexane
hexachlorophene assay
hexadecimal
Hexadnovirus
hexafluorosilicate
    sodium h.
hexamer
hexamethonium bromide
hexamethylenetetramine
hexamethylpararosaniline
hexamethyl violet
Hexamita
hexamitiasis
hexane
hexanitrate
    inositol h.
hexanoic acid
hexaphosphate
    inositol h.
Hexaplex assay
Hexapoda
hexavalent
hexazonium salt
hexokinase method
hexon
    h. antigen
    h. gene
hexopyranose

H

hexosamine
hexosaminidase
    h. A, B
    h. A deficiency
    h. A gene
    total h.
hexose
    h. diphosphate
    h. monophosphate (HMP)
    h. monophosphate pathway
    h. monophosphate shunt
    (HMPS)
hexosephosphate
    h. dehydrogenase
    h. isomerase
hexose-1-phosphate uridyltransferase
hexosephosphoric esters
hexuronate
hexuronic acid
Heymann pattern
HF
    Hageman factor
    heart failure
    hemorrhagic fever
    high flow
    high frequency
H-FABP
    heart fatty acid binding protein
H1F1 antibody
HFAS
    hereditary flat adenoma
    syndrome
HFBA
    heptafluorobutyric anhydride
HFE gene
HFI
    hereditary fructose intolerance
HFLL
    hemosiderotic fibrohistiocytic
    lipomatous lesion
Hfr
    high-frequency recombination
hFSH
    human-derived follicle-stimulating
    hormone
HG
    high grade
Hg
    mercury
Hg2+
    inorganic mercury
HGA
    homogentisic acid
HGA1c
    glycosylated hemoglobin
HgA1c
    glycosylated hemoglobin
Hgb, hgb
    hemoglobin

HGBV
    hepatitis GB virus
HgCN
    mercury cyanide
HGE
    human granulocytic ehrlichiosis
HGF
    hepatocyte growth factor
    hyperglycemic-glycogenolytic
    factor
HGF/SF
    hepatocyte growth factor/scatter
    factor
hGG
    human gamma globulin
hGH
    human growth hormone
    somatotropin
HGPRT
    hypoxanthine guanine
    phosphoribosyltransferase
HGPRT-deficient cell
HGSIL
    high-grade squamous intraepithelial
    lesion
HGV
    hepatitis G virus
HH
    hereditary hemochromatosis
HHA
    hereditary hemolytic anemia
HHb
    hypohemoglobin
    reduced hemoglobin
    unionized hemoglobin
HHC
    hereditary hemochromatosis
HHD
    hypertensive heart disease
HHF-35
    muscle-specific actin
        HHF-35 antibody
        HHF-35 stain
HHLL
    histocytoid hemangioma-like
    lesion
HHT
    hereditary hemorrhagic telangiectasia
HHV
    human herpesvirus 1–8
        HHV 8 antigen
        HHV 8 DNA in sarcoidosis
HI
    hemagglutination inhibition
HIA
    hemagglutination-inhibition
    antibody
5-HIAA
    5-hydroxyindoleacetic acid

hians
>   *Diphyllobothrium h.*

hiatal hernia, hiatus hernia
hiatus hernia (*var. of* hiatal hernia)
hibernating
>   h. gland
>   h. myocardium

hibernica
hibernoma
>   interscapular h.

HIC
>   hepatic iron concentration

Hickey-Hare test
Hicks-Pitney thromboplastin generation test
HID
>   high iron diamine

hidden radiation source
hidebound disease
hidradenitis
>   h. axillaris of Verneuil
>   neutrophilic eccrine h.
>   h. suppurativa

hidradenocarcinoma
hidradenoma, hydradenoma
>   clear cell h.
>   nodular h.
>   h. papilliferum

hidroa
hidrocystoma
>   apocrine h.

hidrosadenitis
hidrotic ectodermal dysplasia
HIER
>   heat-induced epitope retrieval

hierarchical
>   h. clustering
>   h. clustering analysis

HIF
>   hypoxia inducible factor

HIF-1
>   hypoxia inducible factor-1
>   HIF-1 alpha

high
>   h. amplitude swelling
>   h. anion gap acidosis
>   h. birth weight (HBW)
>   h. dosage (HD)
>   h. egg-passage Flury strain rabies vaccine
>   h. electrophoretic mobility
>   h. endothelial
>   h. endothelial postcapillary
>   h. explosive
>   h. eyepoint eyepiece
>   h. flow (HF)
>   h. frequency (HF)
>   h. grade (HG)
>   h. grade dysplasia

h. iron diamine (HID)
h. level
h. magnification
h. mobility group (HMG)
h. molecular weight (HMW)
h. molecular weight cytokeratin (HMW-CK)
h. molecular weight kininogen (HMWK)
h. protein (HP)
H. Pure PCR product purification kit
h. serum-bound iron (HBI)
h. trough concentration
h. vacuum
h. voltage

high-containment BSL4 facility
high-density
>   h.-d. lipoprotein (HDL)
>   h.-d. lipoprotein-cholesterol (HDL-C)

high-dose
>   h.-d. chemotherapy (HDCT)
>   h.-d. tolerance

high-efficiency particulate air (HEPA)
high-endothelial venule (HEV)
high-energy
>   h.-e. bond
>   h.-e. phosphate
>   h.-e. radiofrequency (HERF)

higher bacteria
high-frequency
>   h.-f. recombination (Hfr)
>   h.-f. recombination mutant
>   h.-f. transduction

high-grade
>   h.-g. B-cell lymphoma
>   h.-g. squamous intraepithelial lesion (HGSIL, HSIL)
>   h.-g. TCC

highly complex series of reaction
Highman
>   H. Congo red technique
>   H. method
>   H. method for amyloid

high-output cardiac failure
high-pass filter
high-performance
>   h.-p. chromatofocusing (HPCF)
>   h.-p. ion exchange chromatography (HPIEC)
>   h.-p. liquid
>   h.-p. liquid chromatography (HPLC)
>   h.-p. size exclusion chromatography (HPSEC)

high-power field (HPF)
high-pressure liquid chromatography (HPLC)

H

high-resolution
    h.-r. banding
    h.-r. CT (HRCT)
    h.-r. fingerprint (HRF)
    h.-r. protein electrophoresis
      (HRE)
high-velocity
    h.-v. missile (HVM)
    h.-v. steel-core round
high-voltage
    h.-v. electrophoresis (HVE)
    h.-v. transformer
Higoumenakia sign
HII
    hepatic iron index
Hikojima antigen
hila (*pl. of* hilum)
hilar
    h. cell
    h. cell tumor of ovary
    h. dance
    h. node (HN)
hilar-based fluffy infiltrate
Hildenbrand disease
hilitis
Hill equation
hillock
    axon h.
hilum, *pl.* **hila**
    h. lienis
    h. nodi lymphatici
    h. of lymph node
    h. of ovary
    h. of spleen
    h. ovarii
    h. pulmonis
    h. renalis
    h. splenicum
hilus
    h. cell
    h. dance
Himasthla
hindrance
    steric h.
Hine-Duley phantom
Hines-Bannick syndrome
Hinfl solution
hinge region
hinshawii
    Arizona h.
Hinton test
hinzii
    Bordetella h.
hip
    congenital dislocation of h.
      (CDH)
HIPA
    heparin-induced platelet activation
    assay

HIPAA
    Health Insurance Portability and
      Accountability Act
Hippea maritima
hippei
    Propionispora h.
Hippelates
Hippel disease
Hippel-Lindau
    H.-L. disease
    von H.-L. (VHL)
Hippeutis
Hippobosca
Hippoboscidae
hippocampal sclerosis (HS)
hippocampus
    alveus hippocampi
    alveus of h.
hippocoleae
    Arcanobacterium h.
hippocratic
    h. face
    h. facies
    h. finger
hippocratica
hippocratici
    digiti h.
hippurate
    h. broth
    methenamine h.
hippuratus
    Agromyces h.
hippuria
hippuric
    h. acid
    h. acid crystal
    h. acid excretion test
Hirano body
hiranonis
    Clostridium h.
hirci (*pl. of* hircus)
hircus, *pl.* **hirci**
Hirneola
Hirschfeld disease
hirschfeldii
    Salmonella enteritidis serotype *h.*
hirschii
    Hydrogenophilus h.
Hirschowitz syndrome
Hirsch-Peiffer stain
Hirschsprung-associated enterocolitis
    (HAEC)
Hirschsprung disease (HD)
hirsuta
    Gordonia h.
hirsuties (*var. of* hirsutism)
hirsutism, hirsuties
    amenorrhea and h.
hirtellous

hirthi
    Filaroides h.
hirudin
hirudinaceus
    Macracanthorhynchus h.
Hirudinea
hirudiniasis
hirudinization
Hirudo
    H. aegyptiaca
    H. japonica
    H. medicinalis
His
    H. bundle
    H. disease
    H. isthmus
    H. perivascular space
hispanica
    Arthropsis h.
    Borrelia h.
hispanicus
    Vibrio h.
hispidum
    Gnathostoma h.
Hiss capsule stain
Histalog test
histaminase
histamine
    h. flare test
    h. liberator
    h. receptor blocker
    h. shock
    h. stimulation test
histaminemia
histamine-releasing factor (HRF)
histaminergic
histaminiformans
    Allisonella h.
histaminuria
histangic (*var. of* histoangic)
His-Tawara system
histidase
histidinase
histidine
    h. alpha deaminase
    analog of h. (AHH)
    h. decarboxylase (HDC)
    h. loading test
    urine h.
histidinemia
histidine-rich matrix protein
histidinuria
histidyl
histioblast
histiocyte, histocyte
    cardiac h.
    crescentic h.
    epithelioid h.
    facultative h.

    foamy h.
    gargoylism type of h.
    Gaucher type of h.
    Hand-Schüller-Christian type of h.
    Niemann-Pick type of h.
    von Hansemann h.
histiocyte-rich B-cell lymphoma (HRBCL)
histiocytic
    h. granuloma
    h. leukemia
    h. lymphoma (HL)
    h. medullary reticulosis
    h. necrotizing lymphadenitis (HNL)
    h. phenotype
histiocytoid carcinoma
histiocytoma
    ankle-type fibrous h.
    atypical fibrous h.
    cellular cutaneous fibrous h.
    (CCFH)
    fibrous h.
    generalized eruptive h.
    malignant fibrous h. (MFH)
    superficial malignant fibrous h.
histiocytosis, histocytosis
    kerasin h.
    Langerhans cell h. (LCH)
    lipid h.
    localized h.
    malignant h.
    nodular non-X h.
    nonlipid h.
    regressing atypical h. (RAH)
    sea-blue h.
    sinus h. (SH)
    systemic h.
    h. X
histiogenic
histioid
histioma
histionic
histoangic, histangic
histoblast
histo-blood group antigen
histochemical stain
histochemistry
Histochoice
Histoclad
Histoclear slide processing solution
histocompatibility
    h. antigen
    h. assay
    h. assessment
    h. complex
    h. gene
    h. locus (HL)
    h. molecule
    h. testing
    h. testinghistocompatibility testing

H

histoculture drug response assay
(HDRA)
histocyte (*var. of* histiocyte)
histocytoid hemangioma-like lesion
(HHLL)
histocytologic research
histocytosis (*var. of*
hystiocytosis)
histodiagnosis
histodiagnostic marker
histodifferentiation
Histo-Dx
    histologic diagnosis
Histofine
    H. SAB-PO immunohistochemical
      staining kit
    H. staining method
histofluorescence
histogenesis
histogenetic
histogenous
histogeny
histogram
    cumulative-frequency h.
    frequence-time h.
    h. mode
    two-parameter h.
histography
histoid
    h. leprosy
    h. neoplasm
    h. tumor
histoincompatibility
histologic, histological
    h. accommodation
    h. activity index (HAI)
    h. appearance
    h. chemistry
    h. diagnosis (Histo-Dx)
    h. grading
    h. lesion
    h. pattern
    h. staining
    h. technician (HT)
    h. tumor grade
histological (*var. of* histologic)
histologically detectable iron
(HDI)
histologist
histology
    tumor h.
histolysis
histolytic
histolytica
    Amoeba h.
    Entamoeba h.
    Torula h.
histolyticum
    Clostridium h.

histolyticus
    Bacillus h.
histoma, histioma
histometaplastic
Histomonas meleagridis
histomoniasis
histomorphology
histomorphometry
histone
    h. acetyltransferase
    h. deacetylase
    (HDAC)
    h. protein
histoneurology
histonomy
histonuria
Histopaque-1077
histopathogenesis
histopathology
    acid-fast staining h.
Histophilus somni
histophysiology
Histoplasma
    H. antibody assay
    H. capsulatum capsulatum
    H. capsulatum duboisii
    H. farciminosus
histoplasmin
histoplasmin-latex test
histoplasmoma
histoplasmosis
    African h.
    bronchopulmonary h.
    h. serology
histoprognostic
historadiography
historrhexis
history
    case h.
    heart disease h. (HDH)
histospectroscopy
histotechnologist
histotechnology
histotome
histotomy
histotope
histotoxic
    h. anoxia
    h. hypoxia
histotrophic
histotropic
histozoic
His-Werner disease
HIT
    hemagglutination-inhibition test
    heparin-induced thrombocytopenia
    hypertrophic infiltrative tendinitis
Hitachi
    H. 704, 736, 911 analyzer

H. 747-100 cholesterol analyzer
H. 747 CK/MB analyzer
hitchhiker thumb
HitHunter cAMP enzyme fragment complementation assay
hits
genetic h.
HITT
heparin-induced thrombocytopenia-thrombosis
HIV
human immunodeficiency virus
HIV-2
HIV antibody test
HIV encephalopathy
HIV quantitation
HIV sialadenitis
SI variant of HIV
Hivagen test
HIVAN
human immunodeficiency virus-associated nephropathy
hives
giant h.
HIV-1 serology
HJ
Howell-Jolly
HJ body
Hjärre disease
HK
heat killed
hK2
human kallikrein-2
hK3
human kallikrein-3
HKLM
heat-killed *Listeria monocytogenes*
HL
histiocytic lymphoma
histocompatibility locus
hyperreactio luteinalis
HLA
human leukocyte antigen
HLA allele
HLA BW 54 antigen
HLA class I deficiency
HLA complex
HLA haplotype segregation
HLA sequence in NK repertoire
soluble HLA
HLA typing
HLA-A antigen
HLA-B antigen
HLA-B8 phenotype
HLA-C locus specificity
HLA-D antigen
HLA-DM gene

HLA-DR antigen
HLA-DR3 phenotype
HLDH
heat-stable lactic dehydrogenase
hL-FABP
human liver-type fatty acid-binding protein
HLH
hemophagocytic lymphohistiocytosis
hLH
human luteinizing hormone
hLT
human lymphocyte transformation
hMAM
human mammaglobin
hMAM RNA
HMB
homatropine methylbromide
HMB 45 antibody
HMB 45 antigen
HMB 45 marker
HMD
hyaline membrane disease
HME
human monocytic ehrlichiosis
HMFG-2 antibody
HMG
high mobility group
human menopausal gonadotropin
hydroxymethylglutaryl
HML
human milk lysozyme
hMLH 1 gene
HMO
hypothetical mean organism
HMP
hexose monophosphate
HMPS
hexose monophosphate shunt
HMRU
Hazardous Materials Response Unit
HMS
hypothetical mean strain
HMSAS
hypertrophic muscular subaortic stenosis
HMW
high molecular weight
HMW kininogen
HMW-CK
high molecular weight cytokeratin
HMWK
high molecular weight kininogen
HMWK antibody
HmX
HmX hematology analyzer
HmX H20 hematology system
HN
hereditary nephritis

453

HN (*continued*)
  hilar node
  NATO code for nitrogen mustard
HN1
  NATO code for nitrogen mustard 1
HN2
  NATO code for nitrogen mustard 2
HN3
  NATO code for nitrogen mustard 3
hNIS
  human sodium/iodide symporter
    hNIS gene expression
HNL
  histiocytic necrotizing lymphadenitis
  human neutrophil lipocalin
HNP
  herniated nucleus pulposus
HNPCC
  hereditary nonpolyposis colon
    cancer
  hereditary nonpolyposis colorectal
    cancer
HNSCC
  head and neck squamous cell
    carcinoma
HNSHA
  hereditary nonspherocytic hemolytic
    anemia
HO
  heme oxygenase
hoagii
    Corynebacterium h.
Ho antigen
hobnail
  h. cell
  h. cell metaplasia
  h. liver
  h. nucleus
Hoboken
  H. gemmules
  H. nodule
HOC
  hydroxycorticoid
hoc
hock disease
HOCM
  hypertrophic obstructive
    cardiomyopathy
HO/CO
  heme oxygenase/carbon monoxide
Hodara disease
Hodgkin
  H. and Reed-Sternberg (HRS)
  H. and Reed-Sternberg cell
  H. disease (HD)
  H. granuloma
  lymphocyte-rich classic H.
  H. lymphoma
  H. sarcoma

Hodgson disease
Hoechst dye
Hoesch test
hof
Hofbauer cell
Hoffa disease
Hoffman
  H. test
  H. violet
Hoffmann duct
Hoffmann-Werdnig syndrome
Hofmann bacillus
hofmannii
    Corynebacterium h.
Hofmeister test
hofstadii
    Leptotrichia h.
hog
  h. cholera
  h. cholera serum
  h. cholera vaccine
  h. cholera virus
Hogben test
Hohenbuehelia
holandric
  h. gene
  h. inheritance
holarthritic
holarthritis
Hollande
  H. fixative
  H. fixative/solution
  H. solution
Hollander test
Hollenhorst plaques
Hollerith code
hollisae
    Grimontia h.
    Vibrio h.
hollow cathode lamp
Holmes
  H. alkaline buffer
  H. method
  H. stain
Holmes-Adie syndrome
holmesii
    Bordetella h.
Holmgren-Golgi canal
holmium
holoacardius
  h. acephalus
  h. acormus
  h. amorphus
holocord
holocrine gland
holocyclus
    Ixodes h.
holoendemic disease
holoenzyme

hologynic
    h. gene
    h. inheritance
holomastigote
holometabolous
Holophyra coli
holophytic
holoprosencephaly
holorachischisis
holotelencephaly
holothuriorum
    Salegentibacter h.
holotrichous
holotype
holozoic
holsaticum
    Mycobacterium h.
Holt-Oram syndrome
Holzer method
Holzknecht unit (H)
Homalomyia
homatropine methylbromide (HMB)
homaxial
home
    H. Access hepatitis C Check test
    h. canning
Homén syndrome
homeobox gene
homeodomain
    h. protein
    h. transcription factor
homeomorphous
homeoplasia, homoioplasia
homeoplastic
homeostasis
    immunologic h.
homeostatic
homeotherapeutics (*var. of*
  homeotherapy)
homeotherapy, homeotherapeutics
Homer-Wright rosette
homing
hominis
    Blastocystis h.
    Campylobacter h.
    Cardiobacterium h.
    Coccidium h.
    Debaryomyces h.
    Dermatobia h.
    Enteromonas h.
    Gastrodiscoides h.
    Gastrodiscus h.
    Gastrospirillum h.
    Herpesvirus h. (HVH)
    Isospora h.
    Mycoplasma h.
    Oestrus h.
    poliovirus h.
    Polycytella h.

    Psilorchis h.
    Rhabditis h.
    Saccharomyces h.
    Sarcocystis h.
    Staphylococcus h.
    Taenia h.
    Tetratrichomonas h.
    Trichomonas h.
    Trypanosoma h.
hominivorax
    Cochliomyia h.
homme rouge
homoallele
homobiotin
homocarnosine
homocentric
homochronous inheritance
homocyclic
homocysteine
    h. desulfhydrase
    h. testing
homocystine
    h. testing
    urine h.
homocystinemia
homocystinuria (HCU)
    h. test
homocytotrophic (HCT)
homocytotropic antibody
homodimer
homofermentation
homogametic sex
homogenate
homogeneity
homogeneous
    h. immersion
    h. ligand assay
    h. staining region (HSR)
homogenization
    amphophilic h.
homogenize
homogenote
homogentisate
    h. 1,2-dioxygenase
    h. dioxygenase
    h. oxidase
    h. oxygenase
homogentisic
    h. acid (HGA)
    h. acid test
homogentisuria
homograft rejection
homoioplasia (*var. of* homeoplasia)
homolactic
homolog, homologue
    deltalike 1 h. (DLK1)
    human achaete-scute h. (HASH)
    human mismatch-repair protein MutL
      h. (MLH1)

H

homolog (*continued*)
    human MutS h.
    smoothened h. (SMOH)
homologous
    h. antigen
    h. antiserum
    artificial insemination h. (AIH)
    h. chimera
    h. chromosome
    h. desensitization
    h. graft
    h. hemagglutinin
    h. recombination
    h. series
    h. serotype
    h. serum
    h. serum jaundice
    h. single-pass membrane
      sialoglycoprotein
    h. structure
    h. tumor
homologue (*var. of* homolog)
homology
    DNA h.
    h. of chains
    h. of strands
    h. region
homolysin
homolysis
homolytic cleavage
homomorphic bivalent
homophil
homoplastic graft
homopolymer
homoscedasticity
homotetrameric complex
homothallic
homothallism
homotopic transplantation
homotransplant (*var. of*
  homotransplantation)
homotransplantation, homotransplant
homovanillic
    h. acid (HVA)
    h. acid test
homozygosis (*var. of* homozygosity)
homozygosity, homozygosis
homozygote
homozygous
    h. achondroplasia
    h. alpha thalassemia 1, 2
    h. hemoglobinopathy
    h. hemoglobin S (HbSS)
    h. point mutation
    h. thalassemia
    h. typing cell
homozygous-type hemoglobin disorder
hone
    automatic h.

honei
    Rickettsia h.
honeycomb
    h. fibrosis
    h. lung
    h. macula
    h. ringworm
    h. tetter
honeycombing
    cell h.
    radiologic h.
honeycomb-like space
honey urine
Hong
    H. Kong foot
    H. Kong influenza
    H. Kong toe
Hongia koreensis
Hongiella
    H. halophila
    H. mannitolivorans
    H. marincola
    H. ornithinivorans
hongkongensis
    Actinomyces h.
    Laribacter h.
honing
HOOD
    hereditary osteoonychodysplasia
hood
    fume h.
    laboratory h.
    laminar flow h.
hooded chemical-resistant clothing
hoof-and-mouth disease
Hooke law
Hooker-Forbes test
hooklet
    hydatid h.
hookworm
    American h.
    h. anemia
    h. disease
    dog h.
    European h.
    New World h.
    Old World h.
Hopkins-Cole test
Hoplopsyllus anomalus
Hoppe-Goldflam disease
Hoppe-Seyler test
hordei
    Acarus h.
Hordeivirus
hordeolum
Horie tumor classification
horizontal
    h. cell of Cajal
    h. transmission

Horm collagen reagent
    hormone
horminium
      Salvia h.
Hormoconis
Hormodendrum
      H. carrionii
      H. cladosporioides
      H. compactum
      H. pedrosoi
Hormogoneae
Hormographiella
hormonal
    h. evaluation
    h. imbalance
    h. receptor
    h. therapy
hormone
    adaptive h.
    adenohypophysial h.
    adipokinetic h.
    adrenocortical h. (ACH)
    adrenocorticotropic h. (ACTH)
    adrenomedullary h.
    alpha melanocytic-stimulating h.
    androgenic h.
    anterior pituitary h. (APH)
    antidiuretic h. (ADH)
    antimüllerian h. (AMH)
    Aschheim-Zondek h.
    bovine growth h. (BGH)
    chondrotrophic h.
    chromaffin h.
    chromatophorotropic h.
    corpus luteum h.
    cortical h.
    corticotropin-releasing h. (CRH)
    diabetogenic h.
    ectopic h.
    erythropoietic h.
    estrogenic h.
    fat-mobilizing h.
    female h.
    follicle-stimulating h. (FSH)
    follicle-stimulating hormone releasing
      h. (FSH-RH)
    galactopoietic h.
    gastrointestinal h.
    glycoprotein h.
    gonadotropic h. (GTH)
    gonadotropin-releasing h. (GnRH)
    growth h. (GH)
    growth hormone-inhibiting h.
      (GH-IH)
    growth hormone release inhibiting h.
      (GH-RIH)
    growth hormone-releasing h.
      (GH-RH)
    growth-stimulating h. (GSH)

hepcidin peptide h.
human-derived follicle-stimulating h.
  (hFSH)
human growth h. (hGH)
human luteinizing h. (hLH)
human pituitary follicle-stimulating
  h. (hPFSH)
hypophysiotropic h.
immunoreactive human growth h.
  (IRhGH)
inappropriate antidiuretic h. (IADH)
incretin h.
incretin-mimetic h.
inhibiting h.
inhibitory h.
interstitial cell-stimulating h. (ICSH)
islet h.
juvenile h.
ketogenic h.
lactogenic h.
langerhansian h.
lipolytic h.
luteal h.
luteinizing h. (LH)
luteinizing hormone-releasing h.
  (LH-RH)
lutein-stimulating h. (LSH)
luteotropic h. (LTH)
lymphocyte-stimulating h.
male h.
mammotropic h.
melanocyte-inhibiting h.
melanocyte-stimulating hormone
  release-inhibiting h.
melanocyte-stimulating hormone
  releasing h.
melanophore-stimulating h. (MSH)
neonatal thyroid-stimulating h.
neurohypophysial h.
orchidic h.
ovarian h.
ovine lactogenic h. (OLH)
pituitary glycoprotein h.
pituitary growth h. (PGH)
placental h.
plasma luteinizing h.
posterior pituitary h.
progestational h.
prolactin release-inhibiting h.
prolactin-releasing h. (PRH)
proparathyroid h.
protein h.
prothoracicotropic h.
h. receptor
h. receptor status
regulatory h.
releasing h. (RH)
sex h. (SH)
somatotropic h. (STH)

H

hormone (*continued*)
    somatotropin-releasing h. (SRH)
    steroid h.
    steroidogenic h.
    syndrome of inappropriate secretion
      of antidiuretic h. (SIADH)
    testicular h.
    thyroid-stimulating h.
    thyrotropic h. (TTH)
    thyrotropin-releasing h. (TRH)
    TSH releasing h.
Hormonema dematioides
hormone-releasing
horn
    Ammon h.
    cicatricial h.
    cutaneous h.
    iliac h.
    lateral gray h.
    nail h.
    sebaceous h.
    warty h.
Horner syndrome
hornification
horny
    h. cell
    h. layer of epidermis
    h. layer of nail
horror autotoxicus
horse
    h. antihuman thymus globulin
      (HAHTG)
    h. red blood cell (HRBC)
    h. serum (HS)
    h. serum block
horsefly
horsepox virus
horseradish
    h. peroxidase (HRP)
    h. peroxidase conjugated
      streptavidin-biotin complex
horseshoe
    h. fistula
    h. kidney
horseshoe-shaped nucleus
hortae
Hortaea werneckii
Hortega
    H. cell
    H. neuroglia stain
Horton
    H. disease
    H. syndrome
HOSE
    human ovarian surface epithelial
    HOSE cell
hose
    drench h.
Hospidex microtiter plate

hospita
    Burkholderia h.
hospital
    h. epidemiology
    h. fever
hospital-acquired
    h.-a. gram-negative pneumonia
    h.-a. methicillin-resistant
      Staphylococcus aureus
    h.-a. penetration contact
host
    accidental h.
    alternate h.
    amplifier h.
    dead-end h.
    h. defenses
    definitive h.
    intermediate h.
    natural h.
    h. of predilection
    reservoir h.
    h. response
    h. stroma
    transfer h.
host-parasite relationship
host-range mutation
Hostuviroid
hot
    h. abscess
    h. antigen suicide
    h. cell
    h. gangrene
    h. lesion
    h. looping
    h. nodule
    h. spot
    h. zone
Hotchkiss-McManus PAS technique
Hottentot apron
houghtoni
    Diphyllobothrium h.
hound-dog facies
Hounsfield unit (H)
hour
    milligram h.
    milligram per h. (mg/h)
2-hour
    2-h. postprandial blood sugar
      test
    2-h. postprandial plasma glucose
      test
hourglass
    h. gallbladder
    h. stomach
housefly
Houssay
    H. animal
    H. phenomenon
    H. syndrome

houstonense
Mycobacterium h.
Howard test
Howell
H. prothrombin test
H. unit
Howell-Jolly (HJ)
H.-J. body
Howship lacuna
Hoyer canal
HP
high protein
FlexSure HP
HPA
hybridization protection assay
HPC
hemangiopericytoma
hematopoietic progenitor cell
hyperplastic-like mucosal
change
HPCF
high-performance chromatofocusing
HPF
heparin-precipitable fraction
high-power field
HPFH
hereditary persistence of fetal
hemoglobin
hPFSH
human pituitary follicle-stimulating
hormone
hPG
human pituitary gonadotropin
HPI
Haemophilus parainfluenzae
HPIEC
high-performance ion exchange
chromatography
hPL
human placental lactogen
HPLC
high-performance liquid chromatography
high-pressure liquid chromatography
32 Karat software for HPLC
System Gold HPLC
HPLC water
hPMS2 gene
HPP
hereditary pyropoikilocytosis
HPPA
hydroxyphenylpyruvic acid
HPRC
hereditary papillary renal cell
carcinoma
hPrL
human prolactin
HPRT
hypoxanthine phosphoribosyltransferase
HPRT-deficient cell

HPS
hematoxylin-phloxine-saffron
hemophagocytic syndrome
hypertrophic pyloric stenosis
HPSEC
high-performance size exclusion
chromatography
HPT
hyperparathyroidism
HPV
Haemophilus pertussis vaccine
human papillomavirus
HPV triage
HPVD
hypertensive pulmonary vascular
disease
HPVG
hepatic portal venous gas
H.P. Wright method
HR
hazard ratio
hRAD30 gene
H-ras gene
HRBC
horse red blood cell
HRBCL
histiocyte-rich B-cell lymphoma
HRCT
high-resolution CT
HRE
high-resolution protein electrophoresis
HRF
high-resolution fingerprint
histamine-releasing factor
HRIG
human rabies immune globulin
HRP
horseradish peroxidase
HRPT2 gene
HRS
Hamilton Rating Scale
Hodgkin and Reed-Sternberg
HRS cell
HRSA
Health Resources and Services
Administration
HS
heat-stable
heme synthetase
hereditary spherocytosis
herpes simplex
hippocampal sclerosis
horse serum
Hurler syndrome
HSA
human serum albumin
HSC
hematopoietic stem cell
totipotent HSC

459

HSF1
heat shock factor 1
HSIL
high-grade squamous intraepithelial
lesion
H-SLAP
human stromelysin aggregated
proteoglycan
HSM
hepatosplenomegaly
HSP
heat shock protein
Henoch-Schönlein purpura
HSP 40, 70, 90
HSR
homogeneous staining
region
HSU method
HSV
herpes simplex virus
HSV culture
HSV isolation
HSVE
herpes simplex virus
encephalitis
HT
histologic technician
hypertension
5-HT, 5HT
5-hydroxytryptamine
H-tetanase
HTLV
human T-cell leukemia-lymphoma
virus
HTLV-I
human T-cell lymphotropic virus
type I
HTLV-I antibody
HTLV-1 associated myelopathy
(HAM)
HTLV-II
human T-cell lymphotropic virus
type II
HTLV-III
human T-cell lymphotropic virus
type III
HTN
hypertension
HTP
hydroxytryptophan
HTV
herpes-type virus
HU
heat unit
hemagglutinating unit
hydroxyurea
hyperemia unit
Hu antigen
Huchard disease

Hucker-Conn
H.-C. crystal violet solution
H.-C. stain
Huddleston agglutination test
Huebener-Thomsen-Friedenreich
phenomenon
Hueck ligament
Hüet-Pelger nuclear anomaly
Hüfner equation
Huhner test
hulunbeirensis
Natrialba h.
human
h. ABC transporter family
h. achaete-scute homolog
(HASH)
h. alpha-lactalbumin
h. alpha-lactalbumin made lethal to
tumor cells
h. alpha-1 proteinase inhibitor
h. alveolar macrophage (HAM)
h. androgen receptor gene
(HUMARA)
h. antichimeric antibody
(HACA)
h. antihemophilic factor
antihemophilic plasma h.
h. antimicrobial peptide
h. antimouse antibody (HAMA)
h. antimurine antibody (HAMA)
h. B lymphotropic virus (HBLV)
h. botulinum neurotoxin type A, B,
E, F
h. chorionic gonadotropin (HCG,
hCG)
h. chorionic gonadotropin injection
test
h. chorionic somatomammotropin
(hCSM)
h. dermal microvascular endothelial
cell (HDMEC)
h. diploid cell rabies vaccine
(HDCV)
h. embryo kidney (HEK)
h. embryo lung (HEL)
h. embryonic kidney (HEK)
h. engineering
h. enteric (virus) (HE)
h. epidermal growth receptor 2
(HER-2)
h. erythrocyte agglutination test
(HEAT)
h. flea
h. gamma globulin (hGG)
h. genetic identity testing
h. genome
h. glandular kallikrein 3
h. granulocytic ehrlichiosis (HGE)
h. growth hormone (hGH)

h. growth hormone deficiency
h. growth hormone stimulation test
h. heparanese II
h. herpesvirus 1–8 (HHV)
h. immunodeficiency virus (HIV)
h. immunodeficiency virus-associated nephropathy (HIVAN)
h. immunodeficiency virus culture
h. kallikrein 2 (hK2)
h. kallikrein 3 (hK3)
h. lamin A gene
h. leukemia-associated antigen
h. leukocyte antigen (HLA)
h. liver-type fatty acid-binding protein (hL-FABP)
h. luteinizing hormone (hLH)
h. lymphocyte antigen
h. lymphocyte transformation (hLT)
h. lymphoproliferative disease
h. mammaglobin (hMAM)
h. measles immune serum
h. menopausal gonadotropin (HMG)
h. mesothelial cell membrane (HBME 1)
h. milk factor globulin
h. milk lysozyme (HML)
h. mismatch-repair protein MutL homolog (MLH1)
h. monocytic ehrlichiosis (HME)
h. MutS homolog
h. neutrophil lipocalin (HNL)
h. normal immunoglobulin
h. ovarian surface epithelial (HOSE)
h. papillomavirus (HPV)
h. papillomavirus DNA probe test
h. parvovirus B19
h. pertussis immune serum
h. pituitary follicle-stimulating hormone (hPFSH)
h. pituitary gonadotropin (hPG)
h. placental lactogen (hPL)
h. progenitor cell antigen
h. prolactin (hPrL)
h. rabies immune globulin (HRIG)
h. remains
h. scarlet fever immune serum
h. serum albumin (HSA)
h. sodium/iodide symporter (hNIS)
h. stromelysin aggregated proteoglycan (H-SLAP)
h. T-cell leukemia-lymphoma virus (HTLV)
h. T-cell lymphotropic virus type I (HTLV-I)
h. T-cell lymphotropic virus type II (HTLV-II)
h. T-cell lymphotropic virus type III (HTLV-III)
h. telomerase reverse transcriptase

h. thymus antiserum (HUTHAS)
h. tubercle bacillus
h. umbilical vein endothelial cell (HUVEC)
human-derived
   h.-d. botulism immune globulin
   h.-d. follicle-stimulating hormone (hFSH)
humanus
   Pediculus h.
HUMARA
   human androgen receptor gene
humectant
Humicola
humidifier lung
humilata
   Cellulomonas h.
humiphilum
   Ornithinimicrobium h.
humor
   aqueous h.
   h. aquosus
   Morgagni h.
   ocular h.
   plasmoid h.
   vitreous h.
   h. vitreus
humoral
   h. antibody
   h. hypercalcemia of malignancy
   h. immune response
   h. immunity
   h. pathology
   h. regulator
   h. thymic factor
hump
   h. deposit
   electron-dense h.
Hünermann syndrome
hungatei
   Butyrivibrio h.
   Clostridium h.
hungry bone syndrome
Hunner
   H. cystitis
   H. stricture
   H. ulcer
Hunt
   H. and Hess hand fracture
   H. disease
   H. syndrome
Hunter
   H. glossitis
   H. membrane
   H. syndrome
Hunter-Hurler syndrome
Hunter-Schreger
   H.-S. band
   H.-S. line

H

huntingtin
　h. gene
　h. protein
huntingtin-associated protein 1 (HAP1)
huntingtin-interacting protein 1
Huntington
　H. chorea (HC)
　H. disease (HD)
Hurler
　H. disease
　H. syndrome (HS)
hurloid facies
Hürthle
　H. cell
　H. cell adenocarcinoma
　H. cell adenoma
　H. cell carcinoma
　H. cell metaplasia
　H. cell tumor
HUS
　hemolytic-uremic syndrome
　hyaluronidase unit for semen
Huschke auditory teeth
HUT
　hyperplasia of usual type
Hutchinson
　H. crescentic notch
　H. disease
　H. facies
　H. incisor
　H. mask
　H. melanotic freckle
　H. patch
　H. pupil
　summer prurigo of H.
　H. syndrome
　H. teeth
　H. triad
Hutchinson-Boeck disease
Hutchinson-Gilford
　H.-G. disease
　H.-G. syndrome
Hutchinson-Guilford progeria
Hutchison syndrome
HUTHAS
　human thymus antiserum
Hutinel disease
HUVEC
　human umbilical vein endothelial cell
Huvos grading system
Huxley
　H. layer
　H. membrane
　H. sheath
huygenian eyepiece
Huygens ocular
HV
　herpesvirus

HVA
　homovanillic acid
　　HVA test
HVE
　high-voltage electrophoresis
hveragerdense
　　Thermodesulfobacterium h.
HVH
　Herpesvirus hominis
HVL
　half-value layer
HVM
　high-velocity missile
HVSD
　hydrogen-detected ventricular septal defect
hwajinpoensis
　　Bacillus h.
hyacinthi
　　Acarus rhizoglypticus h.
hyalin
　alcoholic h.
　hematogenous h.
　Laquer stain for alcoholic h.
　Mallory h.
hyalina
　　Hartmannella h.
hyaline, hyaloid
　alcoholic h.
　h. arteriolosclerosis
　h. body of pituitary
　h. capsule
　h. cartilage
　h. cartilage matrix
　h. cell
　h. Civatte body
　h. core
　h. degeneration
　h. globule
　h. leukocyte
　h. material
　h. membrane
　h. membrane disease (HMD)
　h. membrane disease of newborn
　h. necrosis
　h. nephrosclerosis
　h. perisplenitis
　h. plaque
　h. sclerosis
　h. thickening
　h. thrombus
　h. tubercle
　h. urinary cast
hyalinization
hyalinized
　h. core
　h. stroma
hyalinizing
　h. clear cell carcinoma (HCCC)

h. spindle cell tumor with giant
  rosettes
h. trabecular tumor
hyalinosis
  focal segmental glomerular sclerosis
    and h. (FSGSH)
  systemic h.
hyalinuria
hyalocyte
Hyalodendron lignicola
hyalohyphomycosis
hyaloid (*var. of* hyaline)
  h. body
  h. canal
  h. membrane
hyaloidea
  membrana h.
  stella lentis h.
hyaloideus
  canalis h.
hyalomere
Hyalomma
  H. anatolicum
  H. marginatum
  H. variegatum
hyaloplasm, hyaloplasma
  nuclear h.
hyaloplasma (*var. of* hyaloplasm)
hyaloplasmic
hyaloserositis
hyalosome
hyaluronate
hyaluronic acid (HA)
hyaluronidase
  h. collagen
  h. digestion
  h. unit for semen (HUS)
hyaluronoglucosaminidase
hyaluronoglucuronidase
Hyams esthesioneuroblastoma
  classification
H-Y antigen
Hybond
  H. N filter
  H. N+ nylon membrane
hybrid
  h. antibody
  H. Capture 2 (hc2)
  H. Capture 2 (cervical cancer
    screening) device
  H. Capture 2 Chlamydia test
  H. Capture 2 HPV DNA test
  H. Capture system
  h. cell
  h. orbital
  SV40-adenovirus h.
hybridization
  array-based comparative genomic h.
    (aCGH)

cell h.
cellular h.
comparative genome h.
comparative genomic h. (CGH)
competition h.
cross h.
DNA h.
DNA-DNA h.
DNA-RNA h.
Epstein-Barr virus-encoded RNA in
  situ h.
filter h.
fluorescence in situ h. (FISH)
fluorescent in situ h. (FISH)
genotypic blot h.
in situ h.
in-solution h.
liquid-phase h.
liquid (solution) h.
molecular h.
nonisotopic in situ h. (NISH)
nucleic acid h.
h. protection assay (HPA)
quantitative fluorescence in situ h.
  (Q-FISH)
RNA-driven h.
RNA-RNA h.
sandwich h.
saturation h.
sequencing by h. (SBH)
solid-phase h.
solution h.
suppression subtractive h.
hybridize
hybridized probe
hybridoma
  h. antibody
  h. supernatant
  h. technique
Hybritech
  H. free PSA test
  H. Ostase bone metabolism marker
  H. PSA blood test
  H. PSA determination system
hydantoin
hydatid
  alveolar h.
  h. cyst
  h. degeneration
  h. disease (HD)
  h. hooklet
  h. mole
  h. of Morgagni
  osseous h.
  h. polyp
  h. pregnancy
  h. rash
  sessile h.
  Virchow h.

H

hydatidiform mole, hydatid mole
hydatidocele
hydatidoma
hydatidosis
hydatiduria
hydatigena
    Taenia h.
Hydatigera
    H. infantis
    H. taeniaeformis
Hyde disease
Hydnopolyporus
hydradenitis
hydradenoma (*var. of* hidradenoma)
hydralazine lupus
hydranencephaly
hydrargyromania
hydrarthrosis
hydratase
    aconitate h.
    enoyl-coenzyme A h.
    fumarate h.
hydrate
    chloral h.
    sodium h.
hydrated alumina
hydrazide
    isonicotinic acid h.
    thiophen-2-carboxylic acid h.
    (TCH)
hydrazine
    alpha h.
    h. yellow
hydrazine-sensitive factor
hydremia
hydrencephalocele, hydrocephalocele
hydrencephalomeningocele
hydrencephalus
hydride
    antimony h.
    arsenic h.
    arsenious h.
hydroa
    h. aestivale
    h. febrile
    h. vesiculosum
hydroappendix
hydrocalycosis
hydrocarbon
    alicyclic h.
    aliphatic saturated h.
    aliphatic unsaturated h.
    aromatic h.
    carcinogenic h.
    cyclic h.
    polycyclic aromatic h.
    saturated h.
    unsaturated h.
Hydrocarboniphaga effusa

hydrocele
    h. sac
    h. spinalis
hydrocephalic
hydrocephalocele
hydrocephaloid disease
hydrocephalus, hydrocephaly
    communicating h.
    noncommunicating h.
    normal pressure h. (NPH)
hydrocephaly (*var. of* hydrocephalus)
hydrochloric
    h. acid (HCl)
    secreting h.
hydrochloride
    acridine h.
    adiphenine h.
    aminoacridine h.
    arginine h.
    atabrine h.
    chloroguanide h.
    cocaine h.
    colestipol h.
    cyproheptadine h.
    diphenhydramine h.
    doxepin h.
    ethoxazene h.
    hydromorphone h.
    lidocaine h.
    meperidine h.
    methadone h.
    methamphetamine h.
    prazosin h.
    procaine h.
    quinacrine h.
    semicarbazide h.
hydrochlorothiazide (HCT, HCTZ)
hydrocholecystis
hydrocholeresis
hydrocholeretic
hydrocirsocele
hydrocortisone (compound F)
hydrocyanic acid
hydrocyst
hydrocystoma
hydrocytosis
hydroencephalocele (*var. of*
  hydrenencephalocele)
hydrofluoric acid
hydrogel coated slide
hydrogen
    h. acceptor
    h. arsenide
    arseniuretted h.
    h. bacterium
    h. bond
    h. chloride
    h. cyanide (HCN)
    h. electrode

h. exponent
h. fluoride
h. ion
h. ion concentration (pH)
h. peroxide
h. peroxide solution
h. sulfide
hydrogenalis
    Anaerococcus h.
hydrogenase
hydrogenate
hydrogenation
hydrogen-detected ventricular septal defect (HVSD)
Hydrogenimonas thermophila
hydrogeniphila
hydrogeniphilum
    Thermodesulfobacterium h.
hydrogeniphilus
    Caminibacter h.
Hydrogenobacter
    H. hydrogenophilus
    H. subterraneus
Hydrogenobaculum acidophilum
hydrogenolysis
Hydrogenophaga intermedia
hydrogenophilus
    Geobacter h.
    H. hirschii
    Hydrogenobacter h.
Hydrogenothermaceae
Hydrogenothermus marinus
hydrolability
hydrolase
    acetyl-CoA h.
    acid h.
    aminoacyl-tRNA h.
    aryl-ester h.
    diadenosine oligophosphate h.
    L-kynurenine h.
    ubiquitin C-terminal h.
hydrolysate
    casein h.
    lactalbumin h. (LAH)
    protein h.
hydrolysis
    gelatin h.
hydrolytic enzyme
hydrolyze
hydroma
hydromeningocele
hydrometer scale
hydrometrocolpos
hydromicrocephaly
hydromorphone hydrochloride
hydromphalus
hydromyelia
hydromyelocele
hydromyoma

hydronephrosis
hydronephrotic
hydronium ion
hydropericardium
hydroperitoneum, hydroperitonia
hydroperitonia (*var. of* hydroperitoneum)
hydroperoxide
hydrophila
    Aeromonas h.
hydrophilia
hydrophilic
    h. gel
    h. head
hydrophobia
hydrophobica
    Gordonia h.
hydrophobic gel
hydrophobicity
hydrophthalmos
hydropic
    h. abortus
    h. degeneration
    h. fetus
    h. swelling
hydropneumatosis
hydropneumopericardium
hydropneumoperitoneum
hydropneumothorax
hydrops
    h. abdominis
    h. amnii
    h. articuli
    cochlear h.
    endolymphatic h.
    h. fetalis
    h. folliculi
    gallbladder h.
    immune fetal h.
    labyrinthine h.
    nonimmune fetal h.
    h. tubae profluens
Hydropus
hydropyonephrosis
hydroquinone
hydrorchis
hydrosalpinx
hydrosarca
hydrosarcocele
hydrostatic
    h. pressure
    h. test
hydrosyringomyelia
Hydrotaea
hydrotaxis
hydrothermale
    Desulfacinum h.
hydrothermalis
    Desulfovibrio h.
    Halomonas h.

H

hydrothermalis (*continued*)
    Halothiobacillus h.
    Thermomonas h.
hydrothionemia
hydrothionuria
hydrothorax
    chylous h.
    hepatic h.
hydrotomy
hydrotropism
    negative h.
    positive h.
hydrotympanum
hydroureter
hydroxide
    aluminum h.
    h. ion
    potassium h.
hydroxyapatite, hydroxylapatite
    h. assay
    h. exchange procedure
hydroxybenzene
hydroxybenzoicus
    Sedimentibacter h.
hydroxybutyrate
    beta h.
    h. dehydrogenase (HBD, HBDH)
hydroxybutyric
    h. dehydrogenase
    h. test
hydroxychloroquine cardiotoxicity
hydroxycholecalciferol (HCC)
hydroxycobalamin
hydroxycorticoid (HC, HOC)
17-hydroxycorticosteroid
    1.-h. assay
    1.-h. test
17-hydroxycorticosterone
18-hydroxycorticosterone
hydroxyethyl starch
5-hydroxyindoleacetic
    5-h. acid (5-HIAA)
    5-h. acid assay
    5-h. test
hydroxyketone dye
hydroxyl
    h. concentration (pOH)
    h. group
    h. radical
hydroxylapatite (*var. of* hydroxyapatite)
hydroxylase
    dopamine h.
    phenylamine h.
    proline h.
    pyroglutamate h.
    tyrosine h. (TH)
4-hydroxylase
    prolyl 4-h.
21-hydroxylase

hydroxylation
    h. kidney
    h. liver
hydroxylysylpyridinoline
hydroxy-3-methylglutaric acidemia
hydroxymethylglutaryl (HMG)
**3-hydroxy-3-methylglutaryl-CoA
  (HNG-CoA)**
**hydroxyphenylpyruvic acid
  (HPPA)**
hydroxyphenyluria
hydroxyprogesterone
    alpha h.
17-hydroxyprogesterone test
hydroxyproline
    h. assay
    h. index
    h. oxidase
    urinary h.
    urine h.
hydroxyprolinemia
hydroxyprolinuria
hydroxystilbamidine isethionate
5-hydroxytryptamine (5-HT)
hydroxytryptophan (HTP)
    h. decarboxylase
hydroxyurea (HU)
25-hydroxyvitamin D assay
Hydrozoa
hygienic laboratory coefficient
hygroma, hydroma
    h. axillare
    cervical h.
    h. colli cysticum
    cystic h.
    subdural h.
hygrometer
hygrophilous
Hygrophoropsis
hygroscopic
hylemonae
    Clostridium h.
Hylemonella gracilis
Hylemya
    H. antiqua
    H. brassicae
hylic tumor
hyloma
    mesenchymal h.
    mesothelial h.
hymen
    imperforate h.
hymenal tag
Hymenobacter
    H. actinosclerus
    H. aerophilus
    H. roseosalivarius
Hymenochaete
hymenoid

hymenolepiasis
hymenolepidid
Hymenolepididae
Hymenolepis
    H. diminuta
    H. lanceolata
    H. murina
    H. nana
    H. nana fraterna
hymenology
Hymenomycetes
hymenoptera venom
Hymenoscyphus
Hymorphan
hyodysenteriae
    Treponema h.
hyointestinalis
    Campylobacter h.
hyos
    Leptospira h.
Hyostrongylus rubidus
hypalbuminemia
Hypaque
hypazoturia
hyper IgM syndrome
hyperacanthosis
hyperacidity
hyperactive glutamate receptor
hyperacute rejection
hyperadenosis
hyperadiposis, hyperadiposity
hyperadiposity
hyperadrenalism
hyperadrenocorticism
hyperaggregability
hyperalbuminemia
hyperalbuminosa
    polyemia h.
hyperaldosteronemia
hyperaldosteronism
    primary h.
    secondary h.
hyperalimentation
    intravenous h. (IVH)
hyperallantoinuria
hyperalphaglobulinemia
hyperaminoacidemia
hyperaminoaciduria
hyperammonemia (*var. of* ammonemia)
    h. I, II
hyperamylasemia
hyperamylasuria
hyperbaric chamber
hyperbetaalaninemia
hyperbetaglobulinemia
hyperbetalipoproteinemia
hyperbilirubinemia
    congenital h.
    conjugated h. I

    constitutional h.
    h. I, II
    unconjugated h.
hyperbilirubinuria
    obstructive h.
hyperbola
hyperbradykinism
hypercalcemia
    familial hypocalciuric h.
    idiopathic infantile h.
hypercalcemic
    h. crisis
    h. sarcoidosis
    h. uremia
hypercalcinuria (*var. of* hypercalciuria)
hypercalcitoninemia
hypercalcitoninism
hypercalciuria, hypercalcinuria, hypercalcuria
    idiopathic h. (IH, IHC)
hypercalcuria (*var. of* hypercalciuria)
hypercapnia, hypercarbia
hypercapnic
    h. acidosis
    h. encephalopathy
hypercarbia (*var. of* hypercapnia)
hypercardia
hypercellular bone marrow
hypercellularity
    diffuse mesangial h. (DMH)
hyperchloremia
hyperchloremic metabolic acidosis
hyperchlorhydria, hyperhydrochloria
hyperchloruria
hypercholesteremia (*var. of* hypercholesterolemia)
hypercholesterinemia (*var. of* hypercholesterolemia)
hypercholesterolemia, hypercholesteremia, hypercholesterinemia
    essential h.
    familial h. (FH)
hypercholesterolia
hypercholia
hyperchromasia
    epithelial h.
    nuclear h.
hyperchromatic
    h. anemia
    h. cell
    h. macrocythemia
    h. nucleus
hyperchromatin
hyperchromatism
hyperchromatosis
hyperchromemia
hyperchromia
    macrocytic h.

H

hyperchromic
    h. anemia
    h. shift
hyperchylomicronemia
hypercinesia (*var. of* hyperkinesis)
hypercinesis (*var. of* hyperkinesis)
hypercitraturia
hypercoagulability
hypercoagulable
    h. state
    h. state coagulation screen
hypercorticism
hypercortisolism
hypercupremia
hypercupruria
hypercyanotic
hypercythemia
hypercytochromia
hypercytosis
hyperdiploid cell (HDC)
hyperdistention
hyperdiuresis
hyperechoic
hyperelastica
    cutis h.
hyperelastosis cutis
hyperemesis gravidarum
hyperemia
    acute h.
    reactive h. (RH)
    h. unit (HU)
hyperemic
hyperendemic disease
hypereosinophilia
hypereosinophilic syndrome
hyperergia, hypergia
hyperergic encephalitis
hypererythrocythemia
hyperesthetic zone
hyperestrogenism
hyperextensible skin
hyperferremia
hyperfibrinogenemia
hyperfibrinolysis
hyperflexion
hyperfunction
    anterior pituitary h.
hypergammaglobulinemia
    monoclonal h.
    polyclonal h.
hyperganglionosis
hypergastrinemia
hypergenesis
hypergenetic
hypergenitalism
hypergia (*var. of* hyperergia)
hypergic
hyperglobulia, hyperglobulism
hyperglobulinemia

hyperglobulinemic purpura
hyperglobulism (*var. of* hyperglobulia)
hyperglycemia
    nonketotic h.
hyperglycemic
hyperglycemic-glycogenolytic factor (HGF)
hyperglyceridemia
    endogenous h.
    exogenous h.
hyperglycinemia
    ketotic h.
    nonketotic h.
hyperglycinuria
hyperglycosemia
hyperglycosuria
hyperglyoxylemia
hypergonadism
hypergonadotrophic (*var. of* hypergonadotropic)
hypergonadotropic, hypergonadotrophic
hypergranulosis
hyperguanidinemia
hyperhemoglobinemia
hyperheparinemia
hyperhidrosis
hyperhomocysteinemia
hyperhydrochloria (*var. of* hyperchlorhydria)
hyperhydropexis (*var. of* hyperhydropexy)
hyperhydropexy, hyperhydropexis
hyper-IgE syndrome
hyper-IgM syndrome
hyperimmune serum
hyperimmunity
hyperimmunization
hyperimmunoglobulinemia D, E, G, M
hyperindicanemia
hyperinfection
hyperinnervation
    nitrergic h.
hyperinosemia
hyperinosis
hyperinsulinemia (*var. of* hyperinsulinism)
hyperinsulinism, hyperinsulinemia
    islet cell h.
hyperirritability
hyperisotonic
hyperkalemia, hyperkaliemia
hyperkaliemia (*var. of* hyperkalemia)
hyperkaluresis
hyperkaluria
hyperkeratinization
hyperkeratomycosis
hyperkeratosis
    h. congenita
    h. eccentrica
    epidermolytic h.
    h. figurata centrifuga atrophica
    filiform h.

h. filiform
h. follicularis et parafollicularis
h. lenticularis perstans
h. penetrans
hyperkeratotic papilloma
hyperketonemia
hyperketonuria
hyperkinesia (*var. of* hyperkinesis)
hyperkinesis, hyperkinesia, hypercinesis, hypercinesia
hyperleukocytosis
hyperlipemia (*var. of* hyperlipidemia)
hyperlipidemia, hyperlipemia
carbohydrate-induced h.
endogenous h. (EHL)
essential h.
fat-induced h.
hyperlipoproteinemia
familial h. I, II, IIa, IIb
hyperliposis
hyperlithuria
hyperlucent lung
hyperlysinemia type I, II
hyperlysinuria
hypermagnesemia
hypermature
hypermelanosis
hypermenorrhea
hypermetaplasia
hypermethylation
hypermetropia (*var. of* hyperopia)
hypermobility
apomorphine-induced h.
hypermutation
hypermyotrophy
hypernatremia
hypernatremic encephalopathy
hyperneocytosis
hypernephroid
hypernephroma
hyperoncotic
hyperonychia
hyperopia, hypermetropia
latent h.
manifest h.
hyperorchidism
hyperornithinemia
hyperorthocytosis
hyperorthokeratosis
hyperosmolality
hyperosmolar diabetic coma
hyperosmolarity
hyperosmotic
nonketotic h. (NKH)
hyperostosis
h. corticalis deformans
h. corticalis deformans juvenilis
h. corticalis generalisata
diffuse idiopathic skeletal h.

flowing h.
h. frontalis interna
generalized cortical h.
infantile cortical h.
streak h.
hyperostotic spondylosis
hyperoxaluria
hyperpara
hyperparathyroidism
hyperparakeratosis
hyperparasite
hyperparasitism
hyperparathyroidism
primary h.
secondary h.
tertiary h.
hyperperfusion/hyperfiltration injury
hyperperistalsis
ureteral h.
hyperphenylalaninemia
hyperphosphatasemia
hyperphosphatasia
hyperphosphatemia
hyperphosphaturia
hyperphosphorylation of occludin
hyperpigmentation
hyperpituitarism
postpubertal h.
prepubertal h.
hyperplasia
adenoid h.
adenomatous h.
adrenal cortical h.
adrenocortical h.
alveolar pneumocyte h.
antral G-cell h.
apocrine h. (ApoHyp)
atypical adenomatous h. (AAH)
atypical apocrine h.
atypical ductal h. (ADH)
atypical endometrial h.
atypical lobular h. (ALH)
atypical melanocytic h.
basal cell h.
basaloid h.
basophilic h.
benign florid lymphoid h.
benign giant lymph node h.
benign mediastinal lymph node h.
benign prostatic h.
bilateral micronodular adrenal h.
capsular synovial-like h. (CSH)
C-cell h.
clear cell cribriforming h.
columnar cell h.
complex endometrial h.
congenital adrenal h. (CAH)
congenital sebaceous h.
cortical stromal h. (CSH)

H

469

hyperplasia (*continued*)
  corticotroph cell h.
  cutaneous lymphoid h. (CLH)
  cystic endometrial h.
  cystic hypersecretory h.
  cystic prostatic h.
  diffuse h.
  ductal h.
  endometrial h.
  enterochromaffin cell h. (EC)
  enterochromaffin-like cell h.
  eosinophilic h.
  epithelial h.
  erythroid h.
  fibromuscular h.
  flat urothelial h.
  focal epithelial h.
  focal nodular h. (FNH)
  follicular h. (FH)
  foveolar h.
  gingival h.
  glandular h.
  granulocytic h.
  hematopoietic h.
  hypersecretory h.
  intracystic h.
  intraductal h.
  intravascular papillary endothelial h.
  islet cell h.
  lentiginous melanocytic h.
  Leydig cell h.
  lipomelanotic reticuloendothelial
    cell h.
  lobular epithelial h.
  lymph node h.
  lymphoid h.
  mast cell h.
  megakaryocytic h.
  megaloblastic h.
  mesonephric remnant h.
  microglandular h. (MGH)
  micronodular pneumocyte h.
    (MPH)
  myeloid h.
  myointimal h.
  neuronal h.
  neutrophilic h.
  nodular lymphoid h. (NLH)
  nodular mesothelial h.
  nodular regenerative h. (NRH)
  h. of usual type (HUT)
  plasma cell angiofollicular lymph
    node h.
  polypoid h.
  postatrophic h.
  postsclerotic h.
  primary h.
  prostate h.
  pseudoangiomatous h.

  pseudoangiomatous stromal h.
    (PASH)
  pseudocarcinomatous h.
  pseudoepitheliomatous h.
  pseudolactational h.
  pulmonary lymphoid h. (PLH)
  reactive follicular h.
  reserve cell h.
  reticuloendothelial cell h.
  reticulum cell h.
  secondary h.
  senile sebaceous h.
  stromal h.
  stromovascular h.
  Swiss cheese h.
  thyrotroph h.
  transmural lymphoid h.
  verrucous h.
  vulvar squamous h.
  wasserhelle h.
  water-clear cell h.
hyperplasia/metaplasia
  complex atypical h. (CAHM)
hyperplastic
  h. arteriosclerosis
  h. bone marrow
  h. cholecystosis
  h. gland
  h. inflammation
  h. nephrosclerosis
  h. nodular goiter
  h. osteoarthritis
  h. polyp
hyperplastic-like mucosal change (HPC)
hyperploid pattern
hyperploidy
hyperpolarization
hyperpotassemia
hyperprebetalipoproteinemia
**hyperproduction of pituitary
  corticotropin**
hyperproinsulinemia
hyperprolactinemia
hyperproliferation
hyperprolinemia
hyperproteinemia
hyperreactio luteinalis (HL)
hyperreactivity
  bronchial h.
hyperreninemia
hyperreninism
hypersalemia
hypersarcosinemia
hypersecretion
  extreme gastric h.
  glucagon h.
hypersecretory hyperplasia
hypersegmentation
  hereditary h.

leukocytic h.
h. of granulocyte nuclei
hypersegmented
h. granulocyte
h. neutrophil
hypersensitive
hypersensitivity
h. angiitis
contact h.
delayed h.
delayed-type h. (DTH)
immediate h.
h. myocarditis
h. pneumonitis
h. pneumonitis serology
pulmonary h.
h. reaction, type I–IV
tuberculin-type h.
h. vasculitis
hypersensitization
hyperserotonemia
vasculocardiac syndrome of h.
hyperskeocytosis
hypersomia
hypersplenism
hypersplenosis
hypersthenuria
hypersusceptibility
hypertelorism
ocular h.
hypertension (HT, HTN)
arterial h.
benign intracranial h. (BIH)
diastolic h.
essential h. (EH)
Goldblatt h.
idiopathic h.
intracranial h.
malignant h.
mineralocorticoid h.
orthostatic h.
portal h.
primary plexogenic h. (PPHT)
primary pulmonary h. (PPH)
pulmonary artery h.
renal h.
renovascular h.
systolic h.
thrombotic pulmonary h.
hypertensive
h. arteriopathy
h. arteriosclerosis
h. arteriosclerotic heart disease
(HASHD)
h. cardiovascular disease (HCVD)
h. encephalopathy
h. heart disease (HHD)
h. pulmonary vascular disease
(HPVD)

hyperthecosis
stromal h.
testoid h.
hyperthelia
hyperthermia
malignant h.
hyperthrombinemia
hyperthymic
hyperthymism
hyperthymization
hyperthyroidism
hyperthyroiditis
hyperthyroxinemia
hypertonia polycythemica
hypertonica
polycythemia h.
hypertonic hyponatremia
hypertonicity
hypertrichosis
h. lanuginosa acquisita
nevoid h.
hypertriglyceridemia
familial h.
hypertrophia, hypertrophy
hypertrophic
h. amphophil cell
h. arthritis
h. cervical pachymeningitis
h. chronic vulvitis
h. fibrous pachymeningitis
h. gastritis
h. gingivitis
h. hypersecretory gastropathy
h. infiltrative tendinitis (HIT)
h. interstitial neuropathy
h. lichen planus
h. muscular subaortic stenosis
(HMSAS)
h. obstructive cardiomyopathy
(HOCM)
h. polyneuritic-type muscular atrophy
h. pulmonary osteoarthropathy
h. pyloric stenosis (HPS)
h. scar
hypertrophicum
eczema h.
hypertrophicus
lupus h.
hypertrophied chondrocyte
hypertrophy (*var. of* hypertrophia)
adaptive h.
adenoid h.
asymmetric septal h. (ASH)
benign prostatic h. (BPH)
combined ventricular h. (CVH)
compensatory h.
complementary h.
concentric h.
diffuse h.

H

471

hypertrophy (*continued*)
    eccentric h.
    endemic h.
    false h.
    fibrocongestive h.
    focal h.
    functional h.
    hemangiectatic h.
    idiopathic myocardial h.
      (IMH)
    Kupffer cell h.
    left atrial h. (LAH)
    left ventricular h. (LVH)
    lipomatous h.
    myofibrillary h.
    myometrial h.
    numerical h.
    h. of chamber wall
    prostatic h. (PH)
    quantitative h.
    right atrial h. (RAH)
    right ventricular h. (RVH)
    simple h.
    simulated h.
    true h.
    ventricular h.
    vicarious h.
    virginal h.
hypertyrosinemia, Oregon
  type
hyperuremia
hyperuresis
hyperuricemia
hyperuricemic nephropathy
hyperuricosuria
hyperuricuria
hyperurobilinogenemia
hypervaccination
hypervalinemia
hypervariable region
hypervascular
    h. hepatocellular carcinoma
    h. nodule
hypervascularity
    villous capillary h.
hyperventilation syndrome
hyperviscosity syndrome
hypervitaminosis A, D
hypervolemia
hypervolemic hypotonic hyponatremia
hypha
    fungal hyphae
    racquet h.
    spiral h.
hyphal
hyphemia (*var. of* hypovolemia)
Hypholoma
Hyphomicrobiaceae
Hyphomicrobiales

Hyphomicrobium
    H. chloromethanicum
    H. sulfonivorans
Hyphomonas
    H. adhaerens
    H. johnsonii
    H. rosenbergii
Hyphomyces destruens
Hyphomycetes
hyphomycosis
Hyphopichia
Hyphozyma
hypnocyst
hypnotic
hypnotoxin
hypnozoite
hypoacidity
hypoadrenalism
hypoadrenocorticism
    primary h.
    secondary h.
hypoalbuminemia
hypoaldosteronism
hypoaldosteronuria
hypoalphaglobulinemia
hypoalphalipoproteinemia
hypoazoturia
hypobaric
hypobetalipoproteinemia
hypobromous acid
hypocalcemia
hypocalcification
hypocalciuria
hypocapnia, hypocarbia
hypocapnic
hypocarbia (*var. of* hypocapnia)
hypocellularity of bone marrow
hypocellular stroma
hypoceruloplasminemia
    familial h.
hypochloremia
    dilutional h.
hypochloremic
    h. azotemia
    h. metabolic acidosis
hypochlorhydria
hypochlorite
    sodium h.
hypochlorous acid
hypochloruria
Hypochnicium
Hypochnus
hypocholesterinemia (*var. of*
  hypocholesterolemia)
hypocholesterolemia, hypocholesterinemia
hypochondriac region
hypochondriasis
hypochondroplasia
hypochromasia

hypochromatic
hypochromatism
hypochromemia
    idiopathic h.
hypochromia
hypochromic
    h. microcytic anemia
    h. microcytic erythrocyte
    h. shift
hypochrosis
hypocitraturia
hypocomplementemia
hypocomplementemic glomerulonephritis
hypocorticoidism
Hypocrea
hypocretin (HCR)
    h. 1, 2
hypocupremia
hypocythemia
    progressive h.
hypocytosis
Hypoderaeum conoideum
hypoderm
Hypoderma bovis
hypodermatosis
hypodermic
    h. implantation
    h. microscope
hypodermis
hypodermolithiasis
hypodiploid
hypodipsia
    primary h.
hypoeosinophilia
hypoestrogenism
hypoferremia
hypoferric anemia
hypofibrinogenemia
hypofunction
    adrenal h.
hypogaea
    Arachis h.
hypogammaglobinemia (*var. of*
  hypogammaglobulinemia)
hypogammaglobulinemia,
  hypogammaglobinemia
    acquired h.
    common variable h. (CVH)
    primary h.
    secondary h.
    Swiss-type h.
    transient h.
    X-linked infantile h.
hypoganglionosis
hypogenesis
hypoglobulia
hypoglobulinemia
hypoglycemia
    alimentary h.

    leucine h.
    neonatal h.
    postabsorptive h.
    postprandial h.
    profound h.
hypoglycemic
    h. encephalopathy
    h. shock
hypoglycorrhachia
hypogonadism
hypogonadotropic eunuchoidism
hypogranular granulocyte
hypogranulocytosis
hypohemoglobin (HHb)
hypohidrotic ectodermal
  dysplasia
hypohydremia
hypohydrochloria
hypohyloma
hypoinsulinism
hypoisotonic
hypokalemia, hypopotassemia
hypokalemic
    h. alkalosis
    h. diarrhea
    h. nephropathy
    h. nephrosis
    h. periodic paralysis
hypokaluria
hypoleukemia
hypoleydigism
hypolipoproteinemia
hypoliposis
hypolymphemia
hypomagnesemia
hypomelanosis of Ito
hypomethylation
hypomineralization
hypomotility
    esophageal h.
Hypomyces
hyponatremia
    dead-space h.
    drip-arm h.
    euvolemic hypotonic h.
    hypertonic h.
    hypervolemic hypotonic h.
    hypotonic h.
    hypovolemic hypotonic h.
    isotonic h.
hyponatruria
hyponeocytosis
hypooncotic
hypoorthocytosis
hypoparathyroidism
    immunodeficiency with h.
hypoperfusion
    tissue h.
hypopharyngeal diverticulum

H

hypophosphatasia
- congenital h.

hypophosphatemia
- X-linked familial h.

hypophosphatemic rickets

hypophosphaturia

hypophyseal (*var. of* hypophysial)

hypophysectomy

hypophyseoportal system

hypophyseos
- lobus anterior h.
- lobus glandularis h.
- lobus posterior h.

hypophysial, hypophyseal
- h. stalk germinoma
- h. syndrome

hypophysiotropic hormone

hypophysis
- alpha cell of h.
- anterior lobe of h.
- basophil cell of anterior lobe of h.
- beta cell of h.
- h. cerebri
- chromophobe cell of h.
- delta cell of anterior lobe of h.
- posterior lobe of h.
- h. staining procedure

hypophysitis
- lymphocytic h.
- lymphoid h.
- purulent h.

hypopigmentation

hypopigmentation-immunodeficiency disease

hypopituitarism

hypoplasia
- cartilage-hair h. (CHH)
- crypt h.
- enamel h.
- erythroid h.
- focal dermal h.
- granulocytic h.
- hematopoietic h.
- lymphoid h.
- megakaryocytic h.
- oligonephronic h.
- renal h.
- right ventricular h.
- thymic h.

hypoplasminogenemia

hypoplastic
- h. anemia
- h. bone marrow
- h. heart

hypoploid

hypoploidy

hypopotassemia (*var. of* hypokalemia)

hypoproaccelerinemia

hypoproconvertinemia

hypoproteinemia
- prehepatic h.

hypoprothrombinemia

hypopyon

hyporegenerative anemia

hyporeninemia

hyporeninemic

hyposalemia

hyposarca

hyposecretion

hyposegmentation
- leukocytic nuclear h.

hyposegmented granulocyte

hyposensitivity

hyposensitization

hyposialadenitis

hyposkeocytosis

hyposmotic

hypospadias

hyposplenism

hypostasis
- postmortem h.
- pulmonary h.

hypostatic
- h. abscess
- h. congestion
- h. ectasia
- h. pneumonia

hyposthenuria

hypostome

hyposulfite
- sodium h.

hypotension
- orthostatic h.

hypotensive

hypotetraploid cell

hypothalamic gangliocytoma

hypothalamic-pituitary-testicular axis

hypothalamohypophysial
- h. portal system
- h. tract

hypothalamoneurohypophysial system

hypothalamus
- lateral h.

hypothermia

hypothesis
- alternative h.
- autocrine h.
- Benditt h.
- biogenic amine h.
- cardionector h.
- chemiosmotic h.
- encrustation h.
- Haldane h.
- lattice h.
- Lyon h.
- metabolic h.
- monoclonal h.
- omnibus h.

proton-motive h.
h. testing
thrombogenic h.
unitarian h.
wobble h.
hypothetical
    h. mean organism (HMO)
    h. mean strain (HMS)
hypothrombinemia
hypothromboplastinemia
hypothyroid
hypothyroidism
hypothyroxinemia
hypotonia, hypotonus, hypotony
    vasomotor h.
hypotonic hyponatremia
hypotonicity
hypotonus, hypotony
hypotony (*var. of* hypotonia, hypotonus)
hypotransferrinemia
hypotriploid
hypouricemia
hypouricuria
hypoventilation
Hypovirus
hypovitaminosis
hypovolemia, hyphemia
hypovolemic
    h. hypotonic hyponatremia
    h. shock
hypoxanthine
    h. guanine phosphoribosyltransferase
    (HGPRT)
    h. phosphoribosyltransferase (HPRT)
hypoxanthine-aminopterin-thymidine
  (HAT)
hypoxemia

hypoxia
    anemic h.
    histotoxic h.
    hypoxic h.
    h. inducible factor (HIF)
    h. inducible factor 1 (HIF-1)
    ischemic h.
    oxygen affinity h.
    stagnant h.
    tissue h.
hypoxic
    h. anoxia
    h. cell
    h. cell injury
    h. encephalopathy
    h. hypoxia
    h. nephrosis
    h. vasoconstriction
Hypoxylon
hypsiloid cartilage
Hypsizygus
hypsochrome
hypsochromic shift
Hyskon distention medium
hysteratresia
hysteresis loop
hysterical blindness
Hysterolecitha
hysterolith
hysteromyoma
hysterotonin
hystrix
    ichthyosis h.
Hz
    hertz
HZV
    herpes zoster virus

H

I
iodine
I antigen
I band
I blood group
I cell
I disc
I region
^{123}I
iodine-123
^{125}I
iodine-125
^{127}I
iodine-127
^{132}I
iodine-132
Ia antigen
IADH
inappropriate antidiuretic
hormone
IAHA
immune adherence hemagglutination
assay
IAHS
infection-associated hemophagocytic
syndrome
IASD
interatrial septal defect
IAT
invasive activity test
iodine-azide test
iatrogenic
i. agent
i. anemia
i. artifact
i. disease
i. immunosuppression
IB
immune body
inclusion body
Ibaraki virus
IBC
iron-binding capacity
IBD
inflammatory bowel disease
IBD First Step test
IBF
immunoglobulin-binding factor
IBL
immunoblastic lymphadenopathy
IBM
inclusion body myositis
IBR
infectious bovine rhinotracheitis
IBR virus

IBU
International benzoate unit
IBV
infectious bronchitis virus
IBW
ideal body weight
IC
infection control
intermittent claudication
interstitial cystitis
irritable colon
isovolumic contraction
ICA
immunocytochemical assay
intracranial aneurysm
islet cell antibody
ICAM-1
intercellular adhesion molecule-1
ICAO
internal carotid artery occlusion
Icaria
hemoglobin I.
ICC
immunocompetent cell
Indian childhood cirrhosis
ICD
International Classification of Diseases
ICE
iridocorneal endothelial syndrome
ice
i. point
i. water calorics test
iceberg phenomenon
I-cell disease
ICF
intracellular fluid
ICG
indocyanine green
ICG excretion test
Ichnovirus
ichorous pus
ichorrhea
ichthyoacanthotoxism
ichthyohemotoxism
Ichthyophthirius multifiliis
ichthyosarcotoxism
ichthyosis
acquired i.
i. congenita
i. congenita neonatorum
i. fetalis
i. hystrix
i. intrauterina
lamellar i.
i. linguae

ichthyosis (*continued*)
    nacreous i.
    i. palmaris et plantaris
    i. sauroderma
    i. scutulata
    i. sebacea
    i. sebacea cornea
    i. simplex
    i. spinosa
    i. uteri
    i. vulgaris
    X-linked i.
ichthyotic
ichthyotoxin
icing
    i. heart
    i. liver
ICM
    interference-contrast microscopy
ICOD
    infectious cause of death
Icon
    I. Fx
    I. 25 hCG test
    I. II HCG
    I. MicroALB
icosahedral symmetry
ICSH
    International Committee for
      Standardization in Hematology
    interstitial cell-stimulating hormone
ICSI
    intracytoplasmic sperm injection
ICT
    inflammation of connective tissue
    insulin coma therapy
ICt50, ICt$_{50}$
    incapacitating Ct$_{50}$
Ictalurid herpes-like viruses
icteric serum hepatitis (ISH)
icteroanemia
icterogenic spirochetosis
icterohaemorrhagiae
    Leptospira i.
icterohematuric
icterohemoglobinuria
icterohemolytic anemia
icterohemorrhagica
    leptospirosis i.
icterohepatitis
icteroid
icterus
    acquired hemolytic i.
    benign familial i.
    chronic familial i.
    congenital familial i.
    congenital hemolytic i.
    cythemolytic i.
    i. gravis

    i. gravis of newborn
    i. index (ict ind)
    i. index test
    i. interference
    i. melas
    i. neonatorum
    i. praecox
Ictotest reagent tablet
ICW
    intracellular water
ID
    identification
    immunodiffusion
    infecting dose
    infective dose
ID50, ID$_{50}$
    median infectious dose
IDA
    image display and analysis
    iminodiacetic acid
    iron deficiency anemia
Idaeovirus
IDC
    infiltrating ductal carcinoma
    interdigitating dendritic cell
IDCS
    interdigitating dendritic cell sarcoma
IDDM
    insulin-dependent diabetes mellitus
IDDRT
    Infectious Disease Death Review Team
ideal
    i. body weight (IBW)
    i. gas
    i. gas law
    i. solution
identical twins
identification (ID)
    antibody i.
    arthropod i.
    definitive organism i.
    gram-positive i. (GPI)
    hazard i.
    hemoglobin i.
    victim i.
identifier
    biometric i.
identity
    i. pattern
    reaction of i.
    reaction of partial i.
Ide test
idioagglutinin
idiocy
    amaurotic familial i.
    infantile amaurotic familial i.
    late infantile amaurotic familial i.
idiogram
idioheteroagglutinin

idioheterolysin
idioisoagglutinin
idioisolysin
idiolysin
Idiomarina
    I. abyssalis
    I. baltica
    I. fontislapidosi
    I. loihiensis
    I. ramblicola
    I. zobellii
Idiomarinaceae
idiopathic
  i. Bamberger-Marie disease
  i. bone cavity
  i. brachial plexopathy
  i. cardiomyopathy
  i. endomyocardial fibrosis
  i. etiology
  i. fibrous mediastinitis
  i. fibrous retroperitonitis
  i. generalized glycogenosis
  i. hemosiderosis
  i. hypercalciuria (IHC)
  i. hypertension
  i. hypertrophic osteoarthropathy (IHO)
  i. hypertrophic subaortic stenosis (IHSS)
  i. hypochromemia
  i. infantile hypercalcemia
  i. megacolon
  i. mesenteric phlebosclerosis
  i. myelofibrosis
  i. myocardial hypertrophy (IMH)
  i. myocarditis
  i. myxedema
  i. nephrotic syndrome (INS)
  i. Parkinson disease
  i. paroxysmal rhabdomyolysis
  i. pauciimmune necrotizing crescentic glomerulonephritis
  i. pentosuria
  i. pericarditis
  i. polyneuritis
  i. proctitis
  i. pulmonary fibrosis (IPF)
  i. pulmonary hemosiderosis (IPH)
  i. refractory sideroblastic anemia (IRSA)
  i. respiratory distress syndrome (IRDS)
  i. retractile mesenteritis (IRM)
  i. retroperitoneal fibrosis (IRF)
  i. thrombocytopenia
  i. thrombocytopenic purpura (ITP)
  i. warm autoimmune hemolytic anemia

idiopathica
  dermatitis chronica atrophicans i.
  livedo reticularis i.
idiopathy
  toxic i.
idiosyncrasy
idiosyncratic
  i. reaction
  i. sensitivity
idiotope
  set of i.'s
idiotype
  i. antibody
  i. autoantibody
idiotypic
  i. antigen
  i. antigenic determinant
IDI-Strep B test
iditol
  i. dehydrogenase
  i. dehydrogenase assay
IDL
  intermediate-density lipoprotein
IDLH
  immediately dangerous to life or health
ID-Micro typing system
idoxuridine (IDU)
IDR
  intradermal reaction
IDS
  immunity deficiency state
ID-Tag RVP assay
IDU
  idoxuridine
  iododeoxyuridine
iduronic
  i. acid
  i. sulfatase
iduronidase
IE
  immunoelectrophoresis
IED
  improvised explosive device
  incendiary IED
IEF
  isoelectric focusing
  IEF gel electrophoresis
IEM
  immune electron microscopy
IEOP
  immunoelectroosmophoresis
IEP
  immunoelectrophoresis
IF
  immunofluorescence
  interfollicular

IF (*continued*)
    intermediate filament
    intrinsic factor
IFA
    immunofluorescence assay
    indirect fluorescent antibody
IFC
    intrinsic factor concentrate
IFCC
    International Federation of Clinical
      Chemistry
IFE
    immunofixation electrophoresis
Iflavirus
IFN
    interferon
      IFN alpha
      IFN beta
      IFN gamma
IFR
    inspiratory flow rate
IFRA
    indirect fluorescent rabies antibody
      (test)
IFV
    intracellular fluid volume
Ig
    immunoglobulin
IgA
    immunoglobulin A
      IgA endomysial antibody
      IgA globulinemia
      IgA II-HA assay test kit
      IgA immunodeficiency
      IgA myeloma
      IgA nephropathy
      secretory IgA (sIgA)
IgA-antigliadin antibody
IGCN
    intratubular germ cell neoplasia
IGCNU
    intratubular germ cell neoplasia,
      unclassified type
IgD
    immunoglobulin D
      IgD myeloma
IgE
    immunoglobulin E
      IgE antibody
      latex-specific IgE
      IgE myeloma
      specific IgE
      total serum IgE
IgE-mediated disease
IGF-1
    insulinlike growth factor-1
IGF-II antigen
IgG
    immunoglobulin G

      IgG desmoglein-3
      IgG desmoplakin antibody
      IgG index
      IgG index method
      IgG myeloma
      IgG ratio
IgG:albumin ratio
IGH gene
IgM
    immunoglobulin M
      IgM antibody
IgM-RF
    immunoglobulin M-rheumatoid factor
      IgM-RF antibody
Ig-mutated chronic lymphocytic leukemia
ignava
    Cryomorpha i.
    Johnsonella i.
    Tepidimonas i.
Ignavigranum ruoffiae
igne
    erythema ab i.
ignea
    zona i.
Ignicoccus
    I. islandicus
    I. pacificus
ignitability
igniterrae
    Thermus i.
ignition
    i. point
    i. source control
    i. temperature
ignorata
    Nocardia i.
IGPD
    inherited giant platelet disorder
IGSS
    immunogold-silver staining
Ig-unmutated chronic lymphocytic leukemia
IGV
    intrathoracic gas volume
IH
    infectious hepatitis
IHA
    indirect hemagglutination
IHBTD
    incompatible hemolytic blood
      transfusion disease
IHC
    idiopathic hypercalciuria
    immunohistochemical
    immunohistochemistry
IHD
    ischemic heart disease
iheyensis
    Oceanobacillus i.

I

IHO
idiopathic hypertrophic
osteoarthropathy
IHSA
iodinated human serum albumin
IHSS
idiopathic hypertrophic subaortic
stenosis
I/i antigen
IIF
indirect immunofluorescent
IiQ 200 automated urine microscopy analyzer
Ikegami video camera
IL
interleukin
IL test liquid antithrombin
ILA
insulinlike activity
Ilarvirus
ILC
infiltrating lobular
carcinoma
ILD
interstitial lung disease
ischemic leg disease
ischemic limb disease
ileal intussusception
ileitis
backwash i.
Crohn i.
distal i.
postcolectomy i.
prestomal i.
regional i. (RI)
terminal i.
ileocecal intussusception
ileocolic intussusception
ileocolitis ulcerosa chronica
ileojejunitis
ileostomy
Koch i.
ileum
duplex i.
i. duplex
terminal i.
ileus
adynamic i.
dynamic i.
gallstone i.
mechanical i.
meconium i.
spastic i.
i. subparta
ureteral i.
Ilhéus
I. encephalitis
I. fever
I. virus

iliac
i. horn
i. roll
ill
louping i.
ill-defined
illinoisensis
Alkanindiges i.
illness
environmental i.
neuroparalytic i.
respiratory i. (RI)
severity of i.
illucens
Hermetia i.
illudens
Omphalotus i.
illuminance
illumination
critical i.
diffuse i.
Köhler i.
illustris
Lucilia i.
ILNR
intralobar nephrogenic rest
ilocanum
Echinostoma i.
Ilosvay reagent
IL-2 receptor alpha-chain deficiency
ILVEN
inflammatory linear verrucous
epidermal nevus
Ilyobacter insuetus
IM
infectious mononucleosis
intestinal metaplasia
intracellular macroadenoma
IMA
immunometric assay
ima
IMAA
iodinated macroaggregated albumin
I(Ma) antigen
image
confocal i.
i. cytology
i. cytometry
i. display and analysis (IDA)
I. Titer
image-guided
i.-g. breast biopsy
i.-g. core biopsy
imaging
FLM i.
fluorescence lifetime i. (FLM)
in vivo tissue i.
postmortem i.
Imago broth

imatinib
imbalance
    allelic i.
    calcium i.
    chloride i.
    electrolyte i.
    hormonal i.
    magnesium i.
    potassium i.
    sodium i.
    sympathetic i.
imbed
imbibition
imbricata
    tinea i.
imbricate, imbricated
imbricated (*var. of* imbricate)
imbrication line of von Ebner
IMBT
    intestinal mucinous borderline tumor
IMC
    immunohistochemical
Imerslund-Grasbeck syndrome
IMH
    idiopathic myocardial hypertrophy
    myometrial hypertrophy
imidazole
imidazolepyruvic acid
imide
imine
imino acid
iminodiacetic acid (IDA)
iminoglycinuria
imipramine and desipramine assays
Imlach fat-pad
Immage
    I. Anti-DNaseB
    I. immunochemistry system
immature
    i. granulocyte
    i. neutrophil
    i. teratoma
immediate
    i. allergy
    i. contagion
    i. hypersensitivity
    i. hypersensitivity reaction
    i. principle
    i. radiation toxicity
    triage i.
immediately dangerous to life or health (IDLH)
immediate-phase skin response
immediate-spin crossmatch
immersion
    i. foot
    homogeneous i.
    i. microscopy
    i. objective

    oil i.
    i. syndrome
    water i.
immersion-submersion
imminent abortion
immiscible
immite
    Geotrichum i.
immitis
    Coccidioides i.
    Dirofilaria i.
immobilization
    Treponema pallidum i.
immobilized enzyme
immobilizing antibody
immortalization
immotile cilia syndrome
immotility
ImmuKnow immune cell function assay
Immulite
    I. 2000 chemiluminescent analyzer
    I. Dynamic Duo analyzer
    I. 2000 free PSA
    I. free PSA assay
    I. 1000 free PSA test
    I. 2000 free PSA test
    I. free PSA test
    I. 1000, 2000, 2500 immunoassay
        system
    I. 2000 PSA assay
    I. 2500 SMS immunoassay system
    I. 2000 third-generation PSA
    I. third-generation PSA assay
Immu-Mark immunostaining kit
immune
    i. adherence
    i. adherence hemagglutination assay
        (IAHA)
    i. adherence phenomenon
    i. adhesion test
    i. adsorption
    i. agglutination
    i. agglutinin
    i. barrier
    i. body (IB)
    i. clearance
    i. complex
    i. complex assay
    i. complex disease
    i. complex disorder
    i. complex glomerulonephritis
    i. complex glomerulopathy
    i. complex-mediated hypersensitivity
        reaction
    i. complex nephritis
    i. complex nephropathy
    i. cytolysis
    i. deficiency
    i. deviation

i. dysfunction syndrome
i. electron microscopy (IEM)
i. elimination
i. fetal hydrops
i. hemolysin
i. hemolysis
i. inflammation
i. inflammatory reaction
i. interferon
i. lactoglobulin
i. opsonin
i. paralysis
i. precipitation
i. protein
i. rejection of seminoma
i. response (Ir)
i. response gene
i. senescence
i. serum
i. serum globulin
i. surveillance
i. system
i. thrombocytopenia
i. thrombocytopenic purpura
i. tolerance
immune-deposit disease
immune-mediated
i.-m. destruction
i.-m. mechanism
i.-m. process
i.-m. vasculitide
immune-privileged
immune-stimulating complex (ISCOM)
immunifacient
immunity
acquired i.
active i.
adaptive i.
adoptive i.
antibody-dependent i.
antiviral i.
artificial active i.
artificial passive i.
bacteriophage i.
cell-mediated i. (CMI)
cellular i.
combinatorial i.
concomitant i.
cross-protective i.
i. deficiency state (IDS)
general i.
group i.
herd i.
humoral i.
infection i.
innate i.
local i.
maternal i.
natural i.

nonspecific i.
relative i.
specific active i.
specific passive i.
i. substance
immunization
active i.
postexposure i.
preexposure i.
i. reaction poliomyelitis
Rh i.
smallpox i.
immunize
immunizing unit (IU)
immunoadjuvant
immunoadsorbent
immunoadsorption
immunoaffinity
i. chromatography
i. purification
immunoagglutination
immunoalkaline phosphatase stain
immunoamyloidosis
immunoarchitectural appearance
immunoassay
Advia Centaur HBc Total i.
agglutination i.
Architect HBsAg reagent i.
Asserachrom APA i.
chemiluminescent i.
cloned enzyme donor i. (CEDIA)
Cobas Integra Cyclosporine I.
coenzyme-labeled i.
competitive heterogeneous enzyme i.
direct quenching fluorescent i.
DNA-enzyme i. (DEIA)
double antibody i.
Elecsys free PSA i.
Elecsys proBNP i.
Elecsys total PSA i.
electrochemiluminescence i. (ECLIA)
enzyme-enhancement i.
enzyme-multiplied i. (EIA)
i. fecal occult blood test
fluorescence excitation transfer i.
(FETI)
fluorescence polarization i. (FPIA)
fluorescent i. (FIA)
Hemoccult ICT i.
ImmunoCard STAT! rotavirus i.
ImmunoCard STAT! strep A i.
ligand i.
light-scattering i.
lymphocyte transformation i.
MAb-based enzyme i.
microparticle capture enzyme i.
(MEIA)
microparticle enzyme i. (MEIA)
Monolisa Anti-HBc IgM EIA i.

immunoassay (*continued*)
    nephelometric i.
    noncompetitive heterogeneous
      enzyme i.
    nonradioisotopic i.
    OncoChek i.
    Optical I.
    PhiCal fecal calprotectin i.
    radioisotopic i.
    i. reagent
    solid phase i.
    solid phase fluorescence i.
      (SPFIA)
    sperm-ubiquitin tag i. (SUTI)
    substrate-labeled fluorescence i.
      (SLFIA)
    substrate-labeled fluorescent i.
      (SLFIA)
    thin-layer i.
    time-resolved fluorescence i.
    turbidimetric i.
immunobiology
immunoblast
immunoblastic
    i. lymphadenopathy (IBL)
    i. lymphoma
    i. sarcoma
immunoblot test
immunoblotting
Immuno-Brite Fluorospheres
ImmunoCard
    I. STAT! rotavirus immunoassay
    I. STAT! rotavirus test
    I. STAT! strep A immunoassay
immunocatalysis
immunochemical
    i. assay
    i. fecal occult blood test
immunochemistry
    i. reagent
    ultrastructural i.
immunochromatography
    enzyme i. (EIC)
immunocompetence
immunocompetent cell (ICC)
immunocomplex
immunocompromised
immunoconcentration assay
immunoconglutinin
ImmunoCyt cytopathology recurrent
  bladder cancer test
immunocyte
immunocytoadherence
immunocytochemical
    i. assay (ICA)
    i. localization
immunocytochemically
immunocytochemistry
immunocytoma

immunocytopenia
immunodeficiency
    B-cell i.
    combined i.
    common variable i. (CVID)
    i. disease
    IgA i.
    immunoglobulin A i.
    secondary i.
    severe combined i. (SCID)
    i. syndrome
    T-cell i.
    i. with hypoparathyroidism
immunodeficient
immunodepressant
immunodepression
immunodepressor
immunodetection
    HBc antigen i.
immunodiagnosis
immunodiffusion (ID)
    double i.
    Ouchterlony i.
    Oudin i.
    radial i. (RID)
    single i.
    single-diffusion radial i.
ImmunoDip urinary albumin test
immunodominance
ImmunoDOT Mono G, M test kit
Immuno 1 DPD assay
immunoelectroosmophoresis (IEOP)
immunoelectrophoresis (IE, IEP)
    countercurrent i. (CIE, CIEP)
    crossed i.
    double-crossed i.
    factor VIII-crossed i.
    Laurell rocket i.
    reverse i.
    rocket i.
    two-dimensional i.
immunoenhancement
immunoenhancer
immunoenzymometric
    i. assay
    i. staining
immunoferritin
immunofiltration
    analytical i.
    preparative i.
immunofixation
    i. by subtraction
    i. electrophoresis (IFE)
immunofluorescence (IF)
    adenovirus i.
    i. assay (IFA)
    direct i.
    lumpy-bumpy i.
    i. method

i. microscopy
mixed i. (MIF)
i. technique
i. test
immunofluorescent
i. assay
i. assay kit
indirect i. (IIF)
i. stain
i. staining
immunogen
immunogenetic
immunogenic determinant
immunogenicity
immunogenotyping
immunogenum
Mycobacterium i.
immunoglobulin (Ig)
i. A (IgA)
i. A, D, E,G, M test
i. A immunodeficiency
aggregated human i. G (AHuG)
anti-D i.
cerebrospinal fluid i.
chickenpox i.
i. class
i. D (IgD)
i. disorder
i. domain
i. E (IgE)
i. family adhesion protein
i. G (IgG)
i. gene rearrangement
human normal i.
i. M (IgM)
measles i.
monoclonal i.
i. M-rheumatoid factor (IgM-RF)
poliomyelitis i.
quantitative i.
rabies i.
$Rh_o(D)$ i.
secretory i.
i. subclass
i. supergene
surface i. (sIg)
tetanus i.
thyroid-stimulating i. (TSI)
TSH binding inhibitory i.
(TBII)
immunoglobulin-binding factor
(IBF)
immunoglobulinopathy
immunogold
i. electron microscopy
i. labeling
i. probe
immunogold-silver staining
(IGSS)

immunohematology
immunohemolytic anemia
immunohistochemical (IHC, IMC)
i. analysis
i. marker
i. parameter
i. pattern
i. stain
i. stain for T cell
i. staining
i. technique
immunohistochemistry (IHC)
anticytokeratin i.
E-cadherin i.
epithelial marker i.
i. reagent
immunohistofluorescence
immunohistology
qualitative i.
quantitative i.
immunoincompetent
immunoinhibition
immunolabeling
double i.
immunologic, immunological
i. competence
i. deficiency
i. enhancement
i. homeostasis
i. mechanism
i. memory
i. paralysis
i. pregnancy test
i. surveillance
i. tolerance
i. unresponsiveness
immunological (*var. of* immunologic)
immunologically
i. activated cell
i. competent cell
i. privileged site
immunologist
immunology
armchair i.
transplantation i.
immunoluminometric assay
immunomagnetic cell separation
immunomarker
immunometric assay
(IMA)
immunomodulation
immunomodulator
immunomodulatory
i. agent
i. treatment
immunomorphology
immunoparalysis
immunopathogenesis
immunopathology

immunoperoxidase
    i. stain
    i. staining method
    i. technique (IPT)
    i. test
immunophenotype
    myofibroblastic i.
immunophenotypic
    i. signature
    i. study
immunophenotypical
immunophenotyping
    cell surface i.
    flow cytometric i.
    leukemia i.
    lymphoma i.
immunophilin
immunopositivity
    S-100 protein i.
immunopotency
immunopotentiation
immunopotentiator
immunoprecipitation
    automated i. (AIP)
ImmunoPrep reagent system
immunoprofile
immunoproliferative
    i. disorder
    i. small intestinal disease (IPSID)
immunoprophylaxis
immunoradioassayable human chorionic somatomammotropin (IRHCS)
immunoradiometric assay (IRMA)
immunoradiometry
immunoreaction
immunoreactive (IR)
    i. glucagon (IRG)
    i. human growth hormone (IRhGH)
    i. insulin (IRI)
immunoreactivity
    caspase i.
    cytokeratin i.
    cytoplasmic i.
    filaggrin-like i.
    somatostatin-like i. (SLI)
immunoreceptor
    i. tyrosine activation motif (ITAM)
    i. tyrosine inhibitory motif (ITIM)
immunoregulation
    disordered i.
immunoselection
immunosenescence
immunosilent
immunosorbent antibody
immunostain
    BG8 i.
    CD99 i.
    Dako hepatocyte i.
    E-cadherin i.

    MIB1 nuclear i.
    PTEN i.
    S-100 i.
    TDT i.
    thyroid transcription factor 1 i. (TTF-1)
    tryptase i.
immunostainer
    Shandon Cadenza i.
    TechMate 1000 i.
    Ventana automated i.
    Ventana NexES i.
    Ventana TechMate 100 i.
immunostaining
    clusterin i.
    keratin i.
    MyoD1 i.
immunostimulant
immunostimulation
immunosubtraction (ISUB)
immunosuppressant
immunosuppression
    iatrogenic i.
immunosuppressive
immunosurveillance
immunotactoid
    i. glomerulonephritis
    i. glomerulopathy
Immunotech
    I. immunoassay component
    I. immunoassay kit
immunotherapy
    adoptive i.
    biological i.
immunotolerance
immunotransfusion
Immuno-trol cell
immunotyping
ImmuSTRIP HAMA test kit
impact
    i. loading
    I. on-site drug and alcohol test system
    planar i.
    projectile i.
    i. splatter
impacted
    i. feces
    i. fracture
    i. tooth
impaction
    fecal i.
    i. lesion
impaired
    i. clot retraction
    i. utilization of iron
impairment
    functional aerobic i.
impalpable

impatiens
>*Saccharospirillum* i.

impedance
>electrode i.
>output i.

imperfect
>i. fungus
>i. stage
>i. state
>i. yeast

imperfecta
>amelogenesis i.
>dentinogenesis i.
>enamelogenesis i.
>erythrogenesis i.
>osteogenesis i.

Imperfecti
>Fungi I.

imperforate
>i. anus
>i. hymen

imperforation

impermeable junction

impetiginized

impetigo
>bullous i.
>i. contagiosa
>i. neonatorum
>i. vulgaris

impingement syndrome

implant
>buffered i.
>carcinomatous i.
>invasive i.
>noninvasive i.
>silicone breast i. (SBI)
>Zyplast i.

implantation
>i. bleeding
>circumferential i.
>i. cone
>i. cyst
>i. dermoid
>hypodermic i.
>interstitial i.
>i. site
>superficial i.
>i. test (IT)

implosion

importin receptor

impotence, impotency

impotency (*var. of* impotence)

imprecision

impregnation
>silver i.
>Watanabe silver i.

impressio (*var. of* impression)

impression, impressio
>i. cytology

>i. preparation
>rifling i.

imprint
>maternal i.
>touch i.
>Wright-Giemsa stained touch i.

imprinting
>genomic i.

improvement
>quality i. (QI)

improvised explosive device (IED)

impulse sealing

impulsive loading

impurity

IMR
>infant mortality rate

IMT
>inflammatory myofibroblastic tumor

IMViC
>indole, methyl red, Voges-Proskauer, and citrate

IMx analyzer

In
>indium

in
>I. Charge diabetes control system
>i. situ
>i. situ DNA nick end labeling
>i. situ finding
>i. situ hybridization (ISH)
>i. situ nick end labeling
>i. tela
>i. utero (IU)
>i. vacuo
>i. vitro
>i. vitro invasion assay
>i. vitro transcription/translation (IVTT)
>i. vivo
>i. vivo adhesive platelet (IVAP)
>i. vivo compatibility test
>i. vivo tissue imaging

^{111}In
>indium 111

Inaba antigen

inactivate

inactivated
>i. leukocytolytic serum
>i. poliovirus vaccine (IPV)
>i. ricin toxoid vaccine

inactivation
>complement i.
>i. mechanism

inactivator
>anaphylatoxin i.

inactive tuberculosis

INAD
>infantile neuroaxonal dystrophy

inadvertent
- i. inoculation
- i. inoculation of vaccinia virus

inanition

inapparent infection

inappropriate
- i. antidiuretic hormone (IADH)
- i. antidiuretic hormone syndrome
- i. production of erythropoietin

INB
- internuclear bridging

inborn
- i. error of vitamin D metabolism
- i. lysosomal disease

inbreeding
- i. coefficient
- coefficient of i.

Inc Ab

incapacitate

incapacitating
- i. chemical agent
- i. Ct_{50} (ICt_{50})
- i. dose

incaprettamento (ritual ligature strangulation)

incarcerated hernia

incendiary IED

inch
- pounds per square i. (psi)

inchonensis
- *Tsukamurella i.*

incidence
- angle of i.
- i. increase
- i. of hepatocellular carcinoma
- i. rate

incident
- criticality i.
- i. light
- mass casualty i. (MCI)
- mass fatality i.

incineration

incised wound

incisional biopsy

incisor
- Hutchinson i.

incisura, incisure, *pl.* **incisurae**
- i. angularis
- *Anthomyia i.*
- gastric i.

incisurae (*pl. of* incisura)

incisure (*var. of* incisura)
- Lanterman i.
- Schmidt-Lanterman i.

inclusion
- blennorrhea i.
- i. blennorrhea
- i. body (IB)
- i. body disease

- i. body encephalitis
- i. body fibromatosis
- i. body myositis (IBM)
- cell i.
- i. cell
- i. cell disease
- i. conjunctivitis
- i. conjunctivitis virus
- i. cyst
- cytoplasmic i.
- i. dermoid
- Döhle i.
- endothelial tubuloreticular i.
- intranuclear i.
- leukocyte i.
- neural i. (NI)
- neuronal intranuclear i.
- ubiquitinated i.
- viral i.

incognita
- *Oxyuris i.*

incohesive

incompatibility
- ABO i.
- blood i.
- chemical i.
- fetomaternal i.
- Rh i.

incompatible
- i. blood transfusion
- i. blood transfusion reaction
- i. chemical
- i. hemolytic blood transfusion disease (IHBTD)

incompetence, incompetency
- aortic i. (AI)
- mitral i.
- pulmonary i. (PI)
- tricuspid i. (TI)
- valvular i.

incompetency (*var. of* incompetence)

incompetent
- i. aortic valve
- i. cervix
- i. foramen ovale valve
- i. mitral valve
- i. pulmonic valve
- i. tricuspid valve

incomplete
- i. abortion
- i. agglutinin
- i. amnion
- i. amputation
- i. antibody
- i. antigen
- i. compound fracture
- i. conjoined twins
- i. differentiation (cardiac valve)
- i. dislocation

i. dominance
i. fistula
i. hernia
i. muzzle contusion
i. neurofibromatosis
i. penetrance
i. regeneration
i. right bundle-branch block
i. transposition
incongruus
Conidiobolus i.
inconstans
Proteus i.
incontinence, incontinentia
fecal i.
i. of pigment
urinary i.
incontinentia (*var. of* incontinence)
i. pigmenti
i. pigmenti achromians
incorporation of irradiation
increase
absolute cell i.
incidence i.
increased
i. arterial H+
i. basal metabolism
i. capillary fragility
i. erythropoiesis
i. flow
i. metabolism
i. pressure
i. sodium retention
i. specific gravity
i. temperature
i. turbidity
i. urine urobilinogen
i. viscosity
i. volume
increment
incremental
i. line
i. line of von Ebner
increta
placenta i.
incretin hormone
incretin-mimetic hormone
incrustation
incubate
incubation period (IP)
incubative stage
incubator
Sagian 180 CO2 i.
incubatory carrier
incurable
IND
intestinal neuronal dysplasia
IND A, B
indamine dye

indenization
indentation
independence
anchorage i.
independent
i. assortment
i. practice association
i. variable
indeterminate
i. calcification
i. cell adenocarcinoma
i. colitis
i. leprosy
i. pattern
i. range entrance wound
index, *pl.* **indices**
absorbency i.
acidophilic i.
activity i.
amniotic fluid foam stability i.
antitryptic i.
apoptotic i.
Arneth i.
bacteriological i. (BI)
blood indices
body mass i. (BMI)
Breslow tumor i.
Broders tumor i.
burn i. (BI)
carbohydrate metabolism i. (CMI)
cardiac i.
i. case
cephalic i.
cerebrospinal fluid albumin i.
cerebrospinal fluid IgG i.
cerebrospinal fluid-to-serum albumin
i.
chemotherapeutic i. (CI)
chronicity i.
Colour I. (CI)
coronary prognostic i. (CPI)
creatinine height i. (CHI)
crowded cell i.
degenerative i.
development-at-birth i. (DBI)
DNA i. (DI)
endemic i.
eosinophilic i. (EI)
erythrocyte indices
foam stability i. (FSI)
folded-cell i.
free thyroxine i. (FTI, FT_4I)
free/total PSA i.
free triiodothyronine i. (FT_3I)
grid i.
hematopneic i.
hemolytic i.
hepatic iron i. (HII)
histologic activity i. (HAI)

index (*continued*)

hydroxyproline i.
icterus i. (ict ind)
IgG i.
international prognostic i.
International Sensitivity I. (ISI)
iron i.
juxtaglomerular granulation i. (JGI)
karyopyknotic i. (KI)
Ki-67 i.
Knodell histology activity i.
Kovats i.
Krebs leukocyte i.
labeling i.
leukopenic i.
lymphocyte proliferation/regression i.
  (LPI/LRI)
mass i.
maturation i.
mean peroxidase i. (MPXI)
Mentzer MCV i.
metacarpal i.
mitosis-karyorrhexis i. (MKI)
mitotic i.
mitotic activity i. (MAI)
myelofibrosis proliferation/regression
  i. (MPI/MRI)
Nottingham Prognostic I. (NPI)
nucleoplasmic i. (NPI)
i. of refraction
O'Grady prognostic indices
opsonic i.
plasma-cell labeling i.
proliferative i. (PI)
PSA i.
pyknotic i.
red cell indices
refractive i. (RI)
i. register
Reid i.
relative value i. (RVI)
retention i.
reticulocytic production i. (RPI)
saturation i. (SI)
Schilling i.
sedimentation i.
Sertoli cell i. (SCI)
short increment sensitivity i.
  (SISI)
splenic i.
squamous cell i.
staphyloopsonic i.
steroid protein activity i. (SPAI)
stratification i.
thoracic i. (TI)
thyroxine-binding i. (TBI)
time-tension i. (TTI)
topo-II-alpha i.
tuberculoopsonic i.

tubular-fertility i. (TFI)
uricolytic i.
volume i.

India
I. ink capsule stain
I. ink method
I. ink mount
I. ink preparation
I. rubber man syndrome

Indian
I. childhood cirrhosis (ICC)
I. file
I. rat flea

Indianapolis
hemoglobin I.

Indian-file pattern

indica
Pseudomonas i.

indican
metabolic i.
plant i.
i. test

indicanidrosis

indicanuria

indicated
method of collection not i.
  (MOCNI)

indicator
acid-base i.
alizarin i.
Andrade i.
clinical i.
i. culture medium
i. electrode
i. organism
oxidation-reduction i.
i. paper
redox i.
i. system
i. tube

indicator-dilution curve

indices (*pl. of* index)

indicus
Bacillus i.
Deinococcus i.
Thermodesulfatator i.

Indiella

indifferent
i. cell
i. electrode
i. neutrotaxis

indigenous bacterium

indigo (ind)
i. blue
i. calculus
i. carmine

indigo-carmine
i.-c. stain
i.-c. test

indigoferae
    Rhizobium i.
indigoid dye
indigotin
indiguria
indirect
    i. addressing
    i. agglutination
    i. antiglobulin test
    i. assay
    i. bilirubin test
    i. Coombs test
    i. fluorescent antibody (IFA)
    i. fluorescent antibody test
    i. fluorescent rabies antibody (test) (IFRA)
    i. hemagglutination (IHA)
    i. hemagglutination test
    i. hernia
    i. immunofluorescence test
    i. immunofluorescent (IIF)
    i. maternal death
    i. reacting bilirubin
    i. suffocation
    i. transport
indiscriminate lesion
indium (In)
    i. 111 (^{111}In)
    i. 111 chloride
    i. leukocyte scan
    i. 111 trichloride
individual protective equipment (IPE)
indocyanine
    i. green (ICG)
    i. green test
indolacetic acid
indolaceturia
indolaceturic acid
indolelactic acid
indole, methyl red, Voges-Proskauer, and citrate (IMViC)
indole-nitrate broth
indolent ulcer
indolicus
indolifex
    Oceanibulbus i.
indologenes
    Kingella i.
    Suttonella i.
indoluria
indonesiensis
    Acetobacter i.
    Desulfovibrio i.
    Streptomyces i.
indophenol
    i. dye
    i. method
    i. test
indoxyl sulfate

indoxyluria
induced
    i. abortion
    i. allergic encephalomyelitis
    i. allergic neuritis
    i. aspermatogenesis
    i. glomerulonephritis
    i. phagocytosis
    i. sensitivity
    i. thyroiditis
    i. uveitis
inducer cell
inducible
    i. enzyme
    i. nitric oxide synthetase (iNOS)
inducing
    syncytium i. (SI)
inductance
induction
    enzyme i.
    lysogenic i.
    magnetic i.
    negative control enzyme i.
    i. period
    positive control enzyme i.
    sputum i.
    i. therapy
inductive
    i. phase
    i. reactance
inductor
indulin
indulinophil, indulinophile
indulinophile (*var. of* indulinophil)
indurated
induration
    collapse i.
    cyanotic i.
    Froriep i.
    gray i.
    plastic i.
    red i.
indurative myocarditis
induratum
    erythema i.
indusium
industrial
    i. poison
    i. toxicology
INE
    infantile necrotizing encephalomyelopathy
ineffective erythropoiesis
inelastic scattering
Inermicapsifer madagascariensis
inert electrode
inertia
inevitable abortion

inexpectatum
  Albidovulum i.
inf
  infusion
infancy
  chronic pneumonitis of i. (CPI)
  melanotic neuroectodermal tumor of
    i.
  sudden unexpected death in i.
    (SUDI)
  transient hypogammaglobulinemia of
    i.
infant
  i. botulism
  i. death
  low birth weight i. (LBWI)
  i. mortality rate (IMR)
  premature i.
infantarius
  Streptococcus i.
  Streptococcus infantarius subsp. *i.*
infantile
  i. amaurotic familial idiocy
  i. celiac disease
  i. cortical hyperostosis
  i. digital fibromatosis
  i. fibrosarcoma
  i. gastroenteritis
  i. gastroenteritis virus
  i. glaucoma
  i. hemangioma
  i. hepatic hemangioendothelioma
  i. muscular atrophy
  i. myofibromatosis
  i. myxedema
  i. necrotizing encephalomyelopathy
    (INE)
  i. neuroaxonal dystrophy (INAD)
  i. paralysis
  i. polycystic kidney disease
  i. progressive spinal muscular
    dystrophy
  i. purulent conjunctivitis
  i. pyknocytosis
  i. respiratory distress syndrome
  i. SMA
  i. spasm
  i. type coarctation
  i. uterus
infantilis
  poliodystrophia cerebri
    progressiva i.
  roseola i.
infantilism
  tubal i.
infantis
  Bifidobacterium i.
  Hydatigera i.
  Salmonella enteritidis serotype *i.*

infantum
  dermatitis exfoliativa i.
  dermatitis gangrenosa i.
  Leishmania i.
  Leishmania donovani i.
infarct (*var. of* infarction)
  acute i.
  anemic i.
  anterior lateral myocardial i.
    (ALMI)
  anteroseptal myocardial i. (ASMI)
  bile i.
  bland i.
  bone i.
  Brewer i.
  cerebral i.
  digital i.
  embolic i.
  focal i.
  healed i.
  hemorrhagic i.
  microscopic i.
  old i.
  posterior wall i. (PWI)
  pulmonary i.
  recent i.
  red i.
  reddish-brown i.
  ruptured myocardial i.
  septic i.
  thrombotic i.
  uric acid i.
  white i.
  Zahn i.
infarction, infarct
  acute myocardial i. (AMI)
  anterior wall i. (AWI)
  anterior wall myocardial i. (AWMI)
  atrial i.
  bowel i.
  cerebral i. (CI)
  inferior wall myocardial i. (IWMI)
  intestinal i.
  lymph node i.
  maternal floor i.
  mesenteric i.
  myocardial i. (MI)
  nontransmural myocardial i.
  old myocardial i. (OMI)
  postmyocardial i.
  pulmonary i. (PI)
  renal i.
  silent myocardial i.
  subendocardial myocardial i.
  through-and-through myocardial i.
  transmural myocardial i.
infarctive placental dysfunction
infected abortion
infecting dose (ID)

infection
  abortive i.
  airborne i.
  atypical mycobacteria i.
  bacterial i.
  biliary tract i.
  chlamydia i.
  colonization i.
  concurrent i.
  i. control (IC)
  cross i.
  cryptogenic i.
  cutaneous anthrax i.
  cytomegalovirus i.
  dragon worm i.
  droplet i.
  ectothrix i.
  endogenous i.
  enterobacter urinary tract i.
  enterococcus urinary tract i.
  enzootic i.
  Escherichia coli urinary tract i.
  exogenous i.
  exuberant i.
  fever caused by i. (FI)
  focal i.
  foodborne i.
  fusospirochetal i.
  gastrointestinal anthrax i.
  guinea worm i.
  helmintic i.
  herpes simplex virus i.
  i. immunity
  inapparent i.
  inhalational anthrax i.
  intestinal parasitic i.
  klebsiella urinary tract i.
  latent i.
  lower urinary tract i.
  mass i.
  medina worm i.
  meningococcal i.
  meningococcus i.
  mixed i.
  mycobacteria i.
  Mycobacterium avium i.
  mycoplasma i.
  natural focus of i.
  nosocomial i.
  opportunistic i.
  oral i.
  orf i.
  postoperative i.
  proteus urinary tract i.
  providencia urinary tract i.
  pseudomonas urinary tract i.
  puerperal i.
  pulmonary i.
  pyogenic i.
  recurrent bacterial i.
  recurrent hepatitis C virus i.
  recurrent sinus and pulmonary i.
  recurrent upper respiratory tract i.
    (RURTI)
  reservoir of i.
  respiratory syncytial virus i.
  rickettsial i.
  secondary i.
  second-strain i.
  serpent i.
  serratia urinary tract i.
  spinal cord i.
  Staphylococcus aureus urinary tract
    i.
  streptococcal i.
  suppurative i.
  i. surveillance and control program
    (ISCP)
  upper respiratory i. (URI)
  upper respiratory tract i. (URTI)
  urea-splitting bacterial i.
  urinary tract i. (UTI)
  viral respiratory i. (VRI)
  whipworm i.
  zoonotic i.
infection-associated hemophagocytic
  syndrome (IAHS)
infection-immunity
infectiosity
infectiosum
  ecthyma i.
  erythema i.
infectious
  i. agent
  i. anemia
  i. arteritis
  i. arthritis
  i. avian bronchitis
  i. bovine rhinotracheitis (IBR)
  i. bovine rhinotracheitis virus
  i. bronchitis virus (IBV)
  i. bulbar paralysis
  i. canine hepatitis
  i. cause of death (ICOD)
  i. colitis
  i. disease
  I. Disease Death Review Team
    (IDDRT)
  I. Disease Surveillance Information
    System (ISIS)
  i. disorder
  i. ectromelia virus
  i. eczematoid dermatitis
  i. endocarditis
  i. enterocolitides
  i. esophagitis
  i. granuloma
  i. hepatitis (IH)

infectious (*continued*)
    i. hepatitis virus
    i. laryngo-tracheitis-like viruses
    i. mononucleosis (IM)
    i. mononucleosis screening test
    i. myocarditis
    i. myositis
    i. myxoma
    i. nucleic acid
    i. papilloma virus
    i. parotitis
    i. plasmid
    i. polyneuritis
    i. porcine encephalomyelitis
    i. porcine encephalomyelitis virus
    i. wart
    i. waste
infectiousness
infectiva
    polioencephalitis i.
infective
    i. dose (ID)
    i. embolism
    i. endocarditis (IE)
    i. thrombus
infectivity
infectoria
    Lewia i.
inferior
    i. complete closed dislocation
    i. complete compound dislocation
    i. dislocation
    i. displacement
    ductulus aberrans i.
    i. lipodystrophy
    i. olivary nucleus
    i. petrosal sinus sampling
    i. petrosal vein sampling
    tarsus i.
    tela choroidea i.
    i. wall myocardial infarction (IWMI)
infernum
    Desulfacinum i.
infertility screen
infestans
infestation
    saprophytic i.
    trichomonas i.
infidelity
    lineage i.
infiltrate
    acute inflammatory i.
    Assmann tuberculous i.
    brisk i.
    central-patch i.
    eosinophil leukocytic i.
    hilar-based fluffy i.
    inflammatory i.
    infraclavicular i.

    Jessner lymphocytic i.
    leukocytic i.
    lymphocytic inflammatory i.
    lymphoplasmacytic i.
    microscopic inflammatory i.
    monocytic inflammatory i.
    neutrophilic i.
    nonbrisk i.
    plasma cell i.
    plasmacytic i.
    polymorphonuclear leukocytic i.
    polymorphous lymphoid i.
    pulmonary i.
infiltrating
    i. comedocarcinoma
    i. cribriform carcinoma
    i. duct adenocarcinoma
    i. ductal carcinoma (IDC)
    i. lipoma
    i. lobular carcinoma (ILC)
    i. papillary carcinoma
infiltration
    adipose i.
    calcareous i.
    cellular i.
    epituberculous i.
    fatty i.
    gelatinous i.
    glycogen i.
    gray i.
    intratumoral i.
    lipomatous i.
    lymphocytic i.
    lymphoplasmacytic i.
    muconodular i.
    i. of leukemic cell
    sanguineous i.
    tuberculous i.
    tubular i.
infiltrative
    i. disease
    i. fasciitis
    i. margin
    i. ophthalmopathy
infinite
infinitely miscible
infinitesimal
infinity
inflamed ulcer
inflammable
inflammation
    active chronic i.
    acute and chronic i.
    acute hemorrhagic i.
    adhesive i.
    allergic i.
    alterative i.
    atrophic i.
    blennorrhagic i.

bullous granulomatous i.
calcified granulomatous i.
caseating granulomatous i.
caseous i.
catarrhal i.
cavitating i.
chronic active i.
chronic nonspecific i.
circumscribed i.
confluent i.
croupous i.
cystic acute i.
cystic chronic i.
cystic granulomatous i.
degenerative i.
diffuse acute i.
diffuse chronic i.
disseminated i.
erosive i.
exanthematous i.
exudative granulomatous i.
fibrinoid necrotizing i.
fibrinopurulent i.
fibrinous i.
fibrocaseous i.
fibroid i.
follicular i.
gelatinous acute i.
granulomatous i.
hemorrhagic i.
hyperplastic i.
immune i.
interstitial i.
localized i.
lymphoplasmacytic i.
membranous acute i.
multifocal i.
necrotic i.
necrotizing granulomatous i.
neutrophilic i.
nonnecrotizing granulomatous i.
obliterative i.
i. of connective tissue (ICT)
organizing i.
ossifying i.
productive i.
proliferative i.
pseudomembranous acute i.
purulent i.
pustular i.
recurrent i.
respiratory i.
sclerosing i.
serofibrinous i.
serous acute i.
sinusoidal i.
spinal cord i.
subacute i.
suppurative acute i.

suppurative chronic i.
suppurative granulomatous i.
testis i.
transudative i.
ulcerative i.
uremic i.
vesicular acute i.
vesicular granulomatous i.
inflammatoria
crusta i.
inflammatory
i. adenocarcinoma
i. arthritis
i. bowel disease (IBD)
i. carcinoma
i. cavity
i. cell
i. cell debris
i. corpuscle
i. dermatosis
i. disorder
i. edema
i. exudate
i. fibromyxoid tumor
i. fibrosarcoma
i. fistula
i. infiltrate
i. linear verrucous epidermal nevus (ILVEN)
i. lymph
i. macrophage
i. marker
i. mediator
i. membrane
i. myofibroblastic lesion
i. myofibroblastic tumor (IMT)
i. myofibrohistiocytic proliferation
i. myopathy
i. necrosis
i. odontogenic cyst
i. papillary hyperplasia of the palate (IPHP)
i. pelvic disease (IPD)
i. perforation
i. polyp
i. pseudomembrane
i. pseudotumor
i. reaction
i. rheumatism
i. rupture
i. sinus tract
i. transudate
inflation
inflatum
Scedosporium i.
inflatus
Wardomyces i.
inflection, inflexion
point of i.

inflexion (*var. of* inflection)
influenza (flu), flu
    i. A, B, C
    i. A, B titer
    avian i.
    Bacillus influenzae
    equine i.
    Haemophilus influenzae
    Hong Kong i.
    Spanish i.
    swine i.
    i. test
    i. virus
    i. virus culture
    i. virus vaccine
    ZstatFlu rapid diagnostic test for i.
      A and B
***Influenzavirus* A, B, C**
infolding
    VSMC i.
information
    i. retrieval
    i. theory
informed consent
infra
    vide i.
infraclavicular infiltrate
infradian rhythm
infragranular layer
infrared
    i. CO_2 analyzer
    i. microscope
    i. spectrophotometry
      (IRS)
    i. spectroscopy
infrasubspecific
infratemporal fossa
infraumbilical
infundibula (*pl. of* infundibulum)
infundibular
    i. part
    i. stalk
    i. stem
    i. stenosis
infundibularis
infundibuloma
infundibulum, *pl.* **infundibula**
    Choanotaenia i.
    follicular infundibula
infusion (inf)
    brain-heart i. (BHI)
    JAZF1 gene i.
    total-dose i. (TDI)
Infusoria
infusorian
ingestion challenge test
ingestive
ingluviei
    Lactobacillus i.

ingrown
    i. hair
    i. toenail
inguinale
    Epidermophyton i.
    granuloma i.
    hernia uteri i.
    lymphogranuloma i.
    Trichophyton i.
inguinal hernia
inguinalis
    tinea i.
inhae
    Leuconostoc i.
inhalant
    i. antigen
    i. corticosteroid
inhalation
    i. injury
    i. pneumonia
    volatile substance i.
inhalational
    i. anthrax
    i. anthrax infection
    i. botulism
inherent filter
inheritance
    alternative i.
    amphigenous i.
    autosomal dominant i.
    autosomal recessive i.
    biparental i.
    codominant i.
    complemental i.
    cytoplasmic i.
    dominant i.
    extrachromosomal i.
    holandric i.
    hologynic i.
    homochronous i.
    intermediate i.
    maternal i.
    mendelian i.
    mitochondrial i.
    multifactorial i.
    i. pattern
    polygenic i.
    quantitative i.
    quasicontinuous i.
    quasidominant i.
    recessive i.
    sex-linked i.
    supplemental i.
    unit i.
    X-linked dominant i.
    X-linked recessive i.
inherited
    i. albumin variant
    i. cancer

i. disease
i. genetic factor
i. giant platelet disorder (IGPD)

inhibens
Carnobacterium i.

inhibin
i. A
i. antibody
i. expression

inhibiting
i. antibody
i. factor
i. hormone

inhibition
allogeneic i.
allosteric i.
competitive i.
contact i.
enzyme i.
i. factor
fertility i.
hemagglutination i. (HI)
hemagglutinin i. (HAI)
neurogenic i.
RAST i.
i. test
tetrazolium reduction i. (TRI)
tissue thromboplastin i.

inhibitor
alloantibody i.
alpha-2 macroglobulin i.
alpha-1 protease i.
alpha-1 trypsin i.
apoptosis i. (IAP)
i. assay
carbonic anhydrase i.
cell-cycle i.
C1 esterase i. (C1EInh)
cholinesterase i.
coagulation factor i.
cyclin-dependent kinase i. (CDKI)
electron transport i.
enzyme i. (EI)
factor i.
HDAC i.
human alpha-1 proteinase i.
inter-alpha-trypsin i. (ITI)
lupus erythematosus i.
malonate i.
monoamine oxidase i. (MAOI)
noggin protein i.
noncompetitive i.
i. of transcription
oxidative phosphorylation i.
plasminogen activator i. (PAI)
protease i. (PI)
proteinase i.
soybean trypsin i. (SBTI)
tissue factor pathway i. (TFPI)

Trojan horse i.
tryosine kinase i.
trypsin i.
Z-dependent protease i. (ZPI)

inhibitory
i. enzyme
i. hormone
i. mold agar

iniencephaly
In-111, ^{111}In
initial (I)
i. hematuria
i. oliguric phase
i. prognostic score (IPS)
i. segment
i. syphilitic lesion

initialization
initiating agent
initiation
i. codon
i. factor

initio
ab i.

initis
injection
facet joint i.
intracytoplasmic sperm i. (ICSI)
lactated Ringer i.
i. mass
Ringer i.
sensitizing i.

injurious agent
injury
auditory blast i.
avulsion i.
birth i.
blast i.
blunt head i.
cell i.
cold i.
compression i.
crush i.
decompensation i.
decompression i.
diffuse axonal i.
first-degree radiation i.
focal axonal i.
fourth-degree radiation i.
freezing i.
gastrointestinal blast i.
hyperperfusion/hyperfiltration i.
hypoxic cell i.
inhalation i.
miscellaneous blast i.
posterior dislocation i.
primary blast i.
pulmonary blast i.
quaternary blast i.
radiation i.

injury (*continued*)
    red blood cell i.
    reperfusion i.
    reversible i.
    rotator cuff i.
    secondary blast i.
    second-degree radiation i.
    spinal cord i.
    tendon i.
    tertiary blast i.
    third-degree radiation i.
    torsion i.
    transfusion-related acute lung i. (TRALI)
    traumatic brain i. (TBI)
ink
    Waterman blue i.
inkin
    Sarcinosporon i.
    Trichosporon i.
In-Line Strep A test
innate immunity
innatus
    calor i.
inner
    i. circular muscle layer
    i. circumferential lamella
    i. dental epithelium
    i. hair cell
    i. neural layer
    i. phalangeal cell
innervation
    motor i.
innidiation
innocens
    diabetes i.
innocent
    i. bystander cell
    i. tumor
innocuous
innocuum
    Clostridium i.
innominate
innoxious
inochondritis
inoculability
inoculable
inoculate
inoculating loop
inoculation
    inadvertent i.
    i. smallpox
inoculum
Inocybe geophylla
inohanensis
    Nocardia i.
Inonotus
inopectic
inopexia

inopinata
    Erysipelothrix i.
    Scardovia i.
inorganic
    i. acid
    i. chemistry
    i. component
    i. electrolyte
    i. mercury (Hg2+)
    i. phosphate
    i. pyrophosphatase
    i. pyrophosphate
inornata
    Culiseta i.
iNOS
    inducible nitric oxide synthetase
inoscopy
inosemia
inosinate
inosine
    i. cyclohydrolase
    i. dehydrogenase
    i. diphosphate
    i. monophosphate
    i. phosphate
    i. phosphorylase (IP)
    i. pyrophosphorylase
    i. triphosphate (ITP)
inosine-5′-phosphate
inosinic acid
inosita
    melituria i.
inosite-free broth
inosithin neutralization test
inositol
    i. dehydrogenase
    i. hexanitrate
    i. hexaphosphate
    i. niacinate
inosituria
inosuria
inotropic
Inoviridae
Inovirus
inquiline
Inquilinus limosus
inquiry
INR
    International Normalized Ratio
INRatio PT/INR monitoring for patient self-testing
INS
    idiopathic nephrotic syndrome
inscription
    tendinous i.
inscriptio tendinea
insect
    i. bite
    i. virus

Insecta
insectarium
insecticide
>chlorfenthion i.
>fenthion i.
>organochlorine i.
>organophosphate i.

insemination
insensible water loss
insertion
>battledore i.
>i. mutation
>promoter i.
>i. sequence
>velamentous i.

insertional
>i. activity
>i. mutagenesis
>i. translocation

insheathed
insidiosa
>*Erysipelothrix i.*
>*Ralstonia i.*

insidiosum
>*Pythium i.*

insidiosus
>*Triphleps i.*

Insight digital camera
insipidus
>central diabetes i.
>diabetes i.
>nephrogenic diabetes i.
>(NDI)

insol
>insoluble

insolitus
>*Achromobacter i.*

insoluble (insol)
>i. complement-bound aggregate
>i. Prussian blue
>i. salt

in-solution hybridization
insolutum
>*Polypaecilum i.*

inspiratory
>i. flow
>i. flow rate (IFR)
>i. reserve capacity (IRC)
>i. reserve volume (IRV)

inspiratory:expiratory phase ratio
inspissate
inspissated
inspissation
inspissator
INSS
>International Neuroblastoma Staging
>System

instabilis
>*Trichostrongylus i.*

instability
>chromosomal i. (CIN)
>microsatellite i. (MIN)
>nuclear excision repair i. (NIN)
>vasomotor i.

InstaCheck Med+ immunoassay for
drugs of abuse
instantaneous rigor mortis
instant thin-layer chromatography
(ITLC)
Instant-View fecal occult blood test
instar
INSTI HIV-1 rapid antibody test
instillation
institute
>American National Standards I.
>(ANSI)
>National Cancer I. (NCI)
>I. of Virus Preparations

instructive theory
instrument
>Advia 60, 120 automated cell
>counting i.
>Cell-Dyn 1200, 3200, 4000
>automated cell counting i.
>Gen-S automated cell counting i.
>GM i.
>ionizing chamber i.
>MLA-100 coagulation i.
>stereotaxic i.
>STKS automated cell counting i.
>Sysmex CA-6000 coagulation i.

instrumentation
>advanced breast biopsy i.
>(ABBI)

insudate
insudation
>plasmatic i.

insuetus
>*Ilyobacter i.*

insufficiency
>adrenal i.
>adrenocortical i.
>aortic valvular i.
>arterial i.
>circulatory i.
>coronary i. (CI)
>metabolic i.
>mitral i. (MI, MIS)
>ovarian i.
>primary adrenal i.
>pulmonary i.
>renal i.
>respiratory i.
>tricuspid i. (TI)
>uteroplacental i. (UPI)
>velopharyngeal i.
>venous i.

insufficient signal (IS)

insufflation
    cranial i.
    endotracheal i.
    presacral i.
    retroperitoneal gas i.
insula, *pl.* **insulae**
insulae (*pl. of* insula)
insular
    i. carcinoma
    i. sclerosis
insulated gate field effect transistor
insulator
insulin
    i. antagonist
    i. antibody
    atypical i.
    i. clearance (C_{in})
    i. clearance test
    i. coma therapy (ICT)
    crystalline i. (CI)
    crystalline zinc i.
    i. dependent diabetes
    globin i.
    i. hypoglycemia test
    immunoreactive i. (IRI)
    i. lipoatrophy
    i. lipodystrophy
    potassium, glucose, and i.
      (PGI)
    prompt zinc i.
    protamine zinc i.
    i. receptor and signal
      transduction
    i. resistance
    i. sensitivity test (IST)
    i. shock
    i. shock therapy (IST)
    soluble i. (SI)
    i. tolerance test (ITT)
    i. unit (international)
insulinase
insulin-dependent diabetes mellitus
  (IDDM)
insulinemia
insulin-glucose tolerance test
insulinlike
    i. activity (ILA)
    i. growth factor
    i. growth factor-1 (IGF-1)
insulinoma
insulinopenic
insulinotropic
insulitis
Insul-Tote
InSure fecal immunochemical test
insusceptibility
intake and output (I/O)
integer oocyte
Integra chemical analyzer

integral
    i. dose
    i. protein
Integrated Core system
integrating microscope
integration
    genomic i.
    large-scale i.
    medium-scale i.
    plasmid i.
    very large scale i. (VLSI)
integrator
integrin alpha$_1$-beta$_1$
integrity
    sarcolemmal i.
integument
integumentary system
integumentum commune
intense inflammatory reaction
intensely basophilic cytoplasm
intensity
    luminous i.
interacinar
interacinous
interaction
    bacterial-fungal i.
    cell i. (CI)
    cell-cell i.
    CTLA-4 i.
    drug i.
    i. of radiation with matter
    sample i.
interactive processing
inter-alpha-globulin
inter-alpha-trypsin inhibitor (ITI)
interalveolar
    i. pore
    i. septum
interalveolare
    connective tissue septa
    septum i.
interannular segment
interatrial septal defect (IASD)
interband
intercalary
    i. cell
    i. deletion
    i. neuron
intercalate
intercalated
    i. cell of the renal cortex
    i. disc
    i. duct
intercalatum
    Schistosoma i.
intercapillary
    i. cell
    i. glomerulosclerosis
    i. nephrosclerosis

intercarotid body
intercellular
    i. adhesion molecule-1
      (ICAM-1)
    i. bridge
    i. canaliculus of parietal cell
    i. cement
    i. junction
    i. lymph
    i. prickle
Intercept
    I. oral fluid drug testing
    I. platelet system
interchange
interchromosomal aberration
intercommunicating network
intercristal space
intercurrent disease
interdigitale
    Trichophyton i.
    Trichophyton mentagrophytes i.
interdigitating
    i. cell sarcoma
    i. dendritic cell (IDC)
    i. dendritic cell sarcoma (IDCS)
    i. dendritic cell tumor
    i. papillary neoplasm
    i. reticulum cell
interdigitation
    cell membrane i.
interelectrode distance
interface
    air-liquid i.
    alveolar-capillary i.
    dermoepidermal i.
    EIA i.
interfacial canal
interfascicular connective tissue
interference
    anion i.
    background i.
    bacterial i.
    cation i.
    centromere i.
    chemical i.
    chromatid i.
    constructive i.
    destructive i.
    drug i.
    i. filter
    hemolysis i.
    icterus i.
    ionization i.
    i. microscope
    spectral i.
    i. test
interference-contrast microscopy (ICM)
interfering
    defective i. (DI)

interferon (IFN)
    i. alpha (IFN-alpha)
    antigen i.
    i. beta (IFN beta)
    fibroblast i.
    i. gamma (IFN-gamma)
    immune i.
    leukocyte i.
    i. regulatory factor 1 (IRF1)
interferon-9
    recumbant i.-9 (IFN-a)
interfibrillar, interfibrillary
interfibrillary (*var. of* interfibrillar)
interfibrous
interfilamentous
interfollicular (IF)
interganglionic
intergemmal
interglobular
    i. space
    i. space of Owen
interglobulare
    spatia anguli iridocornealis
    spatium i.
    spatia zonularia
interieur
    milieu i.
interindividual CNV
interjectum
    Mycobacterium i.
interkinesis
interlamellar
interleukin (IL)
    i. 1–18
interlobar duct
interlobitis
interlobular
    i. connective tissue septum
    i. duct
    i. ductule
    i. pleurisy
interlobulares
    ductuli i.
interlobularis
    pneumonia i.
intermedia
    alpha thalassemia i.
    Brevundimonas i.
    Hydrogenophaga i.
    Prevotella i.
    thalassemia i.
    Yersinia i.
intermediary
    i. metabolism
    i. system
intermediate
    i. body of Flemming
    i. carcinoma
    i. cell

intermediate (*continued*)
   i. coliform bacteria
   i. disc
   i. filament (IF)
   i. filament protein
   i. host
   i. inheritance
   i. junction
   i. lamella
   malignant teratoma, i. (MTI)
   i. normoblast
   i. part
   i. range entrance wound
   reaction i.
intermediate-density lipoprotein (IDL)
intermedin
   unit of i.
intermedium
intermedius
   Gluconacetobacter i.
   Lutzomyia i.
   Streptococcus i.
intermittent
   i. albuminuria
   i. claudication (IC)
   i. hemoglobinuria
   i. malaria
   i. malarial fever
   i. parasite
   i. sterilization
interna
   hematorrhachis i.
   hyperostosis frontalis i.
   lamina elastica i.
   lamina rara i
   pachymeningitis i.
   theca i.
internal
   i. adhesive pericarditis
   i. carotid artery occlusion
   (ICAO)
   i. carotid stenosis
   i. cavity
   i. conversion
   i. decontamination
   i. elastic lamellae
   i. elastic lamina
   i. elastic membrane
   i. fistula
   i. hemorrhoid
   i. meningitis
   i. pathology
   i. pillar cell
   i. pyocephalus
   i. resistance (IR)
   i. root sheath
   i. standard
   i. storage
   i. telomerase standard (ITAS)

international
   International benzoate unit (IBU)
   International Classification of
     Diseases (ICD)
   International Committee for
     Standardization in Hematology
     (ICSH)
   International Federation of Clinical
     Chemistry (IFCC)
   International Federation of
     Gynecology and Obstetrics
     (FIGO)
   International Neuroblastoma Staging
     System (INSS)
   International Normalized Ratio (INR)
   international prognostic index
   International Prostate Symptom
     Score (IPPS, IPSS)
   International Sensitivity Index (ISI)
   International Society for Heart and
     Lung Transplantation
   International Society for Urological
     Pathology (ISUP)
   International Standards Organization
     (ISO)
   International System of Units (SI)
   International Union of Pure and
     Applied Chemistry
   international unit (IU)
interneuron
internexin
   alpha i.
internodal
   i. pathway
   i. segment
internodale
   segmentum i.
internode
internuclear bridging (INB)
internum
internuncial
   i. cell
   i. neuron
interobserver variability
interocclusal clearance
interoceptive
interoceptor
interosseous cartilage
interpapillary ridge
interphalangeal (IP)
   proximal i. (PIP)
interphase
interphyletic
interplant
interplanting
interpolation
interrod enamel
interrogans
   Leptospira i.

interscapular
    i. gland
    i. hibernoma
intersection
    tendinous i.
intersectio tendinea
intersex syndrome
interspace
interspecific graft
interspersed repeats
interspongioplastic substance
interstice
interstitial
    i. cell of Leydig
    i. cell-stimulating hormone
      (ICSH)
    i. cell tumor of testis
    i. cystitis (IC)
    i. deletion
    i. emphysema
    i. fluid
    i. gastritis
    i. giant cell pneumonia
    i. gland
    i. growth
    i. implantation
    i. inflammation
    i. keratitis
    i. lamella
    i. lung disease (ILD)
    i. mastitis
    i. myositis
    i. nephritis
    i. plasma cell pneumonia
    i. pneumonitis
    i. pulmonary fibrosis
    i. tissue
    i. water (ISW)
interstitium
intertriginis
    Trichophyton i.
intertriginous
intertrigo
intertropical anemia
interval
    asymptomatic i.
    calibration i.
    confidence i. (CI)
    i. estimate
    postmortem i. (PMI)
    reference i. (RI)
    rupture-delivery i. (RDI)
    i. scale
    systolic time i. (STI)
    time i. (TI)
    tolerance i.
intervening sequence
interventricular septal defect
    (IVSD)

intervertebralis
    anulus fibrosus disci i.
    calcinosis i.
intervillositis
    chronic i.
intervillous
    i. fibrin
    i. microabscess
    i. perfusion
    i. space
intestinal
    i. absorption
    i. amebiasis
    i. atresia
    i. botulism
    i. calculus
    i. ceroid deposition
    i. chronic graft-versus-host disease
    i. colic
    i. crypt cell
    i. emphysema
    i. fistula
    i. flora
    i. flow disorder
    i. follicle
    i. gland
    i. heterotopia
    i. infarction
    i. lipodystrophy
    i. lymphangiectasis
    i. malrotation
    i. metaplasia (IM)
    i. mucinous borderline tumor (IMBT)
    i. mucosa
    i. myiasis
    i. necrosis
    i. neuronal dysplasia (IND)
    i. obstruction (IO)
    i. parasite
    i. parasitic infection
    i. phenotype lesion
    i. sand
    i. sepsis
    i. tract carcinoid
    i. villus
intestinale
    Encephalitozoon i.
intestinales (*pl. of* intestinalis)
intestinalis, *pl.* **intestinales**
    Collinsella i.
    Giardia i.
    glandulae intestinales
    Lamblia i.
    Ligula i.
    lipodystrophia i.
    mycosis i.
    pneumatosis cystoides i.
    Retortamonas i.
    Roseburia i.

intestinalis (*continued*)
    Septata i.
    tonsilla i.
    Trichomonas i.
    villi intestinales
intestine
intestinotoxin
intima
    aortic tunica i.
    tunica i.
intimal
    i. cell
    i. fibroelastosis
    i. surface
intimitis
    proliferative i.
intolerance
    cold i.
    exercise i.
    food i.
    fructose i.
    heat i.
    hereditary fructose i.
    (HFI)
    lactose i.
    lysine i.
    lysinuric protein i. (LPI)
    sucrose i.
intoxication
    acid i.
    alcohol i.
    alkaline i.
    anaphylactic i.
    botulism i.
    citrate i.
    ethylene glycol i.
    methanol i.
    neuronal cell i.
    salicylate i.
    septic i.
    serum i.
    TCDD i.
    vitamin A, D i.
    water i.
intraabdominal adhesion
intraacinous
intraarterial
intraauricular
intrabuccal
intracanalicular fibroadenoma
intracapsular ankylosis
intracartilaginous
intracavernous
    i. aneurysm
    i. injection test
intracavitary
intracellular
    i. accumulation
    i. canaliculus

    i. coccobacillus
    i. fluid (ICF)
    i. fluid volume (IFV)
    i. free cholesterol
    i. macroadenoma (IM)
    i. myofibril
    i. NADP
    i. NADPH
    i. parasite
    i. receptor analysis
    i. signal transduction
    effect
    i. thrombosis
    i. toxin
    i. water (ICW)
intracellulare
    Mycobacterium i.
intracerebral hemorrhage
intrachain disulphide bond
intrachange
intrachromosomal aberration
intracisternal
    i. microtubule
    i. space
intracorporeal
intracorpuscular
intracranial
    i. aneurysm (ICA)
    i. hematoma
    i. hemorrhage
    i. hypertension
    i. tumor
intracrine
intracristal space
intracutaneous
    i. allergy testing
    i. reaction
    i. tuberculin skin testing
intracystic
    i. hyperplasia
    i. papillary carcinoma
    i. papillary nodule
    i. papilloma
intracytoplasmic
    i. crystal
    i. glycogen
    i. inclusion cell
    i. lumina
    i. microfilament
    i. microlumen
    i. mucin
    i. sperm injection (ICSI)
    i. vacuole
intradermal, intradermic
    i. allergy testing
    i. nevus
    i. reaction (IDR)
    i. test (IT)
intradermic (*var. of* intradermal)

intraductal
- i. hyperplasia
- i. papillary carcinoma (IPC)
- i. papillary mucinous neoplasia (IPMN, IPNM)
- i. papillary mucinous tumor (IPMT)
- i. papillary projection
- i. papilloma
- i. papillomatosis

intraepidermal
- i. basal cell epithelioma, Borst-Jadassohn type
- i. squamous cell carcinoma

intraepidermic bulla
intraepiphysial
intraepithelial
- i. carcinoma
- i. dyskeratosis
- i. gland
- i. lymphocyte
- i. lymphocytosis
- i. neoplasia

intraesophageal pH test
intrafascicular
intrafilar
intrafusal fiber
intragemmal
intraglandular
intraglobular
intraglomerular crystallization
intrahepatic vascular obstruction
intrahyoid
intralesional
intralobar
- i. nephrogenic rest (ILNR)
- i. reticulation
- i. sequestration

intralobular
- i. duct
- i. ductule
- i. lesion

intramedullary hemolysis
intramembranous
- i. ossification
- i. space

intramucosal loose granuloma
intramural
- i. hematoma
- i. protruding form (IPF)

intraneural nerve ending
intranuclear
- i. inclusion
- i. perichromatin granule
- i. spot

intraobserver variability
intraocular
- i. fluid
- i. foreign body (IOFB)

intraoperative
- i. cell salvage
- i. cytology
- i. touch preparation

intraosseous
intraosteal
intraperitoneal air
IntraPrep permeabilization reagent
intraprotoplasmic
intrapulmonary
- i. hemorrhage
- i. spindle cell thymoma

intrarenal
intrasinusoidal cytokeratin-positive mesothelial cell
Intrasporangiaceae
intrastromal
intratesticular tumor
intrathoracic
- i. extramedullary hematopoiesis
- i. gas volume (IGV)

intratubular
- i. germ cell neoplasia (IGCN)
- i. germ cell neoplasia, unclassified type (IGCNU)

intratumoral (IT)
- i. infiltration
- i. lymph vessel density

intratumor microvessel density
intrauterina
- ichthyosis i.
- rachitis i.

intrauterine
- i. asphyxia
- i. contraceptive device (IUD)
- i. fetal death (IUFD)
- i. fetal transfusion (IVT)
- i. foreign body (IUFB)
- i. growth rate (IUGR)
- i. malnutrition (IUM)

intravasation
intravascular
- i. agglutination
- i. coagulation of blood
- i. coagulation screen
- i. consumption coagulopathy (IVCC)
- i. coronary ultrasound
- i. hemolysis
- i. lymph
- i. mass (IVM)
- i. papillary endothelial hyperplasia
- i. sclerosing bronchioloalveolar tumor (IVBAT)
- i. space

intravenous
- botulism immune globulin i. (human)
- i. glucose tolerance test (IVGTT)
- i. hyperalimentation (IVH)

intravenous (*continued*)
  i. leiomyomatosis (IVL)
  i. tolbutamide tolerance test
    (IVTTT)
intraventricular
  i. conduction defect (IVCD)
  i. hemorrhage (IVH)
intravital
  i. microscopy
  i. stain
intra vitam necrosis
intrinsic
  i. asthma
  i. factor (IF)
  i. factor antibody
  i. factor concentrate (IFC)
  i. pathway
  i. semiconductor
  i. system
  i. tyrosine kinase
**Introl CF Panel I Control DNA quality
  control material**
intron
intron-exon distribution
introversion
intumesce
intumescence
intumescent
intussusception
  colic i.
  double i.
  ileal i.
  ileocecal i.
  ileocolic i.
  jejunogastric i.
  retrograde i.
intussusceptive growth
intussusceptum
intussuscipiens
Inuit traditional food
inulin clearance
inundation fever
InV
  InV allotype
  InV group antigen
invaccination
invadens
  Trichomaris i.
invagination
  plasmalemmal i.
invariant chain
invasin
invasion
  angiolymphatic i.
  benign pheochromocytoma with
    histological i. (BPCHI)
  early i.
  lymphatic vessel i. (LVI)
  lymphovascular i.

  lymphovascular space i. (LVSI)
  melanomatous follicular i.
  regulator of i.
  Rosen criteria for lymphovascular i.
  stage of i.
  stromal i.
  vascular i. (VI)
invasive
  i. activity test (IAT)
  i. aspergillosis
  i. ductal carcinoma
  i. fibrous thyroiditis
  i. implant
  i. lobular carcinoma
  i. mole
  i. papillary carcinoma
  i. squamous cell carcinoma (ISCC)
invasiveness
invermination
inverse anaphylaxis
inverse-square law
inversion
  carbohydrate i.
  chromosomal i.
  heterobrachial i.
  i. of uterus
  overlapping i.
  visceral i.
inversus
  dextrocardia with situs i.
  situs i.
invertase
inverted
  i. follicular keratosis
  i. papilloma
  i. repeat
  i. testis
inverter
inverting enzyme
invert sugar
investigation
  crime scene i.
  CSF morphologic i.
investing tissue
invisible differentiation
invisus
  Dialister i.
Invitrogen TA cloning kit
invocatus
  Brevibacillus i.
involucre (*var. of* involucrum)
involucrin
involucrum, involucre
involuntary muscle
involution
  i. cyst
  i. form
  senile i.
involutus

I

involvement
 central nervous system i.
 focal i.
 lymph node i.
 nodal i.
 NSLN i.
I/O
 intake and output
 I/O device
io
 Automeris i.
IOBeads magnetic beads
Iodamoeba
 I. butschlii
 I. williamsi
iodate
 potassium i.
 i. reaction of epinephrine
iodemia
iodic acid
iodide
 i. assay
 bismuth i.
 potassium mercuric i.
 propidium i.
 radioactive i. (RAI)
 saturated solution of potassium i.
 (SSKI)
 sodium i.
 i. transport defect
iodimetry
iodinated
 i. human serum albumin (IHSA)
 i. macroaggregated albumin
 (IMAA)
 i. thyroglobulin
iodine
 butanol-extractable i. (BEI)
 i. cyst
 i. deficiency
 i. escape peak
 gram i.
 Lugol i.
 i. mumps
 i. number
 i. overload
 plasma inorganic i. (PII)
 propidium i. (PI)
 protein-bound i. (PBI)
 radioactive i. (RAI)
 i. reaction of epinephrine
 serum precipitable i. (SPI)
 serum protein-bound i. (SPBI)
 i. solution
 i. stain
 i. staining
 i. test
 tincture of i.
 i. value

iodine-123 (^{123}I)
iodine-125 (^{125}I)
iodine-127 (^{127}I)
iodine-131 (^{131}I)
 i.-1. thyroid metastatic survey
 i.-1. uptake test
iodine-132 (^{132}I)
iodine-azide test (IAT)
iodine-131-6 beta
 iodomethyl-19-norcholesterol
iodinism
iodinophil, iodinophile
iodinophile (*var. of* iodinophil)
iodinophilous
iodobismuthate
iodochlorhydroxyquin
iodocholesterol
iododeoxyuridine (IDU, IUDR)
5-iododeoxyuridine
iododerma
iodomethyl-19-norcholesterol
 iodine-131-6 beta i.-19-n.
iodometric
iodometry
iodophil granule
iodophilia
iodophor
iodoplatinate
iodotyrosine deiodinase defect
ioduria
IOFB
 intraocular foreign body
iometer
ion
 alkoxide i.
 bicarbonate i.
 calcium i. (Ca2+)
 carbonium i.
 carboxylate i.
 i. channel
 i. concentration
 i. counter
 dipolar i.
 i. disorder
 gram i.
 hydrogen i.
 hydronium i.
 hydroxide i.
 magnesium i. (Mg2+)
 i. microscope
 oxonium i.
 i. pair
ion-exchange
 i.-e. chromatography
 i.-e. column
 i.-e. resin
ionic
 i. bond
 i. charge

ionic (*continued*)
    i. concentration
    i. strength
ionization
    avalanche i.
    i. chamber
    i. constant
    i. interference
    specific i.
ionize
ionized
    i. calcium
    i. calcium assay
ionizing
    i. chamber instrument
    i. radiation
ionogram
ionopherogram
ionophore
ion-selective electrode (ISE)
iontophoresis
    pilocarpine nitrate i.
IOPath immunohistochemistry reagent
iota
    Clostridium perfringens enterotoxin
      i. (CPI)
IOTest monoclonal antibody
IP
    immunoperoxidase
    incubation period
    inosine phosphorylase
    interphalangeal
    isoelectric point
IPA
    isopropyl alcohol
IPC
    intraductal papillary carcinoma
IPD
    inflammatory pelvic disease
IP3 dependent calcium fluctuation
IPE
    individual protective equipment
IPF
    idiopathic pulmonary fibrosis
    intramural protruding form
IPH
    idiopathic pulmonary hemosiderosis
IPHP
    inflammatory papillary hyperplasia of
    the palate
i(12p) marker chromosome
IPMN
    intraductal papillary mucinous neoplasia
IPMT
    intraductal papillary mucinous tumor
IPNM
    intraductal papillary mucinous neoplasia
Ipomoea
Ipomovirus

IPPS
    International Prostate Symptom Score
iproniazid
IPS
    initial prognostic score
ipsefact
IPSID
    immunoproliferative small intestinal
    disease
ipsilateral intraductal carcinoma
IPSS
    International Prostate Symptom Score
IPT
    immunoperoxidase technique
    immunoprecipitation
IPV
    inactivated poliovirus vaccine
IR
    immunoreactive
    internal resistance
Ir
    immune response
iranensis
    Cellulomonas i.
IRC
    inspiratory reserve capacity
IRDS
    idiopathic respiratory distress syndrome
IRF
    idiopathic retroperitoneal fibrosis
IRF1
    interferon regulatory factor 1
IRG
    immunoreactive glucagon
IRHCS
    immunoradioassayable human chorionic
    somatomammotropin
IRhGH
    immunoreactive human growth
    hormone
IRI
    immunoreactive insulin
iridescent virus
iridica
    stella lentis i.
iridis
    ligamentum pectinatum i.
    stratum pigmenti i.
    stroma i.
iridium
iridocapsulitis
iridochoroiditis
iridocorneal endothelial syndrome (ICE)
iridocornealis
    spatia anguli i.
iridocyclitis
    heterochromic i.
    i. septica
iridokeratitis

Iridoviridae
Iridovirus
iris
>   erythema i.
>   i. frill
>   herpes i.

iritis
IRM
>   idiopathic retractile mesenteritis

IRMA
>   immunoradiometric assay

iron (Fe)
>   i. assay
>   bound serum i. (BSI)
>   i. broth
>   decreased serum i.
>   i. deficiency anemia (IDA)
>   i. deposit
>   ferric i.
>   ferrous i.
>   i. hematoxylin
>   i. hematoxylin stain
>   high serum-bound i. (HBI)
>   histologically detectable i. (HDI)
>   impaired utilization of i.
>   i. index
>   low serum-bound i. (LBI)
>   i. overload
>   i. plasma clearance
>   i. protein
>   serum i. (SI)
>   i. stain
>   stainable i.
>   triple sugar i.

iron-binding
>   i.-b. capacity (IBC)
>   i.-b. capacity test

iron-positive pigment demonstration
iron-storage disease
iron-sulfide protein
Irpex
irradiated
>   i. casualty
>   i. CPD blood

irradiation
>   contamination i.
>   i. CVS/CNS syndrome
>   i. damage
>   i. esophagitis
>   external i.
>   i. hematopoietic syndrome
>   incorporation of i.
>   ultraviolet i.
>   ultraviolet blood i. (UBI)

irreducible hernia
irregular
>   i. border colony
>   i. fried egg morphology
>   i. margin

irregularis
>   *Cephaliophora i.*

irreversible
>   i. coma
>   i. damage
>   i. reaction

irreversibly sickled cell (ISC)
irrigation
>   Ringer i.

irritability
irritable
>   i. bowel syndrome
>   i. colon (IC)

irritans
>   *Pulex i.*
>   *Siphona i.*

irritant
>   primary i.

irritation
>   i. cell
>   i. fibroma

irritative lesion
irruption
irruptive
IRS
>   infrared spectrophotometry

IRSA
>   idiopathic refractory sideroblastic
>   anemia

IRV
>   inspiratory reserve volume

Irvine syndrome
IS
>   insufficient signal
>   IS gene
>   mucopolysaccharidosis type IS

Isaacson gastric lymphoma
classification
Isambert disease
Isamine blue
Isaria
Isavirus
ISC
>   irreversibly sickled cell

ISCC
>   invasive squamous cell carcinoma

ischemia
>   basilar artery i.
>   gastrointestinal i.
>   mesenteric i.
>   mucosal i.
>   myocardial i. (MI)
>   i. retinae
>   small bowel i.
>   transient cerebral i. (TCI)

ischemic
>   i. bowel disease
>   i. colitis
>   i. contracture

ischemic (*continued*)
    i. encephalopathy
    i. heart disease (IHD)
    i. hepatitis
    i. hypoxia
    i. leg disease (ILD)
    i. limb disease (ILD)
    i. muscular atrophy
    i. necrosis
ischial tuberosity
ischiopagus
ischiorectal abscess
ISCOM
    immune-stimulating complex
ISCP
    infection surveillance and control
      program
ISE
    ion-selective electrode
isethionate
    hydroxystilbamidine i.
ISH
    icteric serum hepatitis
    in situ hybridization
    EBER ISH
ishikariensis
    Asanoa i.
Ishikawa cell line
ISI
    International Sensitivity Index
ISIS
    Infectious Disease Surveillance
    Information System
island
    blood i.
    bony i.
    CpG i.
    i. disease
    erythroblastic i.
    i. fever
    Langerhans i.'s
    i.'s of Calleja
    i.'s of Langerhans
    i.'s of pancreas
islandicus
    Ignicoccus i.
    Thermodesulfovibrio i.
island-sparing
    i.-s. plaque
    i.-s. plaques
islet
    i. alpha cell
    i. amyloid polypeptide
    i. beta cell
    i. cell adenoma
    i. cell antibody (ICA)
    i. cell antibody screening test
    i. cell carcinoma
    i. cell focal fibrosis

    i. cell hyperinsulinism
    i. cell hyperplasia
    i. cell tumor
    delta cell i.
    i. delta cell
    i. hormone
    i.'s of Calleja
    i.'s of Langerhans
    i. tissue
ISO
    International Standards Organization
    isoenzyme
isoagglutination
isoagglutinin
isoagglutinogen
isoallele
isoallelism
isoallotypic determinant
isoalloxazine
isoanaphylaxis
isoantibody
    platelet i.
isoantigen
    Rh i.
Isobaculum melis
isobar
isobaric
isobuteine
isobutyl alcohol
isobutyric acid
isocellular
isochromatic
isochromatid
    i. break
    i. gap
isochromatophil, isochromatophile
isochromatophile (*var. of*
  isochromatophil)
isochromic anemia
isochromosome
isochronal rhythm
isochronous
isochrous
isocitrate
    i. dehydrogenase
    i. dehydrogenase assay
    i. dehydrogenase test
isocitric
    i. acid
    i. dehydrogenase
IsoCode Stix device
isocortex
isocyanate
isocytolysin
isodactylism
isodesmosine
isodisomy
isoelectric
    i. focusing (IEF)

i. focusing electrophoresis
i. level
i. point
isoenzyme, isozyme
    i. A
    A or B i. of G6PD
    alkaline phosphatase i.
    cerebrospinal fluid lactate
      dehydrogenase i.'s
    creatine kinase i.
    i. electrophoresis
    lactate dehydrogenase i.
    PKC i.
    protein kinase C i.
    Regan i.
    skeletal muscle component of
      cardiac i.'s (MM)
isoerythrolysis
    neonatal i.
isoferritin
    acidic i.
isoflow
    volume of i.
isoform
    beta i.
    Cbfal/Runx2 i.
    epsilon i.
    eta i.
    sigma i.
    zeta i.
isogamy
isogeneic, isogenic
    i. graft
isogenic (*var. of* isogeneic)
isogenous
    i. chondrocyte
    i. group
    i. nest
isograft
isohemagglutination
isohemagglutinin
isohemolysin
isohemolysis
isohydric shift
isohydruria
isohypercytosis
isohypocytosis
isoimmune
    i. antibody
    i. hemolytic anemia
    i. neonatal
    i. neonatal purpura
    i. neonatal thrombocytopenia
isolate
    Towne CMV low passage
      clinical i.
isolated
    i. cleft palate
    i. dextrocardia

    i. dyskeratosis follicularis
    i. gland carcinoma in situ
      (GCIS)
    i. levocardia
    i. parietal endocarditis
    i. proteinuria
    i. sinistrocardia
isolation
    body substance i. (BSI)
    CMV i.
    cytomegalovirus i.
    herpes simplex virus i.
    HSV i.
    i. of nucleic acid
    postexposure i.
Isolator
    I. blood culture system
    I. lysis-centrifugation
      tube
isolectin B4
isoleucine
    urine i.
isoleucyl
isoleucyl-RNA synthetase
isoleukoagglutinin
**Isolex 300i magnetic cell selection
system**
isologous
    i. chimera
    i. graft
isolysin
isolysis
isolytic
isomaltase
isomastigote
isomer
    optical i.
isomerase
    glucosephosphate i.
    hexosephosphate i.
    triosephosphate i.
isomeric transition (IT)
isomerism
    chain i.
    dynamic i.
    functional group i.
    geometric i.
    nuclear i.
    optical i.
    position i.
    spatial i.
    stereochemical i.
    structural i.
isomerization
isometric
isomicrogamete
isomorphic response
isomorphous gliosis
isomuscarine

isoniazid
    i. assay
    i. phenotype test
isonicotinic acid hydrazide
isonormocytosis
isoolomoucine
isoosmolar
isoosmotic
Isopaque
Isoparorchis trisimilitubis
isopathy
isopentane-dry ice bath
isopentane fixative/solution
isophagy
isophil antibody
isophile antigen
isoplastic graft
isopleth
isoprecipitin
isoprene
isoprenoid
isopropanol
    i. assay
    i. precipitation test
isopropyl alcohol (IPA)
Isoptericola variabilis
isopyknic
isopyknotic
isosbestic point
isosensitize
isoserum treatment
isosexual pseudoprecocity
isosmotic
Isospora
    I. belli
    I. bigemina
    I. canis
    I. felis
    I. hominis
    I. rivolta
    I. suis
isosporiasis
isosthenuria
isosulfan blue
isothermal
isothiocyanate
    fluorescein i. (FITC)
    tetramethylrhodamine i.
      (XRITC)
isotone
isotonic
    i. coefficient
    i. hyponatremia
    i. sodium chloride solution
isotope dilution-mass
  spectrometry
isotopic dilution
isotransplantation
isotropic disc

isotype switching
isotypic
isovaleric acid
isovalericacidemia, isovaleric
  acidemia
isovaleryl-CoA dehydrogenase
isovolumic contraction (IC)
isozyme (*var. of* isoenzyme)
israelensis
    Chromohalobacter i.
israelii
    Actinomyces i.
issachenkonii
    Pseudoalteromonas i.
Issatchenkia orientalis
IST
    insulin sensitivity test
    insulin shock therapy
isthmi (*pl. of* isthmus)
isthmus, *pl.* isthmi, isthmuses
    His i.
isthmuses (*pl. of* isthmus)
ISUB
    immunosubtraction
ISUP
    International Society for Urological
      Pathology
ISW
    interstitial water
IT
    implantation test
    intradermal test
    intratumoral
    isomeric transition
itai-itai disease
italicus
    Enterococcus i.
ITAM
    immunoreceptor tyrosine activation
      motif
Itaqui virus
ITAS
    internal telomerase standard
itch
    barber's i.
    Cuban i.
    dhobie i.
    grain i.
    jock i.
    mad i.
    Malabar i.
    prairie i.
    swimmer's i.
    winter i.
iteration
iterative process
Iteravirus
ITI
    inter-alpha-trypsin inhibitor

ITIM
>immunoreceptor tyrosine inhibitory motif

ITLC
>instant thin-layer chromatography

Ito
>I. cell
>hypomelanosis of I. (HI, HMI)
>I. nevus

Ito-Reenstierna test

ITP
>idiopathic thrombocytopenic purpura

I-TRAC Plus transfusion system

ITT
>insulin tolerance test

i-tumor
>intratumoral

IU
>immunizing unit
>international unit

IUD
>intrauterine contraceptive device

IUDR
>iododeoxyuridine

IUFB
>intrauterine foreign body

IUFD
>intrauterine fetal death
>>fetal karyotyping in mid-trimester I.

IUGR
>intrauterine growth rate

IUM
>intrauterine malnutrition

^{131}I uptake test
>iodine-131
>radioactive iodine

IVAP
>in vivo adhesive platelet

IVBAT
>intravascular sclerosing bronchioloalveolar tumor

IVCC
>intravascular consumption coagulopathy

IVCD
>intraventricular conduction defect

Ivemark syndrome

IVGTT
>intravenous glucose tolerance test

IVH
>intravenous hyperalimentation
>intraventricular hemorrhage

IVL
>intravenous leiomyomatosis

IVM
>intravascular mass

ivory exostosis

IVSD
>interventricular septal defect

IVT
>intrauterine fetal transfusion

IVTT
>in vitro transcription/translation
>IVTT assay

IVTTT
>intravenous tolbutamide tolerance test

Ivy
>I. bleeding time test
>I. method
>I. method of bleeding time
>I. template bleeding time

IWMI
>inferior wall myocardial infarction

Ixodes
>*I. bicornis*
>*I. cavipalpus*
>*I. cookei*
>*I. dammini*
>*I. frequens*
>*I. holocyclus*
>*I. pacificus*
>*I. persulcatus*
>*I. rasus*
>*I. ricinus*
>*I. scapularis*
>*I. spinipalpis*

ixodiasis

ixodic

ixodid

Ixodidae

Ixodoidea

J

joule
J chain
hemoglobin J
J receptor
Jaa antigen
Jaa-F11 antigen
jaagsiekte sheep retrovirus
Ja antigen
Jab1
Jun activation domain binding protein 1
Jaccoud
J. arthritis
J. arthropathy
J. syndrome
jacketed high-velocity round
jacksonian epilepsy
Jackson syndrome
Jacobsson method
Jacod syndrome
Jacquemin test
Jadassohn
cyst of J.
J. nevus
Jadassohn-Lewandowski syndrome
Jadassohn-Tièche nevus
jadensis
Alcanivorax j.
Fundibacter j.
Jaffe
J. assay
J. reaction
J. test
Jaffe-Campanacci syndrome
Jaffe-Lichtenstein disease
Jagged1 gene
Jahnke syndrome
jail fever
JAK kinase
Jakob-Creutzfeldt (JC)
J.-C. disease
J.-C. pseudosclerosis
Jakob disease
Jaksch disease
jalaludinii
Mitsuokella j.
Jamaican vomiting sickness
Jamestown Canyon virus
jamilae
Paenibacillus j.
Jamshidi needle
Janet disease
Janeway lesion

Janibacter
J. brevis
J. terrae
janiceps
Jannaschia
J. cystaugens
J. helgolandensis
jannaschii
Thialkalivibrio j.
Jansen disease
Jansky-Bielschowsky disease
Jansky human blood group classification
Janus green B
Japanese
J. B encephalitis (JBE)
J. B encephalitis virus
J. river fever
japonica
Amycolatopsis j.
encephalitis j.
Hirudo j.
Rickettsia j.
Shewanella j.
Tetrasphaera j.
japonicum
Pseudospirillum j.
Rhizobium j.
Schistosoma j.
japonicus
Cellvibrio j.
Debaromyces j.
Thermosipho j.
jar
anaerobic j.
Coplin j.
Jarisch-Herxheimer reaction
Jass staging system
Jatlow-Nadim procedure
Jatropha kurcas
jaundice
acholuric j.
acute febrile j.
black j.
catarrhal j.
cholestatic j.
chronic acholuric j.
chronic familial j.
chronic idiopathic j.
congenital familial nonhemolytic j.
congenital hemolytic j.
familial nonhemolytic j.
hematogenous j.
hemolytic j.
hepatocellular j.
hepatogenous j.

J

jaundice (*continued*)
    homologous serum j.
    leptospiral j.
    malignant j.
    mechanical j.
    nonhemolytic j.
    nonobstructive j.
    obstructive j.
    regurgitation j.
    retention j.
    spherocytic j.
    toxemic j.
javensis
    Streptomyces j.
jaw
    fibrous dysplasia of j.
    lumpy j.
    progonoma of j.
Jaworski
    J. body
    J. corpuscle
    J. test
JAZF1 gene infusion
JBE
    Japanese B encephalitis
JCapetown
JCML
    juvenile chronic myelogenous
    leukemia
jeanselmei
    Exophiala j.
    Fonsecaea j.
Jeanselme nodule
Jeghers-Peutz syndrome
jeikeium
    Corynebacterium j.
jejuense
    Clostridium j.
jejuensis
    Kribbella j.
jejuni
    Campylobacter j.
jejunitis cystica profunda
jejunogastric intussusception
jejunoileitis
jejunostomy
Jellison
    Francisella tularensis biovar J. type
      A, B
jelly
    Wharton j.
**JEM-100CX electron
microscope**
Jendrassik-Grof method
jenensis
    Oerskovia j.
Jenner
    J. method
    J. stain

Jenner-Giemsa stain
Jenner-Kay unit
Jensen
    J. disease
    J. sarcoma
    J. trochanteric fracture
      classification
jensenii
    Lactobacillus j.
    Propionibacterium j.
Jeol
    J. 100 S transmission electron
      microscope
    J. 1200 transmission electron
      microscope
jeotgali
    Bacillus j.
    Psychrobacter j.
Jeotgalibacillus alimentarius
Jeotgalicoccus
    J. halotolerans
    J. pinnipedialis
    J. psychrophilus
Jerne
    J. plaque assay
    J. technique
**Jervell and Lange-Nielsen
syndrome**
Jessner lymphocytic infiltrate
jet lesion
Jeune syndrome
Jewett
    J. and Strong staging
    J. bladder carcinoma
    J. bladder carcinoma classification
      [O, A, B, C, D]
jeyporiensis
    Anopheles j.
JGCT
    juvenile granulosa cell tumor
    juxtaglomerular cell tumor
JGI
    juxtaglomerular granulation index
**J6-HC, J6-MC, J6-MI high capacity
centrifuge**
JH virus
jigger
Jimson weed
jinjuensis
    Pseudomonas j.
jiroveci
    Pneumocystis j.
Jk antigen
JM
    juxtamembrane
JMML
    juvenile myelomonocytic
    leukemia
Jobbins antigen

Job syndrome
jock itch
Jod-Basedow phenomenon
Joest body
johannae
    Gluconacetobacter j.
Johne
    J. bacillus
    J. disease
johnin
Johns Hopkins Center for Civilian Biodefense Studies
Johnson-Dubin syndrome
Johnsonella ignava
johnsonii
    Hyphomonas j.
Johnson-Steven disease
joint
    j. adhesion
    j. calculus
    j. capsule
    Clutton j.
    j. disease
    j. effusion
    j. oil
    J. Task Force for Civil Support (of the Defense Department)
jointed bamboo-rod cellular appearance
Joklik buffer
Jolles test
Jolly body
Jones
    Bence J. (BJ)
    J. methenamine silver stain
    J. method
Jones-Cantarow test
Jonesiaceae
Jonesia dentrificans
Jones-Mote reaction
joostei
    Chryseobacterium j.
Jordan anomaly
jordanis
    Legionella j.
Jores fixative
Joseph syndrome
jostii
    Rhodococcus j.
joule (J)
    J. law
Jourdain disease
journal
    telehealth j.
JRA
    juvenile rheumatoid arthritis
Js antigen
J-sella deformity

J-series prostaglandin
juccuya
Judet epiphysial fracture
jugular gland
juice
    cancer j.
jumbo biopsy
jump
    conditional j.
    unconditional j.
jumper
jumping
    j. disease
    j. gene
Jun activation domain binding protein 1 (Jab1)
juncea
    Filaria j.
junction
    adhering j.
    j. capacitor
    cell j.
    cervical-vaginal j.
    choledochoduodenal j.
    communicating j.
    corneoscleral j.
    corticomedullary j.
    dermal epidermal j.
    electrotonic j.
    esophagogastric j.
    fibronexus j.
    j. field effect transistor
    gap j.
    impermeable j.
    intercellular j.
    intermediate j.
    mucocutaneous j.
    muscle-tendon j.
    myoneural j.
    neuromuscular j.
    j. nevus
    occipitoatlantoaxial j.
    j. potential
    sclerocorneal j.
    squamocolumnar j. (SCJ)
    tight j. (TJ)
    ureteropelvic j.
junctional
    j. complex
    j. cyst
    j. epidermolysis bullosa
    j. epithelium
    j. expansion nodule
    j. nevus
Jung
    J. Autostainer XL
    J. CV 5000 Robotic Coverslipper
    J. muscle
jungle yellow fever

J

Jüngling disease
Junin virus
justifiable abortion
justify
juvenile
    j. angiofibroma
    j. carcinoma
    j. cell
    j. cerebellar astrocytoma
    j. chronic myelogenous leukemia
    (JCML)
    j. cirrhosis
    j. diabetes mellitus
    j. elastoma
    j. fibroadenoma
    j. granulosa cell tumor (JGCT)
    j. hemangiofibroma
    j. hemochromatosis
    j. hormone
    j. hyalin fibromatosis
    j. kyphosis
    j. melanoma
    j. myelomonocytic leukemia
    (JMML)
    j. neutrophil
    j. ossifying fibroma
    j. osteoporosis
    j. Paget disease
    j. palmoplantar fibromatosis
    j. papillomatosis
    j. pernicious anemia
    j. pilocytic astrocytoma
    j. polyp
    j. polyposis coli
    j. polyposis syndrome
    j. rheumatoid arthritis (JRA)
    j. SMA
    j. xanthogranuloma (JXG)
    j. xanthoma
juvenile-onset diabetes
juvenilis
    hyperostosis corticalis deformans j.
    osteochondritis deformans j.
    verruca plana j.
juxtaarticular nodule
juxtacortical
    j. chondroma
    j. osteogenic sarcoma
juxtaglomerular
    j. apparatus
    j. body
    j. cell
    j. cell tumor (JGCT)
    j. complex
    j. granulation index (JGI)
    j. granule
juxtamedullary
juxtamembrane (JM)
juxtanuclear Golgi reactivity
juxtaoral organ of Chievitz
juxtapapillaris
    retinochoroiditis j.
juxtapulmonary-capillary receptor
juxtatumoral stroma
JXG
    juvenile xanthogranuloma

K
Kell blood group
kelvin
lysine
potassium
K and k antigen
K antigen
K cell
proteinase K
K virus

k
constant
kelvin temperature scale

KA
ketoacidosis

Kabatiella
Kabatina
kabure
Kaes
K. feltwork
K. line
Kaes-Bekhterev
K.-B. band
K.-B. layer
K.-B. stripe
Kaffir pox
Kahlbaum disease
Kahler
K. disease
K. law
Kahn test
kaikoae
Psychromonas k.
kainate receptor
Kaiserling
K. fixative
K. method
K. solution
kala azar
kalemia
kaliopenia
kaliopenic
Kalischer disease
kalium
kaliuresis
kaliuretic
kallidin
kallikrein
human k. 2 (hK2)
human k. 3 (hK3)
human glandular k. 3
plasma k.
k. system
kallikrein-inhibiting unit (KIU)
Kallmann syndrome

kaluresis
kaluretic
Kamino body
Kanagawa phenomenon
kanaloae
Vibrio k.
kanamycin
Kandinskii-Clerambault syndrome
kanei
Trichophyton k.
Kangiella
K. aquimarina
K. koreensis
kangri
k. burn carcinoma
k. cancer
Kanner syndrome
Kansas
Hb K.
hemoglobin K.
kansasii
Mycobacterium k.
kaodzera
kaolin
k. partial thromboplastin time (KPTT)
k. pneumoconiosis
kaolin-clotting time
kaolinosis
Kapetanakis purpura
Kaplan-Meier staining method
Kaposi
K. sarcoma
K. sarcoma-like granuloma
K. varicelliform eruption
kaposiform
kappa
k. chain specificity
k. granule
k. light chain
k. opioid receptor (KOR)
karajensis
Halobacillus k.
Karapandzic lip reconstruction flap
32 Karat software for HPLC
Karmen unit (KU)
Karnofsky status
Karnovsky
K. fixative
K. II solution
Kartagener syndrome
kartulisi
Entamoeba k.
karwari
Anopheles k.

K

karyochrome cell
karyoclasis
karyocyte
karyogamy
karyogonad
karyokinesis
karyology
karyolymph
karyolysis
karyolytic
karyomere
karyomicrosome
karyomitome
karyomorphism
karyon
karyophage
karyoplasm
karyoplasmolysis
karyoplast
karyoplastin
karyopyknosis
karyopyknotic index (KI)
karyorrhectic nuclear debris
karyorrhexis
karyostasis
karyotheca
karyotype
    k. aberration
    numerical k.
    spectral k.
    X k.
    XO k.
    XX k.
    XXX k.
    XXY k.
    XY k.
    XYY k.
karyotyping
    digital k.
    spectral k.
karyozoic
Kasabach-Merritt syndrome
Kashin-Bek disease
Kasten
    K. fluorescent Feulgen stain
    K. fluorescent PAS stain
    K. fluorescent Schiff reagent
Kast syndrome
kat
    katal
katacalcin peptide
katal (kat)
Katayama
    K. fever
    K. test
katharometer
Kato thick smear technique
katsuradai
    Heterophyes k.

Katzenstein and Peiper criteria
KAU
    King-Armstrong unit
Kauffman-White Salmonella serotype
  classification
kaustophilus
    Geobacillus k.
Kawasaki disease
kayaii
Kayser disease
Kayser-Fleischer ring
KB
    ketone body
kbp
    kilobase pair
kc
    kilocycle
kcal
    kilocalorie
K-capture
    electron K-c.
KC1 Delta coagulation
  analyzer
KCl
    potassium chloride
KCN
    potassium cyanide
kcps
    kilocycles per second
kDa
    kilodalton
KD antigen
KE
    kinetic energy
Kearns-Sayre syndrome
Kearns syndrome
kedani
    k. disease
    k. fever
    k. mite
K3 EDTA
    menadione
kefirgranum
    Lactobacillus kefiranofaciens subsp.
      k.
Keissleriella
Keith bundle
Keith-Wagener-Barker (KWB)
Keith-Wagener retinal changes
  classification
Kelev strain rabies virus
Kell
    K. antigen
    K. blood group (K)
    K. blood group system
    K. body antibody type
    K. HDN
Kell-Cellano blood group
kellicotti

kellyi
>*Halothiobacillus k.*

keloid
>Addison k.

keloidalis
>folliculitis k.

keloidosis
kelosomia
kelvin (K)
>k. temperature scale (k)
>k. thermometer

Kendall Company Telfa pad
Kennedy syndrome
Kent bundle
Kent-His bundle
kentuckyensis
>*Amycolatopsis k.*

Kenya tick fever
kerasin histiocytosis
keratan sulfate
keratiasis
keratic
keratin
>k. cocktail
>k. filament
>k. immunostaining
>k. pearl
>k. polypeptide
>k. stain
>k. staining
>k. whorl
>wide-spectrum k.

keratiniphila
>*Amycolatopsis k.*
>*Amycolatopsis keratiniphila*
>subsp. *k.*

keratinization
>metaplastic k.

keratinize
keratinized cell
keratinizing
>k. invasive squamous cell carcinoma
>(KISCC)
>k. squamous cell carcinoma
>(KSCC)

keratinocyte
>apoptotic k.
>k. growth factor 2 (KGF2)

keratinophilic
keratinosome
keratinous cyst
keratitic precipitate (KP)
keratitis
>*Acanthamoeba k.*
>acne rosacea k.
>k. bullosa
>k. disciformis
>herpetic k.
>interstitial k.

mycotic k.
reticular k.
sclerosing k.
serpiginous k.
suppurative k.
vascular k.
vesicular k.
zonular k.

keratoacanthoma
keratoacanthosis
keratoangioma
keratoatrophoderma
keratoconjunctivitis
>chronic follicular k.
>epidemic k. (EKC)
>herpetic k.
>k. sicca
>superior limbic k.
>(SLKC)
>virus k.

keratoconus posticus circumscriptus
keratocyst
>odontogenic k. (OKC)

keratocyte
keratoderma
>k. acquisitum
>k. blennorrhagica
>k. climactericum
>k. eccentrica
>lymphedematous k.
>mutilating k.
>k. palmaris et plantaris
>k. plantare sulcatum
>punctate k.
>senile k.
>k. symmetrica

keratodermatitis
keratodes
>erythema k.

keratohyalin
>k. granule
>k. granule of epidermis

keratohyaline alteration
keratohyalin-like granule
keratoid
keratolysis exfoliativa
keratolytic
keratoma
>k. disseminatum
>k. hereditarium mutilans
>k. plantare sulcatum
>senile k.

keratomalacia
keratomycosis
keratonosis
keratopathy
>band k.

keratoplasia
keratose

keratosis
actinic k.
arsenic k.
arsenical k.
k. blennorrhagica
clonal seborrheic k.
k. diffusa fetalis
follicular inverted k.
k. follicularis
follicularis k.
inverted follicular k.
lichenoid k.
nevus follicularis k.
k. nigricans
k. palmaris et plantaris
pilaris k.
preexisting actinic k.
k. punctata
k. rubra figurata
seborrheic k.
k. seborrheica
senile k.
k. senilis
solar k.
tar k.
k. vegetans
keratotic
k. micaceous balanitis
k. papilloma
Kerckring
K. fold
K. valve
kerion
Celsus k.
tinea k.
Kerley A, B lines
Kernia
kernicterus
Kernig meningeal sign
Kernohan
K. malignant astrocytoma grading
K. notch
kern-plasma relation theory
keroid
Kerstersia gyiorum
kerstersii
Comamonas k.
Keshan disease
kestanbolensis
Anoxybacillus k.
ketal
ketimine
aminoethylcysteine k.
keto
k. acid
k. group
ketoacidosis (KA)
alcoholic k.

diabetic k. (DKA)
starvation k.
ketoaciduria
branched chain k.
ketoconazole
Keto-Diastix urine ketone and glucose test
keto-enol tautomer
ketogenesis
ketogenic
k. amino acid
k. corticoid test
k. hormone
k. steroid (KGS)
17-ketogenic
l.-k. steroid
l.-k. steroids assay
ketogenic/antiketogenic ratio
ketoglutarate
alpha k.
Ketogulonicigenium
K. robustum
K. vulgare
ketohexokinase
ketohexose
ketone
k. body (KB)
k. body formation
k. body test
k. body utilization
dimethyl k.
methyl butyl k.
methyl ethyl k. (MEK)
methyl isobutyl k.
ketonemia
ketonimine dye
ketonuria
branched chain k.
ketopentose
ketose
ketosis
ketosteroid (KS)
17-ketosteroid
l.-k. assay
l.-k. fractionation
Ketostix
ketosuria
ketotic hyperglycinemia
ketotransferase
ketotriose
Ketron-Goodman pagetoid reticulosis
Kety-Schmidt method
keV
kiloelectron volt
key
k. enzyme
k. vein
keyhole-limpet hemocyanin (KLH)

KFAB, KFAb
    kidney-fixing antibody
KFD
    Kikuchi-Fujimoto disease
KFS
    Klippel-Feil syndrome
kg
    kilogram
kg-cal
    kilogram-calorie
KGF2
    keratinocyte growth factor 2
KGS
    ketogenic steroid
Khuskia
kHz
    kilohertz
KI
    karyopyknotic index
Ki-1
    Ki-1 antibody
    Ki-1 antigen
Ki-67
    Ki-67 antibody
    Ki-67 antigen
    growth fraction with Ki-67
    Ki-67 immunohistochemical
      well-differentiated gastric carcinoma
      analysis
    Ki-67 immunophenotypic marker
    Ki-67 index
    Ki-67 oncogene
    Ki-67 positive cell
    Ki-67 protein
KIA
    Kliger iron agar
Kibra gene
Kidd
    K. antigen
    K. blood antibody type
    K. blood group
    K. blood group system
kidney
    amyloid k.
    Armanni-Ebstein k.
    arteriolosclerotic k.
    arteriosclerotic k.
    artificial k. (AK)
    Ask-Upmark k.
    atrophic k.
    k. biopsy
    cake k.
    k. cancer
    k. carbuncle
    clear cell sarcoma of the k.
      (CCSK)
    contracted k.
    k. cortex
    cow k.

    crush k.
    cystic k.
    disc k.
    doll's k.
    duplex k.
    dwarf k.
    fatty k.
    flea-bitten k.
    Formad k.
    fused k.
    Goldblatt k.
    granular k.
    guinea pig k. (GPK)
    horseshoe k.
    human embryo k. (HEK)
    human embryonic k. (HEK)
    hydroxylation k.
    malignant rhabdoid tumor of k.
      (MRTK)
    maximal tubular excretory capacity
      of k.'s (T_m)
    medullary sponge k.
    monkey k. (MK)
    mortar k.
    multicystic dysplasia of k. (MCDK)
    multicystic dysplastic k. (MCDK)
    multilocular cystic k.
    nonrotation of k.
    primary African green monkey k.
      (PAGMK)
    k. profile
    putty k.
    pyelonephritic k.
    rabbit k.
    rhabdoid tumor of the k. (RTK)
    rhesus monkey k. (RMK)
    Rose-Bradford k.
    sclerotic k.
    k. stone analysis
    supernumerary k.
    k. transplant rejection
    waxy k.
kidney-fixing antibody (KFAB)
KidneyScreen
    K. At·Home mail-in test
    K. At·Home testing kit
kielensis
    Ahrensia k.
**Kiel non-Hodgkin lymphoma
  classification**
Kienböck
    K. atrophy
    K. disease
Kiernan space
kieselguhr
Ki-FDC1p antibody
Kikuchi
    K. disease
    K. lymphadenitis

K

Kikuchi-Fujimoto
K.-F. disease (KFD)
K.-F. lymphadenitis
Kilham rat virus
killed
heat k. (HK)
k. measles virus vaccine (KMV)
k. vaccine (KV)
killer
k. cell
k. immunoglobulin-like receptor (KIR)
k. lymphocyte
T-natural k. (TNK)
kilobase pair (kbp)
kilocalorie (kca)
kilocycle (kc)
k.'s per second (kcps)
kilodalton (kDa)
kiloelectron volt (keV)
kilogram (kg)
kilogram-calorie (kg-cal)
kilohertz (kHz)
kilohm
Kiloh-Nevin syndrome
kilojoule (kJ)
kilometer (km)
kilonensis
Pseudomonas k.
kilopascal (kPa)
kiloton (kT)
kilovolt (kV)
k. ampere (kVA)
k. peak (kVp)
kilovoltage
kilowatt (kW)
kilowatt-hour (kWh)
Ki-1+ lymphoma
Kimax glassware
kimchii
Lactobacillus k.
Leuconostoc k.
Weissella k.
Kimex
Kimmelstiel-Wilson
K.-W. disease (KW)
K.-W. lesion
K.-W. nodule
K.-W. syndrome
Ki-M1p antibody
Ki-M4p antibody
Kimura disease
kinase
adenosine k.
adenylate k.
anaplastic lymphoma k. (ALK)
aspartate k.
ATR k.

Bruton tyrosine k. (BTK)
cAMP-dependent protein k.
Chk1 k.
Chk2 k.
conserved helix-loop-helix ubiquitous k. (CHUK)
creatine k. (CK)
cyclin-dependent k. (CDK)
cyclin-dependent k. 5 (CDK5)
cyclin-dependent protein k. 1 (Cdk1)
focal adhesion k. (FAK)
k. inhibitory protein (KIP)
intrinsic tyrosine k.
JAK k.
macrocreatine k.
mitochondrial creatine k. (mtCK)
protein k. C (PKC)
protein k. A
pyruvate k. (PK)
receptor tyrosine k.
Ser-Thr k.
serum creatine k. (SCK)
thymidine k.
k. tyrosine
kind
electrode of first k.
electrode of second k.
kindred
kinematic viscosity
Kineococcus radiotolerans
Kineosphaera limosa
kinetic
k. analyzer
k. energy (KE)
k. measurement
kinetics
cell k.
cellular k.
first-order k.
molecular k.
simulation k. (simkin)
tumor cell k.
zero-order k.
kinetochore
kinetocyte
kinetoplasm
kinetoplast
kinetosome
Kinevac
kingae
Kingella k.
Moraxella k.
King-Armstrong unit (KAU)
Kingella
K. denitrificans
Haemophilus, Actinobacillus, Cardiobacterium, Eikenella, K. (HACEK)

K. *indologenes*
K. *kingae*
king's evil
King unit
kinin
plasma k.
k. system
kininogen
high molecular weight k. (HMWK)
HMW k.
low molecular weight k.
kinky hair disease
Kinnier Wilson disease
kinocentrum
kinocilium
kinoplasm
kinoplasmic
Kinsbourne syndrome
Kinyoun carbolfuchsin stain
KIP
kinase inhibitory protein
KIR
killer immunoglobulin-like receptor
Ki-ras mutation
Kirby-Bauer
K.-B. method
K.-B. test
Kirchoff law
Kiricephalus
Kirkland disease
KIR sequence in NK repertoire
Ki-S5 antibody
KISCC
keratinizing invasive squamous cell
carcinoma
Kisenyi sheep disease virus
kissing disease
kit
A1c At·Home testing k.
active total PSA ELISA k.
adenovirus test k.
Aldecount Progenitor Cell
Enumeration k.
Amersham Life Science PCR
product presequencing k.
Amersham Life Science Thermo
Sequenase sequencing k.
Ana-Sal HIV home test k.
ApopTag Plus k.
Architect AUSAB reagent k.
Asserachrom D-Dimer k.
AxSYM CORE HBV antibody
reagent k.
Babystart fertility test k.
BD-CHEK intestinal inflammation k.
Bindazyme ANA Screening
ELISA k.
Bioshaf automated one-step
fertility k.

Boehringer in vitro transcription k.
Boehringer Mannheim DIG-Nucleic
Detection k.
Boehringer Mannheim
DIG-Oligonucleotide Tailing k.
CAS DNA staining k.
Cellquant K.
CEP 12 SpectrumOrange DNA
probe k.
CEP X, Y SpectrumOrange DNA
probe k.
CINtec cytology k.
CINtec histology k.
Coulter Manual CD4 K.
cyanide antidote k.
DakoCytomation EGFR pharmDx
colorectal cancer diagnostic k.
Dako large volume LSAB2 alkaline
phosphatase k.
Diatest diabetes breath test k.
Directigen Flu A + B test k.
Elucigene CF29 analyte-specific
reagent k.
Extract-N-Amp Blood PCR k.
Farrzyme human high avidity
anti-dsNA enzyme immunoassay k.
FertilMARQ male fertility screening
test k.
First Check Ecstasy test k.
Fix and Perm Cell Permeabilization
K.
Fluorognost HIV-1 IFA assay k.
GenePhor DNA silver staining k.
GenSpin gDNA purification k.
Gentra Systems Puregene DNA
isolation k.
Glucatell beta-glucagan blood test k.
Great Smokies Diagnostic
Laboratories intestinal permeability
test k.
HercepTest IHC k.
HerpeSelect type specific IgG
antibody detection k.
High Pure PCR product purification
k.
Histofine SAB-PO
immunohistochemical staining k.
IgA II-HA assay test k.
IgM II-HA assay test k.
Immu-Mark immunostaining k.
ImmunoDOT Mono G, M test k.
immunofluorescent assay k.
Immunotech immunoassay k.
ImmuSTRIP HAMA test k.
Invitrogen TA cloning k.
KidneyScreen At·Home testing k.
Legionella urinary antigen ELISA
test k.
LUA ELISA test k.

kit (*continued*)
    manual CD4 k.
    Melastatin test k.
    MERmaid-Spin k.
    MOM basic k.
    MOM fluorescein k.
    MOM peroxidase k.
    nerve agent antidote k.
      (NAAK)
    PowerPlex 1.2 genetic
      identification k.
    protein S-free k.
    k. protooncogene
    PSA IRMA k.
    Puregene DNA isolation k.
    QIAamp DNA blood biorobot k.
    Qiagen QIAquick gel extraction k.
    QIAquick PCR 96 purification k.
    Quanta Lite ANA ELISA test k.
    Quanta Lite CCP ELISA k.
    Quanta Lite ELISA autoimmune k.
    rapid drug screen multiple drug
      screen standard k.
    Redquant k.
    RLP-Cholesterol Immunoseparation
      Assay k.
    spill control k.
    Staclot Protein S test k.
    STA Liatest D-DI
      coagulation/inflammation test k.
    Staller k.
    Takara Biomedicals One-Step RNA
      PCR k.
    Taq DyeDeoxy Terminator Cycle
      Sequencing k.
    Taq Master Mix k.
    True test k.
    TruGene HIV-1 genotyping k.
    Universal ISH detection k.
    UroVision bladder cancer
      recurrence k.
    Vectastain ABC Elit k.
    Vectastain Universal Elite
      ABC k.
    Vectastain Universal Quick k.
    Vector MOM k.
    Ventana alkaline phosphatase blue
      detection k.
    Vidas total PSA assay k.
    Vielle menopause home test k.
    Vitros HBsAg confirmatory k.
    Wako NEFA test k.
    ZstatFlu test k.
Kitasato broth
kitasatonis
    Lactobacillus k.
Kitasatospora
    K. niigatensis
    K. putterlickiae

Kittrich stain
KIU
    kallikrein-inhibiting unit
kJ
    kilojoule
Kjeldahl
    K. method
    K. procedure
Klatskin tumor classification
Klauder syndrome
Klebanoff reaction
Klebs disease
klebsiella
    K. mobilis
    K. oxytoca
    K. pneumonia
    K. pneumoniae
    K. pneumoniae subsp. *ozaenae*
    K. pneumonia rhinoscleromatis
    k. urinary tract infection
    K. variicola
Klebsielleae
Klebs-Löffler bacillus
Kleihauer
    K. acid elution
    K. stain
    K. test
Kleihauer-Betke
    K.-B. acid elution
    K.-B. stain
    K.-B. test
Klein bacillus
Kleine-Levin syndrome
Klein-Gumprecht shadow nuclei
Klemperer disease
Klenow fragment
KLH
    keyhole-limpet hemocyanin
Kliger iron agar (KIA)
Klinefelter syndrome (KS)
Klinger-Ludwig acid-thionin stain for sex
    chromatin
Klippel disease
Klippel-Feil
    K.-F. deformity
    K.-F. syndrome (KFS)
Klippel-Trenaunay syndrome
Klippel-Trenaunay-Weber
    syndrome
Kloeckera
Klump and Bieth method
Klumpke-Dejerine syndrome
Klumpke paralysis
Klüver-Barrera Luxol fast blue stain
Klüver-Bucy syndrome
Kluyvera
kluyveri
    Clostridium k.
Kluyveromyces

Km
    Km allotype
    Km antigen
km
    kilometer
KMV
    killed measles virus vaccine
knee
    Brodie k.
    dashboard k.
    septic k.
    k. synoviocyte
Knemidokoptes
Kniest syndrome
knife, *pl.* **knives**
    microtome k.
    souvenir k.
knife-rest crystal
knight disease
knives (*pl. of* knife)
knizocyte
knob
    aortic k.
    malarial k.
knock-out (*var. of* knockout)
knockout, knock-out
    gene k.
Knodell histology activity index
Knoellia
    K. sinensis
    K. subterranea
Knoll gland
knot
    false k. (umbilical cord)
    syncytial k.
knotting
    syncytial k.
Knott technique
knowlesi
    Plasmodium k.
Kobelt cyst
Kober test
Köbner phenomenon
Koch
    K. bacillus
    K. ileostomy
    K. law
    K. old tuberculin
    K. phenomenon
    K. postulate
Kocher-Debré-Semelaigne syndrome
Kocher dilation ulcer
kochi
    Plasmodium k.
kochii
    Borrelia k.
Koch-Weeks
    K.-W. bacillus
    K.-W. *Haemophilus*

    hemophilus of K.-W. (*Haemophilus aegypticus*)
Kocuria
    K. marina
    K. polaris
    K. rhizophila
Kodak
    K. Ektachem DT-60 cholesterol analyzer
    K. Ektachem Vitros 250, 750, 950 cholesterol analyzer
Koebner phenomenon
koehlerae
    Bartonella k.
Koenen tumor
Koenig syndrome
Koerber-Salus-Elschnig syndrome
Kogoj
    K. abscess
    pustules of K.
    spongiform pustule of K.
KOH
    potassium hydroxide
    K. preparation
    K. test
Köhler
    K. disease
    K. illumination
Köhlmeier-Degos disease
Kohn
    K. one-step staining technique
    K. pore
koilocyte
koilocytosis
koilocytotic
    k. atypia
    k. cell
koilonychia
KO89-kit antibody
kokoi venom
Kokoskin stain
koleovorans
    Paenibacillus k.
Kölliker
    K. layer
    K. reticulum
Kolliker-Fuse complex
Kolmer
    K. test
    K. test with Reiter protein (KRP)
Koln
    Hb K.
Köln hemoglobin
kongjuensis
    Pseudonocardia k.
koningi
    Scopulariopsis k.
koniocortex
Konzo

K

Koongol virus
Koplik spot
KOR
    kappa opioid receptor
    KOR agonist
Kordia algicida
Korean
    K. hemorrhagic fever
    K. hemorrhagic fever virus
koreense
    Planomicrobium k.
koreensis
    Arthrobacter k.
    Catellatospora k.
    Comamonas k.
    Hongia k.
    Kangiella k.
    Kribbella k.
    Paenibacillus k.
    Pseudomonas k.
    Rhodococcus k.
    Sphingomonas k.
    Weissella k.
Korff fiber
Korsakoff syndrome
Koser citrate broth
koseri
    Citrobacter k.
Koshevnikoff disease
Kossa stain
kostiensis
    Ensifer k.
Kostmann
    K. agranulocytosis
    K. syndrome
Kova Glasstic Slide #10 with
  Grids
Kovalevsky canal
Kovats index
Kowarsky test
Kozakia baliensis
KP
    keratitic precipitate
KP1
    KP1 antibody
    KP1 immunohistochemical reagent
kPa
    kilopascal
KP1/CD68 monoclonal antibody
KPTT
    kaolin partial thromboplastin time
Kr
    krypton
Kr85
    krypton 85
Krabbe
    K. disease
    K. leukodystrophy
    K. syndrome

Krafft point
krajdenii
    Trichophyton k.
kra-kra (*var. of* craw-craw)
K-ras
    K-r. mutation
    K-r. oncogene
KRAS mutation marker
kraurosis vulvae
Krause
    K. end bulb
    K. gland
    K. syndrome
Krauss and Neubecker morphologic
  criteria
KRB
    Krebs-Ringer bicarbonate buffer
Krebs
    K. cycle
    K. leukocyte index
Krebs-Henseleit cycle
    K. ornithine cycle
    K. urea cycle
Krebs-Ringer
    K.-R. bicarbonate buffer
    (KRB)
    K.-R. phosphate (KRP)
    K.-R. solution
Kribbella
    K. antibiotica
    K. flavida
    K. jejuensis
    K. koreensis
    Lachnobacterium K.
    K. sandramycini
    K. solani
kribbensis
    Paenibacillus k.
kriegii
    Oceanobacter k.
kringle
Krishaber disease
Krisovski sign
kristensenii
    Yersinia k.
Krokiewicz test
Krompecher carcinoma
Kronecker stain
KRP
    Kolmer test with Reiter
    protein
    Krebs-Ringer phosphate
Krukenberg
    K. spindle
    K. tumor
    K. vein
krulwichiae
    Bacillus k.
Krumwiede triple sugar agar

krungthepensis
Asaia k.
krusei
Candida k.
Kruskal-Wallis test
krypton (Kr)
k. 85 (Kr85)
KS
ketosteroid
Klinefelter syndrome
KSCC
keratinizing squamous cell
carcinoma
KSOM
potassium simplex optimized medium
HEPES-buffered K.
kT
kiloton
KU
Karmen unit
kubicae
Mycobacterium k.
Kuehneromyces
Kufs disease
Kugelberg-Welander disease
Kühne
K. methylene blue
K. spindle
K. terminal plate
Kuhnt-Junius disease
Kulchitsky cell
kullae
Külz cylinder
Kumba virus
Kümmell disease
Kümmell-Verneuil disease
kummerowiae
Ensifer k.
Sinorhizobium k.
Kunin antigen
Kunitz domain-containing protein
Kunkel
K. syndrome
K. test
kunsanensis
Nocardiopsis k.
Kupffer
K. cell
K. cell hypertrophy
K. cell iron deposition
K. cell sarcoma
kurcas
Jatropha k.
Kurthia
kurtosis

kuru plaque
kururiensis
Burkholderia k.
Kurzrok-Ratner test
kushneri
Halanaerobium k.
Kuskokwim syndrome
Kussmaul
K. disease
K. paralysis
K. respiration
Kussmaul-Kien respiration
Kussmaul-Landry paralysis
Kussmaul-Maier disease
Kuwabara paper
kuzendorf
Salmonella cholerae suis k.
KV
killed vaccine
kV
kilovolt
kilovoltage
kVA
kilovolt ampere
Kveim
K. antigen
K. test
Kveim-Stilzbach
K.-S. antigen
K.-S. test
kVp
kilovolt peak
KW
Keith-Wagener
kW
kilowatt
kwashiorkor
marasmic k.
kwashiorkor-marasmus syndrome
KWB
Keith-Wagener-Barker
kweiyangensis
Anopheles k.
kWh
kilowatt-hour
Kyasanur
K. Forest disease
K. Forest disease virus
kyphoscoliosis
kyphoscoliotic pelvis
kyphosis
juvenile k.
kyphotic pelvis
Kyrle disease
Kytococcus schroeteri

K

L
lethal
leucine
lewisite
light
liter
NATO code for lewisite
   L cell
   L chain
   L dose
   L layer
   L unit of streptomycin

l-
levorotatory

μL
microliter

μl
microliter

L0
limes zero

L1
lewisite 1

L2
lewisite 2

L3
lewisite 3

LA
latex agglutination
lupus anticoagulant
   Staclot LA

La
   L. Brea hepatitis
   L. Crosse virus

LAA
leukocyte ascorbic acid

lab
laboratory

Laband syndrome
Labbé neurocirculatory syndrome
label
affinity l.
ligand-conjugate l.
radioactive l.
l. variable

labeled
l. antigen
l. streptavidin biotin (LSAB)

labeling
cohort l.
double fluorescence l.
hazardous materials l.
immunogold l.
l. index
in situ DNA nick end l.
in situ nick end l.

ligand-conjugate l.
l. of hazardous materials
ruthenium red l.
T-cell antibody l.
TdT-mediated dUTP nick-end l.
   (TUNEL)

labia (*pl. of* labium)
labial
l. gland
l. salivary gland (LSG)
l. salivary gland biopsy

labiales
glandulae l.

labialis
Filaria l.
herpes l.

labile
l. cell
l. element
l. factor
heat l.

labiomycosis
labium, *pl.* **labia**
l. limbi tympanicum laminae spiralis
   ossei
l. limbi vestibulare laminae
labia majus

Labophot-2 microscope
labor
false l.
stages of l.

laboratorian
laboratory (lab)
bacteriology l.
clinical l.
controlled access l.
l. diagnosis
l. hood
LRN BioWatch l.
l. manifestation
national l.
public health l.
QuestDirect direct to
   consumer l.
reference l.
l. reference (LR)
L. Response Network (LRN)
restricted access l.
sentinel l.
venereal disease experimental l.
   (VDEL)
Venereal Disease Research L.
   (VDRL)
virology l.

Labpette FX pipette

L

labranchiae
   Anopheles l.
labrocyte
labstation
   T/T Mega advanced multifunction
   microwave l.
labyrinth
   Ludwig l.
   renal l.
labyrinthica
   otitis l.
labyrinthine
   l. defect (LD)
   l. hydrops
   l. space
Lacazia loboi
Laccaria
lacerated wound
laceration
laceyi
   Streptomyces l.
Lachesis
Lachnellula
Lachnobacterium
   L. bovis
   L. Kribbella
LaChrom HPLC system
lachrymal (*var. of* lacrimal)
laciniae tubae
lacis cell
lack of collagen
lacrimal, lachrymal
   l. calculus
   l. gland
   l. gland tumor
   l. sac tumor
lacrimalis
   glandula l.
lacrimator
lactacidemia
lactacidosis
lactaciduria
lactalbumin hydrolysate
   (LAH)
lactamica
   Neisseria l.
Lactarius
lactase deficiency
lactate
   cerebrospinal fluid l.
   l. dehydrogenase (LD, LDH)
   l. dehydrogenase, aspartate
   aminotransferase, white blood cells
   (LAW)
   l. dehydrogenase assay
   l. dehydrogenase isoenzyme
   l. dehydrogenase isoenzyme
   determination
   l. dehydrogenase test

   l. dehydrogenase virus
   sodium l.
lactated
   l. Ringer injection
   l. Ringer solution (LRS)
lactate-pyruvate ratio (L:P, LPR)
lactatifermentans
   Clostridium l.
lactating adenoma
lactational mastitis
lactea
   macula l.
lacteal
   central l.
   l. cyst
   l. fistula
   l. vessel
lactenin
lactescence
lacteus
   Mycetocola l.
lactic
   l. acid
   l. acid assay
   l. acid bacteria
   l. acidemia
   l. acidosis
   l. dehydrogenase (LD, LDH)
   l. dehydrogenase test
   l. dehydrogenase virus
   (LDV)
lacticacidemia
lactiferi
   ductus l.
   tubuli l.
lactiferous
   l. duct
   l. gland
   l. sinus
lactis
   Paenibacillus l.
Lactobacillaceae
lactobacillary milk
Lactobacilleae
lactobacilli (*pl. of* lactobacillus)
lactobacillus, *pl.* **lactobacilli**
   L. acidipiscis
   L. acidophilus
   L. algidus
   L. amylolyticus
   L. arizonensis
   L. bifidus
   Boas-Oppler l.
   L. brevis
   L. buchneri
   L. bulgaricus
   L. bulgaricus factor
   (LBF)
   L. casei

L. *catenaformis*
L. *coleohominis*
L. *crispatus*
L. *curvatus*
L. *cypricasei*
L. *delbrueckii*
L. *diolivorans*
L. *durianis*
L. *equi*
L. *ferintoshensis*
L. *fermentum*
L. *fornicalis*
L. *frumenti*
L. *fuchuensis*
L. *ingluviei*
L. *jensenii*
L. *kefiranofaciens* subsp. *kefirgranum*
L. *kimchii*
L. *kitasatonis*
L. *leichmannii*
L. *mindensis*
L. *minor*
L. *mucosae*
L. *nagelii*
L. *pantheris*
L. *paracollinoides*
L. *paralimentarius*
L. *perolens*
L. *plantarum*
L. *psittaci*
L. *saerimneri*
L. *salivarius*
L. *spicheri*
L. *thermotolerans*
L. *trichodes*
L. *versmoldensis*

lactobezoar
lactocele
lactoferrin
lactogen
    human placental l. (hPL)
    placental l. (PL)
lactogenic hormone
lactoglobulin
    beta l. (BLG)
    immune l.
lactolyticus
    Anaerococcus l.
lactone dye
lactoperoxidase radioiodination
lactophenol cotton blue stain
lactose
    l. intolerance
    l. tolerance test
lactose-litmus broth
lactoside
    ceramide l.
lactosidosis
lactosuria

lactosyl ceramide
lactotrope adenoma
lactotroph
    pituitary l.
lactotrophic
lacuna, *pl.* **lacunae**
    cartilage l.
    chondrocyte l.
    Howship l.
    osseous l.
    resorption lacunae
lacunae (*pl. of* lacuna)
lacunar
    l. abscess
    l. cell
    l. resorption
lacunaris
    status l.
lacunata
    Moraxella l.
lacune
    vascular l.
lacunule
lacus
    Mycobacterium l.
lacuscaerulensis
    Silicibacter l.
lacusekhoensis
    Nesterenkonia l.
lacusfryxellense
    Clostridium l.
lacustris
    Friedmanniella l.
lacy chromatin pattern
lacZ-tagged cell
LAD
    leukocyte adhesion deficiency
Ladd
    L. band
    L. syndrome
ladder
    180-bp l.
    sequence l.
Ladendorff test
LAE
    left atrial enlargement
Laelaps echidninus
Läennec
    L. disease
    L. pearl
Laënnec cirrhosis
laesa
    functio l.
laeta
    Loxosceles l.
Laetiporus sulphureus
Laetrile
laeve
    chorion l.

L

laevis
> *Xenopus l.*

Lafora
> L. body
> L. disease

lag
> anaphase l.
> nitrogen l.
> l. phase
> l. time

lagena
> *Torulomyces l.*

Lagochilascaris minor

Lagovirus

lagunensis
> *Caldisphaera l.*

LAH
> lactalbumin hydrolysate
> left atrial hypertrophy

lahorensis
> *Ornithodoros l.*

laidlawii
> *Acholeplasma l.*

LAIT
> latex agglutination-inhibition test

laiteuse
> tache l.

LAK
> lymphokine-activated killer cell

lake
> acellular mucus l.
> bile l.
> red cell l.
> subchorial l.
> vascular l.
> venous l.

laked blood agar

Laki-Lorand factor

laky blood

LAL
> *Limulus amoebocyte* lysate

LAL gram-negative bacteria test

Lallemand body

LAM
> lymphangioleiomyomatosis
> lymphangiomyomatosis
> pulmonary LAM

LAMB
> lentigines, atrial myxoma,
> mucocutaneous myxomas, and blue
> nevi
> LAMB syndrome

lambda
> l. carrageenin
> l. chain specificity
> l. light chain

Lambert
> L. canal
> L. law

Lambert-Eaton
> L.-E. myasthenic syndrome (LEMS)
> L.-E. syndrome

Lambl excrescence

lamblia
> *Giardia l.*
> *L. intestinalis*

lambliasis

lambo
> l. lambo

lame foliacée

lamella, *pl.* **lamellae**
> annulate lamellae
> articular l.
> circumferential l.
> concentric l.
> cornoid l.
> elastic lamellae
> external elastic lamellae
> ground l.
> haversian l.
> inner circumferential l.
> intermediate l.
> internal elastic lamellae
> interstitial l.
> outer circumferential l.
> ovigerous l.
> triangular l.
> vitreous l.

lamellae (*pl. of* lamella)

lamellar
> l. body
> l. bone
> l. collagen
> l. granule
> l. ichthyosis
> l. necrosis

lamellate, lamellated

lamellated (*var. of* lamellate)
> l. collection of inspissated
> inflammatory debris
> l. corpuscle

lamellipodium

lamellosa
> corpuscula l.

lamin
> l. A protein
> l. B protein
> l. C protein

lamina, *pl.* **laminae**
> basal l.
> l. basalis choroideae
> basement l.
> basilar l.
> l. basilaris cochleae
> boundary l.
> l. choriocapillaris
> l. choroidea epithelialis
> l. choroidocapillaris

l. cribrosa ossis ethmoidalis
l. cribrosa sclerae
l. densa
dense fibrous l. (DFL)
l. dentata
l. elastica anterior
l. elastica interna
l. elastica posterior
episcleral l.
l. episcleralis
epithelial l.
external elastic l.
l. fibroreticularis
l. fusca sclerae
glomerular basal l.
hepatic laminae
internal elastic l.
labium limbi vestibulare laminae
l. lateralis cartilaginis tubae
  auditivae
l. lateralis cartilaginis tubae
  auditoriae
l. limitans anterior corneae
l. limitans posterior corneae
l. lucida
l. medialis cartilaginis tubae
  auditivae
l. medialis cartilaginis tubae
  auditoriae
l. membranacea cartilaginis tubae
  auditivae
l. muscularis mucosae
l. of Rexed
osseous spiral l.
l. propria (LP)
l. propria mucosae
l. rara
l. rara interna
reticular l.
spiral l.
laminae spiralis ossei
successional l.
l. vasculosa choroideae
l. vitrea
laminae (*pl. of* lamina)
laminar
l. cortical necrosis
l. cortical sclerosis
l. flow burner
l. flow hood
laminariae
Zobellia l.
laminated
l. epithelium
l. thrombus
lamination
laminin
l. antigen
l. chain

l. α5 gene
l. α3β1 gene
l. β2 gene
l. marker
l. receptor
laminitis
l-amino acid oxidase
lamins
lamotrigine
lamp
gas-discharge l.
hollow cathode l.
slit l.
spirit l.
tungsten arc l.
tungsten halogen l.
VisionSaver lab l.
Wood l.
xenon-arc discharge l.
LAMP
lysosomal-associated membrane
  protein
LAMP-1
lysosomal-associated membrane
  protein-1
LAMP-2
lysosomal-associated membrane
  protein-2
Lamprocystis purpurea
Lan antigen
Lancefield
L. classification
L. grouping
L. precipitation test
lanceolata
Drepanidotaenia l.
Hymenolepis l.
lanceolate myxoma
lanceolatus
lance-ovate spot
Lancereaux-Mathieu disease
lancet
l. fluke
Laser l.
Safe-T Lance Plus l.
**Landouzy-Dejerine progressive muscular
dystrophy**
Landouzy disease
Landry
L. disease
L. syndrome
Landry-Guillain-Barré syndrome
Landschutz tumor
land scurvy
Landsteiner classification
Landsteiner-Donath test
Landström muscle
Lane disease
Langdon-Down disease

L

Lange
    L. colloidal gold test
    L. solution
Langendorff apparatus
Langerhans
    L. cell granulomatosis (LCG)
    L. cell histiocytosis (LCH)
    L. granule
    L. islands
    islands of L.
    islets of L.
langerhansian hormone
Langer line
langeroni
    Arthrographis l.
langeronii
    Eremomyces l.
    Pithoascus l.
Langhans
    L. giant cell
    L. layer
    L. stria
    L. type of giant cell reaction
Langley granule
Lang test
lanienae
    Campylobacter l.
Lanosa nivalis
lanosum
    Microsporum l.
Lansing virus
Lanterman
    L. incisure
    L. segment
lanthanide
lanthanoid
lanthanum nitrate
L26 antibody
lanuginosus
    Thermomyces l.
lanugo hair
LAP
    leucine aminopeptidase
    leukocyte alkaline phosphatase
    lymphangiomatous polyp
    lyophilized anterior pituitary
    LAP score
    LAP stain
    LAP test
laparomyositis
laparoscopic renal resection
lapinization
lapinized
Laplace law
Laquer stain for alcoholic hyalin
l-arabinose dehydrogenase
l-arabitol dehydrogenase
laramiense
    Clostridium estertheticum subsp. *l.*

larbish
lardaceous
    l. liver
    l. spleen
large
    l. B-cell lymphoma (LBCL)
    l. calorie (C, Cal)
    l. cell (LC)
    l. deletion
    l. external transformation-sensitive (LETS)
    l. glandular pattern
    l. granular lymphocyte (LGL)
    l. granular lymphocyte leukemia
    l. noncleaved (LNC)
    l. particle sorting module (LPS)
    l. unstained cell (LUC)
    l. vein
    l. vessel hematocrit (LVH)
large-cell
    l.-c. acanthoma
    l.-c. calcifying Sertoli cell tumor (LCCSCT)
    l.-c. immunoblastic lymphoma
    l.-c. neuroendocrine carcinoma (LCNEC)
    l.-c. non-Hodgkin lymphoma (LCNHL)
large-cup forceps
large-needle aspiration biopsy (LNB)
large-scale integration
lari
    Campylobacter l.
Laribacter hongkongensis
Laricifomes
Laron dwarfism
Larrey
    L. cleft
    L. hernia
Larrey-Weil disease
larrymoorei
    Agrobacterium l.
    Rhizobium l.
Larsen
    L. disease
    L. syndrome
Larsen-Johansson disease
larva
    Bacillus larvae
    l. currens
    l. fly
    fly l.
    Lepidoptera l.
    l. migrans
larval
larvicidal
larvicide
larviparous
larviphagic

laryngeae
    glandulae l.
laryngeal
    l. cancer
    l. carcinoma
    l. edema
    l. gland
    l. granuloma
    l. intraepithelial neoplasia (LIN)
    l. intubation trauma
    l. lupus
    l. nodule
    l. papillomatosis
    l. polyp
    l. tonsil
    l. tuberculosis
    l. web
larynges (*pl. of* larynx)
laryngeus
    folliculi lymphatici laryngei
    Mammomonogamus l.
    Syngamus l.
laryngis
    pachyderma l.
    tunica mucosa l.
laryngitis
laryngocele
laryngogram
laryngomalacia
laryngopharyngitis
laryngotracheitis
    avian infectious l.
laryngotracheobronchitis (LTB)
larynx, *pl.* **larynges**
    chondromalacia of l.
    Gussenbauer artificial l.
    lymphatic follicle of l.
LASA
    lipid-associated sialic acid
Lasègue disease
laser
    l. capture microdissection (LCM)
    l. confocal microscopy
    l. diffraction particle size
    L. lancet
    l. microprobe
    l. microscope
    neodymium-yttrium-aluminum-garnet
      l. (Nd-YAG laser)
    Tsunami l.
laser-activated fluorescence
laser-scanning confocal microscopy
LaserTweezer
Lasette
Lash casein hydrolysate-serum
  medium
Lasiodiplodia
Lasiohelea
L-asparaginase therapy

Lassa
    L. hemorrhagic fever
    L. virus
late
    l. cortical T cell
    l. effect poliomyelitis
    l. event
    l. infantile amaurotic familial idiocy
    l. neonatal death
    l. positive component (LPC)
    l. reaction
    l. replicating X chromosome
    l. systolic murmur (LSM)
latency
    distal l.
    l. period (LP)
    terminal l.
latens
    scarlatina l.
latent
    l. allergy
    l. coccidioidomycosis
    l. empyema
    l. heat
    l. hyperopia
    l. infection
    l. iron-binding capacity (LIBC)
    l. membrane protein (LMP)
    l. membrane protein 1 (LMP-1)
    l. membrane protein-1 expression
    l. microbism
    l. period
    l. porphyria
    l. rat virus
    l. stage
latentiation
late-phase response (LPR)
lateral
    l. aberrant thyroid carcinoma
    l. cartilaginous plate
    l. cell membrane
    l. collateral ligament degeneration
    l. epicondylitis
    l. geniculate body
    l. gray horn
    l. hypothalamus
    l. plate of cartilaginous auditory tube
    l. semicircular canal
lateralis
latericius
    Arenibacter l.
lateritium
    sedimentum l.
latex
    l. agglutination (LA)
    l. agglutination-inhibition test (LAIT)
    l. agglutination test
    l. agglutinin
    l. allergy

L

latex (*continued*)
    l. fixation test (LFT)
    l. flocculation test
    l. particle agglutination test
    l. screen
    l. slide agglutination test
latex-specific IgE
lathyrism
lathyrus protein
latina
    Actinomadura l.
lato
    Borrelia burgdorferi sensu l.
Latrodectus
    L. bishopi
    L. geometricus
    L. mactans
LATS
    long-acting thyroid stimulator
    LATS assay
    LATS protector
    LATS test
lattice hypothesis
latum
    condyloma l.
    Diphyllobothrium l.
    Taenia lata
latus
    Bothriocephalus l.
    Dibothriocephalus l.
latyschewii
    Borrelia l.
Lauber disease
laudable pus
Launois-Bensaude syndrome
Launois-Cléret syndrome
Launois syndrome
laurel fever
Laurell
    L. rocket immunoelectrophoresis
    L. technique
Laurence-Biedl syndrome
Laurence-Moon-Bardet-Biedl syndrome
Laurence-Moon-Biedl syndrome
Laurence-Moon syndrome
Lauren classification
Laurén criteria
lauric acid
lauryl sulfate broth
Lauth violet
LAV
    lymphadenopathy-associated virus
lavage
    bronchoalveolar l. (BAL)
    bronchopulmonary l.
    cervicovaginal l.
    ductal l.
    gastric l.
lavamentivorans

Lavdovsky nucleoid
lavender cytoplasm
Laverania
LAW
    lactate dehydrogenase, aspartate aminotransferase, white blood cells
law
    Ambard laws
    Ångström l.
    Avogadro l.
    Baume l.
    Beer l.
    Beer-Boguer l.
    Behring l.
    Bell-Magendie l.
    Bernoulli l.
    Bouguer l.
    Boyle l.
    Charles l.
    Coulomb l.
    Courvoisier l.
    Dalton l.
    Einthoven l.
    Farr l.
    Fick l.
    gas l.
    Gay-Lussac l.
    Graham l.
    Halsted l.
    Hamburger l.
    Hardy-Weinberg l.
    Henry l.
    Hooke l.
    ideal gas l.
    inverse-square l.
    Joule l.
    Kahler l.
    Kirchoff l.
    Koch l.
    Lambert l.
    Laplace l.
    Marfan l.
    mass action l.
    Mendel l.
    l. of mass action
    l. of priority
    Ohm l.
    Planck radiation l.
    Poiseuille l.
    Profeta l.
    Raoult l.
    right-to-know l.
    Snell l.
    Starling l.
    Stefan-Boltzmann l.
    Stokes l.
    Virchow l.
Lawford syndrome
Lawless stain

lawn plate
Lawrence-Seip syndrome
laxa
    cutis l. (CL)
Laxitextum
layer
    ameloblastic l.
    anterior elastic l.
    bacillary l.
    basal cell l.
    Bowman l.
    brown l.
    cambium l.
    Chievitz l.
    choriocapillary l.
    columnar l.
    depletion l.
    enamel l.
    ependymal l.
    epithelial choroid l.
    external pyramidal l.
    fibrous l.
    fusiform l.
    germ l.
    germinative l.
    glycolipid l.
    half-value l. (HVL)
    Henle fiber l.
    Henle nervous l.
    Huxley l.
    infragranular l.
    inner circular muscle l.
    inner neural l.
    Kaes-Bekhterev l.
    Kölliker l.
    L l.
    Langhans l.
    longitudinal l.
    malpighian l.
    membranous l.
    Meynert l.
    molecular cell l.
    Nitabuch l.
    odontoblastic l.
    l. of cerebellar cortex
    l. of cerebral cortex
    l. of retina
    l. of skin
    osteogenetic l.
    plasma l.
    plexiform l.
    polymorphous l.
    posterior elastic l.
    prickle cell l.
    Purkinje cell l.
    pyramidal cell l.
    Sattler elastic l.
    sluggish l.
    spindle-celled l.
    spinous l.
    still l.
    subendocardial l.
    subendothelial l.
    subpapillary l.
    suprabasal cell l.
    Tomes granular l.
    uteroplacental fibrinoid l.
    vascular l.
    ventricular l.
    Weil basal l.
lazarine leprosy
Lazaro
    mal de San L.
lazy leukocyte syndrome
LBCL
    large B-cell lymphoma
LBF
    Lactobacillus bulgaricus factor
LBI
    low serum-bound iron
LBM
    lean body mass
LBW
    low birth weight
LBWI
    low birth weight infant
LC
    large cell
    lethal concentration
    lymphocytic colitis
LCA
    leukocyte common antigen
    LCA antibody
LCAT
    lecithin-cholesterol acyltransferase
    LCAT deficiency
LCCSCT
    large-cell calcifying Sertoli cell tumor
LCFA
    long-chain fatty acid
LCG
    Langerhans cell granulomatosis
LCH
    Langerhans cell histiocytosis
L-chain
    L-c. disease
    L-c. myeloma
LCIS
    lobular carcinoma in situ
LCL
    Levinthal-Coles-Lillie
    lymphocytic leukemia
    lymphocytic lymphosarcoma
    LCL bodies
LCM
    laser capture microdissection
    left costal margin
    lymphatic choriomeningitis

L

LCM (*continued*)
  lymphocytic choriomeningitis
    LCM virus
LCNEC
  large-cell neuroendocrine carcinoma
LCNHL
  large-cell non-Hodgkin lymphoma
LCPUFA
  long-chain polyunsaturated fatty acid
LCR
  ligase chain reaction
LCT
  Leydig cell tumor
  long-chain triglyceride
  lymphocytotoxin
LCt
  lethal concentration
LCt$_{50}$
  lethal Ct$_{50}$
LCTA
  lymphocytotoxic antibody
LCV
  leukocytoclastic vasculitis
  lymphocytic choriomeningitis virus
LD
  labyrinthine defect
  lactate dehydrogenase
  lactic dehydrogenase
  Legionnaire disease
  lethal dose
  living donor
  lymphocyte-defined
LDH
  lactate dehydrogenase
  lactic dehydrogenase
LDHD
  lymphocyte-depleted Hodgkin disease
LDL
  low-density lipoprotein
    LDL cholesterol assay
    LDL direct test prefilled cartridge
LDL-C
  low-density lipoprotein-cholesterol
LD 400 luminescence detector
L$_+$dose (*var. of* L$^+$dose)
LDV
  lactic dehydrogenase virus
LE
  lupus erythematosus
    LE body
    LE cell
    LE cell test
    LE factor
    LE phenomenon
Le
  L. antigen
  L. Veen shunt
leachi
  Haemaphysalis l.

leaching
lead
  l. anemia
  l. assay
  black l.
  l. broth
  l. chromate
  chromate stain for l.
  l. citrate
  l. citrate stain
  l. colic
  l. core high-velocity round
  l. encephalitis
  l. encephalopathy
  l. fixative
  l. gout
  l. hydroxide stain
  l. level
  l. nephropathy
  l. pigmentation
  l. poisoning
  l. snowstorm
  l. stomatitis
leading strand
lead-pipe
  l.-p. colon
  l.-p. rigidity
leaflet
  mitral valve cleft l.
  outer l.
  tricuspid valve cleft l.
leak
  spinal fluid l.
leakage
  vascular l.
lean body mass (LBM)
learning
  distance l.
least splanchnic nerve
leather-bottle stomach
leave-one-out cross-validation analysis
Leber
  L. disease
  L. hereditary optic neuropathy (LHON)
  L. optic atrophy
Lechtheimia corymbifera
lecithin
  amniotic fluid unsaturated l.
lecithinase A
lecithin-cholesterol acyltransferase (LCAT)
lecithin/sphingomyelin ratio (L:S)
LECL
  lymphoepithelioid cell lymphoma
Leclanché cell
Leclercia
lectin
  mannose binding l. (MBL)
  Ulex l.
  l. Ulex europaeus agglutinin I

lectin-binding pathway
lectotype
lectularia
    Acanthia l.
lectularius
    Cimex l.
lectus
    Algibacter l.
Lecythophora
LED
    lupus erythematosus disseminatus
Ledderhose disease
Leder
    L. reaction
    L. stain
Lederer anemia
leech
    American l.
    artificial l.
    medicinal l.
leeching
LEEP
    loop electrosurgical excisional procedure
Leeuwenhoek canal
Lee-White (LW)
    L.-W. clotting test
    L.-W. clotting time method
left
    l. atrial enlargement (LAE)
    l. atrial hypertrophy (LAH)
    l. bundle branch block
    l. costal margin (LCM)
    l. shift
    l. shift (increased band forms on WBC differential)
    l. ventricular enlargement (LVE)
    l. ventricular failure (LVF)
    l. ventricular hypertrophy (LVH)
left-sidedness
    bilateral l.-s.
left-to-right ratio (L:R)
leg
    Barbados l.
    elephant l.
    milk l.
    white l.
Legal
    L. disease
    L. test
Legg-Calvé-Perthes disease
Legg disease
Legg-Perthes disease
legionella
    L. beliardensis
    L. bozemanii
    L. busanensis
    L. drancourtii
    L. drozanskii
    L. dumoffii

    L. fallonii
    L. feeleii
    L. gormanii
    L. gresilensis
    L. jordanis
    L. longbeachae
    L. micdadei
    L. pittsburgensis
    L. pneumophila
    L. pneumophila culture
    L. pneumophila direct fA smear
    L. rowbothamii
    L. taurinensis
    L. urinary antigen (LUA)
    L. urinary antigen ELISA test kit
    L. wadsworthii
Legionellaceae
legionellosis
Legionnaire
    L. disease (LD)
    L. disease antibody
Leica
    L. VT1000 E fully automatic microtome
    L. VT1000 M semi-automatic microtome
leichmannii
    Lactobacillus l.
Leiden
    L. factor
    L. mutation
LeIF
    leukocyte interferon
Leifsonia
    L. aquatica
    L. aurea
    L. cynodontis
    L. naganoensis
    L. poae
    L. rubra
    L. shinshuensis
    L. xyli
    L. xyli subsp. cynodontis
    L. xyli subsp. xyli
Leigh disease
Leiner disease
leiodermia
leiomyoblastoma
leiomyofibroma
leiomyoma, *pl.* **leiomyomas, leiomyomata**
    benign metastasizing l. (BML)
    bizarre l.
    clear cell l.
    l. cutis
    epithelioid l.
    uterine l.
    vascular l.
leiomyomas (*pl. of* leiomyoma)
leiomyomata (*pl. of* leiomyoma)

L

leiomyomatosis
    intravenous l. (IVL)
    l. peritonealis disseminata
leiomyomatous hamartoma
leiomyosarcoma (LMS)
    epithelioid l. (ELMS)
    pleomorphic l.
    uterine l. (ULMS)
Leipzig yellow
Leishman
    L. chrome cell
    L. stain
Leishman-Donovan body
Leishmania
    L. aethiopica
    L. braziliensis braziliensis
    L. braziliensis guyanensis
    L. braziliensis panamensis
    L. caninum
    L. donovani archibaldi
    L. donovani chagasi
    L. donovani donovani
    L. donovani infantum
    L. furunculosa
    L. infantum
    L. mexicana amazonensis
    L. mexicana garnhami
    L. mexicana mexicana
    L. mexicana pifanoi
    L. mexicana venezuelensis
    L. nilotica
    L. peruviana
    L. tropica
    L. tropica major
    L. tropica mexicana
leishmaniasis, leishmaniosis
    American l.
    l. americana
    anergic l.
    cutaneous l.
    lupoid l.
    mucocutaneous l.
    nasooral l.
    nasopharyngeal l.
    pseudolepromatous l.
    l. recidivans
    l. serological test
    l. tegumentaria diffusa
    visceral l.
Leishmaniavirus
leishmanicidal
leishmaniosis (*var. of* leishmaniasis)
leishmanoid
Leisingera methylohalidivorans
Leitz image analysis system
LEL
    lymphoepithelial lesion
LELC
    lymphoepithelioma-like carcinoma

Leloir disease
Leminorella
lemmocyte
lemniscus
lemoignei
lemonnieri
    Saccharomyces l.
lemon sign
LEMS
    Lambert-Eaton myasthenic
    syndrome
    LEMS antibody
Lendrum
    L. inclusion body stain
    L. phloxine-tartrazine stain
Lenègre disease
length
    focal l.
    fragment l.
    greatest l. (GL)
Lenhossek process
Lennert
    L. classification
    L. lesion
    L. lymphoma
Lennox syndrome
lens
    achromatic l.
    l. antigen
    aplanatic l.
    cortex of l.
    l. dislocation
    electron l.
    epithelium of l.
    oil immersion l.
    l. star
lens-induced uveitis
lenta
    Eggerthella l.
    sepsis l.
Lentibacillus salicampi
lenticula
lenticular
    l. opacity
    l. papilla
    l. progressive degeneration
    l. protein
lenticularis
    dermatofibrosis l.
lenticulopapular
lentigines (*pl. of* lentigo)
lentiginosis
lentiginous
    l. melanocytic hyperplasia
    l. melanocytic structure
lentigo, *pl.* **lentigines**
    lentigines, atrial myxoma,
    mucocutaneous myxomas, and blue
    nevi (LAMB)

lentigines, electrocardiographic abnormalities, ocular hypertelorism, pulmonary stenosis, abnormalities of genitalia, retardation of growth, and deafness
l. maligna
l. maligna melanoma
malignant l.
PUVA l.
solar l.
lentigomelanosis
Lentinula
Lentinus
lentis
apparatus suspensorius l.
cortex l.
epithelium l.
fibrae l.
Filaria l.
radii l.
substantia l.
tunica vasculosa l.
Lentisphaera araneosa
Lentisphaerae
Lentisphaerales
Lentivirinae
lentivirus
L.
Lentodium
lentogenic
lentum
Eubacterium l.
lentus
Vibrio l.
Lentzea
L. albida
L. albidocapillata
L. californiensis
L. flaviverrucosa
L. violacea
L. waywayandensis
Lenzites betulina
Lenz syndrome
leonina
Toxascaris l.
leonine facies
leontiasis ossea
Leon virus
LEOPARD syndrome
Lepehne-Pickworth stain
leper
lepidic
Lepidoptera larva
lepidosis
Lepiota
lepirudin
Lepista

Lepore
hemoglobin L. (Hb_{Lepore})
L. thalassemia
leporinum
Arnium l.
Leporipoxvirus
leporis-palustris
Haemaphysalis l.-p.
lepra
l. cell
l. cell organism
l. manchada
leprae
Bacillus l.
Mycobacterium l.
lepraemurium
Mycobacterium l.
leprechaun facies
leprologist
leprology
leproma
lepromatous leprosy
lepromin
l. reaction
l. skin test
leprosarium, leprosery
leprose
leprosery (*var. of* leprosarium)
leprostatic
leprosum
erythema nodosum l. (ENL)
leprosus
leprosy
anesthetic l.
articular l.
l. bacillus
borderline l.
cutaneous l.
dimorphous l.
dry l.
histoid l.
indeterminate l.
lazarine l.
lepromatous l.
Lucio l.
macular l.
Malabar l.
murine l.
mutilating l.
nodular l.
smooth l.
trophoneurotic l.
tuberculoid l.
leprotic
leprous
leptin protein
leptochromatic

L

Leptoconops
leptocyte
leptocytosis
Leptodontium camptobactrum
Leptographium
leptokurtic
leptomeningeal
    l. carcinoma
    l. carcinomatosis
    l. cyst
    l. fibrosis
leptomeninges
leptomeningitis
    basilar l.
leptomonad
Leptomonas
leptonema
Leptoporus
Leptopsylla segnis
leptoscope
Leptosphaeria
Leptosphaerulina
Leptospira
    L. australis
    L. autumnalis
    L. biflexa
    L. canicola
    L. culture
    L. grippotyphosa
    L. hebdomidis
    L. hyos
    L. icterohaemorrhagiae
    L. interrogans
    L. pomona
    L. serodiagnosis
Leptospiraceae
leptospiral jaundice
leptospire
Leptospirillum
    L. ferriphilum
    L. ferrooxidans
    L. thermoferrooxidans
leptospirosis icterohemorrhagica
leptospiruria
leptotene
Leptothrix
Leptotrichia
    L. buccalis
    L. goodfellowii
    L. hofstadii
    L. shahii
    L. trevisanii
    L. wadei
Leptotrombidium
    L. akamushi
    L. deliense
Leptus
Leriche syndrome
Leri pleonosteosis

Leri-Weill
    L.-W. disease
    L.-W. syndrome
Lermoyez syndrome
Leroy disease
Lesch-Nyhan syndrome
Leser-Trélat sign
lesion
    angiocentric immunoproliferative l. (AIL)
    angiocentric lymphoproliferative l.
    angioimmunoproliferative l. (AIL)
    Antopol-Goldman l.
    apocrine l.
    Armanni-Ebstein l.
    Baehr-Lohlein l.
    benign lymphoepithelial l.
    benign proliferative l.
    bird's nest l.
    bone marrow l.
    brain l.
    bull's-eye l.
    Cameron l.
    cavitary l.
    central l.
    coin l.
    cold l.
    collar button l.
    complex sclerosing l.
    Councilman l.
    cryptolytic l.
    diffuse l.
    discrete l.
    dysplasia-associated l.
    Ebstein l.
    encysted papillary l.
    epithelial hyperplastic laryngeal l. (EHLL)
    extracapillary l. (ECL)
    fibroblastic l.
    fibroepithelial l.
    fibrohistiocytic l.
    fibroinflammatory l.
    fibroosseous l.
    fibrosclerosing l.
    gastric phenotype l.
    Ghon primary l.
    Ghon-Sachs primary l.
    granulomatous l.
    gross l.
    gunpowder mark l.
    hemosiderotic fibrohistiocytic lipomatous l. (HFLL)
    high-grade squamous intraepithelial l. (HGSIL, HSIL)
    histocytoid hemangioma-like l. (HHLL)
    histologic l.
    hot l.
    impaction l.

indiscriminate l.
inflammatory myofibroblastic l.
initial syphilitic l.
intestinal phenotype l.
intralobular l.
irritative l.
Janeway l.
jet l.
Kimmelstiel-Wilson l.
Lennert l.
lobular proliferative l.
local l.
Lohlein-Baehr l.
low-grade squamous intraepithelial l.
  (LGSIL, LSIL)
lymphoepithelial l. (LEL)
lymphoplasmacytic l.
lytic l.
macroscopic l.
Mallory-Weiss l.
mass l.
melanocytic l.
molecular l.
mucinous breast l.
myofibroblastic l.
nil l.
nonexophytic l.
noninvasive lobular l.
nonodontogenic l.
Nora l.
null phenotype l.
odontogenic l.
l. of vasculature
onion scale l.
onionskin l.
organic l.
plexiform l.
polar l.
portal tract l.
precancerous l.
precursor l.
prenecrotizing phagocytic l.
primary l.
pseudo-Kaposi l.
Quilty l.
radial sclerosing l.
ring-wall l.
satellite vesicular l.
shagreen l.
skip l.
space-occupying l. (SOL)
spitzoid melanocytic l.
spontaneous l. (SPL)
squamous intraepithelial l. (SIL)
structural l.
synchronous airway l. (SAL)
synchronous mass l.
systemic l.
target l.

total l.
trophic l.
tubulointerstitial l.
tumefactive fibroinflammatory l. (TFL)
tumor-like l.
verrucopapillary external genital l.
wire-loop l.

lesser
  l. omentum
  l. splanchnic nerve
lesteri
  Anopheles l.
LET
  leukocyte esterase test
  linear energy transfer
LETC
  lymphoepithelioma-like thymic
  carcinoma
lethal (L)
  l. anthrax aerosol
  l. coefficient
  l. concentration (LC, LCt)
  l. Ct_{50} (LCt_{50})
  l. dose (LD)
  l. dwarfism
  l. equivalent
  l. factor (LF)
  l. gene
  l. midline granuloma
  l. mutation
  synthetic l.
lethalis
  epidermolysis bullosa l.
lethargica
  encephalitis l.
lethargic encephalitis
LETS
  large external transformation-sensitive
letter bomb
Letterer-Siwe disease
lettingae
  Thermotoga l.
Leu
  leucine
  Leu 1–22 antibody
  Leu 1 antigen
leucin
leucine (L, Leu)
  l. aminopeptidase (LAP)
  l. aminopeptidase test
  l. hypoglycemia
  l. tolerance test
  urine l.
leucinosis
leucinuria
Leucoagaricus
Leucobacter albus
leucocelaenus
  Aedes l.

Leucocoprinus
Leucocytozoon
leucocytozoonosis
leucofuchsin
leucomethylene blue
Leuconostoc
    L. ficulneum
    L. fructosum
    L. gasicomitatum
    L. inhae
    L. kimchii
    L. mesenteroides
leuco patent blue
leucosphyrus
    Anopheles l.
Leucosporidium
Leucostoma
leucotome (*var. of* leukotome)
Leucotrichaceae
leucovorin calcium
leucyl
leucyl-RNA synthetase
leukanemia
leukapheresis
leukasmus
leukemia
    acute biphenotypic l.
    acute granulocytic l. (AGL)
    acute lymphoblastic l. (ALL)
    acute lymphocytic l. (ALL)
    acute megakaryoblastic l.
    acute megakaryocytic l. (M7)
    acute monoblastic l. (AMoL)
    acute monocytic l. (AMoL, M5)
    acute myelocytic l.
    acute myelogenous l.
    acute myeloid l. (AML)
    acute myelomonocytic l. (AMML, M4)
    acute nonlymphocytic l. (ANLL)
    acute promyelocytic l. (APL, M3)
    acute undifferentiated l. (AUL)
    aleukemic granulocytic l.
    aleukemic lymphocytic l.
    aleukemic monocytic l.
    atypical chronic myeloid l. (aCML)
    basophilic l.
    basophilocytic l.
    B-cell acute lymphoblastic l. (B-ALL)
    B-cell chronic lymphocytic l. (B-CLL)
    B-cell precursor lymphoblastic l. (BCP-LBL)
    B-cell prolymphocytic l. (B-PLL)
    bilineal acute l.
    blast cell l.
    chronic cell l.
    chronic eosinophilic l. (CEL)
    chronic granulocytic l. (CGL)
    chronic lymphatic l. (CLL)
    chronic lymphocytic l. (CLL)
    chronic lymphosarcoma l. (CLSL)
    chronic monoblastic l. (CMoL)
    chronic monocytic l. (CMoL)
    chronic myelocytic l. (CML)
    chronic myelogenous l. (CML)
    chronic myeloid l.
    chronic myelomonocytic l. (CMML)
    chronic neutrophilic l.
    chronic prolymphocytic l.
    compound l.
    congenital l.
    l. cutis
    embryonal l.
    eosinophilic l.
    eosinophilocytic l.
    erythroid l.
    erythromyeloblastic l.
    extramedullary myelogenous l.
    feline l.
    granulocytic l.
    hairy cell l. (HCL)
    histiocytic l.
    Ig-mutated chronic lymphocytic l.
    Ig-unmutated chronic lymphocytic l.
    l. immunophenotyping
    l. inhibitory factor (LIF)
    juvenile chronic myelogenous l. (JCML)
    juvenile myelomonocytic l. (JMML)
    large granular lymphocyte l.
    leukemic l.
    leukopenic l.
    lymphatic l.
    lymphoblastic l.
    lymphocytic l. (LCL)
    lymphoid l.
    lymphosarcoma cell l.
    mast cell l.
    mature cell l.
    megakaryocytic l.
    meningeal l.
    micromyeloblastic l.
    mixed cell l.
    mixed lineage l. (MLL)
    monoblastic l.
    monocytic l.
    monomyelocytic l.
    murine l.
    myeloblastic l.
    myelocytic l.
    myelogenic l.
    myelogenous l.
    myeloid l.
    myelomonocytic l.
    Nägeli type of monocytic l.
    natural killer cell l.
    neutrophilic l.
    nonlymphocytic l.

null cell lymphoblastic l.
plasma cell l.
plasmacytic l.
polymorphocytic l.
progranulocytic l.
prolymphocytic l. (PLL)
promyelocytic l. (PML)
putative l.
Rai classification of chronic
  lymphocytic l.
Rieder cell l.
Schilling type of monocytic l.
smoldering l.
splenic l.
stem cell l.
subacute myelomonocytic l.
subleukemic granulocytic l.
subleukemic lymphocytic l.
subleukemic monocytic l.
T-cell acute lymphoblastic l.
  (T-ALL)
T-cell chronic lymphocytic l.
T-cell prolymphocytic l. (T-PLL)
thrombocytic l.
thymic l.
thymus l. (TL)

leukemia-associated inhibitory activity
(LIA)
leukemia/lymphoma
adult T-cell l. (ATLL)
leukemic
l. erythrocytosis
l. leukemia
l. meningitis
l. myelosis
l. reticuloendotheliosis
l. reticulosis
leukemid
leukemogenesis
leukemogenic
leukemoid reaction
Leukeran
leukin
leukoagglutination
EDTA-associated l.
leukoagglutinin test
leukobilin
leukoblast
granular l.
leukoblastosis
leukochloroma
leukocidin
leukocoria, leukokoria
leukocytactic
leukocytal
leukocytaxia, leukocytaxis
leukocytaxis (*var. of* leukocytaxia)
leukocyte
acidophilic l.

l. acid phosphatase stain
l. adherence assay test
l. adhesion deficiency (LAD)
l. adhesion molecule
l. agglutinin
agranular l.
l. alkaline phosphatase (LAP)
l. alkaline phosphatase method
l. alkaline phosphatase score
l. alloantibodies
l. alloimmunization
l. ascorbic acid (LAA)
l. bactericidal assay test
basophilic l. (baso)
l. common antigen (LCA)
l. count
l. cream
cystinotic l.
l. cytochemistry
l. differential count
endothelial l.
eosinophilic l. (eos)
l. esterase
l. esterase test (LET)
fecal l.
filament polymorphonuclear l.
globular l.
granular l.
heterophilic l.
hyaline l.
l. inclusion
l. in feces
l. inhibitory factor
l. interferon (LeIF)
lymphoid l.
mast l.
mononuclear l. (mono)
motile l.
multinuclear l.
neutrophilic l.
nonfilament polymorphonuclear l.
nongranular l.
nonmotile l.
oxyphilic l.
polymorphonuclear l.
polynuclear l.
l. recruitment
segmented l.
stool l.
l. transfusion
transitional l.
l. transmigration
Türk irritation l.
vaginal l.
leukocyte-poor packed red blood cells
leukocyte-reduced
l.-r. platelets
l.-r. red blood cells

L

leukocythemia
leukocytic
  l. crystal
  l. hypersegmentation
  l. infiltrate
  l. margination
  l. marrow
  l. maturation alteration
  l. nuclear hyposegmentation
  l. sarcoma
leukocytoblast
leukocytoclasia
leukocytoclasis
leukocytoclastic
  l. angiitis
  l. vasculitis (LCV)
leukocytogenesis
leukocytoid habit
leukocytolysin
leukocytolysis
leukocytolytic
leukocytoma
leukocytometer
leukocytopenia
leukocytoplania
leukocytopoiesis
leukocytosis
  absolute l.
  agonal l.
  basophilic l.
  digestive l.
  distribution l.
  emotional l.
  eosinophilic l.
  lymphocytic l.
  monocytic l.
  neutrophilic l.
  l. of the newborn
  pure l.
  relative l.
  terminal l.
**leukocytosis-promoting factor
  (LPF)**
leukocytotactic
**leukocytotaxia, positive leukocytotaxia,
  negative leukocytotaxia**
leukocytotoxin
Leukocytozoon
leukocytozoonosis
leukocyturia
leukoderma
  acquired l.
  l. acquisitum centrifugum
leukodystrophy
  Alexander l.
  globoid cell l.
  Krabbe l.
  metachromatic l. (MLD)
  metachromatic-type l.

  spongy degenerative-type l.
  sudanophilic l.
leukoencephalitis (LEAP, LEC)
  acute epidemic l.
  acute hemorrhagic l. (AHLE)
  subacute sclerosing l.
leukoencephalopathy
  cerebral autosomal dominant
    arteriopathy with subcortical
    infarcts and l. (CADASIL)
  megaloencephalic l.
  multifocal progressive l.
  progressive multifocal l. (PML)
  subcortical arteriosclerotic l.
leukoerythroblastic
  l. anemia
  l. reaction
leukoerythroblastosis
leukogram
leukokeratosis
leukokinetic
leukokinetics
leukokinin
leukokoria (*var. of* leukocoria)
leukokraurosis
leukolymphosarcoma
leukolysin
leukolysis
leukolytic
leukoma
leukomyelopathy
leukon
leukonecrosis
leukonychia
leukoparakeratosis
leukopathia, leukopathy
  acquired l.
leukopathy (*var. of* leukopathia)
leukopedesis
leukopenia
  autoimmune l.
  basophilic l.
  eosinophilic l.
  lymphocytic l.
  monocytic l.
  neutrophilic l.
leukopenic
  l. factor
  l. index
  l. leukemia
  l. myelosis
leukophagocytosis
leukophlegmasia dolens
leukophoresis
leukoplakia
  oral hairy l. (OHL)
  proliferative verrucous l. (PVL)
  l. vulva
leukoplakic vulvitis

leukopoiesis
leukopoietic
leukopoietin
leukoreduction
    poststorage l.
    prestorage l.
    universal l.
leukorrhea
leukosarcoma
leukosarcomatosis
leukosis
    avian l.
    enzootic bovine l.
    fowl l.
Leukosporidium
leukostasis
Leukostat stain
leukotactic assay
leukotaxia
leukotaxine
leukotaxis
leukotic
leukotome, leucotome
leukotoxin
leukotriene A, B, C, D
leukotriene-dependent erythroid
  differentiation
Leukovirus
LeuM1
    L. antibody
    L. antigen
    L. immunoperoxidase stain
LeuM3 antibody
LeuM5 antibody
Leung stain
leuprolide acetate
Levaditi
    L. method
    L. stain
levan
Levay antigen
Lev disease
level
    antibiotic l.
    barbiturate l.
    biosafety l. (BSL)
    biosafety l. 1 (BSL1)
    biosafety l. 2 (BSL2)
    biosafety l. 3 (BSL3)
    biosafety l. 4 (BSL4)
    blood calcium l.
    blood cholesterol l.
    ceruloplasmin l.
    cidal l.
    Clark l.
    confidence l.
    critical staining l.
    DNA adduct l.
    ethanol l.

    high l.
    isoelectric l.
    lead l.
    low l.
    minimal bactercidal l. (MBL)
    l. of agreement
    plasma-acetaminophen l.
    salicylate l.
    serum drug l.
    signal l.
    significance l.
    sweat chloride l.
    therapeutic drug l.
    whole-blood mercury l.
Levey-Jennings chart
Lévi disease
Levine
    L. alkaline Congo red stain
    L. EMB agar
Levinea
    L. amalonatica
    L. diversus
    L. malonatica
Levine-Rosai tumor classification
Levinson test
Levinthal-Coles-Lillie (LCL)
Leviviridae
Levivirus
levocardia
    isolated l.
levodopa
levorotatory (*l*-, L)
levothyroxine (T$_4$)
levulosemia
levulose tolerance test
levulosuria
Lévy-Roussy syndrome
Lewandowski
    nevus elasticus of L.
Lewandowski-Lutz disease
Lewia infectoria
Lewis
    L. acid
    L. antibody (Le)
    L. antigen
    L. base
    L. blood group
    L. lung tumor
    L. phenomenon
    sialyl L. X (SLex)
lewisi
    Trypanosoma l.
lewisite (L)
    l. 1 (L1)
    l. 2 (L2)
    l. 3 (L3)
    NATO code for l. (L)
Lewis-X blood group antigen
Lewy body

L

lexingtonensis
>*Amycolatopsis l.*

Leyden
>L. crystal
>L. disease
>hemophilia B L.

Leyden-Mobius syndrome

Leydig
>L. cell adenóma
>L. cell hyperplasia
>L. cell tumor (LCT)
>L. interstitial cell
>interstitial cell of L.

Leydig-Sertoli cell tumor

LF
>lethal factor
>limit of flocculation
>LF protein

Lf
>limes flocculation
>Lf dose

L_fdose (*var. of* Lf dose)

LFT
>latex fixation test
>liver function tests
>localized fibrous tumor

l-fucose

LGD
>low-grade dysplasia

LGESS
>low-grade endometrial stromal sarcoma

LGL
>large granular lymphocyte

l-glyceric aciduria

LGSIL
>low-grade squamous intraepithelial lesion

LGV
>lymphogranuloma venereum

LGV-TRIC
>lymphogranuloma venereum-trachoma inclusion conjunctivitis

L-H
>lymphocytic-histiocytic
>>L. cell

LH
>luteinizing hormone
>LH 755 hematology Workcell
>LH 500, 750, 1500 series hematology analyzer

Lhermitte-Duclos disease

Lhermitte-McAlpine syndrome

l-histidine ammonia-lyase

LHM
>lymphohistiocytoid mesothelioma

LHMT
>low-range heparin management
>LHMT test

LHON
>Leber hereditary optic neuropathy

LHPC
>lipomatous hemangiopericytoma

LH-RF
>luteinizing hormone-releasing factor

LH-RH
>luteinizing hormone-releasing hormone

l-hydroxyacyl coenzyme A

LIA
>leukemia-associated inhibitory activity

Liacopoulos phenomenon

Liaison Borrelia burgdorferi assay

libanotica
>*Actinocorallia l.*

LIBC
>latent iron-binding capacity

liberae
>terminationes nervorum l.

liberator
>histamine l.
>L. universal locking stylet

Libertella

Libman-Sacks
>L.-S. disease
>L.-S. endocarditis
>L.-S. syndrome

library
>cDNA l.
>gene l.

LIBS
>ligand-induced binding site

LIC
>limiting isorrheic concentration

lichen
>l. amyloidosis
>l. annularis
>l. aureus
>l. myxedematosus
>l. nitidus
>l. planopilaris (LPP)
>l. planus
>l. sclerosus et atrophicus
>l. sclerosus of vulva
>l. scrofulosorum
>l. simplex chronicus
>l. striatus

lichenification

licheniformis
>*Bacillus l.*

lichenization

lichenoid
>l. eczema
>l. interface dermatitis
>l. keratosis

lichenoides

Lichtheim
>L. disease
>L. syndrome

LID
low iron diamine
Liddle syndrome
lidocaine
l. assay
l. hydrochloride
l-iduronidase
Lieberkuhn
crypts of L.
Lieberkühn
L. follicles
L. glands
Liebermann-Burchard
L.-B. reaction
L.-B. test
Liebermeister
L. furrow
L. groove
lien
l. accessorius
l. mobilis
l. succentorius
lienalis
folliculi lymphatici lienales
Onchocerca l.
lienis
hilum l.
porta l.
pulpa l.
sinus l.
tunica fibrosa l.
tunica propria l.
lienomedullary
lienomyelogenous
Liesegang
L. phenomenon
L. ring
LIF
leukemia inhibitory factor
life
average l.
fetal l.
mean effective l.
quality of l.
l. table
technologic l.
L. Technologies TRIzol
reagent
useful l.
Li-Fraumeni cancer syndrome
ligament
Arantius l.
gingivodental l.
hammock l.
Hueck l.
ligamenta (*pl. of* ligamentum)
ligamentum, *pl.* **ligamenta**
l. anulare bulbi
l. pectinatum

l. pectinatum anguli
l. pectinatum iridis
l. spirale cochleae
ligand
addressing l.
l. assay
Fas l. (FasL, Fas-L)
l. immunoassay
receptor activator of nuclear factor
kappa B l. (RANKL)
ligand-activated transcription factor
ligand-conjugate
l.-c. label
l.-c. labeling
ligand-dependent dimerization
ligand-gated channel
ligandin
ligand-induced binding site (LIBS)
ligase
l. chain reaction (LCR)
l. detection reaction
DNA l.
polynucleotide l.
ubiquitin l.
ligation-dependent amplification
light (L)
l. band
black l.
l. cell of thyroid
l. chain
l. chain class-restricted B cell
l. chain deposition disease
l. chain Fanconi syndrome
l. green SF yellowish
incident l.
l. meromyosin
l. micrograph
l. microscope
l. microscopy (LM)
l. pipe
polarized l.
l. reaction (LR)
stray l.
strobe l.
ultraviolet l.
visible l.
l. water
Wood l.
LightCycler system
lighter layer of fibrin
light-scattering immunoassay
light-staining
l.-s. apical cytoplasm
l.-s. granule
Lightwood syndrome
Lignac
L. disease
L. syndrome
Lignac-Fanconi syndrome

L

ligneous
l. struma
l. thyroiditis
lignicola
Hyalodendron l.
lignieresii
Actinobacillus l.
lignoceric acid
ligroin
Ligula intestinalis
lilacinus
Paecilomyces l.
Lillie
L. allochrome connective tissue stain
L. allochrome method
L. azure-eosin stain
L. ferrous iron stain
L. hematoxylin
L. sulfuric acid Nile blue stain
limb-girdle muscular dystrophy
limbic encephalitis
limb lipodystrophy
limbus
l. corneae
l. penicillatus
l. striatus
limen
difference l. (DL)
limes
l. flocculation (Lf)
l. reacting (Lr)
l. zero (L_0)
limicola
Flavobacterium l.
Propionivibrio l.
limimaris
Desulfomonile l.
limit
assimilation l.
l. check
critical l.
l. dextrin
l. dextrinosis
explosive l.
gas storage l.
Hayflick l.
l. of flocculation (LF)
l. of resolution
quantum l.
saturation l.
storage l.
tolerance l.
within normal l.'s (WNL)
limitans
membrana l.
limitation
limitations
container size l.

limited scleroderma
limiting
l. isorrheic concentration (LIC)
l. layer of cornea
l. membrane of retina
l. reactant
limnaea
Gillisia l.
limnaeum
Chlorobaculum l.
limnaeus
Thialkalicoccus l.
Limnatis nilotica
limnemia
limnemic
limneticum
Ferribacterium l.
Limnobacter thiooxidans
limnology
Limnoperdon
limnophilus
Brevibacillus l.
limosa
Kineosphaera l.
limosum
Eubacterium l.
limosus
Inquilinus l.
limulus
l. amebocyte lysate assay
L. *amoebocyte* lysate (LAL)
l. lysate test
L. *polyphemus*
LIN
laryngeal intraepithelial neoplasia
lincomycin
Linda
Mycobacterium paratuberculosis L.
lindane
lindaniclasticus
Rhodanobacter l.
Lindau
L. disease
L. tumor
Lindau-von Hippel disease
lindemanni
Sarcocystis l.
Lindner body
lindoensis
Echinostoma l.
line
accretion l.
Amici l.
Baillarger l.
Beau l.
BeWo choriocarcinoma cell l.
Blaschko l.
cell l.
cement l.

cleavage l.
D l.
delay l.
dentate l.
Eberth l.
emission l.
equipotential l.
established cell l.
l. filter
germ l.
glioblastoma cell l.
grid l.
Gubler l.
Haller l.
Head l.
Hensen l.
Hunter-Schreger l.
incremental l.
Ishikawa cell l.
Kaes l.
Kerley A, B l.'s
Langer l.
LoVo human colorectal cancer
cell l.
M l.
Muehrcke l.
l. number
l. of demarcation
l. of Retzius
l.'s of Zahn
Ohngren l.
Owen l.
Raji cell l.
Reid base l. (RBL)
resonance l.
Retzius l.
Schreger l.
l. spectrum
tender l.
l. test
Ullmann l.
Wegner l.
WiDr human colorectal cancer
cell l.
Z l.
Zahn l.
linea, *pl.* **lineae**
lineae albicantes
lineae atrophicae
l. pectinata canalis analis
l. splendens
lineae (*pl. of* linea)
lineage
l. infidelity
l. marker
ulcer associated cell l. (UACL)
linear
l. acceleration
l. amplifier

l. attenuation coefficient
l. deposition
l. discriminant algorithm
l. energy transfer (LET)
l. fracture
l. IgA bullous disease in
children
l. sebaceous nevus syndrome
l. ulcer
linearis
morphea l.
linearity check
linens
Staphylococcus equorum subsp. *l.*
line-spread function
Lineweaver-Burk equation
Lingelsheimia anitrata
lingua, *pl.* **linguae**
anthracosis linguae
folia linguae
frenulum linguae
ichthyosis linguae
tunica mucosa linguae
linguae (*pl. of* lingua)
lingual
l. crypt
l. follicle
l. goiter
l. papilla
l. tonsil
lingualis
folliculi linguales
tonsilla l.
Linguatula
L. rhinaria
L. serrata
linguatuliasis
Linguatulidae
linguloides
Diphyllobothrium l.
lini
Pseudomonas l.
lining cell
linin network
linitis plastica
linkage
l. analysis
chromosomal l.
l. disequilibrium
l. group
l. map
linnaean system of nomenclature
Linognathus
linoleate
linoleic acid
linolenic acid
linolic acid
Linstowiidae
liotrix

L

lip
    cleft l.
    pseudocolloid of l's.
    rhombic l.
liparocele
lipase
    l. assay
    clearing factor l.
    lipoprotein l. (LPL)
    l. 105 stain
    l. test
    triacylglycerol l.
lipedema
lipemia
    absorptive l.
    alimentary l.
    diabetic l.
    postprandial l.
    l. retinalis
lipemic
lipid
    l. A
    accumulation of complex l.'s
    anisotropic l.
    l. assay
    Ciaccio-positive l.
    l. degeneration
    l. depletion
    l. embolism
    extracellular aggregate alteration l.
    fecal l.'s
    l. histiocytosis
    l. metabolism
    l. nephrosis
    Niemann-Pick l.
    nuclear aggregate l.
    l. peroxidation
    l. peroxidation of intracellular
      membrane
    l. pigment
    l. pneumonia
    l. profile
    l. proteinosis
    l. stain
    stool l.'s
    l. storage disease
    l. synthesis (LS)
    l. test
    l. transport disorder
    l. vesicle-encapsulated hemoglobin
lipid-associated
    l.-a. sialic acid
    l.-a. sialic acid in plasma
lipidemia
lipidized glioma
lipid-linked glycoconjugate
lipidosis
    cerebroside l.
    glycolipid l.

    sphingomyelin l.
    stellate-cell l.
    sulfatide l.
lipid-rich neoplastic cell
lipiduria
Lipi+Plus
    L. direct HDL assay
    L. direct LDL assay
lipoarthritis
lipoatrophia
    l. annularis
    l. circumscripta
lipoatrophic diabetes
lipoatrophy
    insulin l.
lipoblastic lipoma
lipoblastoma
lipoblastomatosis
lipocalidus
    Syntrophothermus l.
lipocalin
    human neutrophil l. (HNL)
lipocele
lipochitooligosaccharide
lipochondral degeneration
lipochondrodystrophy
lipochoristoma
lipochrome
    l. pigment
    l. pigmentation
LipoClear
    L. Plus lipemia clearing reagent
    L. reagent tube
lipocortin enzyme
lipocrit
lipocyte
lipodystrophia
    l. intestinalis
    l. progessiva superior
lipodystrophy
    congenital total l.
    inferior l.
    insulin l.
    intestinal l.
    limb l.
    mesenteric l.
    progressive l.
lipoedema
lipofibroma
lipofuscin
    l. accumulation
    ceroid l.
    l. granule
    l. pigment
lipofuscinosis
lipogenesis
lipogenic
lipogranuloma
lipogranulomatosis

disseminated l.
Farber l.
lipoic acid
lipoid
  l. degeneration
  l. dermatoarthritis
  l. dystrophy
  Forssman l.
  l. granuloma
  l. nephrosis (LN)
  l. pneumonia
  l. proteinosis
  l. thesaurismosis
lipoidica
  necrobiosis l.
lipoidosis
lipolysis regulation
lipolysosome
lipolytic
  l. enzyme
  l. hormone
lipolytica
  Aequorivita l.
lipoma
  l. annulare colli
  l. arborescens
  atypical l.
  l. capsulare
  l. cavernosum
  chondroid l.
  fetal fat cell l.
  l. fibrosum
  fibrous spindle cell l.
  infiltrating l.
  lipoblastic l.
  l. myxomatodes
  l. ossificans
  l. petrificans
  pleomorphic l.
  l. sarcomatodes
  l. sarcomatosum
  soft tissue l.
  spindle cell l.
  telangiectatic l.
lipomatodes
  nevus l.
lipomatoid
lipomatosa
  macrodystrophia l.
lipomatosis
  encephalocraniocutaneous l.
  mediastinal l.
  multiple symmetric l.
  l. neurotica
  l. of nerve
lipomatosum
  myxoma l.
lipomatosus
  nevus l.

lipomatous
  l. hemangiopericytoma (LHPC)
  l. hypertrophy
  l. infiltration
  l. myxoma
  l. polyp
lipomelanic reticulosis
lipomelanin
lipomelanotic
  l. reticuloendothelial cell hyperplasia
  l. reticulosis
lipomeningocele
lipomucopolysaccharidosis
Lipomyces
lipomyelomeningocele
Liponyssoides
Liponyssus
lipopeliosis
lipopenia
lipopenic
lipophage
lipophagia granulomatosis
lipophagic
  l. granuloma
  l. intestinal granulomatosis
lipophagy
lipophanerosis
lipophilic dye
lipophilum
  Mycoplasma l.
lipophyllodes tumor
lipopolysaccharide (LPS, OXK)
  l. extract
  OX2 l.
  OX19 l.
Lipoprint
  L. cholesterol subfraction test system
  L. LDL subfraction test
lipoprotein (LP)
  l. a (LpA)
  acetylated low-density l. (AcLDL)
  alpha l.
  l. assay
  beta l.
  l. chylomicron
  l. electrophoresis (LPE)
  l. electrophoresis test
  high-density l. (HDL)
  intermediate-density l. (IDL)
  l. lipase (LPL)
  l. lipase deficiency
  low-density l. (LDL)
  oxidized low density l. (oxLDL)
  l. phenotyping
  l. polymorphism
  very-high-density l. (VHDL)
  very-low-density l. (VLDL)
  l. X (LpX)

L

lipoprotein-associated phospholipase A2
lipoprotein-cholesterol
    l.-c. fractionation
    high-density l.-c. (HDL-C)
    low-density l.-c. (LDL-C)
lipoproteinemia
liposarcoma
    dedifferentiated l.
    myxoid l.
liposis
liposome
Lipotena cervi
Lipothrixvirus
lipotoxin
lipotrophic
lipotropic
lipotropin (LPH)
lipotropy
lipovaccine
lipoxenous
lipoxeny
lipoxin
lipoxygenase
    l. enzyme
    l. pathway
lipoxygenase-induced apoptosis
lipping
Lipschtz cell
Lipschütz
    L. body
    L. disease
    L. ulcer
lipuria
lipuric
liquefaciens
    Aerobacter l.
    Aeromonas l.
    Enterobacter l.
    Moraxella l.
    Serratia l.
liquefacient
liquefaction
    l. degeneration
    l. necrosis
liquefactive
    l. degeneration
    l. necrosis
liquefy
Liquichek
    L. hematology-16 control
    L. hematology control (A)
    L. hematology control (C)
    L. immunology control
    L. qualitative urine toxicology control
    L. reticulocyte control and stain
    L. sedimentation rate control
    L. ToRCH Plus control

    L. urine toxicology control C2, C3, S1, S2 low opiate
liquid
    Altmann l.
    l. chromatography
    combustible l.
    Cotunnius l.
    l. crystal
    high-performance l.
    l. human serum
    l. junction potential
    l. scintillation counter
    l. scintillation counting
    l. scintillator
    l. (solution) hybridization
liquidation
    enzymatic l.
liquid-in-glass thermometer
liquid-liquid
    l.-l. chromatography
    l.-l. junction potential
liquid-phase
    l.-p. hybridization
    l.-p. hybridization protection assay
liquid-solid chromatography
liquiform
liquor
    l. cerebrospinalis
    l. cotunnii
    meconium-stained l.
    Morgagni l.
    l. puris
Lisch nodule
Lison-Dunn
    L.-D. method
    L.-D. stain
lissamine rhodamine B 200
Lissauer paralysis
lissencephalia, lissencephaly
lissencephalic
lissencephaly (*var. of* lissencephalia)
list
    l. mode
    l. structure
Listerella parodoxa
Listeria
    L. denitrificans
    L. grayi
    L. monocytogenes
listeriosis
liter (L)
    milligram per l. (mg/L)
    millimole per l. (mmol/L)
    l. per minute (L/min, Lpm)
literal
lithiasis conjunctivae
lithic acid
lithium
    l. assay

l. carbonate
l. carmine
heparin l.
l. tungstate
lithium-drifted detector
Lithobius
lithocholate
lithocholic acid
lithogenesis, lithogeny
lithogenic
lithogenous
lithogeny (*var. of* lithogenesis)
lithoid
lithonephritis
lithopedion, lithopedium
lithopedium (*var. of* lithopedion)
lithotripsy, lithotrity
lithotrity (*var. of* lithotripsy)
lithotroph
lithotrophica
    Nautilia l.
lithotrophicum
    Balnearium l.
    Sulfurovum l.
lithuresis
lithureteria
lithuria
litmus
    l. paper
    l. whey
litoralis
    Bacteriovorax l.
    Oceanisphaera l.
    Thiocapsa l.
    Ulvibacter l.
litorea
    Alteromonas l.
Little disease
littoral
    l. cell
    l. cell angioma
Littré gland
littritis
live
    l. oral poliovirus vaccine
    rubella virus vaccine, l.
livedo
    lupus l.
    postmortem l.
    l. racemosa
    l. reticularis
    l. reticularis idiopathica
    l. reticularis symptomatica
    l. telangiectatica
    l. vasculitis
livedoid
liver
    l. acinus
    l. battery

l. cancer
l. cell adenoma
l. cell carcinoma
l. cell necrosis
l. cyst
l. failure
fatty l.
l. flocculation test
l. fluke
frosted l.
l. function
l. function tests (LFT)
l. grooves
hobnail l.
hydroxylation l.
icing l.
l. kidney microsomal (LKM)
lardaceous l.
nutmeg l.
l. palm
polycystic l.
portal lobule of l.
l. profile
l. rot
septal fibrosis of l.
sugar-icing l.
wandering l.
waxy l.
yellow atrophy of l.
liver-derived sex steroid-binding globulin
liver-pancreas (LP)
lividity
    postmortem l.
living donor (LD)
livingstonensis
    Shewanella l.
livor mortis
lixiviation
LJM
    Lowenstein-Jensen medium
Ljubljana classification
l1307K gene mutation
LKM
    liver kidney microsomal
    LKM antibody
L-kynurenine hydrolase
L-L factor
LLL
    localized leishmania lymphadenitis
LLM
    localized leukocyte mobilization
Lloyd reagent
l-lysine:NAD$^+$ oxidoreductase
LM
    light microscopy
LMC
    lymphocyte-mediated cytotoxicity
    LMC assay

L

LMD
low molecular weight dextran
L/min
liter per minute
LMP
latent membrane protein
low malignant potential
LMP-1
latent membrane protein 1
LMS
leiomyosarcoma
LMW
low molecular weight
LMWD
low molecular weight dextran
LMX1B gene
LN
lipoid nephrosis
lobular neoplasia
lymph node
LN1 antibody
LN2 antibody
LNB
large-needle aspiration biopsy
LNC
large noncleaved
LNGFR
low-affinity nerve growth factor
receptor
LN-met
lymph node metastasis
LN3 monoclonal antibody
LNPF
lymph node permeability
factor
loa
Filaria l.
load
l. factor
magnum l.
viral l.
loading
l. buffer
l. dose
impact l.
impulsive l.
salt l.
lobar
l. cerebral atrophy
l. pneumonia
l. pulmonary atrophy
l. sclerosis
lobatum
hepar l.
lobe
succenturiate l.
lobectomy
sleeve l.
lobi (*pl. of* lobus)

lobitis
Loboa loboi
Lobo disease
loboi
Lacazia l.
Loboa l.
Trichosporon l.
Lobomyces
lobomycosis
lobopodium
Lobstein
L. disease
L. ganglion
L. syndrome
lobster-claw deformity
lobular
l. adenocarcinoma
l. cancerization
l. carcinoma
l. carcinoma in situ (LCIS)
l. disarray
l. epithelial hyperplasia
l. glomerulonephritis
l. neoplasia (LN)
l. panniculitis
l. pattern
l. phenotype
l. pneumonia
l. proliferation
l. proliferative lesion
lobulation
fetal l.
lobule
classic liver l.
ear l.
hepatic l.
l. of epididymis
l. of testis
l. of thymus
primary pulmonary l.
renal cortical l.
respiratory l.
secondary pulmonary l.
thyroid l.
lobulet, lobulette
lobulette (*var. of* lobulet)
lobuli (*pl. of* lobulus)
lobulitis
lymphocytic l.
lobulocentricity
lobulocentric pattern
lobulus, *pl.* **lobuli**
l. corticalis renalis
lobuli epididymidis
lobuli glandulae mammariae
lobuli glandulae thyroideae
l. hepatis
lobuli testis
lobuli thymi

lobus, *pl.* **lobi**
l. anterior hypophyseos
lobi glandulae mammariae
l. glandularis hypophyseos
l. nervosus
l. posterior hypophyseos
local
l. anaphylaxis
l. anemia
l. cementoosseous dysphasia (LOCD)
l. death
l. deposition of hemosiderin
l. exhaust ventilation
l. glomerulonephritis
l. immunity
l. lesion
l. reaction
l. recurrence
l. replication
l. skin memory
localization
immunocytochemical l.
l. needle
l. suture
localized
l. black eschar
l. fibroma
l. fibrous tumor (LFT)
l. histiocytosis
l. inflammation
l. leishmania lymphadenitis (LLL)
l. leukocyte mobilization (LLM)
l. mucinosis
l. nodular tenosynovitis
l. osteitis fibrosa
l. peritonitis
l. plaque formation (LPF)
l. Schwartzman reaction
l. scleroderma
locant
location
storage l.
LOCD
local cementoosseous dysphasia
loci (*pl. of* locus)
locisalis
Halobacillus l.
Locke-Ringer solution
Locke solution
lock-in amplifier
lockout
criticality l.
locomotive cell
locoregional
loculated
l. architecture
l. empyema

loculation
loculus
locus, *pl.* **loci**
l. ceruleus
cis-acting l.
developmental endothelial l. 1 (DEL1)
four l.
histocompatibility l. (HL)
major histocompatibility l.
microsatellite l.
l. niger
LOD
logarithm of odds
LOD score
Lodderomyces elongisporus
Loeb deciduoma
loessense
Rhizobium l.
Loevit cell
Loewenthal reaction
Löffler
L. blood culture medium
L. blood serum
L. caustic stain
L. coagulated serum medium
L. disease
L. endocarditis
L. methylene blue
L. myocarditis
L. serum agar
L. syndrome I, II
logarithm
common l.
napierian l.
l. of odds (LOD)
logarithmic
l. amplifier
l. curve
l. phase
log dilution
logic
logical record
logit transformation
lognormal distribution
LOH
loss of heterozygosity
LOH assay
Lohlein-Baehr lesion
loiasis
loihiensis
Idiomarina l.
Loktanella
L. fryxellensis
L. salsilacus
L. vestfoldensis
Lomentospora
lomustine
London force

L

long
l. arm of chromosome
L. coefficient
L. formula
l. incubation hepatitis
l. terminal repeat sequence (LTR)
l. tract
l. tract sign
long-acting thyroid stimulator (LATS)
longbeachae
Legionella l.
long-chain
l.-c. fatty acid (LCFA)
l.-c. polyunsaturated fatty acid (LCPUFA)
l.-c. triglyceride (LCT)
longicatena
Actinocorallia l.
Dorea l.
longifusum
Trichophyton l.
longior
Tyroglyphus l.
longipalpis
Lutzomyia l.
longirostratum
Exserohilum l.
longispicularis
Trichostrongylus l.
longispiculata
Nematodirella l.
Longispora albida
longissimespiculata
Nematodirella l.
longitudinal
l. fold
l. layer
l. layer of muscular tunic
l. section
long-range wound
long-segment Hirschsprung disease
long-spacing
segment l.-s. (SLS)
long-term
l.-t. potentiation (LTP)
l.-t. treatment with aspirin
longus
Erythrobacter l.
lookback process
loop
capillary l.
l. diuretic
l. electrosurgical excisional procedure (LEEP)
feedback l.
feed forward l.
flow volume l.
gamma l.
Granit l.

hairpin l.
hysteresis l.
inoculating l.
nephronic l.
l. of Henle
looped fluid
looping
hot l.
loop-o-gram
loose
l. contact wound
l. skin
Looser-Milkman syndrome
Lophodermium
Lophophora
lophotrichous
Lorain
L. disease
L. dwarfism
Lorain-Lévi syndrome
lordoscoliosis
lordosis
lordotic
l. albuminuria
l. pelvis
lorgnette
main en l.
loricrin
Losch nodule
loss
allele-specific l.
allelic l.
blood l. (BL)
conductive hearing l.
eddy-current l.
estimated blood l. (EBL)
fractional allelic l.
insensible water l.
occult blood l.
l. of expression and prognosis
l. of heterozygosity (LOH)
recurrent fetal l. (RFL)
third-space fluid l.
transepidermal water l. (TWL)
lost to followup (LTF)
Lou Gehrig disease
Louis-Bar syndrome
Louisiana pneumonia
louping
l. ill
l. ill virus
louse
body l.
chicken l.
crab l.
dog l.
head l.
pubic l.
sucking l.

louse-borne
    l.-b. relapsing fever
    l.-b. typhus
lousiness
lousy
lova
    Dracunculus l.
lovaniensis
    Acetobacter l.
Lovelace (*var.* of Boothby, Lovelace, Bulbulian)
LoVo human colorectal cancer cell line
low
    l. birth weight (LBW)
    l. birth weight infant (LBWI)
    l. density lipoprotein receptor
    l. egg-passage vaccine
    l. explosive
    l. grade astrocytoma
    l. iron diamine (LID)
    l. level
    l. magnification
    l. malignant potential (LMP)
    l. molecular weight (LMW)
    l. molecular weight dextran (LMD, LMWD)
    l. molecular weight kininogen
    l. order
    l. probability, high consequence event (LPHC)
    l. protein
    l. serum-bound iron (LBI)
low-actinic glass
low-affinity nerve growth factor receptor (LNGFR)
low-compliance bladder
low-density
    l.-d. lipoprotein (LDL)
    l.-d. lipoprotein-cholesterol (LDL-C)
Lowe
    L. disease
    L. syndrome (LS)
Löwenberg
    L. canal
    L. scala
Lowenstein-Jensen
    L.-J. agar
    L.-J. medium (LJM)
    L.-J. plate
Löwenstein process
Lowenthal test
lower
    l. anal canal
    l. motor neuron (LM)
    l. nephron nephrosis
    l. ring
    l. urinary tract infection
Lowe-Terrey-MacLachlan syndrome
low-fiber diet

low-frequency transduction
low-grade
    l.-g. angiosarcoma
    l.-g. dysplasia (LGD)
    l.-g. endometrial stromal sarcoma (LGESS)
    l.-g. fibromyxoid sarcoma
    l.-g. squamous intraepithelial lesion (LGSIL, LSIL)
    l.-g. TCC
Lown-Ganong-Levine syndrome
low-pass filter
low-power field (LPF)
low-range heparin management (LHMT)
low-risk tumor (LRT)
low-temperature
    l.-t. antigen retrieval (LTAR)
    l.-t., heat-mediated antigen retrieval (LTHMAR)
low-voltage
    l.-v. fast (LVF)
    l.-v. focus (LVF)
    l.-v. high-resolution scanning electron microscopy (LV-HRSEM)
low-volume air thermal cycle format
Loxosceles
    L. laeta
    L. reclusa
Loxotrema ovatum
L:P
    lactate-pyruvate ratio
LP
    lamina propria
    latency period
    lipoprotein
    liver-pancreas
    low protein
    lumbar puncture
    lymphocyte predominant
    lymphoid plasma
    LP antigen
LPA
    lysophosphatidic acid
LpA
    lipoprotein a
LPC
    late positive component
LPD
    lymphoproliferative disease
LPE
    lipoprotein electrophoresis
LPF
    leukocytosis-promoting factor
    localized plaque formation
    low-power field
    lymphocytosis-promoting factor
LPH
    lipotropin
L-phase variant

L

LPHC
> low probability, high consequence event

LPHD
> lymphocyte-predominant Hodgkin disease

LPI
> lysinuric protein intolerance

LPI/LRI
> lymphocyte proliferation/regression index

LPL
> lipoprotein lipase
> lymphoplasmacytoid lymphoma

Lpm
> liter per minute

LPP
> lichen planopilaris

LPR
> lactate-pyruvate ratio
> late-phase response

LPS
> large particle sorting module
> lipopolysaccharide

LPT
> lymphocyte-predominant thymoma

LPV
> lymphotropic papovavirus

LpX
> lipoprotein X

LQTS Finnish founder mutation

L:R
> left-to-right ratio

LR
> laboratory reference
> light reaction

Lr
> limes reacting

L$_r$dose (*var. of* Lr dose)

Lr dose, L$_r$dose, L$_r$dose

LRN
> Laboratory Response Network
> LRN BioWatch laboratory

LRP
> luciferase reporter mycobacteriophage
> LRP assay

LRS
> lactated Ringer solution

LRT
> low-risk tumor

LS
> leiomyosarcoma
> lipid synthesis
> Lowe syndrome
> lymphosarcoma

LSA
> lymphosarcoma
> LSA 6500 liquid scintillation counting system

> LSA 100Q/200/230 series laser diffraction particle size analyzer
> LSA 13 320 series laser diffraction particle size analyzer

LSAB
> labeled streptavidin biotin

LSAB2 multistep detection system

l-saccharopine

LSA/RCS
> lymphosarcoma-reticulum cell sarcoma

LSD
> lysergic acid diethylamide

L-selectin

LSG
> labial salivary gland
> LSG biopsy

LSH
> lutein-stimulating hormone

LSIL
> low-grade squamous intraepithelial lesion

LSM
> late systolic murmur

L:S ratio

LST
> lysis, storage, and transportation
> LST buffer

l-sulfoiduronate sulfatase

LT
> lymphotoxin

LTA4
> epoxide leukotriene L.

LTAR
> low-temperature antigen retrieval

LTB
> laryngotracheobronchitis

LTF
> lost to followup

LTH
> luteotropic hormone

LTHMAR
> low-temperature, heat-mediated antigen retrieval

LTP
> long-term potentiation

LTR
> long terminal repeat sequence

LUA
> Legionella urinary antigen
> LUA ELISA test kit

Lu antigen

Lubarsch
> L. crystal
> crystal of L.

LUC
> large unstained cell

Lucas-Championnière disease

lucent

lucentense
  Haloferax l.
lucentensis
  Thalassospira l.
Lucetina
Lucey-Driscoll syndrome
lucida
  lamina l.
lucidum
  stratum l.
luciferase reporter mycobacteriophage (LRP)
luciferensis
  Bacillus l.
Lucilia
  L. caesar
  L. illustris
  L. sericata
Lucio
  L. leprosy
  L. leprosy phenomenon
Lucké
  L. adenocarcinoma
  L. carcinoma
  L. virus
lückenschädel
Lücke test
ludipueritiae
  Teichococcus l.
Ludwig
  L. angina
  L. labyrinth
Luebering-Rapaport pathway
Luer lock glass syringe
lues
  L. III
luetic
  l. aneurysm
  l. aortitis
Luft
  L. disease
  L. potassium permanganate
    fixative
Lugol
  L. iodine
  L. iodine solution
  L. stain
Lukes-Butler
  L.-B. histologic subclassification
  L.-B. Hodgkin disease classification
  L.-B. non-Hodgkin lymphoma
    classification
Lukes-Collins non-Hodgkin lymphoma classification
Luki aspirating tube
lumbago
lumbar
  l. appendicitis
  l. canal stenosis

  l. puncture (LP)
  l. spondylosis
lumbosacral (LS)
  l. myelopathy
  l. radiculopathy
lumbrical
lumbricidal
lumbricide
lumbricoid
lumbricoides
  Ascaris l.
lumbricosis
lumbricus
lumen, *pl.* **lumina, lumens**
  acinar l.
  Fluhmann l.
  intracytoplasmic lumina (ICL)
  residual l.
lumens (*pl. of* lumen)
lumiaggregation
  platelet l.
lumican
lumina (*pl. of* lumen)
luminal pattern
luminescence
luminescent
luminometer
luminometry
luminophore
luminous
  l. flux
  l. flux density
  l. intensity
Lumi-Phos solution
lumpy
  l. jaw
  l. skin disease
lumpy-bumpy
  l.-b. deposit
  l.-b. immunofluorescence
Luna-Ishak stain
lunar
lunata
  Curvularia l.
lunate
lung
  acinic cell tumor of l.
  l. aspiration
  l. biopsy
  bird-breeder's l.
  bird-fancier's l.
  black l.
  blast l.
  busulfan l.
  butterfly l.
  l. cancer
  l. carcinoid
  l. carcinoma
  cheese worker's l.

L

lung (*continued*)
    collier's l.
    eosinophilic l.
    eosinophilic granuloma of l. (EGL)
    l. fluke
    honeycomb l.
    human embryo l. (HEL)
    humidifier l.
    hyperlucent l.
    malt-worker's l.
    maple bark stripper's l.
    mason's l.
    miner's l.
    mushroom-worker's l.
    pizza l.
    rheumatoid l.
    rudimentary l.
    l. section
    shock l.
    silo-filler's l.
    thresher's l.
    l. tumor
    l. unit
    uremic l.
    welder's l.
    woodworker's l.
lunger disease
lungworm
lunotriquetral
Lunyo virus
lupi
    Spirocerca l.
lupiform
lupinine
lupinosa
    porrigo l.
lupoid
    l. hepatitis
    l. leishmaniasis
    l. ulcer
luposa
    tuberculosis cutis l.
lupous
lupus
    l. anticoagulant (LA)
    l. anticoagulant positive control
    l. band test
    cerebral l.
    chilblain l.
    chronic discoid l.
    l. erythematosus (LE)
    l. erythematosus cell
    l. erythematosus disseminatus (LED)
    l. erythematosus inhibitor
    l. erythematosus profundus
    hydralazine l.
    l. hypertrophicus
    laryngeal l.
    l. livedo

    l. lymphaticus
    l. mutilans
    neonatal l.
    l. nephritis
    l. panniculitis
    l. papillomatosus
    l. pernio
    l. pleuritis
    l. psoriasis
    l. sclerosus
    l. sebaceous
    l. serpiginosus
    subacute cutaneous l.
    l. superficialis
    l. tuberculosus
    l. tumidus
    l. verrucosus
    l. vulgaris
lurida
    Amycolatopsis l.
    Amycolatopsis orientalis
      subsp. *l.*
luridiscabiei
    Streptomyces l.
lusatiensis
    Defluvibacter l.
Luschka
    L. cystic gland
    L. duct
    foramen of L.
    L. tonsil
Luse body
lusitana
    Aquicella l.
lusitaniae
    Clavispora l.
lusitanum
    Herbaspirillum l.
lusoria
    dysphagia l.
lutea
    macula l.
    Pseudomonas l.
luteae
    fovea centralis maculae l.
luteal
    l. cell
    l. cyst
    l. hormone
Luteimonas mephitis
lutein cell
luteinalis
    hyperreactio l. (HL)
luteinization
luteinize
luteinized follicular cyst
luteinizing
    l. hormone (LH)
    l. hormone assay

l. hormone-releasing factor (LH-RF)
l. hormone-releasing hormone (LH-RH)
l. hormone secretion
l. principle
l. tumor
luteinoma
lutein-stimulating hormone (LSH)
luteireticuli
    Streptomyces l.
Lutembacher syndrome
Luteococcus
    L. peritonei
    L. sanguinis
luteogenic
luteola
    Auchmeromyia l.
luteolum
    Brevibacterium l.
    Chlorobium l.
luteolus
    Agromyces l.
    Arthrobacter l.
luteolysis
luteolytic
luteoma
    pregnancy l.
    stromal l.
luteotropic hormone (LTH)
luteotropin
Luteovirus
lutetiensis
    Streptococcus l.
lutetium
luteum
    atretic corpus l.
    l. cell
    corpus l.
    cystic corpus l.
    punctum l.
luteus
    Micrococcus l.
Lutheran
    L. blood antibody type
    L. blood group
    L. blood group system
luti
    Psychrobacter l.
    Ruminococcus l.
lututrin
Lutzomyia
    L. flaviscutellata
    L. intermedius
    L. longipalpis
    L. peruensis
Lutz-Splendore-Almeida disease
luxation
Luxol fast blue stain
luxury perfusion

luxus heart
Luys
    L. body syndrome
    L. segregator
LVE
    left ventricular enlargement
LVF
    left ventricular failure
    low-voltage fast
    low-voltage focus
LVH
    large vessel hematocrit
    left ventricular hypertrophy
LV-HRSEM
    low-voltage high-resolution scanning electron microscopy
LVI
    lymphatic vessel invasion
LVSI
    lymphovascular space invasion
LW
    Lee-White
Lw antigen
lwoffi
    Acinetobacter calcoaceticus l.
lwoffii
    Achromobacter l.
LX4201 clinical system
LXi 725 clinical system
LX20, LX200, LX2000 PRO clinical system
l-xylulose
    l-x. dehydrogenase
    l-x. reductase
l-xylulosuria
Ly antigen
lyase
    adenylosuccinate l.
    argininosuccinate l.
Lyb antigen
lycopenemia
lycoperdonosis
Lycoperdon perlatum
lycophora
lye
Lyell
    L. disease
    L. syndrome
LYG
    lymphomatoid granulomatosis
LYM
    lymphoma
Lymantria
Lyme
    L. borreliosis
    L. disease
    L. disease serology
    L. neuroborreliosis
Lymnaea

L

lymph
　　aplastic l.
　　blood l.
　　l. capillary
　　l. cell
　　l. cord
　　l. corpuscle
　　corpuscular l.
　　croupous l.
　　dental l.
　　l. embolism
　　euplastic l.
　　fibrinous l.
　　l. filtration
　　l. gland
　　glycerinated l.
　　inflammatory l.
　　intercellular l.
　　intravascular l.
　　l. node (LN)
　　l. node biopsy
　　l. node cancer
　　l. node hyperplasia
　　l. node infarction
　　l. node involvement
　　l. node metastasis (LN-met)
　　l. node permeability factor (LNPF)
　　l. node puncture
　　l. node sectioning
　　l. nodule
　　plastic l.
　　l. scrotum
　　l. sinus
　　l. space
　　tissue l.
　　vaccine l.
　　l. varix
lymphaden
lymphadenitis
　　acute suppurative l.
　　cytomegalovirus l.
　　dermatopathic l.
　　hemorrhagic thoracic l.
　　herpes simplex l.
　　histiocytic necrotizing l. (HNL)
　　Kikuchi l.
　　Kikuchi-Fujimoto l.
　　localized leishmania l. (LLL)
　　mediastinal l.
　　mesenteric l.
　　postvaccinial l.
　　regional granulomatous l.
　　tuberculosis l.
　　tuberculous l.
lymphadenoid goiter
lymphadenoma
lymphadenomatosis
lymphadenopathy
　　angioimmunoblastic l.

　　dermatopathic l.
　　immunoblastic l. (IBL)
　　shotty l.
　　silicone l.
　　sinus histiocytosis with massive l. (SHML)
　　l. syndrome
　　syphilitic l.
lymphadenopathy-associated virus (LAV)
lymphadenosis
　　benign l.
　　malignant l.
lymphadenovarix
lymphangeitis
lymphangiectasia (*var. of* lymphangiectasis)
lymphangiectasis, lymphangiectasia
　　cavernous l.
　　congenital pulmonary l. (CPL)
　　cystic l.
　　intestinal l.
　　simple l.
lymphangiectatic
lymphangiectatica
　　pachyderma l.
lymphangiectodes
lymphangiitis
lymphangioendothelial sarcoma
lymphangioendothelioma
lymphangiogram
lymphangioleiomyomatosis (LAM)
　　pulmonary l.
lymphangiology
lymphangioma
　　l. capillare varicosum
　　l. cavernosum
　　l. circumscriptum
　　l. cysticum
　　l. superficium simplex
　　l. tuberosum multiplex
　　l. xanthelasmoideum
lymphangiomatosis
　　pulmonary l.
lymphangiomatous polyp (LAP)
lymphangiomyomatosis (LAM)
lymphangiophlebitis
lymphangiosarcoma
lymphangitis
　　l. carcinomatosa
　　epizootic l.
　　l. epizootica
lymphapheresis
lymphatic
　　l. angina
　　l. cancer
　　l. choriomeningitis (LCM)
　　l. corpuscle

l. dissemination theory of
endometriosis
l. duct
l. dyscrasia
l. edema
l. endothelial hyaluronan receptor
(LYVE1)
l. filariasis
l. follicle
l. follicle of larynx
l. leukemia
l. mapping
l. nevus
l. sarcoma
l. sinus
l. stroma
l. tissue
l. tracking
l. vessel invasion (LVI)

lymphatica
anemia l.
Filaria l.
telangiectasia l.

lymphatici
cortex nodi l.
hilum nodi l.

lymphaticum
angioma l.

lymphaticus
folliculus l.
lupus l.
nevus l.
nodulus l.
nodus l.
status l.
varix l.

lymphatitis
lymphatolysis
lymphatolytic
lymphectasia
lymphedema
congenital l.
hereditary l.
l. praecox
primary l.

lymphedematous keratoderma
lymphemia
lymphoadenoma
lymphoblast
lymphoblastic
l. leukemia
l. lymphoma
l. lymphosarcoma
l. plasma cell

lymphoblastoid
lymphoblastoma
giant follicular l.

lymphoblastosis
lymphocele

lymphocerastism
Lymphocryptovirus
lymphocutaneous sporotrichosis
lymphocyst
Lymphocystivirus
lymphocytapheresis
lymphocyte
activated l.
l. activation
atypical l.
B l.
binucleated l.
l. blastogenic factor
bronchial l.
bronchiolar l.
cytologic T l. (CTL)
Downey-type l.
l. function associated antigen
helper T l.
l. homing receptor
intraepithelial l.
killer l.
large granular l. (LGL)
mantle-zone l.
l. marker assay
l. microcytotoxicity assay
l. mitogenic factor
monocytoid l. (ML)
neoplastic l.
nodular poorly differentiated l.
(NPDL)
null l.
plasmacytoid l.
l. predominant
l. proliferation/regression index
(LPI/LRI)
reactive l.'s
Rieder l.
small l. (SL)
splenic lymphoma with villous l.
(SLVL)
l. subset
l. subset enumeration
l. subset panel
suppressor T l.
T l.
l. transfer test
l. transformation
l. transformation immunoassay
l. transformation test
transformed l.
tumor-infiltrating l. (TIL)
vacuolated l.
Willemze type A l.

lymphocyte-activating factor
lymphocyte-defined (LD)
**lymphocyte-depleted Hodgkin disease
(LDHD)**
lymphocyte-mediated cytotoxicity (LMC)

L

lymphocyte-predominant
l.-p. Hodgkin disease (LPHD)
l.-p. thymoma (LPT)
lymphocyte-rich classic Hodgkin
lymphocyte-stimulating hormone
lymphocyte-transforming factor
lymphocythemia
lymphocytic
l. adenohypophysitis
l. blood cell
l. choriomeningitis (LCM)
l. choriomeningitis virus (LCV)
l. colitis (LC)
l. cuffing
l. enterocolitis
l. gastritis
l. hypophysitis
l. infiltration
l. inflammatory infiltrate
l. interstitial pneumonia (LIP)
l. interstitial pneumonitis (LIP)
l. leukemia (LCL)
l. leukemia marker panel
l. leukemoid reaction
l. leukocytosis
l. leukopenia
l. lobulitis
l. lymphoma
l. lymphosarcoma (LCL)
l. marrow
l. series
l. thymoma
l. thyroiditis
l. transformation
l. vasculitis
lymphocytic-histiocytic (L-H)
lymphocytoblast
lymphocytolysis
lymphocytoma
lymphocytopenia
lymphocytopoiesis
lymphocytorrhexis
lymphocytosis
intraepithelial l.
neutrophilic l.
lymphocytosis-promoting factor (LPF)
lymphocytotoxic antibody (LCTA)
lymphocytotoxicity
lymphocytotoxin
lymphoderma perniciosa
lymphoepithelial lesion (LEL)
lymphoepithelioid cell lymphoma (LECL)
lymphoepithelioma
lymphoepithelioma-like
l.-l. carcinoma (LELC)
l.-l. thymic carcinoma (LETC)
lymphogenesis
lymphogenic

lymphogenous
l. embolism
l. metastasis
lymphoglandula
lymphogranuloma
l. benignum
l. inguinale
l. malignum
Schaumann l.
venereal l.
l. venereum (LGV)
l. venereum antigen
l. venereum titer
l. venereum-trachoma inclusion
conjunctivitis (LGV-TRIC)
l. venereum virus
lymphogranulomatosis
Miyagawanella l.
lymphohematopoiesis
lymphohematopoietic
lymphohistiocytic vasculitis
lymphohistiocytoid mesothelioma (LHM)
lymphohistiocytosis
familial erythrophagocytic l. (FEL)
familial hemophagocytic l. (FHL, FHLH, FMLH)
hemophagocytic l. (HLH)
lymphoid
l. aggregate
l. aplasia
l. corpuscle
l. cuffing
l. follicle
l. hemoblast of Pappenheim
l. hyperplasia
l. hypophysitis
l. hypoplasia
l. interstitial pneumonia (LIP)
l. leukemia
l. leukocyte
l. monoclonal antibody
l. neoplasm
l. nodule
l. organ
l. plasma (LP)
l. polyp
l. progenitor cell
l. series
l. stem cell
l. tumor
lymphoidei
medulla nodi l.
lymphoidocyte
lymphoid-rich effusion
lymphokine
lymphokine-activated killer cell
lympholeukocyte
lymphology
lymphoma (LYM)

acute lymphoblastic leukemia
  secondary to Burkitt l.
adult T-cell l. (ATL)
anaplastic large cell l. (ALCL)
angiocentric T-cell l.
angioimmunoblastic l. (AIL)
angioimmunoblastic T-cell l. (AIL
angiotrophic l.
B-cell l. (BCL)
B-cell chronic lymphocytic
  leukemia/small lymphocytic l.
B-cell non-Hodgkin l. (B-NHL)
biphenotypic l.
blastoid variant of mantle cell l.
  (BMCL)
blastoma mantle cell l. (BMCL)
Burkitt l. (BL)
Burkitt-like l.
centroblastic l.
centrocytic l.
centrocytic/mantle-cell l. (CC/MCL)
classic Hodgkin l. (CHL)
composite l.
cutaneous l.
cutaneous B-cell l. (CBCL)
cutaneous T-cell l. (CTCL)
diffuse histocytic l. (DHL)
diffuse large B-cell l. (DLBCL)
diffuse large cell l. (DLCL)
diffuse poorly differentiated l.
  (DPDL)
diffuse small cleaved cell l.
discordant l.
endemic Burkitt l. (eBL)
enteropathy-associated T-cell l.
extranodal marginal zone l.
floral variant of follicular l. (FFL)
follicle-cell l.
follicle center l. (FCL)
follicular l. (FL)
giant follicle l.
giant follicular l.
gray zone l.
high-grade B-cell l.
histiocyte-rich B-cell l. (HRBCL)
histiocytic l. (HL)
Hodgkin l.
immunoblastic l.
l. immunophenotyping
Ki-1+ l.
large B-cell l. (LBCL)
large-cell immunoblastic l.
large-cell non-Hodgkin l. (LCNHL)
Lennert l.
lymphoblastic l.
lymphocytic l.
lymphoepithelioid cell l. (LECL)
lymphoplasmacytic l.
lymphoplasmacytoid l. (LPL)

lymphosarcoma-type malignant l.
macrofollicular l.
malignant l. (ML)
MALT l.
mantle cell l. (MCL)
mantle cell lymphocytic l.
mantle zone l. (MZL)
marginal zone l. (MZL)
marginal zone B-cell l. (MZBCL)
marginal zone cell l. (MZL)
Mediterranean l.
microvillus l.
mixed large- and small-cell
  non-Hodgkin l. (MNHL)
monocytoid B-cell l.
mucosa-associated lymphoid tissue l.
  (MALToma)
nasal angiocentric T-cell l. (NATL)
nasal T/NK-cell l.
natural killer cell l.
NK l.
nodal marginal zone B-cell l.
nodular histiocytic l.
nonepidermotropic primary cutaneous
  T-cell l.
non-Hodgkin l. (NHL)
non-MALT l.
null cell l.
null-type non-Hodgkin l.
plaque-stage cutaneous T-cell l.
plasmacytoid l.
polymorphic B-cell l.
poorly differentiated lymphocytic l.
  (PDLL)
postthymic T-cell l. (PTCL)
prethymic lymphoblastic l.
primary bone l. (PBL)
primary central nervous system l.
  (PCNSL)
primary cutaneous anaplastic large
  cell l.
primary cutaneous CD30+ large
  T-cell l.
primary effusion l. (PEL)
primary gastric l.
pulmonary MALT l.
respiratory angiocentric l.
Revised European-American L.
  (REAL)
small cell malignant l. (SCML)
small lymphocytic l. (SLL)
small noncleaved cell, non-Burkitt l.
SNCC l.
SNCC Burkitt l.
SNCC non-Burkitt l.
splenic marginal zone l. (SMZL)
stem cell l.
T-cell l.
T-cell rich B-cell l. (TCRBCL)

L

lymphoma (*continued*)
 T-natural killer cell l.
 U-cell l.
 undifferentiated l. (UL)
 Waldeyer ring l.
 well-differentiated lymphocytic l.
  (WDLL)
 Western-type intestinal l.
lymphomagenesis
lymphoma/leukemia
 adult T-cell l.
lymphomatoid
 l. granulomatosis (LYG)
 l. papulosis
 l. polyposis
lymphomatosa
 angina l.
 struma l.
lymphomatosis
 avian l.
 fowl l.
 ocular l.
 visceral l.
lymphomatosum
 adenocystoma l.
 cystadenoma l.
lymphomatous
lymphomyeloma
lymphomyxoma
lymphopathia venereum
lymphopenia
 CD4 l.
lymphopenic thymic dysplasia
lymphophagocytosis
lymphophilum
 Propionibacterium l.
 Propionimicrobium l.
lymphoplasmacytic
 l. infiltrate
 l. infiltration
 l. inflammation
 l. lesion
 l. lymphoma
 l. response
 l. synovitis
lymphoplasmacytoid
 l. cell
 l. lymphoma (LPL)
lymphoplasmapheresis
lymphopoiesis
 B cell l.
lymphopoietic
lymphoproliferative
 l. disease (LPD)
 l. disorder
 l. syndrome
 X-linked l. (XLP)
lymphoreticular
 l. aggregate

 l. cancer
 l. disease
 l. disorder
 l. malignancy
 l. neoplasia
 l. system
lymphoreticulosis
 benign inoculation l.
lymphorrhagia (*var. of* lymphorrhea)
lymphorrhea, lymphorrhagia
lymphorrhoid
lymphosarcoma (LSA)
 l. cell leukemia
 follicular l. (FLSA)
 lymphoblastic l.
 lymphocytic l. (LCL)
 reticulum cell l.
**lymphosarcoma-reticulum cell sarcoma
 (LSA/RCS)**
lymphosarcomatosis
lymphosarcoma-type malignant lymphoma
lymphoscintigraphy
lymphosis
lymphostatic verrucosis
lymphotoxicity
lymphotoxin (LT)
lymphotropic papovavirus (LPV)
lymphovascular
 l. invasion
 l. space invasion (LVSI)
lymphuria
Lynch
 L. II syndrome
 L. syndrome tumor
lyoenzyme
Lyon hypothesis
lyonization
lyonize
lyophilization
lyophilize
lyophilized anterior pituitary (LAP)
Lyophyllum
LyP
 lymphomatoid papulosis
LYP gene
Lyphochek
 L. anemia control
 L. fertility control
 L. hypertension markers control
 L. maternal serum control
 L. tumor marker control
 L. whole blood control
Lyponyssus
Lys
 lysine
lysate
 Limulus amoebocyte l. (LAL)
lyse
lysemia

lysergic
>l. acid
>l. acid diethylamide (LSD)
>l. acid diethylamide assay

lysin
>beta l.

lysine (K, Lys)
>l. dehydrogenase
>l. intolerance
>l. ketoglutarate reductase

lysine-iron agar
lysinemia
lysine-2-oxoglutaryl reductase
lysing
>l. agent
>l. reagent

lysinogen
lysinogenic
lysinuria
lysinuric protein intolerance (LPI)
lysis
>l. buffer
>bystander l.
>clot l.
>colloid-osmotic l.
>differential cell l.
>dilute blood clot l. (DBCL)
>diluted whole blood clot l.
>euglobulin clot l. (ECL)
>fibrin plate l.
>follicle l. (Fl)
>gamma phage l.
>preferential l.
>lysis, storage, and transportation (LST)

Lysobacteraceae
Lysobacterales
lysochrome
lysogen
lysogenesis
lysogenic
>l. bacterium
>l. induction
>l. strain

lysogenicity
lysogenization
lysogeny
lysokinase

lysolecithin
lysophosphatidate
lysophosphatide
lysophosphatidic acid (LPA)
lysophosphatidyl choline
lysophosphatidylethanolamine
lysophospholipase
lysosomal
>l. protease
>l. storage disease
>l. trafficking regulator protein (LYST)

lysosomal-associated
>l.-a. membrane protein (LAMP)
>l.-a. membrane protein-1 (LAMP-1)
>l.-a. membrane protein-2 (LAMP-2)

lysosome
>angulated l.
>definitive l.
>Golgi endoplasmic reticulum l. (GERL)
>primary l.
>secondary l.

lysostaphin
lysotype
lysozyme
>l. assay
>egg-white l. (EWL)
>human milk l. (HML)
>l. test
>urine l.

lysozymuria
lyssa
Lyssavirus
LYST
>lysosomal trafficking regulator protein

lysyl
lysyl-bradykinin
lysylpyridinoline
Lyt antigen
Lythoglyphopsis
lytica
>*Cellulophaga l.*

lytic lesion
Lytta
LYVE1
>lymphatic endothelial hyaluronan receptor

L

MΩ
  megohm
m
  meter
mμ
  millimicron
M
  molar
    M antigen
    M band
    M cell
    M colony
    M component
    M concentration
    M line
    M phase
    M protein
    M spike
μm
  micrometer
M0
  acute myeloblastic leukemia without
    localized differentiation
  no cancer spread to other organs
  no evidence of distant metastases
M1
  acute myeloblastic leukemia without
    maturation
  myeloblast
M2
  acute myeloblastic leukemia with
    maturation
  promyelocyte
M3
  acute promyelocytic leukemia
M4
  acute myelomonocytic leukemia
M5
  acute monocytic leukemia
  metamyelocyte
M5a
  acute monocytic leukemia without
    differentiation
M5b
  acute monocytic leukemia with
    differentiation
M6
  acute erythroleukemia
M7
  acute megakaryocytic leukemia
  polymorphonuclear neutrophil
MA
  metastatic adenocarcinoma
  monomorphic adenoma
  muscle actin

mA
  milliampere
MAA
  macroaggregated albumin
maanshanensis
    Rhodococcus m.
MAb, mAb
  monoclonal antibody
    MAb 12C3
MAb-based enzyme immunoassay
MAC
  membrane attack complex
  Mycobacterium avium-intracellulare
    complex
Macaca
Mac387 antibody
MacCallum patch
Macchiavello stain
MacConkey
    M. agar
    M. broth
macedonicum
macedonicus
    Streptococcus gallolyticus subsp. *m.*
macerated
    m. fetus
    m. stillbirth
maceration
macestii
    Desulfomicrobium m.
MacFarlane serum method
Machado-Guerreiro test
Mache unit (MU)
machine
    m. error
    Rosys Plato Gene M.
    Sakura Seiki Autosmear automatic
      smear m.
    Select-a-Fuge microcentrifuge m.
    suicide m.
    Ventana ES slide processor m.
Machlomovirus
Machupo virus
MacKenzie syndrome
Macleod
    M. rheumatism
    M. syndrome
Macluravirus
maclurin
macmurdoensis
    Sporosarcina m.
MacNeal tetrachrome blood stain
Macracanthorhynchus hirudinaceus
macrencephalia (*var. of* macrencephaly)
macrencephaly, macrencephalia

M

macroadenoma
  intracellular m. (IM)
macroaggregate
macroaggregated albumin (MAA)
macroamylase
macroamylasemia
macroanatomic
macroangiopathic
macroarray
Macrobdella decora
macrobiote
macroblast
macrocephala
  Acrocarpospora m.
macrocephalia (*var. of* macrocephaly)
macrocephalic, macrocephalous
macrocephalous (*var. of* macrocephalic)
macrocephaly, macrocephalia
macrochemistry
macrochilia
macrochylomicron
macrocolon
macroconidium
macrocranium
macrocreatine kinase
macrocryoglobulin
macrocryoglobulinemia
macrocyst
macrocytase
macrocyte
  oval m.
macrocythemia
  hyperchromatic m.
macrocytic
  m. achylic anemia
  m. anemia of pregnancy
  m. hyperchromia
macrocytosis
macrodentium
  Treponema m.
Macroduct
  M. coil
  M. collecting system
  M. system for sweat stimulation
    and collection
macrodystrophia lipomatosa
macroencephalon
macroerythroblast
macroerythrocyte
macrofollicular
  m. adenoma
  m. lymphoma
  m. variant
macrogamete
macrogametocyte
macrogamont
macrogamy
macrogastria
macrogenitosomia

m. praecox
m. praecox suprarenalis
macroglia cell
macroglobulin
  alpha m.
  alpha-2 m.
  m. assay
macroglobulinemia
  essential m.
  Waldenström m. (WM)
macroglossia
macrogoltabida
  Sphingopyxis m.
macrogyria
macrohomology
Macrohyporia
macro-Kjeldahl method
macrolabia
Macrolepiota
macroleukoblast
macrolide antibiotic
macromastia, macromazia
macromazia (*var. of* macromastia)
macromelanosome
macromerozoite
macrometastasis
macromethod of Wintrobe
macromolecular
macromolecule
Macromonas
  M. bipunctata
  M. mobilis
macromonocyte
macromyeloblast
macronodular
macronormoblast
macronormochromoblast
macronucleolus
macronucleus
  eosinophilic m.
macroorchidism
macroovalocyte
macroparasite
macropathology
macrophage
  activated m.
  m. activation factor (MAF)
  m. agglutination factor (MAggF)
  alveolar m.
  armed m.
  associated m.
  bone marrow m.
  m. chemotactic and activating factor
    (MCAF)
  m. chemotactic factor (MCF)
  m. colony stimulating factor (M-CSF)
  m. density
  fixed m.
  foamy m.

free m.
m. growth factor
Hansemann m.
hemosiderin-laden m.'s
human alveolar m. (HAM)
inflammatory m.
m. inflammatory protein (MIP)
m. inhibiting factor (MIF)
m. migration inhibition factor
m. migration inhibition test
modified m.
monocyte m.
m. phagocytosis
m. presented antigen result
pulmonary alveolar m. (PAM)
starry-sky m.
system of m.'s
tingible-body m.
transmigration m.
von Hansemann m.
macrophage-derived growth factor
macrophagocyte
macrophases
system of m.
Macrophoma
Macrophomina
macrophotography
digital m.
macropolycyte
macroprolactinoma
macropromyelocyte
macrorchis
Prosthogonimus m.
macroreticulocyte
macroscopic
m. agglutination
m. lesion
macroscopy
macrosigmoid
macrosis
macrosomia
macrospore
Macrosporium tomato
macrosporoidium
Stemphylium m.
macrostomia
macrothrombocyte
macrotrabeculae
macrovascular hemolysis
macrovesicular
m. fat droplet
m. steatosis
mactans
Latrodectus m.
macula, *pl.* **maculae**
m. adherens
m. albida
m. atrophica
m. cerulea

m. communicans
m. communis
m. cribrosa
m. densa
m. flava
m. germinativa
m. gonorrhoica
honeycomb m.
m. lactea
m. lutea
mongolian m.
neuroepithelium of m.
m. pellucida
m. retinae
m. sacculi
Saenger m.
m. tendinea
m. utriculi
maculae (*pl. of* macula)
macular, maculate
m. amyloidosis
m. atrophy
m. eruption
m. erythema
m. fan
m. leprosy
m. star
maculate (*var. of* macular)
maculatum
Amblyomma m.
atrophoderma m.
maculatus
Anopheles m.
Maculavirus
macule
maculipennis
Anopheles m.
maculoerythematous
maculopapular eruption
maculosa
dermatitis atrophicans m.
madagascariensis
Inermicapsifer m.
Taenia m.
madarosis
madder
Maddrey discriminant function
Madelung
M. disease
M. neck
mad itch
Madura
M. boil
M. foot
madurae
Actinomadura m.
Streptomyces m.
Madurella
M. grisea

M

Madurella (*continued*)
    M. mycetomi
maduromycetoma
maduromycosis
maduromycotic mycetoma
maedi virus
MAF
    macrophage activation factor
    metanephric adenofibroma
Maffucci
    M. disease
    M. syndrome
MAFP
    methylarachidonyl fluorophosphonate
MAG
    multifocal atrophic gastritis
magadiensis
    Halomonas m.
    Tindallia m.
magaldrate
magenta
    acid m.
    basic m.
    m. I–III
    m. O
MAggF
    macrophage agglutination factor
maggot
    Congo floor m.
    rat-tail m.
Magitot disease
magna
    coxa m.
    Fascioloides m.
    Finegoldia m.
magnesium (Mg)
    m. ammonium phosphate
    m. assay
    m. imbalance
    m. ion (Mg2+)
    m. oxide (MgO)
    m. test
    urine m.
magnesium-activated ATPase
magnetic
    m. core
    m. core memory
    m. field
    m. field strength
    m. flux
    m. induction
    m. moment
    m. susceptibility
    m. tape
magneticus
    Desulfovibrio m.
magnetization
magnifica
    Wohlfahrtia m.

magnification (X)
    high m.
    low m.
    medium m.
magnifier
    Omnivue illuminated m.
magnitude
    signed m.
magnivelare
    Tricholoma m.
magnocellular hypothalamic neuron
magnum load
magnus
    M. and de Kleijn neck reflex
    Diplococcus m.
MAHA
    microangiopathic hemolytic anemia
Mahaim fiber
Maher disease
MAI
    mitotic activity index
    Mycobacterium avium-intracellulare
main
    m. en griffe
    m. en lorgnette
    m. site of airway resistance
maintenance
    minichromosome m.
MAIPA
    monoclonal antibody-specific immobilization of platelet antigen
maitriensis
    Planococcus m.
Majocchi
    M. disease
    M. granuloma
    M. purpura
major
    m. agglutinin
    m. basic protein (MBP)
    beta thalassemia m.
    m. breakpoint region (MBR)
    ductus sublingualis m.
    m. gene
    glandula vestibularis m.
    m. GU-AG spliceosome
    m. histocompatibility antigen (MHA)
    m. histocompatibility complex (MHC)
    m. histocompatibility locus
    Leishmania tropica m.
    m. outer membrane protein (MOMP)
    Plantago m.
    thalassemia m.
    m. tranquilizer
    variola m.
majus
    Habronema m.
    labia m.

maker
>   Geometric Data Miniprep
>   slide m.
MAK6 immunohistochemical reagent
Malabar
>   M. itch
>   M. leprosy
malabarica
malabsorption
>   m. disease
>   m. disorder
>   m. syndrome
malachite
>   m. green
>   m. green broth
>   m. green stain
malacia
malacic
malacoplakia, malakoplakia
>   m. vesicae
malacosis
malacotic
maladie de Roger
malakoplakia (*var. of* malacoplakia)
malaria
>   algid m.
>   benign tertian m.
>   bilious remittent m.
>   bovine m.
>   double tertian m.
>   falciparum m.
>   m. film test
>   gastric algid m.
>   hemolytic m.
>   hemorrhagic m.
>   intermittent m.
>   *malariae m.*
>   malignant tertian m.
>   ovale m.
>   quartan m.
>   quotidian m.
>   remittent m.
>   m. smear
>   tertian m.
>   therapeutic m.
>   vivax m.
malariacidal
malariae
>   *m. malaria*
>   *Plasmodium m.*
malarial
>   m. cachexia
>   m. deposition pigment
>   m. dysentery
>   m. fever
>   m. hemoglobinuria
>   m. knob
>   m. parasite
>   m. pigment deposition

>   m. pigment stain
>   m. rosette
malariology
malarious
malar rash
Malassez disease
Malassezia
>   *M. furfur*
>   *M. ovalis*
>   *M. pachydermatis*
malate dehydrogenase
malathion
malaya
>   microfilaria m.
Malayan
>   M. filariasis
>   M. pit viper venom
malayanum
>   *Echinostoma m.*
malayensis
>   *Schistosoma m.*
malayi
>   *Brugia m.*
>   *Wuchereria m.*
malaysiensis
>   *Angiostrongylus m.*
Malbranchea
mal de San Lazaro
maldigestive disease
MALDIMS
>   matrix-assisted laser desorption and
>   ionization mass spectrometry
MALDI-TOF
>   matrix-assisted laser desorption
>   ionization time-of-flight
>   MALDI-TOF mass spectrometry
Maldonado-San Jose stain
male
>   m. castration
>   m. frog test
>   m. hormone
>   m. pseudohermaphrodite
>   m. reproductive system
>   m. rudimentary uterus
>   m. sex chromatin pattern
>   m. toad test
>   m. Turner syndrome
>   47,XYY m.
malformation
>   Arnold-Chiari m.
>   arteriovenous m. (AVM)
>   cardiac valvular m.
>   cardiovascular m.
>   cavernous m. (CM)
>   cerebrovascular m. (CVM)
>   chromosome dicentric m.
>   congenital cardiovascular m.
>   cutaneous m.
>   cystic adenomatoid m.

M

malformation (*continued*)
    Dandy-Walker m.
    dicentric m.
    Dieulafoy m.
    Ebstein m.
    genitourinary m.
    spinal cord vascular m.
    m. syndrome
    vascular m.
malfunction
Malherbe
    M. calcifying epithelioma
    calcifying epithelioma of M.
    M. disease
Malibu disease
malic
    m. acid
    m. dehydrogenase (MDH)
maligna
    cynanche m.
    lentigo m.
    scarlatina m.
    struma m.
    variola m.
malignancy
    B-cell m.
    borderline m.
    gland-forming m.
    hematolymphoid m.
    hematopoietic m.
    humoral hypercalcemia of m.
    lymphoreticular m.
    postthymic m.
malignancy-related ascites
malignant
    m. adenoma
    m. ameloblastoma
    m. anemia
    m. atrophic papulosis
    m. breast tumor
    m. bubo
    m. carbuncle
    m. carcinoid syndrome
    m. cartilaginous tumor
    m. dyskeratosis
    m. edema
    m. endocarditis
    m. endovascular papillary angioendothelioma
    m. ependymoma
    m. fibrous histiocytoma (MFH)
    m. giant cell tumor (MGCT)
    m. glioma
    m. granuloma
    m. hepatoma
    m. histiocytosis
    m. Hodgkin and Reed-Sternberg cell
    m. hypertension

    m. hyperthermia
    m. intratubular germ-cell neoplasia (MITGCN)
    m. jaundice
    m. lentigo
    m. lentigo melanoma
    m. lymphadenosis
    m. lymphoma (ML)
    m. melanoma in situ
    m. melanoma staging
    m. meningioma
    m. mesenchymoma
    m. mesothelioma
    m. mixed mesodermal tumor (MMMT)
    m. mixed müllerian tumor (MMMT)
    m. mixed tumor (MMT)
    m. myoepithelioma
    m. neoplasm
    m. nephrosclerosis
    m. neurilemmoma
    m. paraganglioma (MPG)
    m. peripheral nerve sheath tumor (MPNST)
    m. plasma cell tumor
    m. pleural effusion
    m. primary pheochromocytoma (MPPC)
    m. pustule
    m. rhabdoid tumor (MRT)
    m. rhabdoid tumor of kidney (MRTK)
    m. rhabdoid tumor of soft tissue (MRTS)
    m. schwannoma
    m. smallpox
    m. synovioma
    m. teratoma, intermediate (MTI)
    m. teratoma, trophoblastic (MTT)
    m. teratoma, undifferentiated (MTU)
    m. tertian fever
    m. tertian malaria
    m. thymoma
    m. transformation
    m. triton tumor (MTT)
    m. trophoblastic teratoma (MTT)
    m. vascular tumor
maligni
    Bacillus oedematis m.
malignum
    Eurotium m.
    lymphogranuloma m.
Malin syndrome
Mali syndrome
Mall
mallei
    Actinobacillus m.
    Bacillus m.
    Burkholderia m.
    Malleomyces m.

malleinization
mallein test
Malleomyces
    M. mallei
    M. pseudomallei
    M. whitmori
malleosa
    pneumonia m.
mallet finger
Mallophaga
Mallory
    M. aniline blue stain
    M. body
    M. collagen stain
    M. hyalin
    M. iodine stain
    M. phloxine stain
    M. phosphotungstic acid
    M. phosphotungstic acid hematoxylin
      stain
    M. stain for *Actinomyces*
    M. stain for hemofuchsin
    M. trichrome stain
    M. triple stain
Mallory-Weiss
    M.-W. lesion
    M.-W. syndrome
    M.-W. tear
Malmejde test
malmoense
    Mycobacterium m.
Malmö protocol
malnutrition
    intrauterine m. (IUM)
    protein-calorie m. (PCM)
malocclusion
malonate inhibitor
malonatica
    Levinea m.
malondialdehyde concentrate
Maloney leukemia virus
malonic acid
malonitrile
    chlorobenzylidene m.
malononitrile
    NATO code for o-chlorobenzylidene
      m. (CS)
malonyl coenzyme A
malorum
    Acetobacter m.
malperfusion
    placental m.
malpighian
    m. body
    m. body of spleen
    m. capsule
    m. cell
    m. corpuscle
    m. gland

    m. glomerulus
    m. layer
    m. nodule
    m. rete
    m. stratum
    m. tuft
malpighii
    stratum m.
malposition
malrotation
    intestinal m.
MALT
    mucosa-associated lymphoid tissue
    MALT lymphoma
malt
    m. agar
    m. extract broth
Malta fever
maltaromaticum
    Carnobacterium m.
Maltese cross
MALToma
maltophilia
    Pseudomonas m.
    Stenotrophomonas m.
    Xanthomonas m.
maltose
maltosuria
malt-worker's lung
malum
    m. articulorum senilis
    m. coxae senile
Mamastrovirus
mamelonated
mamelonation
mamelonné
    état m.
mamillary duct
mammaglobin
    human m. (hMAM)
Mammalian Prions
mammaria, *pl.* **mammariae**
    glandula m.
    lobi glandulae mammariae
    lobuli glandulae mammariae
mammariae (*pl. of* mammaria)
mammary
    m. actinomycosis
    m. aspiration specimen (MAS)
    m. aspiration specimen cytology test
      (MASCT)
    m. calculus
    m. cysticercosis
    m. duct
    m. duct ectasia
    m. dysplasia
    m. fistula
    m. gland
    m. intraepithelial neoplasia

M

mammary (*continued*)
    m. Paget disease
    m. tumor virus (MTV)
mammilla
mammillitis
    bovine herpes m.
    bovine ulcerative m.
    bovine vaccinia m.
mammitis
mammographic microcalcification
Mammomonogamus laryngeus
mammosomatotroph cell
mammosomatotropic adenoma
Mammotome biopsy system
mammotroph
mammotrophin (*var. of* mammotropin)
mammotropic hormone
mammotropin, mammotrophin
management
    automation initiative in laboratory
        m.
    component m.
    critical incident stress m. (CISM)
    low-range heparin m. (LHMT)
manager
    Cholesterol M.
Manan needle
manchada
    lepra m.
manchette
Manchurian hemorrhagic fever
Mancini
    M. iodine stain
    M. method
mandelate
    methenamine m.
mandelii
    Pseudomonas m.
Mandelin reagent
mandibuloacral dysostosis
mandibulofacial
    m. dysostosis
    m. dysotosis syndrome
    m. dysplasia
mandibulooculofacial
    m. dysmorphia
    m. dysmorphism
    m. syndrome
mandibulooculofacialis
    dyscephalia m.
mandrake root
mandrillaris
    Balamuthia m.
maneuver
    Valsalva m.
manganese
    m. assay
    m. poisoning
    m. toxicity

manganic
manganism
manganous
manganoxidans
    Caldimonas m.
mange
    sarcoptic m.
mangiferae
    Dothiorella m.
    Nattrassia m.
manifesta
    spina bifida m.
manifestation
    abnormal clinical m.
    extraintestinal m.
    laboratory m.
manifest hyperopia
manifesting heterozygote
manifold
    Visiprep solid-phase extraction
        vacuum m.
mannan
manner
    bimodal m.
mannitol fermentation
mannitolilytica
    Ralstonia m.
mannitolivorans
    Hongiella m.
Mann methyl blue-eosin stain
mannoheptulosuria
mannoprotein
mannose binding lectin (MBL)
mannose-6-phosphate (Man6P)
mannosidase
    alpha m.
mannosidosis
Mann-Whitney rank sum statistic
manometric flame
MANOVA
    multivariate analysis of variance
man-o'-war
    Portuguese m.-o.-w.
Man6P
    mannose-6-phosphate
    Man6P recognition marker
Manson
    M. blood fluke
    M. disease
Mansonella
    M. demarquayi
    M. ozzardi
    M. perstans
    M. streptocerca
    M. tucumana
mansonelliasis
mansoni
    Bothriocephalus m.
    Diphyllobothrium m.

Oxyspirura m.
Schistosoma m.
Spirometra m.
Mansonia
mansonii
Cladosporium m.
Zygosporium m.
mansonoides
Bothriocephalus m.
Diphyllobothrium m.
Spirometra m.
Mantel-Cox
M.-C. method
M.-C. procedure
M₁antigen, Mᵍantigen, Mᶜantigen, M₂antigen
M₂antigen (*var. of* M₁antigen)
mantle
m. cell lymphocytic lymphoma
m. cell lymphoma (MCL)
m. sclerosis
m. zone
m. zone lymphoma (MZL)
mantle-zone lymphocyte
Mantoux
M. conversion
M. diameter (MD)
M. pit
M. skin test
manual
m. CD4 kit
m. optic planimeter
manus
tinea m.
manuum
tinea m.
MAP
megaloblastic anemia of pregnancy
mitogen-activated protein
map
chromosome m.
cytogenetic m.
genetic m.
linkage m.
memory m.
restriction m.
tumor m.
m. unit
maple
m. bark stripper's disease
m. bark stripper's lung
m. syrup urine disease (MSUD)
maplike skull
mapping
epitope m.
gene m.
genetic m.

lymphatic m.
site-specific biopsy m.
maprotiline
MAPSS
multiangle polarized scatter separation
maquilingensis
Caldivirga m.
Marafivirus
Maragiliano body
Marañón syndrome
marantic
m. atrophy
m. endocarditis
m. thrombosis
m. thrombus
marasmic, marantic
m. kwashiorkor
m. thrombosis
m. thrombus
Marasmius
marasmus
marble
m. bone
m. bone disease
Marboran
Marburg
M. agent
M. virus
M. virus disease
Marburg-like viruses
marcescens
Serratia m.
march
m. albuminuria
m. anemia
M. disease
m. hemoglobinuria
Marchand
M. adrenal
M. rest
M. wandering cell
Marchesani syndrome
Marchi
M. fixative
M. reaction
M. stain
Marchiafava-Bignami disease
Marchiafava-Micheli
M.-M. anemia
M.-M. syndrome
marcid
Marcus Gunn syndrome
Marcy agent
Marek
M. disease
M. disease virus (MDV)
M. herpesvirus disease (MDHV)
Marek's disease-like viruses

M

Marfan
  M. disease
  M. law
  M. syndrome
Margarinomyces
margaritifer
  Tepidiphilus m.
Margaritispora
Margaropus winthemi
margin
  corneal m.
  infiltrative m.
  irregular m.
  left costal m. (LCM)
  outer m.
  placental disc m.
  sclerotic m.
  seared wound m.
  slitlike m.
  true mucosal m.
marginal
  m. excision (ME)
  m. granulocyte pool (MGP)
  m. ulcer
  m. zone (MZ)
  m. zone B-cell lymphoma (MZBCL)
  m. zone cell lymphoma (MZL)
  m. zone lymphoma
marginated chromatin
marginating pool
margination
  leukocytic m.
marginatum
  Clinostomum m.
  eczema m.
  erythema m.
  Hyalomma m.
Margolis syndrome
maricaloris
  Pseudoalteromonas m.
Marie
  M. disease
  M. syndrome
Marie-Bamberger
  M.-B. disease
  M.-B. syndrome
Marie-Robinson syndrome
Marie-Strümpell disease
Marie-Tooth disease
marihuana (*var. of* marijuana)
marijuana, marihuana
marimammalium
  Actinomyces m.
marina
  Alteromonas m.
  Anisakis m.
  Blastopirellula m.
  Cobetia m.
  Kocuria m.

  Nitrosomonas m.
  Pseudomonas m.
  Psychromonas m.
  Roseospira m.
  Thiocapsa m.
marincola
  Hongiella m.
  Psychrobacter m.
marine protein concentrate (MPC)
Marinesco-Garland syndrome
Marinesco-Sjögren syndrome
mariniglutinosa
  Pseudoalteromonas m.
marinintestina
  Shewanella m.
marinisedimentorum
  Reinekea m.
Marino and Muller-Hermelink (MMH)
marinum
  Aeromicrobium m.
  Mycobacterium m.
  plasma m.
marinus
  Bacteriovorax m.
  Dethiosulfovibrio m.
  Hydrogenothermus m.
  Prochlorococcus marinus subsp. *m.*
  Serinicoccus m.
Marion disease
marioni
  Heterodera m.
maris
  Williamsia m.
marisflavi
  Bacillus m.
  Halomonas m.
marismortui
  Chromohalobacter m.
  Salibacillus m.
  Virgibacillus m.
maritima
  Hippea m.
  Woodsholea m.
maritimum
  Tenacibaculum m.
maritimus
  Planococcus m.
  Psychrobacter m.
  Thermodiscus m.
Marituba virus
Marjolin ulcer
mark
  port-wine m.
  m. sense reader
  strawberry m.
  tape m.
  tide m.
  Unna m.

marker
allotypic m.
annexin A1 m.
B-cell m.
biliary progenitor m.
candidate tumor m.
CD15 m.
CD205 m.
CDX2 immunohistochemical m.
cell surface m.
chromosomal m.
m. chromosome
chromosome 14q tumor m.
CK7 m.
clusterin m.
C-myc m.
collagen m.
DEC-205 m.
DNA m.
endocrine m.
endothelial m.
enzyme m.
fecal m.
fibrohistiocytic m.
m. gene
genetic m.
GLUT-1 m.
HBV DNA m.
H-CD m.
histodiagnostic m.
HMB 45 m.
Hybritech Ostase bone
 metabolism m.
immunohistochemical m.
inflammatory m.
Ki-67 immunophenotypic m.
KRAS mutation m.
laminin m.
lineage m.
Man6P recognition m.
mesothelioma m.
MIB1 cell proliferation m.
microsatellite m.
molecular m.
myogen m.
myoid m.
Nanog gene m.
N-cadherin m.
neuroendocrine m.
N-myc m.
nonlineage m.
oncofetal m.
Ostase biochemical m.
Ostase bone metabolism m.
polymorphic genetic m.
progenitor m.
proliferation m.
rapid intraoperative quantitative
 RT-PCR assessment of tumor m.

RCC m.
m. rescue
rhabdomyosarcoma m.
S-100 m.
single copy gene m.
smooth muscle m.
supernumerary m.
surface m.
tau molecular m.
T-cell m.
T-helper/inducer subset m.
T-suppressor/cytotoxic
 subset m.
tumor m.
tumor progression m.
utrophin m.
VEGFR3 m.
WT-1 m.

marking
coarse m.

markovian texture

Marme reagent

marmoratus
status m.

marmoset virus

marmot

Maroteaux-Lamy syndrome

Marquis reagent

marrow
aplastic bone m.
basophilic m.
bone m. (BM)
m. cavity
m. cell
empty m.
eosinophilic m.
erythrocytic m.
m. fibrosis
hypercellular bone m.
hyperplastic bone m.
hypocellularity of
 bone m.
hypoplastic bone m.
leukocytic m.
lymphocytic m.
Maximow stain for
 bone m.
mesodermal bone m.
monocytic m.
neutrophilic m.
red bone m.
m. reticulin
reticulocytic m.
yellow bone m.

marrow-lymph gland

MARSA
methicillin and aminoglycoside-resistant
 Staphylococcus aureus

Marseilles fever

marsh
    M. disease
    m. fever
Marshall
    M. Hall facies
    M. method
    M. syndrome
Marshallagia marshalli
marshalli
    Alcaligenes m.
    Marshallagia m.
Marshall-Marchetti (MM)
Marsonnina
Martin
    M. broth
    M. disease
Martininia
Martin-Lester agar
Martinotti cell
martius
    m. scarlet blue (MSB)
    m. yellow
Martorell syndrome
MAS
    mammary aspiration specimen
    McCune-Albright syndrome
mA-s
    milliampere-second
Masaoka
    M. classification
    M. staging criteria
    M. thymic cancer staging
      system
maschaladenitis
maschaloncus
MASCT
    mammary aspiration specimen cytology
    test
masculinae
    glandulae urethrales m.
masculinization
    ovarian m.
masculinovoblastoma
mask
    BLB m.
    escape m.
    HEPA filter m.
    Hutchinson m.
    m. of pregnancy
    tropical m.
masked
    m. message
    m. virus
masking
    epitope m.
Mason-Pfizer monkey virus
mason's lung
MASP
    MBL-associated serine protease

maspin
    m. nuclear staining
    m. stain
mass
    m. action law
    atomic m.
    m. attenuation coefficient
    body m. (BM)
    carbon gelatin m.
    m. casualty incident (MCI)
    circumscribed m.
    m. concentration
    critical m.
    cul-de-sac m.
    decrease in bone m.
    dysplasia-associated m.
    dysplasia-associated lesion or m.
      (DALM)
    erythrocyte m. (EM)
    exchangeable m.
    m. fatality incident
    fat-free m. (FFM)
    filar m.
    m. fragmentography
    m. index
    m. infection
    injection m.
    intravascular m. (IVM)
    lean body m. (LBM)
    m. lesion
    mediastinal m.
    m. memory
    m. miniature radiography
      (MMR)
    molecular m.
    m. number
    m. pinocytosis
    red blood cell m. (RBCM)
    red cell m. (RCM)
    m. spectrograph
    m. spectrometer
    m. spectrometry (MS)
    m. spectroscopy
    m. storage
    unit of m.
    whorled m.
massa, *pl.* **massae**
massae (*pl. of* massa)
mass-casualty weapon (MCW)
massiliae
    Rickettsia m.
massiliensis
    Afipia m.
    Bosea m.
massive
    m. collapse
    m. embolus
    m. hepatic necrosis (MHN)
    m. pulmonary hemorrhage

m. transfusion
m. vitreous retraction (MVR)
Masson
M. argentaffin stain
M. body
M. humid meningioma
M. pseudoangiosarcoma
M. trichrome method
M. trichrome stain
M. tumor
Masson-Fontana
M.-F. ammoniacal silver stain
M.-F. ammoniac silver stain
M.-F. method
MAST
multiple antigen stimulation test
multithread allergosorbent test
mast
m. cell
m. cell degranulation test
m. cell disease
m. cell hyperplasia
m. cell leukemia
m. cell positive tryptase and chymase (MCTC)
m. cell sarcoma
m. cell staining
m. cell tryptase
m. cell tryptase positive chymase negative (MCT)
m. cell tumor
m. leukocyte
mastadenitis
mastadenoma
Mastadenovirus
mastatrophia (*var. of* mastatrophy)
mastatrophy, mastatrophia
mastauxe
mastectomy
Halsted m.
master
m. file
m. gland
M. 2-step test
mastic test
Mastigomyces
Mastigophora
mastigophorous
mastigote
mastitis
acute m.
bovine m.
chronic cystic m.
cystic m.
fibrocystic m.
gargantuan m.
glandular m.
granulomatous m.
interstitial m.

lactational m.
m. neonatorum
plasma cell m.
puerperal m.
retromammary m.
submammary m.
suppurative m.
mastocyte
mastocytogenesis
mastocytoma
mastocytosis
mastoidea
otitis m.
mastoiditis
Mastomys natalensis
mastoncus
mastopathy
cystic m.
diabetic m.
fibrocystic m.
Mastophora
mastoplasia, mazoplasia
mastoscirrhus
Mastrevirus
matching
CREG m.
mater
dura m.
material
Advia Centaur HBc IgM control m.
biological matrix reference m.'s
biuret-reactive m. (BRM)
calibration m.
certified reference m.
chromatin m.
coarse m.
control m.
Cotasil silicone slide coating m.
cross-reacting m. (CRM)
diastase-resistant m.
eosinophilic proteinaceous granular m.
explosive m.
extracellular m. (ECM)
fibrin-like proteinaceous m.
fluorescent m.
gonadotropin-inhibitory m. (GIM)
m. graft
granular osmiophilic m. (GOM)
hazardous m.
hyaline m.
Introl CF Panel I Control DNA quality control m.
labeling of hazardous m.'s
matrix reference m.'s
neurosecretory m. (NSM)
primary reference m.
proteinaceous matrix m.
reactive m.

M

585

material (*continued*)
 reference m.
 m. safety data sheet (MSDS)
 secondary reference m.'s
 simulated matrix reference m.'s
 vasodepressor m. (VDM)
 vasoexcitor m. (VEM)
 weapons-grade nuclear m.
maternal
 m. age
 m. antibody
 m. cotyledon
 m. floor infarction
 m. immunity
 m. imprint
 m. inheritance
 m. meiotic nondisjunction
 m. polyhydramnios
 m. serum alpha-fetoprotein (MSAFP)
 m. urine estriol
maternal-fetal hemorrhage
mathematical genetics
Mathieu disease
mating
 assortative m.
 consanguineous m.
 negative assortative m.
 positive assortative m.
 random m.
matrass
matrical, matricial
matrices (*pl. of* matrix)
matricial (*var. of* matrical)
matrilineal
matrilysin
matritensis
 Citeromyces m.
matrix, pl. matrices
 bone m.
 m. calculus
 cartilage m.
 cell m.
 cytoplasmic m.
 m. effect
 extracellular m. (ECM)
 fibrin m.
 groove of nail m.
 hyaline cartilage m.
 m. metalloproteinase (MMP)
 m. metalloproteinase 1 (MMP 1)
 m. metalloproteinase 2 (MMP 2)
 mitochondrial m.
 m. mitochondrialis
 myxochondroid m.
 myxocollagenous m.
 myxoid m.
 osteoid m.
 m. reference m.'s
 territorial m.

 m. vesicle
matrix-assisted
 m.-a. laser desorption and ionization mass spectrometry (MALDIMS)
 m.-a. laser desorption ionization time-of-flight (MALDI-TOF)
matrix-producing carcinoma
matruchotii
 Corynebacterium m.
matter
 interaction of radiation with m.
 sclerosis of white m.
 white m.
mattheei
 Schistosoma m.
maturate
maturation
 accelerated villous m.
 acute myeloblastic leukemia with m. (M2)
 acute myeloblastic leukemia without m. (M1)
 m. arrest
 m. B cell
 m. division
 hematopoietic m.
 m. index (MI)
 m. of gonadal structure
 trilinear m.
mature
 m. abnormal chorion
 m. abnormal placenta
 m. adipocyte
 m. bacteriophage
 m. B cell
 m. cell leukemia
 m. neutrophil
 m. ovarian follicle
 m. spermatozoon
 m. teratoma
maturity
 fetal lung m. (FLM)
 m. onset diabetes of the young (MODY)
maturity-onset diabetes (MODM)
Maunier-Kuhn disease
maura
 Halomonas m.
Maurer
 M. cleft
 M. dot
Mauriac syndrome
Mauthner sheath
MAV
 multinucleated atypia of the vulva
Maxcy disease
maxillary gland
maxillectomy cavity
maxillitis

maximal
- m. acid output
- m. growth temperature
- m. Histalog test
- m. inspiratory flow rate (MIFR)
- m. midexpiratory flow (MMEF)
- m. midexpiratory flow rate (MMEFR)
- m. midflow rate (MMFR)
- m. permissible dose (MPD)
- m. sustained ventilatory capacity (MSVC)
- m. tubular excretory capacity of kidneys (T_m)
- m. tubular reabsorption of glucose (T_{mg})

Maximow stain for bone marrow

maximum
- m. expiratory flow (MEF)
- m. expiratory flow rate (MEFR)
- m. expiratory flow volume (MEFV)
- m. impurities reagent
- m. inhibiting dilution (MID)
- m. inspiratory flow (MIF)
- m. inspiratory pressure (MIP)
- m. permissible concentration (MPC)
- m. temperature (T-MAX, T-max, T_{max})
- m. thermometer
- m. urea clearance
- m. urinary concentration (MUC)
- m. voluntary ventilation (MVV)

Maxisorp microtiter plate
Max-Joseph space
MAXM hematology flow cytometer
maxwell (Mx)
Mayaro virus
maydis
- *Ustilago m.*

Mayer
- M. acid alum hematoxylin stain
- M. hemalum
- M. hemalum stain
- M. hematoxylin
- M. hematoxylin stain
- M. mucicarmine stain
- M. mucihematein stain

Mayer-Rokitansky-Küster syndrome
mayfly
May-Grünwald-Giemsa stain
May-Grünwald stain
May-Hegglin
- M.-H. anomaly
- M.-H. body

mazamorra
mazoplasia (*var. of* mastoplasia)
Mazzoni corpuscle
mazzottii
- *Borrelia m.*

Mazzotti test
M5b
- acute monocytic leukemia with differentiation

MB
- methylene blue
- microbiological assay

Mb
- myoglobin

MB1
- monoclonal antibody M.

mbar
- millibar

MBAS
- methylene blue active substance

MBC
- minimal bactericidal concentration

MbCO
- carbon dioxide myoglobin
- myoglobin

MBD
- methylene blue dye
- minimal brain damage
- minimal brain dysfunction

MBL
- mannose binding lectin
- minimal bactercidal level

MBL-associated serine protease (MASP)
MbO2
- deoxyhemoglobin

MBP
- major basic protein
- myelin basic protein
  - MBP assay

MBR
- major breakpoint region

MB-Redox system
MBT
- mucinous borderline tumor

MC
- medullary carcinoma
- mixed cellularity

mC
- millicoulomb

MCA
- microcarcinoma
- multichannel analyzer

MCAF
- macrophage chemotactic and activating factor

MCAG
- multiple colloid adenomatous goiter

M^{c}antigen (*var. of* M$_1$antigen)
McArdle disease
McArdle-Schmid-Pearson disease
MCB
- membranous cytoplasmic body

MCBR
- minimum concentration of bilirubin

M

MCC
    minimum complete-killing concentration
    mutated in colon cancer
    Mycobacterium phlei cell wall DNA
      complex
    MCC gene

mcC
    microcoulomb

McCarey-Kaufman (M-K)
    M.-K. medium

McCune-Albright syndrome (MAS)

MCD
    mean cell diameter
    mean corpuscular diameter
    medullary cystic disease
    multiple carboxylase deficiency

MCDK
    multicystic dysplasia of kidney
    multicystic dysplastic kidney

McEwen point

MCF
    macrophage chemotactic factor

MCFA
    medium-chain fatty acid

mcg
    microgram

MCH
    mean cell hemoglobin
    mean corpuscular hemoglobin

MCHC
    mean cell hemoglobin concentration
    mean corpuscular hemoglobin
      concentration

MCHD
    mixed cellularity Hodgkin disease

MCI
    mass casualty incident
      trauma MCI

mCi
    millicurie

mCi-hr
    millicurie-hour

McKrae herpes simplex virus strain

mcL
    microliter

MCL
    mantle cell lymphoma

McLean-Maxwell disease

McLeod blood phenotype

McMaster technique

mcmeekinii
    Planomicrobium m.

mcmol, μmol
    micromole

McNeer gastric carcinoma classification

McNemar test

MCP
    mitotic control protein
    monocyte chemoattractant protein

MCP 1
    monocyte chemoattractant protein 1

McPhail test

MCR
    metabolic clearance rate
    minor cluster region
    mutation cluster region

M-CSF
    macrophage colony stimulating factor

MCT
    mast cell tryptase positive chymase
      negative
    mean circulation time
    mean corpuscular thickness
    medium-chain triglyceride
    mucinous cystic tumor

MCTC
    mast cell positive tryptase and
      chymase

MCTD
    mixed connective tissue disease

MCV
    mean cell volume
    mean corpuscular volume
    molluscum contagiosum virus

MCVr
    reticulocyte mean corpuscular
      volume

MCW
    mass-casualty weapon

MD
    Mantoux diameter
    moderately differentiated
    muscular dystrophy

Md
    mendelevium

MDA
    methylenedioxyamphetamine
    multiple displacement amplification
      MDA in WGA

MDC
    minimum detectable concentration

MDF
    mean dominant frequency
    myocardial depressant factor

MDH
    malic dehydrogenase

MDHV
    Marek herpesvirus disease

MDMA
    methylenedioxymethamphetamine

mDNA
    mitochondrial deoxyribonucleic acid

MDNCF
    monocyte-derived neutrophil
      chemotactic factor

MDR
    multidrug resistance
    multiple drug resistance

MDR1
> multidrug resistance 1
> > MDR1 transporter

MDS
> myelodysplastic syndrome
> > MDS system

MDT
> median detection threshold

MDTR
> mean diameter-thickness ratio

MDUO
> myocardial disease of unknown origin

M:E
> myeloid-erythroid ratio

ME
> marginal excision
> medical examiner

MEA
> measles virus vaccine
> multiple endocrine adenomatosis

meal
> test m.

mean
> m. cell diameter (MCD)
> m. cell hemoglobin (MCH)
> m. cell hemoglobin concentration (MCHC)
> m. cell threshold
> m. cell volume (MCV)
> m. circulation time (MCT)
> m. circulatory hematocrit
> m. corpuscular diameter (MCD)
> m. corpuscular hemoglobin (MCH)
> m. corpuscular hemoglobin concentration (MCHC)
> m. corpuscular thickness (MCT)
> m. corpuscular volume (MCV)
> m. diameter-thickness ratio (MDTR)
> m. dominant frequency (MDF)
> m. dose per unit cumulated activity
> m. effective life
> m. follicle size
> m. generation time
> m. hemolytic dose (MHD)
> m. nuclear area (MNA)
> m. peroxidase index
> m. platelet volume (MPV, MVP)
> m. platelet volume nomogram
> m. square deviation
> m. time between failures
> m. tubular diameter (MTD)

measles
> m. antibody
> atypical m.
> m. convalescent serum
> German m.
> m. immune globulin (human)
> m. immunoglobulin
> m., mumps, and rubella (MMR)
> m., mumps, and rubella vaccine
> m. pneumonitis
> three-day m.
> tropical m.
> m. virus
> m. virus pneumonia
> m. virus vaccine (MEA)

measly

measurable
> not m. (NM)

measurement
> blood volume m.
> carbon dioxide combining power m.
> end-point m.
> kinetic m.
> oxygen saturation m.
> right anterior m. (RAM)
> total exchangeable potassium m.

measuring pipette

meat fiber

MEBMM
> mixed epithelial papillary cystadenoma of borderline malignancy of müllerian type

MEC
> mucoepidermoid carcinoma

5-MeC
> 5-methylcytosine

mechanical
> m. agent
> m. asphyxia
> m. displacement
> m. diuretic
> m. fragility
> m. ileus
> m. jaundice
> m. styptic
> m. vector
> m. ventilation

mechanic's hand

mechanism
> autoimmune m.
> compensatory m.
> countercurrent m.
> defense m.
> extravascular migratory metastasis m.
> Frank-Starling m.
> hapten m.
> immune-mediated m.
> immunological m.
> inactivation m.
> ping-pong m.

mechanocyte

mechanoreceptor

mechlorethamine (HN$_2$)

mecillinam

Mecistocirrus

Meckel
> M. cave

M

Meckel (*continued*)
    M. diverticulum
    M. plane
    M. syndrome
Meckel-Gruber syndrome
Mecke reagent
meconium
    m. aspiration
    m. ileus
    m. periorchitis
    m. peritonitis
    m. stain
meconium-stained liquor
MED
    minimal erythema dose
media (*pl. of* medium)
mediae
    cellulae ethmoidales m.
medial
    m. arteriosclerosis
    m. calcification
    m. cartilaginous plate
    m. cystic necrosis
    m. epicondylitis
    m. necrosis of aorta
    m. plate of cartilaginous auditory
      tube
    m. preoptic nucleus
median
    m. bar of Mercier
    m. curative dose (CD_{50})
    m. detection threshold (MDT)
    m. effective dose (ED_{50})
    m. eminence
    m. fatal dose (FD_{50})
    m. infectious dose (ID_{50})
    m. lethal dose
    m. rhomboid glossitis (MRG)
    m. tissue culture dose (TCD_{50})
    m. tissue culture infective dose
      ($TCID_{50}$)
    m. unbiased estimate
mediastinal
    m. elastofibroma
    m. fibrosis
    m. lipomatosis
    m. lymphadenitis
    m. mass
    m. pericarditis
    m. shadow
    m. yolk sac tumor (MYST)
mediastinitis
    hemorrhagic m.
    idiopathic fibrous m.
    sclerosing m.
mediastinopericarditis
mediastinum
    extraosseous plasmacytoma of the
      m. (EPM)

mediate
    m. agglutination
    m. contagion
mediated conversion
mediation
mediator
    m. cell
    chemical m.
    inflammatory m.
    vasoactive m.
medicae
    Ensifer m.
medical
    m. bacteriology
    m. equipment set (MES)
    m. examiner (ME)
    m. food
    m. genetics
    m. internal radiation dose
      (MIRD)
    m. laboratory technician
    m. mycology
    m. pathology
    m. radiology
    m. record
    m. review officer (MRO)
    m. technologist (MT)
    m. treatment facility (MTF)
medicamentosa
    dermatitis m.
    struma m.
medication-related diarrhea
medicinal
    m. leech
    m. scarlet red
medicinalis
    Hirudo m.
medicine
    systematized nomenclature of m.
      (SNOMED)
medicolegal autopsy
medina worm infection
Medin disease
medinensis
    Dracunculus m.
    Filaria m.
mediocanellata
    Taenia m.
medionecrosis
    m. aortae idiopathica cystica
    cystic m.
    m. of the aorta
mediterranea
    Pseudomonas m.
Mediterranean
    M. anemia
    M. fever
    M. hemoglobin E disease
    M. lymphoma

mediterranei
  Amycolatopsis m.
  Nocardia m.
mediterraneus
  Desulfobulbus m.
  Sulfitobacter m.
medium, *pl.* **media**
  Acanthamoeba m.
  active m.
  aerotitis media
  aortic tunica media
  aqueous mounting m.
  Balamuth aqueous egg yolk
    infusion m.
  Balamuth culture m.
  bilateral otitis media (BOM)
  Boeck-Drbohlav-Locke egg-serum m.
  Bordet-Gengou culture m.
  brain-heart infusion broth m.
  Bruns glucose m.
  m. chocolatization
  chocolatization of blood culture m.
  cholesterol-free m.
  chopped meat m.
  clearing m.
  Columbia m.
  contrast m.
  Cryo-Gel embedding m.
  culture m.
  Czapek-Dox m.
  defined culture m.
  dermatophyte test m. (DTM)
  Diamond TYM m.
  dispersion m.
  dispersive m.
  DTPA-Lys(40)-Exendin 4
    radio-labeled imaging m.
  Eagle basal m.
  Eagle essential m.
  Eagle minimum essential m.
    (EMEM)
  enrichment m.
  Epon tissue-embedding m.
  Farrant m.
  m. frequency (MF)
  Glycergel mounting m.
  glycerol gelatin m.
  Hyskon distention m.
  m. incisural space
  indicator culture m.
  Lash casein hydrolysate-serum m.
  Löffler blood culture m.
  Löffler coagulated serum m.
  Lowenstein-Jensen m. (LJM)
  m. magnification
  McCarey-Kaufman m.
  Michel transport m.
  minimum essential m. (MEM)
  M-K m.

  motility test m.
  mounting m.
  Nickerson m.
  NNN culture m.
  nonpermissive culture m.
  nutrient m.
  OF m.
  otitis media (OM)
  oxidation-fermentation m.
  potassium simplex optimized m.
    (KSOM)
  PVA lacto-phenol m.
  radiopaque m.
  Rees culture m.
  refracting m.
  RPMI-1640 contrast m.
  Sabouraud m.
  scala media
  secretory otitis media
  selective m.
  separating m.
  serous otitis media
  sodium chloride culture m.
  sorbitol-MacConkey m.
  support m.
  suppurative chronic otitis
    media
  tellurite m.
  Thayer-Martin m.
  thioglycolate m.
  tissue culture m. (TCM)
  Tobie, von Brand, and Mehlman
    diphasic m.
  transport m.
  tunica media
  TY1-S-33 m.
  TYSGM-9 m.
  m. vein
  von Apathy gum syrup m.
  Weinman m.
  Wickersheimer m.
  xylene-soluble mounting m.
medium-chain
  m.-c. fatty acid (MCFA)
  m.-c. triglyceride (MCT)
medium-scale integration
Medlar body
medorrhea
medulla, *pl.* **medullae**
  adrenal m.
  m. glandulae suprarenalis
  m. nodi lymphoidei
  m. of hair shaft
  m. of lymph node
  m. ossium
  m. ossium flava
  m. ossium rubra
medullae (*pl. of* medulla)
medullar

M

medullare
 osteoma m.
medullaris
 substantia m.
medullary
 m. adenocarcinoma
 m. carcinoma (MC)
 m. carcinoma cell
 m. carcinoma of breast
 m. carcinoma of thyroid
 m. chemoreceptor
 m. chromaffinoma
 m. cord
 m. cystic disease (MCD)
 m. ducts of Bellini
 m. fibrosarcoma
 m. histiocytic reticulosis
 m. interstitial cell
 m. membrane
 m. necrosis
 m. ray
 m. renal carcinoma (MRC)
 m. sarcoma
 m. serotonergic network deficiency
 m. sheath
 m. sinus
 m. sponge kidney
 m. substance
 m. T cell
 m. thymoma
 m. thyroid carcinoma (MTC)
medullated nerve fiber
medullation
medullization
medulloarthritis
medulloblast
medulloblastoma
 desmoplastic m.
 melanotic m.
medulloepithelial cell
medulloepithelioma
 adult m.
medullomyoblastoma
medullovasculosa
 zona m.
medusa, *pl.* **medusae**
 caput medusae
 M. head
medusae (*pl. of* medusa)
MEF
 maximum expiratory flow
MEFR
 maximum expiratory flow rate
MEFV
 maximum expiratory flow volume
MEG
 megakaryocyte
megabladder
megacaryoblast (*var. of* megakaryoblast)

megacaryocyte (*var. of* megakaryocyte)
megacephalia (*var. of* megacephaly)
megacephaly, megacephalia
megacin
Megacollybia
megacolon
 aganglionic m.
 chronic idiopathic m.
 congenital m.
 m. congenitum
 idiopathic m.
 toxic m.
megacycle
megacystic syndrome
megacystis
megadolichocolon
megaelectron volt (MeV)
megaesophagus
megagamete
megahertz (MHz)
megakaryoblast, megacaryoblast
megakaryocyte (MEG), megacaryocyte
 basophilic m.
 bizarre m.
 colony-forming unit granulocyte, erythrocyte, monocyte, and m. (CFU-GEMM)
 granulocyte, erythrocyte, monocyte, and m. (GEMM)
 m. growth and development factor (MGDF)
megakaryocytic
 m. aplasia
 m. blood cell
 m. emperipolesis
 m. hyperplasia
 m. hypoplasia
 m. leukemia
 m. myelosis
 m. precursor
megakaryocytopoiesis
megakaryopoiesis
megalencephaly, megaloencephaly
megaloblast
 basophilic m.
 orthochromatic m.
 polychromatophilic m.
megaloblastic
 m. anemia
 m. anemia of pregnancy (MAP)
 m. erythropoiesis
 m. hyperplasia
megaloblastoid
megaloblastosis
megalocephalia (*var. of* megalocephaly)
megalocephaly, megalocephalia
megalocystis
megalocyte
megalocythemia

megalocytic anemia
megalocytosis
megaloencephalic leukoencephalopathy
megaloencephalon
megaloencephaly (*var. of* megalencephaly)
megaloenteron
megalogastria
megalohepatia
megalokaryocyte
Megalopyge
megalosplenia
megalosplenica
    erythrocytosis m.
megalospore
megaloureter, megaureter
megalourethra
megamerozoite
megamitochondria
meganucleus
megapoietin
megarectum
Megaselia
megasigmoid
Megasphaera
megaspore
megastoma
    Habronema m.
megaterium
    Bacillus m.
megathrombocyte
Megatrichophyton
megaureter, megaloureter
megaurethra (*var. of* megalourethra)
megavolt (MV)
megavoltage
meglumine
megninii
    Trichophyton m.
megohm (MΩ)
megoxycyte
megoxyphil, megoxyphile
megoxyphile (*var. of* megoxyphil)
MEIA
    microparticle capture enzyme
      immunoassay
    microparticle enzyme immunoassay
meibomian
    m. cyst
    m. gland
    m. stye
meibomianitis (*var. of* meibomitis)
meibomitis, meibomianitis
Meige disease
Meigs syndrome
Meinicke
    M. test
    M. turbidity reaction (MTR)
meiocyte
meiosis

meiotic
    m. nondisjunction
    m. phase
    m. recombination
Meissel stain
Meissner
    M. corpuscle
    M. plexus
meissnerian differentiation
MEK
    methyl ethyl ketone
mekongi
    Schistosoma m.
Melan
    M. A/MART-1 antibody
    M. A/MART-1 antigen
Melan-A (MART-1) gene
melanemia
melaniferous phagocyte
melanimon
    Aedes m.
melanin
    artificial m.
    m. bleaching method
    factitious m.
    m. pigmentation
    smoky m.
    m. staining method
    m. test
melaninogenica
    Prevotella m.
melaninogenicus
    Bacteroides m.
melanism
melanoacanthoma
melanoameloblastoma
melanoblast
melanoblastoma
melanocarcinoma of anus
melanocortin
melanocyte-inhibiting hormone
melanocyte specific MITF (MITF-M)
melanocyte-stimulating
    m.-s. hormone inhibiting factor
      (MIF)
    m.-s. hormone release-inhibiting
      hormone
    m.-s. hormone releasing factor
      (MRF)
    m.-s. hormone releasing hormone
melanocytic
    m. lesion
    m. nevus
melanocytosis
melanodendrocyte
melanodermatitis
melanodermic
melanogenemia
melanogenesis

M

melanogen test
melanoglossia
melanoid
Melanoides
melanokeratosis
Melanolestes picipes
melanoleukoderma
melanoma
 acral lentiginous m.
 amelanotic mucosal m.
 angiotropic m.
 anorectal m.
 m. antigen-encoding gene family
 benign juvenile m.
 Cloudman m.
 cutaneous malignant m. (CMM)
 desmoplastic m.
 epidermotropic metastatic malignant
  m. (EMMM)
 epithelioid cell m.
 halo m.
 Harding-Passey m.
 m. in situ
 juvenile m.
 lentigo maligna m.
 malignant lentigo m.
 minimal deviation m.
 mucosal lentiginous m.
 multifocal choroidal m.
 nodular m.
 ocular m.
 oral-sinonasal m.
 spindle cell m.
 Spitz-like m.
 subungual m.
 superficial spreading m.
 uveal m.
 verrucous m.
melanomatosis
 meningeal m.
melanomatous follicular invasion
Melanomma
melanonychia
melanopathy
melanophage
melanophagocyte
melanophore
melanophore-stimulating hormone (MSH)
melanoplakia
Melanoporia
melanosarcoma
melanosis
 m. circumscripta precancerosa
 m. coli
 m. corii degenerativa
 mucosal m.
 neurocutaneous m.
 oculodermal m.
 primary acquired m.

 Riehl m.
 vagabond's m.
melanosome
 giant m.
melanotic
 m. ameloblastoma
 m. carcinoma
 m. freckle
 m. medulloblastoma
 m. neuroectodermal tumor
 m. neuroectodermal tumor of
  infancy
 m. pigment
 m. progonoma
 m. prurigo
 m. schwannoma
 m. stool
 m. whitlow
melanotroph
melanotropic cell
melanura
 Culiseta m.
melanuria
melanuric
MELAS
 mitochondrial encephalopathy, lactic
  acidosis, and strokelike episodes
  MELAS syndrome
melas
 icterus m.
melasma universale
Melastatin test kit
melatonin
Melchior syndrome
meleagridis
 Amoeba m.
 Histomonas m.
Meleda disease
melena
Meleney
 M. gangrene
 M. ulcer
melicera, meliceris
meliceris (*var. of* melicera)
meliloti
 Ensifer m.
melioidosis
 Whitmore m.
melis
 Isobaculum m.
melitensis
 Brucella m.
melitis
melitose
melituria
 glycosuric m.
 m. inosita
 nondiabetic glycosuric m.
Melkersson-Rosenthal syndrome

Melkersson syndrome
mellis
> *Saccharomyces m.*

mellitus
> diabetes m.
> insulin-dependent diabetes m.
> (IDDM)
> juvenile diabetes m. (JDM)
> noninsulin-dependent diabetes m.
> (NIDDM)

Melnick-Needles syndrome
Meloidae
Meloidogyne
melonis
> *Sphingomonas m.*

melon seed body
melophagium
> *Trypanosoma m.*

Melophagus
melorheostosis
melting
> m. point (MP)
> m. temperature (Tm)

MEM
> minimum essential medium

membrana, *pl.* **membranae**
> m. adventitia
> m. basalis ductus semicircularis
> m. basilaris
> m. carnosa
> m. choriocapillaris
> m. cordis
> m. decidua
> m. fibrosa capsulae articularis
> m. fusca
> m. granulosa
> m. hyaloidea
> m. limitans
> m. limitans gliae
> m. mucosa
> m. pituitosa
> m. preformativa
> m. propria ductus semicircularis
> m. pupillaris
> m. reticularis organi spiralis
> m. serosa
> m. statoconiorum
> m. synovialis
> m. tectoria ductus cochlearis
> m. tympani
> m. versicolor
> m. vestibularis ductus cochlearis
> m. vitellina
> m. vitrea

membranacea
> placenta m.

membranaceous
membranae (*pl. of* membrana)
membranaefaciens

membranate
membrane
> acellular basement m.
> air bleb m.
> alveolodental m.
> antiglomerular basement m.
> (anti-GBM)
> artificial rupture of m.'s (ARM)
> asymmetric unit m.
> m. attack complex (MAC)
> basement m.
> basolateral m.
> Bichat m.
> m. bone
> Bowman m.
> Bruch m.
> Brunn m.
> canalicular m.
> m. capacitance
> cell m.
> Corti m.
> croupous m.
> cytoplasmic m.
> Debove m.
> decidual m.
> deciduous m.
> Descemet m.
> diphtheritic m.
> drum m.
> Duddell m.
> elastic m.
> enamel m.
> epithelial basement m.
> erythrocyte m.
> false m.
> fenestrated m.
> Fielding m.
> m. filter
> m. filter technique
> glassy m.
> glomerular basement m. (GBM)
> Henle fenestrated elastic m.
> human mesothelial cell m.
> Hunter m.
> Huxley m.
> hyaline m.
> hyaloid m.
> Hybond N+ nylon m.
> inflammatory m.
> internal elastic m.
> lateral cell m.
> lipid peroxidation of intracellular m.
> medullary m.
> mitochondrial m.
> mucous m.
> Nitabuch m.
> nitrocellulose m.
> nuclear m.
> m. of tympanum

M

membrane (*continued*)
    olfactory m.
    osmiophilic cell surface m.
    otolithic m.
    outer mitochondrial m.
    pituitary m.
    placental m.
    plasma m.
    postsynaptic m.
    m. potential
    premature rupture of (fetal) m.'s (PROM)
    presynaptic m.
    proligerous m.
    prolonged rupture of fetal m.'s (PRFM)
    prophylactic m.
    m. protein
    Puchtler-Sweat stain for basement m.'s
    pyogenic m.
    radiate layer of tympanic m.
    Reissner m.
    rupture of m.'s (ROM)
    Ruysch m.
    schneiderian m.
    Schultze m.
    semipermeable m.
    serous m.
    m. sidedness
    m. skeleton
    spiral m.
    statoconial m.
    subsurface basement m.
    Sure Blot m.
    synovial m.
    torocyte m.
    m. trafficking
    m. transport
    trophoblastic cell m.
    tubular basement m. (TBM)
    tympanic m.
    m. type 1–6
    undulating m.
    unit m.
    vaginal synovial m.
    vasculosyncytial m.
    vestibular m.
    vitreous m.
    Volkmann m.
    yolk m.
membrane-bound receptor analysis
membrane-coating granule
membranelle
membraniform
membranocartilaginous
membranoid
membranoproliferative glomerulonephritis (MPGN)

membranous
    m. acute inflammation
    m. cisternae
    m. cochlea
    m. cytoplasmic body (MCB)
    m. deciduitis
    m. glomerulonephritis (MGN)
    m. layer
    m. lupus nephritis
    m. nephropathy (MN)
    m. ossification
    m. pattern
    m. pharyngitis
    m. pregnancy
Memnoniella echinata
memory
    m. B, T cell
    cache m.
    core m.
    immunologic m.
    local skin m.
    magnetic core m.
    m. map
    mass m.
    scratch-pad m.
MEN
    multiple endocrine neoplasia
    MEN syndrome, type 1, 2, 2a, 2b, 3
menadione
menaquinone
Mendel-Bekhterev sign
mendelevium (Md)
mendelian
    m. character
    m. genetics
    m. inheritance
Mendel law
Mendosicutes
Ménétrier
    M. disease
    M. syndrome
Mengert shock syndrome
Menghini needle
Mengo
    M. encephalitis
    M. virus
Ménière
    M. disease
    M. syndrome
menin
meningeal
    m. carcinoma
    m. carcinomatosis
    m. hernia
    m. leukemia
    m. melanomatosis
    m. sarcoma
    m. sarcomatosis

meninges (*pl. of* meninx)
meningioangiomatosis
meningioma
    anaplastic m.
    angiomatous m.
    clear cell m.
    cutaneous m.
    fibroblastic m.
    malignant m.
    Masson humid m.
    meningothelial m.
    mucinous m.
    nonanaplastic invasive m.
    orbital m.
    psammomatous m.
    spinal m.
    suprasellar m.
meningiomatosis
    diffuse m.
meningismus
meningitic streak
meningitidis
    Neisseria m.
meningitis
    amebic m.
    anthrax m.
    aseptic m.
    bacterial m.
    basilar m.
    Candida m.
    cerebrospinal m.
      (CSM)
    cryptococcal m.
    enteroviral m.
    epidural m.
    external m.
    hemorrhagic m.
    internal m.
    leukemic m.
    meningococcal m.
    Mollaret m.
    mycotic m.
    neoplastic m.
    occlusive m.
    otitic m.
    plague m.
    pyogenic m.
    serous m.
    subacute m.
    syphilitic m.
    torular m.
    tuberculous m.
      (TBM)
    viral m.
meningoblastoma
    fibroblastic m.
meningocele
meningocerebral cicatrix
meningocerebritis

meningococcal
    m. infection
    m. meningitis
meningococcemia
meningococcin
meningococcus
    m. conjunctivitis
    m. infection
meningocyte
meningoencephalitis
    acute fulminating primary amebic m.
    acute primary hemorrhagic m.
    amebic m.
    biundulant m.
    eosinophilic m.
    herpetic m.
    mumps m.
    primary amebic m.
    syphilitic m.
meningoencephalocele
meningoencephalomyelitis
meningoencephalopathy
    carcinomatous m.
meningomyelitis
meningomyelocele
meningomyeloradiculitis
Meningonema peruzzii
meningoosteophlebitis
meningoradiculitis
meningosepticum
    Chryseobacterium m.
    Flavobacterium m.
meningothelial meningioma
meninguria
meninx, *pl.* meninges
meniscal
    m. degeneration
    m. tear
meniscitis
meniscocyte
meniscocytosis
meniscus
    degenerated m.
    tactile m.
    m. tactus
Menkes syndrome
menometrorrhagia
menopausal
    m. gonadotropin
    m. syndrome
menopause
    delayed m.
    m. home test
Menopon
menorrhagia
menostasia (*var. of* menostasis)
menostasis, menostasia, menostaxis
menostaxis (*var. of* menostasis)

M

menstrual
  m. colic
  m. cycle
  m. sclerosis
  m. stage
mentagrophytes
  Trichophyton m.
  Trichophyton mentagrophytes m.
Mentha
Mentzer MCV index
Menzies melanoma diagnosis method
meperidine hydrochloride
mephenytoin
mephitis
  Luteimonas m.
meprobamate assay
mEq
  milliequivalent
MER
  methanol-extruded residue
merbromin
mercaptan
mercaptoacetic acid
mercaptomerin sodium
mercaptopurine
mercaptopyrazidopyrimidine (MPP)
Mercier
  median bar of M.
Merck new fuchsin stain
mercocresol
mercurialism
mercurial thermometer
mercuric
  m. conjugate
  m. cyanide
  m. fixative
mercurous
mercury (Hg)
  m. assay
  m. cyanide (HgCN)
  inorganic m. (Hg2+)
  methyl m.
  millimeter of m. (mmHg)
  m. poisoning
mercury-wetted relay
Merfluor DFA *Cryptosporidium/Giardia*
  detection procedure
meridiana
  Pseudomonas m.
meridiei
  Desulfosporosinus m.
meridional fiber of ciliary muscle
Meripilus
Merismodes
merispore
meristematic
meristic variation
Merkel
  M. cell tumor

M. corpuscle
M. tactile cell
M. tactile disc
Merkel-Ranvier cell
merlin gene
MERmaid-Spin kit
Mermis nigrescens
mermithid
Mermithidae
Mermithoidea
merocrine gland
merogenesis
merogenetic, merogenic
merogenic (*var. of* merogenetic)
merogony
  diploid m.
meromelia
meromicrosomia
meromyosin
  heavy m. (HMM)
  light m. (LMM)
meront
merorachischisis, merorrhachischisis
merorrhachischisis (*var. of*
  merorachischisis)
merosporangium
merotomy
merozoite antigen
merozygote
mersalyl
  m. exchange assay
  m. exchange method
Merulius
Merzbacher-Pelizaeus disease
MES
  medical equipment set
MESA
  microsurgical epididymal sperm aspiration
  myoepithelial sialadenitis
mesameboid
mesangial
  m. cell
  m. deposit
  m. IgA nephropathy
  m. lupus nephritis
  m. proliferative glomerulonephritis
  m. ring
mesangiocapillary glomerulonephritis
mesangiolysis
mesangioproliferative glomerulonephritis
mesangium
  extraglomerular m.
mesaortitis
mesaraic (*var. of* mesenteric)
mesareic (*var. of* mesenteric)
mesarteritis
mesaxon
mescal
mescaline

mesectic
mesencephalic reticular formation (MRF)
mesencephalitis
mesenchyma
mesenchymal
    m. cell
    m. chondrosarcoma
    m. differentiation
    m. epithelium
    m. hamartoma
    m. hyloma
    m. neoplasia
    m. neoplasm
    m. stroma
    m. tissue
    m. tumor
mesenchyme
    myxoid m.
    splanchnic m.
mesenchymoma
    benign m.
    malignant m.
mesenteric, mesaraic, mesareic
    m. adenitis
    m. fibromatosis
    m. gland
    m. infarction
    m. ischemia
    m. lipodystrophy
    m. lymphadenitis
    m. panniculitis
    m. phlebosclerosis
    m. thrombosis
    m. vascular obstruction
mesenteritis
    idiopathic retractile m. (IRM)
mesenteroides
    Leuconostoc m.
mesenteron
mesentery
MESF
    molecule of equivalent soluble
    fluorochrome
meshwork
    trabecular m.
mesnili
    Chilomastix m.
mesoappendiceal
mesoappendix
mesobacterium
mesoblast
    extraembryonic m.
    primitive m.
mesoblastic nephroma
mesocardia
Mesocestoides
    M. corti
    M. variabilis
Mesocestoididae

mesocolic
meso compound
mesocricetorum
    Helicobacter m.
mesodermal bone marrow
mesoderm cell
Mesogastropoda
mesogenic
mesoglia
mesoglial cell
mesolepidoma
mesolimbic dopaminergic system
mesolymphocyte
mesomelia
mesomelic dwarfism
mesometanephric carcinoma
mesometritis
meson
mesonephric
    m. adenocarcinoma
    m. cyst
    m. remnant
    m. remnant hyperplasia
    m. rest
    m. tissue
    m. tubule
mesonephroi (*pl. of* mesonephros)
mesonephroid tumor
mesonephroma
mesonephros, *pl.* mesonephroi
mesoneuritis
    nodular m.
mesophaeum
    Hebeloma m.
mesophil, mesophile
mesophila
    Glaciecola m.
mesophile (*var. of* mesophil)
mesophilica
    Pseudomonas m.
mesophilic bacterium
mesophilicum
    Methylobacterium m.
mesophilum
    Tenacibaculum m.
mesophilus
    Gelidibacter m.
mesophlebitis
mesophragma
mesosigmoiditis
mesosome
mesothelial
    m. cell
    m. cyst
    m. hyloma
    m. sarcoma
mesothelial/monocytic incidental cardiac
  excrescence (MICE)
mesothelin

M

mesothelioma
    benign m.
    fibrous m.
    lymphohistiocytoid m. (LHM)
    malignant m.
    m. marker
    pleural m.
    sarcomatoid m.
mesothelium
Mesozoa
message
    masked m.
messeae
    Anopheles m.
messenger ribonucleic acid (mRNA)
messinensis
    Oleiphilus m.
mesylate
    deferoxamine m.
    ergoloid m.
MET
    metabolic equivalent
metabiosis
metabisulfite test
metabolic
    m. acidosis
    m. alkalosis
    m. antagonism
    m. antagonist
    m. bone disease
    m. clearance rate (MCR)
    m. coma
    m. craniopathy
    m. detoxification
    m. disorder
    m. encephalopathy
    m. equivalent (MET)
    m. hypothesis
    m. indican
    m. insufficiency
    m. mucinosis
    m. pathway
    m. pool
    m. stone disease
    m. storage disease
    m. syndrome
metabolism
    aerobic m.
    anaerobic m.
    basal m.
    copper m.
    divalent ion m. (DIM)
    drug m.
    first-pass m.
    glucose m.
    inborn error of vitamin D
      m.
    increased m.
    increased basal m.

    intermediary m.
    lipid m.
    propionate m.
metabolite
    arachidonic acid m.
    cyanohydrin m.
    PredictRx m.'s
    Pro-PredictRx m.
    reactive oxygen m. (ROM)
metabolizable
metabolome
metabolomic
metacarpal index
metacarpophalangeal (MP)
metacentric
metacercaria
metacestode
metachromasia
    alpha m.
    beta m.
    gamma m.
metachromatic
    m. body
    m. dye
    m. granule
    m. leukodystrophy (MLD)
    m. stain
    m. stain test
metachromaticogranularis
    substantia m.
metachromatic-type leukodystrophy
metachromatism
metachroming
metachromophil, metachromophile
metachromophile (*var. of* metachromophil)
metachronal rhythm
metachronous
    m. carcinoma
    m. collagenous colitis
    m. seeding
metachrosis
metacryptozoite
metagenesis
metagglutinin
metaglobulin
metagonimiasis
Metagonimus
    M. ovatus
    M. yokogawai
metal
    alkali m.
    alkaline earth m.
    m. fume fever
    heavy m.
    m. oxide semiconductor field effect
      transistor
    m. sol
metal-catalyzed pseudoperoxidation
metaldehyde

metallic
    m. bond
    m. foreign body (MFB)
    m. thermometer
metallicus
    Nocardiopsis m.
metallidurans
    Ralstonia m.
    Wautersia m.
metallireducens
    Desulfitobacterium m.
metalloenzyme
metalloflavoprotein
metallophil cell
metallophilia
metalloprotease
    a disintegrin and m. (ADAM)
metalloprotein
metalloproteinase
    m. 1
    matrix m. (MMP)
    matrix m. 1 (MMP 1)
    matrix m. 2 (MMP 2)
    m. transcription
metalloproteinase-1
    tissue inhibitor of m.-1 (TIMP-1)
metalloproteinase-2
    tissue inhibitor of m.-2 (TIMP-2)
metalloproteinase-3
    tissue inhibitor of m.-3 (TIMP-3)
metalloscopy
metallothionein concentrate
metal-to-metal contact
metamere
metameric
metamerism
metamorphosis
    fatty m.
    retrograde m.
    syringomatous m.
metamyelocyte
    basophilic m.
    eosinophilic m.
    neutrophilic m.
metanephric
    m. adenofibroma (MAF)
    m. adenoma
    m. adenosarcoma
    m. stromal tumor
    m. tubule
metanephrine
    m. assay
    m. test
    urine m.
metanephrogenic tissue
metaneutrophil, metaneutrophile
metaneutrophile (*var. of* metaneutrophil)
metanil (*var. of* metaniline)

metaniline, metanil
    m. yellow
metaphase
    m. cell
    m. chromosome
    m. plate
metaphosphate
    potassium m.
metaphosphoric acid
metaphyseal (*var. of* metaphysial)
metaphysial, metaphyseal
    m. dysostosis
    m. dysplasia
metaphysis
metaphysitis
metaplasia
    agnogenic myeloid m.
    apocrine m.
    atypical squamous m. (ASM)
    autoparenchymatous m.
    Barrett m.
    bronchiolar m.
    cardia intestinal m. (CIM)
    cartilaginous m.
    celomic m.
    chondroid m.
    chondromyxoid m.
    ciliated m.
    columnar m.
    decidual m.
    embryonal m.
    endothelial m.
    eosinophilic cell m.
    epidermoid m.
    glandular m.
    goblet cell m.
    heterologous m.
    hobnail cell m.
    Hürthle cell m.
    intestinal m. (IM)
    mucinous m.
    myelofibrosis with myeloid m. (MMM)
    myeloid m. (MM)
    myelosclerosis with myeloid m.
    oncocytic m.
    osseous m.
    peribronchial m.
    primary myeloid m.
    pseudopyloric m.
    pyloric gland m.
    secondary myeloid m.
    smooth muscle m.
    squamous m.
    symptomatic myeloid m.
    tuboendometrioid m.
metaplasis
metaplasm
metaplastic
    m. anemia

M

metaplastic (*continued*)
    m. carcinoma
    m. cell
    m. columnar epithelium
    m. keratinization
    m. ossification
    m. polyp
Metapneumovirus
metapyrone
Metarhizium
metarubricyte
metastable state
metastases (*pl. of* metastasis)
metastasis, *pl.* **metastases**
    biochemical m.
    calcareous m.
    contralateral axillary m.
    distal m.
    distant organ m.
    hematogenous m.
    lymph node m. (LN-met)
    lymphogenous m.
    no evidence of distant metastases (M0)
    occult m.
    (primary) tumor, (regional lymph) nodes, (remote) metastases (TNM)
    pulsating m.
    satellite m.
    skip m.
metastasis-free survival
metastasize
metastatic
    m. abscess
    m. adenocarcinoma (MA)
    m. bone survey
    m. calcification
    m. carcinoid syndrome
    m. carcinoma
    m. cascade
    m. cluster
    m. focus
    m. hepatocellular carcinoma (HCC)
    m. malignant pheochromocytoma (MMPC)
    m. mumps
    m. neoplasm
    m. panniculitis
    m. pneumonia
    m. thermometer
    m. tumor
metastrongyle
Metastrongylus
    M. apri
    M. elongatus
metatroph
metatrophic
metatropic
metatypical carcinoma
metavinculin

Metavirus
Metazoa
metazoan parasite
metazoonosis
Metchnikoff theory
met-enkephalin
    methionine-enkephalin
meteori
    Agrobacterium m.
meteorism
meter (m)
    count rate m.
    d'Arsonval m.
    HemoSite hemoglobin m.
    neutron m.
    oxygen saturation m. (OSM)
    rate m.
    survey m.
meter-kilogram-second (MKS, mks)
    m.-k.-s. system
    m.-k.-s. unit
MeterPlus
    Triage M.
methacrylate
    butyl m.
    glycol m.
    m. resin
methacycline
methadone
    m. assay
    m. hydrochloride
methallenestril
methamphetamine hydrochloride
methanal
methandrostenolone
methane
Methanobacteria
Methanobacteriaceae
Methanobacteriales
Methanobacterium
Methanocaldococcaceae
Methanococcaceae
Methanococcales
Methanococci
Methanococcus
Methanocorpusculaceae
methanol
    m. assay
    m. fixative
    m. intoxication
    m. poisoning
    m. test
methanol-extruded residue (MER)
methanolica
    Pseudomonas m.
Methanomicrobiaceae
Methanomicrobiales
Methanoplanaceae
Methanopyraceae

Methanopyrales
Methanopyri
Methanosaetaceae
Methanosarcinaceae
Methanosarcinales
Methanospirillaceae
Methanothermaceae
Methanothermea
methaqualone assay
metHb
    methemoglobin
methemalbumin (MHA)
    m. assay
methemalbuminemia
methemalbuminuria
methemoglobin (metHb)
    m. reductase
    stroma-free m.
methemoglobinemia
    acquired m.
    congenital m.
    enterogenous m.
    hereditary enzymatic-type m.
    primary m.
    secondary m.
    toxic m.
methemoglobinuria
methenamine
    m. hippurate
    m. mandelate
    m. silver
    m. silver stain
methicillin and aminoglycoside-resistant
Staphylococcus aureus (MARSA)
methicillin-resistant
    m.-r. coagulase-negative
      Staphylococcus (MRCNS)
    m.-r. *Staphylococcus aureus* (MRSA)
methicillin-susceptible
    m.-s. coagulase-negative
      Staphylococcus (MSCNS)
    m.-s. *Staphylococcus aureus*
      (MSSA)
methimazole
methine dye
methionine
    m. malabsorption syndrome
    N-formyl m.
    m. synthase
    m. test
methionine-enkephalin (met-enkephalin)
methionyl
methionyl-RNA synthetase
methisazone
methocycline
method
    ABC staining m.
    Abell-Kendall m.
    AccuProbe m.

acid anhydride m.
acid-fast staining m.
acridine orange m.
aequorin recombinant m.
agar diffusion m.
AgNOR m.
alkaline phosphatase m.
Altmann-Gersh m.
AMeX processing and embedding m.
amidohydrolase m.
analytic m.
antialkaline phosphatase m.
Ashby differential agglutination m.
Astrup m.
axon staining m.
Ayoub-Shklar m.
bacterial agar m.
bacterial antigen detection m.
Baker Sudan black m.
Bang m.
Barnett-Bourne acetic alcohol-silver
  nitrate m.
Barrnett-Seligman
  dihydroxydinaphthyl disulfide m.
Barrnett-Seligman indoxyl
  esterase m.
Barroso-Moguel and Costero
  silver m.
Baumgartner m.
Beaver direct smear m.
Bence Jones protein m.
bench m.
Benedict m.
Bengston m.
Bennett sulfhydryl m.
Bennhold Congo red m.
Bensley aniline-acid fuchsin-methyl
  green m.
benzo sky blue m.
Berg chelate removal m.
bicinchoninic acid m. (BCA)
Bielschowsky m.
Billheimer m.
bioluminescent m.
biotin-streptavidin-alkaline
  phosphatase m.
biotin-streptavidin detection m.
biotin-streptavidin-peroxidase m.
black periodic acid m.
Bloch m.
Bodian m.
Borchgrevink m.
Born m.
bread-loaf m.
Brecher-Cronkite m.
Breen and Tullis m.
Cajal gold sublimate m.
Cajal uranium silver m.
Caldwell-Moloy m.

M

method (*continued*)

Camp-Gianturco radiography m.
Caraway m.
carbolfuchsin-methylene blue staining m.
cellophane tape m.
cell separation m.
Chang aniline-acid fuchsin m.
Chiffelle and Putt m.
chloranilate m.
chloride m.
cholesterol staining m.
chromate m.
chrome alum hematoxylin-phloxine m.
chromolytic m.
Ciaccio m.
Clark-Collip m.
clean-catch collection m.
cobaltinitrite m.
Coblentz test m.
Colcher-Sussman x-ray pelvimetry m.
collagen staining m.
colorimetric m.
constitutive heterochromatin m.
cooled-knife m.
copper sulfate m.
Craigie tube m.
Credé m.
Crippa lead tetraacetate m.
cysteic acid m.
Dacie m.
Dale-Laidlaw clotting time m.
Dane m.
definitive m.
diazo staining m.
Dick m.
Dieterle m.
diffusion m.
digitonin m.
dilute blood clot lysis m.
disc sensitivity m.
double antibody m.
Duke m.
dyed starch m.
enzymatic digestion m.
enzyme demonstration m.
esterase staining m.
Fahey and McKelvey m.
fibrin degradation product m.
fibrinogen m.
field m.
Fite m.
fixed sediment m.
fixed-time m.
flat substrate m.
Folin and Wu m. (FW, FWM)
Fontana-Masson staining m.
Foot reticulin m.

formaldehyde-induced fluorescence m.
formalin-ether sedimentation m.
freeze-cleave m.
freeze-etch m.
freeze-fracture-etch m.
frozen section m.
FW m.
Gallyas m.
Gerota m.
Giemsa m.
Girard m.
glass-bead retention m.
glucose oxidase m.
glycerin m.
gram m.
Granger m.
Grimelius argyrophil stain m.
Grocott-Gomori methenamine silver m.
guanidine isothiocyanate m.
Hall pterygium m.
Hammerschlag m.
Harris staining m.
Heublein m.
heuristic m.
hexokinase m.
Highman m.
Histofine staining m.
Holmes m.
Holzer m.
H.P. Wright m.
HSU m.
IgG index m.
immunofluorescence m.
immunoperoxidase staining m.
India ink m.
indophenol m.
Ivy m.
Jacobsson m.
Jendrassik-Grof m.
Jenner m.
Jones m.
Kaiserling m.
Kaplan-Meier staining m.
Kety-Schmidt m.
Kirby-Bauer m.
Kjeldahl m.
Klump and Bieth m.
Lee-White clotting time m.
leukocyte alkaline phosphatase m.
Levaditi m.
Lillie allochrome m.
Lison-Dunn m.
MacFarlane serum m.
macro-Kjeldahl m.
Mancini m.
Mantel-Cox m.
Marshall m.

Masson-Fontana m.
Masson trichrome m.
melanin bleaching m.
melanin staining m.
Menzies melanoma diagnosis m.
mersalyl exchange m.
micro-Astrup m.
micro-Kjeldahl m.
Miles-Misra m.
Millipore m.
ModAMeX section m.
Monte Carlo m.
Movat pentachrome m.
myelin staining m.
myoglobin identification m.
Nichols m.
Nikiforoff m.
Nuclepore m.
m. of Cleary
m. of collection not indicated
  (MOCNI)
m. of Shiiki
Ouchterlony m.
Pisano m.
Pizzolato peroxide-silver m.
plasma thrombin clot m.
Ploton staining m.
point counting m.
polyvinyl alcohol fixative m.
protein separation m.
Puchtler alkaline Congo red m.
Puchtler Sirius red m.
push-wedge m.
PVA fixative m.
Quicgel m.
Quick m.
Rees-Ecker m.
reference m.
Rideal-Walker m.
RNAzol B RNA extraction m.
Sahli m.
Salzman m.
Sanger DNA sequencing m.
Schick m.
Scotch tape m.
SEM freeze-fracture m.
SEREX m.
Shaffer-Hartmann m.
Sheather sugar flotation m.
Simplate heterotrophic plate
  count m.
solochrome azurine staining m.
Somogyi m.
special reference m.
Stovall-Black m.
streptavidin-biotin peroxidase m.
suction m.
Sweet m.
template bleeding time m.

thermodilution m.
Thoms m.
Tietz-Fiereck m.
two-slide m.
ultropaque m.
Van Slyke and Cullen m.
von Clauss m.
von Kossa m.
Warthin-Starry m.
Welker m.
Whipple m.
Wilson m.
Wintrobe and Landsberg m.
Wintrobe sedimentation rate m.
Ziehl-Neelsen m.
ZSR m.
methodology
methotrexate
  m. poisoning
methoxychlor
methoxyhydroxymandelic acid
  (MOMA)
methoxy-4-hydroxymandelic acid test
methyl
  m. acetate
  m. alcohol poisoning
  m. aldehyde
  m. blue
  m. bromide
  m. butyl ketone
  m. chloroform
  m. cyanoacrylate
  m. demeton
  m. ethyl ketone (MEK)
  m. green
  m. green-pyronin stain
  m. isobutyl ketone
  m. mercury
  m. orange
  m. parathion
  m. red (MR)
  m. red test
  m. red, Voges-Proskauer (MR-VP)
  m. red, Voges-Proskauer broth
  m. violet
  m. yellow
methylarachidonyl fluorophosphonate
  (MAFP)
methylation
  DNA m.
  m. pattern diversity
methylbenzene
methylbromide
  homatropine m. (HMB)
methylbutane fixative/solution
3-methylcrotonylglycinuria
methylcytosine
5-methylcytosine (5-MeC)
methyldichloroarsine

M

methyldopa
    alpha m.
methylene
    m. azure
    m. blue (MB)
    m. blue active substance (MBAS)
    m. blue dye (MBD)
    m. blue stain
    m. blue test
    m. chloride
    m. dichloride
    m. violet
    m. white
methylenedioxyamphetamine (MDA)
3,4-methylenedioxyamphetamine assay
methylenedioxymethamphetamine (MDMA)
methylenetetrahydrofolate reductase (MTHFR)
methylenophil, methylenophile
methylenophile (*var. of* methylenophil)
methylenophilic, methylenophilous
methylenophilous (*var. of* methylenophilic)
methylisobutylketone
methylmalonic
    m. acid
    m. acidemia
    m. aciduria
methylmalonyl-CoA decarboxylase
methylmercaptan
methylmorphine
methylnitrosourea
Methylobacterium
    M. fujisawaense
    M. mesophilicum
    M. organophilum
    M. radiotolerans
    M. rhodesianum
    M. rhodinum
    M. zatmanii
Methylococcaceae
methylohalidivorans
    Leisingera m.
methylotrophus
    Arthrobacter m.
methylovorans
    Albibacter m.
methylparaben
methylphenidate (MPH)
methylphenylethylhydantoin (MPEH)
1-methyl-4-phenyl-1,2,3,6-tetrahydropyridine (MPTP), 6-tetrahydropyridine
methylphosphonofluoridate
    NATO code for nerve agent cyclohexyl m. (GF)

methylphosphonothioate
    NATO code for nerve agent O-ethyl S-[2-(diethylamino)ethyl] m. (VM)
methylprednisdone pulse therapy (MPPT)
5-methylresorcinol
methylrosaniline chloride
methyltetrahydrofolate
methylthymol blue
methyltransferase
    tetrahydropteroylglutamate m.
4-methylumbelliferyl phosphate (MUP)
methyprylon assay
MetMb
    metmyoglobin
metMb
    metmyoglobin
metmyoglobin (metMb, MetMb)
Metopirone test
Metopium
Metorchis
metoxenous
metoxeny
Metra
    M. BAP assay
    M. DPD test
    M. PYD assay
metraterm
metratrophia (*var. of* metratrophy)
metratrophy, metratrophia
metria
metric
    m. data
    m. system
metritis
metrocyte
metrofibroma
metrolymphangitis
metromalacia
metromalacoma, metromalacosis
metromalacosis (*var. of* metromalacoma)
metronidazole assay
metroperitoneal fistula
metroperitonitis
metropolitan medical response system (MMRS)
metrorrhagia
metrosalpingitis
metrotrophic test
mets
    metastases
    metastasis
metschnikovii
    Vibrio m.
Metschnikowia
Mett, Mette
    M. test tube
    M. unit
Mette (*var. of* Mett)
metyrapone stimulation test

MeV
    megaelectron volt
    million electron volts
mevalonate
mevinphos
Mexican
    M. hat cell
    M. hat corpuscle
mexicana
    Actinomadura m.
    Leishmania mexicana m.
    Leishmania tropica m.
mexicanus
    Desulfovibrio m.
    Streptomyces m.
Mexico
    albumin M.
mexiletine
Meyenburg
    M. complex
    M. disease
Meyenburg-Altherr-Uehlinger syndrome
meyerae
    Actinomadura m.
Meyer-Betz syndrome
Meyer disease
Meyer-Schwickerath and Weyers syndrome
Meynert
    M. cell
    M. layer
Meynet node
MF
    medium frequency
    mossy fiber
    mycosis fungoides
    myelin figure
mF
    millifarad
M'Fadyean stain
MFB
    metallic foreign body
MFF
    metal fume fever
MFH
    malignant fibrous histiocytoma
MFO system
MF/SS
    mycosis fungoides/Sézary syndrome
Mg
    magnesium
Mg2+
    magnesium ion
MGAB
    mucous gland adenoma of bronchus
Mg agglutinin
    milligram
Mᵍ antigen (*var. of* M₁ antigen)

MGC
    multinucleated giant cell
MGCT
    malignant giant cell tumor
    mixed germ cell tumor
MGDF
    megakaryocyte growth and development factor
mg/dL
    milligram per deciliter
MGH
    microglandular hyperplasia
mg/h
    milligram per hour
MG-intermedius
MGIT
    mycobacteria growth indicator tube
        Bactec MGIT 960
mg/L
    milligram per liter
MGN
    membranous glomerulonephritis
MgO
    magnesium oxide
        MgO nanoparticle
MGP
    marginal granulocyte pool
MGUS
    monoclonal gammopathy of undetermined significance
    monoclonal gammopathy of unknown significance
mH
    millihenry
MHA
    major histocompatibility antigen
    methemalbumin
    microangiopathic hemolytic anemia
    microhemagglutination assay
    mixed hemadsorption
MHA-TP
    microhemagglutination assay-*Treponema pallidum*
MHC
    major histocompatibility complex
        MHC I/calreticulin complex
        MHC molecule
        MHC restriction
MHD
    mean hemolytic dose
    minimum hemolytic dose
MHN
    massive hepatic necrosis
MHz
    megahertz
MI
    mitral insufficiency
    myocardial infarct
    myocardial infarction

M

Mi-2 antigen
MIB1
    MIB1 antibody
    MIB1 antigen
    MIB1 cell proliferation marker
    MIB1 nuclear immunostain
MIBB
    minimally invasive breast biopsy
Mibelli
    M. angiokeratoma
    M. disease
    M. porokeratosis
MIC
    minimal inhibitory concentration
    minimal isorrheic concentration
    minimum inhibitory concentration
MIC2
    MIC2 antibody
    MIC2 oncogene
MICA
    mirror-image complementary antibody
micaceous
mica pneumoconiosis
micdadei
    Legionella m.
    Tatlockia m.
mice (*pl. of* mouse)
MICE
    mesothelial/monocytic incidental cardiac excrescence
micelle
    ferruginous m.'s
Michaelis-Gutmann body
Michaelis-Menten equation
Michel
    M. deformity
    M. transport medium
Micral
    M. chemstrip
    M. urine dipstick test
micranatomy
micrencephalia (*var. of* micrencephaly)
micrencephalous
micrencephaly, micrencephalia, microencephaly
micro
    microscopic
microabscess
    intervillous m.
    Munro m.
microabsorption spectroscopy
microacinar architectural pattern
microadenoma
microaerophila
    Thioalkalispira m.
microaerophile
microaerophilic streptococcus
microaerophilum
    Propionibacterium m.

microaggregate filter
MicroALB
    Icon M.
microalbinuria
microalbumin
    m. immunoturbidimetric assay
    m. test
microalbuminuria
microaleuriospore
microammeter
microampere
microanalysis
    energy dispersive x-ray m.
microanalytical EDS analysis
microanatomic
microanatomist
microanatomy
microaneurysm
    Charcot-Bouchard m.
    retinal m.
microangiopathic
    m. hemolytic
    m. hemolytic anemia (MAHA, MHA)
microangiopathy
    diabetic m.
    thrombotic m. (TMA)
microangioscopy
Microanthomyces alpinus
microarray
    Affymetrix U133A oligonucleotide m.
    DNA m.
    m. expression profiling assay
    resequencing m.
    tissue m. (TMA)
Microascus trigonosporus
micro-Astrup method
Microbacteriaceae
Microbacterium
Microbank cryopreservative
microbar (μbar)
microbe
microbeam
    P.A.L.M. ultraviolet laser m.
microbial
    m. antagonism
    m. associate
    m. genetics
    m. persistence
    m. variation
    m. vitamin
microbic dissociation
microbicidal
microbicide
microbid
Microbilharzia variglandis
microbioassay
microbiological assay (MB)

microbiologic assay
microbiologist
    National Registry of M.'s
microbiology
    m. automation
    m. identification system
microbiotic
microbism
    latent m.
microblast
microbody
microbore test
Microbotryum
microbroth
microburet
microcalcification
    mammographic m.
microcapillary bed
microcarcinoma (MCA)
microcell
microcentrifuge
    Microfuge 18 m.
    Microfuge 22R refrigerated m.
    MicroPrep 2 m.
microcentrum
microcephalia (*var. of* microcephaly)
microcephaly, microcephalia
    encephaloclastic m.
    schizencephalic m.
microchemical balance
microchemistry
microchimerism
MicroChisel
    Eppendorf M.
microchromosome
Micrococcaceae
Micrococcales
Micrococceae
Micrococcineae
micrococcus
    M. conglomeratus
    M. luteus
    M. varians
microcolitis
microcolony
microcolumn chromatography
micro(computerized)tomography
microconidium
microcoulomb
microcrypt
    atrophic m.
microcrystalline
microcurie (μCi)
microcurie-hour (μCi-hr)
microcyst
Microcystis aeruginosa
microcyte
microcythemia
microcytic

    m. erythrocyte
    m. hypochromic anemia
microcytosis
microdeletion syndrome
microdensitometer
microdentium
    Treponema m.
microdeposit
microdiffusion analysis
microdissection
    laser capture m.
MicroDissector
    Eppendorf M.
microdochectomy
Microdochium
microdrepanocytic
    m. anemia
    m. disease
microdrepanocytosis
microdysgenesia
microelectrophoresis
microencephaly (*var. of* micrencephaly)
microenvironment
microerythrocyte
microevolution
microfarad (μF)
microfibril
microfilament
    intracytoplasmic m.
    subplasmalemmal m.
microfilaremia
microfilaria
    Brugia microfilariae
    m. diurna
    m. malaya
microfilariasis
microflora
Microflow test
microfluorodensitometry
microfold cell
microfollicular
    m. adenoma
    m. goiter
    m. pattern
microfuge
    M. 18 microcentrifuge
    M. 22R refrigerated microcentrifuge
    m. tube
microgamete
microgametocyte
microgamont
microgamy
microglandular
    m. adenosis
    m. hyperplasia (MGH)
    m. pattern
microglia
    activated m.
    m. cell

M

microgliacyte
microglial
    m. cell
    m. nodule
microglioma
microgliomatosis
microgliosis
microglobulin
    beta-2 m.
    serum beta-2 m.
microglossia
micrognathia with peromelia
microgram (mcg)
micrograph
    acoustic m.
    electron m.
    light m.
    scanning electron m. (SEM)
micrographia (*var. of* micrography)
micrography, micrographia
microgyria
microhemagglutination
    m. assay (MHA)
    m. assay-*Treponema pallidum*
    (MHA-TP)
microhemagglutination-*Treponema*
***pallidum* test**
microhematocrit
    m. centrifugation
    m. concentration
microhenry (μH)
microhistology
microhm ($\mu\Omega$)
microhomology
microimmunofluorescence test
microincineration
microincinerator
microinfarct
microinjection
microinjector
microinvasion
microinvasive carcinoma
microiontophoretically applied
micro-Kjeldahl method
microlesion
microleukoblast
microliter (μL, mcL)
microlith
microlithiasis
    pulmonary alveolar m. (PAM)
micrology
microlumen
    intracytoplasmic m.
microlymphocytotoxicity
    m. assay
    double-fluorescence m.
    m. test
micromanipulation
micromanipulator

micromati
    Flavobacterium m.
micromegakaryocyte
micromelia
micromelica
    rachitis fetalis m.
micromelic dwarfism
micromerozoite
micrometastases (*pl. of* micrometastasis)
micrometastasis, *pl.* **micrometastases**
    carcinomatous m.
micrometastatic
    m. disease
    m. vascular deposit
micrometer (μm)
    caliper m.
    filar m.
    ocular m.
    slide m.
micromethod
    buffy coat m.
micrometry
micromillimeter (μmm)
micromolar concentration
micromole
Micromonosporaceae
Micromonospora purpurea
Micromonosporineae
micromyeloblast
micromyeloblastic leukemia
micron (μ)
microneedle
Micronema
microneme
micronodular
    m. pneumocyte hyperplasia
    (MPH)
    m. stromal endometriosis
micronodularity
    regenerative m.
micronucleus
microorganism
micropapillary
    m. component (MPC)
    m. serous carcinoma (MPSC)
micropapilloma
microparasite
microparticle
    m. capture enzyme immunoassay
    (MEIA)
    m. enzyme immunoassay (MEIA)
    procoagulant platelet-derived m.
microparticulate
micropathology
microphage
microphagocyte
microphotograph
microphthalmia
    progeria with m.

microphthalmia-associated transcription factor (MITF)
micropinocytosis
micropinocytotic vesicle
micropipet (*var. of* micropipette)
micropipette, micropipet
microplania
microplasia
microplethysmography
micropolygyria
Micropolyspora faeni
micropore filter technique
microprecipitation test
micropredation
micropredator
MicroPrep 2 microcentrifuge
microprobe
    electron m.
    laser m.
    Raman m.
microprocessor
microprogram
microprolactinoma
    pituitary m.
micropromyelocyte
microprotein
micropyle
microrefractometer
microRNA
    m. molecule
    m. signature
microroentgen
micros
microsatellite
    m. analysis
    m. instability (MIN)
    m. locus
    m. marker
    m. polymorphism
microscope
    acoustic m.
    analytical electron m. (AEM)
    beta ray m.
    BHTU m.
    binocular m.
    capillary m.
    cellular debris centrifuge polarizing m.
    centrifuge m.
    color-contrast m.
    comparator m.
    comparison m.
    compound m.
    dark-field m.
    dark-ground m.
    dissecting m.
    electron m. (EM)
    field of m.
    fluorescence m.

    fluorescent m.
    flying spot m.
    hypodermic m.
    infrared m.
    integrating m.
    interference m.
    ion m.
    JEM-100CX electron m.
    Jeol 100 S transmission electron m.
    Jeol 1200 transmission electron m.
    Labophot-2 m.
    laser m.
    light m. (LM)
    Nomarski m.
    Olympus BH2 m.
    opaque m.
    polarizing m.
    projection x-ray m.
    reflecting m.
    Rheinberg m.
    scanning electron m. (SEM)
    schlieren m.
    simple m.
    stereoscopic m.
    stroboscopic m.
    television m.
    transmission electron m. (TEM)
    trinocular m.
    ultrasonic m.
    ultraviolet m.
    x-ray m.
    Zeiss Axiophot fluorescent m.
    Zeiss Axioplan m.
    Zeiss Axioskop m.
    Zeiss LSM-10 laser m.
    Zeiss transmission electron m.
microscopic, microscopical
    m. agglutination
    m. anatomy
    m. appearance
    m. colitis
    m. field
    filter paper m. (FPM)
    m. hematuria
    m. infarct
    m. inflammatory infiltrate
    m. polyangiitis
    m. section
    m. thymoma
microscopical (*var. of* microscopic)
microscopy
    atomic force m. (AFM)
    bright-field m.
    clinical m.
    confocal m.
    confocal laser scan m. (CLSM)
    cryoelectron m.
    dark-field m.

M

microscopy (*continued*)
deconvolution fluorescence m.
electron m. (EM)
epifluorescence m.
FLM m.
fluorescence m.
fluorescent m.
immersion m.
immune electron m. (IEM)
immunofluorescence m.
immunogold electron m.
interference-contrast m. (ICM)
intravital m.
laser confocal m.
laser-scanning confocal m.
light m. (LM)
low-voltage high-resolution scanning electron m. (LV-HRSEM)
polarized m.
scanning electron m. (SEM)
scanning probe m. (SPM)
scanning transmission electron m.
scanning tunneling m. (STM)
transmission electron m. (TEM)
urine m.
video time-lapse m.
widefield capillary m.
microsecond (μs)
microsection
microslide
microsomal
m. enzyme
m. enzyme system
liver kidney m. (LKM)
m. thyroid antibody
m. thyroid antibody test
microsome
microspectrophotometry
microspectroscope
microspectroscopy
Fourier transform infrared m. (FTIR)
Microsphaeraceae
Microsphaeropsis
microsphere
aggregated m.
FocalCheck m.
trisacryl gelatin m.
microspherocyte
microspherocytosis
microsplanchnic
microsplenia
Microspora
Microsporasida
microspore
Microsporida
microsporidian
microsporidiosis, microsporidiasis
Microsporidium

microsporon
Audouin m.
microsporosis
Microsporum
M. audouinii
M. canis
M. canis distortum
M. felineum
M. ferrugineum
M. fulvum
M. furfur
M. gallinae
M. gypseum
M. lanosum
M. nanum
M. persicolor
M. vanbreuseghemi
M. vanbreuseghemii
microsteatosis
microstoma
Habronema m.
microstomia
microsurgical epididymal sperm aspiration (MESA)
microsyringe
Microtatobiotes
microtear
microthrombocytopenia
X-linked m.
microthrombus
microti
Babesia m.
Mycobacterium m.
Mycoplasma m.
microtiter plate
microtome
cold m.
freezing m.
m. knife
Leica VT1000 E fully automatic m.
Leica VT1000 M semi-automatic m.
rocker m.
rocking m.
rotary m.
sliding m.
Stadie-Riggs m.
microtomization
microtomy
microtonometer
microtoxicity assay
Microtrombidium
microtubule
axon containing m.
m. in cilia
intracisternal m.
microtubule-associated protein
Microtus
microunit
microvascular

microvenular hemangioma
microvesicle
microvesicular
microvessel
    m. count (MVC)
    decidual m.
    m. density (MVD)
microvilli (*pl. of* microvillus)
microvillus, *pl.* **microvilli**
    brush-border m.
    m. inclusion disease
    m. lymphoma
    stubby m.
Microviridae
Microvirus
microvivisection
microvolt (μV)
microwatt (μW)
microwave fixation
microxyphil
microzoon
micrurgical
Micrurus
MID
    maximum inhibiting dilution
    minimal infecting dose
    minimum infective dose
mid
    middle
Midas II automated stainer
midbody
midbrain
    red nucleus of m.
midcarpal
midcervical region
middle
    m. cell
    m. ear adenoma
    m. lobe syndrome
    m. molecule
    m. piece
Middlebrook
    M. agar
    Bacto M.
    M. broth
Middlebrook-Dubos hemagglutination test
midge
midget bipolar cell
midkine protein
midline
    m. lethal granuloma
    m. malignant reticulosis granuloma
    m. shift
midstream urinalysis
midterminal spore
midthoracic region
midzonal necrosis
Mielke bleeding time
Miescher

    M. elastoma
    M. granulomatosis
    M. syndrome
miescheriana
    Sarcocystis m.
MIF
    macrophage inhibiting factor
    maximum inspiratory flow
    melanocyte-stimulating hormone
     inhibiting factor
    migration inhibition factor
    mixed immunofluorescence
    MIF test
MIFC
    minimally invasive follicular
     carcinoma
MIFR
    maximal inspiratory flow rate
migraine
    familial hemiplegic m. (FHM,
     FMH)
migrans
    Agamonematodum m.
    cutaneous larva m.
    erythema m. (EM)
    erythema chronicum m. (ECM)
    larva m.
    ocular larva m.
    spiruroid larva m.
    thrombophlebitis m.
    visceral larva m.
migrating
    m. abscess
    m. bullet
    m. thrombophlebitis
migration
    m. inhibition factor (MIF)
    m. inhibition test
migration-inhibitory
    m.-i. factor
    m.-i. factor test
migratory
    m. cell
    m. pneumonia
    m. polyarthritis
Mikulicz
    M. cell
    M. disease
    M. syndrome
mild silver protein
Miles-Misra method
milia (*pl. of* milium)
miliaria
    apocrine m.
    m. profunda
    m. rubra
    sebaceous m.
miliaris
    variola m.

M

miliary

    m. abscess
    m. aneurysm
    m. embolism
    m. fever
    m. tuberculosis

milieu interieur

military

    m. nerve agent
    m. operation

milium, *pl.* **milia**

    colloid m.
    m. cyst

milk

    acidophilus m.
    m. anemia
    m. cyst
    m. duct
    m. factor
    m. gland
    lactobacillary m.
    m. leg
    m. spot

milk-alkali syndrome

milker's

    m. nodes
    m. nodule
    m. nodule virus

Milkman syndrome

milkpox

milky

    m. ascites
    m. spot
    m. urine

mill

    Retsch MM200 mixer m.

Millard-Gubler

    M.-G. paralysis
    M.-G. syndrome

Miller-Dieker syndrome

Miller ocular disc

miller's asthma

Millex-GS plasma filter

milliamperage

milliampere (mA)

milliampere-second (mA-s)

millibar (mbar)

millicoulomb (mC)

millicurie (mCi)

millicurie-hour (mCi-hr)

milliequivalent (mEq)

millifarad (mF)

Milligan trichrome stain

milligram (mg)

    m. hour
    m. percent
    m. per deciliter (mg/dL)
    m. per hour (mg/h)
    m. per liter (mg/L)

millihenry (mH)

millijoule (mJ)

millikatal (mkat)

millilambert

milliliter (mL)

millimeter

    cubic m. (cmm, cu mm, mm^3)
    m. of mercury (mmHg)

millimicrocurie (mμc)

millimicrogram (mμg)

millimicron (mμ)

millimolar

millimole (mmol)

    m. per liter (mmol/L)

millinormal (mN)

million electron volts (MeV)

milliosmole (mOsm)

millipede

Millipore

    M. filter
    M. filtration
    M. method

millirad (mrad)

millirem (mrem)

milliroentgen (mR)

millisecond (ms, msec)

milliunit (mU)

millivolt (mV)

milliwatt (mW)

Millonig

    M. phosphate buffer
    M. phosphate-buffered formalin fixative

Millon-Nasse test

Millon reagent

Mills disease

Mills-Reincke phenomenon

milnei

    Culicoides m.

milosensis

    Filobacillus m.

Milroy disease

Miltenberger antigen

Milton disease

Mima polymorpha

mimicus

    Vibrio m.

MIN

    microsatellite instability

Minamata disease

minatitlanensis

    Bosea m.

mindensis

    Lactobacillus m.

mineral

    m. crystal
    m. nutrient
    m. oil aspiration

m. oil foreign body
m. oil granuloma
ultrastructural morphology of
bone m.
mineralization
mineralocorticoid
m. deficiency
m. hypertension
m. receptor
miner's
m. asthma
m. lung
mini
m. Hype-Wipe bleach towelette
m. scissors
miniature scarlet fever
miniblock
minicell
minichromosome
m. maintenance
m. maintenance protein
minima
Taenia m.
minimal
m. bactercidal level (MBL)
m. bactericidal concentration
(MBC)
m. brain damage (MBD)
m. brain dysfunction (MBD)
m. deviation melanoma
m. erythema dose (MED)
m. growth temperature
m. hemolytic unit
m. infecting dose (MID)
m. inhibitory concentration (MIC)
m. isorrheic concentration
(MIC)
m. lethal concentration (MLC)
m. lethal dose
m. morbidostatic dose (MMD)
m. reacting dose (MRD)
m. residual disease (MRD)
triage m.
minimal-change
m.-c. disease
m.-c. nephrotic syndrome
minimally
m. invasive breast biopsy
(MIBB)
m. invasive follicular carcinoma
(MIFC)
minimum
m. bactericidal concentration
m. bactericidal concentration test
m. complete-killing concentration
(MCC)
m. concentration of bilirubin
(MCBR)
m. detectable concentration (MDC)

m. dose causing death or
malformation of 100% of fetuses
(T/LD_{100})
m. essential medium (MEM)
m. hemolytic dose (MHD)
m. infective dose (MID)
m. inhibitory concentration (MIC)
m. lethal concentration
m. lethal dose (MLD)
m. mission-oriented protective
posture (MOPP)
m. mycoplasmacidal concentration
(MPC)
m. temperature
m. thermometer
minimus
Anopheles m.
Scopulariopsis m.
minipool (MP)
m. NAT
m. nucleic acid testing
mink
enteritis of m.
m. enteritis virus
Minkowski-Chauffard syndrome
minocycline
minor
m. agglutinin
m. AU-AC spliceosome
beta thalassemia m.
m. cluster region (MCR)
M. disease
m. epilepsy
m. histocompatibility antigen
m. histocompatibility complex
Lactobacillus m.
Lagochilascaris m.
Streptococcus m.
thalassemia m.
m. tranquilizer
variola m.
Weissella m.
minores
ductus sublinguales m.
glandulae vestibulares m.
Minot-von Willebrand syndrome
minus
Spirillum m.
m. strand
minuta
Plasmodium vivax m.
minute (min)
count per m. (cpm)
cycle per m. (c/min)
liter per m. (Lpm)
revolutions per m. (rpm)
m. volume (MV)
minutisporangium
Cryptosporangium m.

M

minutissima
minutissimum
> *Corynebacterium m.*
> *Nocardia m.*

minutum
> *Eubacterium m.*

mionectic
miostagmin reaction
MIP
> macrophage inflammatory
> protein
> maximum inspiratory pressure

mirabilis
> *Proteus m.*

miracidium
Mirchamp sign
MIRD
> medical internal radiation dose

Mirex
miricola
> *Chryseobacterium m.*

Mirizzi syndrome
miroungae
> *Facklamia m.*

mirror-image
> m.-i. cell
> m.-i. complementary antibody
> (MICA)

miscarriage
miscellaneous blast injury
miscibility
miscible
> infinitely m.

mismatch
> m. repair (MMR)
> m. repair gene
> V/Q m.

missed abortion
missense mutation
missile
> high-velocity m. (HVM)
> m. wound

missplicing
mistranslation
mitchellae
> *Aedes m.*

Mitchell disease
mite
> grain itch m.
> harvest m.
> kedani m.
> predaceous m.
> red m.
> trombiculid m.
> m. typhus

MITF
> microphthalmia-associated transcription
> factor
> melanocyte specific MITF (MITF-M)

MITF-M
> melanocyte specific MITF

MITGCN
> malignant intratubular germ-cell
> neoplasia

miticidal
miticide
mitis
> prurigo m.
> *Streptococcus m.*

mitochondrial
> m. aggregation
> m. antibody
> m. complex II
> m. creatine kinase (mtCK)
> m. crista alteration
> m. cytochrome oxidase
> m. deoxyribonucleic acid (mDNA)
> m. disorder
> m. encephalopathy, lactic acidosis,
> and strokelike episodes
> (MELAS)
> m. enzyme desmolase
> m. inheritance
> m. matrix
> m. matrix alteration
> m. membrane
> m. membrane alteration
> m. myopathy
> m. pyruvate dehydrogenase
> m. sheath
> m. toxin

mitochondrialis
> matrix m.

mitogen
> m. assay
> pokeweed m. (PWM)

mitogen-activated protein (MAP)
mitogenesis
mitogenetic
mitogenic factor
mitokinetic
mitoplasm
mitosis
> abnormal m.
> three-part m.

mitosis-karyorrhexis index (MKI)
mitotic
> m. activity index (MAI)
> m. arrest
> m. chromosome
> m. control protein (MCP)
> m. count
> m. cycle
> m. figure
> m. index
> m. period
> m. poison
> m. rate

m. spindle
m. spindle assembly checkpoint
m. spindle defect
MitoTracker Red CMXRos
Mitovirus
mitoxantrone
mitral
m. atresia
m. cell
m. incompetence
m. incompetency and stenosis
m. insufficiency
m. regurgitation
m. valve
m. valve calcification
m. valve cleft leaflet
m. valve prolapse
(MPV, MVP)
Mitrophora
Mitsuda
M. antigen
M. reaction
mitsuokai
Catenibacterium m.
Mitsuokella jalaludinii
Mittendorf dot
mixed
m. acid fermentation
m. agglutination
m. agglutination reaction
m. agglutination test
m. anemia
m. calculus
m. cell leukemia
m. cellularity (MC)
m. cellularity Hodgkin disease
(MCHD)
m. chancre
m. connective tissue disease
(MCTD)
m. cryoglobulinemia
m. cryoglobulin syndrome
m. dust pneumoconiosis
m. epithelial-mesenchymal tumor
m. epithelial papillary cystadenoma
of borderline malignancy of
müllerian type (MEBMM)
m. epithelial tumor
m. function oxidase system
m. germ cell tumor (MGCT)
m. glioma
m. hemadsorption (MHA)
m. hemoglobinopathy
m. hepatocellular carcinoma
m. immunofluorescence (MIF)
m. infection
m. large- and small-cell
non-Hodgkin lymphoma (MNHL)
m. leukocyte culture (MLC)

m. lineage leukemia (MLL)
m. lymphocyte culture (MLC)
m. lymphocyte culture assay
m. lymphocyte culture reaction
m. lymphocyte culture test
m. lymphocyte reaction (MLR)
m. lymphocyte-tumor culture
(MLTC)
m. mesodermal tumor
m. thalassemia
m. thrombus
m. tumor of skin
m. venous
m. venous blood
mixing
mixoploid
developmental m.
proliferative m.
mixoploidy
mixotrophic
mixture
dextrose solution m. (DSM)
dichloropropene-dichloropropane m.
racemic m.
Ringer m.
toxoid-antitoxoid m. (TAM)
mixtus
Cellvibrio m.
Miyagawa body
Miyagawanella
M. lymphogranulomatosis
M. ornithosis
M. pneumoniae
M. psittaci
Miyasato disease
Miyoshi myopathy
mJ
millijoule
M-K
McCarey-Kaufman
M-K medium
MK
monkey kidney
MK protein
mkat
millikatal
MKI
mitosis-karyorrhexis index
MKS
meter-kilogram-second
MKS system
MKS unit
mks
meter-kilogram-second
M:L
monocyte-lymphocyte ratio
ML
malignant lymphoma
monocytoid lymphocyte

M

mL
    millilambert
    milliliter
MLA-100 coagulation instrument
MLC
    minimal lethal concentration
    mixed leukocyte culture
    mixed lymphocyte culture
    mixed lymphocyte culture
      assay
        MLC assay
        MLC test
MLD
    metachromatic leukodystrophy
    minimum lethal dose
MLH1
    human mismatch-repair protein MutL
      homolog
        MLH1 gene
M1-like viruses
MLL
    mixed lineage leukemia
MLR
    mixed lymphocyte reaction
MLTC
    mixed lymphocyte-tumor culture
MLV
    Moloney leukemogenic virus
    mouse leukemia virus
MM
    Marshall-Marchetti
    Miyoshi myopathy
    multiple myeloma
    myeloid metaplasia
    skeletal muscle component of cardiac
      isoenzymes
        MM band
        MM virus
mm3
    cubic millimeter
MMA
    monomethylarsonic acid
MMD
    minimal morbidostatic dose
    moyamoya disease
MMEF
    maximal midexpiratory flow
MMEFR
    maximal midexpiratory flow rate
MMFR
    maximal midflow rate
MMH
    Marino and Muller-Hermelink
      MMH osteogenic classification
mmHg
    millimeter of mercury
MMM
    myelofibrosis with myeloid metaplasia
    myeloid metaplasia with myelofibrosis

MMMT
    malignant mixed mesodermal tumor
    malignant mixed müllerian tumor
mmol
    millimole
mmol/L
    millimole per liter
MMP
    matrix metalloproteinase
MMP1
    matrix metalloproteinase 1
MMP2
    matrix metalloproteinase 2
MMPC
    metastatic malignant pheochromocytoma
MMR
    mass miniature radiography
    measles, mumps, and rubella
    mismatch repair
      MMR gene
MMRS
    metropolitan medical response system
MMT
    malignant mixed tumor
MMTV
    mouse mammary tumor virus
M3 muscarinic acetylcholine receptor
mN
    millinormal
MNA
    mean nuclear area
mnemonic code
MNHL
    mixed large- and small-cell
      non-Hodgkin lymphoma
MNP
    malignant neoplasm
MNSs blood group
MO
    myositis ossificans
mobile
    Alkalispirillum m.
    Aminobacterium m.
    Anaerobaculum m.
    m. chilling unit
    cor m.
    m. gene
    m. phase
mobilis
    Klebsiella m.
    lien m.
    Macromonas m.
    Tistrella m.
mobility
    electrophoretic m.
    high electrophoretic m.
mobilization
    localized leukocyte m. (LLM)
    m. test

mobilizing agent
Mobiluncus
Möbius
    M. disease
    M. syndrome
MOC31 monoclonal antibody
MOCNI
    method of collection not indicated
modal centromere copy number
ModAMeX
    modified acetone methylbenzoate
    xylene
      ModAMeX section method
mode
    decay m.
    histogram m.
    list m.
model
    Cox proportional hazards regression m.
    fluid mosaic m.
    generalized linear mixed m. (GLMM)
    geometrical m.
    hairpin-mediated polymerase
      slippage m.
    polymerase slippage m.
    unequal crossing over m.
modeling
    finite element m.
moderate dysplasia or high grade
moderately differentiated (MD)
moderator band
Modestobacter multiseptatus
modification
    racemic m.
    Rye m.
modified
    m. acetone methylbenzoate xylene
      (ModAMeX)
    m. acid-fast stain
    m. amino acid
    m. macrophage
    m. Masaoka thymic cancer staging
      system
    m. red blood cell
    m. smallpox
    m. Steiner stain
    m. TM agar
    m. zinc sulfate centrifugal flotation
      technique
modifier
modifying gene
modiolus
MODM
    maturity-onset diabetes
modular
modulate
modulation (mod)
    antigenic m.
    m. transfer function

module (mod)
    large particle sorting m. (LPS)
modulus
MODY
    maturity onset diabetes of the
    young
moesin
Mogibacterium
    M. diversum
    M. neglectum
    M. pumilum
    M. timidum
Mohr pipette
moiety
    ceramide m.
    fucosyl m.
    heme m.
    sialyl m.
moist
    m. desquamation
    m. gangrene
    m. necrosis
    m. papule
    m. wart
Mokola virus
mol
    mole
μmol
    micromole
molal
molality
molar (M)
    m. absorptivity
    m. concentration
    m. heat capacity
    m. pregnancy
    m. villi
    m. weight
molarity
mold
    Cryo rubber m.
    pink bread m.
mole (mol)
    blood m.
    Breus m.
    carneous m.
    complete m.
    cystic m.
    false m.
    fleshy m.
    m. fraction
    grape m.
    hairy m.
    hydatid m.
    hydatidiform m.
    invasive m.
    m. of glucose
    spider m.
    vesicular m.

M

molecular
- m. allelotyping
- m. anemia
- m. assay
- m. biology
- m. cell layer
- m. chaperone
- m. characterization
- m. cloning
- m. cytogenetic analysis
- m. disease
- m. dispersion
- m. distillation
- m. epidemiology
- m. exclusion chromatography
- m. genetics
- m. hybridization
- m. kinetics
- m. layer of cerebellum
- m. layer of cerebral cortex
- m. lesion
- m. marker
- m. mass
- m. pathology
- m. resistance testing
- m. sieve
- m. sieve chromatography
- m. staging
- m. typing
- m. weight (MW)

moleculare
- stratum m.

molecularly targeted therapy

molecule
- accessory m.
- adhesion m.
- carcinoembryonic antigen-related cell adhesion m. 1 (CEACAM1)
- CD m.
- cell adhesion m. (CAM)
- cell-cell adhesion m.
- cell-substrate adhesion m.
- CI m.
- costimulatory m.
- E-cadherin calcium-dependent m.
- endothelial-leukocyte adhesion m. (E-LAM)
- histocompatibility m.
- leukocyte adhesion m.
- microRNA m.
- middle m.
- neuron cell adhesion m.
- m. of equivalent soluble fluorochrome (MESF)
- signaling m.
- U1 snRNA m.
- U2 snRNA m.
- U4 snRNA m.

U5 snRNA m.
U6 snRNA m.

molecule-1
- intercellular adhesion m.-1 (ICAM-1)
- vascular cell adhesion m.-1 (VCAM-1)

molenkampi
- *Prosthodendrium m.*

mole fraction (molfr)

molinativorax
- *Gulosibacter m.*

Molisch test

Moll
- adenocarcinoma of M.
- M. gland

Mollaret meningitis

molle
- fibroma m.

Möller-Barlow disease

Mollicutes

Mollisia fusca

mollities

mollusc (*var. of* mollusk)

mollusciformis
- verruca m.

Molluscipoxvirus

molluscous animal

molluscum
- m. body
- m. contagiosum
- m. contagiosum virus (MCV)
- m. corpuscle
- m. fibrosum
- m. fibrosum gravidarum
- m. sebaceum virus
- m. verrucosum

mollusk, mollusc

Moloney
- M. leukemogenic virus (MLV)
- M. sarcoma virus (MSV)
- M. test

Molotov cocktail

Molten disease

molybdate
- ammonium m.

molybdenum

molybdic

molybdites
- *Chlorophyllum m.*

MOM
- mouse-on-mouse
- MOM basic kit
- MOM fluorescein kit
- MOM peroxidase kit

MOMA
- methoxyhydroxymandelic acid

moment
- dipole m.
- magnetic m.

momentum

MOMP
major outer membrane protein
Monacrosporium
monad
Monakow
M. bundle
M. fascia
M. stria
M. syndrome
monamide
monaminergic
monaminuria
monarthritis
Monascus
monaxonic
Mönckeberg
M. arteriosclerosis
M. degeneration
M. medial calcification
M. medial calcific sclerosis
Mondor disease
Monera
moneran
Monge disease
mongol
mongolian
m. macula
m. spot
mongolism
mongoloid
Moniezia
M. benedeni
M. expansa
monilated
monilethrix
Monilia albicans
Moniliaceae
monilial esophagitis
moniliasis pneumonia
Moniliella
moniliform
moniliforme
Eubacterium m.
Fusarium m.
moniliformis
Armillifer m.
Haverhillia m.
M. moniliformis
Streptobacillus m.
Monilinia
monitor
air m.
Amplicor CMV M.
chemical agent m. (CAM)
Crit-Line fluid m.
Sof-Tact glucose m.
monitoring
atmospheric m.
fetal oxygen saturation m.

therapeutic drug m. (TDM)
monitorization
monkey
m. B virus
m. kidney (MK)
monkeypox virus
mono
monocyte
mononuclear leukocyte
mononucleosis
Acceava Mono
monoallelic
monoamine oxidase inhibitor
monoaminodicarboxylic acid
**monoaminomonocarboxylic
acid**
monoaminuria
monoamniotic placenta twins
monoassociated
monobactam
monobasic
m. acid
m. potassium phosphate
m. sodium phosphate
monoblast
monoblastic leukemia
Monocelis
monocentric
monocephalus
m. tetrapus dibrachius
m. tripus dibrachius
monochorionic
m. diamniotic placenta
m. diamniotic placenta twins
m. monoamniotic placenta
monochroic
monochromatic
monochromatism
monochromatophil, monochromatophile
monochromatophile (*var. of*
monochromatophil)
monochromator
monochromic
monochromophil, monochromophile
monochromophile (*var. of* monochromophil)
Monocillium
monoclonal
m. antibody (MAb)
m. antibody MB1
m. antibody-specific immobilization
of platelet antigen (MAIPA)
m. antiepithelial membrane
antigen
m. band
m. B-cell pattern
m. free light chain
m. gammopathy
m. gammopathy of undetermined
significance (MGUS)

M

monoclonal (*continued*)
    m. gammopathy of unknown significance (MGUS)
    m. hypergammaglobulinemia
    m. hypothesis
    m. immunoglobulin
    m. M spike
    m. paraprotein
    m. peak
    m. protein
    m. tumor
monoclonality
monocular function
monocyte (mono)
    m. chemoattractant protein (MCP)
    m. chemoattractant protein 1 (MCP 1)
    m. chemotactic protein 1
    m. function test
    m. macrophage
    plasmacytoid m.
monocyte-derived neutrophil chemotactic factor (MDNCF)
monocyte-lymphocyte ratio (M:L)
monocyte-macrophage system
monocytic
    m. angina
    m. blood cell
    m. inflammatory infiltrate
    m. leukemia
    m. leukemoid reaction
    m. leukocytosis
    m. leukopenia
    m. marrow
    m. neoplasia
    m. precursor cell
monocytogenes
    m. bacterium
    heat-killed Listeria m. (HKLM)
    Listeria m.
monocytoid
    m. B-cell lymphoma
    m. cell
    m. lymphocyte (ML)
monocytopenia
monocytopoiesis
monocytosis
    avian m.
monodermal teratoma
monodermoma
Monodictys nigrosperma
Mono-Diff test
monoenoic fatty acid
monoethylglycinexylidide
monofluorophosphate
    sodium m.
monogenesis

monogenetic
monogenic character
monogenous
monoglyceride
monoglycosylated
monohistiocytic series
monohydric alcohol
monohydrochloride
    arginine m.
monohydrolase
    orthophosphoric ester m.
monoinfection
monoiodotyrosine
monokine
monolayer
    cell m.
monoleptic fever
Monolisa Anti-HBc IgM EIA immunoassay
monolocular
monomastigote
monomelica
    osteosis eburnisans m.
monomer
    fibrin m.
    globular m.
monomeric actin
monomethylarsonic acid (MMA)
monomicrobic
monomorphic adenoma (MA)
monomorphism
monomorphous
monomyelocytic leukemia
monomyositis
Mononchus
mononeme
mononeural, mononeuric
mononeuric (*var. of* mononeural)
mononeuritis multiplex
mononeuropathy multiplex
mononuclear
    m. cell
    m. leukocyte (mono)
    m. phagocyte
    m. phagocyte system (MPS)
    m. Reed-variant (MRV)
mononucleate
mononucleosis (mono)
    infectious m. (IM)
    posttransfusion m. (PTM)
    spot test for infectious m.
mononucleotide
    flavin m. (FMN)
    m. repeat
monooxygenase
    beta m.
    dopamine m.
monopenia

monophasic (MP)
    m. choriocarcinoma
    m. synovial sarcoma (MSS)
    m. wave
monophosphate
    adenosine m. (AMP)
    adenosine 3′,5′-cyclic m. (cAMP)
    concentration of adenosine m.
    cyclic adenosine m. (cAMP)
    cyclic guanosine m.
    cytidine m. (CMP)
    deoxyadenosine m. (dAMP)
    deoxycytidine m.
    deoxyguanosine m. (dGMP)
    deoxyuridine m. (dUMP)
    guanosine m. (GMP)
    hexose m. (HMP)
    inosine m.
    thymidine m.
    uridine m.
    xanthosine m.
3′,5′-monophosphate
monophyletic theory
monophyletism
monoplasmatic
monoplast
monoplastic
monoploid
monopolar
MonoPrep Pap test
monoptychial
monorecidive chancre
monosaccharide
Monoscreen test
monosodium
    m. glutamate (MSG)
    m. urate
    m. urate crystal
monosome
monosomic cell
monosomy
    mosaic autosomal m.
    m. X
monospecific direct Coombs test
Monosporium apiospermum
Monospot test
Monostichella
Monosticon Dri-Dot test
Monostoma
monostome
monostotic fibrous dysplasia
monostratal
monosynaptic bipolar cell
monotherapy
Monotospora
monotreme
Monotricha
monotrichate
monotrichous

monotypic effect
monounsaturated
Mono-Vacc test
monovalent antiserum
monoxenic culture
monoxenous
monoxide
    carbon m. (CO)
    diffusing capacity for carbon m.
      (D_{CO}, DCO)
    diffusing capacity of lung for
      carbon m. (DLCO)
    heme oxygenase/carbon m.
      (HO/CO)
monoxime
    diacetyl m.
monozoic
monozygosity
monozygotic twins
Monsel solution
monstrocellular sarcoma of Zulch
montana
    Rickettsia m.
montanus
    Diamanus m.
Monte Carlo method
montefiorense
    Mycobacterium m.
Montenegro skin test
montevideo
    Salmonella enteritidis serotype *m.*
    M. unit (MU)
Montgomery
    M. follicle
    M. tubercle
montoyai
montpellierensis
    Veillonella m.
Montreal platelet syndrome (MPS)
moorei
    Solobacterium m.
mooreparkense
    Corynebacterium m.
Moore syndrome
mop bipolar cell
MOPP
    minimum mission-oriented protective
    posture
Morand foot
moraviensis
    Enterococcus m.
Morax-Axenfeld
    M.-A. bacillus
    M.-A. diplococcus
    diplococcus of M.-A.
Moraxella
    M. anatipestifer
    M. bovis
    M. catarrhalis

Moraxella (*continued*)
    M. conjunctivitis
    M. kingae
    M. lacunata
    M. liquefaciens
    M. nonliquefaciens
    M. osloensis
    M. phenylpyruvica
Moraxellaceae
morbidity rate
morbility
morbilli
morbilliform rash
morbillivirus
    equine m. (Hendra virus)
morbillorum
    Diplococcus m.
    Gemella m.
    Streptococcus m.
morbus
Morchella
mordant solution
mordens
mordicans
morelense
    Sinorhizobium m.
Morel-Kraepelin disease
Morel syndrome
Morerastrongylus costaricensis
Morgagni
    M. column
    M. cyst
    M. disease
    M. hernia
    M. humor
    hydatid of M.
    M. liquor
    M. nodule
    M. prolapse
    M. sphere
    M. syndrome
Morgagni-Adams-Stokes syndrome
Morgagni-Stewart-Morel syndrome
Morgan bacillus
Morganella morganii
morgani
    Chordodes m.
morganii
    Morganella m.
    Proteus m.
morgue
    m. capability
    m. operations
    m. service
moriens
    ultimum m.
morin
Moritella
    M. abyssi

    M. profunda
    M. viscosa
Moritellaceae
Mörner test
Morococcus cerebrosus
morphallactic regeneration
morphea
    m. acroterica
    m. alba
    m. guttata
    m. herpetiformis
    m. linearis
    m. pigmentosa
    m. profundus
morphine assay
morphodifferentiation
morphogenesis
morphologic, morphological
    m. abnormality
    m. criteria
    m. element
    m. feature
morphological (*var. of* morphologic)
    m. analysis
morphology
    blood smear m.
    clear cell m.
    colony m.
    epithelioid m.
    irregular fried egg m.
    red blood cell m.
    syncytial m.
    vascular m.
morphometric analysis
morphometry
morphon
Morquio
    M. disease
    M. syndrome
Morquio-Brailsford syndrome
Morquio-Ullrich
    M.-U. disease
    M.-U. syndrome
morrhuate
    sodium m.
Morris syndrome
Morrow Brown needle
morselize
morsitans
    Glossina m.
mors thymica
mortality rate (MR)
mortar kidney
Mortierella wolfii
mortiferum
    Fusobacterium m.
mortification
mortified

mortis
  instantaneous rigor m.
  livor m.
  rigor m.
Morton
  M. disease
  M. neuroma
  M. syndrome
mortuary science
morula
morular
morule
  m. formation
  squamous m.
Morvan
  M. disease
  M. syndrome
mosaic
  m. autosomal monosomy
  m. fungus
  m. pattern
  ring m.
  Schmorl m.
  m. wart
mosaicism
  confined placental m. (CPM)
  diploid m.
  germline m.
  triploid m.
  trisomy 8 m.
  45,X/46,XY m.
Moschcowitz disease
moscoviensis
  Nitrospira m.
Mosenthal test
MOSF
  multiple-organ system failure
Mosher
  M. air cell
  air cell of M.
moshkovskii
  Entamoeba m.
Mosler diabetes
mOsm
  milliosmole
mosquitocidal
mosquitocide
Moss classification
mosselii
  Pseudomonas m.
Mosse syndrome
mossii
  Dysgonomonas m.
mossy
  m. cell
  m. fiber
  m. foot
mote
  blood m.

moth-eaten pattern
mother
  m. cell
  m. cyst
moth patch
motif
  antigen receptor activation m.
    (ARAM)
  immunoreceptor tyrosine activation
    m. (ITAM)
  immunoreceptor tyrosine inhibitory
    m. (ITIM)
motile
  m. cell
  m. cilia
  m. leukocyte
  m. rod
  m. serum
motilin
motility
  m. test
  m. test medium
  tumor cell m.
motion
  active range of m. (AROM)
  brownian m.
  range of m. (ROM)
motoneuron (*var. of* motor neuron)
motor
  m. axon
  m. axon twig
  m. cell
  m. end plate
  m. endplate
  m. innervation
  m. neuron
  m. neuron disease
MOTT
  mycobacteria other than tubercle
Mott
  M. bacilli
  M. cell
mottled
  m. enamel
  m. erythema
mottling
  reddish-blue m.
Motulsky dye reduction test
moulage
Mounier-Kuhn syndrome
mount
  India ink m.
  wet m.
mountant
mounting medium
mouse, *pl.* **mice**
  cancer-free white m. (CFWM)
  m. encephalomyelitis virus
  m. hepatitis virus

M

mouse (*continued*)
    m. leukemia virus (MLV)
    m. mammary tumor virus
      (MMTV)
    New Zealand mice
    m. parotid tumor virus
    pneumonia virus of mice (PVM)
    m. poliomyelitis virus
    m. thymic virus
    transgenic mice
    m. unit (MU)
    m. uterine unit (MUU)
mouse-on-mouse (MOM)
mousepox virus
**mouse-specific lymphocyte antigen
(MSLA)**
mouth
    m. fistula
    glass-blower's m.
    scabby m.
    sore m.
    tapir m.
    trench m.
movable, moveable
    m. heart
    m. testis
Movat
    M. pentachrome method
    M. pentachrome stain
moveable (*var. of* movable)
movement
    ameboid m.
    m. artifact (MA)
    brownian m.
    doll's eye m.
    euglenoid m.
    nonrapid eye m. (NREM)
    streaming m.
moving-boundary electrophoresis
moving phase
Mowry colloidal iron stain
moyamoya disease (MMD)
MP
    melting point
    minipool
      MP NAT
MPC
    marine protein concentrate
    maximum permissible concentration
    micropapillary component
    minimum mycoplasmacidal
      concentration
MPD
    maximal permissible dose
    myeloproliferative disease
MPE
    malignant pleural effusion
MPEH
    methylphenylethylhydantoin

MPG
    malignant paraganglioma
MPGN
    membranoproliferative
      glomerulonephritis
MPH
    micronodular pneumocyte hyperplasia
MPIF1
    myeloid progenitor inhibitory factor 1
MPI/MRI
    myelofibrosis proliferation/regression
      index
MPNST
    malignant peripheral nerve sheath tumor
MPO
    myeloperoxidase
MPP
    mercaptopyrazidopyrimidine
MPPC
    malignant primary pheochromocytoma
MPPT
    methylprednisdone pulse therapy
MPS
    mononuclear phagocyte system
    Montreal platelet syndrome
    mucopolysaccharide
MPSC
    micropapillary serous carcinoma
MPTP
    1-methyl-4-phenyl-1,2,3,6-
      tetrahydropyridine
MPV
    mean platelet volume
    mitral valve prolapse
MPXI
    mean peroxidase index
MR
    methyl red
    mortality rate
mR
    milliroentgen
mrad
    millirad
Mrakia
MRC
    medullary renal carcinoma
MRC-5 human diploid fibroblast cell
MRCNS
    methicillin-resistant coagulase-negative
      Staphylococcus
MRD
    minimal reacting dose
    minimal residual disease
mrem
    millirem
MRF
    melanocyte-stimulating hormone
     releasing factor
    mesencephalic reticular formation

Mrf4 gene

MRG
median rhomboid glossitis

mRNA
messenger ribonucleic acid

MRO
medical review officer

MRP
multidrug resistance protein

MRSA
methicillin-resistant *Staphylococcus aureus*

MRT
malignant rhabdoid tumor

MRTK
malignant rhabdoid tumor of kidney

MRTS
malignant rhabdoid tumor of soft tissue

MRV
mononuclear Reed-variant

MR-VP
methyl red, Voges-Proskauer
MR-VP broth

MS
mass spectrometry
mucosubstance
multiple sclerosis
myeloid sarcoma

ms
millisecond
musculoskeletal

MS-1
MS-1 agent
MS-1 hepatitis

MS-2
MS-2 agent
MS-2 hepatitis

MSA
muscle-specific actin
MSA antibody

MSAFP
maternal serum alpha-fetoprotein

M-Saskatoon
hemoglobin M-S.

MSB
martius scarlet blue
MSB trichrome stain

MSCNS
methicillin-susceptible coagulase-negative *Staphylococcus*

MSDS
material safety data sheet

msec
millisecond

MSG
monosodium glutamate

MSH
melanophore-stimulating hormone

MSH2 gene

MSH6 gene

MSLA
mouse-specific lymphocyte antigen

MSS
monophasic synovial sarcoma

MSSA
methicillin-susceptible *Staphylococcus aureus*

MSTS
Musculoskeletal Tumor Society

MSTS
MSTS score
MSTS staging system

MSU
monosodium urate
monosodium urate crystal
MSU crystal

MSUD
maple syrup urine disease

MSV
Moloney sarcoma virus
murine sarcoma virus

MSVC
maximal sustained ventilatory capacity

MT
antimetallothionein antibody
medical technologist

MTB
Mycobacterium tuberculosis

MTC
medullary thyroid carcinoma

mtCK
mitochondrial creatine kinase

MTD
mean tubular diameter

mtDNA
mitochondrial deoxyribnucleic acid

MTF
medical treatment facility

MTHFR
methylenetetrahydrofolate reductase

MTI
malignant teratoma, intermediate
MTI antibody

MTND2 gene

MTND5 gene

MTR
Meinicke turbidity reaction

MTT
malignant teratoma, trophoblastic
malignant triton tumor
malignant trophoblastic teratoma

MTTA gene

MTU
malignant teratoma, undifferentiated

MTV
mammary tumor virus

M

MU
    Mache unit
    Montevideo unit
    mouse unit
mU
    milliunit
mu
    milliunit
      mu antigen
      mu heavy chain disease
MUC
    maximum urinary concentration
mucase
mucescens
    Salipiger m.
MUC4 expression
MUC1 gene derived glycoprotein assay
Mucha disease
Mucha-Habermann
    M.-H. disease
    M.-H. syndrome
MUCI antibody
mucicarmine stain
mucid
muciferous
muciform
mucigen granule
mucigenous
mucihematein
mucilaginosa
    Rhodotorula m.
    Rothia m.
mucilaginosus
    Stomatococcus m.
mucilaginous gland
mucilloid
    psyllium hydrophilic m.
mucin
    allergic m.
    basophilic m.
    m. clot test
    m. depletion
    intracytoplasmic m.
    polymorphic epithelial m. (PEM)
mucin-depleted mucoepidermoid carcinoma
mucinemia
mucin-4 gene
muciniphila
    Akkermansia m.
mucinogen granule
mucinoid degeneration
mucinosa
    alopecia m.
mucinosis
    cutaneous dermal m.
    cutaneous focal m.
    follicular m.
    localized m.

    metabolic m.
    reticular erythematous m. (REM)
    secondary m.
mucinous
    m. adenocarcinoma
    m. adenoma
    m. atrophy
    m. borderline tumor (MBT)
    m. breast lesion
    m. bronchioloalveolar carcinoma
    m. cyst
    m. cystadenocarcinoma
    m. cystadenoma
    m. cystic tumor (MCT)
    m. degeneration
    m. ductal ectasia
    m. meningioma
    m. metaplasia
    m. stroma
    m. tubular and spindle cell carcinoma
mucinuria
muciparous gland
muciphage
mucitis
Muckle-Wells syndrome
mucoalbuminous cell
mucobuccal fold
mucocele
    orbital m.
    sinus m.
mucociliary
mucoclasis
mucocutaneous
    m. junction
    m. leishmaniasis
    m. lymph node syndrome
mucoenteritis
mucoepidermoid
    m. carcinoma (MEC)
    m. tumor
mucoepithelial dysplasia
mucohyaline stroma
mucoid
    m. adenocarcinoma
    m. colony
    m. medial degeneration
mucoides
    Trichosporon m.
Mucolexx
mucolipidosis
    m. type I–IV
muconodular infiltration
mucopeptide
mucopolysaccharidase
mucopolysaccharide (MPS)
    acid m. (AMP)
    m. stain
    m. staining
    m. storage disease

stromal m.
sulfated acid m. (SAM)
m. test
mucopolysaccharidosis
m. subgroup
m. type I
m. type IS
m. type IVA, B
m. type I–VIII
mucopolysacchariduria
mucoprotein
m. assay
Tamm-Horsfall m. (THM)
m. test
mucopurulent exudate
mucopus
Mucoraceae
mucormycosis
pulmonary m.
mucoroides
Aspergillus m.
Mucor racemosus
mucosa, *pl.* **mucosae**
fundic m.
gastric m.
glandula m.
intestinal m.
Lactobacillus mucosae
lamina muscularis mucosae
lamina propria mucosae
membrana m.
muscularis mucosae (MM)
mucosae nasi
Neisseria m.
olfactory m.
oxyntocardiac m.
regio respiratoria tunicae mucosae
respiratory m.
Roseomonas m.
tunica m.
mucosa-associated
m.-a. lymphoid tissue (MALT)
m.-a. lymphoid tissue lymphoma
mucosae (*pl. of* mucosa)
mucosal
m. disease
m. disease virus
m. ischemia
m. lentiginous melanoma
m. melanosis
m. neuroma
m. neuroma syndrome
m. prolapse syndrome
m. ridge
m. tunic
mucosanguineous, mucosanguinolent
mucosanguinolent (*var. of*
mucosanguineous)
mucoserous cell

mucositis
plasma cell m.
mucosubstance (MS)
mucosulfatidosis
mucosum
Treponema m.
mucosus
Diplococcus m.
mucous
m. acinus
m. carcinoid
m. cast
m. colitis
m. connective tissue
m. cyst
m. gland adenoma of bronchus (MGAB)
m. gland of auditory tube
m. membrane
m. neck cell
m. papule
m. patch
m. plaque
m. plug
m. polyp
m. sheath of tendon
m. thread
mucoviscidosis
mucro
m. cordis
m. sterni
mucron
Mucuna
mucus
m. extravasation
fecal m.
m. retention
m. secreting cervical gland
stool m.
muddy brown urinary cast
mud fever
Muehrcke line
Mueller-Hinton
M.-H. agar
M.-H. broth
Muellerius capillaris
Muir-Torre syndrome
mukohataei
Halomicrobium m.
mulberry calculus
Mulder test
mule-spinner's cancer
muliebris
corpus spongiosum urethrae m.
dartos m.
mu-like viruses
Müller
M. capsule
M. fiber
M. fixative

M

Müller (*continued*)
    M. muscle
    M. radial cell
Muller-Hermelink
    M.-H. histological criteria
    Marino and M.-H. (MMH)
müllerian
    m. adenosarcoma
    M. duct
    M. rest
    m. tumor
multiangle polarized scatter separation (MAPSS)
multiblock
    m. technique
    tissue m.
multicapsular
multicellular
multicentric
    m. occurrence
    m. reticulohistiocytosis
multiceps
    M. multiceps (Taenia multiceps)
    M. serialis
    Taenia m.
multichannel analyzer (MCA)
multiclonal
multicolored FISH
multicolor FISH analysis
multicore disease
multicystic
    m. ameloblastoma
    m. dysplasia of kidney (MCDK)
    m. dysplastic kidney (MCDK)
multidot pattern
multidrug
    m. resistance (MDR)
    m. resistance 1 (MDR1)
    m. resistance protein (MRP)
multifactorial
    m. inheritance
    m. inherited disease
multifiliis
    Ichthyophthirius m.
multifocal
    m. atrophic gastritis (MAG)
    m. choroidal melanoma
    m. eosinophilic granuloma
    m. fibrosis
    m. inflammation
    m. osteitis fibrosa
    m. progressive leukoencephalopathy
multiformatter
multiforme
    erythema m.
    glioblastoma m.
multiformis
    Haverhillia m.
    prurigo chronica m.

multiform layer of cerebral cortex
multiglandular
multiinfarct dementia
multiinfection
multilamellar body
multilaminar primary follicle
multilobar, multilobate, multilobed
multilobate (*var. of* multilobar)
    m. placenta
multilobated
multilobed (*var. of* multilobar)
multilobular
multilocular
    m. adipose tissue
    m. cystic kidney
    m. fat
    m. hydatid cyst
multilocularis
    Echinococcus m.
multiloculate hydatid cyst
multilocus variable number (tandem repeat) analysis
Multimek 96/384
multimeter
multimodal peak
multinodal
multinodular goiter
multinuclearity
    hereditary erythroblastic m.
multinuclear leukocyte
multinucleated
    m. atypia of the vulva (MAV)
    m. cell
    m. giant cell (MGC)
    m. osteoclast
multinucleosis
multiorgan dysfunction
multipapillosa
multiparameter flow cytometry
multipartial
multipartita
    Nakamurella m.
    placenta m.
multiphasic screening
multipixel spectral analysis
multiple
    m. access
    m. adenoma
    m. adenomatous polyps
    m. allele
    m. antigen stimulation test (MAST)
    m. biotin-avidin amplification
    m. carboxylase deficiency (MCD)
    m. chemical sensitivity
    m. colloid adenomatous goiter (MCAG)
    m. displacement amplification (MDA)
    m. drug resistance (MDR)

m. endochondromatosis
m. endocrine adenomatosis (MEA)
m. endocrine neoplasia (MEN)
m. endocrinoma
m. endocrinopathy
m. epiphysial dysplasia
m. event curve
m. exostosis
m. hamartoma syndrome
m. idiopathic hemorrhagic sarcoma
m. intestinal polyposis
m. lentigines syndrome
m. level sectioning
m. lymphomatous polyposis
m. marker screen
m. mucosal neuroma syndrome
m. myeloma (MM)
m. myelomatosis
m. myositis
m. organ dysfunction syndrome
m. osteochondromas
m. puncture tuberculin skin testing
m. puncture tuberculin test
m. sclerosis (MS)
m. self-healing squamous epithelioma
m. serositis
m. stage random sample
m. stain
m. symmetric lipomatosis
m. system atrophy
m. tumor
multiple-organ system failure (MOSF)
multiplex
dysostosis m.
dysplasia epiphysialis m.
hemangioendothelioma tuberosum m.
lymphangioma tuberosum m.
mononeuritis m.
mononeuropathy m.
myeloma m.
myelomatosis m.
m. reverse transcription PCR
enzyme hybridization assay
steatocystoma m.
trichoepithelioma papillosum m.
multiplexed fluorescent microsphere
immunoassay for TH1, TH2 cytokines
multiplication
vegetative m.
multiplicative growth
multiplier
multiploid adenoma
multiploidy
DNA m.
multipolar
m. cell
m. motor neuron
m. spindle
multipotent

multipuncture tuberculin skin test
multiresinivorans
Pseudomonas m.
multirule Shewhart procedure
multiseptatus
Modestobacter m.
Multisizer 3 Coulter counter
Multistix
multisynaptic
multithread allergosorbent test (MAST)
multitrichous
multivalent vaccine
multivariate
m. analysis
m. analysis of variance (MANOVA)
multivesicular body
multivorans
Dehalospirillum m.
Salana m.
Sulfurospirillum m.
multiwire proportional chamber
multocida
mummification necrosis
mummified cell
mumps
m. antibody titer
iodine m.
m. meningoencephalitis
metastatic m.
m. sensitivity test
m. serology
m. skin test antigen
m. virus
m. virus culture
m. virus vaccine
Munchmeyer disease
Munich tumor classification system
munition
smoke-producing m.
Munro
M. abscess
M. microabscess
MUP
4-methylumbelliferyl phosphate
mural
m. aneurysm
m. cell
m. endocarditis
m. nodule
m. thrombus
muralis
Citricoccus m.
Georgenia m.
Halomonas m.
muramic acid
muramidase
Murchison-Sanderson syndrome
murein
Murex *Candida albicans* **CA50 test**

M

murexide
muriatic acid
Muricauda ruestringensis
Muricoccus roseus
muriform
murina
    Hymenolepis m.
    Taenia m.
murine
    m. hepatitis
    m. leprosy
    m. leukemia
    m. sarcoma virus (MSV)
    m. typhus
muris
    Actinomyces m.
    Brachybacterium m.
muris-ratti
    Actinomyces m.-r.
murliniae
    Citrobacter m.
murmur
    ejection m. (EM)
    late systolic m. (LSM)
Muromegalovirus
murorum
    Gliomastix m.
Murphy-Pattee test
Murray
    M. Valley encephalitis (MVE)
    M. Valley rash
Murutucu virus
Musca domestica
muscae
    Habronema m.
muscaria
    Amanita m.
muscarine
muscarinic
    m. effect
    m. receptor
muscarinism
Muscidae
muscle
    m. actin (MA)
    m. action potential
    arrector pili m.
    m. biopsy
    m. bundle
    cardiac m.
    m. contractile protein
    dartos m.
    dilator pupillae m.
    m. epithelium
    m. fascicle
    genioglossus m.
    m. hemoglobin
    involuntary m.
    Jung m.

    Landström m.
    meridional fiber of ciliary m.
    Müller m.
    m. of heart
    red m.
    Reisseisen m.
    Rouget m.
    m. serum
    skeletal m.
    smooth m.
    m. spindle
    striated m.
    unstriated m.
    white m.
muscle-specific actin (MSA)
muscle-tendon
    m.-t. attachment
    m.-t. junction
musculamine
muscular
    m. atrophy
    m. cushion
    m. dystrophy (MD)
    m. fibril
    m. rheumatism
    m. rigidity
    m. subaortic stenosis
    m. tissue
    m. tunic
muscularis
    m. externa
    fibrae obliquae tunicae m.
    m. mucosae
    tunica m.
musculoaponeurotic fibromatosis
Musculoskeletal Tumor Society (MSTS)
musculotropic
musculus skeleti
mushroom
    angel of death m.
    m. poisoning
mushroom-worker's lung
mustard
    m. gas
    NATO code for distilled (neat) sulfur m.
    NATO code for impure sulfur m. (H)
    NATO code for nitrogen m. (HN)
    NATO code for nitrogen m. 1 (HN1)
    NATO code for nitrogen m. 2 (HN2)
    NATO code for nitrogen m. 3 (HN3)
mustard-induced burn
mustargen

Musto stain
mutabilis
mutagen
    chromosomal m.
mutagenesis
    insertional m.
mutagenic
mutagenicity test
mutans
    Streptococcus m.
mutant
    conditional-lethal m.
    conditionally lethal m.
    core promoter m.
    escape m.
    m. gene
    HFR m.
    high-frequency recombination m.
    precore m.
    suppressor-sensitive m.
    temperature-sensitive m.
mutarotation
mutase
    diphosphoglycerate m.
    2,3-diphosphoglycerate m.
    S-methylmalonyl-CoA m.
mutated
    m. crypt
    m. in colon cancer (MCC)
mutation
    addition-deletion m.
    amber m.
    auxotrophic m.
    BRAF m.
    BRAF V600E m.
    m. burden
    clear plaque m.
    m. cluster region (MCR)
    cold-sensitive m.
    conditional lethal m.
    constitutive m.
    deletion m.
    dominant negative m.
    feedback inhibition m.
    forward m.
    frameshift m.
    GATA3 gene m.
    genetic m.
    genome m.
    germ-time m.
    Ha-ras m.
    heterozygous point m.
    homozygous point m.
    host-range m.
    insertion m.
    Ki-ras m.
    K-ras m.
    Leiden m.
    lethal m.

    I1307K gene m.
    LQTS Finnish founder m.
    missense m.
    NOD2/CARD15 m.
    nonsense m.
    ochre m.
    p53 m.
    PDGFRA gene m.
    pleiotropic m.
    point m.
    prothrombin G20210A m.
    prothrombin II m.
    rapid-lysis m.
    m. rate
    reverse m.
    semilethal m.
    sex-reversed m.
    silent m.
    somatic point m.
    spontaneous m.
    subvital m.
    suppressor m.
    temperature-sensitive m.
    transition m.
    transversion m.
    t-s m.
    ultraviolet light-induced m.
mutational analysis
mutator gene
mutilans
    arthritis m.
    keratoma hereditarium m.
    lupus m.
    rhinopharyngitis m.
mutilating
    m. keratoderma
    m. leprosy
    m. wound
Mutinus
mutL **gene**
muton
mutS **gene**
mutualism
mutualist
MUU
    mouse uterine unit
muzzle
    m. abrasion
    m. contusion
muzzled sperm
MV
    megavolt
    minute volume
Mv
    mendelevium
MVC
    microvessel count
MVD
    microvessel density

M

MVE
 Murray Valley encephalitis
 MVE virus
MVP
 mean platelet volume
 mitral valve prolapse
MVR
 massive vitreous retraction
MVV
 maximum voluntary ventilation
mW
 milliwatt
Mx
 maxwell
Myá disease
myalgia
 cervical m.
 epidemic m.
myasis
myasthenia gravis
myasthenic crisis
myatrophy
mycelial
 m. fungus
 m. pathogen
mycelian
Myceligenerans xiligouense
mycelioid
Myceliophthora
mycelium
 aerial m.
 nonseptate m.
 septate m.
Myceloblastanon
Mycena
mycete
mycetism, mycetismus
 m. cerebralis
 m. choliformis
 m. nervosa
mycetismus (*var. of* mycetism)
Mycetocola
 M. lacteus
 M. saprophilus
 M. tolaasinivorans
mycetogenetic, mycetogenic
mycetogenic (*var. of* mycetogenetic)
mycetogenous
mycetoides
 Corynebacterium m.
mycetoma
 actinomycotic m.
 Bouffardi black m.
 Bouffardi white m.
 Brumpt white m.
 Carter black m.
 eumycotic m.
 Exophiala m.
 maduromycotic m.

 Nicolle white m.
 Vincent white m.
mycetomi
 Madurella m.
MY-10 clone stain
MycoAKT latex bead agglutination test
mycobacteria (*pl. of* mycobacterium, Mycobacterium)
Mycobacteriaceae
mycobacterial
 m. adjuvant
 m. DNA in sarcoidosis
Mycobacteriales
mycobacteriophage
 luciferase reporter m. (LRP)
mycobacteriosis
mycobacterium, *pl.* **mycobacteria**
 M. africanum
 M. avium
 M. avium infection
 M. avium-intracellulare (MAI)
 M. avium-intracellulare complex (MAC)
 M. avium serovar 1–29
 M. balnei
 Battey-type m.
 M. boenickei
 M. botniense
 M. bovis
 M. bovis BCG strain
 M. bovis subsp. *caprae*
 M. butyricum
 M. canariasense
 M. caprae
 M. chelonae subsp. *abscessus*
 M. chimaera
 mycobacteria culture
 M. doricum
 M. elephantis
 M. flavescens
 M. fortuitum
 M. fortuitum-chelonae
 M. frederiksbergense
 M. gastri
 M. genavense
 M. gordonae
 group I-IV mycobacteria
 mycobacteria growth indicator tube (MGIT)
 M. haemophilum
 M. heckeshornense
 M. holsaticum
 M. houstonense
 M. immunogenum
 mycobacteria infection
 M. interjectum
 M. intracellulare
 M. kansasii

M. kubicae
M. lacus
M. leprae
M. lepraemurium
M. malmoense
M. marinum
M. microti
M. montefiorense
M. neworleansense
M. nonchromogenicum
nonphotochromogenic mycobacteria
nontuberculous mycobacteria (NTM, NTMB)
mycobacteria other than tubercle (MOTT)
M. palustre
M. parascrofulaceum
M. paratuberculosis
M. paratuberculosis Linda
M. parmense
M. phlei
M. phlei cell wall DNA complex (MCC)
M. pinnipedii
M. psychrotolerans
Runyon mycobacteria (group I–IV)
M. saskatchewanense
scotochromogenic mycobacteria
M. scrofulaceum
M. septicum
M. shottsii
M. simiae
M. smegmatis
M. szulgai
M. terrae
M. triviale
M. tuberculosis (MTB)
M. ulcerans
M. vanbaalenii
M. xenopi
mycobactin
mycobiotic agar
Mycocandida
Mycocentrospora acerina
mycocide
Mycococcus
mycoderma
  Saccharomyces m.
mycodermatitis
mycogastritis
Mycogone
Mycokluyveria
mycolic acid
mycologist
mycology
  medical m.
mycomyringitis
myc oncogene

mycophage
Mycoplana
M. bullata
M. dimorpha
mycoplasma
M. agar
M. agassizii
M. alligatoris
M. buccale
M. faucium
M. fermentans
M. gallisepticum
genital m.
M. genitalium
M. granularum
M. haemocanis
M. haemofelis
M. haemomuris
M. hominis
m. infection
M. lipophilum
M. microti
M. orale
M. pneumoniae
M. primatum
M. pulmonis
M. salivarium
M. serology
M. suis
M. testudineum
T-strain m.
M. wenyonii
mycoplasmal pneumonia
Mycoplasmataceae
Mycoplasmatales
mycopus
mycoses (*pl. of* mycosis)
mycoside
mycosis, *pl.* **mycoses**
  allergic bronchopulmonary m. (ABPM)
  m. cutis chronica
  m. fungoides (MF)
  m. fungoides dèmblee
  m. fungoides/Sézary syndrome (MF/SS)
  Gilchrist m.
  m. intestinalis
  opportunistic m.
  superficial m.
  systemic m.
Mycosphaerella
mycostatic
mycotic
  m. abscess
  m. aneurysm
  m. keratitis
  m. meningitis
  m. prostatitis

M

mycotica
    otitis m.
Mycotoruloides
mycotoxicosis
mycotoxin
    T2 m.
    trichothecene m.
    weaponized T2 m.
Mycotypha
mycovirus
*myc*protooncogene
mydriasis
myelapoplexy
myelatelia
myelauxe
myelemia
myelin
    m. basic protein (MBP)
    m. body
    m. degeneration
    m. figure (MF)
    neurokeratin network of
      dissolved m.
    m. sheath
    m. staining method
    Weigert stain for m.
myelinated
    m. nerve
    m. nerve fiber
myelination, myelinization
myelinic degeneration
myelinization (*var. of* myelination)
myelinogenesis
myelinolysis
    central pontine m.
myelinosis
    central pontine m.
myelitis
    acute necrotizing m.
    acute transverse m.
    ascending m.
    bulbar m.
    concussion m.
    demyelinated m.
    Foix-Alajouanine m.
    funicular m.
    postinfectious m.
    postvaccinal m.
    subacute necrotizing m.
    systemic m.
    transverse m.
myeloablative therapy
myeloarchitectonics
myeloblast
myeloblastemia
myeloblastic
    m. leukemia
    m. protein
myeloblastoma

myeloblastosis
    avian m.
myelocele
myelocyst
myelocystic
myelocystocele
myelocystomeningocele
myelocyte
    m. A, B, C
    basophilic m.
    eosinophilic m.
    neutrophilic m.
myelocythemia
myelocytic
    m. crisis
    m. leukemia
    m. leukemoid reaction
myelocytoma
myelocytomatosis
myelocytosis
myelodiastasis
myelodysplasia
myelodysplastic syndrome (MDS)
myelofibrosis
    m. anemia
    chronic idiopathic m. (CIMF)
    idiopathic m.
    myeloid metaplasia with m.
      (MMM)
    primary m.
    m. proliferation/regression index
      (MPI/MRI)
    m. with myeloid metaplasia
myelogenesis
myelogenetic, myelogenic
myelogenic (*var. of* myelogenetic)
    m. leukemia
    m. osteopathy
    m. sarcoma
myelogenous
    m. callus
    m. leukemia
myelogone, myelogonium
myelogonium (*var. of* myelogone)
myeloic
myeloid
    m. depression
    m. hyperplasia
    m. leukemia
    m. metaplasia (MM)
    m. metaplasia with myelofibrosis
      (MMM)
    m. metaplasia with polycythemia
      vera (PCV-M)
    m. progenitor inhibitory factor 1
      (MPIF1)
    m. reticulosis
    m. sarcoma (MS)
    m. series

m. stem cell
m. tissue
myeloid-erythroid ratio (M:E)
myeloidosis
myelokathexis
myeloleukemia
myelolipoma
myelolymphocyte
myelolysis
myeloma
Bence Jones m.
m. cast nephropathy
m. cell
endothelial m.
giant cell m.
IgA m.
IgD m.
IgE m.
IgG m.
L-chain m.
multiple m. (MM)
m. multiplex
nonsecretory m.
plasma-cell m.
plasmacytic m.
m. protein
myelomalacia
angiodysgenetic m.
myelomatosis
multiple m.
m. multiplex
myelomeningitis
myelomeningocele
myelomonocyte
myelomonocytic leukemia
myelonencephalitis
myelopathic
m. anemia
m. polycythemia
myelopathy
carcinomatous m.
cervical m.
compressive m.
diabetic m.
HTLV-1 associated m.
  (HAM)
lumbosacral m.
transverse m.
vascular m.
myeloperoxidase (MPO)
m. deficiency
m. H_2O_2 halide system
m. stain
m. system
myelopetal
myelophthisic anemia, myelopathic anemia
myelophthisis
myeloplast

myelopoiesis
extramedullary m.
myelopoietic
myeloproliferative
m. disease (MPD)
m. disorder
m. syndrome
myeloradiculitis
myeloradiculodysplasia
myeloradiculopolyneuronitis
myelorrhagia
myelorrhaphy
myelosarcoma
myelosarcomatosis
myeloschisis
myelosclerosis with myeloid metaplasia
myelosis
aleukemic m.
erythremic m.
funicular m.
leukemic m.
leukopenic m.
megakaryocytic m.
nonleukemic m.
subleukemic m.
myelostimulatory theory
myelosuppression
myelosyringosis
myelotoxic
myenteric
m. nerve
m. plexus
myenteron
myf3 gene
myf4 gene
myf5 gene
MYH9
myosin heavy chain 9
MYH9 gene
Myhre syndrome
myiasis
cutaneous m.
facial m.
gastric m.
genitourinary m.
intestinal m.
nasal m.
sanguivorous m.
Mylar capacitor
myleran
MYO
myoglobin
myoadenylate
m. deaminase
m. deaminase deficiency
myoarchitectonic
myoatrophy
myoblast
myoblastoid carcinoma

M

myoblastoma
    granular cell m.
myoblastomatoid carcinoma
myocardial
    m. anoxia
    m. bridge
    m. damage
    m. depressant factor (MDF)
    m. disease
    m. disease of unknown origin
      (MDUO)
    m. endocrine cell
    m. infarction (MI)
    m. infarction in dumbbell
      form
    m. infarction in H-form
    m. ischemia
    m. scarring
myocarditis
    bacterial m.
    drug-induced m.
    Fiedler m.
    fragmentation m.
    fulminant m.
    giant cell m.
    hypersensitivity m.
    idiopathic m.
    indurative m.
    infectious m.
    Löffler m.
    rheumatic m.
    toxic m.
    viral m.
myocardium
    hibernating m.
    stunned m.
myocardosis
myocele
myocelialgia
myocelitis
myocellulitis
myocerosis
myochondroblast
myoclonica
    dyssynergia cerebellaris m.
myoclonic epilepsy
myocyte
    Anitschkow m.
    cardiac m.
    m. disarray
    Purkinje m.
    m. stretch
myocytoma
MyoD
    myogenic regulatory
    MyoD family of genes
    MyoD gene family
    MyoD protein
MyoD1

    MyoD1 immunostaining
    MyoD1 regulatory gene
myodegeneration
myodemia
myodiastasis
myoelastic
myoendocarditis
myoepithelial
    m. carcinoma
    m. cell
    m. sialadenitis (MESA)
myoepithelioma
    malignant m.
myoepithelium
    neoplastic m.
myofascial syndrome
myofascitis
myoferlin
myofiber
myofibril
    intracellular m.
    m. necrosis
myofibrilla
myofibrillar
myofibrillary hypertrophy
myofibroblast
    stromal m.
myofibroblastic
    m. differentiation
    m. immunophenotype
    m. lesion
    m. mammary stromal tumor
    m. proliferation
myofibroblastoma
myofibrohistiocytic
myofibroma
myofibromatosis
    infantile m.
myofibrosis cordis
myofibrositis
myofilament
    thick m.
    thin m.
myogenesis
myogenetic, myogenic
myogenic (*var. of* myogenetic)
    m. cell
    m. paralysis
    m. regulatory (MyoD)
myogenin protein
myogen marker
myogenous
myoglobin (MYO)
    m. A, B, C, D, E, G, H
    carbon dioxide m. (MbCO)
    m. cardiac diagnostic test
    m. clearance test
    m. identification method
    m. stain

myoglobinemia
myoglobinuria
    acute paroxysmal m.
myoglobinuric
    m. nephropathy
    m. nephrosis
myoglobulin
myoglobulinuria
myohemoglobin
myoid
    m. cell
    m. marker
    m. marker expression
myo-inositol
myointimal
    m. hyperplasia
    m. proliferation
myoischemia
myokerosis
myokinase
myolemma
myolipoma
myolysis
    cardiotoxic m.
myoma
myomalacia
myomatous polyp
myomelanosis
myometrial hypertrophy (IMH)
myometritis
myometrium
myomitochondrion
myon
myonecrosis
    clostridial m.
    myonecrosis, myoglobinuria, renal
      failure
myoneme
myoneural junction
myoneuroma
myonosus
myopachynsis
myopathic
myopathy
    alcoholic m.
    carcinomatous m.
    centronuclear m.
    congenital m.
    corticosteroid m.
    distal m.
    endocrine m.
    inflammatory m.
    mitochondrial m.
    Miyoshi m. (MM)
    myotubular m.
    nemaline m.
    rod m.
    thyrotoxic m.
myopericarditis

myopericytoma
myoperitonitis
myophagocytosis
myophosphorylase deficiency glycogenosis
myoplasm
myopodin gene
myoporoides
    Duboisia m.
myorrhexis
myosalpingitis
myosarcoma
myosclerosis
myosin
    m. binding protein C
    m. cross-bridge
    m. filament
    m. heavy chain 9 (MYH9)
    m. phosphatase
    skeletal-muscle m.
    m. stain
myosis
    endolymphatic stromal m.
myositic
myositis
    clostridial m.
    epidemic m.
    m. fibrosa
    inclusion body m.
    infectious m.
    interstitial m.
    multiple m.
    m. ossificans (MO)
    m. ossificans circumscripta
    m. ossificans progressiva
    proliferative m.
    m. sine dermatitides
myospherulosis
myostroma
myotenositis
myotonia
myotonic dystrophy (DM)
myotonin protein kinase gene
myotube
myotubular myopathy
myotubule
Myoviridae
myriapod
Myriapoda
myringa
myringitis
    bullous m.
myringomycosis
myrinx
Myriodontium
myristic acid
myrmecia
    m.
Myrothecium
mysophilia

MYST
mediastinal yolk sac tumor
mystax
Ascaris m.
Toxocara m.
myxadenitis
myxadenoma
myxedema
m. heart
idiopathic m.
infantile m.
pituitary m.
pretibial m.
myxedematoid
myxedematosus
lichen m.
myxedematous
myxemia
myxochondrofibrosarcoma
myxochondroid matrix
myxochondroma
Myxococcaceae
Myxococcales
Myxococcidium stegomyiae
myxocollagenous matrix
myxocyte
myxofibroma
myxofibrosarcoma
myxohyaline degeneration
myxoid
m. change
m. cyst
m. degeneration
m. fibroma
m. liposarcoma
m. matrix
m. mesenchyme
m. neurofibroma
m. stroma
m. synovial sarcoma
myxolipoma
myxoliposarcoma
myxoma
atrial m.
cardiac m. (CM)

cystic m.
m. enchondromatosum
endochondromatous m.
erectile m.
m. fibrosum
infectious m.
lanceolate m.
m. lipomatosum
lipomatous m.
nerve sheath m. (NSM)
odontogenic m.
m. sarcomatosum
sinonasal m.
vascular m.
myxomatodes
carcinoma m.
fibroma m.
lipoma m.
myxomatosis
cardiac valve m.
m. virus
myxomatous degeneration
myxomycete
Myxomycetes
myxoneuroma
myxopapillary ependymoma
myxopapilloma
myxosarcoma
Myxospora
myxospore
Myxosporea
Myxosporidia
Myxotrichum
myxovirus
Myxozoa
Myzomyia
Myzorhynchus
MZ
marginal zone
MZBCL
marginal zone B-cell lymphoma
MZL
mantle zone lymphoma
marginal zone (cell)
lymphoma

N
- asparagine
- newton
- normal
  - N antigen

n
- haploid genome

N0
- no lymph nodes containing cancer cells

NA
- nasopharyngeal angiofibroma
- neutralizing antibody
- nodular amyloidoma

NAA
- N-acetylaspartate acid

NAAK
- nerve agent antidote kit

nabothian
- n. cyst
- n. follicle

N-acetylaspartate acid (NAA)
N-acetyl-B-hexosaminidase
N-acetylcysteine
N-acetylgalactosamine
N-acetylgalactosamine-4-sulfatase
N-acetylgalactosamine-6-sulfatase
N-acetylglucosamine
N-acetylglucosamine-6-sulfatase
N-**acetylmannosamine**
N-**acetylmuramic acid**
N-**acetylneuraminic**
NaCl
- sodium chloride

NaCN
- sodium cyanide

nacreous ichthyosis
N-**acylsphingosine**
NAD
- nicotinamide adenine dinucleotide

NADH
- nicotinamide adenine dinucleotide
  - NADH control
  - NADH dehydrogenase
  - NADH methemoglobin reductase

nadir
Nadi reaction
NADP
- nicotinamide adenine dinucleotide phosphate
  - intracellular NADP

NADPH
- nicotinamide adenine dinucleotide phosphate
  - intracellular NADPH
  - NADPH oxidase

Nadsonia
Naegleria fowleri
Naemacyclus
Naemospora
naeslundii
- *Actinomyces n.*

naevoid (*var. of* nevoid)
naevus (*var. of* nevus)
NAF
- neutrophil activating factor

Naffziger syndrome
NAFLD
- nonalcoholic fatty liver disease

nagana
naganoensis
- *Leifsonia n.*

Nagao enzyme
nagasakiensis
- *Thermaerobacter n.*

Nägele pelvis
Nägeli
- N. syndrome
- N. type of monocytic leukemia

nagelii
- *Lactobacillus n.*

Nageotte cell
Nagler reaction
nail
- n. bomb
- cornified layer of n.
- germinative layer of n.
- n. horn
- horny layer of n.
- n. plate
- ringworm of nails
- shell n.
- sinus of n.
- yellow n.

nail-patella syndrome
Nairobi
- N. sheep disease
- N. sheep disease virus

Nairovirus
NAIT
- neonatal alloimmune thrombocytopenia

naive cell
Nakamurellaceae
Nakamurella multipartita
Nakanishi stain
naked virus
Nalgene
- N. capsule filter
- N. freezer storage rack
- N. PETG media bottle

nalidixic acid

N

NAME
    nevi, atrial myxoma, myxoid
    neurofibroma, and ephelides
    NAME syndrome
name
    generic n.
Namibia
    sulfur pearl of N.
namibiensis
    Actinomadura n.
    Gordonia n.
    Thiomargarita n.
nana
    Endolimax n.
    Entamoeba n.
    Hymenolepis n.
    Taenia n.
NANB
    non-A, non-B hepatitis
    NANB hepatitis
nanism
Nannizzia
NanoChip
    N. molecular biology workstation
    N. test for factor V Leiden
        single-nucleotide polymorphism
nanocurie (nCi)
Nanoduct neonatal sweat analysis system
nanoemulsion
    surfactant n.
nanofarad (nF)
Nanog gene marker
nanogram (ng)
nanoliter (nL)
nanomelia
nanometer (nm)
nanomole (nmol)
nanoparticle
    MgO n.
Nanophyetus salmincola
nanoprobe
Nanoprobes
    N. GoldEnhance reagent
    N. Nanogold reagent
nanosecond (ns, nsec)
Nanovirus
nanukayami
nanum
    Microsporum n.
NAP
    neutrophil activating protein
    nucleic acid panel
    NAP bacteria differentiation test
    NAP hepatitis B virus quantitative
        panel
    NAP modified LRP assay
nape nevus
naphtha
    coal tar n.

naphthalenivorans
    Polaromonas n.
naphthalenovorans
naphthol
    alpha n.
    n. ASBI phosphate stain
    n. AS-D chloracetate (NASDCA)
    beta n.
    n. poisoning
    n. pyronine
    n. yellow S
**naphthol-AS-D-chloracetate esterase
    (NASDCE)**
naphthophila
    Thermotoga n.
Napier formol-gel test
napierian logarithm
napkin ring tumor
NAPP
    nerve agent pyridostigmine pretreatment
    NAPP tablet set
narcosis
    carbon dioxide n.
    nitrogen n.
narcotic
    n. antagonist
    n. blockade
NARES
    nonallergic rhinitis with eosinophilia
nares (*pl. of* naris)
naris, *pl.* **nares**
    nares swab anthrax spore test
Narnavirus
NARP
    neurogenic muscle weakness, ataxia,
        and retinitis pigmentosa
narugense
    Thermodesulfobium n.
nasal
    n. allergic disorder
    n. angiocentric T-cell lymphoma
        (NATL)
    n. cytology
    n. gland
    n. glioma
    n. myiasis
    n. polyp
    n. smear
    n. T/NK-cell lymphoma
nasales
    glandulae n.
NASBA
    nucleic acid sequence based
        amplification
    nucleic acid sequence based analysis
nascent
NaSCN
    sodium thiocyanate
    NaSCN exchange assay

nasdae
>Brevundimonas *n.*

NASDCA
>naphthol AS-D chloracetate

NASDCE
>naphthol-AS-D-chloracetate esterase
>NASDCE stain

NASH
>nonalcoholic steatohepatitis

nasi
>cancrum n.
>granulosis rubra n.
>mucosae n.
>tunica mucosa n.

nasicola
>Actinomyces *n.*

Nasik vibrio

nasimurium
>Rothia *n.*

nasiphocae
>Arthrobacter *n.*

Naskapi
>albumin N.

nasogastric
nasolabial cyst
nasooral leishmaniasis
nasopalatal
nasopalatine duct cyst
nasopharyngeal (NP)
>n. angiofibroma (NA)
>n. aspirate
>n. carcinoma (NPC)
>n. culture
>n. leishmaniasis
>n. swab

nasopharyngitis
nasopharynx
nasosinusitis
nasus
NAT
>nucleic acid amplification test
>NAT for HCV and HIV-1 in blood
>donation
>minipool NAT
>MP NAT

natalensis
>Mastomys *n.*

natans
>Sphaerotilus *n.*

national
>N. Accrediting Agency for Clinical
>Laboratory Sciences
>N. Biomonitoring Program (NBP)
>N. Bladder Cancer Collaborative
>Group (NBCCG)
>N. Cancer Data Base (NCDB)
>N. Cancer Institute (NCI)
>N. Committee for Clinical
>Laboratory Standards (NCCLS)

>N. Council of Health Laboratory
>Services (NCHLS)
>N. Electronic Disease Surveillance
>System (NEDSS)
>n. examination
>N. Immunization Program (NIP)
>N. Institute for Occupational Safety
>and Health (NIOSH)
>N. Institutes of Health (NIH)
>n. laboratory
>N. Medical Response Team (NMRT)
>N. Notifiable Diseases Surveillance
>System (NNDSS)
>N. Pharmaceutical Stockpile (NPS)
>N. Registry of Microbiologists
>N. Wilms Tumor Study

native albumin
NATL
>nasal angiocentric T-cell lymphoma

NATO
>North Atlantic Treaty Organization
>NATO code
>NATO code for an extremely toxic
>persistent nerve agent (no common
>chemical name)
>NATO code for arsine (SA)
>NATO code for chloracetophenone
>(CS)
>NATO code for
>1-chloroacetophenone (CN)
>NATO code for cyanogen chloride
>(CNCl$_2$)
>NATO code for cyclosarin (GF)
>NATO code for
>dibenz(b,f)-1:4-oxazepine (CR)
>NATO code for diphenylaminearsine
>(adamsite)
>NATO code for
>diphenylaminochloroarsine (adamsite)
>NATO code for distilled (neat)
>sulfur mustard
>NATO code for HCN (AC)
>NATO code for impure sulfur
>mustard (H)
>NATO code for lewisite (L)
>NATO code for military obscurant
>smoke (zinc oxide and
>hexachloroethane, grained aluminum)
>NATO code for nerve agent cyclohexyl
>methylphosphonofluoridate (GF)
>NATO code for nerve agent
>isopropyl ethylphosphonofluoridate
>(GE)
>NATO code for nerve agent O-ethyl
>S-[2-(diethylamino)ethyl]
>ethylphosphonothioate (VE)
>NATO code for nerve agent O-ethyl
>S-[2-(diethylamino)ethyl]
>methylphosphonothioate (VM)

N

NATO (*continued*)
  NATO code for nerve agent
  O,O-diethyl S-[2-(diethylamino)ethyl]
  phosphonothioate (VG)
  NATO code for nitrogen mustard
  (HN)
  NATO code for nitrogen mustard 1
  (HN1)
  NATO code for nitrogen mustard 2
  (HN2)
  NATO code for nitrogen mustard 3
  (HN3)
  NATO code for nonpersistent nerve
  agent
  NATO code for o-chlorobenzylidene
  malononitrile (CS)
  NATO code for persistent nerve
  agent
  NATO code for phosgene (choking
  gas)
  NATO code for phosgene oxime
  (CX)
  NATO code for QNB (BZ)
  NATO code for riot control agent
  bromobenzylcyanide (CA)
  NATO code for sarin (GB)
  NATO code for soman (GD)
  NATO code for tabun (GA)
natremia, natriemia
Natrialba
  N. aegyptia
  N. chahannaoensis
  N. hulunbeirensis
  N. taiwanensis
natriemia (*var. of* natremia)
Natrinema versiforme
natriuresis
natriuretic agent
Natronobacterium
  nitratireducens
natronolimnaea
  Dietzia n.
Nattrassia mangiferae
natural
  n. agglutinin
  n. antibody
  n. death
  n. dye
  n. focus of infection
  n. hemolysin
  n. host
  n. immunity
  n. killer cell
  n. killer cell leukemia
  n. killer cell lymphoma
  n. killer cell-stimulating factor
  (NKSF)
  n. selection
Naucoria

nausea
  epidemic n.
Nauta stain
Nautiliaceae
Nautiliales
Nautilia lithotrophica
navarrensis
  Roseospira n.
navicular
  n. arthritis
  n. cell
navicularis
  fossa n.
naviforme
  Fusobacterium n.
NB
  neuroblastoma
NBCCG
  National Bladder Cancer Collaborative
  Group
NBCCS
  nevoid basal cell carcinoma syndrome
NBP
  National Biomonitoring Program
NBS
  Nijmegen breakage syndrome
  normal blood serum
NBT
  nitroblue tetrazolium
  NBT dye
  NBT reduction assay
  NBT test
NBTE
  nonbacterial thrombotic endocarditis
NC
  neural crest
n:c
  nuclear-to-cytoplasmic ratio
NCA
  nonspecific cross-reacting antigen
N-cadherin marker
NCCLS
  National Committee for Clinical
  Laboratory Standards
NCDB
  National Cancer Data Base
NCF
  neutrophil chemotactic factor
NCHLS
  National Council of Health Laboratory
  Services
NCI
  National Cancer Institute
nCi
  nanocurie
NCL-ARm monoclonal antibody
NCL-ARp polyclonal antibody
NCL-ER-LH2 monoclonal antibody
NCL-PCR monoclonal antibody

ND
    neonatal death
    nondisabling
      ND virus
NDA
    no data available
    no demonstrable antibodies
NDFP
    nodular and diffuse fibrous
      proliferation
NDI
    nephrogenic diabetes insipidus
NDP
    net dietary protein
NDV
    Newcastle disease virus
Nd-YAG laser
Ne
    norepinephrine
nealsonii
    Bacillus n.
neapolitanus
    Halothiobacillus n.
neavei
    Simulium n.
Nebraska calf scours virus
nebulizer
    ultrasonic n. (USN)
nebulous urine
NEC
    necrotizing enterocolitis
Necator americanus
necatoriasis
necessitatis
    empyema n.
neck
    buffalo n.
    bull n.
    Madelung n.
    potato tumor of n.
    radiation-induced sarcoma of the
      head and n. (RISHN)
    TFL of head and n.
    webbed n.
necrobiosis
    n. lipoidica
    n. lipoidica diabeticorum
    superficial ulcerating rheumatoid n.
necrobiotic
    n. granuloma
    n. xanthogranuloma
necrocytosis
necrogenica
    verruca n.
necrogenic wart
necrogenous
necrogranulomatous
necrolysis
    toxic epidermal n. (TEN)

necrolytic migratory erythema (NME)
necroparasite
necropathy
necrophilic
necrophorum
    Fusobacterium n.
necrophorus
    Actinomyces n.
    Bacillus n.
    Fusiformis n.
    Sphaerophorus n.
necropolis
    Virgibacillus n.
necropsy, necroscopy
necroscopy (*var of* necropsy)
necrose
necroses (*pl. of* necrosis)
necrosis, *pl.* **necroses**
    acidophilic n.
    acute inflammatory n.
    acute massive liver n.
    acute tubular n. (ATN)
    aseptic n.
    avascular n. (AVN)
    bile duct n.
    bone aseptic n.
    bridging hepatic n.
    cardiac cell n.
    caseation n.
    caseous n.
    central n.
    central hemorrhagic n. (CHN)
    centrilobular n.
    cheesy n.
    coagulation n.
    coagulative n.
    colliquative n.
    comedo n.
    confluent hepatic n.
    contraction band n.
    cortical n.
    cystic medial n. (CMN)
    cytodegenerative n.
    cytotoxic n.
    diffuse n.
    dirty n.
    ductular piecemeal n.
    enzymatic fat n.
    enzymic fat n.
    epiphysial aseptic n.
    fat n.
    fibrinoid n.
    focal n.
    gangrenous n.
    geographic n.
    hepatocellular n.
    hyaline n.
    inflammatory n.
    intestinal n.

N

necrosis (*continued*)
  intra vitam n.
  ischemic n.
  lamellar n.
  laminar cortical n.
  liquefaction n.
  liquefactive n.
  liver cell n.
  massive hepatic n. (MHN)
  medial cystic n.
  medullary n.
  midzonal n.
  moist n.
  mummification n.
  myofibril n.
  postpartum pituitary n.
  progressive emphysematous n.
  pseudolaminar n.
  radiation n.
  radium n.
  renal cortical n.
  renal medullary n.
  renal papillary n.
  satellite cell n.
  sclerosing hyaline n.
  septic n.
  simple n.
  spotty lobular n.
  submassive confluent n.
  suppurative n.
  tissue n.
  total n.
  n. tumor
  tumor n.
  villous ischemic n.
  Zenker n.
  zonal n.
  zone n.
necrospermia
necrosteon, necrosteosis
necrosteosis (*var. of* necrosteon)
necrotic
  n. adipocyte
  n. cirrhosis
  n. cyst
  n. focus
  n. inflammation
  n. pseudoxanthomatous nodule
    (NPN)
necroticans
  enteritis n.
necrotisans
necrotizing
  n. angiitis
  n. arteriolitis
  n. bronchopneumonia
  n. encephalitis
  n. encephalomyelopathy
  n. enterocolitis (NEC)

  n. factor
  n. fasciitis (NF)
  n. funisitis
  n. glomerulonephritis
  n. granulomatous inflammation
  n. lobar pneumonia
  n. pancreatitis
  n. papillitis
  n. sarcoid granulomatosis (NSG)
  n. sialometaplasia
  n. ulcerative gingivitis (NUG)
  n. ulcerative gingivostomatitis
  n. vasculitis
necrotomy
Necrovirus
nectariphilum
  Catellibacterium n.
Nectria
Nectriopsis
NED
  no evidence of disease
NEDD8 gene
NEDSS
  National Electronic Disease
  Surveillance System
needle
  n. aspiration cytology
  Bard n.
  Becton-Dickinson n.
  Crown n.
  n. culture
  Jamshidi n.
  localization n.
  Manan n.
  Menghini n.
  Morrow Brown n.
  Surecut n.
  Tru-Cut n.
  Wang n.
  Wyeth bifurcated n.
Neer shoulder fracture I–III
Neethling virus
Neftel disease
neg
  negative
negative (neg)
  n. anergy
  n. assortative mating
  n. base excess
  beta-lactamase n.
  n. catalyst
  n. control enzyme induction
  n. control repression
  n. cytotaxis
  D^u n.
  false n.
  mast cell tryptase positive chymase
    n. (MCT)
  n. neutrotaxis

n. phase
n. predictive value (NPV)
Rh n.
n. stain
n. strand virus
n. variation (NV)
negative-pressure room
negevensis
    Simkania n.
Negibacteria
Negishi virus
neglectum
    Mogibacterium n.
Negri
    N. body
    N. corpuscle
neidei
    Bacillus n.
Neisser
    diplococcus of N.
    N. stain
Neisseria
    anaerobic *N.*
    N. caviae
    N. flava
    N. flavescens
    N. gonorrhoeae
    N. gonorrhoeae culture
    N. gonorrhoeae smear
    N. lactamica
    N. meningitidis
    N. mucosa
    N. ovis
    N. perflava
    N. sicca
    N. subflava
Neisseriaceae
Neisser-Wechsberg phenomenon
Nelson
    N. syndrome
    N. tumor
Nelson-Salassa syndrome
nemaline
    n. myopathy
    n. rod
nemathelminth
Nemathelminthes
nematicidal, nematocidal
nematicide, nematocide
nematization
nematoblast
nematocidal (*var. of* nematicidal)
nematocide (*var. of* nematicide)
Nematoda
nematode
nematodiasis
Nematodirella
    N. longispiculata
    N. longissimespiculata

Nematodirus
nematoid
nematologist
nematology
Nematoloma
Nematomorpha
nematophilus
nematosis
nematospermia
Nematospora
neoangiogenesis
neoantigens
Neoascaris vitulorum
neoautoimmune disease
Neobacteria
neocaledoniensis
    Nocardia n.
Neochlamydia hartmannellae
Neochordodes
Neocosmospora
neocyte
    donor n.
neocytosis
neodymium-yttrium-aluminum-garnet laser (Nd-YAG laser)
neoepitope
    cytokeratin n.
neoformans
    Cryptococcus n.
    Debaryomyces n.
    Filobasidiella n.
    Saccharomyces n.
neoformation
neoformative
neogenesis
Neohendersonia
neomembrane
neomort
neomycin assay agar
neonatal
    n. alloimmune thrombocytopenia (NAIT)
    n. anemia
    n. apnea
    n. autoimmune thrombocytopenia
    n. biliary function
    n. bilirubin
    n. calf diarrhea virus
    n. cerebrovascular accident (n. CVA)
    n. cholestasis workup
    n. death (ND, NND)
    n. gastrointestinal hemorrhage
    n. hemochromatosis
    n. hepatitis
    n. herpes
    n. hypoglycemia
    n. isoerythrolysis
    isoimmune n.

N

neonatal (*continued*)
- n. lupus
- n. necrotizing enterocolitis
- n. nesidioblastosis
- n. respiratory distress syndrome
- n. screening
- n. testing
- n. thymectomy
- n. thyroid-stimulating hormone
- n. thyroid-stimulating hormone test

neonatorum
- anemia n.
- anoxia n.
- atelectasis n.
- blennorrhea n.
- conjunctivitis n.
- dermatitis exfoliativa n.
- edema n.
- encephalitis n.
- erythema n.
- erythroblastosis n.
- ichthyosis congenita n.
- icterus n. (IN)
- impetigo n.
- mastitis n.
- ophthalmia n.
- sclerema n.

neopathy

neoplasia
- B-cell n.
- cervical intraepithelial n. (CIN)
- ductal intraepithelial n. (DIN)
- gestational trophoblastic n.
- intraductal papillary mucinous n. (IPMN)
- intraepithelial n.
- intratubular germ cell n. (IGCN)
- laryngeal intraepithelial n. (LIN)
- lobular n.
- lymphoreticular n.
- malignant intratubular germ-cell n. (MITGCN)
- mammary intraepithelial n.
- mesenchymal n.
- monocytic n.
- multiple endocrine n. (MEN)
- preinvasive urothelial n.
- prostatic intraepithelial n. (PIN)
- pulmonary mucinous cyst n.
- trophoblastic n.
- vaginal intraepithelial n.
- vascular n.
- vulvar intraepithelial n. (VIN)

neoplasm
- adipocytic n.
- adnexal n.
- adrenal n.
- astrocytic n.
- B-cell n.
- benign n.
- clear cell n.
- epithelial n.
- epithelioid soft-tissue n. (ESTN)
- germ cell n.
- hematodermic n.
- hematologic malignant n.
- histoid n.
- interdigitating papillary n.
- lymphoid n.
- malignant n. (MNP)
- mesenchymal n.
- metastatic n.
- nervous system n.
- oncocytic papillary n.
- prostatic intraepithelial n. (PIN)
- pseudopapillary n.
- renal epithelioid oxyphilic n. (REON)
- respiratory system n.
- Revised European-American Classification of Lymphoid N.'s
- sebaceous n.
- spinal n.
- stromal cell n.
- stromal-epithelial n.
- synchronous n.
- trophoblastic n.
- urothelial n.

neoplastic
- n. arachnoiditis
- n. disease
- n. element
- n. epidermal cell
- n. epithelium
- n. hematopoietic tissue
- n. lymphocyte
- n. meningitis
- n. myoepithelium
- n. proliferation
- n. theory

neoprecipitin test (NPT)

neopterin

neorickettsia
- *N. helmintheca*
- *N. risticii*
- *N. sennetsu*

Neosartorya fischeri

Neospora caninum

neoteny

Neotestudina rosatii

neotissue

Neotrombicula autumnalis

neotype

neovascularization
- choroidal n. (CNV)

nepalensis
- *Staphylococcus n.*

nephelometer

nephelometric
    n. immunoassay
    n. inhibition assay (NIA)
nephelometry
    rate n.
nephradenoma
nephrectasia
nephrectasis
nephredema
nephrelcosis
nephridium
nephritic
    n. calculus
    n. factor
    n. syndrome
nephritides (*pl. of* nephritis)
nephritis, *pl.* **nephritides**
    acute interstitial n. (AIN)
    allergic interstitial n. (AIN)
    analgesic n.
    antibasement membrane n.
    antikidney serum n.
    bacterial n.
    chronic interstitial n. (CIN)
    crescentic n.
    diffuse proliferative lupus n.
    Ellis types 1, 2 n.
    familial n.
    focal proliferative lupus n.
    glomerular n.
    n. gravidarum
    hemorrhagic n.
    hereditary n. (HN)
    immune complex n.
    interstitial n.
    lupus n. (LN)
    membranous lupus n.
    mesangial lupus n.
    nephrotoxic n. (NTN)
    nephrotoxic serum n. (NTSN)
    radiation n.
    salt-losing n.
    scarlatinal n.
    serum n.
    shunt n.
    subacute n.
    suppurative n.
    syphilitic n.
    transfusion n.
    tuberculous n.
    tubulointerstitial n.
    uranium n.
nephritogenic
nephroblastoma
    cystic partially differentiated n. (CPDN)
nephrocalcinosis
nephrocystosis
nephrogenetic, nephrogenic

nephrogenic (*var. of* nephrogenetic)
    n. adenoma
    n. diabetes insipidus (NDI)
    n. rest (NR)
nephrogenous ascites
nephrohydrosis
nephrolith
nephrolithiasis
nephrolysin
nephrolysis
nephrolytic
nephroma
    congenital mesoblastic n. (CMN)
    cystic n.
    embryonal n.
    mesoblastic n.
nephromalacia
nephromegaly
nephron
nephronic loop
nephronophthisis (*var. of* nephrophthisis)
nephropathia (*var. of* nephropathy)
    n. epidemica
nephropathic
nephropathy, nephropathia
    acute uric acid n.
    Alport hereditary n.
    analgesic n.
    Balkan n.
    Bence Jones cast n.
    chronic pyelonephritis/reflux n.
    C1q n.
    Danubian endemic familial n.
    diabetic n.
    gout n.
    gouty n.
    hemoglobinuric n.
    heroin-associated n.
    human immunodeficiency virus-associated n. (HIVAN)
    hyperuricemic n.
    hypokalemic n.
    IgA n.
    IgM n.
    immune complex n.
    lead n.
    membranous n.
    mesangial IgA n.
    myeloma cast n.
    myoglobinuric n.
    reflux n.
    sickle cell n.
    thin basement membrane n.
    tubulointerstitial n. (TIN)
nephrophthisis, nephronophthisis
    familial n.
    familial juvenile n. (FJN)
nephroptosia (*var. of* nephroptosis)
nephroptosis, nephroptosia

N

nephropyelitis
nephropyosis (*var. of* pyonephrosis)
nephrosclerosis
    arterial n.
    arteriolar n.
    benign n. (BNS)
    hyaline n.
    hyperplastic n.
    intercapillary n.
    malignant n.
    senile n.
nephrosclerotic
nephrosis
    acute n.
    amyloid n.
    bile n.
    cholemic n.
    familial n.
    hemoglobinuric n.
    hypokalemic n.
    hypoxic n.
    lipid n.
    lipoid n. (LN)
    lower nephron n.
    myoglobinuric n.
    osmotic n.
    toxic n.
    tubular n.
    vacuolar n.
nephrospasia (*var. of*
  nephrospasis)
nephrospasis, nephrospasia
nephrostogram
nephrotic syndrome (NS)
nephrotoxic
    n. antibody (NTAB)
    n. nephritis (NTN)
    n. serum
    n. serum nephritis
      (NTSN)
nephrotoxin
nephrotuberculosis
Nepovirus
neptunia
    Halomonas n.
neptuniae
    Devosia n.
neptunius
    Vibrio n.
Nernst equation
nerve
    n. agent
    n. agent antidote kit (NAAK)
    n. agent pyridostigmine pretreatment
      (NAPP)
    Auerbach n.
    n. cell
    n. cell body
    n. ending

    n. fascicle
    n. fiber
    n. ganglion
    n. growth factor (NGF)
    n. growth factor antiserum
    hemorrhoidal n.
    least splanchnic n.
    lesser splanchnic n.
    lipomatosis of n.
    myelinated n.
    myenteric n.
    obturator n.
    n. papilla
    postganglionic sympathetic n.
    n. root
    n. sheath (NS)
    n. sheath myxoma (NSM)
    n. sheath tumor
    nerves synapsing
nervea
    tunica n.
nervi (*pl. of* nervus)
nervosa
    anorexia n.
    foramina n.
    mycetism n.
    rhinitis n.
nervosum
    vaccinia n.
nervosus
    lobus n.
    status n.
nervous
    n. system neoplasm
    n. tissue
nervus, *pl.* **nervi**
nesidioblast
nesidioblastoma
nesidioblastosis
    focal n.
    neonatal n.
nesidiodysplasia
nesslerization
nesslerize
Nessler reaction
nest
    Brunn epithelial n.
    cell n.
    cribriform n.
    epithelial n.
    isogenous n.
    tumor n.
    von Brunn n.
Nesterenkonia
    N. halotolerans
    N. lacusekhoensis
    N. xinjisis
NET
    neuroendocrine tumor

net
- Chiari n.
- chromidial n.
- n. dietary protein (NDP)
- n. protein ratio (NPR)
- n. protein utilization (NPU)

Netherton syndrome
N-ethylmaleimide-sensitive-factor (NSF)
N-ethylmaleimide-sensitive fusion protein
N-ethyl-N-(2-hydroxy-3-sulfopropyl)-3, 5-dimethoxyaniline
nettle gas
network
- chromatin n.
- Cooperative Human Tissue N.
- cytokine n.
- Health Alert N. (HAN)
- intercommunicating n.
- Laboratory Response N. (LRN)
- linin n.
- neural n. (NN)
- neurokeratin n.
- probabilistic neural n. (PNN)
- Purkinje n.
- subpapillary n.
- trabecular n.
- tubovesicular n.

Neubauer hemocytometer
Neufeld
- N. capsular swelling
- N. reaction

Neumann
- N. cell
- N. disease
- N. sheath

neu-oncogene
neural
- n. crest (NC)
- n. crest cell
- n. cyst
- n. inclusion (NI)
- n. layer of retina
- n. network (NN)
- n. rosette
- n. tube defect

neuralgic amyotrophy
neuraminic acid
neuraminidase digestion
neuraminoglycoprotein
- alpha-2 n.

neurapraxia
neurasthenia, neurosthenia
neuraxis
neuraxon, neuraxone
neuraxone (*var. of* neuraxon)
neuregulin (NRG)
- n. protein
- n. 1 (protein)
- n. 2 (protein)
- n. 3 (protein)
- n. 4 (protein)

neurepithelial (*var. of* neuroepithelial)
neurepithelium
neuridine
neurilemma, neurolemma
- n. cell

neurilemmitis
neurilemmoma, neurolemmoma
- acoustic n.
- ameloblastic n.
- Antoni type A, B n.
- malignant n.

neurilemoma
neurilemosarcoma
neurility
neurimotility
neurimotor
neurinoma (*var. of* neuroma)
neurite
- dystrophic n.

neuritic
- n. atrophy
- n. plaques

neuriticum
- atrophoderma n.

neuritis
- adventitial n.
- allergic n.
- branchial n.
- experimental allergic n.
- induced allergic n.
- optic n.

neuroacanthosis
neuroallergy
neuroarthropathy
neuroastrocytoma
neuroblast
- sympathetic n.

neuroblastic
neuroblastoma (NB)
- olfactory n. (ONB)

neuroborreliosis
- Lyme n.

neurocalcin immunoreactive neuron
neurochitin
neurochoroiditis
neurocognition
neurocristic hamartoma
neurocristopathy
neurocutaneous
- n. melanosis
- n. phacomatosis syndrome

neurocyte
neurocytology
neurocytolysis
neurocytoma
- central n.

N

neuroD
- transcription factor n.

neurodegeneration

neurodegenerative disorder

neurodendrite

neurodendron

neurodermatitis

neuroectodermal tumor

neuroectoderm-derived cell

neuroencephalomyelopathy

neuroendocrine
- n. differentiation
- n. ductal carcinoma in situ
- n. marker
- n. transducer cell
- n. tumor (NET)

neuroendocrine-type feature in adrenal cortical adenoma

neuroendocrinology

neuroepidemiology

neuroepithelial, neurepithelial
- n. body
- n. cell

neuroepithelioma

neuroepithelium, neurepithelium
- n. of ampullary crest
- n. of macula

neurofiber

neurofibril in cytoplasm

neurofibrillar

neurofibrillary
- n. degeneration (tau)
- n. tangle

neurofibroma
- myxoid n.
- plexiform n.
- storiform n.

neurofibromatosis (NF)
- abortive n.
- central type n.
- incomplete n.

neurofibromin gene

neurofibrosarcoma

neurofilament
- n. protein (NFP)
- n. triplet polypeptide (NFP)

neuroganglion

neurogenesis

neurogenetic (*var. of* neurogenic)

neurogenic, neurogenetic, neurogenous
- n. arthropathy
- n. bladder
- n. inhibition
- n. muscle weakness, ataxia, and retinitis pigmentosa (NARP)
- n. muscular atrophy (NMA)
- n. sarcoma
- n. shock

neurogenous (*var. of* neurogenic)

neuroglia
- n. cell
- nuclei of n.
- Weigert stain for n.

neurogliacyte

neuroglial cell

neurogliomatosis

neurohemal

neurohistology

neurohormone

neurohumoral factor

neurohypophysial hormone

neurohypophysis

neuroid melanocytic structure

neuroimaging

neuroinflammation

neurokeratin
- n. network
- n. network of dissolved myelin

neurolemma (*var. of* neurilemma)

neurolemmoma (*var. of* neurilemmoma)

neuroleptic malignant syndrome

neuroleukin

neurological cell

neurolymphomatosis gallinarum

neurolysin

neuroma, neurinoma, *pl.* **neuromata, neuromas**
- acoustic n.
- amputation n.
- n. cutis
- false n.
- fibrillary n.
- Morton n.
- mucosal n.
- plexiform n.
- n. telangiectodes
- traumatic n.
- Verneuil n.

neuromalacia

neuromas (*pl. of* neuroma)

neuromata (*pl. of* neuroma)

neuromatosa
- elephantiasis n.

neuromatosis

neuromedin B

neuromelanin

neuromelaninogenesis

neuromesenchyme

neuromuscular
- n. choristoma
- n. junction
- n. junction testing
- n. spindle
- n. system disease

neuromyelitis

neuromyopathy
- carcinomatous n.

neuromyositis

neuron, neurone
  alpha motor n.
  autonomic motor n.
  balloon n.
  bipolar n.
  n. cell adhesion molecule
  cytoplasm of n.
  dopaminergic n.
  fetal n.
  gamma motor n.
  ganglionic motor n.
  intercalary n.
  internuncial n.
  lower motor n.
  magnocellular hypothalamic n.
  motor n.
  multipolar motor n.
  neurocalcin immunoreactive n.
  nucleus of motor n.
  n. of myenteric nerve plexus
  POMC n.
  postganglionic motor n.
  preganglionic motor n.
  pseudounipolar n.
  quisqualate activated n.
  red n.
  somatic motor n.
  survival motor n. (SMN)
  tangle-bearing n.
  tangle-free n.
  unipolar n.
  upper motor n.
  vicinal n.
  visceral motor n.
neuronal
  n. cell intoxication
  n. choristoma
  n. chromatolysis
  n. hyperplasia
  n. intermediate filament inclusion
    disease (NIFID)
  n. intestinal dysplasia
  n. intranuclear inclusion
  n. lipofibromatous hamartoma
  n. nodular heterotopia
  n. perikarya
neuron-associated class III
  beta-tubulin
neurone (*var. of* neuron)
neuronevus
neuronophage
neuronophagia, neuronophagy,
  neuronophagy
neuronophagy (*var. of* neuronophagia)
neuron-specific
  n.-s. enolase (NSA, NSE)
  n.-s. esterase (NSE)
neurooncology
neuroparalytic illness

neuropathic
  n. albuminuria
  n. arthritis
neuropathologist
neuropathology
neuropathy
  amblyopia n.
  amyloid n.
  diabetic n.
  dysproteinemic n.
  entrapment n.
  hereditary sensory radicular n.
  hypertrophic interstitial n.
  Leber hereditary optic n. (LHON)
  Nigerian nutritional ataxic n.
  organophosphate-induced delayed n.
    (OPIDN)
  retrobulbar n.
  subacute myelooptic n. (SMON)
  n. target esterase (NTE)
  tropical ataxic n. (TAN)
  vincristine n.
  vitamin B12 n.
neuropeptide
  anorexigenic n.
  substance P n.
  n. Y (NPY)
neurophysin
neuropil, neuropile, neuropile
neuropile (*var. of* neuropil)
neuropilin
neuroplasm
neuroplasticity
neuroplexus
neuropodion
neuroprogenitor cell
neuroretinitis
neuroretinopathy
neurosarcocleisis
neurosarcoidosis
neurosarcoma
neuroschwannoma
neurosclerosis
neurosecretion
neurosecretory
  n. cell
  n. granule (NSG)
  n. material (NSM)
  n. substance
neurospongium
Neurospora
neurosthenia (*var. of* neurasthenia)
neurosyphilis
neurotendinous
  n. organ
  n. spindle
neurothekeoma
  cellular n.
neurothekoma

N

neurothele
neurotica
    lipomatosis n.
neurotization
neurotome
neurotoxin
    Clostridium botulinum n. type A, B, C1, D, E, F, G
    human botulinum n. type A, B, E, F
    potent protein n.
neurotransmitter
neurotransporter receptor
neurotrauma
neurotrophic
    n. atrophy
    n. factor
    n. factor receptor
    n. tyrosine kinase receptor, type 1 (NTRK1)
neurotrophin
neurotropic virus
neurotubule
neurovaccine
neurovascular hamartoma
neurovirus
neurovisceral storage disorder
Neusser granule
neutral
    n. buffered formalin fixative
    n. lipid storage disease
    n. protamine Hagedorn (NPH)
    n. red
    n. stain
neutralization
    n. test (NT)
    viral n.
neutralizing antibody (NA)
neutrinimicus
    Streptacidiphilus n.
neutriphila
    Halorhodospira n.
neutron
    n. exposure
    n. meter
    n. personnel dosimeter
    slow n.
    n. source
    thermal n.
neutropenia
    cyclic n.
    drug-induced n.
    familial cyclic n.
neutropenic angina
neutrophil, neutrophile
    n. activating factor (NAF)
    n. activating protein (NAP)
    band n.

    n. chemotactant factor
    n. chemotactic factor (NCF)
    filamented n.
    n. functional disorder
    giant n.
    n. granule
    hypersegmented n.
    immature n.
    juvenile n.
    n. killing activity
    mature n.
    polymorphonuclear n. (PMN)
    rod n.
    segmented n. (seg)
    stab n.
    transmigration n.
neutrophile (*var. of* neutrophil)
neutrophilia
    giant n.
neutrophilic
    n. chemotactic factor
    n. cryptitis
    n. dermatosis
    n. eccrine hidradenitis
    n. hyperplasia
    n. infiltrate
    n. inflammation
    n. leukemia
    n. leukocyte
    n. leukocytosis
    n. leukopenia
    n. lymphocytosis
    n. marrow
    n. metamyelocyte
    n. myelocyte
    n. pleocytosis
    n. promyelocyte
neutrophilopenia
neutrophilous
neutrotaxis
    indifferent n.
    negative n.
    positive n.
nevi (*pl. of* nevus)
nevocarcinoma
nevocellular nevus
nevocyte
nevocytic nevus
nevoid, naevoid
    n. basal cell carcinoma syndrome (NBCCS)
    n. elephantiasis
    n. hypertrichosis
nevolipoma
nevomelanocyte
nevous
nevoxanthoendothelioma
Nevskiaceae

nevus, naevus, *pl.* **nevi**
  acquired n.
  acral n.
  agminate n.
  n. anemicus
  n. angiomatodes
  apocrine n.
  n. arachnoideus
  n. araneus
  nevi, atrial myxoma, myxoid
    neurofibroma, and ephelides
    (NAME)
  atypical melanocytic n. (AMN)
  balloon cell n.
  basal cell n.
  Becker n.
  Blitz nevi
  blue rubber bleb n.
  capillary n.
  n. cavernosus
  n. cell
  cellular blue n. (CBN)
  Clark n.
  comedo n.
  n. comedonicus
  compound n.
  congenital melanocytic nevi (CMN)
  connective tissue n.
  deep penetrating n. (DPN)
  dermal n.
  dysplastic n.
  n. elasticus of Lewandowski
  epidermal dermal n.
  epidermic-dermic n.
  epithelioid cell n.
  faun tail n.
  flame n.
  n. flammeus
  n. follicularis keratosis
  giant blue n.
  giant hairy n.
  giant pigmented n.
  halo n.
  inflammatory linear verrucous
    epidermal n. (ILVEN)
  intradermal n.
  Ito n.
  Jadassohn n.
  Jadassohn-Tièche n.
  junction n.
  junctional n.
  lentigines, atrial myxoma, mucocutaneous
    myxomas, and blue nevi (LAMB)
  n. lipomatodes
  n. lipomatosus
  lymphatic n.
  n. lymphaticus
  melanocytic n.

  nape n.
  nevocellular n.
  nevocytic n.
  nodal n.
  organoid n.
  Ota n.
  n. pigmentosus
  n. pilosus
  sebaceous n.
  n. sebaceus (NS)
  spider n.
  n. spilus
  spindle cell n.
  Spitz n.
  spongy n.
  strawberry n.
  Sutton n.
  systematized n.
  n. unius lateris
  UV-irradiated n.
  vascular n.
  n. venosus
  verrucous n.
new
  n. fuchsin
  n. growth
  n. methylene blue
  N. World hookworm
  N. World screwworm
  N. Zealand mice
newborn
  ABO hemolytic disease of the n.
  alloimmune hemolytic disease of n.
  n. aspiration
  bullous impetigo of n.
  n. crossmatch
  hemolytic anemia of n.
  n. hemolytic disease
  hemolytic disease of n.
  n. hemorrhagic disease
  hemorrhagic disease of n. (HDN)
  hyaline membrane disease of n.
  icterus gravis of n.
  leukocytosis of the n.
  n. pneumonitis virus
  respiratory distress syndrome of n.
  n. respiratory syndrome
  n. screen
  subcutaneous fat necrosis of n.
Newcastle
  N. disease
  N. disease virus (NDV)
  N. virus disease (NVD)
Newcastle-Manchester bacillus
Newcomer fixative
newly formed vessel
neworleansense
  Mycobacterium n.

N

newport
  Salmonella enteritidis serotype *n.*
newton (N)
  N. law of cooling
nexin
nexin-II
  protease n.-I.
nexus, *pl.* **nexus**
Nezelof
  N. syndrome
  N. type of thymic alymphoplasia
NF
  neurofibromatosis
nF
  nanofarad
NFA-I
  normal fecal antigen
NFB
  nonfermentative bacillus
NF-1 gene
NF2 gene
NF-kappa B protein
N_5-formyl FH$_4$
N-formyl methionine
NFP
  neurofilament protein
  neurofilament triplet polypeptide
NG
  nasogastric
ng
  nanogram
NGB
  neurogenic bladder
NGC
  nongynecologic cytopathology
NGF
  nerve growth factor
  nerve growth factor antiserum
    NGF antiserum
NGU
  nongonococcal urethritis
NHC
  nonhistone chromosomal
    NHC protein
NHL
  non-Hodgkin lymphoma
NHPA
  no histopathologic abnormality
NHS
  normal horse serum
  normal human serum
NI
  neural inclusion
Ni
  nickel
NIA
  nephelometric inhibition assay
niacinate
  inositol n.

niacin test
niche
  ecologic n.
  enamel n.
Nichols
  N. method
  N. reagent
nickel (Ni)
  n. dermatitis
  n. grid
  Raney n.
Nickerson
  N. medium
  N. medium smear
Nickerson-Kveim
  N.-K. test
  N.-K. test reaction
Nicklès test
Nicolas-Favre disease
Nicolle
  Novy, MacNeal, and N. (NNN)
  N. stain for capsules
  N. white mycetoma
nicolli
  Spelotrema n.
Nicol prism
Nicotiana
nicotinamide
  n. adenine dinucleotide (NAD, NADH)
  n. adenine dinucleotide diaphorase control
  n. adenine dinucleotide diaphorase stain
  n. adenine dinucleotide phosphate (NADP, NADPH)
  n. adenine dinucleotide phosphate oxidase
nicotine test
nicotinic acid
nidal
NIDDM
  noninsulin-dependent diabetes mellitus
nidi (*pl. of* nidus)
Nidoko disease
nidulans
  Aspergillus n.
  Emericella n.
nidus, *pl.* **nidi**
Nieden disease
Niemann disease
Niemann-Pick
  N.-P. cell
  N.-P. disease (NPD)
  N.-P. disease type C, tau pathology class I
  N.-P. lipid
  N.-P. type of histiocyte
Niesslia

NIFID
 neuronal intermediate filament inclusion disease
niger
 Aspergillus n.
 locus n.
 nucleus n.
 Rhizopus n.
Nigerian nutritional ataxic neuropathy
nigeriense
 Trypanosoma n.
nighttime salivary cortisol test
nigra
 cataracta n.
 dermatosis papulosa n.
 pityriasis n.
 substantia n.
 tinea n.
nigrescens
 Mermis n.
nigricans
 acanthosis n.
 Corynebacterium n.
 keratosis n.
 pseudoacanthosis n.
 Rhizopus n.
nigrificans
 Desulfotomaculum n.
nigripalpus
 Culex n.
nigrities
nigromaculis
 Aedes n.
nigrosin, nigrosine
nigrosine (*var. of* nigrosin)
nigrosperma
 Monodictys n.
Nigrospora sphaerica
nigrum
 tapetum n.
NIH
 National Institutes of Health
nihonkaiense
 Diphyllobothrium n.
niigatensis
 Kitasatospora n.
 Nocardia n.
Nijmegen breakage syndrome (NBS)
Nikiforoff method
Nikolsky sign
Nikon microprocessor-controlled camera
nil
 n. disease
 n. lesion
Nile
 N. blue
 N. blue A
 N. blue fat stain
nilotica

 Leishmania n.
 Limnatis n.
NIN
 nuclear excision repair instability
ninhydrin reaction
ninhydrin-Schiff
 n.-S. reaction
 n.-S. stain for proteins
NIOSH
 National Institute for Occupational Safety and Health
NIOX nitric oxide monitoring system
NIP
 National Immunization Program
nipple
 n. adenoma
 n. arranged in a ring
 n. discharge cytology
 erosive adenomatosis of n.
nipponica
 Entamoeba n.
nipponicum
 Gnathostoma n.
Nippostrongylus
Nipride
NIS
 sodium-iodine symporter
NISH
 nonisotopic in situ hybridization
nishinomiyaensis
 Dermacoccus n.
nisin
Nissl
 N. body
 N. degeneration
 N. granule
 N. stain
 N. substance
 N. substance alteration
nit
Nitabuch
 N. fibrin
 N. layer
 N. membrane
 N. stria
nitida
 Gordonia n.
nitidus
 lichen n.
nitrate
 n. agar
 n. broth
 cold silver n.
 lanthanum n.
 potassium n.
 n. reduction test
 silver n.
 sodium n.
 n. utilization test

N

nitratireducens
　　Garciella n.
　　Halobiforma n.
　　Natronobacterium n.
　　Thialkalivibrio n.
Nitratireductor aquibiodomus
nitratis
　　Thialkalivibrio n.
nitrativorans
　　Comamonas n.
nitrergic hyperinnervation
nitric
　　n. acid
　　n. acid test
　　n. oxide (NO)
　　n. oxide synthase (NOS)
nitrifying bacterium
nitrile
　　propane n.
nitrite
　　sodium n.
　　n. test
nitritireducens
　　Stenotrophomonas n.
nitritoid reaction
nitrituria
nitroaniline poisoning
Nitrobacter
　　N. hamburgensis
　　N. vulgaris
Nitrobacteraceae
nitroblue
　　n. tetrazolium (NBT)
　　n. tetrazolium dye
　　n. tetrazolium dye reduction
　　　assay
　　n. tetrazolium stain
　　n. tetrazolium test (NBT test)
nitrocellulose membrane
Nitrocystis
nitro dye
nitroferricyanide
　　sodium n.
nitrogen
　　alkali-soluble n. (ASN)
　　alpha amino n.
　　amino acid n. (AAN)
　　n. balance
　　blood urea n. (BUN)
　　n. dilution
　　n. distribution
　　n. equivalent
　　fecal n.
　　n. lag
　　n. narcosis
　　nonprotein n. (NPN)
　　n. partition
　　serum urea n. (SUN)
　　stool n.

　　undetermined n.
　　urea n. (UN)
　　urinary n.
　　urine urea n. (UUN)
nitrogen-fixing
nitrogenous
nitroguajacolicus
　　Arthrobacter n.
nitropropiol test
3-nitroproprionic acid (3NP)
nitroprusside (NP)
　　sodium n.
　　n. test
nitroreducens
　　Diaphorobacter n.
nitrosa
　　Nitrosomonas n.
nitrosamine
nitroso dye
nitroso-indole-nitrate test
Nitrosomonas
　　N. aestuarii
　　N. eutropha
　　N. halophila
　　N. marina
　　N. nitrosa
　　N. oligotropha
　　N. ureae
nitrosothiol
nitrosourea agent
Nitrospina gracilis
Nitrospira moscoviensis
nitrous acid
nivalis
　　Lanosa n.
niveiscabiei
　　Streptomyces n.
niveum
　　Trichophyton n.
NIXIE
　　numeric indicator experimental
　　number 1
　　NIXIE tube
njovera
NK
　　N. clonal diversity
　　N. lymphoma
NK1-C3 antibody
NKH
　　nonketotic hyperosmotic
NKHG
　　nonketotic hyperglycinemia
NKSF
　　natural killer cell-stimulating factor
NLH
　　nodular lymphoid hyperplasia
N-linked glycosylation
nL
　　nanoliter

NLT
  normal lymphocyte transfer
    test
NM
  not measurable
nm
  nanometer
NMA
  neurogenic muscular atrophy
NMDA
  N-methyl-D-aspartase
    NMDA receptor agonist
    NMDA receptor antagonist
NME
  necrolytic migratory erythema
N-methylacetamide
N-methyl-D-aspartase (NMDA)
N-methylformamide
N1-methylnicotinamide (NMN)
N′-methylnicotinamide
NMID
  N-terminal mid fragment
N-MID
    N-MID osteocalcin ELISA
    N-MID osteocalcin ELISA test
NMN
  N1-methylnicotinamide
  normetanephrine
nmol
  nanomole
NMP
  nuclear matrix protein
NMP22 BladderChek test
NMRT
  National Medical Response Team
N-myc
    N-m. amplification
    N-m. marker
    N-m. oncogene
NN
  neural network
NND
  neonatal death
N,N-dimethylacetamide
N,N-dimethylformamide
NNDSS
  National Notifiable Diseases
  Surveillance System
NNN
  Novy, MacNeal, and Nicolle
    NNN culture medium
NO
  nitric oxide
no
    n. cancer spread to other organs
    (M0)
    n. data available (NDA)
    n. demonstrable antibodies (NDA)
    n. evidence of disease (NED)

n. evidence of distant metastases
  (M0)
n. evidence of primary tumor (T0)
n. histopathologic abnormality
  (NHPA)
n. lymph nodes containing cancer
  cells (N0)
n. mineral component
n. reflow phenomenon
n. serious abnormality (NSA)
n. significant abnormality (NSA)
n. significant defect (NSD)
n. significant deviation (NSD)
n. significant difference (NSD)
n. significant disease (NSD)
n. specific type (NST)
Noack syndrome
Noble stain
Nocard bacillus
Nocardia
  N. abscessus
  N. africana
  N. alba
  N. asiatica
  N. asteroides
  N. beijingensis
  N. brasiliensis
  N. caishijiensis
  N. calcarea
  N. cerradoensis
  N. culture
  N. cummidelens
  N. cyriacigeorgica
  N. dacryolith
  N. farcinica
  N. fluminea
  N. ignorata
  N. inohanensis
  N. mediterranei
  N. minutissimum
  N. neocaledoniensis
  N. niigatensis
  N. nova
  N. orientalis
  N. otitidiscaviarum
  N. paucivorans
  N. pigrifrangens
  N. pseudovaccinii
  N. puris
  N. sienata
  N. soli
  N. tenerifensis
  N. testacea
  N. transvalensis
  N. veterana
  N. vinacea
  N. yamanashiensis
Nocardiaceae
nocardioform actinomycete

N

Nocardioidaceae
Nocardioides
    N. albus
    N. aquaticus
    N. aquiterrae
    N. ganghwensis
Nocardiopsaceae
Nocardiopsis
    N. aegyptia
    N. alkaliphila
    N. composta
    N. dassonvillei
    N. dassonvillei subsp. *albirubida*
    N. exhalans
    N. halotolerans
    N. kunsanensis
    N. metallicus
    N. salina
    N. trehalosi
    N. tropica
    N. umidischolae
    N. xinjiangensis
nocardiosis
nocere
    primum non n.
noctalbuminuria
nocturnal penile tumescence test
nodal
    n. involvement
    n. marginal zone B-cell lymphoma
    n. nevus
    n. tissue
NOD2/CARD15
    NOD2/CARD15 mutation
    PRO-GenoLogix NOD2/CARD15
node
    Auerbach n.
    Babès n.
    Bouchard n.
    cortex of lymph n.
    delphian n.
    Dürck n.
    germinal center of lymph n.
    Haygarth n.
    Heberden n.
    hemal n.
    hemolymph n.
    Hensen n.
    hilar n. (HN)
    hilum of lymph n.
    lymph n. (LN)
    medulla of lymph n.
    Meynet n.
    milker's n.'s
    nonsentinel lymph n. (NSLN, NSN)
    normal lymph n.
    n. of Cloquet
    n. of Ranvier
    Osler n.

    portal lymph n.
    Ranvier n.
    regional lymph n.
    Rosenmüller n.
    Rotter n.
    SA n.
    sentinel lymph n. (SLN)
    shotty n.
    signal n.
    singer's n.
    syphilitic n.
    Troisier n.
    Virchow n.
Nod factor
NOD2 gene
nodi (*pl. of* nodus)
nodosa
    arteritis n.
    arthritis n.
    polyarteritis n. (PAN, PN)
    salpingitis isthmica n.
    trichorrhexis n.
    vasitis n.
nodose
    n. ganglion
    n. rheumatism
nodositas
nodosity
nodososetosus
    Arachnomyces n.
nodosum
    amnion n.
    erythema n. (EN)
nodosus
    Bacteroides n.
    Dichelobacter n.
nodous, nodular, nodulate, nodulated
nodular (*var. of* nodous)
    n. adenosis
    n. amyloidoma (NA)
    n. amyloidosis
    n. and diffuse fibrous proliferation (NDFP)
    n. arteriosclerosis
    n. blastema
    n. body
    n. calcific aortic stenosis
    n. colloid goiter
    n. embryo
    n. fasciitis
    n. glomerulosclerosis
    n. hidradenoma
    n. histiocytic lymphoma
    n. hyperplastic goiter
    n. leprosy
    n. lymphocyte-rich Hodgkin disease
    n. lymphoid hyperplasia (NLH)
    n. melanoma
    n. mesoneuritis

n. mesothelial hyperplasia
n. nonsuppurative panniculitis
n. non-X histiocytosis
n. palmar fibromatosis
n. panencephalitis
n. paragranuloma (NP)
n. poorly differentiated lymphocyte (NPDL)
n. prurigo
n. regenerative hyperplasia (NRH)
n. sclerosing Hodgkin disease (NSHD)
n. sclerosis (NS)
n. subepidermal fibrosis (NSF)
n. syphilid
n. tuberculid
n. vasculitis

nodulare
Trichophyton n.
Trichophyton mentagrophytes n.

nodularis
prurigo n.

nodulate (var. of nodous)
nodulated (var. of nodous)
nodulation
nodule
adenomatoid cystic papillary n.
aggregated lymphatic n.
apple jelly n.
Arantius n.
Aschoff n.
Babès n.
Caplan n.
cold n.
Dalen-Fuchs n.
discrete n.
dysplastic n.
elastotic n.
endometrial stromal n. (ESN)
fibrocalcific n.
fibrosiderotic n.
fibrous n.
Gamna-Gandy n.
Gandy-Gamna n.
gastric lymphoid n.
germinal center of lymphatic n.
Hoboken n.
hot n.
hypervascular n.
intracystic papillary n.
Jeanselme n.
junctional expansion n.
juxtaarticular n.
Kimmelstiel-Wilson n.
laryngeal n.
Lisch n.
Losch n.
lymph n.
lymphoid n.

malpighian n.
microglial n.
milker's n.
Morgagni n.
mural n.
necrotic pseudoxanthomatous n. (NPN)
primary n.
reactive spindle cell n. (RSCN)
rheumatic n.
rheumatoid n.
sarcoma-like mural n. (SLMN)
satellite n.
Schmorl n.
secondary n.
siderotic n.
silicotic n.
singer's n.
Sister Mary Joseph n.
spindle cell n.
splenic lymph n.
subcutaneous n.
vocal fold n.

Nodulisporium
nodulous
nodulus
n. caroticus
n. lymphaticus

nodus, pl. **nodi**
cortex nodi lymphatici
hilum nodi lymphatici
n. lymphaticus
nodi lymphoidei axillares
nodi lymphoidei coeliaci
nodi lymphoidei inguinales profundi
nodi lymphoidei inguinales superficiales

nogabecina
Amycolatopsis keratiniphila subsp. n.

noggin protein inhibitor
noguchi
Noguchia
N. granulosis
N. granulosus

Nomarski
N. microscope
N. optics

nomenclature
binary n.
binomial n.
chromosome n.
Fisher-Race n.
linnaean system of n.
n. of tumor

nomogram
acid-base n.
Andrews n.
blood volume n.
cartesian n.

N

nomogram (*continued*)
    mean platelet volume n. (MPV nomogram)
    Radford n.
    Rumack-Matthew n.
    Siggaard-Andersen alignment n.
nomograph
non-A
    n.-A hepatitis
    n.-A, non-B
    n.-A, non-B hepatitis (NANB)
nonadherent cell
nonagglutinating vibrio
nonalcoholic
    n. fatty liver disease (NAFLD)
    n. steatohepatitis (NASH)
nonallergic
    n. rhinitis
    n. rhinitis with eosinophilia (NARES)
non-Alzheimer dementia
nonanaplastic invasive meningioma
non-B
    n.-B hepatitis
    non-A, n.-B
nonbacterial
    n. gastroenteritis virus
    n. thrombotic endocarditis (NBTE)
    n. verrucous endocarditis
nonbirefringent
nonbrisk infiltrate
non-Burkitt lymphoma
nonbursate
noncardiogenic pulmonary edema
noncaseating granuloma
noncellular
nonchromaffin
    n. paraganglia
    n. paraganglioma
nonchromogenicum
    Mycobacterium n.
noncleaved
    n. follicular center cell
    large n. (LNC)
noncollagenous pneumoconiosis
noncommunicating hydrocephalus
noncompetitive
    n. assay
    n. heterogeneous enzyme immunoassay
    n. inhibitor
nonconjugative plasmid
nonconsanguineous
noncornifying form
noncorrosive
noncystic mucinous carcinoma
nondiabetic glycosuric melituria
nondisabling (ND)
    nonsymptomatic, n. (NSND)

nondiscrete bands
nondisease
nondisjunction
    maternal meiotic n.
    meiotic n.
nondissecting aortic aneurysm
nonelectrolyte
nonenveloped RNA virus
nonepidermotropic primary cutaneous T-cell lymphoma
nonesterified fatty acid
nonexophytic lesion
non-FCC
    nonfollicular center cell
nonfermentative bacillus (NFB)
nonfilament polymorphonuclear leukocyte
nonfilarial chylothorax
nonflagellated vegetative cell
nonfluorescent acetoxymethyl ester
nonfollicular center cell (non-FCC)
nonfunctional factor VIII-related gene
nongermline band
nonglomerular hematuria
nongonococcal urethritis (NGU)
nongranular leukocyte
nongynecologic cytopathology (NGC)
non-heat-extracted antigen
nonhematogenous
nonhemolytic
    n. jaundice
    n. streptococcus
non-HFE-related hemochromatosis
nonhistone
    n. chromosomal (NHC)
    n. chromosomal protein
non-Hodgkin lymphoma (NHL)
nonideal solution
nonimmune
    n. agglutination
    n. fetal hydrops
    n. hemolysis
    n. hemolytic anemia
    n. serum
nonimmunity
noninfectious
noninfiltrating lobular carcinoma
noninflammatory edema
noninsulin-dependent diabetes mellitus (NIDDM)
noninvasive (NIV)
    n. implant
    n. lobular lesion
nonionic detergent
nonisolated proteinuria
nonisotopic
    n. gel detection system
    n. in situ hybridization (NISH)
nonketotic
    n. hyperglycemia

n. hyperglycinemia (NKHG)
n. hyperosmolar syndrome
n. hyperosmotic (NKH)
nonlactose-fermenting bacterium
nonlamellar bone
nonleukemic myelosis
nonleukoreduced red cell
nonlineage
n. marker
n. specific transmembrane
glycoprotein
nonlipid histiocytosis
nonliquefaciens
Moraxella n.
Pseudomonas n.
nonlymphocytic leukemia
non-MALT
nonmucosa-associated lymphoid tissue
non-MALT lymphoma
nonmedullated fiber
nonmegaloblastic anemia
nonmelanocytic pigmentation
nonmelanosomal vesicle
nonmembrane-bound nucleolus
nonmotile
n. bacteria
n. leukocyte
n. organism
nonmucinous adenocarcinoma
nonmucosa-associated lymphoid tissue (non-MALT)
nonmyelinated
nonmyloidotic fibrillary glomerulopathy
nonmyogenous tumor
nonnecrotizing
n. granuloma
n. granulomatous inflammation
Nonne-Milroy disease
Nonne-Milroy-Meige syndrome
nonneoplastic
non-nephrotic range proteinuria
Nonne test
nonnucleated
nonobstructive jaundice
nonoccluded virus
nonodontogenic
n. cyst
n. lesion
nonoemulsion disinfectant
Nonomuraea
N. dietziae
N. roseoviolacea subsp. carminate
nonossifying fibroma
nonparametric
nonparatrabecular
nonpathogenic
nonpenicillinase-producing *Staphylococcus* **epidermidis**
nonpermissive culture medium

nonpersistent agent
nonphotochromogenic mycobacteria
nonprecipitable antibody
nonprecipitating antibody
nonprotein
n. nitrogen (NPN)
n. nitrogen test
nonradioisotopic immunoassay
nonrandom pattern
nonrapid eye movement (NREM)
nonreactive (NR)
n. pattern
nonrelapsing
n. colitis
n. disease
nonrenal
n. azotemia
n. death (NRD)
nonreplicating cell
nonreplicative state
nonrespiratory alkalosis
nonresponder tolerance
nonrotation of kidney
nonsecretor
nonsecretory myeloma
nonseminomatous germ cell tumor (NSGCT)
nonsense
n. mutation
n. triplet
nonsentinel lymph node (NSLN)
nonseptate mycelium
nonsister chromatid
nonsmall
n. cell cancer (NSCC)
n. cell lung cancer (NSCLC)
nonspecific (NS)
n. anergy
n. bronchial reactivity (NSBR)
n. cross-reacting antigen (NCA)
n. esterase (NSE)
n. granulomatous orchitis (NSGO)
n. granulomatous prostatitis
n. hepatocellular abnormality
n. immunity
n. interstitial pneumonia (NSIP)
n. interstitial pneumonia/fibrosis
n. interstitial pneumonitis (NSIP)
n. protein
n. system
n. therapy
n. urethritis (NSU)
n. viral syndrome
nonspore-forming bacterium
nonsteroidal antiinflammatory (NSAID)
nonstress test (NST)
nonstructural
n. gene
n. protein 3

N

nonsuppressible insulinlike activity (NSILA)
nonsymptomatic, nondisabling (NSND)
nonsyndromal dysplasia
nonsyndromic
nontoxic goiter (NTG)
nontransmural myocardial infarction
nontreponemal antibody test
nontropical sprue
nontuberculous mycobacteria (NTM)
nontyepable
nontyphoidal infectious colitis
nonulcer dyspepsia
nonunion fracture
nonvascular
nonviable
nonviral hepatitis
Noonan syndrome
NOR
   nucleolar organizing region
   nucleolus organizing region
     NOR banding
Nora lesion
Nordau disease
norepinephrine (Ne)
   urine n.
norimbergensis
normal (N)
   n. animal
   n. anion gap acidosis
   n. antibody
   n. antithrombin
   n. antitoxin
   n. blood serum (NBS)
   n. body temperature
   n. cholesteremic xanthomatosis
   n. complement of cells
   diphtheria toxin n. (DTN)
   n. fecal antigen (NFA-I)
   n. horse serum (NHS)
   n. human plasma
   n. human serum (NHS)
   n. human serum albumin
   n. lymph node
   n. lymphocyte transfer test (NLT)
   n. opsonin
   n. plasma (NP)
   n. pressure hydrocephalus (NPH)
   n. rabbit serum (NRS)
   n. RB protein
   n. reference serum (NRS)
   n. replication
   n. single dose (NSD)
   n. term pregnancy
   n. thymus
   n. toxin

   upper limits of n. (ULN)
   n. value
normal-AG metabolic acidosis
normetanephrine
   urine n.
normoblast
   acidophilic n.
   basophilic n.
   intermediate n.
   orthochromatic n.
   orthochromatophilic n.
   polychromatic n.
   polychromatophilic n.
normoblastic
normoblastosis
normocalcemia
normocellular bone marrow specimen
normochromia
normochromic anemia
normocomplementemia
normocyte
normocytic
   n. anemia
   n. erythrocyte
normocytosis
normoerythrocyte
normoglycemia
normoglycemic glycosuria
normokalemia, normokaliemia
normokalemic periodic paralysis
normokaliemia (*var. of* normokalemia)
normolipemic xanthoma planum
normoplasia
normotensive
normovolemia
Norovirus
Norris corpuscle
North
   N. American blastomycosis
   N. Atlantic Treaty Organization (NATO)
Northern
   N. blot analysis
   N. blot technique
   N. blot test
norvegicus
   Enterovibrio n.
norwalk
   N. agent
   N. disease
   N. virus *(Norovirus)*
Norymberski procedure
NOS
   nitric oxide synthase
   not otherwise specified
nose
   cleft n.
   dog n.

olfactory region of tunica mucosa of n.
Nosema corneum
Nosematidae
nosepiece
nosocomial
  n. anemia
  n. infection
  n. pneumonia
nosocomialis
nosologic drift
nosomycosis
nosophyte
Nosopsyllus fasciatus
nosotoxic
nosotoxin
Nostocales
nostras
  elephantiasis n.
nostrum
  elephantiasis verrucosa n.
not
  n. measurable (NM)
  n. otherwise specified (NOS)
  n. recorded (NR)
  n. resolved (NR)
  n. significant (NS)
  n. statistically significant (NSS)
  n. sufficient (NS)
  n. sufficient quantity (NSQ)
notanencephalia
notation
  scientific n.
notatum
notch
  Hutchinson crescentic n.
  Kernohan n.
  N. receptor
Notch3 gene polymorphism in ischemic cerebrovascular disease
notencephalocele
notencephalus
Nothopanus
notification
  death n.
notochord
notochordal sheath
Notoedres cati
NoTox formalin substitute solution
Nottingham
  N. histologic grade
  N. modification of Scarff-Bloom-Richardson grading
  N. Prognostic Index (NPI)
nova
  N. Celltrak 12 hematology analyzer
  Nocardia n.

novae-caledoniae
  Ascotricha n.-c.
novalis
  Bacillus n.
Novapath HIV-1 immunoblot tester
novel
  n. coronavirus
  n. microbiology test
  n. toxicology test
novella
  Starkeya n.
Novelli stain
noverca
  Opisthorchis n.
Novirhabdovirus
novobiosepticus
  Staphylococcus hominis n.
Novosphingobium
  N. aromaticivorans
  N. capsulatum
  N. hassiacum
  N. pentaromativorans
  N. rosa
  N. stygium
  N. subarcticum
  N. subterraneum
  N. tardaugens
Novy
  Novy, MacNeal, and Nicolle (NNN)
  N. rat disease
novyi
  Clostridium n.
noxa
NP
  nasopharyngeal
  neuropathology
  nodular paragranuloma
  normal plasma
  nucleoprotein
  NP antigen
N+P
  STA Liatest control N+P
3NP
  3-nitroproprionic acid
NPC
  nasopharyngeal carcinoma
NPD
  Niemann-Pick disease
NPDL
  nodular poorly differentiated lymphocyte
NPG
  BactiSwab NPG
NPH
  neutral protamine Hagedorn
  normal pressure hydrocephalus
NPI
  Nottingham Prognostic Index
  nucleoplasmic index

N

NPN
  necrotic pseudoxanthomatous
    nodule
  nonprotein nitrogen
NPR
  net protein ratio
n-propanol
NPS
  National Pharmaceutical Stockpile
NPT
  neoprecipitin test
NPU
  net protein utilization
NPV
  negative predictive value
NR
  nephrogenic rest
  nonreactive
  not recorded
  not resolved
  nucleotide residue
N-ras gene
NRBC
  nucleated red blood cell
NRD
  nonrenal death
NREM
  nonrapid eye movement
NRG
  neuregulin
NRG1
    NRG1 alpha
    NRG1 beta
NRG2
    NRG2 alpha
    NRG2 beta
NRH
  nodular regenerative hyperplasia
NRS
  normal rabbit serum
  normal reference serum
NS
  nephrotic syndrome
  nerve sheath
  nevus sebaceus
  nodular sclerosis
  nonspecific
  not significant
  not sufficient
ns
  nanosecond
NSA
  neuron-specific enolase
  no serious abnormality
  no significant abnormality
NSAID
  nonsteroidal antiinflammatory
NSBR
  nonspecific bronchial reactivity

NSCC
  nonsmall cell cancer
NSCLC
  nonsmall cell lung cancer
NSD
  normal single dose
  no significant defect
  no significant deviation
  no significant difference
  no significant disease
NSE
  neuron-specific enolase
  neuron-specific esterase
  nonspecific esterase
    NSE stain
nsec
  nanosecond
NSF
  N-ethylmaleimide-sensitive-factor
  nodular subepidermal fibrosis
NSG
  necrotizing sarcoid granulomatosis
  neurosecretory granule
NSGCT
  nonseminomatous germ cell tumor
NSGO
  nonspecific granulomatous orchitis
NSHD
  nodular sclerosing Hodgkin disease
NSILA
  nonsuppressible insulinlike activity
NSIP
  nonspecific interstitial pneumonia
  nonspecific interstitial pneumonitis
NSLN
  nonsentinel lymph node
    NSLN involvement
NSM
  nerve sheath myxoma
  neurosecretory material
NSND
  nonsymptomatic, nondisabling
NSQ
  not sufficient quantity
NSS
  not statistically significant
NST
  nonstress test
  no specific type
NSU
  nonspecific urethritis
N5 submicron particle size analyzer
NT
  neutralization test
NTAB
  nephrotoxic antibody
Ntaya virus
NTE
  neuropathy target esterase

N-telopeptide (NTx)
    cross-linked N-t.
N-terminal
    N-t. fragment
    N-t. mid fragment (NMID)
    N-t. prohormone brain natriuretic peptide (NT-proBNP)
n-**tetracosanoic acid**
NTG
    nontoxic goiter
NTM
    nontuberculous mycobacteria
NTN
    nephrotoxic nephritis
NT-proBNP
    N-terminal prohormone brain natriuretic peptide
NTRK1
    neurotrophic tyrosine kinase receptor, type 1
NTSN
    nephrotoxic serum nephritis
NTx
    N-telopeptide
nubecula
nubinhibens
    Roseovarius n.
nuchal
    n. fibrocartilaginous pseudotumor
    n. fibroma
    n. hemangioma
    n. rigidity
nuclear
    n. aggregate lipid
    n. antibody
    n. aplasia
    n. bag
    n. bag fiber
    n., biological, and chemical
    n., biological, chemical (mass-casualty weapon)
    n. chain
    n. chain fiber
    chemical, biological, radiological or n. (CBRN)
    n. crystalline aggregate
    n. dust
    n. envelope
    n. envelope of spermatid
    n. excision repair instability (NIN)
    n. fast red stain
    n. grade
    n. groove
    n. heterochromatin
    n. hyaloplasm
    n. hyperchromasia
    n. inclusion body
    n. isomerism
    n. lipid aggregate

n. magnetic resonance spectroscopy
n. matrix protein (NMP)
n. membrane
n. membrane alteration
n. mitotic apparatus (NuMA)
n. palisading
n. polarity
n. pore
n. pore alteration
n. pore complex
n. profile diameter
n. proliferation marker pKi67
n. pseudoinclusion
n. pseudostratification
n. pyknosis
n. sap
n. sap alteration
n. shape alteration
n. signal
n. size alteration
n. spindle
n. staining
n. unrest
n. wreath cell
nuclear-cytoplasmic
    n.-c. ratio
    n.-c. ratio alteration
nuclear-to-cytoplasmic ratio
nucleated red blood cell (NRBC)
nucleation
    heterogeneous n.
nucleatum
    Fusobacterium n.
nuclei (*pl. of* nucleus)
nucleic
    n. acid amplification test (NAT)
    n. acid amplification testing
    n. acid chip technology
    n. acid detection
    n. acid hybridization
    n. acid panel (NAP)
    n. acid probe
    n. acid sequence based amplification (NASBA)
    n. acid sequence based analysis (NASBA)
    n. acid sequencing
    n. acid test
nucleiform
nucleocapsid
nucleochylema
nucleochyme
nucleocytoplasmic fractionation
nucleoid
    Lavdovsky n.
nucleolar
    n. organizing region (NOR)
    n. pattern
    n. RNAs

N

nucleolar-associated chromatin
nucleolar-nuclear ratio
nucleoliform
nucleolin
nucleoloid
nucleolonema
  wandering n.
nucleolus
  nonmembrane-bound n.
  organization of the n.
  n. organizing region (NOR)
nucleomegaly
nucleomicrosome
Nucleophaga
nucleophagocytosis
nucleophile
nucleophosphoprotein
nucleoplasm
nucleoplasmic index (NPI)
Nucleopolyhedrovirus
nucleoprotein (NP)
nucleoreticulum
Nucleorhabdovirus
nucleorrhexis
nucleosidase
nucleoskeleton
nucleosome
nucleotidase
  5′ n.
5′ nucleotidase
nucleotide
  cyclic n.
  diphosphopyridine n. (DPN, DPNH)
  n. polymerase
  pyridine n.
  n. residue (NR)
  n. sequencing
nucleotidylexotransferase
  DNA n.
nucleotidyltransferase
  DNA n.
  RNA n.
nucleotoxin
Nucleopore
  N. filter
  N. method
nucleus, *pl.* **nuclei**
  n. accumbens
  arcuate n.
  Balbiani n.
  band-shaped n.
  n. basalis of Ganser
  Bekhterev n.
  bland n.
  Cajal interstitial n.
  caudate n.
  cerebriform n.
  cigar-shaped n.
  Clarke dorsal n.

  dentate n.
  diploid n.
  droplet nuclei
  eccentric n.
  Edinger-Westphal n.
  fissured n.
  folded n.
  hobnail n.
  horseshoe-shaped n.
  hyperchromatic n.
  hypersegmentation of granulocyte
    nuclei
  inferior olivary n.
  Klein-Gumprecht shadow
    nuclei
  medial preoptic n.
  n. niger
  nuclei of chondrocyte
  n. of motor neuron
  nuclei of neuroglia
  oligodendroglial n.
  Orphan Annie eye n.
  pleomorphic n.
  popcorn nuclei
  presegmented n.
  prominent n.
  pyknotic nuclei
  raisinoid n.
  reniform n.
  Schwann n.
  segmentation n.
  shadow n.
  smudged n.
  sole n.
  sperm n.
  stripped n.
  supraoptic n.
  trophic n.
  vesicular n.
  wrinkled n.
nucleus-to-cytoplasm ratio
NucliSens
  N. CMV assay
  N. HIV-1 QT assay
Nuel space
NUG
  necrotizing ulcerative
    gingivitis
Nuhn gland
nuisance fistula
null
  n. allele
  n. cell
  n. cell adenoma
  n. cell lymphoblastic
    leukemia
  n. cell lymphoma
  n. cell population
  n. lymphocyte

n. phenotype
n. phenotype lesion
null-point potentiometer
null-type non-Hodgkin lymphoma
NuMA
nuclear mitotic apparatus
NuMA gene
number
acid n.
atomic n.
Avogadro n.
CI n.
complex n.
CT n.
dibucaine n. (DN)
diploid n.
DNA copy n.
fluoride n.
haploid n.
iodine n.
line n.
mass n.
modal centromere copy n.
numeric indicator experimental n. 1
  (NIXIE)
oxidation n.
random n.
real n.
Reynolds n.
turnover n.
numbering
stereospecific n.
numerical
n. aperture
n. hypertrophy
n. karyotype
n. taxonomy
numeric indicator experimental number
1 (NIXIE)
numerous mucosal folds
nummiform
nummular
n. dermatitis
n. eczema
n. sputum

nummulation
NuPAGE Bis-Tris gel
nurse cell
Nutiliaceae
nutmeglike appearance
nutmeg liver
nutricium
foramen n.
nutricius
canalis n.
nutriens
nutrient
n. agar
n. broth
n. canal
n. foramen
n. medium
mineral n.
vehiculated n.
nutrition
total parenteral n. (TPN)
nutritional
n. anemia
n. cirrhosis
n. recovery syndrome
Nuttallia
NV
negative variation
NVD
Newcastle virus disease
nyctalopia
Nyctotherus
nymph
nymphal
nymphearum
Dichotomophthoropsis n.
nymphitis
nympholabial
nymphoncus
Nyssorhynchus
nystagmus
positional alcohol n. (PAN)
nystatin assay agar
NZ
enzyme

N

O

O agglutination
O agglutinin
O antibody
O antigen
O colony

O₂

oxygen

OA

osteoarthritis

OAAD

ovarian ascorbic acid depletion
OAAD test

O-acyl-transferase

OAD

obstructive airway disease

o-aminoazotoluene

OAP

osteoarthropathy

oasthouse urine disease

oat

o. cell
o. cell carcinoma

oatmeal-tomato paste agar

OAV

oculoauriculovertebral
OAV syndrome

OB

osteoblastoma

Obermayer test

Obermeier spirillum

Obermüller test

obesity

central o.
exogenous o.

Obesumbacterium proteus

obidoxime therapy

OBIS albicans rapid colorimetric test

object

o. code
o. glass
o. program
test o.

objective

achromatic o.
aplanatic o.
apochromatic o.
dry o.
flat-field o.
fluorite o.
immersion o.
semiapochromatic o.

obligate

o. aerobe
o. anaerobe

o. autotroph
o. coccobacillus
o. osteogenic transcription factor
o. parasite

oblique

o. fracture

obliterans

arteriosclerosis o.
arteritis o.
balanitis xerotica o.
bronchiolitis fibrosa o.
bronchitis o.
endangiitis o.
endarteritis o.
thromboangiitis o. (TAO)

obliterating

o. arteritis
o. endarteritis

obliteration

fibrous o.

obliterative

o. arachnoiditis
o. bronchiolitis
o. bronchitis
o. endarteritis
o. hepatocavopathy
o. inflammation
o. pericarditis
o. pleuritis

obnubilate

obnubilation

oboediens

Gluconacetobacter o.

OBS

organic brain syndrome

observation

censored o.

obsolescent glomerulus

obstetric, obstetrical

o. catastrophe
o. panel

obstetrical (*var. of* obstetric)

obstetrics

International Federation of
Gynecology and O. (FIGO)

obstipation

obstructed testis

obstruction

ball-valve o.
biliary o.
bladder neck o. (BNO)
bronchiole o.
chronic airway o. (CAO)
closed loop o.
common bile duct o.

O

obstruction (*continued*)
    complete o.
    extrahepatic o. (EHO)
    intestinal o. (IO)
    intrahepatic vascular o.
    mesenteric vascular o.
    renal o.
    salivary duct o.
    site of venous o.
    ureteropelvic junction o.
    (UPJO)
    ureterovesical o.
    urethral o.
    urinary o.
    vena cava o.
obstructive
    o. airway disease (OAD)
    o. appendicitis
    o. atelectasis
    o. cirrhosis
    o. diverticulitis
    o. emphysema
    o. hyperbilirubinuria
    o. jaundice
    o. lung disease
    o. sleep apnea
    o. uropathy
obstruent
OBT
    occult blood test
    FlexSure OBT
obtecta
obturating embolism
obturation
obturator
    o. canal
    o. crest
    o. foramen
    o. hernia
    o. nerve
    o. vein
obturbans
    Armigeres o.
obvelata
    Syphacia o.
obvelatus
    Cosmocephalus o.
OC
    oleoresin capsicum
    organ confined
occidentalis
    Dermacentor o.
occipitoatlantoaxial junction
occlude
occluded virus
occludens
    zonula o.
occludin
    hyperphosphorylation of o.

occlusion
    aortic o.
    carotid artery o.
    coronary o.
    internal carotid artery o.
    (ICAO)
    retinal artery o.
    thrombotic o.
    o. time (OT)
    venous o.
occlusive meningitis
occult
    o. bleeding
    o. blood
    o. blood loss
    o. blood test (OBT)
    o. carcinoma
    o. metastasis
    o. nodular heterotopia
occulta
    spina bifida o.
occupational
    o. hypersensitivity pneumonitis
    o. lung disease
    O. Safety and Health Administration
    (OSHA)
occurrence
    multicentric o.
oceanense
    Desulfofrigus o.
Oceanibulbus indolifex
Oceanicaulis alexandrii
Oceanicola
    O. batsensis
    O. granulosus
Oceanimonas
    O. baumannii
    O. doudoroffii
Oceanisphaera litoralis
Oceanithermus
    O. desulfurans
    O. profundus
Oceanobacillus iheyensis
Oceanobacter kriegii
Oceanospirillum
ocellus
OCG
    oral cholecystogram
ochraceum
    Haliangium o.
    Simulium o.
    Virgisporangium o.
ochraceus
    Aspergillus o.
    Bacteroides o.
ochratoxin
ochre mutation
Ochrobactrum
    O. gallinifaecis

O. grignonense
O. tritici
Ochroconis
Ochromyia anthropophaga
ochronosis
ochronotic
    o. arthritis
    o. pigment
OCT
  ornithine carbamoyltransferase
  oxytocin challenge test
    OCT freezing compound
octal
octamer-binding transcription
factor 4
octane
octanoic acid
octavius
    Anaerococcus o.
Octosporomyces
octreotide scintigraph
octulosonic acid
ocular
    o. cicatricial pemphigoid
  compensating o.
    o. cytology
    o. grid
    o. humor
  Huygens o.
    o. hypertelorism
    o. inflammatory disease
    (OID)
    o. larva migrans
    o. lymphomatosis
    o. melanoma
    o. micrometer
    o. muscle dystrophy (OMD)
  Ramsden o.
    o. reticle
  widefield o.
ocular-mucous membrane syndrome
oculi (*pl. of* oculus)
oculoauriculovertebral (OAV)
    o. dysplasia
oculobuccogenital syndrome
oculocerebral syndrome
oculocerebrorenal syndrome
oculocutaneous albinism
oculodentodigital (ODD)
    o. dysplasia
    o. syndrome
oculodermal melanosis
oculoencephalic angiomatosis
oculogenitalis
    Chlamydia o.
oculoglandular tularemia
oculomandibulodyscephaly
oculomandibulomelic (OMM)
oculomycosis

oculovertebral
    o. dysplasia
    o. syndrome
oculus, *pl.* **oculi**
    Dracunculus oculi
    tapetum oculi
    tunica albuginea oculi
    tunica externa oculi
    tunica vasculosa oculi
OD
  optical density
  outside diameter
ODD
  oculodentodigital
    ODD syndrome
odditis
    foreign body o.
    primary o.
    stenosing o.
odds
    logarithm of o. (LOD)
O-diethyl S-[2-(diethylamino)ethyl]
  phosphonothioate
Odland body
ODN
  oligodeoxynucleotide
odontoameloblastoma
odontoblastic
    o. layer
    o. tissue
odontoblast process
Odontobutis
odontoclast
odontogenesis
odontogenic
    o. cyst
    o. epithelium
    o. fibroma
    o. fibrosarcoma
    o. ghost cell tumor
    o. keratocyst (OKC)
    o. lesion
    o. myxoma
odontology
    forensic o.
odontolyticus
    Actinomyces o.
odontoma
    ameloblastic o.
    complex o.
    compound o.
    fibroameloblastic o.
odorans
    Alcaligenes o.
odoratism
odorifer
odoriferous gland
odorimutans
    Anaerovorax o.

O

odysseyi
> Bacillus *o.*

Oe
> oersted

oedematiens
> Bacillus *o.*

oedipodis
> Brackiella *o.*

Oedocephalum

Oerskovia
> *O. enterophila*
> *O. jenensis*
> *O. paurometabola*

oersted (Oe)

Oesophagostomum
> *O. apiostomum*
> *O. bifurcum*
> *O. brevicaudum*
> *O. brumpti*
> *O. columbianum*
> *O. dentatum*
> *O. georgianum*
> *O. quadrispinulatum*
> *O. radiatum*
> *O. stephanostomum*
> *O. venulosum*

Oestridae
oestrids
oestrosis
Oestrus
> *O. hominis*
> *O. ovis*

OF
> Ovenstone factor
> oxidation-fermentation
> OF medium

OFB
> oval fat body
> OFB cast

OFD
> oral-facial-digital
> orofaciodigital
> OFD syndrome 1–8

office
> Epidemiology Program O.
> (EPO)
> O. of Emergency Preparedness
> O. of National Statistics (ONS)
> Public Health Practice Program O.
> (PHPPO)

officer
> medical review o. (MRO)
> radiation protection o. (RPO)

officinalis
> poxvirus o.

Ofuji disease
Ogawa antigen
Ogilvie syndrome
O'Grady prognostic indices

OGTT
> oral glucose tolerance test

Oguchi disease
oguniense
> Pyrobaculum *o.*

Ohara disease
O₂Hb
> oxyhemoglobin
> O_2Hb fraction

17-OH corticoid test
OHL
> oral hairy leukoplakia

Ohm law
ohmmeter
ohne Hauch
Ohngren line
OHP
> oxygen under high pressure

OHS
> ovarian hyperstimulation
> syndrome

o-**hydroxyphenylacetic acid**
OIA
> Optical ImmunoAssay
> CdTOX A OIA
> Chlamydia OIA
> GC OIA
> Strep B OIA

OID
> ocular inflammatory
> disease
> GC OID

oidia (*pl. of* oidium)
Oidiodendron cerealis
Oidiomycetes
oidiomycin
oidiomycosis
oidium, *pl.* oidia
oid-oid disease
OIF
> oil immersion field

oil
> anise o.
> bergamot o.
> cedar o.
> chenopodium o.
> clove o.
> croton o.
> o. cyst
> distilled o.
> o. embolism
> essential o.
> ethiodized o.
> eucalyptus o.
> fatty o.
> fixed o.
> flaxseed o.
> fog o. (SGF2)
> o. gland

o. immersion
o. immersion field
  (OIF)
o. immersion lens
o. in water (O/W)
joint o.
origanum o.
red o.
o. red O stain
safflower o.
sandalwood o.
santal o.
sesame o.
silicone o.
o. tumor
turpentine o.
o. vaccine
volatile o.
water in o. (W/O)
oil-aspiration pneumonia
oil-water ratio (O:W)
oily granuloma
ointment
BAL o.
Okavirus
Okazaki segment
OKC
odontogenic keratocyst
okeanokoites
Planomicrobium o.
okhotskensis
Psychrobacter o.
Okibacterium fritillariae
OKT
Ortho-Kung T cell
OKT-9 antibody
okuhidensis
Bacillus o.
OLB
open lung biopsy
OLC
oligodendroglia-like cell
old
o. infarct
o. myocardial infarction
  (OMI)
o. thrombus
o. tuberculin (OT)
O. World hookworm
O. World screwworm
oleaginous
oleandomycin
olearia
olearium
Sporobacterium o.
oleate
Oleavirus
olecranarthropathy
olefin

oleic
o. acid
o. acid I-125
o. acid uptake test
Oleiphilaceae
Oleiphilus messinensis
Oleispira antarctica
oleivorans
Thalassolituus o.
oleogranuloma
oleoma
oleoresin
aspidium o.
o. capsicum (OC)
olfactoriae
glandulae o.
olfactorius
bulbus o.
olfactory
o. bulb
o. epithelium
o. esthesioneuroblastoma
o. gland
o. glomerulus
o. membrane
o. mucosa
o. neuroblastoma (ONB)
o. organ
o. receptor cell
olfactus
organum o.
OLGC
osteoclast-like giant cell
OLH
ovine lactogenic hormone
Oligella urethralis
oligemia
oligemic
oligoadenylate synthetase
oligoastrocytoma
oligoclonal
o. band
o. banding
oligocystic
oligocythemia
oligodactylia (*var. of* oligodactyly)
oligodactyly, oligodactylia
oligodendria
oligodendroblast
oligodendroblastoma
oligodendrocyte
oligodendrogenic cell
oligodendroglia
o. cell
o. stain
o. staining
oligodendroglial
o. nucleus
o. tumor

O

oligodendroglia-like cell (OLC)
oligodendroglioma
>anaplastic o.
>pleomorphic o.
oligodeoxynucleotide (ODN)
oligodynamic
oligofermentans
>*Streptococcus o.*
oligo-1,6-glucosidase
oligohydramnios
oligomeganephronia
oligomenorrhea
oligomer
>allele-specific o.
>toxic soluble o.
oligomeric plasmid
oligomerization
oligonephronic hypoplasia
oligonucleotide
>allele-specific o.
>enzyme-labeled o.
>o. genomic array
>o. primer
>o. probe
oligonucleotide-primed
>degenerate o.-p. (DOP)
oligopeptide
oligophrenia
Oligoporus
oligosaccharide
oligospermatism (*var. of* oligospermia, oligozoospermia)
oligospermia, oligospermatism
oligospora
>*Arthobotrys o.*
oligosynaptic
oligotropha
>*Nitrosomonas o.*
oligotrophic
oligotyping
oligozoospermatism
oligozoospermia, oligospermia, oligospermatism, oligozoospermatism
oliguresia (*var. of* oliguria)
oliguresis (*var. of* oliguria)
oliguria, oliguresis, oliguresia
olivapovliticus
>*Alkalibacterium o.*
olivary eminence
olivocerebellar atrophy
olivopontocerebellar atrophy
olleyana
>*Shewanella o.*
Ollier disease
Ollulanus tricuspis
Olmer disease
olomoucine
ol res
Olsenella

>*O. profusa*
>*O. uli*
olympian forehead
Olympus
>O. AU5200 cholesterol analyzer
>O. BH2 microscope
OM
>otitis media
OMD
>ocular muscle dystrophy
omega
Omegatetravirus
Omenn syndrome
omenta (*pl. of* omentum)
omentitis
omentovolvulus
omentum, *pl.* omenta
>greater o.
>lesser o.
OMI
>old myocardial infarction
omicron
omitis
OMM
>oculomandibulomelic
>OMM syndrome
omnibus hypothesis
Omnifix
omnivorum
>*Flavobacterium o.*
Omnivue illuminated magnifier
OMPA
>otitis media, purulent, acute
omphalelcosis
omphalitis
omphalocele
omphalomesenteric duct remnant
omphalophlebitis
Omphalospora
Omphalotus illudens
Omsk
>O. hemorrhagic fever
>O. hemorrhagic fever virus
OMT
>ovarian mucinous tumor
ONB
>olfactory neuroblastoma
Onchocerca
>*O. caecutiens*
>*O. cervicalis*
>*O. lienalis*
>*O. volvulus*
onchocerciasis
onchocerciasis-type filariasis
onchocercid
Onchocercidae
Oncocerca
OncoChek immunoassay
oncocyte

oncocytic
    o. adenoma
    o. carcinoma
    o. cell
    o. epithelium
    o. hepatocellular tumor
    o. metaplasia
    o. papillary cystadenoma
    o. papillary neoplasm
    o. transformation
oncocytoma
    renal o.
oncofetal
    o. activation
    o. antigen
    o. marker
    o. protein
oncogene
    Abelson o.
    bcl-2 o.
    c-abl o.
    c-fos o.
    c-kit o.
    c-*myc* o.
    cyclin D1 o.
    erb A o.
    erb B, B-2 o.
    o. expression
    fms o.
    HER-2/neu o.
    Ki-67 o.
    K-ras o.
    MIC2 o.
    myc o.
    N-myc o.
    p16 o.
    ras o.
    retroviral o.
oncogenesis
oncogenic
    o. human papillomavirus
    o. virus
oncogenous
oncoides
oncologist
oncology
oncolysis
oncolytic
oncoma
Oncomelania
Oncometrics Imaging Cyto-Savant image analyzer
oncophora
    Cooperia o.
oncoplastic carcinoma
oncoprotein
    o. antigen
    c-erb-B2 o.
    c-myc o.

Oncor
    O. antifade mounting solution
    O. Inform HER2/neu gene
        amplification detection system
Oncorhynchus
oncornavirus
oncosis
oncosphere
oncotic pressure
oncotropic
Oncovirinae
oncovirus
on-demand system
one-sided alternative
one-stage
    o.-s. factor assay
    o.-s. prothrombin time
    o.-s. prothrombin time test
one-step
    O.-S. hCG combo test
    o.-s. nested PCR (OSNP)
one-tailed test
one-tube nested PCR
onion
    o. body
    o. scale lesion
onionskin
    o. change
    o. lesion
o-**nitrophenyl-beta-D-galactopyranoside (ONPG)**
o-**nitrophenyl beta galactosidase**
onkinocele
Onnia
onocytoma
ONPG
    o-nitrophenyl-beta-D-galactopyranoside
    ONPG test
ONS
    Office of National Statistics
Onthophagus
ontogeny
OnTrak TestTcard drug testing device
onychatrophia, onychatrophy
onychatrophy (*var. of* onychatrophia)
onychia
Onychocola canadensis
onychoheterotopia
onycholysis
onychoma
onychomycosis
onychoosteodysplasia
onychophosis
onychorrhexis
O'nyong-nyong
    O.-n. fever
    O.-n. fever virus
onyx (*var. of* unguis)
onyxitis

O

OO
osteoid osteoma
OOC
orthokeratinized odontogenic
cyst
oocyst
oocyte
integer o.
oogenesis
oogonium
ookinete
oolemma
oomycosis
oophoritic cyst
oophoritis
oophorocystosis
oophoroma
oophoron
oophorosalpingitis
oophorus
cumulus o.
oosome
Oospora granulosa
oosporangium
oospore
Oosporidium
ootheca
ootid
ootype
O&P
ova and parasites
O&P test
OP
osmotic pressure
opaca
Wohlfahrtia o.
opacity
corneal o. (CO)
ground glass o.
lenticular o.
opalescent
opalgia
Opalski cell
opaque
o. colony
o. microscope
OPCP
orthocresolphthalein
complex
OPD4 antibody
open
o. circuit
o. lung biopsy (OLB)
o. reading frame (ORF)
o. tuberculosis
open-angle glaucoma
opera-glass hand
operating
o. cycle

o. system
o. time
operation
o. code
comparison o.
military o.
morgue o.'s
serial o.
symmetry o.
operational amplifier
operator
o. certification
o. gene
operculated
operculum
operon
arabinose o.
lac o.
tra o.
Ophiostoma
Ophiovirus
ophryogenes
ulerythema o.
Ophryoscolecidae
ophthalmia
gonococcal o.
gonorrheal o.
o. neonatorum
spring o.
sympathetic o.
ophthalmica
zona o.
ophthalmicus
herpes zoster o. (HZO)
ophthalmitis
sympathetic o.
ophthalmobium
Agamodistomum o.
**ophthalmomandibulomelic
dysplasia**
ophthalmomycosis
ophthalmomyiasis
ophthalmopathy
infiltrative o.
thyroid o.
ophthalmoplegia
**ophthalmoplegic-type progressive
muscular dystrophy**
ophthalmosteresis
ophthalmovascular choke
opiate
o. assay
Liquichek urine toxicology control
C2, C3, S1, S2 low o.
OPIDN
organophosphate-induced delayed
neuropathy
opioid peptide
opisthomastigote

opisthorchiasis
opisthorchid
Opisthorchiidae
Opisthorchioidea
Opisthorchis
    O. felineus
    O. noverca
    O. sinensis
    O. viverrini
opisthorchosis
opisthotonos, opisthotonus
opisthotonus (*var. of* opisthotonos)
Opitutus terrae
Opitz
    O. disease
    O. GBBB syndrome
opium
Oppenheim
    O. disease
    O. syndrome
Oppenheim-Urbach disease
opportunistic
    o. infection
    o. mycosis
    o. pathogen
opsin
opsinogen
opsoclonus-myoclonus
    o.-m. diarrhea
    o.-m. syndrome
opsonic
    o. action
    o. index
opsonin
    bacterial o.
    common o.
    immune o.
    normal o.
    o. receptor
    specific o.
    thermolabile o.
    thermostable o.
opsonization
    bacterial o.
opsonizing antibody
opsonocytophagic
opsonometry
opsonophilia
opsonophilic
optic, optical
    o. atrophy
    geometric optics
    o. nerve disease
    o. nerve glioma
    o. neuritis
    Nomarski optics
    o. papillitis
optical (*var. of* optic)
    o. allachesthesia

    o. density (OD)
    o. glass
    O. ImmunoAssay (OIA)
    o. isomer
    o. isomerism
    o. light scatter
    o. purity
    o. rotary dispersion (ORD)
    o. rotation
optici
    spatium intervaginale subarachnoidale
      nervi o.
    stratum ganglionare nervi o.
OptiClone monoclonal antibody
OptiLyse lysing reagent
Optima
    O. L-XP, L-90 K, LE-80 K
      preparative ultracentrifuge
    O. Max, Max-E, TLX personal
      benchtop ultracentrifuge
optimal growth temperature
OptiMax immunostaining system
optimization
    automated assay o. (AAO)
    Sagian automated assay o.
optimized robot for chemical analysis
(ORCA)
optimizing compiler
optimum temperature
Optochin susceptibility test
optomeninx
Opus cardiac troponin I assay
OPV
    oral poliovirus vaccine
orae (*pl. of* ora)
oral
    o. actinomycosis
    o. cavity
    o. cavity cytology
    o. cholecystogram (OCG)
    o. flora
    o. glucose tolerance test
      (OGTT)
    o. hairy leukoplakia (OHL)
    o. infection
    o. lactose tolerance test
    o. pathology
    o. poliovirus vaccine (OPV)
    o. smear
orale
    Desulfomicrobium o.
    Mycoplasma o.
    Treponema o.
oral-facial-digital (OFD)
oralis
    Bacteroides o.
    Prevotella o.
OralScreen
    O. 3-panel oral fluids test

O

OralScreen (*continued*)
    O. rapid oral fluid screening and test device
    O. 4 substance abuse test
oral-sinonasal melanoma
orange
    acridine o. (AO)
    ethyl o.
    o. G
    methyl o.
    o. peel corneal appearance
    Victoria o.
OraQuick rapid HIV-1 antibody test
OraSure HIV-1 oral specimen collection device
OraTest oral cancer test
orbiculare
    Pityrosporum o.
orbital
    o. cellulitis
    o. cyst
    o. fracture
    o. hemangiopericytoma
    hybrid o.
    o. meningioma
    o. mucocele
    o. trauma
    o. tumor
orbitopathy
    thyroid o.
Orbivirus
ORCA
    optimized robot for chemical analysis
    ORCA Robot
orcein
    acetic o.
    acid o.
    o. stain
orchella
orchiatrophy
orchica
    adiposis o.
orchidic hormone
orchiditis (*var. of* orchitis)
orchidoblastoma
orchidopexy (*var. of* orchiopexy)
orchidoptosis
orchidorrhaphy (*var. of* orchiopexy)
orchiepididymitis
orchil
orchioblastoma
orchiocele
orchioncus
orchiopexy, orchidopexy, orchidorrhaphy
orchitic
orchitis, orchiditis
    autoimmune o.

    granulomatous o.
    nonspecific granulomatous o. (NSGO)
orcini
    Diphyllobothrium o.
orcinol test
ORD
    optical rotary dispersion
order
    low o.
ordinal variable
ordinary smallpox
ordinate
orellanus
    Cortinarius o.
Orenia
    O. salinaria
    O. sivashensis
orexigenic factor
orexin A, B peptide
ORF
    open reading frame
orf
    o. infection
    o. virus
organ
    accessory o.
    o. and tissue procurement organization
    annulospiral o.
    Chievitz o.
    o. confined (OC)
    Corti o.
    o. culture
    digestive o.
    enamel o.
    end o.
    floating o.
    Golgi tendon o.
    gustatory o.
    lymphoid o.
    neurotendinous o.
    no cancer spread to other o.'s (M0)
    o. of smell
    o. of taste
    olfactory o.
    o. perfusion
    principal target o.
    ptotic o.
    reticular membrane of spinal o.
    sense o.
    spiral o.
    subcommissural o.
    supernumerary o.
    target o.
    tendon o.
    o. tolerance dose (OTD)
    vestibular o.
    wandering o.

o. xenotransplantation
Zuckerkandl o.

organelle
cell o.
cytoplasmic o.

organic
o. acid
o. anion-dicarboxylate/tricarboxylate exchanger
o. anion-X exchanger
o. brain syndrome (OBS)
o. cation
o. chemistry
o. chloroarsine
o. contracture
o. disease
o. dust toxic syndrome
o. lesion
o. phosphate
o. radical (R)
o. solvent

organification defect

organism
Arizona o.
boxcar o.
calculated mean o. (CMO)
Campylobacter-like o. (CLO)
catalase-negative o.
catalase-positive o.
o. characteristic
demonstration of o.
facultative o.
hypothetical mean o. (HMO)
indicator o.
lepra cell o.
nonmotile o.
pleuropneumonia-like o. (PPLO)
Ricketts o.
unusual isolates/fastidious o.'s
Vincent o.

organivorans
Halomonas o.

organization
International Standards O. (ISO)
North Atlantic Treaty O. (NATO)
o. of the nucleolus
organ and tissue procurement o.
Professional Standards Review O. (PSRO)
World Health O. (WHO)

organized
o. hematoma
o. old thrombotic residue
o. pneumonia
o. thrombus

organizer
procentriole o.

organizing
o. inflammation
o. pneumonitis

organochlorine
o. insecticide
o. pesticide

organogenesis

organoid
o. arrangement
o. growth pattern
o. nevus
o. thymoma
o. tumor

organoma

organometallic compound

organophilum
Methylobacterium o.

organophosphate
o. compound
o. insecticide
o. pesticide

organophosphate-induced delayed neuropathy (OPIDN)

organophosphorous
toxic o.

organosilicon compound

organotaxis

organothiophosphate compound assay

organotroph

organotropic bacterium

organotropism

organotypic feature

organ-specific antigen

organum
o. gustus
o. olfactus
organa sensuum
o. spirale
o. tactus

Orgaran

Oribacterium sinus

Oriboca virus

oricola
Actinomyces o.

Oriental
O. blood fluke
O. hemoptysis
O. lung fluke
O. lung fluke disease
O. ringworm
O. sore

orientalis
Acetobacter o.
Dermacentroxenus o.
Issatchenkia o.
Nocardia o.
Pseudomonas o.
Trichostrongylus o.

Orientia tsutsugamushi

O

orientis
>   *Desulfosporosinus o.*

orifice
>   golf hole ureteral o.

orificialis
>   tuberculosis cutis o.

origanum oil

origin
>   amyloid of immunoglobulin o. (AIO)
>   amyloid of unknown o. (AUO)
>   anomalous o.
>   fever of undetermined o. (FUO)
>   fever of unknown o. (FUO)
>   hematopoietic cell o.
>   myocardial disease of unknown o. (MDUO)
>   ovarian sex cord-stromal o.
>   pyrexia of unknown o. (PUO)
>   tumor of germ cell o.

Orion
>   O. electrode
>   O. skin electrode for chloride

oris
>   *Bacteroides o.*
>   cancrum o.
>   *Filaria hominis o.*
>   glandulae o.
>   pachyderma o.
>   *Prevotella o.*
>   tunica mucosa o.

orisratti
>   *Streptococcus o.*

orleanensis
>   *Acetobacter o.*

Ormond disease

ornate

ornithine
>   o. aminotransferase
>   o. carbamoyltransferase (OCT)
>   o. carbamoyltransferase assay
>   o. carbamoyltransferase deficiency
>   o. decarboxylase
>   o. transcarbamoylase (OTC)
>   o. transcarbamoylase deficiency

ornithinemia

ornithine-oxo-acid aminotransferase

Ornithinimicrobium humiphilum

ornithinivorans
>   *Hongiella o.*

ornithinolytica
>   *Raoultella o.*

ornithinuria

Ornithobilharzia

Ornithodoros
>   *O. coriaceus*
>   *O. erraticus*
>   *O. hermsi*
>   *O. lahorensis*

O. moubata complex
O. pappilipes
O. parkeri
O. rudis
O. savigni
O. talaje
O. tholozani
O. turicata
O. venezuelensis
O. verrucosus

Ornithonyssus

ornithosis
>   *Miyagawanella o.*
>   o. virus

orodigitofacial dysostosis

orofaciodigital (OFD)

oropharyngeal
>   o. anthrax
>   o. tularemia

oropharynx

Oropouche virus

orosomucoid

orotate phosphoribosyltransferase

orotic
>   o. acid
>   o. aciduria

orotidine-5'-phosphate decarboxylase

orotidylate decarboxylase

Oroya fever

orphan
>   O. Annie eye nucleus
>   chicken embryo lethal o. (CELO)
>   enteric cytopathogenic bovine o. (ECBO)
>   enteric cytopathogenic dog o. (ECDO)
>   enteric cytopathogenic human o. (ECHO)
>   enteric cytopathogenic monkey o. (ECMO)
>   enteric cytopathogenic swine o. (ECSO)
>   o. virus

orseillin BB

Ortalidae

Orth
>   O. fixative
>   O. fluid
>   O. solution
>   O. stain

orthoaminoazotoluene

Orthobunyavirus

orthochromatic
>   o. megaloblast
>   o. normoblast

orthochromatophilic normoblast

orthochromophil, orthochromophile

orthochromophile (*var. of* orthochromophil)

orthocresolphthalein complex (OPCP)

orthocytosis
orthodromic
Orthohepadnavirus
orthoiodohippurate
orthokeratinized odontogenic cyst (OOC)
orthokeratosis
orthokeratotic sparing
Ortho-Kung T cell (OKT)
Orthomune antibody
Orthomyxoviridae
orthomyxovirus
orthophosphoric
    o. acid
    o. ester monohydrolase
orthopnea
Orthopodomyia
Orthopoxvirus
Orthoptera
orthoptic transplantation
Orthoreovirus
Orthorrhapha
orthostatic
    o. albuminuria
    o. hypertension
    o. hypotension
    o. proteinuria
Ortho Summit donor screening system
orthotolidine
orthotopic liver transplant
orthovanadate
    sodium o.
Ortolani sign
oryzae
    Azospira o.
    Helminthosporium o.
    Pyricularia o.
    Rhizopus o.
    Xanthomonas o.
Oryzavirus
OS
    osteosarcoma
    overall survival
Os
    osmium
OSA
    osteosarcoma
osazone test
OSBT
    ovarian serous borderline tumor
oscheitis
oschelephantiasis
oscheohydrocele
oscillation
oscillator
Oscillatoriales
Oscillochloridaceae
oscilloscope
    storage o.
Oscillospiraceae

osculum
Osgood-Schlatter disease
OSHA
    Occupational Safety and Health
    Administration
Osler
    O. disease
    O. erythema
    O. node
Osler-Vaquez disease
Osler-Weber-Rendu
    O.-W.-R. disease
    O.-W.-R. syndrome
osloensis
    Moraxella o.
OSM
    oxygen saturation meter
Osm
    osmole
osmic
    o. acid
    o. acid fixative
osmicate
osmication, osmification
osmification (*var. of* osmication)
osmiophilic cell surface membrane
osmiophobic
osmium (Os)
    o. tetroxide
    o. tetroxide stain
osmoceptor (*var. of* osmoreceptor)
osmolal
    o. clearance
    o. gap
osmolality
    calculated serum o.
    fecal o.
    stool o.
    urine o.
osmolar
    o. clearance (Cosm)
    o. gap
osmolarity
osmole (Osm)
osmometer
    freezing point depression o.
    vapor pressure depression o.
    Vapro vapor pressure o.
osmometry
osmophil, osmophilic
osmophile
osmophilic (*var. of* osmophil)
Osmoporus
osmoreceptor, osmoceptor
osmosis
osmotic
    o. clearance
    o. coefficient
    o. diuretic

O

osmotic (*continued*)
 o. fragility
 o. fragility test
 o. hemolysis
 o. nephrosis
 o. pressure (OP)
 o. shock
OSNP
 one-step nested PCR
ossea
 leontiasis o.
ossei
 canales semicircularis o.
 labium limbi tympanicum laminae
  spiralis o.
 laminae spiralis o.
ossein, osseine
osseine (*var. of* ossein)
osseocartilaginous
osseomucin
osseous, osteal
 o. ankylosis
 o. cell
 o. hydatid
 o. hydatid cyst
 o. lacuna
 o. metaplasia
 o. polyp
 o. spiral lamina
 o. tissue
ossicle
 Andernach o.
ossicular
 o. chain disruption
 o. damage
ossiferous
ossificans
 lipoma o.
 myositis o. (MO)
ossification
 endochondral o.
 intramembranous o.
 membranous o.
 metaplastic o.
 point of o.
 primary center of o.
 primary point of o.
 secondary center
  of o.
 secondary point of o.
 zone o.
ossificationis
 punctum o.
ossific center
ossiform
ossify
ossifying
 o. fibroma
 o. inflammation

ossium
 fibrogenesis imperfecta o.
 fragilitas o.
 medulla o.
 substantia compacta o.
 xanthoma generalisata o.
Ostase
 O. biochemical marker
 O. bone metabolism marker
osteal
ostealgia
osteanagenesis
osteanaphysis
ostein, osteine
osteine (*var. of* ostein)
osteitic
osteitis
 caseous o.
 central o.
 o. condensans
 condensing o.
 cortical o.
 o. deformans
 dissecting o.
 o. fibrosa
 o. fibrosa circumscripta
 o. fibrosa cystica
 o. fibrosa disseminata
 hematogenous o.
 sclerosing o.
 o. tuberculosa multiplex cystica
ostemia
ostempyesis
osteoanagenesis
osteoarthritis (OA)
 hyperplastic o.
osteoarthropathy (OAP)
 hypertrophic pulmonary o.
 idiopathic hypertrophic o. (IHO)
 pneumogenic o.
 pulmonary o.
 secondary hypertrophic o. (SHO)
osteoblastic
 o. osteosarcoma
 o. response
osteoblastoma (OB)
osteoblast proliferation fluorometric assay
osteocalcin
osteocarcinoma
 central o.
osteocartilaginous exostosis
osteochondral
osteochondritis
 o. deformans juvenilis
 o. deformans juvenilis dorsi
 o. dissecans
 syphilitic o.
osteochondrodystrophia deformans
osteochondrodystrophy

osteochondrogenic cell
osteochondroma
    multiple o.'s
osteochondromatosis
    synovial o.
osteochondrosarcoma
osteochondrosis
osteochondrous
osteoclasia (*var. of* osteoclasis)
osteoclasis, osteoclasia
osteoclast
    o. activating factor
    bone-resorbing o.
    multinucleated o.
osteoclastic
    o. factor assay
    o. reaction
    o. resorption
osteoclast-like giant cell
  (OLGC)
osteoclastoma
osteocollagenous fiber
osteocystoma
osteocyte
osteodentin
osteodermatopoikilosis
osteodermatous
osteodermia
osteodiastasis
osteodysplastica
    geroderma o. (GO)
osteodysplasty
osteodystrophia (*var. of* osteodystrophy)
osteodystrophy, osteodystrophia
    Albright hereditary o.
    renal o.
osteoectasia
osteofibroma
osteofibrosis
osteofibrous dysplasia of Campanacci
osteogen
osteogenesis
    o. imperfecta
    o. imperfecta congenita
    o. imperfecta tarda
osteogenetic (*var. of* osteogenic)
    o. fiber
    o. layer
osteogenic, osteogenetic
    o. cell
    o. sarcoma
    o. tissue
osteogenous
osteogeny
OsteoGram bone density test
osteohalisteresis
osteohypertrophy
osteoid
    o. matrix

    o. osteoma (OO)
    o. tissue
osteolathyrism
osteolipochondroma
osteolysis
osteolytic
osteoma
    o. cutis
    fibrous o.
    giant osteoid o.
    o. medullare
    osteoid o. (OO)
    o. spongiosum
osteomalacia
    senile o.
osteomalacic pelvis
Osteomark NTx point-of-care
  device
osteomatoid
osteomesopyknosis
osteomyelitis
    Garré sclerosing o.
    pyogenic o.
    tuberculous o.
osteomyelodysplasia
osteomyelofibrotic
  syndrome
osteomyelosclerosis
osteon, osteone
osteoncus
osteone (*var. of* osteon)
osteonecrosis
osteonectin
osteoonychodysplasia
    hereditary o. (HOOD)
osteopathia
    o. condensans
    o. striata
osteopathy
    alimentary o.
    disseminated condensing o.
    myelogenic o.
osteopenia
osteoperiostitis
osteopetrosis
    o. acroosteolytica
    o. gallinarum
osteopetrotic
osteophage
osteophlebitis
osteophyma
osteophyte
osteoplaque
osteoplast
osteoplastic
osteoplastica
    tracheopathia o.
osteopoikilosis
osteopontin

osteoporosis
  o. circumscripta
  o. circumscripta cranii
  juvenile o.
  posttraumatic o.
  traumatic o.
osteoporotic
osteoprogenitor cell
osteopulmonary arthropathy
osteoradionecrosis
Osteosal osteoporosis test
osteosarcoma (OS)
  central o.
  chondroblastoma-like o.
  extraskeletal o.
  osteoblastic o.
  telangiectatic o.
  undifferentiated o.
    (UOS)
osteosclerosis congenita
osteosclerotic anemia
osteosis
  o. cutis
  o. eburnisans
    monomelica
osteospongioma
osteosteatoma
osteothrombosis
Ostertagia
ostia (*pl. of* ostium)
ostiomeatal complex
ostitic
ostium, *pl.* **ostia**
Ostor study
ostracea
  psoriasis o.
ostraceous
ostraviensis
  Cellvibrio o.
Ostrum-Furst syndrome
Ostwald-Folin pipette
Ostwald viscosimeter
OT
  occlusion time
  old tuberculin
otalgia
Ota nevus
Ot antigen
OTC
  ornithine transcarbamoylase
  oxytetracycline
OTD
  organ tolerance dose
other (diagnoses)
otitic
  o. abscess
  o. meningitis
otitidis-caviarum
  Nocardia o.-c.

otitis
  Alloiococcus o.
  o. desquamativa
  o. diphtheritica
  o. externa
  o. labyrinthica
  o. mastoidea
  o. media (OM)
  o. media, purulent, acute (OMPA)
  o. mycotica
  o. sclerotica
otoacariasis
otobiosis
Otobius
otocerebritis
otoconia
otocyst
Otodectes
otodectic
otoencephalitis
otolith
otolithic membrane
O-toluidine
otomandibular
  o. dysostosis
  o. syndrome
Otomyces
  O. hageni
  O. purpureus
otomycosis
otopharyngeal tube
otorrhagia
otorrhea
otosalpinx
otosclerosis
  cochlear o.
ototoxic drug
ototoxicity
  aminoglycoside o.
OTR
  Ovarian Tumor Registry
Otto
  O. disease
  O. pelvis
Ottowia thiooxydans
Ouchterlony
  O. double diffusion
  O. immunodiffusion
  O. method
  O. technique
  O. test
Oudemansiella
Oudin immunodiffusion
Ourmiavirus
outer
  o. circumferential lamella
  o. hair cell
  o. leaflet
  o. margin

o. mitochondrial membrane
o. phalangeal cell

outlet
right ventricle double o.

outlier

output
basal acid o. (BAO)
o. capacitor
carbon dioxide o. (V_{CO_2})
CO_2 o.
decreased cardiac o.
o. impedance
intake and o.
maximal acid o.

outside diameter (OD)

ova (*pl. of* ovum)

Ovabloc device

oval
o. corpuscle
o. fat body (OFB)
o. macrocyte
o. subterminal spore
o. window (OW)

ovalbumin

ovale
foramen o.
o. malaria
Pityrosporum o.
Plasmodium o.
Pseudeurotium o.

ovalis
fenestra o.
Malassezia o.

ovalocyte

ovalocytic anemia

ovalocytosis

oval-shaped goblet cell

ovaria (*pl. of* ovarium)

ovarian
o. agenesis
o. ascorbic acid depletion (OAAD)
o. borderline tumor
o. cancer
o. cancer biomarker
o. carcinoma
o. cyst
o. dysfunction
o. failure
o. follicle
o. granulosa cell tumor
o. hormone
o. hyperstimulation syndrome (OHS)
o. insufficiency
o. masculinization
o. mucinous tumor (OMT)
o. pregnancy
o. serous borderline tumor (OSBT)
o. sex cord-stromal origin
o. sex cord tumor

o. teratoma
o. torsion
o. tubular adenoma
O. Tumor Registry (OTR)
o. tumor triage test
o. varicocele

ovaricus
cumulus o.

ovarii
cortex o.
hilum o.
Pseudomyxoma o.
stratum granulosum o.
stroma o.
struma o.

ovarioabdominal pregnancy

ovarioncus

ovariosalpingitis

ovaritis

ovarium, *pl.* **ovaria**

ovary
dermoid cyst of o.
hilar cell tumor of o.
hilum of o.
polycystic o. (PCO)
rete cyst of o.
stroma of o.

ovatum
Loxotrema o.

ovatus
Metagonimus o.

oven
Bio-Rad H2500 microwave o.

Ovenstone factor (OF)

over
unequal crossing o.

overall survival (OS)

overdominance

overexposure
dental o.

overexpressing

overexpression
HER-2/neu o.
protein o.

overflow

overgrowth
small-intestine bacterial o.

overhydration

overlap
spectral o.
o. syndrome

overlapping inversion

overload
circulatory o.
dysmetabolic iron o.
iodine o.
iron o.

overpressure

overshoot

O

overwhelming postsplenectomy
  sepsis
overwintering
ovigerous lamella
ovine
    o. lactogenic hormone (OLH)
    o. progressive pneumonia
ovinia
oviposit
oviposition
ovipositor
ovis
    Cysticercus o.
    Neisseria o.
    Oestrus o.
    Streptococcus o.
    Taenia o.
    Tetratrichomonas o.
    Trichomonas o.
ovoid bacterium
ovoides
    Trichosporon o.
ovolarviparous
ovolyticum
    Tenacibaculum o.
ovotestes (*pl. of* ovotestis)
ovotestis, *pl.* ovotestes
OvuKIT
ovular
ovulational sclerosis
ovulation test
ovule
ovulum
ovum, *pl.* ova
    ova and parasite
      examination
    ova and parasites (O&P)
    blighted o.
    cleavage of o.
OvuQUICK
O/W
    oil in water
O:W
    oil-water ratio
OW
    oval window
Owen
    contour line of O.
    interglobular space of O.
    O. line
owl
    o. eye
    o. eye cell
owl-eye appearance
Owren disease
oxalate
    ammonium o.
    calcium o. (CO)
    o. calculus

double o.
potassium o.
urine o.
oxalatica
    Ralstonia o.
    Wautersia o.
oxalemia
oxalic
    o. acid
    o. acid assay
    o. acid stain
Oxalicibacterium flavum
oxalism
oxaloacetate decarboxylase
oxaloacetic acid
oxalosis
oxaluria
oxazin, oxazine
    o. dye
oxazine (*var. of* oxazin)
Oxford unit
Oxi
    oximeter
    oximetry
oxidant
    o. stress
    total o.
oxidase
    aldehyde o.
    coproporphyrinogen o.
    cytochrome o.
    d-amino acid o.
    glucose o.
    glycerol-3-phosphate o. (GOI)
    homogentisate o.
    hydroxyproline o.
    l-amino acid o.
    mitochondrial cytochrome o.
    NADPH o.
    nicotinamide adenine dinucleotide
      phosphate o. (NADPH)
    p-hydroxyphenylpyruvate o.
    proline o.
    protoporphyrinogen o.
    o. reaction
    sulfite o.
    o. test
    xanthine o. (XO)
oxidase-induced acute hemolytic
  anemia
oxidation
    beta o.
    fatty acid o.
    o. number
    o. state
oxidation-fermentation (OF)
    o.-f. medium
    o.-f. test
oxidation-reducing potential

oxidation-reduction (redox)
:   o.-r. indicator
:   o.-r. reaction

oxidative
:   o. energy
:   o. phosphorylation
:   o. phosphorylation inhibitor
:   o. phosphorylation uncoupler
:   o. stress

oxide
:   aluminum o.
:   ethylene o.
:   ferric o.
:   magnesium o. (MgO)
:   nitric o. (NO)
:   sulfur o.
:   vitamin K_1 o.
:   zinc o.

oxidize

oxidized
:   o. glutathione (GSSG)
:   o. low density lipoprotein (oxLDL)

oxidizer

oxidizing
:   o. agent
:   o. detergent
:   o. gas

oxidoreductase
:   l-lysine:NAD^+ o.

oxime
:   o. antidote
:   NATO code for phosgene o. (CX)

oximeter (Oxi)
:   AVOXimeter 4000 CO o.
:   carbon monoxide o. (CO-oximeter)

oximetry (Oxi)
:   arterial blood o.
:   pulse o.

OXK
:   lipopolysaccharide

oxLDL
:   oxidized low density lipoprotein

OX2 lipopolysaccharide
OX19 lipopolysaccharide
oxo acid
oxobutyric acid
oxoglutarate dehydrogenase
oxoglutaric acid
oxoisovalerate dehydrogenase
oxolinic acid
oxonium ion
5-oxoproline
4-oxoproline reductase
5-oxoprolinuria
oxoprolinuria
oxosteroid reductase
oxovanadate
:   potassium bisperoxo o. V

ox-warble disease

oxyacoia, oxyakoia
oxyakoia (var. of oxyacoia)
oxyaphia
oxybate
:   sodium o.

oxybiotin
oxycephalia (var. of oxycephaly)
oxycephalic, oxycephalous
oxycephalous (var. of oxycephalic)
oxycephaly, oxycephalia
oxychloride
:   carbon o.

oxychromatic
oxychromatin
oxyclinae
:   Desulfovibrio o.

oxygen (O_2)
:   o. acceptor
:   o. affinity anoxia
:   o. affinity hypoxia
:   alveolar-arterial o.
:   o. analyzer
:   o. capacity of blood
:   cerebral metabolic rate of o. (CMRO)
:   concentration of total o. (CtO_2)
:   o. consumption
:   o. content of blood
:   o. effect
:   forced inspiratory o.
:   fractional concentration of inspired o. (FIO_2)
:   fraction of inspired o.
:   o. half-saturation pressure of hemoglobin
:   o. poisoning
:   o. quotient (QO_2)
:   rapid recompression-high pressure o. (RR-HPO)
:   o. saturation
:   o. saturation measurement
:   o. saturation meter (OSM)
:   o. tension
:   o. under high pressure (OHP)
:   o. uptake
:   o. utilization coefficient

oxygenase
:   heme o. (HO)
:   homogentisate o.

oxygenase-1
:   heme o.-1 (HO1)

oxygenated hemoglobin
oxygenation
:   extracorporeal membrane o. (ECMO)
:   o. of tissue

oxygenator
oxygen-derived free radical
oxygen-hemoglobin dissociation curve
oxygen-modified polystyrene

O

oxyhemoglobin (HbO_2, O_2Hb)
oxyhemogram
oxyhemograph
oxyntic
    o. cell
    o. gland
oxyntocardiac mucosa
oxyphil, oxyphile, oxyphile
    o. adenoma
    o. cell
    o. chromatin
    o. granule
    o. inclusion body
oxyphile (*var. of* oxyphil)
oxyphilic
    o. cell
    o. endometrioid adenocarcinoma
    o. leukocyte
    o. papillary carcinoma
Oxyphotobacteria
oxypolygelatin
oxypurinol
Oxyspirura mansoni
oxysporum
    Fusarium o.
oxytalan
    o. fiber
    o. fiber stain

oxytetracycline
oxytoca
    Klebsiella o.
oxytocin
    brain o.
    o. challenge test (OCT)
    synthesize o.
    unit of o.
Oxytrema
Oxyurata
oxyuriasis
oxyuricide
oxyurid
Oxyuridae
Oxyuris
    O. incognita
    O. vermicularis
Oxyuroidea
ozaenae
    Klebsiella pneumoniae subsp. *o.*
Oz antigen
ozone
ozonization
ozonolysis
Ozzard filaria
ozzardi
    Filaria o.
    Mansonella o.

P
    face of polyhedron
    plasma
    pressure
    probability
      P antigen
      P blood group
      P cell
      P value

p16
      p16 gene
      p16 oncogene

p24
      p24 HIV antigen
      p24 protein

p53
      p53 gene
      p53 immunohistochemical breast
        cancer analysis
      p53 mutation
      p53 tumor suppressor

PA
    pleomorphic adenoma
    protective antigen
      PA protein

Pa
    protactinium

Paas disease

PAB, PABA
    p-aminobenzoic acid

pacchionian
      p. body
      p. corpuscle
      p. gland
      p. granulation

pacefollower

pacemaker
      p. check
      p. twiddler's syndrome
      wandering p.

P/ACE MDQ series capillary
  electrophoresis system

Pacheco parrot disease virus

pachnodae
      Promicromonospora p.
      Xylanimicrobium p.

pachometer (*var. of* pachymeter)

pachyacria

pachyblepharon

pachyblepharosis

pachycephalic, pachycephalous

pachycephalous (*var. of* pachycephalic)

pachycephaly

pachycheilia, pachychilia

pachychilia (*var. of* pachycheilia)

pachychromatic

pachydactylous

pachydactyly

pachyderma
      p. laryngis
      p. lymphangiectatica
      p. oris
      p. verrucosa
      p. vesicae

pachydermatis
      Malassezia p.

pachydermatocele

pachydermatosis

pachydermatous

pachydermia

pachydermic

pachydermoperiostosis

pachyglossia

pachygyria

pachyhymenia

pachyhymenic

pachyleptomeningitis

pachylosis

pachymenia

pachymenic

pachymeningitis
      adhesive chronic p.
      chronic adhesive p.
      p. externa
      fibrous hypertrophic p.
      hemorrhagic p.
      hypertrophic cervical p.
      hypertrophic fibrous p.
      p. interna
      pyogenic p.

pachymeningopathy

pachymeter, pachometer

pachynema

pachynsis

pachyntic

pachyonychia congenita

pachyperiostitis

pachyperitonitis

pachypleuritis

pachysalpingitis

pachysalpingoovaritis

Pachysolen tannophilus

pachysomia

pachytene

pachyvaginalitis

pachyvaginitis cystica

pacifica
      Cellulophaga p.
      Plesiocystis p.
      Rheinheimera p.

P

pacifica (*continued*)
    Shewanella p.
    Wuchereria p.
pacificensis
    Psychrobacter p.
pacificum
    Carboxydibrachium p.
    Diphyllobothrium p.
pacificus
    Ignicoccus p.
    Ixodes p.
pacinian corpuscle
pacinii
    Vibrio p.
pacinitis
pack
    Vitros Immunodiagnostic Products
      anti-HBc reagent p.
package
    dual-in-line p.
    push p.
packed
    p. cell volume (PCV)
    p. human blood cells
    p. red blood cells
packet
packing ratio
paclitaxel
PACONA technique
pad
    Kendall Company Telfa p.
    protein p.
padenii
    Chlamydoabsidia p.
padwickii
    Trichoconis p.
Padykula-Herman stain for myosin ATPase
Paecilomyces lilacinus
paecilomycosis
Paederus
Paenibacillus
    P. agarexedens
    P. agaridevorans
    P. antarcticus
    P. azoreducens
    P. borealis
    P. brasilensis
    P. chinjuensis
    P. chitinolyticus
    P. cookii
    P. daejeonensis
    P. ehimensis
    P. favisporus
    P. glycanilyticus
    P. graminis
    P. granivorans
    P. jamilae
    P. koleovorans

    P. koreensis
    P. kribbensis
    P. lactis
PAF
    platelet-activating factor
    platelet-aggregating factor
    pulmonary arteriovenous fistula
PAF-AH
    platelet-activating factor acetylhydrolase
PAG
    protein A gold
PAGE
    polyacrylamide gel electrophoresis
    2D PAGE
pagetoid foam cell
PAGMK
    primary African green monkey
    kidney
PAH, PAHA
    p-aminohippuric acid
    pulmonary artery hypertension
PAI
    plasminogen activator inhibitor
painting
    chromosome p.
pair
    base p. (bp)
    conjugate acid-base p.'s
    conjugate redox p.
    electron p.
    ion p.
    kilobase p. (kbp)
pairing
    base p.
    exchange p.
    somatic p.
palate
    cleft p.
    inflammatory papillary hyperplasia of
      the p. (IPHP)
    isolated cleft p.
palaticanis
    Gemella p.
palatina
    tonsilla p.
palatinae
    glandulae p.
palatopharyngis
    Amycolatopsis p.
palearctica
    Yersinia enterocolitica subsp. p.
pale cytoplasm
paleopneumoniae
    Diplococcus p.
palisading
    nuclear p.
pallens
    Enterococcus p.
    Prevotella p.

palleroniana
    Pseudomonas p.
pallescens
    Curvularia p.
pallida
    Spirochaeta p.
    Trombicula p.
pallidipes
    Glossina p.
pallidula
    Glaciecola p.
pallidum
    microhemagglutination
     assay-*Treponema p.*
     (MHA-TP)
    Treponema p.
pallidus
    Synosternus p.
palm
    liver p.
palmaris
    verruca p.
palmitatis
    Desulfuromonas p.
palmitoyltransferase
    carnitine p. 2 (CPT2)
P.A.L.M. ultraviolet laser microbeam
palpalis
    Glossina p.
palpebralis
    Filaria p.
palpebrarum
    tunica conjunctiva p.
    xanthelasma p.
    xanthoma p.
palsy
    bulbar p.
    cerebral p. (CP)
    facial p.
    progressive bulbar p.
    progressive dystonic p.
    progressive supranuclear p.
     (PSP)
    pseudobulbar p.
    Saturday night p.
paludicola
    Propionicimonas p.
palustre
    Mycobacterium p.
palustris
    Trichococcus p.
PAM
    pulmonary alveolar macrophage
    pulmonary alveolar microlithiasis
p-**aminobenzoate**
    potassium p-a.
p-**aminobenzoic acid (PAB, PABA)**
p-**aminodimethylaniline**

p-**aminohippurate**
    p-a. clearance (C_{pah})
    p-a. clearance test
    sodium p-a.
p-**aminohippuric acid (PAH, PAHA)**
p-**aminosalicylate**
    potassium p-a.
p-**aminosalicylic acid (PAS)**
PAN
    polyarteritis nodosa
    positional alcohol nystagmus
panamensis
    Leishmania braziliensis p.
panbronchiolitis
    diffuse p. (DPB)
pancreas
    aberrant p.
    accessory p.
    anular p.
    Baggenstoss change in p.
    beta cell of p.
    cystic fibrosis of p.
     (CFP)
    delta cell of p.
    exocrine p.
    islands of p.
pancreaticum
    Eurytrema p.
pancreaticus
    ductus p.
    hemosuccus p.
pancreatitis
    acute hemorrhagic p.
    calcifying p.
    chronic fibrosing p.
    hemorrhagic p.
    necrotizing p.
    relapsing p.
pancytopenia
    autoimmune p.
    congenital p.
    Fanconi p.
panel
    basic metabolic p.
     (BMP)
    British Testicular Tumour P.
     (BTTP)
    chemistry p. (chem)
    lymphocyte subset p.
    lymphocytic leukemia
     marker p.
    NAP hepatitis B virus
     quantitative p.
    nucleic acid p. (NAP)
    obstetric p.
    Profile-ER drugs of abuse
     screening p.
    QuestTest diagnostic p.

P

panel (*continued*)
    Triage Cardiac p.
    urine drug p. (UDP)
panencephalitis
    nodular p.
    subacute sclerosing p. (SSPE)
panhypopituitarism
    generalized p.
    postpubertal p.
    prepubertal p.
panmyelosis
panniculitis
    A1AT deficiency p.
    alpha$_1$ antitrypsin deficiency p.
    cytophagic histiocytic p.
    factitial p.
    lobular p.
    lupus p.
    mesenteric p.
    metastatic p.
    nodular nonsuppurative p.
    relapsing febrile nodular p.
    septal p.
pannorus
    Geomyces p.
pannus
    degenerative p.
    glaucomatous p.
PANSS
    positive and negative symptom scale
pantherina
    Amanita p.
pantheris
    Lactobacillus p.
p27 antigen
P54 antigen
PAP
    primary atypical pneumonia
    pulmonary alveolar proteinosis
papain
    Wako 1% crude p.
papaya
    Carica p.
papayae
    Erwinia p.
paper
    alkannin p.
    azolitmin p.
    blue litmus p.
    chemical agent detector p.
    Congo red p.
    filter p. (FP)
    indicator p.
    Kuwabara p.
    litmus p.
    probability p.
    red litmus p.
    test p.
    Whatman p.

papilla, *pl.* **papillae**
    acoustic p.
    circumvallate papillae
    clavate p.
    conical shaped filiform papillae
    dermal p.
    excavatio p.
    excavatio papillae
    exophytic p.
    filiform p.
    filiform papillae
    foliate p.
    foliate papillae
    fungiform papillae
    fungiform p.
    hair p.
    lenticular p.
    lingual p.
    nerve p.
    renal papillae
    tactile p.
    vallate p.
    vascular p.
papillae (*pl. of* papilla)
papillare
    corpus p.
papillaris
    foveola p.
papillary stroma
papilliferum
    hidradenoma p.
    syringocystadenoma p.
papillitis
    anal p.
    necrotizing p.
    optic p.
papilloma
    basal cell p.
    canine oral p.
    choroid plexus p.
    duct p.
    ductal p.
    fibroepithelial p.
    hard p.
    hyperkeratotic p.
    intracystic p.
    intraductal p.
    inverted p. (IP)
    keratotic p.
    rabbit p.
    schneiderian p.
    Shope p.
    soft p.
    squamous cell p.
    transitional cell p.
    urothelial p.
    verrucous p.
    villous p.

papillomatosis
>church spire p.
>confluent and reticulate p.
>florid oral p.
>intraductal p.
>juvenile p.
>laryngeal p.
>recurrent respiratory p. (RRP)
>subareolar duct p.

papillomatosus
>lupus p.

papillomavirus
>human p. (HPV)
>oncogenic human p.

papio
>herpesvirus p. 2

papovavirus
>lymphotropic p. (LPV)

PAPP-A
>pregnancy-associated plasma protein A

PAPP-B
>pregnancy-associated plasma protein B

Pappenheim
>lymphoid hemoblast of P.

pappilipes
>*Ornithodoros p.*

papule
>Gottron p.
>moist p.
>mucous p.
>prurigo p.

papulosis
>bowenoid p. (BP)
>lymphomatoid p. (LyP)
>malignant atrophic p.

papyraceus
>fetus p.

PAR
>protease-activated receptor

para-**aminosalicylate**
>sodium p.-a.

paraaortica
>corpora p.

Paracoccus haeundaensis
paracollinoides
>*Lactobacillus p.*

paradoxa
>ectasia ventriculi p.

paradoxus
>*Thialkalivibrio p.*

parafaecalis
>*Alcaligenes faecalis* subsp. *p.*

paraffin
>bismuth iodoform p. (BIP)

paraffin-embedded
>formalin-fixed p.-e. (FFPE)

paraffinivorans
>*Gordonia p.*

parafollicularis
>hyperkeratosis follicularis et p.

parafulva
>*Pseudomonas p.*

paraganglia
>nonchromaffin p.

paraganglioma
>aorticopulmonary p. (APPG)
>aorticosympathetic p.
>benign p. (BPG)
>chromaffin p.
>malignant p. (MPG)
>nonchromaffin p.
>sclerosing p.

paragranuloma
>nodular p. (NP)

parahaemolyticus
>*Haemophilus p.*
>*Vibrio p.*

parainfluenzae
>*Haemophilus p.*

paralimentarius
>*Lactobacillus p.*

paralyses (*pl. of* paralysis)
paralysis, *pl.* **paralyses**
>acute atrophic p.
>Brown-Sequard p.
>Cruveilhier p.
>curariform p.
>Dejerine-Klumpke p.
>descending flaccid p.
>diaphragm p.
>familial periodic p.
>fowl p.
>Gubler p.
>hypokalemic periodic p.
>immune p.
>immunologic p.
>immunological p.
>infantile p.
>infectious bulbar p.
>Klumpke p.
>Kussmaul p.
>Kussmaul-Landry p.
>Lissauer p.
>Millard-Gubler p.
>myogenic p.
>normokalemic periodic p.
>postdormital p.
>Pott p.
>Ramsay Hunt p.
>Remak p.
>rucksack p.
>tick p.
>Todd p.
>vasomotor p.
>vocal cord p.
>Volkmann ischemic p.

P

paralysis (*continued*)
    Weber p.
    writer's p.
paramesonephric duct
parameter
    immunohistochemical p.
    practice p.
paranuclear vacuole
parapertussis
    Acinetobacter p.
    Bordetella p.
    Haemophilus p.
paraphrophilus
    Haemophilus p.
paraprotein
    monoclonal p.
parapsilosis
    Candida p.
paraputrificum
    Clostridium p.
parascrofulaceum
    Mycobacterium p.
parasite
    accidental p.
    duodenal p.
    extracellular p.
    facultative p.
    intermittent p.
    intestinal p.
    intracellular p.
    malarial p.
    metazoan p.
    obligate p.
    ova and p.'s (O&P)
    protozoan p.
    smear preparation and staining for
      blood parasites
    spurious p.
    string test for duodenal p.
    temporary p.
parasitica
    achromia p.
parasiticus
    Aspergillus p.
    dipygus p.
    epigastrius p.
    Rhizoglyphus p.
parasitovorax
    Cheyletiella p.
parathion
    methyl p.
parathyroid
    water-clear cell of p.
parathyroidea
    glandula p.
paratropicalis
    Haemophilus p.
paratuberculosis
    Mycobacterium p.

paratyphi
    Salmonella p.
    Salmonella enteritidis serotype
      p. A
typhoid, paratyphoid A, and
  p. B
paraurethrales
    ductus p.
pardinum
    Tricholoma p.
parenchyma
    placental p.
paresis
    general p. (GP)
parietography
    gastric p.
Park
    hemoglobin M Hyde P.
parkeri
    Borrelia p.
    Ornithodoros p.
parmense
    Mycobacterium p.
parodoxa
    Listerella p.
paronychia
    herpetic p.
parooensis
    Skermanella p.
paroophori
    ductuli p.
    tubuli p.
parotidea
    glandula p.
parotideus
    ductus p.
parotidis
    socia p.
parotis
    glandula p.
parotitides
    epidemic p.
parotitis
    infectious p.
    postoperative p.
    punctate p.
part
    infundibular p.
    intermediate p.
particle
    alpha p.
    beta p.
    bone marrow p.
    charged p.
    chromatin p.
    Dane p.
    DI p.
    elementary p.
    gelatin sponge p.

glycogen p.
gold p.
remanantlike lipoprotein p. (RLP)
ridge of intramembranous p.
stick-and-ball-shaped virion p.
Zimmermann elementary p.

particles-cholesterol
remnantlike lipoprotein p.-c.
(RLP-C)

particulate
settled p.
suspended p.

partition
nitrogen p.

parva
Emmonsia parva p.

parvula
Veillonella p.

parvum
Aquabacterium p.
Chlorobaculum p.
Chrysosporium p.
Corynebacterium p.
Cryptosporidium p.
Diphyllobothrium p.
Eubacterium p.
Haplosporangium p.
Roseospirillum p.
Treponema p.
Ureaplasma p.

parvus
Acinetobacter p.

PAS
p-aminosalicylic acid
pulmonary artery stenosis

PASCC
pseudovascular adenoid squamous cell
carcinoma

PASH
pseudoangiomatous stromal hyperplasia

passage
blind p.
bouton en p.
egg p.
serial p.

passularum
Carpoglyphus p.

pasteurianum
Clostridium p.

pasteurianus
Streptococcus p.
Streptococcus gallolyticus subsp. *p.*

pasteurii
Sporosarcina p.
Trichococcus p.

pastorianus
Saccharomyces p.

pastoris
Prochlorococcus marinus subsp. *p.*

patch
CF indicator system chloride p.
Dacron p.
gray p.
herald p.
Hutchinson p.
MacCallum p.
moth p.
mucous p.
salmon p.
shagreen p.
soldier's p.
white p.

patella, *pl.* **patellae**
chondromalacia patellae

patellae (*pl. of* patella)
patent ductus arteriosus
path
pathogen
antiplant p.
class A, B, C, D p.
foodborne p.
mycelial p.
opportunistic p.
plant p.
waterborne p.

pathogen-free
specific p.-f. (SPF)

pathogenicity
bacterial p.

pathologic
characteristic p.

pathologist
College of American P.'s
World Health
Organization/International Society
of Urologic P.'s

pathology
ageing (hippocampal region, patients
over 75 years), tau p. class I
anatomic p.
anatomical p.
Armed Forces Institute of P. (AFIP)
cellular p.
clinical p.
comparative p.
dental p.
Down syndrome tau p.
experimental p.
functional p.
general p.
geographic p.
Gerstmann-Straussler-Scheinker
disease (Indiana kindred), tau
p. class I
humoral p.
internal p.
International Society for Urological
P. (ISUP)

P

697

pathology (*continued*)
    medical p.
    molecular p.
    Niemann-Pick disease type C, tau p. class I
    oral p.
    posteencephalitic parkinsonism, tau p. class I
    posttransplant biopsy p.
    Society for Pediatric P. (SPP)
    solidistic p.
    special p.
    surgical p.
    Systematized Nomenclature of P. (SNOP)
    tau p. class I
    tau protein p.
    World Association of Societies of P. (WASP)
pathophysiologic features
pathway
    activation of the coagulation p.'s
    alternative complement p.
    amphibolic p.
    biosynthetic p.
    classical complement p.
    coagulation p.
    cortisol synthesis p.
    critical p.
    Embden-Meyerhof p.
    Entner-Doudoroff p.
    extrinsic p.
    hexose monophosphate p.
    internodal p.
    intrinsic p.
    lectin-binding p.
    lipoxygenase p.
    Luebering-Rapaport p.
    metabolic p.
    polyol p.
    reentrant p.
    transcellular p.
    tumor suppressor p.
    ubiquitin-protease p.
    wnt signaling transduction p.
patient
    contaminated p.
pattern
    acinar p.
    angiocentric p.
    angiodestructive p.
    angled soot p.
    arborizing p.
    architectural p.
    basaloid growth p.
    basket-weave p.
    biphasic p.
    blue cell p.
    canalicular p.

    carcinoid-like architectural p.
    chicken-wire p.
    clear cell p.
    cribriform growth p.
    cross striation p.
    cytoplasmic p.
    diffuse p.
    double phenotypic p.
    euploid-polyploid p.
    fascicular p.
    female sex chromatin p.
    filiform growth p.
    filigree p.
    finely stippled chromatin p.
    fingerprint p.
    follicular p.
    full house p.
    fused glandular p.
    gel electrophoresis p.
    gene expression p.
    Gleason p.
    growth p.
    hemangiopericytomatous growth p.
    herringbone p.
    heterogeneous p.
    Heymann p.
    histological p.
    hyperploid p.
    identity p.
    immunohistochemical p.
    indeterminate p.
    Indian-file p.
    inheritance p.
    lacy chromatin p.
    large glandular p.
    lobular p.
    lobulocentric p.
    luminal p.
    male sex chromatin p.
    membranous p.
    microacinar architectural p.
    microfollicular p.
    microglandular p.
    monoclonal B-cell p.
    mosaic p.
    moth-eaten p.
    multidot p.
    nonrandom p.
    nonreactive p.
    nucleolar p.
    organoid growth p.
    plasmalemmal p.
    plywood p.
    polka dot p.
    polyclonal p.
    protein expression p.
    pseudoalveolar p.
    pseudomantle zone p.

pseudopapillary p.
punctate p.
quiltlike p.
receptogram p.
reticular growth p.
rim p.
scalloped p.
Schmincke p.
secretory p.
Sertoli-like p.
short fascicular growth p.
single-dot p.
skin reaction p.
small glandular p.
solid p.
solid growth p.
speckled p.
spindle cell fascicular p.
squamoid p.
starburst p.
starry sky p.
storiform p.
syringomatous growth p.
targetoid p.
trabecular p.
tubulocystic growth p.
tubulopapillary architectural p.
variant p.
vesicular chromatin p.
whorled storiform p.
XX/XY sex chromosome p.
Zellballen p.

paucimobilis
Pseudomonas p.
paucivorans
Brevibacterium p.
Dolosicoccus p.
Fusibacter p.
Nocardia p.
paucula
Wautersia p.
pauli
Solirubrobacter p.
paurometabola
Oerskovia p.
Tsukamurella p.
paurometabolica
Saccharomonospora p.

PB
protein binding
Pb
barometric pressure
PBC
primary biliary cirrhosis
PBD
proliferating bile ductules
proliferative breast disease
PBG
porphobilinogen

PBG-D
porphobilinogen deaminase
PBG-S
porphobilinogen synthase
PBI
protein-bound iodine
PBL
primary bone lymphoma
P-50 blood gas
PBS
prune belly syndrome
PBT4
protein-bound thyroxine
Pbxl gene
PC
plasma cell
platelet count
PCA
prostatic adenocarcinoma
PCB
polychlorinated biphenyl
PCC
prothrombin complex concentration
PCD
posterior corneal deposit
pCEA
polyclonal carcinoembryonic antigen
PCG
plasma cell granuloma
PCH
plasma cell hepatitis
pulmonary capillary hemangiomatosis
PCHA
proliferating cell nuclear antigen
PCHE
pseudocholinesterase
PCI
pneumatosis cystoides intestinalis
PCM
protein-calorie malnutrition
PCNA
proliferating cell nuclear antigen
PCNSL
primary central nervous system
  lymphoma
PCO
polycystic ovary
pCO2, pCO$_2$
arterial pCO$_2$
PCR
plasma clearance rate
polymerase chain reaction
  allele-specific PCR (A-PCR)
  DOP PCR
  one-step nested PCR (OSNP)
  one-tube nested PCR
  real-time reverse-transcriptase
    PCR
  TaqMan real-time PCR

P

PCR (*continued*)
    two-step nested PCR
      (TSNP)
    two-tube nested PCR
PCR-RFLP
    polymerase chain reaction-restriction
    fragment length polymorphism
PCR-SSCP
    polymerase chain reaction-single-strand
    conformation polymorphism
PCT
    porphyria cutanea tarda
    prothrombin consumption time
PCV
    packed cell volume
    polycythemia vera
PCV-M
    myeloid metaplasia with polycythemia
    vera
PD
    plasma defect
    poorly differentiated
PDC
    pyruvate dehydrogenase complex
PDCD4
    programmed cell death 4 gene
4p deletion syndrome
PDGF
    platelet-derived growth factor
PDGF-B gene
PDGFR-A
    PDGFR-A gene
    PDGFR-A gene mutation
PDGFR-β gene
***p*-dichlorobenzene**
PDLL
    poorly differentiated lymphocytic
    lymphoma
PDM
    polydimethylsiloxane
PE
    pulmonary edema
    pulmonary embolism
peak
    absorption p.
    biclonal p.
    coincidence sum p.
    iodine escape p.
    kilovolt p. (kVp)
    monoclonal p.
    multimodal p.
    unimodal p.
pealeana
    Shewanella p.
pearl
    amyl nitrite p.'s
    epidermic p.
    epithelial p.
    keratin p.

    Läennec p.
    squamous p.
pecorum
    Chlamydophila p.
pect
pectinata
    Cooperia p.
    zona p.
pectinatum
    ligamentum p.
pectinolytica
    Aeromonas salmonicida subsp. *p.*
pectinovorum
    Treponema p.
pectoris
    angina p. (AP)
pediculi
    Rickettsia p.
Pediculus humanus
pedis
    dermatomycosis p.
    tinea p.
    Trichophyton p.
pedrosianum
    Trichosporon p.
pedrosoi
    Acrotheca p.
    Fonsecaea p.
    Hormodendrum p.
PEEP
    positive end-expiratory pressure
PEG
    percutaneous endoscopic gastrostom
    polyethylene glycol
peg
    rete p.
    wide rete p.
pekingensis
    Rhodocista p.
PEL
    primary effusion lymphoma
pelagi
    Fulvimarina p.
pellet
    platelet p.
    tissue p.
pelletieri
    Actinomadura p.
    Streptomyces p.
pellucida
    macula p.
    zona p.
pelophilus
    Geobacter p.
    Propionibacter p.
    Propionivibrio p.
pelvic adhesion
pelvis
    beaked p.

caoutchouc p.
frozen p.
hardened p.
kyphoscoliotic p.
kyphotic p.
lordotic p.
Nägele p.
osteomalacic p.
Otto p.
Prague p.
pseudoosteomalacic p.
rachitic p.
Rokitansky p.
rostrate p.
rubber p.
scoliotic p.
spider p.
split p.
spondylolisthetic p.
TCC of renal p.
pelviureteroradiography (*var. of* pyelography)
PEM
polymorphic epithelial mucin
pemphigoid
benign mucosal p.
Brunsting-Perry p.
bulbous p.
bullous p.
cicatricial p.
ocular cicatricial p.
pemphigosa
variola p.
pemphigus
benign familial p.
benign mucous membrane p.
familial benign p.
pendrin protein
pendulum
cor p.
penetrance
complete p.
incomplete p.
reduced p.
penetrans
Dermatophilus p.
hyperkeratosis p.
Pulex p.
Sarcopsylla p.
Tunga p.
penicillatum
Trichosporon p.
penicillatus
limbus p.
penicillin
potassium p. G (KPG)
potassium phenoxymethyl p.
unit of p.

penis
corpus spongiosum p.
pennivorans
Fervidobacterium p.
pentacarboxyporphyrin
urine p.
pentad
Reynolds p.
pentaromativorans
Novosphingobium p.
pentobarbital
sodium p.
pentosetest
Bial p.
pentosuria
alimentary p.
essential p.
idiopathic p.
primary p.
PEP
postexposure prophylaxis
pepsin
proteolytic enzyme p.
peptic
peptidase
cytoplasmic p.
peptide
amyloid-β p. (AB)
anionic neutrophil activating p. (ANAP)
antigenetic p.
atrial natriuretic p. (ANP)
bombesin p.
C p. (CP)
calcitonin gene-related p. (CGRP)
cyclic citrullinated p. (CCP)
gastric inhibitory p. (GIP)
gastrin releasing p. (GRP)
hepcidin p.
human antimicrobial p.
katacalcin p.
N-terminal prohormone brain natriuretic p. (NT-proBNP)
opioid p.
orexin A, B p.
POMC-derived anorexic p.
prohormone B-type natriuretic p. (proBNP)
proopiomelanocortin-related p.
PTC p.
small p.
trefoil p.
vasoactive intestinal p. (VIP)
peptidivorans
Clostridium p.
peptidolytica
Pseudoalteromonas p.
PER
protein efficiency ratio

perborate
sodium p.
percent
milligram p.
p. transmittance
5 percent dextrose in water (D₅W, D5W)
perchlorate
potassium p.
percreta
placenta p.
percutaneous endoscopic gastrostom (PEG)
perflava
Neisseria p.
perfoliata
Anoplocephala p.
perfoliatum
Echinostoma p.
perforans
Trichophyton tonsurans p.
perforata
zona p.
perforatae
habenulae p.
perforation
bowel p.
duodenal ulcer p. (DUP)
esophageal p.
inflammatory p.
perfringens
Clostridium p.
perfusion
Ca2+-free p.
intervillous p.
luxury p.
organ p.
pulmonary p.
periarteritis
syphilitic p.
peribronchial metaplasia
pericardiaci
villi p.
pericardii
concretio p.
synechia p.
pericarditis
adherent p.
adhesive p.
bacterial p.
bread and butter p.
carcinomatous p.
chronic constrictive p.
constrictive p.
fibrinous p.
fungal p.
hemorrhagic p.
idiopathic p.
internal adhesive p.

mediastinal p.
obliterative p.
postmyocardial infarction p.
postpericardiotomy p.
posttraumatic p.
purulent p.
rheumatic p.
serofibrinous p.
suppurative p.
tuberculous p.
uremic p.
viral p.
pericardium
adherent p.
bread-and-butter p.
empyema of p.
shaggy p.
perichondritis
relapsing p.
pericyte
Rouget p.
Zimmermann p.
periductal stroma
perifollicular
cutaneous p.
perikarya
neuronal p.
perilymphaticus
ductus p.
perineum
watering-can p.
perinuclear
prominent p.
period
eclipse p.
effective refractory p. (ERP)
gap₀ p.
gap₁ p.
gap₂ p.
incubation p. (IP)
induction p.
latency p. (LP)
latent p.
mitotic p.
prepatent p.
refractory p. (RP)
relative refractory p. (RRP)
synthesis p.
periorchitis
meconium p.
periosteum
alveolar p.
peripancreatic adipose tissue
perisplenitis
hyaline p.
perithelium
Eberth p.
peritoneales
villi p.

peritonei
 gliomatosis p.
 Luteococcus p.
 pseudomyxoma p. (PP)
 tunica serosa p.
peritonitis
 adhesive p.
 benign paroxysmal p.
 bile p.
 chemical p.
 chyle p.
 circumscribed p.
 diaphragmatic p.
 diffuse acute p.
 feline infectious p.
 fibrinohemorrhagic p.
 fibrinous p.
 fibrocaseous p.
 gas p.
 general p.
 gonococcal p.
 localized p.
 meconium p.
 productive p.
 secondary bacterial p.
 septic p.
 spontaneous bacterial p. (SBP)
 tuberculous p.
perlatum
 Lycoperdon p.
perles
 amyl nitrite p.
permanganate
 potassium p.
permeability
 vascular p.
permeability-inducing
 bacterial p.-i. (BPI)
perniciosa
 lymphoderma p.
pernio
 erythema p.
 lupus p.
perolens
 Lactobacillus p.
peromelia
 micrognathia with p.
peroxidase
 benzidine method for myoglobin p.
 concanavalin A-horseradish p.
 Dako Envision system p.
 endogenous p.
 glutathione p.
 horseradish p. (HRP)
 s-ABC p.
peroxidation
 lipid p.
peroxide
 acyl p.

 alkyl p.
 hydrogen p. (HP)
peroxyacetic acid
peroxydisulfate
 ammonium p.
persarum
 Dracunculus p.
persica
 Borrelia p.
 Cellulomonas p.
persicolor
 Microsporum p.
 Trichophyton p.
persicus
 Argas p.
persistence
 microbial p.
persistent vitelline duct
perstans
 Acanthocheilonema p.
 acrodermatitis p.
 Dipetalonema p.
 erythema p.
 erythema dyschromicum p.
 hyperkeratosis lenticularis p.
 Mansonella p.
 telangiectasia macularis eruptiva p.
 urticaria p.
 xanthoerythrodermia p.
persulcatus
 Ixodes p.
PERT
 program evaluation and review technique
pertenue
 Treponema p.
perturbation
 cell-cycle p.
pertussis
 Bacillus p.
 Bordetella p.
peruana
 verruca p.
 verruga p.
peruensis
 Lutzomyia p.
peruviana
 Leishmania p.
peruzzii
 Meningonema p.
pest
 fowl p.
 swine p.
pesticide
 chlorinated hydrocarbon p.
 cyclodiene hydrocarbon p.
 organochlorine p.
 organophosphate p.
pestilence
 great p.

P

pestis
  Bacillus p.
  Yersinia p.
PET
  predominantly epithelial thymoma
  preeclamptic toxemia
  pulmonary endodermal tumor
petechia, *pl.* **petechiae**
  Tardieu petechiae
petechiae (*pl. of* petechia)
PETG
  polyethylene terephthalate
petrificans
  lipoma p.
  urethritis p.
petrii
  Bordetella p.
petrophila
  Thermotoga p.
peyerianum
  agmen p.
PFA
  platelet function analyzer
PFC
  plaque-forming cell
PFGC
  pseudofollicular growth center
PFGE
  pulsed field gradient gel
    electrophoresis
p-**fluorophenylalanine**
PFP
  platelet-free plasma
PFT
  pulmonary function test
PFU
  plaque-forming unit
PG
  prostaglandin
  proteoglycan
  pyoderma gangrenosum
PG1
  prostaglandin 1
PG2
  prostaglandin 2
PG3
  prostaglandin 3
PGD
  preimplantation genetic diagnosis
  pure gonadal dysgenesis
PGDR
  plasma glucose disappearance
    rate
p15 gene
PGH
  pituitary growth hormone
PGI
  potassium, glucose, and insulin
P-glycoprotein

PGP
  postgamma proteinuria
  protein gene product
PgR
  progesterone receptor
PGTR
  plasma glucose tolerance rate
PH
  prostatic hypertrophy
pH
  hydrogen ion concentration
    blood pH
    fecal pH
    scalp pH
    stool pH
PHA
  pulse height analyzer
phacidiomorpha
  Didymella p.
phaeomuriformis
  Sarcinomyces p.
phage
  beta p.
  defective p.
  temperate p.
phagocyte
  alveolar p.
  endothelial p.
  globuliferous p.
  melaniferous p.
  mononuclear p.
  sessile p.
phagocytophila
  Ehrlichia p.
phagocytophilum
  Anaplasma p.
phagocytosis
  frustrated p.
  induced p.
  macrophage p.
  spontaneous p.
  vacuole alteration p.
phagolysosome
  acidified p.
phalanx
  tufted p.
phalloides
  Amanita p.
phanerosis
  fatty p.
phantom
  Hine-Duley p.
  tissue-compatible plastic p.
pharmacology
  sympathetic p.
pharyngeales
  glandulae p.
pharyngealis
  tonsilla p.

pharyngis
  tunica mucosa p.
pharyngitis
  atrophic p.
  croupous p.
  follicular p.
  gangrenous p.
  glandular p.
  granular p.
  membranous p.
phase
  aqueous p.
  blastic p.
  catabolic flow p.
  cell cycle S p.
  continuous p.
  disperse p.
  ebb p.
  eclipse p.
  exponential p.
  G_0 p.
  G_1 p.
  G_2 p.
  inductive p.
  initial oliguric p.
  lag p.
  logarithmic p.
  M p.
  meiotic p.
  mobile p.
  moving p.
  negative p.
  platelet p.
  positive p.
  previtellogenic p.
  proliferative p.
  radial melanoma growth p.
  S p.
  stationary p.
  synaptic p.
  synthesis p.
  vertical melanoma growth p.
phaseoliforme
  Trichophyton p.
PHAT
  pleomorphic hyalinizing angiectatic tumor
phenobarbital
  sodium p.
phenolica
  Desulfobacula p.
  Pseudoalteromonas p.
phenomenon
  adhesion p.
  anarchic p.
  Anderson p.
  Arias-Stella p.
  Arthus p.
  atavistic p.

Azzopardi p.
Bordet-Gengou p.
cold-agglutination p.
Danysz p.
dawn p.
Debré p.
dedifferentiation p.
Denys-Leclef p.
d'Herelle p.
Donath-Landsteiner p.
Ehrlich p.
erythrocyte adherence p.
Felton p.
generalized Shwartzman p.
Gengou p.
halisteresis p.
Hamburger p.
Hektoen p.
Houssay p.
Huebener-Thomsen-Friedenreich p.
iceberg p.
immune adherence p.
Jod-Basedow p.
Kanagawa p.
Köbner p.
Koch p.
Koebner p.
LE p.
Lewis p.
Liacopoulos p.
Liesegang p.
Lucio leprosy p.
Mills-Reincke p.
Neisser-Wechsberg p.
no reflow p.
pink teeth p.
proliferation-dependent p.
prozone p.
quellung p.
Raynaud p.
reclotting p.
red cell adherence p.
Sanarelli p.
Sanarelli-Shwartzman p. (SSP)
satellite p.
Schultz-Charlton p.
second-set p.
Soret p.
Splendore-Hoeppli p.
starry sky p.
Theobald Smith p.
Twort p.
Twort-d'Herelle p.
wavefront p.
phenotype
  adenocarcinoma p.
  ayr p.
  ayw p.
  Bombay p.

P

phenotype (*continued*)
    CpG island methylator p. (CIMP)
    endocrine p.
    epithelioid p.
    exocrine p.
    Gerbich-negative p.
    histiocytic p.
    HLA-B8 p.
    HLA-DR3 p.
    lobular p.
    McLeod blood p.
    null p.
    prune belly p.
    RER^+ p.
    rhabdoid p.
    secretor p.
    p. V
    p. VA
    p. VAD
    p. VAM
    p. VD
phenotyping
    alpha$_1$ antitrypsin p.
    lipoprotein p.
phenylacetica
    Thauera p.
phenylalanine
    formyl methionyl leucyl p. (fMLP)
    serum p.
    urine p.
phenylamine hydroxylase
phenylcarbinol
    benzoyl p.
phenylethylbarbiturate
    sodium p.
phenylhydrazone
    trifluorocarbonylcyanide p. (FCCP)
phenylpyruvica
    Moraxella p.
phenytoin
    sodium p.
pheochromocytoma
    benign p. (BPC)
    malignant primary p. (MPPC)
    metastatic malignant p. (MMPC)
pheresis
    granulocyte p.
PHG
    pulmonary hyalinizing granuloma
PhiCal fecal calprotectin immunoassay
philippina
    Taenia p.
philippinensis
    Capillaria p.
    Filaria p.
philomiragia
    Francisella p.
PHLA
    postheparin lipolytic activity

phlebitis
    adhesive p.
    puerperal p.
    septic p.
    sinus p.
phlebosclerosis
    idiopathic mesenteric p.
    mesenteric p.
phlebotomum
    Bunostomum p.
phlebotomy
    therapeutic p.
phlegmasia
    cellulitic p.
    thrombotic p.
phlegmon
    diffuse p.
    emphysematous p.
    gas p.
phlei
    Mycobacterium p.
phlogistica
    crusta p.
phocae
    Atopobacter p.
phoeniculicola
    Enterococcus p.
phosgene
    NATO code for p. (choking gas)
phosphatase
    acid p. (ACP)
    alkaline p. (AP)
    alkaline phosphatase antialkaline p. (APAAP)
    antibody placental alkaline p. (anti-PLAP)
    bisphosphoglycerate p.
    cupric ion-inhibited acid p.
    diphosphoglycerate p.
    fractionated alkaline p.
    heat-stable alkaline p. (HSAP)
    leukocyte alkaline p. (LAP)
    myosin p.
    placental alkaline p. (PLAP)
    prostate specific acid p. (PSAP)
    serine/threonine protein p.
    serum alkaline p. (SAP)
    tartrate inhibited acid p.
    tartrate-resistant acid p. (TRAcP, TRAP)
    tartrate-resistant leukocyte acid p.
    thermostable alkaline p.
    tissue-nonspecific alkaline p. (TNAP)
    total serum prostatic acid p. (TSPAP)
5′-phosphate
    deoxyadenosine 5′-p.
    deoxycytidine 5′-p.

deoxyguanosine 5′-p.
deoxyuridine 5′-p.
guanosine 5′-p.

7-phosphate
sedoheptulose 7-p.

phosphate
acid p.
adenosine 3′,5′-cyclic p. (cAMP)
aluminum p.
ammonium magnesium p.
basic calcium p. (BCP)
calcium p.
carbamyl p.
creatine p.
deoxyguanosine p.
deoxyuridine p.
dibasic potassium p.
dihydroxyacetone p. (DAP)
diisopropyl p. (DIP)
dimethyldichlorovinyl p. (DDVP)
dolichol p.
dried sodium p.
effervescent sodium p.
guanosine 3′,5′-cyclic p.
high-energy p.
inorganic p.
inosine p.
Krebs-Ringer p. (KRP)
magnesium ammonium p.
4-methylumbelliferyl p. (MUP)
monobasic potassium p.
monobasic sodium p.
nicotinamide adenine dinucleotide p. (NADP, NADPH)
organic p.
potassium dihydrogen p.
primaquine p.
sodium acid p.
sodium cellulose p.
tartrate resistant acid p.
tribasic potassium p.
tricresyl p.
tri-o-cresyl p.
triple p.
undecaprenol p.

phosphatidylcholine
amniotic fluid desaturated p.
desaturated p. (DSPC)

phosphatonin protein

phosphide
zinc p.

phosphitoxidans
Desulfotignum p.

3′-phosphoadenosine 5′-phosphosulfate
6-phospho-d-gluconate
6-phospho-d-gluconolactone
2-phospho-d-glycerate

3-phospho-d-glycerate
phosphodiesterase
sphingomyelin p.

phosphoethanolamine
urine p.

phosphofluoridate
diisopropyl p.

6-phosphofructokinase
3-phosphoglyceraldehyde
phosphokinase
creatine p. (CPK)
serum creatine p. (SCPK)

phospholipase
glycosylphosphatidylinositol specific p. D
cytosol p. A2 (cPLA2)
lipoprotein-associated p. A2

phospholipid
amniotic fluid primary p.

phosphonothioate
NATO code for nerve agent O,O-diethyl S-[2-(diethylamino)ethyl] p. (VG)

4′-phosphopantetheine
5-phosphoribosyl-1-amine
phosphoribosyltransferase
hypoxanthine p. (HPRT)
hypoxanthine guanine p. (HGPRT)
orotate p.

phosphorus
red p. (RP)
white p. (WP)
yellow p.

phosphorylase
glycogen p.
inosine p.
purine nucleoside p. (PNP)

phosphorylation
oxidative p.
substrate level p.
tyrosine p.

3-phosphoserine
5′-phosphosulfate
3′-phosphoadenosine 5.-p.

photo
gamma p.

photograph
forensic p.

photometer
double-beam p.
filter p.
flame p.

photometry
flame p.

photomicrograph
selected p.

photomicrography
digital p.
through-the-eyepiece p.

P

photophoresis
    extracorporeal p.
PHP
    pseudohypoparathyroidism
    pyridoxalated
    hemoglobin-polyoxyethylene
PHPPO
    Public Health Practice Program Office
p-**hydroxybenzoic acid**
p-**hydroxyphenyllactic acid**
p-**hydroxyphenylpyruvate**
    p-h. dioxygenase
    p-h. oxidase
p-**hydroxyphenylpyruvic acid**
phyllode
    cystosarcoma p.
phymatum
    Burkholderia p.
P16-hypermethylation
physalifora
    ecchordosis p.
physellae
    Trichobilharzia p.
physics
    health p.
phytate
    sodium p.
phytofermentans
    Clostridium p.
PI
    proliferative index
    propidium iodine
    protease inhibitor
    pulmonary incompetence
    pulmonary infarction
PIA
    plasma insulin activity
picipes
    Melanolestes p.
pickettii
    Ralstonia p.
pictor
    Aspergillus p.
picturae
    Brevibacterium p.
    Virgibacillus p.
PID
    plasma iron disappearance
PIDT
    plasma iron disappearance time
PIE
    pulmonary infiltration and eosinophilia
    pulmonary interstitial emphysema
piece
    end p.
    Fab p.
    Fc p.
    middle p.
    principal p.

piedra
    black p.
    white p.
Pierini
    atrophoderma of Pasini
    and P.
piezophila
    Colwellia p.
PIF
    prolactin-inhibiting factor
    proliferation inhibitory factor
pifanoi
    Leishmania mexicana p.
piger
    Desulfovibrio p.
pigment
    anthracotic p.
    bile p.
    bilharzial deposition p.
    brown hemoglobin-derived p.
    calculous p.
    ceroid p.
    cirrhosis p.
    epithelial p.
    formalin p.
    hematogenous p.
    hepatogenous p.
    incontinence of p.
    lipid p.
    lipochrome p.
    lipofuscin p.
    malarial deposition p.
    melanotic p.
    ochronotic p.
    pseudomelanosis p.
    respiratory p.
    urine blood p.
    wear-and-tear p.
    yellow-brown wear and
    tear p.
pigmentation
    arsenic p.
    bismuth p.
    exogenous p.
    hematin p.
    hematoidin p.
    hemofuscin p.
    hemoglobin p.
    lead p.
    lipochrome p.
    melanin p.
    nonmelanocytic p.
    porphyrin p.
    wear-and-tear p.
pigmenti
    incontinentia p.
pigmentosa
    dermatopathia p.
    morphea p.

neurogenic muscle weakness, ataxia, and retinitis p. (NARP)
retinitis p.
urticaria p.

pigmentosum
atrophoderma p.
xeroderma p. (XDP, XP)

pigmentosus
nevus p.

pigrifrangens
Nocardia p.

pigs
virus pneumonia of p.

PII
plasma inorganic iodine

pilar, pilary
p. cyst
p. sheath acanthoma
p. tumor of scalp

pilaris
p. keratosis
pityriasis rubra p. (PRP)

pilary (*var. of* pilar)

pile
sentinel p.

pileous gland
piliate
Pilidae
piliferous cyst
piliform
pilimiction
pilin
pillar
p. cell
p. cell of Corti
Corti p.

pill esophagitis
pill-induced esophagitis
Pilobolus
pilocarpine nitrate iontophoresis
pilocystic
pilocytic astrocytoma
Piloderma
piloid astrocytoma
pilomatricoma, pilomatrixoma
pilomatrix carcinoma
pilomatrixoma (*var. of* pilomatricoma)
pilomotor fiber
pilonidal
p. cyst
p. fistula
p. sinus

pilorum
cruces p.

pilosa
Cavernicola p.

pilosebaceous
pilosus
nevus p.

PiMM genotype
PiMZ genotype
PIN
prostatic intraepithelial neoplasia
prostatic intraepithelial neoplasm

PIN-1
prostatic intraepithelial neoplasia, mild dysplasia or low grade

PIN-2
prostatic intraepithelial neoplasia, moderate dysplasia or high grade

PIN-3
prostatic intraepithelial neoplasia, severe dysplasia or high grade

pinacyanol
pinch
devil's p.

Pindborg tumor
pineal
p. body
p. cell
p. cyst
p. germinoma
p. gland
p. secretory rate

pineale
chief cell of corpus p.
corpus p.

pinealocyte
pinealoma
ectopic p.
extrapineal p.

pinealopathy
pineapple test
pineoblastoma
pineocytoma
pineocytomatous rosette
pine wood test
ping-pong
p.-p. bone
p.-p. mechanism

pinguecula, pinguicula
pinguicula (*var. of* pinguecula)
pink
p. bread mold
p. cytoplasm
p. puffer (PP)
p. puffer emphysema
p. teeth phenomenon

p16INK4A gene
pinkeye
Pinkus disease
pinnipedialis
Jeotgalicoccus p.

pinnipedii
Mycobacterium p.

pinocyte
pinocytosis
mass p.

pinocytotic
    p. vesicle
    p. vessel
pinosome
pinpoint hemorrhage
pinta
pintae
    Treponema p.
pinus
pinworm preparation
pioepithelium
pion
Piophila casei
PIP
    proximal interphalangeal
pipe
    p. bomb
    light p.
piperatus
    Boletus p.
piperazine
pipe-smoker's cancer
pipestem
    p. artery
    p. cirrhosis
    p. fibrosis
pipet (*var. of* pipette)
pipette, pipet
    air-displacement p.
    blowout p.
    Eppendorf Repeater Pro p.
    graduated p.
    HandyStep electronic repeating p.
    Labpette FX p.
    measuring p.
    Mohr p.
    Ostwald-Folin p.
    positive-placement p.
    serologic p.
    SoftGrip p.
    TC p.
    TD p.
    transfer p.
    volumetric p.
    washout p.
pipiens
    Culex p.
Piptocephalis
Piptoporus
Pirenella
Piricauda
piriform, pyriform
    p. sinus carcinoma
Piroplasma
Piroplasmida
piroplasmosis
Pirquet
    P. cutaneous tuberculin test
    P. reaction

PIS
    pulmonary intimal sarcoma
Pisano method
pisciphila
    Exophiala p.
Piscirickettsia salmonis
pisiform
pisiformis
    Taenia p.
Pisolithus
pisotriquetral
pistol
    starter p.
PIT
    plasma iron turnover
pit
    central p.
    clathrin-coated p.
    gastric p.
    Mantoux p.
    shuffle p.
    tubular p.
pitcher's elbow
pitch wart
pitch-worker's cancer
pith
Pithoascus langeronii
Pithomyces
pit-1 protein
PITR
    plasma iron turnover rate
Pitres section
pitting edema
Pitt-Rogers-Danks syndrome
pittsburgensis
    Legionella p.
Pittsburgh
    P. pneumonia
    P. pneumonia agent
    P. variant
pituicyte
pituicytoma
pituitaria
    glandula p.
pituitary
    p. adamantinoma
    p. adenoma
    p. ameloblastoma
    p. basophilia
    p. basophilism
    p. dwarf
    p. dwarfism
    p. dysfunction
    p. endocrine disorder
    p. function test
    p. gland
    Glenner-Lillie stain for p.
    p. glycoprotein hormone
    p. gonadotropic failure

p. gonadotropin
p. growth hormone (PGH)
hyaline body of p.
p. lactotroph
lyophilized anterior p. (LAP)
p. membrane
p. microprolactinoma
p. myxedema
posterior p.
p. stalk
p. stalk section
p. tumor
pituitary-like
anterior p.-l. (APL)
pituitosa
membrana p.
Sphingomonas p.
pityriasic
pityriasis
p. alba
p. capitis
p. lichenoides chronica
p. lichenoides et varioliformis acuta
(PLEVA)
p. nigra
p. rosea
p. rubra
p. rubra pilaris (PRP)
p. versicolor
Pityrosporum
P. furfur
P. orbiculare
P. ovale
P. versicolor
PIVKA
protein induced by vitamin K antagonist
pivotal transcription factor
pixel
pizza lung
Pizzolato peroxide-silver method
PK
Prausnitz-Küstner test
pyruvate kinase
PK deficiency
PK reaction
PKC
protein kinase C
PKC isoenzyme
PK110 centrifuge
PKD
polycystic kidney disease
proteinase K digestion
pKi67
nuclear proliferation marker p.
p57 KIP^2 expression
PKU test
PL
placebo
placental lactogen

PLA2
agonist-induced activation of
PLA2
PLAC coronary heart disease test
placebo (PL)
placei
Haemonchus p.
placenta, *pl.* **placentae,** *pl.* **placentas**
ablatio placentae
abruptio placentae
p. accreta
battledore p.
bilobate p.
p. circummarginata
circummarginate p.
circumvallate p.
dichorionic diamniotic p.
duplex p.
p. fenestrata
fenestrated p.
p. increta
mature abnormal p.
p. membranacea
monochorionic diamniotic p.
monochorionic monoamniotic p.
multilobate p.
p. multipartita
p. percreta
premature abnormal p.
prematurely separated p.
premature separation of p.
p. previa
p. previa abortion
p. spuria
p. succenturiata
p. triloba
trilobate p.
p. tripartita
twin p.
p. twins
placentae (*pl. of* placenta)
placental
p. abruption
p. alkaline phosphatase (PLAP)
p. and fetoplacental function tests
p. barrier
p. biopsy
p. disc margin
p. dysfunction
p. dysmaturity
p. hemangioma
p. hormone
p. lactogen (PL)
p. malperfusion
p. membrane
p. parenchyma
p. polyp
p. residual blood volume (PRBV)
p. site nodule and plaque (PSNP)

P

placental (*continued*)
    p. site trophoblastic tumor (PSTT)
    p. steroid sulfatase deficiency
    p. thrombosis
    p. transmogrification
    p. tuberculosis
placentas (*pl. of* placenta)
placentation
    p. bleeding
    circumvallate p.
    extrachorial p.
placentitis
placentoma
placentomegaly
plagarumbelli
    Diplococcus p.
plagiocephaly
Plagiorchiidae
Plagiorchioidea
Plagiorchis
plague
    p. aerosol
    p. bacillus
    black p.
    bubonic p.
    cattle p.
    cellulocutaneous p.
    duck p.
    fowl p.
    hemorrhagic p.
    p. meningitis
    pneumonic p.
    primary septicemic p.
    rabbit p.
    septicemic p.
    p. serum
    sylvatic p.
    urban p.
    p. vaccine
plakins
plakoglobin
plamare
    xanthoma striatum p.
plan
    Bioterrorism Readiness P.
    p. of care (POC)
plana (*pl. of* planum)
planar impact
Planck (*h*)
    P. constant (h)
    P. radiation law
Planctobacteria
Planctomycea
Planctomycetaceae
Planctomycetales
plane
    cleavage p.
    focal p.

    Meckel p.
    symmetry p.
    tangential p.
    p. wart
planimeter
    manual optic p.
plankter
plankton
planktonic
Planktothricoides raciborskii
planocellular
Planococcaceae
Planococcus
    P. alkanoclasticus
    P. antarcticus
    P. maitriensis
    P. maritimus
    P. psychrophilus
    P. rifietoensis
Planomicrobium
    P. koreense
    P. mcmeekinii
    P. okeanokoites
Planomonospora
planopilaris
    lichen p.
Planorbarius
planorbid
Planorbidae
Planorbis
plant
    p. agglutinin
    p. antitoxin
    p. estrogen
    p. indican
    p. pathogen
    p. protease test (PPT)
    p. toxin
    p. virus
Plantago major
plantar
    p. fascia fibromatosis
    p. wart
plantaris
    ichthyosis palmaris et p.
    keratoderma palmaris et p.
    keratosis palmaris et p.
    pustulosis palmaris et p.
    tylosis palmaris et p.
    verruca p.
plantarum
    Lactobacillus p.
Plantibacter flavus
planticola
    Raoultella p.
planum, *pl.* **plana**
    coxa plana
    normolipemic xanthoma p.
    p. semilunatum

verruca plana
xanthoma p.

planuria

planus

atrophic lichen p.
bullous lichen p.
hypertrophic lichen p.
lichen p. (LP)

PLAP

placental alkaline phosphatase

plaque

p. adhesion
amyloid p.
atheromatous p.
attachment p.'s
bacterial p.
beta-amyloid p.
cerebellar amyloid p.
dental p.
desmoplastic p.
endocardial p.
fibrofatty p.
Hollenhorst p.'s
hyaline p.
island-sparing p.'s
island-sparing p.
kuru p.
mucous p.
neuritic p.'s
placental site nodule and p. (PSNP)
pleural p.
Redlich-Fisher miliary p.'s
p. rupture
senile p.'s
talc p.'s
p. technique

plaque-forming

p.-f. cell (PFC)
p.-f. cell assay
p.-f. unit (PFU)

plaque-stage cutaneous T-cell lymphoma

plasm

plasma (P), plasm

p. accelerator globulin
p. activation
adsorbed p.
p. amino acid screening
p. ammonia
antihemophilic p.
antilymphocyte p. (ALP)
anti-*Pseudomonas* human p.
p. atrial natriuretic factor
p. bicarbonate
blood p.
p. blood cell
p. calcitonin
p. cell (PC)
p. cell angiofollicular lymph node
hyperplasia

p. cell antigen
p. cell dyscrasia
p. cell granuloma (PCG)
p. cell hepatitis (PCH)
p. cell infiltrate
p. cell leukemia
p. cell mastitis
p. cell mucositis
p. cell pneumonia
p. cell vulvitis
p. clearance
p. clearance rate (PCR)
p. clot solubility assay
p. clotting factor
p. clotting time
p. colloid oncotic pressure
p. cortisol test
cryoprecipitate-depleted p.
p. defect (PD)
p. depletion
p. DNA
p. exchange
extracellular p.
p. factor X
p. fibrinogen
p. fibronectin
fresh frozen p. (FFP)
frozen p. (FP)
p. glucagon
p. glucose disappearance rate
(PGDR)
p. glucose tolerance rate (PGTR)
p. hemoglobin test
p. inorganic iodine (PII)
p. insulin activity (PIA)
p. iodoprotein disorder
p. iron disappearance (PID)
p. iron disappearance time (PIDT)
p. iron turnover (PIT)
p. iron turnover rate (PITR)
p. kallikrein
p. kinin
p. labile factor
p. layer
lipid-associated sialic acid in p.
(LASA-P)
p. luteinizing hormone
lymphoid p. (LP)
p. marinum
p. membrane
p. membrane bleb
normal p. (NP)
normal human p.
p. oncotic pressure (POP)
platelet-free p. (PFP)
platelet-poor p. (PPP)
platelet-rich p. (PRP)
p. progesterone
p. protein

P

plasma (*continued*)
    p. protein fraction (PPF)
    p. protein profile
    psoralen-treated pooled p.
    p. renin activity (PRA)
    salted p.
    SD p.
    single-donor p.
    p. sodium (P_{Na})
    p. stain
    p. substitute
    p. therapy
    p. thrombin clot method
    p. thrombin time
    p. thromboplastin antecedent (PTA)
    p. thromboplastin antecedent
      deficiency
    p. thromboplastin component (PTC)
    p. thromboplastin factor (PTF)
    p. thromboplastin factor B
    p. triglyceride
    urea nitrogen or p.
    p. volume (PV)
    p. volume expander
plasma-acetaminophen level
plasmablast
plasma-cell
    p.-c. labeling index
    p.-c. myeloma
plasmacrit test
plasmacyte
plasmacytic
    p. blood cell
    p. infiltrate
    p. leukemia
    p. myeloma
    p. tumor
plasmacytoblast
plasmacytoid
    p. differentiation
    p. lymphocyte
    p. lymphoma
    p. monocyte
plasmacytoma, plasmocytoma
    extramedullary solitary p. (EMP)
    extraosseous p.
plasmacytosis
plasmagene
plasmalemma
plasmalemmal
    p. invagination
    p. pattern
plasmalogen
plasmal reaction
plasmapheresis
plasmarrhexis
plasmatic
    p. insudation
    p. stain

plasmatogamy (*var. of* plasmogamy)
Plasmavirus
plasmic stain
plasmid
    bacteriocinogenic p.
    conjugative p.
    F p.
    p. fingerprinting
    infectious p.
    p. integration
    nonconjugative p.
    oligomeric p.
    R p.
    resistance p.
    rough p.
    p. transfer
    transmissible p.
    p. vector
plasmin
    p. coagulation
    p. prothrombin conversion factor
      (PPCF)
plasminogen
    p. activator
    p. activator deficiency
    p. activator inhibitor (PAI)
    p. activator inhibitor assay
    p. activator inhibitor I, II
plasminogen-plasmin activator
  system
plasminokinase
plasminoplastin
plasmocrine vacuole
plasmocyte
plasmocytic leukemoid
  reaction
plasmocytoma (*var. of*
  plasmacytoma)
plasmodial
Plasmodiidae
Plasmodium
    P. aethiopicum
    P. berghei
    P. brazilianum
    P. cynomolgi
    P. falciparum
    P. knowlesi
    P. kochi
    P. malariae
    P. ovale
    P. pleurodyniae
    P. vivax
    P. vivax minuta
Plasmodromata
plasmogamy, plastogamy,
  plasmatogamy
plasmogen
plasmoid humor
plasmolysis

plasmolytic
plasmolyze
plasmon
plasmoptysis
plasmorrhexis
plasmoschisis
plasmosin
plasmotomy
plasmotropic
plasmotropism
plasmotype
plasmozyme
plastic
    p. bronchitis
    p. corpuscle
    p. induration
    p. lymph
    p. pleurisy
    p. section stain
plastica
    linitis p.
plasticity
    adult stem cell p.
plasticizer
plastid
    blood p.
plastogamy (*var. of* plasmogamy)
plate
    Abbé test p.
    blood agar p. (BAP)
    chorionic p.
    colorimetric microtiter p. (CMP)
    cough p.
    counting p.
    Covalink MicroElisa culture p.
    p. culture
    decidual p.
    ductal p.
    DyNA block 1000 microtiter p.
    Dynex Immulon 1B microtiter p.
    end p.
    epiphysial p.
    flood p.
    foot p.
    growth p.
    Hospidex microtiter p.
    Kühne terminal p.
    lateral cartilaginous p.
    lawn p.
    Lowenstein-Jensen p.
    Maxisorp microtiter p.
    medial cartilaginous p.
    metaphase p.
    microtiter p.
    motor end p.
    nail p.
    polar p.'s
    pour p.
    Pro-Bind U-Bottom microfilter p.

    Sensititre *Streptococcus pneumoniae*
     HPB susceptibility p.
    spiral p.
    spread p.
    streak p.
    tarsal p.'s
    theoretical p.
    p. thrombosis
platelet
    acquired qualitative disorders of p.'s
    p. actomyosin
    p. adhesion test
    p. adhesiveness test
    p. agglutination
    p. agglutinin
    p. aggregation
    p. aggregation test
    p. antiaggregant
    p. antibody
    apheresis p.
    p. autoantibody
    Bizzozero p.
    p. cofactor
    p. concentrate
    p. count (PC)
    p. defect (PLD)
    p. distribution width
    p. factor 1–4
    p. fibrinogen receptor GPIIb IIIa
    p. function analyzer (PFA)
    p. function test
    giant p.
    p. GPIIb/IIIa
    hemolysis, elevated liver enzymes,
     and low p.'s (HELLP)
    in vivo adhesive p. (IVAP)
    p. isoantibody
    leukocyte-reduced p.'s
    p. lumiaggregation
    p. membrane glycoprotein
    p. neutralization procedure
    p. pellet
    p. phase
    p. phospholipid complex
    p. plug
    p. receptor GPIIb IIIa
    p. retention test
    p. satellitism
    single-donor p.'s
    p. sizing
    spent p.
    splenic sequestration of p.'s
    p. survival test
    p. thrombosis
    p. thrombus
    p. tissue factor
    p. transfusion
    vacuolated p.
    p. von Willebrand receptor GP1b

P

platelet-activating
    p.-a. factor (PAF)
    p.-a. factor acetylhydrolase
    (PAF-AH)
platelet-aggregating factor (PAF)
platelet-associated bacteremia
**platelet-derived growth factor
  (PDGF)**
platelet-free plasma (PFP)
plateletpheresis
platelet-poor
    p.-p. blood (PPB)
    p.-p. plasma (PPP)
platelet-refractory state
platelet-rich plasma (PRP)
platelet-type von Willebrand disease
platelike
**PlateTrak automated microplate
  processing system**
platform
    Rapid Analyte Measurement P.
    (RAMP)
plating density
platinosis
platinum group
platybasia
platycyte
platyhelminth
Platyhelminthes
platykurtic
Platynosomum fastosum
platys
    Anaplasma p.
plauti-vincentii
    Fusobacterium p.-v.
PLC
  pleomorphic lobular carcinoma
PLCIS
  pleomorphic lobular carcinoma in situ
  of the breast
PLD
  platelet defect
pleated sheet
plebeius
    Vaginulus p.
plecoglossicida
    Pseudomonas p.
plectonemic coil
Plectosphaerella cucumerina
Plectrovirus
Pleiochaeta
pleiomorpha
    Acrocarpospora p.
pleiotropia (*var. of* pleiotropy)
pleiotropic mutation
pleiotropy, pleiotropia
Pleistophora
pleocellular
pleochroic

pleochroism
pleochromatic
pleochromatism
pleocytosis
  neutrophilic p.
pleokaryocyte
pleomorpha
    Cryptomyces p.
pleomorphic
  p. adenoma (PA)
  p. binucleated giant cell
  p. fibroma
  p. hyalinizing angiectatic tumor
    (PHAT)
  p. leiomyosarcoma
  p. lipoma
  p. lobular carcinoma (PLC)
  p. lobular carcinoma in situ of the
    breast (PLCIS)
  p. mononucleated giant cell
  p. nucleus
  p. oligodendroglioma
  p. rhabdomyosarcoma
  p. sarcoma
  p. xanthoastrocytoma (PXA)
pleomorphism
  cytonuclear p.
pleonosteosis
  Leri p.
Pleospora herbarum
plerocercoid
plerocercus
Plesiocystis pacifica
Plesiomonas shigelloides
pleural
  p. biopsy
  p. calculus
  p. effusion
  p. fibrin ball
  p. fibroma
  p. fibrosis
  p. fluid
  p. fluid examination
  p. friction rub
  p. mesothelioma
  p. plaque
  p. tuberculosis
  p. villi
pleurales
  villi p.
pleurisy
  adhesive p.
  benign dry p.
  costal p.
  diaphragmatic p.
  dry p.
  encysted p.
  epidemic benign dry p.
  fibrinous p.

hemorrhagic p.
interlobular p.
plastic p.
productive p.
proliferating p.
pulmonary p.
purulent p.
sacculated p.
serofibrinous p.
serous p.
suppurative p.
visceral p.
wet p.
pleuritic
pleuritis
acute fibrinous p.
fibrinous acute p.
lupus p.
obliterative p.
reactive eosinophilic p. (REP)
pleuritogenous
Pleurocapsales
Pleuroceridae
pleurodesis
pleurodynia
epidemic p.
pleurodyniae
Plasmodium p.
pleurogenous
pleurohepatitis
pleurolith
pleuropericarditis
Pleurophoma pleurospora
Pleurophragmium
pleuropneumonia
contagious bovine p.
pleuropneumonia-like organism
(PPLO)
pleuropulmonary blastoma
pleurorrhea
pleurospora
Pleurophoma p.
Pleurotellus
Pleurotus
PLEVA
pityriasis lichenoides et varioliformis
acuta
plexiform
p. fibrohistiocytic tumor of
childhood
p. layer
p. lesion
p. neurofibroma
p. neuroma
p. schwannoma
p. unicystic ameloblastoma
Plexiglas
plexitis
brachial p.

plexogenic
p. pulmonary
p. pulmonary arteriopathy
plexopathy
idiopathic brachial p.
plexosarcoma
plexus, *pl.* **plexus, plexuses**
Auerbach p.
Batson p.
choroid p.
Henle p.
Meissner p.
myenteric p.
neuron of myenteric nerve p.
plexuses (*pl. of* plexus)
PLGA
polymorphous low-grade
adenocarcinoma
PLH
pulmonary lymphoid hyperplasia
plica, *pl.* **plicae**
plicae ciliares
plicae circulares
plicae circulares intestini tenuis
spiral p.
plicae (*pl. of* plica)
plicate
plicatilis
Spirochaeta p.
Plicatura
P1-like viruses
P2-like viruses
P4-like viruses
P22-like viruses
Plimmer body
PLL
prolymphocytic leukemia
ploidy
p. analysis
DNA p.
plot
Scatchard p.
time-series p.
Ploton staining method
plotter
PLS
prostaglandin-like substance
PLT
psittacosis-lymphogranuloma venereum
trachoma
PLT group virus
plucked-chicken appearance
plug
adherent p.
carpet tack follicular keratotic p.
Dittrich p.
Ecker p.
fibrin-linked platelet p.
fibrous p.

P

plug (*continued*)
  mucous p.
  platelet p.
  primary platelet p.
  Traube p.
plumbism
plumboporphyria
Plummer
  P. adenoma
  P. disease
Plummer-Vinson syndrome
plumose
plump cell
pluranimalium
  Arcanobacterium p.
pluricentric blastoma
pluriglandular adenomatosis
plurihormonal adenoma
plurilobulated shape
plurilocular
plurinuclear
pluriorificialis
  ectodermosis erosiva p.
pluripotent, pluripotential
  p. hematopoietic stem cell
  p. myeloid stem cell
  p. primitive mesodermal cell
pluripotential (*var. of* pluripotent)
  p. basal cell
  p. hemopoietic stem cell
  p. stromal cell
pluriresistant
plus
  Decal P.
  p. strand
Pluteus
plutonium
plymuthica
  Serratia p.
plywood pattern
PLZF
  promyelocytic leukemia zinc finger
PM
  polymorphic
  postmortem
PMB
  polymorphonuclear basophil
PMC
  pseudomembranous colitis
PMD
  primary myocardial disease
  progressive muscular dystrophy
PME
  polymorphonuclear eosinophil
PMEC
  pseudomembranous enterocolitis
***p*-methoxyamphetamine assay**
PMF
  progressive massive fibrosis

PMI
  postmortem interval
PML
  progressive multifocal
    leukoencephalopathy
  promyelocytic leukemia
PMLS
  primary mediastinal large cell
    lymphoma with sclerosis
PMMA
  polymethylmethacrylate
PMN
  polymorphonuclear neutrophil
PMP
  postmenopausal
    PMP woman
PMP22 gene
PMR
  polymorphic reticulosis
  proportionate morbidity ratio
  proportionate mortality ratio
PMS
  postmitochondrial supernatant
  pregnant mare serum
PMSG
  pregnant mare serum gonadotropin
PMS-1, -2 gene
PMT
  pseudosarcomatous myofibroblastic
    tumor
PN
  pneumonia
  polyarteritis nodosa
  pyelonephritis
PNA probe
PNEC
  pulmonary neuroendocrine cell
PNET
  primitive neuroectodermal
    tumor
pneumarthrosis
pneumatic
pneumatinuria (*var. of* pneumaturia)
pneumatization
pneumatocele
pneumatoides
  cystitis p.
pneumatosis
  p. cystoides intestinalis
    (PCI)
  p. intestinalis cystica
pneumaturia, pneumatinuria
pneumobacillus
  Friedländer p.
pneumocephalus
pneumococcal
  p. pneumonia
  p. polysaccharide
  p. vaccine

pneumococcemia
pneumococcidal
pneumococcolysis
pneumococcosuria
pneumococcus
pneumoconioses (*pl. of* pneumoconiosis)
pneumoconiosis, pneumokoniosis, *pl.*
  pneumoconioses
    antimony p.
    bauxite p.
    coal worker's p. (CWP)
    endogenous p.
    fuller' s earth p.
    graphite p.
    hematite p.
    kaolin p.
    mica p.
    mixed dust p.
    noncollagenous p.
    polyvinyl chloride p.
    rheumatoid p.
    p. siderotica
    talc p.
    titanium dioxide p.
    tungsten carbide p.
pneumocystiasis
Pneumocystis
    P. carinii
    P. carinii pneumonia
    P. fluorescence
    P. jiroveci
    P. pneumoniae
pneumocystosis
pneumocyte
    granular p.
    type 1 p.
    type 2 p.
pneumoderma
pneumogenic osteoarthropathy
pneumohemopericardium
pneumohemothorax
pneumohydroperitoneum
pneumohydrothorax
pneumohypoderma
pneumokoniosis (*var. of* pneumoconiosis)
pneumolith
pneumolithiasis
pneumomalacia
pneumomediastinum
pneumomycosis, pneumonomycosis
pneumonectomy evaluation
pneumonia (PN)
    Acinetobacter p.
    acute gelatinous p.
    acute interstitial p. (AIP)
    alcoholic p.
    anaerobic p.
    anthrax p.
    aspiration p.

atypical primary p.
Bacteroides p.
bronchial p.
bronchiolitis obliterans organizing p.
  (BOOP)
Candida p.
caseous p.
central p.
chemical p.
chlamydial p.
chronic eosinophilic p. (CEP)
confluent p.
core p.
cryptogenic organizing p. (COP)
desquamative interstitial p. (DIP)
diffuse interstitial p.
p. dissecans
double p.
Eaton agent p.
Enterobacter p.
eosinophilic p.
Escherichia coli p.
exogenous lipid p.
fibrinous acute lobar p.
focal p.
Friedländer bacillus p.
fungal p.
gangrenous p.
gelatinous acute p.
giant cell interstitial p. (GIP)
glanders p.
Haemophilus influenzae p.
Hecht p.
hemorrhagic lobar p.
hospital-acquired gram-negative p.
hypostatic p.
inhalation p.
p. interlobularis
p. interlobularis purulenta
interstitial giant cell p.
interstitial plasma cell p.
Klebsiella p.
lipid p.
lipoid p.
lobar p.
lobular p.
Louisiana p.
lymphocytic interstitial p. (LIP)
lymphoid interstitial p. (LIP)
p. malleosa
measles virus p.
metastatic p.
migratory p.
moniliasis p.
mycoplasmal p.
necrotizing lobar p.
nonspecific interstitial p. (NSIP)
nosocomial p.
oil-aspiration p.

P

pneumonia (*continued*)
  organized p.
  ovine progressive p.
  Pittsburgh p.
  plasma cell p.
  pneumococcal p.
  Pneumocystis carinii p.
  primary atypical p. (PAP)
  primary influenza virus p.
  Proteus p.
  pseudomonal p.
  Q fever p.
  rheumatic p.
  secondary eosinophilic p.
  septic p.
  severe atypical p.
  staphylococcal p.
  streptococcal p.
  suppurative p.
  tularemia p.
  p. tularemia
  tularemic p.
  unresolved lobar p.
  uremic p.
  usual interstitial p. (UIP)
  ventilator-associated p.
  viral p.
  p. virus of mice (PVM)
  wandering p.
  white p.
  woolsorter's p.
pneumoniae
  Bacillus p.
  Chlamydia p.
  Chlamydophila p.
  Diplococcus p.
  Klebsiella p.
  Miyagawanella p.
  Mycoplasma p.
  Pneumocystis p.
  Streptococcus p.
pneumonia/fibrosis
  nonspecific interstitial p.
pneumonic
  p. plague
  p. tularemia
pneumonitis
  Ascaris p.
  aspiration p.
  chemical p.
  desquamative interstitial p. (DIP)
  eosinophilic p.
  herpes p.
  hypersensitivity p.
  interstitial p.
  lymphocytic interstitial p. (LIP)
  measles p.
  nonspecific interstitial p. (NSIP)
  occupational hypersensitivity p.

  organizing p.
  pulmonary p.
  radiation p.
  rheumatic p.
  uremic p.
  usual interstitial p. (UIP)
  p. virus
pneumonocyte
  granular p.
pneumonomoniliasis
pneumonomycosis (*var. of* pneumomycosis)
Pneumonyssus simicola
pneumoparotitis
pneumoperitoneum
pneumoperitonitis
pneumophila
  Legionella p.
pneumopleuritis
pneumoretroperitoneum
pneumoscrotum
pneumoserothorax
pneumosintes
  Bacteroides p.
  Dialister p.
pneumothoraces (*pl. of* pneumothorax)
pneumothorax (PT), *pl.* **pneumothoraces**
  spontaneous p.
  therapeutic p.
pneumotropica
Pneumovirus
pneumovirus
p-**nitro-alpha-acetylamino-beta-hydroxy-**
  propiophenone
p-**nitrophenylic acid**
p-**nitrosulfathiazole**
PNN
  probabilistic neural network
pnomenusa
PNP
  purine nucleoside phosphorylase
  PNP deficiency
p80NPM/ALK antibody
PNU
  protein nitrogen unit
P:O
  ratio of number of ATPs produced to
  number of atmospheric oxygen
  molecules converted to water
Po
  polonium
poae
  Leifsonia p.
POC
  plan of care
  point of care
PocketChem
  P. UA
  P. UA analyzer
pocket dosimeter

pocketed calculus
POCT
    point-of-care testing
poculum
POD
    polycystic ovary disease
podagra
podarthritis
podedema
Pod1 gene
poditis
podocalyxin
    p. gene
    p. protein
podocyte foot process
podophyllin resin
podoplanin
    p. expression
    p. staining
Podospora
Podoviridae
poeciloides
    Eubacterium p.
Po$_2$electrode
POEMS
    polyneuropathy, organomegaly, endocrinopathy, monoclonal gammopathy, and skin changes
    POEMS syndrome
POES
    polyoxyethylene stearate
    POES additive
Pogonomyrmex
POG surgicopathologic staging system
POGTD
    primary ovarian gestational trophoblastic disease
pOH
    hydroxyl concentration
poietin
POIK
    poikilocyte
poikiloblast
poikilocyte (POIK)
    tail p.
poikilocythemia
poikilocytosis
poikiloderma
    p. atrophicans and cataract
    p. atrophicans vasculare
    p. congenitale
    p. of Civatte
poikilodermatomyositis
poikilothrombocyte
point
    Boas p.
    boiling p. (bp)
    clinical end p.
    cold rigor p.

    p. counting method
    p. de repere (point of reference)
    end p.
    equivalence p.
    p. estimate
    freezing p. (FP)
    Griffith p.
    growing p.
    ice p.
    ignition p.
    isoelectric p.
    isosbestic p.
    Krafft p.
    McEwen p.
    melting p. (MP)
    p. mutation
    p. of care (POC)
    p. of care INR testing
    p. of inflection
    p. of ossification
    radix p.
    Ramond p.
    Robson p.
    set p.
    Staller p.
    Sudeck p.
    thermal death p.
    triple p.
pointed
    p. condyloma
    p. wart
pointer variable
pointes
    torsade de p.
point-of-care testing (POCT)
Poirier gland
poise
Poiseuille
    P. law
    P. space
poison
    P. Control Center
    industrial p.
    mitotic p.
poisoning
    acetanilid p.
    amobarbital p.
    antimony p.
    arsenic p.
    aspirin p.
    benzene p.
    blood p.
    carbon disulfide p.
    carbon monoxide p.
    carbon tetrachloride p.
    chloroform p.
    cyanide p.
    desquamative interstitial p.
    enzymatic p.

P

poisoning (*continued*)
 ethyl alcohol p.
 ethylene glycol p.
 food p.
 heavy metal p.
 lead p.
 manganese p.
 mercury p.
 methanol p.
 methotrexate p.
 methyl alcohol p.
 mushroom p.
 naphthol p.
 nitroaniline p.
 oxygen p.
 salmonella p.
 scombroid p.
 systemic p.
 tetrachloroethane p.
 thallium p.
Poisson distribution
Poisson-Pearson formula
poker spine
pokeweed mitogen (PWM)
Poland syndrome
polar
 p. anemia
 p. body
 p. cell
 p. compound
 p. coordinates
 p. globule
 p. lesion
 p. plates
polarimeter
polarimetry
polaris
 Glaciecola p.
 Kocuria p.
polarity
 cell p.
 nuclear p.
polarizability
polarization fluoroimmunoassay
polarize
polarized
 p. light
 p. microscopy
polarizer
polarizing microscope
polarogram
polarography
Polaromonas naphthalenivorans
polecki
 Entamoeba p.
Polerovirus
pol gene
Polhemus-Schafer-Ivemark syndrome
policeman

 p. glass stirring rod
 rubber p.
 p. tip
 p. transfer tool
polio
 poliomyelitis
polioclastic
poliodystrophia cerebri progressiva infantilis
poliodystrophy
 progressive cerebral p.
polioencephalitis infectiva
poliomyelitis (polio)
 acute anterior p.
 acute bulbar p.
 anterior acute p.
 p. I–III titer
 p. immune globulin (human)
 immunization reaction p.
 p. immunoglobulin
 late effect p.
 p. vaccine
 p. virus
 virus p.
poliovirus
 p. hominis
 p. vaccine
Polistes
polka
 p. dot pattern
 p. fever
polkissen of Zimmermann
Pollacia
pollen
 p. antigen
 p. extract
Pollenia
pollenosis (*var. of* pollinosis)
pollinosis, pollenosis
polocyte
polonica
 Bilharziella p.
polonium (Po)
polster
 Sanderson p.
polyA
 polyadenylic acid
 polyA tail
polyacrylamide
 p. gel
 p. gel electrophoresis (PAGE)
polyadenitis
polyadenopathy
polyadenosis
polyadenylate tail
polyadenylation
polyadenylic acid (polyA)
poly-ADP-ribose-polymerase enzyme

polyagglutination
polyamide
polyamine
polyamine-methylene resin
polyanetholsulfonate
Polyangiaceae
polyangiitis
    microscopic p.
polyanion
polyarteritis nodosa
  (PAN, PN)
polyarthritis
    p. chronica
    p. chronica villosa
    epidemic p.
    migratory p.
    p. rheumatica acuta
    vertebral p.
polybasic acid
polyblast
polyC
    polycytidylic acid
polycarbonate
polycationic dye
polycentric
Poly-Chem automated
  chemistry-immunoassay system
polychlorinated
    p. biphenyl (PCB)
    p. biphenyl assay
polychondritis
    chronic atrophic p.
    relapsing p.
polychromasia
polychromatia
polychromatic
    p. cell
    p. normoblast
polychromatocyte
polychromatocytosis
polychromatophil, polychromatophile
    p. cell
polychromatophile (*var. of*
  polychromatophil)
polychromatophilia
polychromatophilic
    p. erythroblast
    p. megaloblast
    p. normoblast
    p. rubricyte
polychromatosis
polychrome
    p. methylene blue
    p. methylene blue stain
polychromemia
polychromia
polychromophil
polychromophilia
polyclave

polyclonal
    p. activator
    p. anticarcinoembryonic antigen
    p. antiplacental antibody
    p. anti-S-100 protein
    p. carcinoembryonic antigen
    (pCEA)
    p. gammopathy
    p. hypergammaglobulinemia
    p. lymphoid proliferation
    p. pattern
    p. prolactin antibody
    p. tumor
polyclonality
polycomb group
polycyclic aromatic hydrocarbon
polycystic
    p. change
    p. kidney disease (PKD)
    p. liver
    p. liver disease
    p. ovary (PCO)
    p. ovary disease (POD)
    p. ovary syndrome
    p. renal disease
polycystin-1
Polycytella hominis
polycythemia
    absolute p.
    compensatory p.
    familial p.
    p. hypertonica
    myelopathic p.
    relative p.
    p. rubra
    p. rubra vera (PRV)
    secondary p.
    smoker's p.
    splenomegalic p.
    p. vera (PCV, PV)
polycythemica
    hypertonia p.
    polyemia p.
polycytidylic acid (polyC)
polycytokeratin
polycytosis
polydactyly
polydeoxyribonucleotide
  synthetase
polydermatomyositis
Polydesmus
polydimethylsiloxane (PDM)
polydysplasia
polydystrophia
polydystrophic dwarfism
polydystrophy
    pseudo-Hurler p.
polyelectrolyte
polyembryony

P

polyemia
    p. aquosa
    p. hyperalbuminosa
    p. polycythemica
    p. serosa
polyendocrine
    p. adenomatosis
    p. autoimmune disease
polyendosporus
    Anaerobacter p.
polyene antibiotic
polyenoic acid
polyester resin
polyether sulfone filters
polyethylene
    p. glycol (PEG)
    p. glycol precipitation assay
    p. terephthalate (PETG)
polygenic inheritance
polyglandular
polyglutamine
    p. disease
    p. expansion disorder
polygon
    frequency p.
polygonal cell
polygyny
polygyria
polyhedral
    p. body
    p. cell
polyhedron
    face of p. (P)
polyhelminthism
PolyHeme blood substitute
polyhydramnios
    maternal p.
polyhydric alcohol
polyisoprenivorans
    Gordonia p.
polykaryocyte
    Warthin-Finkeldey-type p.
polykaryon
polyleptic fever
polylysine
polymastia, polymazia
polymastigote
polymazia (*var. of* polymastia)
polymer
    addition p.
    condensation p.
    polymethylmethacrylate p.
    rod-shaped p.
    vinyl p.
polymerase
    p. chain reaction (PCR)
    p. chain reaction amplification
    p. chain reaction-based identity
      testing

    p. chain reaction-restriction fragment
      length polymorphism (PCR-RFLP)
    p. chain reaction-single-strand
      conformation polymorphism
      (PCR-SSCP)
    DNA p.
    nucleotide p.
    Promega Taq DNA p.
    RNA p.
    p. slippage
    p. slippage model
    Taq deoxyribonucleic acid p. (taq
      DNA polymerase)
polymerization
    actin-filament p.
    cytoskeletal p.
polymerization-dependent amplification
polymerize
polymetaphosphate
polymethine dye
polymethylmethacrylate (PMMA)
    p. cement
    p. polymer
polymicrobial culture
polymicrogyria
polymicrolipomatosis
polymitus
polymorph
polymorpha
    Mima p.
polymorphe
    erythema p.
polymorphic
    p. B-cell lymphoma
    p. epithelial mucin (PEM)
    p. genetic marker
    p. light eruption
    p. reticulosis (PMR)
polymorphism
    balanced p.
    cleavase fragment length p.
      (CFLP)
    lipoprotein p.
    microsatellite p.
    NanoChip test for factor V Leiden
      single-nucleotide p.
    polymerase chain reaction-restriction
      fragment length p. (PCR-RFLP)
    polymerase chain
      reaction-single-strand conformation
      p. (PCR-SSCP)
    restriction fragment length p.
      (RFLP)
    single nucleotide p. (SNP)
    single-stranded conformation p.
      (SSCP)
polymorphocellular
polymorphocyte
polymorphocytic leukemia

polymorphonuclear
    p. basophil (PMB)
    p. eosinophil (PME)
    filament p.
    p. granulocyte
    p. leukocyte
    p. leukocytic infiltrate
    p. neutrophil (PMN)
    p. neutrophil chemotactic factor
polymorphonuclear-lymphocyte ratio
polymorphous
    p. dermatitis
    p. eruption
    p. layer
    p. low-grade adenocarcinoma (PLGA)
    p. lymphoid infiltrate
polymyalgia
    p. arteritica
    p. rheumatica
polymyopathy
    alcoholic p.
polymyositis
polymyxa
    Bacillus p.
polymyxin
    p. B sulfate
    p. E
    p. test agar
polynesic
polynesiensis
    Aedes p.
polyneural
polyneuritic-type hypertrophic muscular atrophy
polyneuritiformis
    heredopathia atactia p. (HAP)
polyneuritis
    acute idiopathic p.
    idiopathic p.
    infectious p.
polyneuropathy
    chronic inflammatory demyelinating p. (CIDP)
    polyneuropathy, organomegaly, endocrinopathy, monoclonal gammopathy, and skin changes (POEMS)
polynuclear
    p. leukocyte
polynucleate
polynucleolar
polynucleosis
polynucleotide ligase
polyol
    p. dehydrogenase
    p. pathway
polyolefin
polyoma virus
Polyomavirus

polyonchosis (*var. of* polyoncosis)
polyoncosis, polyonchosis
    cutaneomandibular p.
polyorchidism (*var. of* polyorchism)
polyorchism, polyorchidism
polyostotic fibrous dysplasia
polyovular ovarian follicle
polyoxyethylene stearate (POES)
polyp
    adenomatous p.
    aural p.
    bladder p.
    bleeding p.
    bronchial p.
    cardiac p.
    cellular p.
    cervical p.
    choanal p.
    cholesterol p.
    cloacogenic p.
    cockscomb p.
    colon p.
    colorectal p.
    Cronkhite-Canada p.
    cystic p.
    decidual p.
    endometrial p.
    familial juvenile p. (FJP)
    fibrinous p.
    fibroepithelial p.
    fibrous p.
    fleshy p.
    gallbladder p.
    gastric p.
    gelatinous p.
    granulomatous p.
    hamartomatous p.
    hydatid p.
    hyperplastic p.
    inflammatory p.
    juvenile p.
    laryngeal p.
    lipomatous p.
    lymphangiomatous p. (LAP)
    lymphoid p.
    metaplastic p.
    mucous p.
    multiple adenomatous p.'s
    myomatous p.
    nasal p.
    osseous p.
    placental p.
    postinflammatory p.
    regenerative p.
    retention p.
    serrated colorectal p.
    sessile p.
    small intestine p.
    sporadic adenomatous p. (SAP)

P

polyp (*continued*)
    umbilical p.
    vascular p.
    villous p.
    vocal fold p.
Polypaecilum insolutum
polyparasitism
polypeptide
    adrenocorticotropic p. (ACTP)
    amylin p.
    p. coding
    gastric inhibitory p. (GIP)
    islet amyloid p. (IAPP)
    keratin p.
    neurofilament triplet p.
     (NFP)
    TnC p.
    TnI p.
    TnT p.
    vasoactive intestinal p. (VIP)
polyphaga
    Acanthamoeba p.
polyphase
polyphasic wave
polyphemus
    Limulus p.
polyphenism
polyphenotypia
polyphenotypic profile
polypheny
polyphosphoric acid
polyphyletic theory
polyphyletism
polypiform (*var. of* polypoid)
polyplasmia
Polyplax
Polyplis
polyploid
polyploidy
polypnea
polypoid, polypiform
    p. adenocarcinoma
    p. adenoma
    p. cystitis
    p. excrescence
    p. hyperplasia
    p. intraluminal projection
polyporous
Polyporus
polyposa
    enteritis p.
    gastritis cystica p.
polyposis
    attenuated familial adenomatous p.
    p. coli
    familial p.
    familial adenomatous p. (FAP)
    familial intestinal p.
    lymphomatoid p.

    multiple intestinal p.
    multiple lymphomatous p.
polypous
    p. endocarditis
    p. gastritis
polypropylene
polyptychial
polypus
polypyrrylmethane
polyradiculitis
polyradiculoneuritis
polyradiculoneuropathy
polyradiculopathy
polyribosome
    disaggregation of membrane-bound
     p.'s
polysaccharide
    cryptococcal p.
    pneumococcal p.
    specific soluble p.
polysaccharolyticum
    Thermoanaerobacterium p.
polyserositis
    familial paroxysmal p.
    familial recurrent p.
polysialic acid
polysinusitis
polysomaty
polysome
polysomic
polysomy
polysorbate
polyspermia (*var. of* polyspermy)
polyspermism (*var. of* polyspermy)
polyspermy, polyspermia,
  polyspermism
Polysphondylium
polysplenia syndrome
Polystictus
polystyrene
    oxygen-modified p.
polysynaptic
Polytech 2000 laboratory information
  system
polytendinitis
polytene chromosome
polyteny
polytetrafluoroethylene
polytopic effect
polytoxicomania
polytoxicomaniac syndrome
polytypic
polyU
    polyuridylic acid
polyunsaturated fatty acid (PUFA)
polyunsaturated-to-saturated fatty acids
  ratio (P:S)
polyurethane (PU)
polyuric

polyuridylic acid (polyU)
polyvalent
    p. allergy
    p. antiserum
    p. serum
    p. vaccine
polyvesicular
    p. vitelline
    p. vitelline tumor
polyvinyl
    p. alcohol (PVA)
    p. alcohol fixative method
    p. chloride (PVC)
    p. chloride pneumoconiosis
polyvinylpyrrolidone
polyvisceral echinococcosis
polyzoic
Pomatiopsis
pombe
    Schizosaccharomyces p.
POMC
    proopiomelanocortin
    POMC neuron
POMC-derived anorexic peptide
pomeroyi
    Silicibacter p.
    Vibrio p.
pomona
    Leptospira p.
pomorum
    Alicyclobacillus p.
Pomovirus
Pompe disease
ponceau de xylidine
Poncet disease
Ponfick shadow
ponos
Pontamine sky blue stain
Pontiac fever
pontiacus
    Sulfitobacter p.
pontile, pontine
pontine (*var. of* pontile)
    p. angle tumor
    cerebellar p.
pontis
    basis p.
pontomedullary
pool
    circulating p.
    circulating granulocyte p. (CGP)
    gene p.
    marginal granulocyte p. (MGP)
    marginating p.
    metabolic p.
    rapidly miscible p. (RMP)
    total blood granulocyte p.
    (TBGP)
    vaginal p.

pooled
    p. blood serum
    p. estimate
poorly
    p. compliant bladder
    p. differentiated (PD)
    p. differentiated carcinoma
    p. differentiated lymphocytic
    lymphoma (PDLL)
POP
    plasma oncotic pressure
popcorn
    p. cell
    p. nuclei
popliteal aneurysm
pop-off technique
popper
    amyl nitrite p.
population
    p. biology
    p. cytogenetics
    disomic p.
    p. dispersion
    p. genetics
    null cell p.
    p. sample (PS)
    tumor cell p.
por1 adenocarcinoma
por2 adenocarcinoma
porcelain gallbladder
porcina
    Hespellia p.
porcine
    p. adenovirus
    p. hemagglutinating encephalomyelitis
    virus
    p. transmissible gastroenteritis
porcinum
    Bifidobacterium thermacidophilum
    subsp. *p.*
porcinus
    Enterococcus p.
porcupine skin
pore, porus
    alveolar p.
    gustatory p.
    interalveolar p.
    Kohn p.
    nuclear p.
    slit p.
    sweat p.
    taste p.
porencephalia (*var. of* porencephaly)
porencephalic, porencephalous
porencephalitis
porencephalous (*var. of* porencephalic)
porencephaly, porencephalia
Porges-Meier test
Porges-Salomon test

P

Poria
Porifera
pork tapeworm
porocarcinoma
porocele
porocephaliasis
Porocephalidae
Porocephalus
    P. armillatus
    P. clavatus
    P. constrictus
    P. denticulatus
poroconidium
porokeratosis
    actinic p.
    disseminated superficial actinic p.
      (DSAP)
    Mibelli p. (MP)
poroma
    eccrine p.
Poronia
porosis
    cerebral p.
porosity
porospore
porotic
porous
porphin, porphine
porphine (*var. of* porphin)
porphobilinogen (PBG)
    p. deaminase (PBG-D)
    p. deaminase deficiency
    p. synthase (PBG-S)
    p. synthase assay
    p. synthase deficiency
    p. test
    urine p.
porphyria
    acquired hepatic p.
    acute intermittent p. (AIP)
    chemical p.
    congenital erythropoietic p. (CEP)
    p. cutanea tarda (PCT)
    p. cutanea tarda hereditaria
    erythrohepatic p.
    erythropoietic p.
    hepatic p.
    hepatoerythropoietic p. (HEP)
    latent p.
    South African-type p.
    symptomatic p.
    variegate p.
porphyrin
    alpha p.
    p. assay
    erythropoietic p.
    fecal p.
    fractionated erythrocyte p.
    p. pigmentation

    stool p.
    p. synthesis
    p. test
    urine p.
porphyrinuria, porphyruria
Porphyrobacter
    P. cryptus
    P. sanguineus
Porphyromonas
    P. asaccharolytica
    P. catoniae
porphyruria (*var. of* porphyrinuria)
porrigo
    p. favosa
    p. furfurans
    p. lupinosa
    p. scutulata
porta
    p. lienis
    p. pulmonis
    p. renis
portal
    p. canal
    p. cirrhosis
    p. fibrosis
    p. hypertension
    p. lobule of liver
    p. lymph node
    p. pyemia
    p. system
    p. tract
    p. tract lesion
    p. triad
    p. vein (PV)
    p. vein thrombosis (PVT)
    p. venous pressure
portal-systemic encephalopathy (PSE)
Porter-Silber (PS)
    P.-S. chromogen (PSC)
    P.-S. chromogen test
    P.-S. reaction
Porteus maze test
Porthetria
portion
    excretory p.
    secretory p.
Portland
    P. cell
    hemoglobin P.
Portmann classification
Portuguese man-o'-war
portulacae
    Dichotomophthora p.
port-wine
    p.-w. mark
    p.-w. stain
porus (*var. of* pore)
    p. gustatorius
    p. sudoriferus

Posada disease
Posadasia
Posada-Wernicke disease
Posibacteria
positional
p. alcohol nystagmus (PAN)
p. asphyxia
position isomerism
positive
p. and negative symptom scale (PANSS)
p. anergy
p. assortative mating
beta-lactamase p.
p. cell
p. control enzyme induction
p. control repression
p. cytotaxis
cytotoxicity negative, absorption p. (CYNAP)
D" p.
p. end-expiratory pressure (PEEP)
false p.
p. neutrotaxis
p. phase
p. predictive value (PPV)
predictive value p.
p. pressure
Rh p.
p. stain
uniformly p. (UP)
variably p. (VP)
weakly p. (WP)
p. whiff test
positive-placement pipette
positive-pressure test
positivity/negativity
positron
p. annihilation
p. beta decay
Pospiviroid
post
status post (s/p)
postabsorptive
p. hypoglycemia
p. state
postatrophic hyperplasia
postauricular
postcapillary
high endothelial p.
p. venule
postchromation
postchroming
postcolectomy ileitis
postcurettage reparative change
postdiction
postdormital paralysis
postductal coarctation of aorta

posteencephalitic parkinsonism, tau pathology class I
posterior
p. cell
p. centriole
p. corneal deposit (PCD)
p. dislocation injury
p. elastic layer
p. incisural space
p. iridolenticular synechiae
lamina elastica p.
p. limiting layer of cornea
p. lobe of hypophysis
p. pituitary
p. pituitary hormone
p. semicircular canal
sinus intercavernosi anterior et p.
p. spinal sclerosis
p. subcapsular cataract (PSC)
p. urethritis
p. wall infarct (PWI)
posteriores
cellulae ethmoidales p.
postexposure
p. immunization
p. isolation
p. prophylaxis (PEP)
postgamma proteinuria (PGP)
postganglionic
p. motor neuron
p. sympathetic nerve
postgastrectomy dumping syndrome
postgonococcal urethritis
posthemorrhagic anemia
postheparin lipolytic activity (PHLA)
posthepatitic cirrhosis
posthitis
postholith
posthypocapnia
Postia
postinfectious
p. allergic encephalitis
p. encephalomyelitis
p. glomerulonephritis
p. myelitis
postinflammatory
p. polyp
p. pseudotumor
p. pulmonary fibrosis
postmaturity
postmenopausal (PMP)
p. atrophy
p. bleeding
p. syndrome
postmitochondrial supernatant (PMS)
postmitotic cell
postmordant
postmordanting

postmortem (PM, post)
    p. aerosol-producing procedure
    p. angiography
    p. autolysis
    p. bleeding
    p. clot
    p. dental x-ray
    p. examination
    p. hypostasis
    p. imaging
    p. interval (PMI)
    p. livedo
    p. lividity
    p. pustule
    p. rigidity
    p. specimen
    p. suggillation
    p. thrombus
    p. tubercle
    p. wart
postmyocardial
    p. infarction (PMI)
    p. infarction pericarditis
postnecrotic cirrhosis
postobstructive diuresis
postop
    postoperative
postoperative (postop)
    p. clipped aneurysm
    p. congestion
    p. infection
    p. parotitis
    p. repair
postpartum (PP)
    p. hemorrhage (PPH)
    p. pituitary necrosis
    p. thyroiditis
postpericardiotomy pericarditis
postprandial (PP)
    p. blood sugar (PPBS)
    p. glucose
    p. hypoglycemia
    p. lipemia
postprimary tuberculosis
postpubertal
    p. hyperpituitarism
    p. panhypopituitarism
postpump syndrome (PPS)
postpyknotic
postradiation dysplasia (PRDX)
postrema
    area p.
postremoval and postfixation shrinkage
postrenal
    p. albuminuria
    p. azotemia
postrubella syndrome
postsclerotic hyperplasia
poststenotic dilation

poststorage leukoreduction
poststreptococcal glomerulonephritis (PSGN)
postsynaptic membrane
postthymic
    p. malignancy
    p. T-cell lymphoma (PTCL)
posttransfusion
    p. hepatitis (PST, PTH)
    p. mononucleosis (PTM)
    p. purpura (PTP)
posttransplant
    p. biopsy pathology
    p. lymphoproliferative disease (PTLD)
    p. lymphoproliferative disorder (PTLD)
posttraumatic
    p. epilepsy
    p. osteoporosis
    p. pericarditis
postulate
    Ehrlich p.
    Koch p.
postulated pathogenetic factor
postural
    p. albuminuria
    p. proteinuria
posture
    minimum mission-oriented protective p. (MOPP)
postvaccinal
    p. encephalitis
    p. myelitis
postvaccination
    p. allergic encephalitis
    p. encephalomyelitis (PVEM)
postvaccinial lymphadenitis
postvagotomy syndrome
potable
Potamidae
Potamon
potassium (K)
    p. acetate
    p. acidosis
    p. acid tartrate
    p. alkalosis
    p. alum
    p. aspartate and magnesium aspartate
    p. assay
    p. bicarbonate
    p. bichromate
    p. bisperoxo oxovanadate V
    p. bitartrate
    p. bromide
    p. carbonate
    p. chlorate
    p. chloride (KCl)

p. citrate
p. cyanide (KCN)
p. dichromate
p. dihydrogen phosphate
p. EDTA (K3 EDTA)
fecal p.
p. ferricyanide
p. glucaldrate
p. gluconate
potassium, glucose, and insulin (PGI)
glucose, insulin, and p. (GIK)
p. glycerophosphate
p. guaiacolsulfonate
p. hydroxide (KOH)
p. hydroxide test
p. imbalance
p. iodate
p. mercuric iodide
p. metabisulfate stain
p. metaphosphate
p. nitrate
p. oxalate
p. *p*-aminobenzoate
p. *p*-aminosalicylate
p. penicillin G (KPG)
p. perchlorate
p. permanganate
p. permanganate stain
p. phenoxymethyl penicillin
p. simplex optimized medium (KSOM)
p. sodium tartrate
p. sorbate
stool p.
p. sulfate
p. thiocyanate
total body p. (TBK)
urine p.
potassium-42
potassium-sparing diuretic
potato
p. dextrose agar
p. tumor of neck
potato-blood agar
Potebniamyces
potential
amyloidogenic p.
atypical polypoid adenomyofibroma of low malignant p. (APA-LMP)
cervical somatosensory evoked p.
decomposition p.
diffusion p.
Donnan p.
electric p.
electrode p. (E)
p. energy

fast action p.
giant cell tumor of low malignant p. (GCT-LMP)
half-wave p.
junction p.
liquid junction p.
liquid-liquid junction p.
low malignant p. (LMP)
membrane p.
muscle action p.
oxidation-reducing p.
redox p.
reduction p.
resting membrane p.
smooth muscle tumor of uncertain malignant p. (SMTUMP)
standard electrode p.
standard reduction p.
undetermined malignant p. (UMP)
visual evoked p.
zeta p.
zoonotic p.
potentiation
long-term p. (LTP)
potentiometer
direct-reading p.
null-point p.
slide-wire p.
potentiometric titration
potentiometry
potent protein neurotoxin
Potexvirus
potomania
beer drinker's p.
Pott
P. abscess
P. aneurysm
P. disease
P. paralysis
Potter
P. disease
P. facies
P. syndrome
Potter-Bucky grid
Potter-Elvehjem handheld tissue grinder
potter's asthma
Potyvirus
pouch
p. culture
endodermal pharyngeal p.
Hartmann p.
p. of Douglas
Rathke p.
p. syndrome
pouchitis
diversion p.
preclosure p.
short-strip p.

P

Poulet disease
poultry handler's disease
pounds per square inch (psi)
pour plate
povidone
povidone-iodine
Powassan
    P. encephalitis
    P. virus
powder
    black p.
power
    p. amplifier
    apparent p.
    carbon dioxide combining p.
    p. resistor
    resolving p.
    p. supply
PowerPlex 1.2 genetic identification kit
pox
    Kaffir p.
    sheep p.
Poxviridae
poxvirus officinalis
P&P
    prothrombin and proconvertin
      P&P test
PP
    pink puffer
    postpartum
    postprandial
    prothrombin-proconvertin
    protoporphyrin
    pseudomyxoma peritonei
PPA
    primary pulmonary adenoma
PPAR gamma protein
PPB
    platelet-poor blood
PPBS
    postprandial blood sugar
PPCA
    proserum prothrombin conversion accelerator
PP-CAP
    PP-CAP H. pylori IgA assay
    PP-CAP IgA enzyme immunoassay test
PPCF
    plasmin prothrombin conversion factor
PPD
    purified protein derivative
      PPD skin test
PPD-S
    purified protein derivative-standard
ppENK gene
PPF
    plasma protein fraction

PPH
    postpartum hemorrhage
    primary pulmonary hypertension
p22phox gene
PPHP
    pseudopseudohypoparathyroidism
PPHT
    primary plexogenic hypertension
PPLO
    pleuropneumonia-like organism
PPNAD
    primary pigmented nodular adrenocortical disease
pPNET
    primitive peripheral neuroectodermal tumor
^{32}P-postlabeling assay
PPP
    platelet-poor plasma
PPR
    Price precipitation reaction
PPRE
    putative peroxisome proliferator response element
PPS
    postpump syndrome
PPT
    plant protease test
ppt
    precipitate
PPV
    positive predictive value
PR
    progesterone receptor
Pr
    prism
PRA
    plasma renin activity
    progesterone receptor assay
practice parameter
Prader bead standard
Prader-Willi syndrome
PRAD1 gene
P-radiolabeled DNA probe fragment
praeacuta
    Tissierella p.
praeacutus
    Bacteroides p.
praecox
    dementia p.
    icterus p.
    lymphedema p.
    macrogenitosomia p.
Prague pelvis
prairie itch
pralidoxime chloride
praseodymium
Prasinovirus

PRA-Stat enzyme linked immunosorbent assay
pratensis
>   *Agreia p.*
>   *Subtercola p.*
Prauserella
>   *P. alba*
>   *P. halophila*
>   *P. rugosa*
prausnitzii
>   *Faecalibacterium p.*
>   *Fusobacterium p.*
Prausnitz-Kustner
>   P.-K. antibody
>   P.-K. reaction
Prausnitz-Küstner test (PK)
prazosin hydrochloride
PRBV
>   placental residual blood volume
PRCA
>   pure red cell aplasia
PRCC-TFE3 fusion gene
PRDX
>   postradiation dysplasia
preadaptation
preadenomatous
preadipocyte factor (Pref-1)
prealbumin
>   p. test
>   thyroxine-binding p. (TBPA)
preamplifier
preanalytic error
pre-B cell
prebetalipoprotein
precancer
precancerosa
>   melanosis circumscripta p.
precancerous
>   p. dysplasia
>   p. lesion
>   p. melanosis of Dubreuilh
precatorius
>   *Abrus p.*
precaution
>   barrier isolation p.
>   droplet p.'s
>   universal p.'s
prechroming
preChx
>   preoperative chemotherapy
precipitant
precipitate (ppt)
>   alum p.
>   keratitic p. (KP)
precipitated
precipitating antibody
precipitation
>   double antibody p.
>   hapten inhibition of p.

immune p.
>   p. test
>   tuberculin p. (TP)
precipitin
>   p. curve
>   p. reaction
>   p. test
>   tube p. (TP)
precipitinogen, precipitogen
precipitinogenoid
precipitogen (*var. of* precipitinogen)
precipitoid
precipitophore
precision
>   P. QI-D handheld blood glucose test
>   p. resistor
Precision-G handheld blood glucose test
preclosure pouchitis
precocious
>   p. adrenarche
>   p. pseudopuberty
>   p. puberty
precocity
precollagenous fiber
preconfluent cell
precore mutant
precornified cell
precursor
>   abnormally localized immature p. (ALIP)
>   alkaline phosphatase, tissue-nonspecific isozyme protein p. (AP-TNAP)
>   p. cell
>   erythroid p.
>   p. lesion
>   megakaryocytic p.
precursory cartilage
predaceous mite
predecidual alteration
predeposit autologous transfusion
prediabetes
prediction
>   antibody specificity p. (ASP)
predictive
>   p. value
>   p. value positive (PVP)
predictor of patient survival
PredictRx metabolites
predilection
>   host of p.
predispose
predisposing
>   p. cause
>   p. factor
predisposition
>   rhabdoid p.
prednisone

P

predominant
  p. cell
  lymphocyte p. (LP)
predominantly epithelial thymoma (PET)
preductal coarctation of aorta
preeclampsia (PE, preE)
preeclamptic toxemia
preeruptive
preexisting actinic keratosis
preexposure immunization
Pref-1
  preadipocyte factor
preferential lysis
preformativa
  membrana p.
preganglionic motor neuron
Pre-Gen 26 colorectal cancer test
pregnancy
  aborted ectopic p.
  acute fatty liver of p.
  p. cell
  cornual p.
  corpus luteum of p.
  p. cycle
  ectopic p. (EP)
  exochorial p.
  extrauterine p.
  hydatid p.
  p. luteoma
  macrocytic anemia of p.
  mask of p.
  megaloblastic anemia of p. (MAP)
  membranous p.
  molar p.
  normal term p.
  ovarian p.
  ovarioabdominal p.
  ruptured ectopic p.
  p. test
  toxemia of p.
  tubal p.
  p. urine (PU)
  voluntary interruption of p. (VIP)
pregnancy-associated
  p.-a. plasma protein A (PAPP-A)
  p.-a. plasma protein B (PAPP-B)
pregnanediol
  p. assay
  urine p.
pregnanetriol
  urine p.
pregnant
  p. mare serum (PMS)
  p. mare serum gonadotropin (PMSG)
pregnenolone
pregranulosa cell
prehepatic hypoproteinemia

prehormone
prehyoid gland
preictal
preimplantation genetic diagnosis (PGD)
preinvasive urothelial neoplasia
Preiser disease
Preisz-Nocard bacillus
prekallikrein
P-related blood group
preleukemia
prelymphoma
prelytic sphere
premammary abscess
premature
  p. abnormal placenta
  p. infant
  p. rupture
  p. rupture of (fetal) membranes (PROM)
  p. senility syndrome
  p. separation of placenta
prematurely separated placenta
prematurity
  fetal p.
  retinopathy of p. (ROP)
premeal glucose
premelanosome
premonocyte
premorbid
premunition
premunitive
premutation allele
premyeloblast
premyelocyte
prenatal
  p. diagnosis
  p. screening
prenecrotizing phagocytic lesion
preneoplastic
prenyl group
preoperative
  p. chemotherapy (preChx)
  p. radiotherapy (preRx)
preosteoblast
preovulatory
prep
  preparation
preparation (prep)
  allergenic protein p.
  biomechanical p.
  broken cell p.
  cell block p.
  cervicovaginal smear p.
  commercial insulin p.
  corrosion p.
  cytologic filter p.
  heart-lung p.
  impression p.

India ink p.
Institute of Virus P.'s
intraoperative touch p.
KOH p.
pinworm p.
ThinPrep cytologic p.
touch p.
Trichomonas p.
Vidiera NsP nucleic sample p.
wet p.

preparative
p. immunofiltration
p. ultracentrifugation
prepare (prep)
preparedness
Office of Emergency P.
prepatent period
PrepPlus series workstation
preproprotein
prepubertal
p. hyperpituitarism
p. panhypopituitarism
preputial
p. calculus
p. gland
preputiale
sebum p.
preputiales
glandulae p.
preputii
smegma p.
prepyloric atresia
prerenal
p. albuminuria
p. azotemia
preRx
preoperative radiotherapy
presacral insufflation
presbycardia
presbyopia
presegmented nucleus
presenile
p. dementia with tangles and
calcifications
p. spontaneous gangrene
presentation
antigen p.
compound p.
preservative
PreservCyt fixative
prespermatogonia
pressor
p. amine
p. base
p. substance
pressure (P)
altered intravascular hydrostatic p.
altered intravascular osmotic p.
arterial p.

p. atrophy
barometric p. (Pb)
blood p. (BP)
p. catapulting
central venous p.
cerebrospinal fluid p.
colloidal osmotic p. (COP)
colloid oncotic p. (COP)
continuous distending p. (CDP)
p. differential
end-systolic p. (ESP)
hydrostatic p.
increased p.
maximum inspiratory p. (MIP)
oncotic p.
osmotic p. (OP)
oxygen under high p. (OHP)
plasma colloid oncotic p.
plasma oncotic p. (POP)
portal venous p.
positive p.
positive end-expiratory p. (PEEP)
pulmonary p.
pulse p.
screen filtration p. (SFP)
selection p.
standard temperature and p.
systemic arterial p. (SAP)
p. urticaria
vapor p.
venous p.
pressure-demand SCBA
pressure-volume curve
prestomal ileitis
prestorage leukoreduction
presumptive
p. diagnosis
p. heterophil test
p. testing
presuppurative
presynaptic
p. membrane
p. vesicle
presyncope
prethymic lymphoblastic lymphoma
pretibial myxedema
pretoriensis
Amycolatopsis p.
pretreatment
nerve agent pyridostigmine p.
(NAPP)
Preussia
prevalence rate
prevention
preventive
p. treatment
previa
placenta p.
vasa p.

P

previous value check
previtellogenesis
previtellogenic phase
Prevotella
    P. bivia
    P. denticola
    P. disiens
    P. enoeca
    P. heparinolytica
    P. intermedia
    P. melaninogenica
    P. oralis
    P. oris
    P. pallens
    P. salivae
    P. shahii
    P. tannerae
prevotii
    Anaerococcus p.
PreVue *Borrelia burgdorferi* antibody
  detection assay
prezone
PRF
    prolactin-releasing factor
PRFM
    prolonged rupture of fetal membranes
PRH
    prolactin-releasing hormone
priapism
priapitis
Price-Jones curve
Price precipitation reaction (PPR)
prickle
    p. cell
    p. cell layer
    intercellular p.
prick test
primaquine
    p. phosphate
    p. sensitivity
primaquine-sensitive anemia
primarium
    punctum ossificationis p.
primarius
    folliculus ovaricus p.
primary
    p. acquired melanosis
    p. active transport
    p. adrenal insufficiency
    p. African green monkey kidney
    (PAGMK)
    p. agammaglobulinemia
    p. amebic meningoencephalitis
    p. amenorrhea
    p. amine
    p. amyloidosis (AL)
    p. atelectasis
    p. atypical pneumonia (PAP)
    p. biliary cirrhosis (PBC)

p. blast injury
p. bone lymphoma (PBL)
p. bone tumor
p. bubo
p. cardiomyopathy
p. cementum
p. center of ossification
p. central nervous system lymphoma
  (PCNSL)
p. coccidioidomycosis
p. coil
p. cold agglutinin disease
p. color
p. complex
p. constriction
p. contamination
p. cutaneous anaplastic large cell
  lymphoma
p. cutaneous CD30+ large T-cell
  lymphoma
p. effusion lymphoma (PEL)
p. embryonic cell
p. endocardial sclerosis
p. erythroblastic anemia
p. explant culture
p. fibrinogenolysis syndrome
p. fibrinolysis
p. fibromyalgia syndrome
p. gastric lymphoma
p. glaucoma
p. granule
p. herpetic stomatitis
p. hyperaldosteronism
p. hyperoxaluria, type 1
p. hyperparathyroidism
p. hyperplasia
p. hypoadrenocorticism
p. hypodipsia
p. hypogammaglobulinemia
p. immune response
p. influenza virus pneumonia
p. irritant
p. Ki-1 lymphoma of brain
p. lesion
p. lymphedema
p. lymphoid follicle
p. lysosome
p. mediastinal large cell lymphoma
  with sclerosis (PMLS)
p. methemoglobinemia
p. myelofibrosis
p. myeloid metaplasia
p. myocardial disease (PMD)
p. nodule
p. odditis
p. ossification center
p. ovarian follicle
p. ovarian gestational trophoblastic
  disease (POGTD)

p. pentosuria
p. pigmented nodular adrenocortical disease (PPNAD)
p. platelet plug
p. plexogenic hypertension (PPHT)
p. point of ossification
p. pulmonary adenoma (PPA)
p. pulmonary hypertension (PPH)
p. pulmonary lobule
p. pyoderma
p. reaction
p. reference material
p. refractory anemia
p. rejection
p. renal calculus
p. renal tubular acidosis
p. repair
p. salivary CCC
p. sclerosing cholangitis (PSC)
p. septicemic plague
p. sequestrum
p. sex character
p. spermatocyte
p. standard
p. structure
p. thrombocythemia
p. thymic carcinoma (PTC)
p. transcript
p. trisomy
p. trisomy 18
p. tuberculosis
p. union
(primary) tumor, (regional lymph) nodes, (remote) metastases (TNM)
primatum
   Mycoplasma p.
primed lymphocyte typing
primer
   oligonucleotide p.
   semi-nester p.
primerite
primidone assay
priming
   T-cell p.
primite
primitia
   Treponema p.
primitive
   p. erythroblast
   p. mesoblast
   p. neuroblastic cell
   p. neuroectodermal tumor (PNET)
   p. peripheral neuroectodermal tumor (pPNET)
   p. reticular cell
   p. small-cell thoracopulmonary tumor
primitive-looking cell

primordial
   p. cyst
   p. dwarf
   p. germ cell
   p. ovarian follicle
   p. sex cell
primordium
primulin
primum non nocere
principal
   p. cell
   p. focus
   p. piece
   p. target organ
principle
   antianemic p.
   Bernoulli p.
   Fick p.
   follicle-stimulating p.
   hematinic p.
   immediate p.
   luteinizing p.
   prothrombin-converting p.
   proximate p.
   ultimate p.
   uncertainty p.
Pringle disease
print culture
printed circuit
Prinzmetal angina
prion
   p. disease
   fungal p.'s
   mammalian p.'s
   p. protein (PrP, PrPSc)
   p. protein cerebral amyloid angiopathy
prion-transmitted disease
Prionurus
priority
   law of p.
prism (Pr)
   adamantine p.
   enamel p.
   Nicol p.
prismata adamantina
prismatic follicular cell
pristanic acid
private antigen
privileged site
PRL
   prolactin
proaccelerin
proacrosomal granule
proactivator
   C3 p.
proatherogenic capacity
probabilistic neural network (PNN)

probability (P)
    conditional p.
    p. distribution
    p. paper
    significance p.
probable error
probacteriophage
    defective p.
proband
probe
    alpha p.
    amplified p.
    antisense p.
    ASO p.
    biotin-labeled p.
    biotinylated DNA p.
    CD44v6-specific p.
    centromere enumeration p. (CEP)
    chemiluminescent p.
    cycling p.
    cytochemical p.
    direct p.
    DNA p.
    dual color p.
    fluorescent p.
    genomic p.
    gun-needle p.
    hybridized p.
    immunogold p.
    nucleic acid p.
    oligonucleotide p.
    PNA p.
    radioactive p.
    reverse line p.
    sequence specific oligonucleotide p.
      (SSOP)
    Vidas p.
    viral p.
    Vysis p.
    YAC p.
Pro-Bind U-Bottom microfilter plate
probiosis
probiotic
probit transformation
proBNP
    prohormone B-type natriuretic peptide
probolurus
    Trichostrongylus p.
Probstymayria vivipara
procainamide assay
procaine hydrochloride
procalcitonin
Procandida
procapsid
Procarbazine
procarboxypeptidase
Procaryotae (*var. of* Prokaryotae)
procaryote (*var. of* prokaryote)
procaryotic (*var. of* prokaryotic)

procedure
    Bradford microassay p.
    Cherry-Crandall p.
    Clontech gene expression profiling
      p.
    concentration p.
    Cryptosporidium diagnostic p.
    falling drop p.
    flow cytometric platelet counting p.
    Gomori-Takamatsu p.
    helminth identification p.
    hydroxyapatite exchange p.
    hypophysis staining p.
    Jatlow-Nadim p.
    Kjeldahl p.
    loop electrosurgical excisional p.
      (LEEP)
    Mantel-Cox p.
    Merfluor DFA
      Cryptosporidium/*Giardia*
      detection p.
    multirule Shewhart p.
    Norymberski p.
    platelet neutralization p.
    postmortem aerosol-producing p.
    protein A-Sepharose column p.
    salting-out p.
    Sheather sugar flotation p.
    standard operating p. (SOP)
    Tiselius p.
    TTI p.
    Vindelov p.
    Westgard multirule p.
procentriole organizer
procercoid
Procerovum varium
process
    apical p.
    apoptotic p.
    astrocytic foot p.
    axonal p.
    p. control
    cytoplasmic p.
    dendritic cytoplasmic p.
    epithelial foot p.
    evidence gathering p.
    filiform p.
    foot p.
    granulomatous p.
    immune-mediated p.
    iterative p.
    Lenhossek p.
    lookback p.
    Löwenstein p.
    odontoblast p.
    podocyte foot p.
    psoralen-mediated p.
    styloid p.
    ThinPrep slide p.

Tomes p.
vasculoocclusive p.
processing
    antigen p.
    automatic tissue p.
    interactive p.
    RNA p.
    tissue p.
processor
    Sakura Finetek Tissue-Tek VIP
      300E automatic tissue p.
    ThinPrep p.
processus
    p. ferreini
    p. vaginalis
Prochloraceae
Prochlorales
Prochlorococcus
    P. marinus subsp. *marinus*
    P. marinus subsp. *pastoris*
Prochlorotrichaceae
procidentia
Procleix HIV-1/HCV Assay
procoagulant platelet-derived
  microparticle
procollagen alpha1(I) gene
proconvertase
proconvertin
    prothrombin and p. (P&P)
proctatresia
proctectasia
proctencleisis
proctitis
    allergic p.
    chronic ulcerative p.
    idiopathic p.
proctocele
proctocolitis
    diversion p.
proctodeal
proctodeum
proctopolypus
proctoptosis
proctosigmoiditis
proctostenosis
procyonis
    Baylisascaris p.
prodigiosin
prodromal stage
prodrome, prodromus
prodromus (*var. of* prodrome)
product
    advanced glycation end p. (AGE)
    anthrax-contaminated animal p.
    B-domain-deleted rFVIII p.
    cleavage p.
    concentration-time p. (Ct)
    contact activation p.
    cross p.

decay p.
dot p.
end p.
ERGIC-53 gene p.
fibrin breakdown p.
fibrin degradation p. (FDP)
fibrin/fibrinogen degradation p.
  (FDP)
fibrinogen breakdown p. (FBP)
fibrinogen degradation p. (FDP)
fibrinogen split p.
fibrinolytic split p.
fibrin-split p.
fission p.
gene p.
Pro-PredictRx diagnostic p.
protein gene p. (PGP)
scalar p.
solubility p.
spallation p.
substitution p.
vector p.
waste p.
production
    carbon dioxide p.
    CO_2 p.
    ectopic hormone p.
    excessive heat p. (EHP)
    purulent sputum p.
production-defect anemia
productive
    p. inflammation
    p. peritonitis
    p. pleurisy
productus
proenzyme
proerythroblast
proerythrocyte
Professional Standards Review
  Organization (PSRO)
Profeta law
profibrinolysin
Profichet
    P. disease
    P. syndrome
proficiency
    p. sample
    p. survey
    p. testing
profile
    Astra blood chemistry p.
    biochemical p.
    biophysical p.
    cell volume p. (CVP)
    chemistry p. (chem)
    fatty acid p.
    fetal biophysical p.
    kidney p.
    lipid p. (LIP P)

P

profile (*continued*)
  liver p.
  p. of gene expression
  plasma protein p.
  polyphenotypic p.
  test p.
Profile-ER
  P.-E. drugs of abuse screening
   panel
  P.-E. one-step qualitative drug test
Profile-II ER drug screening device
profiling
  gene expression p.
  transcriptional p.
profluens
  hydrops tubae p.
profound hypoglycemia
profunda
  colitis cystica p.
  gastritis cystica p.
  jejunitis cystica p.
  miliaria p.
  Moritella p.
  Psychromonas p.
profundi
  nodi lymphoidei inguinales p.
profundus
  Caminibacter p.
  lupus erythematosus p.
  morphea p.
  Oceanithermus p.
profusa
  Olsenella p.
Progen antibiotic solution
progenitalis
  herpes p.
progenitor
  p. cell
  p. marker
PRO-GenoLogix NOD2/CARD15
progeny
progeria
  Hutchinson-Guilford p.
  p. with cataract
  p. with microphthalmia
progeroid
progestagenic change
progestational
  p. agent
  p. hormone
progesteroid
progesterone
  plasma p.
  p. receptor (PgR, PR)
  p. receptor assay (PRA)
  p. unit (international)
progestin
progestogen
proglottid

proglottis
prognathia (*var. of* prognathism)
prognathism, prognathia
prognosis (Px)
  loss of expression and p.
prognostic
  p. criteria
  p. factor
  p. role
prognosticator
progonoma
  melanotic p.
  p. of jaw
program
  Bioterrorism Preparedness and
   Response P.
  CAP sweat analysis proficiency
   testing p.
  p. evaluation and review technique
   (PERT)
  infection surveillance and control p.
   (ISCP)
  National Biomonitoring P. (NBP)
  National Immunization P. (NIP)
  object p.
  Q-Probes p.
  Q-Tracks p.
  safety p.
  Shelf-Life Extension P. (SLEP)
  survey p.
programmed
  p. cell death
  p. cell death 4 gene (PDCD4)
programming
  temperature p.
progranulocyte
progranulocytic leukemia
progravid
progressiva
  fibrodysplasia ossificans p.
  granulomatosis disciformis chronica
   et p.
  myositis ossificans p.
progressive
  p. bacterial synergistic gangrene
  p. bulbar palsy
  p. cerebellar dyssynergia
  p. cerebral poliodystrophy
  p. cleavage
  p. contraction of wound
  dyssynergia cerebellaris p.
  p. dystonic palsy
  p. emphysematous necrosis
  p. hypocythemia
  p. impairment of renal function
  p. lipodystrophy
  p. massive fibrosis (PMF)
  p. multifocal leukoencephalopathy
   (PML)

p. muscular dystrophy (PMD)
p. pigmentary dermatosis
p. pneumonia virus
p. spinal muscular atrophy (PSMA)
p. staining
p. subcortical encephalopathy
p. supranuclear palsy (PSNP, PSP)
p. supranuclear palsy, tau pathology class II
p. systemic sclerosis (PSS)
p. transformation of germinal center (PTGC)
p. vaccinia
prohormone B-type natriuretic peptide (proBNP)
proinflammatory
p. cytokine
p. signal
proinsulin
project
Chempack P.
Early Surveillance P. (ESP)
projectile
exiting p.
fragmenting p.
p. impact
yawing p.
projection
cytoplasmic p.
Fischer p.
hair-like filamentous p.
intraductal papillary p.
polypoid intraluminal p.
transmandibular p.
p. x-ray microscope
Prokaryotae, Procaryotae
prokaryote, procaryote
prokaryotic, procaryotic
prolactin (PRL)
p. cell
chorionic growth hormone p. (CGP)
human p. (hPrL)
p. receptor
p. release-inhibiting hormone
p. test
p. unit (international)
prolactin-inhibiting factor (PIF)
prolactinoma
prolactin-producing adenoma
prolactin-releasing
p.-r. factor (PRF)
p.-r. hormone (PRH)
prolapse
mitral valve p. (MVP)
Morgagni p.
Proleukin
proleukocyte
proliferans
endarteritis p.

retinitis p.
Trichophyton p.
proliferate
proliferating
p. bile ductules (PBD)
p. cell nuclear antigen (PCHA, PCNA)
p. endarteritis
p. focus
p. pillar tumor
p. pleurisy
p. systematized angioendotheliomatosis
p. thymolipoma
proliferation
bizarre parosteal osteochondromatous p. (BPOP)
cell p.
p. center
cholangiolar p.
p. cyst
diffuse mesangial p.
fibrogenic p.
glandular p.
inflammatory myofibrohistiocytic p.
p. inhibitory factor (PIF)
lobular p.
p. marker
myofibroblastic p.
myointimal p.
neoplastic p.
nodular and diffuse fibrous p. (NDFP)
p. of fibroblast
polyclonal lymphoid p.
pseudosarcomatous myofibroblastic p.
reactive ductal p.
T-cell p.
tumor-assisted lymphoid p. (TALP)
proliferation-dependent phenomenon
proliferative, proliferous
p. activity
acute p.
p. breast disease (PBD)
p. bronchiolitis
p. chronic arthritis
p. cyst
p. disorder
p. endometrium
p. fasciitis
p. glomerulonephritis
p. glomerulopathy
p. index (PI)
p. inflammation
p. intimitis
p. mixoploid
p. myositis
p. phase
p. stage

P

proliferative (*continued*)
    p. synovitis
    p. verrucous leukoplakia (PVL)
proliferous (*var. of* proliferative)
    p. cyst
proliferum
    Sparganum p.
prolificans
    Scedosporium p.
proligerous
    p. disc
    p. membrane
proligerus
    discus p.
proline
    p. dehydrogenase
    p. hydroxylase
    p. oxidase
    urine p.
prolinemia
proline-2-oxoglutarate dioxygenase
prolinuria
prolixus
    Rhodnius p.
prolongation
    APTT p.
prolonged
    p. bleeding time
    p. coagulation time
    p. estrogen stimulation
    p. rupture of fetal membranes
    (PRFM)
prolyl 4-hydroxylase
prolymphocyte cell
prolymphocytic leukemia (PLL)
PROM
    premature rupture of (fetal) membranes
promastigote
promegakaryoblast
promegakaryocyte
promegaloblast
Promega Taq DNA polymerase
prometaphase banding
promethium
Promicromonospora
    P. aerolata
    P. pachnodae
    P. vindobonensis
Promicromonosporaceae
prominent
    p. nucleus
    p. perinuclear
promiscuous antigen receptor gene rearrangement
promoblast
promonocyte
promoter
    cancer p.
    eosinophil stimulation p. (ESP)

    p. insertion
    transcriptional p.
    tumor p.
promoting agent
promotion
promotor region
prompt zinc insulin
promyelocyte
    basophilic p.
    eosinophilic p.
    neutrophilic p.
promyelocytic
    p. leukemia (PML)
    p. leukemia protein
    p. leukemia zinc finger (PLZF)
Pronase antigen
pronephroi (*pl. of* pronephros)
pronephros, *pl.* **pronephroi**
    glomerulus of p.
pronormoblast
pronucleus
proof
    constructive p.
    existence p.
proopiomelanocortin (POMC)
proopiomelanocortin-related peptide
prooxidant
propagating
    p. nuclear reaction
    p. thrombosis
propagation
propagule
propane nitrile
propanoic acid
1-propanol
2-propanol
proparathyroid hormone
propenal
propepsin
proper
    esophageal gland p.
    p. substance
properdin
    p. assay
    p. deposit
    p. factor A, B, D, E
    p. system
property
    aerobiological p.
prophage
    defective p.
prophase
prophlogistic
prophobilinogen
prophylactic
    p. membrane
    p. serum
    p. treatment
prophylaxes (*pl. of* prophylaxis)

prophylaxis, *pl.* **prophylaxes**
   active p.
   chemical p.
   postexposure p. (PEP)
propidium
   p. iodide
   p. iodide solution
   p. iodine
   p. iodine stain
propionate
   p. carboxylase
   p. metabolism
   sodium p.
Propionibacteriaceae
propionibacterial DNA in sarcoidosis
Propionibacterineae
Propionibacterium
   P. acnes
   P. australiense
   P. avidum
   P. freudenreichii
   P. granulosum
   P. jensenii
   P. lymphophilum
   P. microaerophilum
   P. propionicus
Propionibacter pelophilus
propionic
   p. acid
   p. acidemia
   p. aciduria
propionica
   Arachnia p.
   Smithella p.
Propionicimonas paludicola
propionicus
   Propionibacterium p.
Propionimicrobium lymphophilum
Propionispira arboris
Propionispora
   P. hippei
   P. vibrioides
propionitrile
Propionivibrio
   P. limicola
   P. pelophilus
propionyl-CoA carboxylase
proplasia
proplasmacyte
proportional
   p. count
   p. counter
proportionate
   p. morbidity ratio (PMR)
   p. mortality ratio (PMR)
propositus
propoxur
propoxyphene assay
propranolol assay

Pro-PredictRx
   P.-P. diagnostic product
   P.-P. diagnostic test
   P.-P. Enzact
   P.-P. metabolite
   P.-P. TPMT
propria, *pl.* **propriae**
   gastric lamina p.
   lamina p.
   tunica p.
propriae (*pl. of* propria)
proprioceptor
proprius
   sacculus p.
proprotein
proptosis
propyl alcohol
propylene glycol
prorubricyte
proscolex
proscription
Pro-Scrub
   Zila P.-S.
prosecretion granule
prosection
prosector's
   p. tubercle
   p. wart
proserum prothrombin conversion accelerator (PPCA)
prosodemic
p-**rosolic acid**
prosopalgia
prosopectasia
prosoplasia
ProSpec
   BN P.
ProSpecT *Clostridium difficile* **toxin A microplate assay**
prospective study
prostacyclin
prostaglandin (PG)
   p. 1 (PG1)
   p. 2 (PG2)
   p. 3 (PG3)
   p. A, B
   p. D_2
   p. E_1, E_2
   p. endoperoxide
   p. F_1 alpha
   p. F_2 alpha
   p. G_2
   p. H_2
   p. I_2
   J-series p.
   p. test
prostaglandin-like substance (PLS)
prostanoic acid
prostanoid

P

prostata
prostatae
  substantia glandularis p.
  substantia muscularis p.
prostate
  p. cancer
  p. gland
  p. gland biopsy
  p. hyperplasia
  p. needle core biopsy
  p. seed
  p. specific acid phosphatase (PSAP)
  p. stem cell antigen (PSCA)
  transurethral resection of p. (TURP)
prostate-specific
  p.-s. antigen (PSA)
  p.-s. membrane antigen
prostatic
  p. adenocarcinoma (PCA)
  p. adenoma
  p. calculus
  p. duct
  p. ductule
  p. fluid
  p. hypertrophy (PH)
  p. intraepithelial neoplasia (PIN)
  p. intraepithelial neoplasia, mild
    dysplasia or low grade (PIN-1)
  p. intraepithelial neoplasia, moderate
    dysplasia or high grade (PIN-2)
  p. intraepithelial neoplasia, severe
    dysplasia or high grade (PIN-3)
  p. intraepithelial neoplasm (PIN)
  p. tumor
prostatica
  glandula p.
prostatici
  ductuli p.
  ductus p.
prostatitic
prostatitis
  allergic granulomatous p.
  bacterial p.
  mycotic p.
  nonspecific granulomatous p.
  tuberculous p.
  xanthogranulomatous p.
prostatocystitis
prostatolith
prostatomegaly
prostatovesiculitis
Prosthenorchis elegans
prostheses (*pl. of* prosthesis)
prosthesis, *pl.* **prostheses**
  Bjork-Shiley mitral p.
  p. rupture
prosthetic group
Prosthodendrium molenkampi
Prosthogonimus macrorchis

prosurvival protein
prot
  protein
protactinium (Pa)
Protac venom
protamine
  p. sulfate
  p. sulfate assay
  p. sulfate test
  p. titration test
  p. zinc insulin
protanomaly
protanopia, protanopsia
protanopsia (*var. of* protanopia)
Protargol stain
proteamaculans
  Serratia p.
protean
protease
  binding protein p. (BPP)
  calcium-activated neutral p.
  calpain family of p.
  CD p.
  p. inhibitor (PI)
  lysosomal p.
  MBL-associated serine p. (MASP)
  p. nexin-II
  regeneration-associated muscle p.
    (RAMP)
  slow-moving p. (SMP)
  tricorn p.
protease-activated receptor (PAR)
protect
  DNA/RNA P.
protected catheter brush
protectin
protection
  critical infrastructure p. (CIP)
  radiation p.
  p. test
protective
  p. antigen (PA)
  p. osmatic barrier
  p. protein
protector
  LATS p.
Proteeae
protein (PR, prot)
  p. A
  A68 p.
  accumulation of p.
  activated p. C (APC)
  activator p. 1 (AP1)
  acute phase p.
  acyl carrier p.
  ADAM p.
  ADAMTS 13 p.
  p. A gold (PAG)
  p. A gold complex technique

AL p.
ALK p.
alpha fodrin p.
amyloid p. A
amyloid beta p.
amyloid precursor p. (APP)
androgen-binding p. (ABP)
antiapoptotic p.
anticoagulant p.
anti-S-100 p.
antiviral p.
Apaf-1 adaptor p.
p. A-Sepharose column procedure
band 3 p.
Bax p.
bcl-2 p.
bcl-X$_L$ p.
BCR-ABL hybrid p.
Bence Jones p.
p. binding (PB)
BJ p.
BPI p.
p. breakdown
p. buffer
p. C
calbindin p.
calcium-sensing receptor p. (CASR)
Caldesmon cell p.
cAMP response element binding p.
  (CREB)
carbonic anhydrase-related p.
  (CA-RP)
carrier p.
caspase p.
p. catabolism
catabolite activator p.
C4b-binding p. (C4BP)
CD p.
cell-cycle inhibitory p.
cell-surface p.
cell-to-cell adherent p.
cerebrospinal fluid myelin basic p.
cerebrospinal fluid total p.
channel-forming integral p. (CHIP-1)
p. characterization system
conjugated p.
constitutive p.
copper storage p.
corticosteroid-binding p.
C-reactive p. (CRP)
CREB binding p. (CBP)
cullin family p.
cyclin D1 p.
cyclin-dependent p.
cystinosin p.
cytochrome C p.
cytoskeletal p.
cytoskeleton-associated p.
cytotoxic p.

death-associated p. (DAP)
p. defect
p. deficiency anemia
p. denaturation
derived p.
desmosomal p.
dietary p.
dipeptidyl peptidase IV p. (DPPIV)
disintegrin p.
doppel p.
dysferlin p.
EF p.
p. efficiency ratio (PER)
elastin-binding p.
p. electrolyte
p. electrophoresis
endothelial immunoglobin family
  adhesion p.
enhanced green fluorescent p.
  (EGFP)
eosinophilic cationic p. (ECP)
eosinophil p. X (EPX)
estrogen receptor p. (ERP)
excitotoxin p.
p. expression pattern
extracellular matrix p.
FAA p.
FAC p.
F-actin binding p.
FAS-associated death domain p.
  (FADD)
Fas-Fas ligand p.
fatty acid-binding p. (FABP)
F-box p.
p. fever
FHIT p.
fibrinolytic p.
fibrous p.
FLICE-like inhibitory p. (FLIP)
foreign p.
p. fractionation
fusion p.
G p.
GCDFP-15 p.
p. gene product (PGP)
glial fibrillary acidic p. (GFAP)
gliofibrillary acidic p.
globular p.
green fluorescence p. (GFP)
gross cystic disease fluid p.
  (GCDFP)
p. G Sepharose
GTPase-activating p.
guanyl-nucleotide-binding p.
hamartin p.
HAX p.
Hb1 - Hb4 p.
HBx p.
HDJ1 p.

P

protein (*continued*)

heart fatty acid binding p. (H-FABP)
heat-labile p.
heat shock p. (HSP)
helicase p.
helix-loop-helix p.
HER-2 p.
HER-2/neu p.
heterologous p.
high p. (HP)
histidine-rich matrix p.
histone p.
homeodomain p.
p. hormone
human liver-type fatty acid-binding p. (hL-FABP)
huntingtin p.
huntingtin-associated p. 1 (HAP1)
huntingtin-interacting p. 1 (HIP1)
p. hydrolysate
immune p.
immunoglobulin family adhesion p.
p. induced by vitamin K antagonist (PIVKA)
integral p.
intermediate filament p.
iron p.
iron-sulfide p.
Jun activation domain binding p. 1 (Jab1)
Ki-67 p.
p. kinase A
p. kinase C (PKC)
p. kinase C isoenzyme
kinase inhibitory p. (KIP)
Kolmer test with Reiter p. (KRP)
Kunitz domain-containing p.
lamin A p.
lamin B p.
lamin C p.
latent membrane p. (LMP)
latent membrane p. 1 (LMP-1)
lathyrus p.
lenticular p.
leptin p.
LF p.
low p. (LP)
lysosomal-associated membrane p. (LAMP)
lysosomal trafficking regulator p. (LYST)
M p.
macrophage inflammatory p. (MIP)
major basic p. (MBP)
major outer membrane p. (MOMP)
membrane p.
microtubule-associated p. (MAP)
midkine p.

mild silver p.
minichromosome maintenance p.
mitogen-activated p. (MAP)
mitotic control p. (MCP)
MK p.
monoclonal p.
monocyte chemoattractant p. (MCP)
monocyte chemoattractant p. 1 (MCP 1)
monocyte chemotactic p. 1
multidrug resistance p. (MRP)
muscle contractile p.
myelin basic p. (MBP)
myeloblastic p.
myeloma p.
MyoD p.
myogenin p.
myosin binding p. C
net dietary p. (NDP)
N-ethylmaleimide-sensitive fusion p.
neuregulin p.
neurofilament p. (NFP)
neutrophil activating p. (NAP)
NF-kappa B p.
NHC p.
ninhydrin-Schiff stain for p.'s
p. nitrogen unit (PNU)
nonhistone chromosomal p.
nonspecific p.
nonstructural p. 3
normal RB p.
nuclear matrix p. (NMP, NMP-22)
oncofetal p.
p. overexpression
p24 p.
PA p.
p. pad
pendrin p.
phosphatonin p.
pit-1 p.
plasma p.
podocalyxin p.
polyclonal anti-S-100 p.
PPAR gamma p.
pregnancy-associated plasma p. A (PAPP-A)
pregnancy-associated plasma p. B (PAPP-B)
prion p. (PrPSc)
promyelocytic leukemia p.
prosurvival p.
protective p.
p. purification
p. quotient
R p.
Rad3-related p.
RanBP p.
Rb tumor suppressor p.

reactive p. (RP)
regulator of G protein signaling p.
  5 (RGS5)
respiratory p.
retinoblastoma p.
retinol-binding p. (RBP)
rgp120 p.
rhoptry p.
ribonuclear p. (RNP)
p. S
S-100 p.
SAA p.
SCA p. (SCA)
scaffolding p.
selenium binding p. (SBP)
p. separation method
p. S-free kit
Shh p.
sHLA p.
p. shock
p. shock therapy
simple p.
sodium-iodide transport p.
soluble HLA p.
soluble NSF attachment p.
  (SNAP)
sterol carrier p.
stress p.
structural p.
surfactant p. A, B, C
survivin p.
synaptopodin p.
p. synthesis
Tamm-Horsfall p.
tau p.
p. test
thrombus precursor p.
thyroxine-binding p.
  (TBP)
titin p.
total p. (TP)
total serum p. (TSP)
transmembrane p.
tropomyosin-binding p.
p. truncation assay
p. truncation test
tumor-suppressor p.
p. turnover
p. tyrosine kinase activity
unwinding p.
Vav1 signal transducer p.
VEGF-related p.
vimentin p.
vinculin p.
virus VP1 capsid p.
vitamin K dependent plasma p.
whey acidic p.
Wiskott-Aldrich syndrome p.
  (WASP)

wnt-1-induced secreted p. 1
  (WISP1)
WRN p.
p. X-PO4
Y-box binding p. (YB1)
zinc finger p.
ZO-1 p.
protein-1
  lysosomal-associated membrane p.-1
    (LAMP-1)
protein-2
  lysosomal-associated membrane p.-2
    (LAMP-2)
proteinaceous
  p. fluid
  p. matrix material
proteinase
  aspartic p.
  Bothrops atrox serine p.
  p. inhibitor
  p. K
  p. K buffer
  p. K digestion
  Sigma Tween p.
  Staphylococcus aureus neutral p.
protein-binding
  competitive p.-b. (CPB)
protein-bound
  p.-b. iodine (PBI)
  p.-b. iodine assay
  p.-b. iodine test
  p.-b. iodine-131 test
  p.-b. thyroxine (PBT4)
protein-calorie malnutrition (PCM)
ProteinChip
  P. Biomarker DU, PA system
  P. System Series 4000
    biomarker/assay system
  P. test
proteinemia
  Bence Jones p.
14-3-3 protein family
protein-lipid bilayer
protein-losing enteropathy
proteinosis
  alveolar p.
  lipid p.
  lipoid p.
  pulmonary alveolar p. (PAP)
protein-protein binding assay
proteinuria
  Bence Jones p.
  gestational p.
  isolated p.
  nonisolated p.
  non-nephrotic range p.
  orthostatic p.
  postgamma p. (PGP)
  postural p.

P

Proteobacteria
proteoglycan (PG)
    p. aggregate
    agrin p.
    chondroitin sulfate p. (CSPG)
    heparan sulfate p.
    human stromelysin aggregated p.
     (H-SLAP)
proteolipid
proteolysis
proteolytic
    p. degradation
    p. digestion
    p. enzyme
    p. enzyme pepsin
proteolytica
    Pseudomonas p.
proteolyticum
    Trichosporon p.
proteolyticus
    Psychrobacter p.
    Vibrio p.
proteome analysis
ProteomeLab
    P. DU, PA 800 protein
     characterization system
    P. PF 2D protein fractionation
     system
    P. XL-A, XL-I protein
     characterization system
proteomic
proteomics
Proteomyces
Proteomyxidia
proteose
proteosome
proteosuria
proteus
    p.
    Amoeba p.
    Bacillus p.
    p. group
    P. inconstans
    P. mirabilis
    P. morganii
    Obesumbacterium p.
    P. OX2 antigen
    P. OX19 antigen
    P. OXK antigen
    P. pneumonia
    P. rettgeri
    P. stuartii
    P. syndrome (PS)
    p. urinary tract infection
    Vibrio p.
    P. vulgaris
protheses (*pl. of* prothesis)
prothesis, *pl.* **protheses**
prothionamide

prothoracicotropic hormone
prothrombase
prothrombin
    p. accelerator
    p. and proconvertin (P&P)
    p. and proconvertin test
    p. complex
    p. complex concentration
     (PCC)
    component A of p.
    p. consumption test
    p. consumption time (PCT)
    p. deficiency
    p. G20210A mutation
    p. gene
    p. gene 20210A
    p. II mutation
    p. time (pro time, pro-time, PT)
    p. time test
prothrombinase
prothrombin-converting principle
prothrombinogen
prothrombinopenia
prothrombin-proconvertin (PP)
prothrombokinase factor
prothrombotic
proticity
protic solvent
protime
    ProTime INR test device
    ProTime microcoagulation
     system
    ProTime prothrombin time test
     system
pro time, pro-time
    prothrombin time
protirelin
protist
Protista
protistologist
protistology
protium
Protoarchaea
Protobacterieae
protobe
protobiology
protocol
    heat antigen retrieval p.
    Malmö p.
    standardized p.
    telomerase repeat amplification p.
     (TRAP)
    telomeric repeat amplification p.
     (TRAP)
protocoproporphyria hereditaria
Protoctista
Protocult test
protodiastolic
protoerythrocyte

protofibril
protofilament
protogonoplasm
protoleukocyte
protomerite
protometrocyte
protomyofibroblast
proton
  p. acceptor
  p. acid
  p. donor
  p. pump
  p. spectroscopy
  p. tautomer
protonephridium
proton-motive hypothesis
protonophore FCCP
protooncogene
  bcl-2 p.
  c-erb-B2 p.
  c-kit p.
  erb B p.
  kit p.
protoplasm
  totipotential p.
protoplasmatic (*var. of* protoplasmic)
protoplasmic, protoplasmatic
  p. astrocyte
  p. astrocytoma
protoplasmolysis
protoplast fusion
protoporphyria
  erythropoietic p. (EPP)
protoporphyrin (PP)
  p. assay
  erythrocyte zinc p.
  free erythrocyte p. (FEP,
    FEPP)
  p. test
  zinc p. (ZPP)
protoporphyrinogen
  p. oxidase
  p. oxidase deficiency
protoporthyrinuria
protospore
Protostrongylus rufescens
Prototheca
  P. ciferrii
  P. filamenta
  P. segbwema
  P. stagnora
  P. wickerhamii
  P. zopfii
protothecosis
prototrophic
prototype
protozoa (*pl. of* protozoon)
protozoal dysentery
protozoan parasite

protozoiasis
protozoicide
protozoologist
protozoology
protozoon (*pl. of* protozoa)
protozoophage
protransglutaminase
protriptyline assay
protrusio acetabulum
protrusion
  synovial villus p.
protuberance
  Rokitansky p.
protuberans
  dermatofibrosarcoma p. (DFSP)
  fibrosarcomatous variant of
    dermatofibrosarcoma p.
    (FS-DFSP)
  fibrous dysplasia p.
protumorigenic
proud flesh
proventriculus
providencia
  P. alcalifaciens
  P. providenciae
  P. rettgeri
  P. stuartii
  p. urinary tract infection
providenciae
  Providencia p.
provirus
provisional
  p. callus
  p. cortex
provitamin
provocation
  subcutaneous/sublingual p.
  p. typhoid
provocative
  p. chelation test
  p. diagnosis
  p. Wassermann test
Prowazek-Greeff body
prowazeki
  Copromastix p.
prowazekii
  Rickettsia p.
Prower factor
Prower-Stuart factor
proximal
  p. centriole
  p. femur
  p. interphalangeal (PIP)
proximate
  p. cause
  p. principle
prozone
  p. phenomenon
  p. reaction

P

PRP
    pityriasis rubra pilaris
    platelet-rich plasma
PrP
    prion protein
PrPSc
    prion protein
pruinosum
    Sporotrichum p.
prune
    p. belly
    p. belly phenotype
    p. belly syndrome (PBS)
    p. juice expectoration
    p. juice sputum
prurigo
    p. aestivalis
    p. agria
    Besnier p.
    p. chronica multiformis
    p. ferox
    p. gestationis
    melanotic p.
    p. mitis
    nodular p.
    p. nodularis
    p. of Hebra
    p. papule
    p. simplex
pruritus
Prussak fiber
Prussian
    P. blue
    P. blue iron stain
prussiate
prussic acid
PRV
    polycythemia rubra vera
Prymnesiovirus
P:S
    polyunsaturated-to-saturated fatty acids
    ratio
PS
    population sample
    Porter-Silber
    pyloric stenosis
PSA
    prostate-specific antigen
      complexed PSA
      PSA density (PSAD)
      Immulite 2000 free PSA
      Immulite 2000 third-generation PSA
      PSA index
      PSA IRMA kit
PSAD
    prostate-specific antigen density
psalterial cord
psammocarcinoma
    serous p.

Psammolestes
psammoma
    p. body
    Virchow p.
psammomatous
    p. calcification
    p. meningioma
psammomatous-melanotic schwannoma
psammous
PSAP
    prostate specific acid phosphatase
PSC
    Porter-Silber chromogen
    pluripotential stem cell
    primary sclerosing cholangitis
PSCA
    prostate stem cell antigen
PSE
    portal-systemic encephalopathy
Pselaphephilia
P-selectin glycoprotein
pseudacromegaly
pseudalbuminuria
Pseudallescheria boydii
pseudallescheriasis
Pseudaminobacter
    P. defluvii
    P. salicylatoxidans
Pseudamphistomum truncatum
pseudarthrosis, pseudoarthrosis
Pseudeurotium ovale
pseudinoma
pseudoacanthosis nigricans
pseudoachondroplasia
pseudoachondroplastic spondyloepiphysial
  dysplasia
pseudoacini
pseudoacinus
pseudoagglutination
pseudoainhum
pseudoalbuminuria
pseudoalcaligenes
    Pseudomonas p.
pseudoaldosteronism
pseudoallele
Pseudoalteromonadaceae
Pseudoalteromonas
    P. agarivorans
    P. aliena
    P. distincta
    P. elyakovii
    P. issachenkonii
    P. maricaloris
    P. mariniglutinosa
    P. peptidolytica
    P. phenolica
    P. ruthenica
    P. sagamiensis
    P. tetraodonis

P. *translucida*
P. *ulvae*
pseudoalveolar pattern
pseudoanaphylactic shock
pseudoanaphylaxis
pseudoanemia
pseudoaneuploidy
pseudoaneurysm
pseudoangiomatous
    p. hyperplasia
    p. stromal hyperplasia (PASH)
pseudoangiosarcoma
    Masson p.
pseudoangiosarcomatous carcinoma
Pseudoarachniotus
pseudoarthrosis (*var. of* pseudarthrosis)
pseudobacillus
pseudobacterium
pseudobile canaliculus
pseudobowenoid change
pseudobulbar palsy
Pseudobutyrivibrio
    P. *ruminis*
    P. *xylanivorans*
pseudocapillarization
pseudocarcinomatous
    p. change
    p. hyperplasia
pseudocartilage
pseudocartilaginous
pseudocast
pseudocelom
Pseudochaetosphaeronema
pseudocholesteatoma
pseudocholinesterase (PCHE)
    p. deficiency
pseudochromhidrosis
pseudochylothorax
pseudochylous ascites
pseudocirrhosis
Pseudoclavibacter helvolus
Pseudoclitocybe
pseudoclonality
Pseudococcidioides
Pseudocochliobolus
pseudocolloid of lips
pseudocowpox virus
pseudocoxalgia
pseudo-Cushing state
pseudocyesis
pseudocylindroid
pseudocyst
pseudodecidual
pseudodiphtheria
pseudodiphtheriticum
    Corynebacterium p.
pseudodiploid
pseudodiverticulum
pseudodysentery

pseudoepitheliomatous
    p. change
    p. hyperplasia
pseudoepithelium
pseudoerysipelas
pseudoexfoliation
pseudo-Felty syndrome
pseudofollicle
pseudofollicular
    p. appearance
    p. growth center (PFGC)
    p. proliferation center
Pseudofusarium
pseudo-Gaucher cell
pseudogland
pseudoglanders
pseudoglomerulus
pseudoglucosazone
pseudogout
pseudo-Graefe sign
pseudo-gunpowder stippling
pseudogynecomastia
Pseudohansfordia
Pseudohazis
pseudohematuria
pseudohermaphrodite
    female p.
    male p.
pseudohermaphroditism
    dysgenetic male p. (DMPH)
    female p. (FPH)
pseudohernia
pseudoheterotopia
pseudo-Hurler polydystrophy
pseudohydrocephaly
pseudohydronephrosis
pseudohyperparathyroidism
pseudohyperplasia
pseudohypertrophic
pseudohypertrophy
pseudohypha
pseudohypoglycemia
pseudohypokalemia
pseudohyponatremia
pseudohypoparathyroidism (PHP)
pseudoinclusion
    nuclear p.
pseudointraligamentous
pseudoinvasion
pseudoinvasive appearance
pseudoisochromatic
pseudo-Kaposi lesion
pseudolactational hyperplasia
pseudolaminar necrosis
pseudolepromatous leishmaniasis
pseudoleukemica
    anemia infantum p.
pseudolipoblast
pseudolipoma

P

pseudolipomatosis
pseudolithiasis
pseudolobule
pseudolymphocyte
pseudolymphocytic choriomeningitis virus
pseudolymphoma
    cutaneous p.
    p. of Spiegler-Fendt
    Saltzstein p.
    Spiegler-Fendt p.
pseudolymphomatous folliculitis
pseudolysogenic strain
pseudolysogeny
pseudomalignancy
pseudomallei
    Actinobacillus p.
    Bacillus p.
    Burkholderia p.
    Malleomyces p.
    Pseudomonas p.
pseudomamma
pseudomantle zone pattern
pseudomelanosis
    p. coli
    p. duodeni
    p. pigment
pseudomembrane
    fibrinous p.
    inflammatory p.
pseudomembranous
    p. acute inflammation
    p. bronchitis
    p. colitis (PMC)
    p. enterocolitis (PMEC)
    p. gastritis
pseudometaplasia
pseudometastatic
Pseudomicrodochium
pseudomonad
Pseudomonadaceae
Pseudomonadales
Pseudomonadeae
Pseudomonadineae
pseudomonal pneumonia
pseudomonas
    P. acidovorans
    P. aeruginosa
    P. alboprecipitans
    P. alcaligenes
    P. alcaliphila
    P. brassicacearum
    P. brenneri
    P. cannabina
    P. cedrina
    P. cepacia
    P. chloritidismutans
    P. congelans
    P. costantinii
    P. cremoricolorata

P. diminuta
P. extremorientalis
P. fluorescens
P. fragi
P. frederiksbergensis
P. grimontii
P. indica
P. jinjuensis
P. kilonensis
P. koreensis
P. lini
P. lutea
P. maltophilia
P. mandelii
P. marina
P. mediterranea
P. meridiana
P. mesophilica
P. methanolica
P. mosselii
P. multiresinivorans
P. nonliquefaciens
P. orientalis
P. palleroniana
P. parafulva
P. paucimobilis
P. plecoglossicida
P. proteolytica
P. pseudoalcaligenes
P. pseudomallei
P. psychrophila
P. psychrotolerans
P. putida
P. rhizosphaerae
P. salomonii
P. selective agar
P. stutzeri
P. syncyanea
P. testosteroni
P. thermotolerans
P. thivervalensis
P. trivialis
P. umsongensis
P. urinary tract infection
P. vesicularis
Pseudomonilia
pseudomosaicism
pseudomucinous
    p. cyst
    p. cystadenocarcinoma
    p. cystadenoma
    p. degeneration
pseudomyasthenic syndrome
pseudomycelium
Pseudomycoderma
pseudomyiasis
pseudomyxoma
    P. ovarii
    p. peritonei (PP)

Pseudonectria
pseudoneoplasm
pseudoneuroma
pseudoneutrophilia
Pseudonocardia
    P. *alaniniphila*
    P. *alni*
    P. *antarctica*
    P. *aurantiaca*
    P. *benzenivorans*
    P. *chloroethenivorans*
    P. *kongjuensis*
    P. *spinosispora*
    P. *xinjiangensis*
    P. *yunnanensis*
    P. *zijingensis*
Pseudonocardiaceae
Pseudonocardineae
pseudoosteomalacia
pseudoosteomalacic pelvis
pseudopalisading
pseudopapillary
    p. neoplasm
    p. pattern
pseudoparakeratosis
pseudoparasite
pseudoparenchyma
pseudo-Pelger-Hüet change
pseudoperiodic
pseudoperoxidation
    metal-catalyzed p.
Pseudophaeotrichum
pseudophlegmon
    Hamilton p.
pseudophyllid
Pseudophyllidea
pseudophyllidean
pseudoplatelet
pseudopod flow
pseudopodium
pseudopolycythemia
pseudopolydystrophy
pseudopolyp
pseudopolyposis
pseudoprecocious puberty
pseudoprecocity
    isosexual p.
pseudopseudohypoparathyroidism
  (PPHP)
pseudopseudolymphoma
pseudopuberty
    precocious p.
pseudopunctipennis
    Anopheles p.
pseudopyloric metaplasia
pseudorabies virus
Pseudoramibacter alactolyticus
pseudoreaction
pseudoreplica

pseudorheumatism
Pseudorhodobacter ferrugineus
pseudorosette
pseudorubella
pseudosarcoma botryoides
pseudosarcomatous
    p. carcinoma
    p. cell
    p. fasciitis
    p. fibromyxoid tumor
    p. myofibroblastic proliferation
    p. myofibroblastic tumor (PMT)
    p. stroma
pseudosclerosis
    Jakob-Creutzfeldt p.
    Westphal-Strümpell p.
pseudoscutellaris
    Aedes scutellaris p.
pseudoseizure
pseudoseptum
pseudosmallpox
pseudospiralis
    Trichinella p.
Pseudospirillum japonicum
Pseudostertagia bullosa
pseudostoma
pseudostratification
    nuclear p.
pseudostratified columnar epithelium
pseudosynovium
pseudotattooing
Pseudoterranova decipiens
pseudothalidomide syndrome
Pseudothelphusa
pseudothrombocytopenia
    EDTA-dependent p.
pseudotortuosum
    Eubacterium p.
pseudotrichinosis
pseudotropicalis
    Candida p.
pseudotruncus arteriosus
pseudotubercle
pseudotuberculosis
    p. bacillus
    Corynebacterium p.
    Streptobacillus p.
    Yersinia p.
pseudotubular degeneration
pseudotumor
    calcifying fibrous p.
    cerebri p.
    fibrous p.
    inflammatory p.
    nuchal fibrocartilaginous p.
    postinflammatory p.
    spindle cell p.
    xanthomatous p.
pseudo-Turner syndrome

P

pseudounipolar
    p. cell
    p. neuron
pseudouridine excretion
pseudovaccinii
    Nocardia p.
pseudovacuole
pseudovariola
pseudovascular adenoid squamous cell carcinoma (PASCC)
pseudoventricle
Pseudovirus
pseudo-von Willebrand disease
pseudoxanthoma
    p. cell
    p. elasticum (PXE)
pseudoxanthomatous transformation
Pseudoxanthomonas
    P. broegbernensis
    P. taiwanensis
Pseudozyma
PSFR assay
PSGN
    poststreptococcal glomerulonephritis
psi
    pounds per square inch
Psilobotrys
psilocin
Psilocybe
psilocybin
Psilorchis hominis
psittaci
    Chlamydia p.
    Chlamydophila p.
    Lactobacillus p.
    Miyagawanella p.
psittacicida
    Volucribacter p.
psittacosis
    p. inclusion body
    p. titer
    p. virus
psittacosis-lymphogranuloma
    p.-l. venereum trachoma (PLT)
    p.-l. venereum-trachoma group
PSMA
    prostate-specific membrane antigen
PSNP
    placental site nodule and plaque
psoas abscess
psoralen-mediated process
psoralen-treated pooled plasma
psorelcosis
psorenteritis
Psorergates
psoriasiform dermatitis
psoriasis
    p. arthropica
    Barber p.

    buccal p.
    exfoliative p.
    lupus p.
    p. ostracea
    pustular p.
    rupioides p.
    von Zumbusch p.
    p. vulgaris
psoriatic arthritis
Psorophora
Psoroptes
PSP
    progressive supranuclear palsy
PSRO
    Professional Standards Review Organization
PSS
    progressive systemic sclerosis
PST
    posttransfusion hepatitis
PSTT
    placental site trophoblastic tumor
Psychoda alternata
Psychodidae
psychogenetic (*var. of* psychogenic)
psychogenic, psychogenetic
    p. purpura
    p. seizure
psychogeriatric
psychological autopsy
psychomotor epilepsy
psychosine
psychraerophilum
    Bifidobacterium p.
psychralcaliphila
    Dietzia p.
Psychrobacter
    P. arenosus
    P. faecalis
    P. fozii
    P. jeotgali
    P. luti
    P. marincola
    P. maritimus
    P. okhotskensis
    P. pacificensis
    P. proteolyticus
    P. submarinus
psychrodurans
    Bacillus p.
Psychroflexus
    P. gondwanensis
    P. torquis
    P. tropicus
Psychromonadaceae
Psychromonas
    P. antarctica
    P. arctica

P. *kaikoae*
P. *marina*
P. *profunda*
psychrophil (*var. of* psychrophile)
psychrophila
  Desulfotalea *p.*
  Pseudomonas *p.*
  Sporosarcina *p.*
psychrophile, psychrophil
psychrophilic bacterium
psychrophilum
  Clostridium *p.*
  Cryobacterium *p.*
psychrophilus
  Jeotgalicoccus *p.*
  Planococcus *p.*
psychrotolerans
  Bacillus *p.*
  Mycobacterium *p.*
  Pseudomonas *p.*
psyllium hydrophilic mucilloid
PT
  pneumothorax
  prothrombin time
PTA
  plasma thromboplastin antecedent
    PTA deficiency
    PTA stain
PTAH stain
PTC
  plasma thromboplastin component
  primary thymic carcinoma
    PTC deficiency
    PTC peptide
PTCH receptor
PTCL
  postthymic T-cell lymphoma
PTE
  pulmonary thromboembolism
PTED
  pulmonary thromboembolic disease
PTEN
    PTEN immunostain
    PTEN tumor suppressor gene
pteridine
pterin
pteroic acid
pteronyssinus
  Dermatophagoides *p.*
pteroylglutamic acid
pteroylpolyglutamate
pterygium
  congenital p.
  p. syndrome
Pterygodermatites dipodomis
pterygoid chest
Pterygota
PTF
  plasma thromboplastin factor

PTGC
  progressive transformation of germinal
  center
PTH
  posttransfusion hepatitis
    PTH assay
PTLD
  posttransplant lymphoproliferative
  disease
  posttransplant lymphoproliferative
  disorder
PTM
  posttransfusion mononucleosis
ptomaine
ptomainemia
ptosed
ptosis
ptotic organ
PTP
  posttransfusion purpura
p-(trifluoromethoxy)phenylhydrazone
PTT
  prothrombin time
PTT-LA reagent
ptyalocele
Ptychogaster
ptyocrinous
PU
  polyurethane
  pregnancy urine
puberty
  delayed p.
  precocious p.
  pseudoprecocious p.
pubic
  p. louse
  p. tuberosity
pubis
public
  p. antigen
  p. health bacteriology
  p. health laboratory
  P. Health Practice Program Office
  (PHPPO)
Puccinia
  P. *glumarum*
  P. *graminis*
Puchtler
  P. alkaline Congo red
  method
  P. Sirius red method
Puchtler-Sweat
  P.-S. stain
  P.-S. stain for basement
  membranes
  P.-S. stain for hemoglobin and
  hemosiderin
PUE
  pyrexia of unknown etiology

P

puerperal
- p. eclampsia
- p. fever
- p. hematoma
- p. infection
- p. mastitis
- p. phlebitis
- p. septicemia
- p. thrombosis

puerperia (*pl. of* puerperium)
puerperium, *pl.* **puerperia**
PUFA
- polyunsaturated fatty acid

puffball
puffer
- pink p. (PP)

pulcherrima
- *Capronia p.*

pulchrum
- *Gongylonema p.*

Pulex
- *P. cheopis*
- *P. fasciatus*
- *P. irritans*
- *P. penetrans*
- *P. serraticeps*

pulicicide, pulicide
Pulicidae
pulicide (*var. of* pulicicide)
pullulans
- *Aureobasidium p.*
- *Pullularia p.*
- *Trichosporon p.*

Pullularia pullulans
pullulate
pullulation
pulmolith
pulmonale
- cor p.
- glomus p.

pulmonalis
- *Trichomonas p.*

pulmonary
- p. accumulation
- p. acinus
- p. actinomycosis
- p. adenomatosis
- p. agent
- p. alveolar macrophage (PAM)
- p. alveolar microlithiasis (PAM)
- p. alveolar proteinosis (PAP)
- p. alveolus
- p. angiomyolipoma
- p. anthrax
- p. arteriovenous fistula (PAF)
- p. artery hypertension
- p. artery stenosis (PAS)
- p. aspergillosis
- p. atresia

- p. blast injury
- p. blastoma
- p. blastomycosis
- p. blood flow
- p. bulla
- p. capacity test
- p. capillary blood volume
- p. capillary hemangiomatosis (PCH)
- p. dirofilariasis
- p. distomiasis
- p. docimasia
- p. dysmaturity syndrome
- p. edema (PE)
- p. embolism (PE)
- p. endodermal tumor
- p. eosinophilia
- p. fibrosis
- p. function test (PFT)
- p. glomangiosis
- p. hamartoma
- p. heart disease
- p. hemosiderosis
- p. hyalinizing granuloma (PHG)
- p. hypersensitivity
- p. hypostasis
- p. incompetence (PI)
- p. infarct
- p. infarction (PI)
- p. infection
- p. infiltrate
- p. infiltration and eosinophilia (PIE)
- p. infundibular stenosis
- p. insufficiency
- p. interstitial emphysema (PIE)
- p. intimal sarcoma (PIS)
- p. LAM
- p. lymphangioleiomyomatosis
- p. lymphangiomatosis
- p. lymphoid hyperplasia (PLH)
- p. MALT lymphoma
- p. mucinous cyst neoplasia
- p. mucormycosis
- p. neuroendocrine cell (PNEC)
- p. osteoarthropathy
- p. perfusion
- p. pleurisy
- plexogenic p.
- p. pneumonitis
- p. pressure
- p. resistance (Rp)
- p. sarcoidosis
- p. surfactant
- p. thromboembolic disease (PTED)
- p. thromboembolism (PTE)
- p. trunk
- p. tuberculosis
- p. vascular disease
- p. veno-occlusive disease
- p. venous congestion (PVC)

pulmonary-renal
  syndrome
pulmonic incompetence
pulmonicola
pulmonis
  alveoli p.
  hilum p.
  Mycoplasma p.
  porta p.
  Tsukamurella p.
pulmonitis
pulp, pulpa
  artery of p.
  dental p.
  dentinal p.
  putrescent p.
  red p.
  splenic p.
  splenic red p.
  tooth p.
  white p.
pulpa (*var. of* pulp)
  p. dentis
  p. lienis
  p. splenica
pulpar cell
pulpefaction
pulpiform
pulpitis
  putrescent p.
pulposus
  herniated nucleus p.
    (HNP)
pulpy
pulsating
  p. empyema
  p. metastasis
pulse (P, p)
  electromagnetic p. (EMP)
  p. height analyzer (PHA)
  p. oximetry
  p. pressure
pulsed
  p. field gel electrophoresis
  p. field gradient gel electrophoresis
    (PFGE)
pulseless disease
pulsellum
pulsion diverticulum
pultaceous
pulverulenta
  cataracta centralis p.
pulvinar
  p. gliosis
  p. sign
pumilum
  Mogibacterium p.
pumilus
  Bacillus p.

pump
  chloroquine p.
  proton p.
punch
  p. biopsy
  replicate p.
punctata
  Aeromonas p.
  chondrodysplasia p.
  chondrodystrophia congenita p.
  Cooperia p.
  dysplasia epiphysialis p.
  keratosis p.
punctate
  p. abrasion
  p. basophilia
  p. hemorrhage
  p. keratoderma
  p. nitrate residue
  p. parotitis
  p. pattern
punctation
punctiform
punctum
  p. luteum
  p. ossificationis
  p. ossificationis primarium
  p. ossificationis secundarium
  p. vasculosum
puncture
  femoral p.
  lumbar p.
  lymph node p.
  skin p.
  suprapubic p. (SP)
  transethmoidal p.
punicea
  Glaciecola p.
puniciscabiei
  Streptomyces p.
Punjab
  hemoglobin D P.
punjatensis
  Ceratophyllus p.
Puntius
PUO
  pyrexia of unknown origin
pupa, *pl.* **pupae**
pupae (*pl. of* pupa)
pupil
  Adie p.
  Argyll Robertson p.
  Hutchinson p.
pupilla, *pl.* **pupillae**
  dilator pupillae
pupillae (*pl. of* pupilla)
pupillaris
  membrana p.
pupiparous

P

pure
    p. antiandrogen
    chemically p. (CP)
    p. culture
    p. gonadal dysgenesis
    p. leukocytosis
    p. red cell agenesis
    p. red cell anemia
    p. red cell aplasia (PRCA)
    p. tumor
Puregene DNA isolation kit
purification
    immunoaffinity p.
    protein p.
    Wizard MagneSil plasmid p.
    Wizard SV 96 plasmid p.
purified
    affinity p.
    p. protein derivative (PPD)
    p. protein derivative of tuberculin
    p. protein derivative skin test
    p. protein derivative-standard (PPD-S)
puriform
purine
    p. analogue
    p. and pyrimidine bases
    p. bodies test
    p. nucleoside phosphorylase (PNP)
    p. nucleoside phosphorylase
      deficiency
purinemia
purinergic receptor translocation
  assessment
puris
    liquor p.
    Nocardia p.
purity
    optical p.
    radiochemical p.
    radionuclidic p.
Purkinje
    P. cell
    P. cell layer
    P. corpuscle
    P. fiber
    P. myocyte
    P. network
    P. system
puromucous
purple
    bromcresol p.
purpura
    allergic p.
    anaphylactoid p.
    p. angioneurotica
    p. annularis
    p. annularis telangiectodes
    autoimmune thrombocytopenic p.
    cachectic p.

    fibrinolytic p.
    p. fulminans
    p. hemorrhagica
    Henoch p.
    Henoch-Schönlein p. (HSP)
    hyperglobulinemic p.
    idiopathic thrombocytopenic p. (ITP)
    immune thrombocytopenic p.
    isoimmune neonatal p.
    Kapetanakis p.
    Majocchi p.
    p. of Doucas
    posttransfusion p. (PTP)
    psychogenic p.
    Schönlein p.
    thrombocytopenic p. (TP)
    thrombotic thrombocytopenic p. (TTP)
    Waldenström p.
purpurascens
    Epicoccum p.
purpurea
    Claviceps p.
    Digitalis p.
    Lamprocystis p.
    Micromonospora p.
purpureum
    Trichophyton p.
purpureus
    Otomyces p.
    Rhinoestrus p.
purpuric
purpurin
    alizarin p.
purpurinuria
purpuriparous
Purtscher disease
purulence, purulency
purulency (*var. of* purulence)
purulent
    p. debris
    p. encephalitis
    p. hypophysitis
    p. inflammation
    p. pericarditis
    p. pleurisy
    p. sputum production
    p. synovitis
purulenta
    pneumonia interlobularis p.
    thromboarteritis p.
puruloid
purvisi
    Cyclodontostomum p.
pus
    anchovy sauce p.
    blue p.
    burrowing p.
    p. cell
    cheesy p.

p. corpuscle
curdy p.
green p.
ichorous p.
laudable p.
sanious p.
p. tube
pushchinoensis
   Anoxybacillus p.
push package
push-pull amplifier
push-wedge method
pusilla
   Terasakiella p.
pusillum
pustular
p. bacterid
p. inflammation
p. psoriasis
p. vasculitis
pustule
anthrax malignant p.
malignant p.
p.'s of Kogoj
postmortem p.
shotty p.
pustulosa
pustulosis
p. palmaris et plantaris
p. vacciniformis acuta
putative
p. leukemia
p. peroxisome proliferator response
element (PPRE)
putida
   Pseudomonas p.
putidum
   Treponema p.
Putnam-Dana syndrome
putredinis
   Alistipes p.
   Bacteroides p.
putrefaciens
   Alteromonas p.
putrefaction
putrescent
p. pulp
p. pulpitis
putrescentiae
   Tyrophagus p.
putrescine
putrid throat
putridus
putterlickiae
   Kitasatospora p.
putty kidney
PUVA
PUVA lentigo
PUVA treatment

puzzle
blood p.'s
PV
plasma volume
polycythemia vera
PVA
polyvinyl alcohol
PVA fixative
PVA fixative method
PVA lacto-phenol medium
PVC
polyvinyl chloride
pulmonary venous congestion
PVD
pulmonary vascular disease
PVEM
postvaccination encephalomyelitis
PVL
proliferative verrucous
leukoplakia
PVM
pneumonia virus of mice
PVM virus
PVOD
pulmonary veno-occlusive disease
PVP
predictive value positive
PVT
portal vein thrombosis
PWI
posterior wall infarct
PWM
pokeweed mitogen
Px
pneumothorax
prognosis
prophylaxis
PXA
pleomorphic xanthoastrocytoma
PXE
pseudoxanthoma elasticum
PXF
pseudoexfoliation
pyarthrosis
Pycnidiella
pycnodysostosis (*var. of* pyknodysostosis)
Pycnoporus
pycnus
   Bacillus p.
pyelectasia (*var. of* pyelectasis)
pyelectasis, pyelectasia
pyelitic
pyelitis
p. cystica
p. glandularis
pyelocaliectasis
pyelocystitis
pyelography, pelviureteroradiography
retrograde p.

P

pyelonephritic kidney
pyelonephritis (PN)
    acute p.
    ascending p.
    chronic p. (CPN)
    diffuse p.
    xanthogranulomatous p. (XPN)
pyelonephrosis
pyeloureterectasis
pyemia
    cryptogenic p.
    portal p.
pyemic
    p. abscess
    p. embolism
Pyemotes tritici
Pyemotidae
pyencephalus
pyesis
Pygidiopsis summa
pygomelus
pygopagus
pyknocyte
pyknocytosis
    infantile p.
pyknodysostosis, pycnodysostosis
pyknometer
pyknometry
pyknomorphic (*var. of* pyknomorphous)
pyknomorphous, pyknomorphic
pyknosis
    nuclear p.
pyknotic
    p. cell
    p. index
    p. nuclei
Pyle disease
pylemphraxis
pylephlebectasis
pylephlebitic abscess
pylephlebitis
pylethrombophlebitis
pylethrombosis
pylori
    Acceava *Helicobacter p.*
    Campylobacter (Helicobacter) p.
    coccoid *Helicobacter p.*
    Helicobacter p. (*H. pylori*)
pyloric
    p. gland
    p. gland metaplasia
    p. stenosis (PS)
pyloricae
    glandulae p.
pyloristenosis, pylorostenosis
pyloritis
pyloroduodenitis
pyloroptosia (*var. of* pyloroptosis)
pyloroptosis, pyloroptosia

pylorostenosis (*var. of* pyloristenosis)
Pym fever
pyocele
pyocelia
pyocephalus
    circumscribed p.
    external p.
    internal p.
pyocin
pyocolpos
pyocyanase
pyocyaneus
    Bacillus p.
pyocyanic
pyocyanin
pyocyanogenic
pyocyanolysin
pyocyst
pyocyte
pyoderma
    chancriform p.
    p. gangrenosum (PG)
    primary p.
    secondary p.
    p. vegetans
pyodermatitis
pyodermatosis
pyogen
pyogenes
    Corynebacterium p.
    Staphylococcus p.
    Streptococcus p.
pyogenesis
pyogenetic (*var. of* pyogenic)
pyogenic, pyogenetic, pyogenous
    p. abscess
    p. bacterium
    p. cholangitis
    p. fever
    p. granuloma
    p. infection
    p. membrane
    p. meningitis
    p. osteomyelitis
    p. pachymeningitis
    p. salpingitis
pyogenica
    encephalitis p.
pyogenicum
    granuloma p.
pyogenous (*var. of* pyogenic)
pyogranulomatous
pyohemia
pyoid
pyometra
pyometritis
pyometrium
pyomyositis
pyonephritis

pyonephrolithiasis
pyonephrosis, nephropyosis
pyopericarditis
pyopericardium
pyoperitoneum
pyoperitonitis
pyopoiesis
pyopoietic
pyopyelectasis
pyorrhea
pyosalpinx
pyosemia, pyospermia
pyosepticemia
pyosis
pyospermia (*var. of* pyosemia)
pyostatic
pyostomatitis vegetans
pyothorax
pyoureter
pyoverdin
pyoxanthin
pyoxanthose
pyramid
    Ferrein p.
pyramidal
    p. cell
    p. cell layer
    p. disease
pyramidally
pyran
pyranose
pyranoside
pyrazinamide
Pyrazus
pyrenemia
Pyrenochaeta romeroi
pyrenoid
Pyrenophora
pyrethrin
pyrethrum
Pyrex glassware
pyrexia
    p. of unknown etiology (PUE)
    p. of unknown origin (PUO)
Pyricularia oryzae
pyridine
    alum-precipitated p. (APP)
    p. nucleotide
pyridinivorans
    Rhodococcus p.
pyridoxalated
    p. hemoglobin-polyoxyethylene
      (PHP)
    p. stroma-free hemoglobin solution
pyridoxal-5′-phosphate
pyridoxamine
pyridoxic acid
pyridoxine
pyridoxine-responsive anemia

pyriform (*var. of* piriform)
pyriformis
    Tetrahymena p.
pyrimethamine assay
pyrimidine
    p. base
    p. dimerization
Pyro
    pyrophosphate
Pyrobaculum
    P. arsenaticum
    P. oguniense
pyroborate
    sodium p.
pyrocarbonate
    diethyl p. (DEPC)
Pyrodictiaceae
pyrogallol
pyrogallolphthalein
pyrogen
pyrogenes
    Toxoplasma p.
pyrogenic toxin
pyroglobulin
pyroglobulinemia
pyroglutamase
pyroglutamate hydroxylase
pyroglutamicaciduria
pyrolysis
pyronin B, G, Y
pyronine
    naphthol p.
pyroninophilia
pyroninophilic blast cell
pyrophosphatase
    inorganic p.
pyrophosphate
    coenzyme thiamine p.
    inorganic p.
    sodium p.
pyrophosphohydrolase
    ATP p.
    ectonucleotide p.
pyrophosphoric acid
pyrophosphorylase
    inosine p.
pyropoikilocytosis
    hereditary p. (HPP)
pyroracemic acid
pyrosequencing
pyrosulfite
    sodium p.
pyrotoxin
pyrrhol cell
pyrrol
    p. blue
    p. blue stain
    p. cell
pyrrole

P

pyrrolidone carboxylate
pyrroline-5-carboxylate
    p.-5-c. dehydrogenase
    p.-5-c. reductase
pyruvate
    p. carboxylase
    p. dehydrogenase complex
    (PDC)
    p. kinase (PK)
    p. kinase assay
    p. kinase deficiency

pyruvativorans
    Eubacterium p.
pyruvic
    p. acid
    p. acid assay
Pythium insidiosum
pythogenesis
pythogenic
pythogenous
pyuria
    sterile p.

Q

Q band
Q banding
Q beta replicase
Q disc
Q fever
Q fever endocarditis
Q fever pneumonia
Q fever titer

Q10
temperature coefficient

QA
quality assurance

Qa antigen

QB
total body clearance
whole blood

Q-banding stain

Q-band technique

Q-beta replicase system

QC
quality control

16q chromosome

Q-enzyme

QF
quality factor

QFD
quartz fiber dosimeter

Q-FISH
quantitative fluorescence in situ
hybridization

QI
quality improvement

QIAamp DNA blood biorobot kit

Qiagen QIAquick gel extraction kit

QIAquick PCR 96 purification kit

QNB
3-quinuclidinyl benzilate
NATO code for QNB (BZ)

QNS
quantity not sufficient

QO₂
oxygen quotient

QOL
quality of life

QP
quanti-Pirquet reaction

Q-Prep workstation

Q-Probes program

QS
quantitation standard

Q-Tracks program

quadrant
right lower q.

4 quadrant biopsy

quadrata
Haloarcula q.

quadratic function

quadratum
caput q.

Quadricoccus australiensis

quadrigeminal

quadrilobata
Taenia q.

quadrimaculatus
Anopheles q.

quadriplegia
areflexic q.

quadripolar

quadriradial

quadrispinulatum
Oesophagostomum q.

quadrivalent

quail bronchitis virus

qualitative
q. analysis
q. fecal fat test
q. immunohistology
Q. Platform Immunoassay Device
(QuPID)
q. staging of breast cancer
q. urine myoglobin dipstick test

quality
q. assurance (QA)
q. control (QC)
q. control chart
q. control serum
q. factor (QF)
q. improvement (QI)
q. of life (QOL)

quantasome

quantatrope

QuantiFERON-TB test

quantile

quantimeter

quanti-Pirquet reaction (QP)

quantitation
HIV q.
q. standard (QS)
q. test

quantitative
q. analysis
q. fluorescence in situ hybridization
(Q-FISH)
q. hypertrophy
q. immunoglobulin
q. immunohistology
q. inheritance
q. trait

quantity
  q. not sufficient (QNS)
  not sufficient q. (NSQ)
quantum
  q. limit
  Quanta Lite ANA ELISA test kit
  Quanta Lite CCP ELISA kit
  Quanta Lite ELISA autoimmune
    kit
  q. yield
Quaranfil virus
quarantine
quark
quarta
  crista q.
quartan
  q. fever
  q. malaria
quarti
  tela choroidea ventriculi q.
quartile
quartum
  Eubacterium q.
quartz fiber dosimeter (QFD)
quasicontinuous inheritance
quasidiploid
quasidominance
quasidominant inheritance
quasispecies
quaternary
  q. amine
  q. blast injury
  q. structure
  q. syphilis
Quebec platelet disorder
Queckenstedt test
Queensland tick fever
quellung
  q. phenomenon
  q. reaction
  q. test
quenching
  fluorescence q.
quercetin
quercicolus
  Dendrosporobacter q.
**QuestDirect direct to consumer
  laboratory**
question
  agent in q.
QuestTest diagnostic panel
queue
Queyrat
  erythroplasia of Q.
Quicgel method
Quick
  Q. method
  Q. Slide automated stainer
  Q. tourniquet test

quickvue
  Q. Advance *Gardnerella vaginalis*
    test
  Q. Advance pH and amines
    test
  Q. *Chlamydia* test
  Q. *H. pylori* gII test
  Q. iFOB test
  Q. influenza test
  Q. 1 step *Helicobacter pylori*
    test
  Q. UrinChek 10+ urine test
QuickVue+
  Q. infectious mononucleosis
    test
  Q. One-Step hCG Combo
quiet hip disease
quiltlike pattern
Quilty lesion
quinacrine
  q. banding
  q. chromosome banding stain
  q. hydrochloride
quinaldine red
Quincke
  Q. disease
  Q. edema
quinckeanum
  Trichophyton mentagrophytes q.
quinhydrone electrode
quinidine assay
quinine
  q. assay
  q. carbacrylic resin
  q. carbacrylic resin test
quinivorans
  Serratia q.
Quinlan test
quinoline dye
quinolinic acid
quinolinium dye
quinone
quinovose
Quinquaud disease
quinquefasciatus
  Culex q.
quinquevalent
quinsy
quint.
  fifth
quintana
  Bartonella q.
  Rochalimaea q.
quintum
  Eubacterium q.
3-quinuclidinyl benzilate (QNB)
quisqualate activated neuron
quisquiliarum
  Cerasibacillus q.

quotidian
    q. fever
    q. malaria
quotient
    albumin q.
    blood q.
    caloric q.
    cerebral glucose oxygen q. (CG:OQ)
    circadian q. (CQ)

    oxygen q. (QO_2)
    protein q.
    rachidean q.
    reaction q.
    respiratory q.
QuPID
    Qualitative Platform Immunoassay
    Device
    QuPID pregnancy test

R
    organic radical
    Réaumur scale
    regression coefficient
    Rinne test
        R antigen
        R banding
        R colony
        R determinant
        R factor
        R pilus
        R plasmid
        R protein
2R
        chromotrope 2R
R-250
        Coomassie brilliant blue
        R-250
RA
    rheumatoid arthritis
        RA cell
        RA latex fixation test
rabbit
        r. aorta-contracting substance
        r. blood agar
        r. fever (tularemia)
        r. fibroma
        r. fibroma virus
        r. kidney
        r. papilloma
        r. plague
        r. test
rabbitpox virus
rabid
rabies
        r. immune globulin
        r. immunoglobulin
        r. vaccine
        r. virus
raccoon eyes
RACE
        rapid antigen uptake into the cytosol
        enterocytes
        RACE cell
racemase
racemate
racemic
        r. aerosol
        r. mixture
        r. modification
racemization
racemosa
        livedo r.
racemose
        r. aneurysm

        r. gland
        r. hemangioma
racemosum
        angioma venosum r.
        Syncephalastrum r.
racemosus
        Mucor r.
rachidean quotient
rachischisis
rachitic
        r. pelvis
        r. rosary
rachitis
        r. fetalis
        r. fetalis annularis
        r. fetalis micromelica
        r. intrauterina
        r. uterina
raciborskii
        Planktothricoides r.
rack
        Nalgene freezer storage r.
racket (*var. of* racquet)
racquet, racket
        r. hypha
        r. shaped
RAD
        radian
        right axis deviation
rad
        radiation absorbed dose
Radford nomogram
radial
        r. aplasia-thrombocytopenia
        r. aplasia-thrombocytopenia syndrome
        r. diffusion
        r. immunodiffusion (RID)
        r. melanoma growth phase
        r. scar
        r. sclerosing lesion
        r. styloid tendovaginitis
        r. symmetry
radian (RAD)
radiant energy
radiata
        corona r.
radiate
        r. crown
        r. layer of tympanic membrane
radiation
        r. absorbed dose (rad)
        alpha r.
        r. anemia
        background r.
        beta r.

radiation (*continued*)
    braking r.
    Bremsstrahlung r.
    r. chimera
    r. colitis
    r. counter
    r. cystitis
    r. damage
    r. dermatitis
    r. dermatosis
    r. dispersal device
      (RDD)
    r. effect
    electromagnetic r.
    r. emergency area
      (REA)
    r. enteritis
    r. enterocolitis
    r. fibroblast
    r. gastritis
    general r.
    r. hazard
    r. injury
    ionizing r.
    r. measuring unit
    r. necrosis
    r. nephritis
    r. pneumonitis
    r. protection
    r. protection officer
      (RPO)
    r. sickness
    r. survey
    r. therapy
    ultraviolet r.
radiative capture
radiatum
    Oesophagostomum r.
radiatus
    Strongylus r.
radical
    cyanide r. (CN-)
    free r.
    hydroxyl r.
    organic r. (R)
    oxygen-derived free r.
    r. scavenger
radices (*pl. of* radix)
radicicola
    Heterodera r.
radicidentis
    Actinomyces r.
radicular cyst
radiculitis
    cervical r.
radiculoganglionitis
radiculomeningomyelitis
radiculomyelopathy
radiculoneuropathy

radiculopathy
    lumbosacral r.
radii (*pl. of* radius)
radioactive
    r. challenge
    r. concentration
    r. constant
    r. decay
    r. drug
    r. equilibrium
    r. fibrinogen uptake test
    r. iodide (RAI)
    r. iodide uptake test
    r. iodinated human serum albumin
      (RIHSA)
    r. iodinated serum albumin (RISA)
    r. iodine (RAI)
    r. iodine uptake (RIU)
    r. iodine uptake test
    r. label
    r. probe
    r. waste
radioactivity
    unknown r.
radioallergosorbent
    r. assay
    r. assay test (RAST)
radioassay
    C1q r.
radioautography
radiobacter
    Rhizobium r.
radiobiology
radiocalcium uptake
radiochemical purity
radiochromatogram
radiocolloid tracer
radiodense
radiodensity
radiodermatitis
radioenzymatic assay (REA)
radiofrequency
    high-energy r. (HERF)
radiography
    body-section r.
    breast specimen r.
    chest r.
    mass miniature r. (MMR)
    specimen r.
    stereoscopic r.
radiohumeral bursitis
radioimmunoassay (RIA)
    r. automation
    sandwich r.
    solid-phase r.
radioimmunodiffusion
radioimmunoelectrophoresis
radioimmunoprecipitation (RIP)
    r. assay (RIPA)

radioimmunosorbent test (RIST)
radioiodinated
    r. fatty acid (RIFA)
    r. serum albumin (RISA)
radioiodination
    lactoperoxidase r.
radioisotope renal excretion test
radioisotopic
    r. culture
    r. immunoassay
radiolabeled
radiolatum
    Trichophyton r.
radioligand assay
radiologic, radiological
    r. honeycombing
radiological (*var. of* radiologic)
    r. agent
    chemical, biological, and r.
      (CBR)
radiology
    forensic r.
    medical r.
radiolucency
    central r.
    soap-bubble r.
radiolysis
radiometer
radiometric antibody detection
Radiomyces
radionecrosis
radionucleotide ventriculography
radionuclide
    r. body burden
    transuranic r.
radionuclidic purity
radiopaque medium
radiopharmaceutical
radioreceptor assay (RRA)
radioresistant
radioresistens
    Acinetobacter r.
radioresponsiveness
radiosensitivity
    r. of specialized cell
    r. test (RST)
radiostable water
radiostrontium
radiotherapy, radiation therapy
    chemotherapy and r.
      (chemrad)
    preoperative r. (preRx)
radiotolerans
    Kineococcus r.
    Methylobacterium r.
radium necrosis
radius, *pl.* **radii**
    radii lentis
    r. of resolution

    r. of view
    thrombocytopenia-absent r. (TAR)
radix, *pl.* **radices**
    r. pili
    r. point
radon
Rad3-related protein
RADS
    reactive airways dysfunction syndrome
RAE
    right artial enlargement
RAEB
    refractory anemia with excess of blasts
RAEBT
    refractory anemia with excess blasts
      in transition
Raeder paratrigeminal syndrome
RAF
    rheumatoid arthritis factor
Raffaelea
raffinose
ragocyte cell
RAG-1, -2 recombinase enzyme system
RAH
    regressing atypical histiocytosis
    right atrial hypertrophy
RAI
    radioactive iodide
    radioactive iodine
      RAI test
Rai
    R. classification of chronic
      lymphocytic leukemia
    R. classification of CLL
    R. staging
RAIG1 family receptor
Raillietiella
Raillietina
    R. celebensis
    R. demerariensis
raillietiniasis
rain
    yellow r.
Rainier
    hemoglobin R.
raised colony
raisinoid nucleus
RAIU
    radioactive iodine uptake
Raji
    R. cell
    R. cell line
    R. cell radioimmune assay
Ralstonia
    R. campinensis
    R. insidiosa
    R. mannitolilytica
    R. metallidurans
    R. oxalatica

R

Ralstonia (*continued*)
    R. *pickettii*
    R. *respiraculi*
    R. *syzygii*
    R. *taiwanensis*
RAM
    right anterior measurement
Raman
    R. microprobe
    R. spectroscopy
Ramaria
ramblicola
    Idiomarina r.
Rambourg
    R. chromic acid-phosphotungstic
    acid stain
    R. periodic acid-chromic
    methenamine-silver stain
ramex
rami (*pl. of* ramus)
Ramichloridium
ramification
ramify
Ramlibacter
    R. *henchirensis*
    R. *tataouinensis*
Ramond point
ramosa
    Absidia r.
ramose, ramous
ramosum
    Clostridium r.
ramous (*var. of* ramose)
RAMP
    Rapid Analyte Measurement Platform
    regeneration-associated muscle protease
    RAMP anthrax test
    RAMP biological test system
    RAMP botulinum toxin test
    RAMP heart attack test
    RAMP myoglobin test
    RAMP ricin test
    RAMP smallpox test
    RAMP West Nile Virus test
Ramsay
    R. Hunt paralysis
    R. Hunt syndrome
Ramsden
    R. eyepiece
    R. ocular
Ramularia destructiva
ramus, *pl.* **rami**
ranae
    Aeromonas hydrophila subsp. *r.*
ranarum
    Basidiobolus r.
Ranavirus
RanBP protein
rancid

rancidification
rancidity
random
    r. access immunoassay system
    r. amplified polymorphic DNA
    analysis (RAPD)
    r. coil
    r. error
    r. genetic drift
    r. mating
    r. number
    r. number generator
    r. plasma glucose test
    r. sample
    r. urine specimen
    r. variable
random-donor platelet concentrate
randomization
randomize
Raney nickel
range
    r. of motion (ROM)
    semiinterquartile r.
rangeli
    Trypanosoma r.
Rangoon beggar's disease
Ranikhet disease
Rank
    Rankine temperature scale
rank
    r. correlation coefficient
    r. sum test
ranked data
Ranke formula
Rankine
    R. temperature scale (Rank)
    R. thermometer
RANKL
    receptor activator of nuclear factor
    kappa B ligand
Ranson
    R. acute pancreatitis criteria
    R. pyridine silver stain
RANTES
    regulated on activation, normal T
    expressed and secreted
    RANTES cycle
ranular cyst
Ranvier
    R. cross
    R. disc
    R. node
    node of R.
    R. segment
Raoultella
    R. *ornithinolytica*
    R. *planticola*
    R. *terrigena*
Raoult law

RAPD
random amplified polymorphic DNA analysis
raphe
Raphidascaris
rapid
r. ACTH test
R. ANA II test
R. Analyte Measurement Platform (RAMP)
r. antigen uptake into the cytosol enterocytes (RACE)
r. corticotropin test
r. drug screen multiple drug screen standard kit
r. drug screen on-site drug screening
R. flu A&B test
r. frozen section technique
r. grower
r. intraoperative quantitative RT-PCR assessment of tumor marker
r. microsatellite analysis
R. One lateral flow immunoassay test
R. One single dipstick system
R. One single drug screen dipstick
r. plasma reagin (RPR)
r. plasma reagin circle card test (RPR-CT)
r. recompression-high pressure oxygen (RR-HPO)
r. serum amylase test
r. susceptibility assay (RSA)
r. urease test (RUT)
rapidly
r. miscible pool (RMP)
r. progressive glomerulonephritis (RPGN)
rapid-lysis mutation
RapidVUE particle shape and size analyzer
RapiTex
R. ASO latex agglutination test
R. Hp test
Rapoport test
Rappaport
R. acinus
R. acinus zone 1
R. acinus zone 3
R. classification
Rapp-Hodgkin syndrome
rapture of the deep
raptus
status r.
rara
lamina r.
rare
r. base cutters

r. clostridial strain of *Clostridium argentinense*
r. clostridial strain of *Clostridium baratii*
R. Donor File
r. earth element
rarefaction
bone r.
Rarobacteraceae
RARS
refractory anemia with ringed sideroblasts
retinoic acid receptor
RAS
renal artery stenosis
reticular activating system
ras
r. cascade
r. gene
r. gene family
r. oncogene
r. signal
rash
antitoxin r.
astacoid r.
black currant r.
butterfly r.
hydatid r.
malar r. (MR)
morbilliform r.
Murray Valley r.
serum r.
socks and gloves petechial r.
Rasmussen aneurysm
RAST
radioallergosorbent assay test
RAST inhibition
rasus
Ixodes r.
rat
black house r.
ship r.
r. tapeworm
r. unit (RU)
r. virus (RV)
Wistar r.
rat-bite
r.-b. disease
r.-b. fever
rate
acid secretion r.
age-adjusted r.
age-specific r.
albumin excretion r. (AER)
aldosterone excretion r. (AER)
aldosterone secretion r. (ASR)
aldosterone secretory r. (ASR)
amebic prevalence r. (APR)
attack r.

R

rate (*continued*)
    basal apoptotic r.
    basal metabolic r. (BMR)
    basal secretory flow r. (BSFR)
    bone formation r. (BFR)
    case fatality r.
    cause-specific death r.
    cerebral cortex perfusion r. (CPR)
    cerebral metabolic r. (CMR)
    cerebrospinal fluid IgG synthesis r.
    circulation r.
    r. constant
    corrected sedimentation r. (CSR)
    cortisol production r. (CPR)
    cortisol secretion r. (CSR)
    count r.
    crude r.
    decay r.
    dose r.
    error r.
    erythrocyte sedimentation r. (ESR)
    failure r.
    flotation r.
    flow r. (FR)
    glomerular filtration r. (GFR)
    incidence r.
    infant mortality r. (IMR)
    inspiratory flow r. (IFR)
    intrauterine growth r. (IUGR)
    maximal inspiratory flow r. (MIFR)
    maximal midexpiratory flow r.
      (MMEFR)
    maximal midflow r. (MMFR)
    maximum expiratory flow r.
      (MEFR)
    metabolic clearance r. (MCR)
    r. meter
    mitotic r.
    morbidity r.
    mortality r. (MR)
    mutation r.
    r. nephelometry
    pineal secretory r.
    plasma clearance r. (PCR)
    plasma glucose disappearance r.
      (PGDR)
    plasma glucose tolerance r. (PGTR)
    plasma iron turnover r. (PITR)
    prevalence r.
    reaction r.
    red cell iron turnover r.
    renin-release r. (RRR)
    Rourke-Ernstein sedimentation r.
    secondary attack r.
    secretion r. (SR)
    sedimentation r. (sed rate, SR)
    somnolent metabolic r. (SMR)
    specific r.
    standardized r.

    testosterone production r. (TPR)
    tumor mitotic r.
    Westergren sedimentation r.
    Wintrobe sedimentation r.
    work metabolic r. (WMR)
    zeta sedimentation r. (ZSR)
ratellina
    Grisonella r.
Rathayibacter
    R. caricis
    R. festucae
Rathke
    R. bundle
    R. cleft cyst
    R. pouch
    R. pouch tumor
rathouisi
    Fasciolopsis r.
rating
    reactivity hazard r.
ratio
    absolute terminal innervation r.
    acid-base r. (A:B)
    activity r.
    adenine-thymine/guanine-cytosine r.
    adenosine 5′-diphosphate/adenosine
      triphosphate r.
    AE1:AE3 antibody r.
    alanine aminotransferase:aspartate
      aminotransferase r.
    amniotic fluid lecithin/sphingomyelin
      r.
    amylase/creatinine clearance r. (A:C,
      ACCR)
    base r.
    bile duct-to-portal space r. (BD/BS)
    body hematocrit to venous
      hematocrit r. (BH:VH)
    bound-free r. (B:F)
    branching r.
    BUN/creatinine r.
    cell-fat r.
    cholesterol/phospholipid r. (C:P)
    common mode rejection r. (CMRR)
    conversion r.
    crude mortality r. (CMR)
    cumulated activity r.
    cytoplasmic r.
    de Ritis r.
    desmin ensheathment r. (DER)
    dextrose nitrogen r. (DN)
    fluorescein-to-protein r. (F:P)
    free T_4 r.
    functional terminal innervation r.
    glucose-nitrogen r. (G:N)
    granulocyte/erythroid r. (G:E)
    grid r.
    hazard r. (HR)
    helper/suppressor cell r.

R

IgG r.
IgG:albumin r.
inspiratory:expiratory phase r.
International Normalized R. (INR)
ketogenic/antiketogenic r.
lactate-pyruvate r. (L:P)
lecithin/sphingomyelin r. (L:S)
left-to-right r. (L:R)
mean diameter-thickness r. (MDTR)
monocyte-lymphocyte r. (M:L)
myeloid-erythroid r. (M:E)
net protein r. (NPR)
nuclear-cytoplasmic r.
nuclear-to-cytoplasmic r. (n:c)
nucleolar-nuclear r.
nucleus-to-cytoplasm r.
r. of number of ATPs produced to
number of atmospheric oxygen
molecules converted to water
(P:O)
oil-water r. (O:W)
packing r.
polymorphonuclear-lymphocyte r.
polyunsaturated-to-saturated fatty
acids r. (P:S)
proportionate morbidity r. (PMR)
proportionate mortality r. (PMR)
protein efficiency r. (PER)
resin-uptake r. (RUR)
reversed albumin-globulin r.
r. scale
selectivity r.
signal to noise r. (S:N)
stalk to basilar artery r.
standard morbidity r. (SMR)
standard mortality r. (SMR)
stimulation r. (SR)
therapeutic r.
thyroid hormone binding r.
(THBR)
thyroid-to-serum r. (TSR)
T_4/TBG r.
urine-plasma r. (U:P)
ventilation-perfusion r.
RatioVision
AttoFluor R.
ratkowskyi
Algoriphagus r.
rat-tail maggot
ratti
Enterococcus r.
Rattus
raubitschekii
Trichophyton r.
Rauscher leukemia virus
RAV
Rous-associated virus
ray
beta r.

cathode r.
corresponding r.
delta r.
gamma r.
grenz r.
medullary r.
Rayer disease
Raymond-Cestan syndrome
Raynaud
R. disease (RD)
R. phenomenon
RB
Renaut body
RB1
retinoblastoma gene
RB1 alteration
RB1 protein transcription factor
RBA
rose bengal antigen
R-banding stain
RBC
red blood cell
e-positive RBCs
RBC-ChE
red blood cell cholinesterase
RBC/hpf
red blood cells per high-power field
RBCM
red blood cell mass
RBCV
red blood cell volume
RBE
relative biological effectiveness
RBL
Reid base line
RBP
retinol-binding protein
RC
resistor capacitor
RC circuit
R-cadherin gene
RCBV
regional cerebral blood volume
RCC
red cell count
renal cell carcinoma
RCC marker
RCC-CC
clear cell renal cell carcinoma
RCF
red cell folate
relative centrifugal force
RCM
red cell mass
RcoF
ristocetin cofactor
RcoF unit
RCS
reticulum cell sarcoma

RCV
   red cell volume
RD
   Raynaud disease
   resistance determinant
   reticular dysgenesis
Rd
   rutherford
RDD
   radiation dispersal device
   Rosai-Dorfman disease
RDE
   receptor-destroying enzyme
RDI
   rupture-delivery interval
rDNA
   recombinant DNA
   ribosomal DNA
RDS
   respiratory distress syndrome
RDW
   red cell distribution width
RDWr
   reticulocyte distribution width
RE
   regional enteritis
REA
   radiation emergency area
   radioenzymatic assay
   restriction endonuclease analysis
reabsorb
reabsorption
   tubular r.
Reach & Roll cart
reactance
   capacitive r.
   inductive r.
reactant
   acute phase r. (APR)
   limiting r.
reacting
   limes r. (Lr)
reaction
   accelerated r.
   acid r.
   acrosome r.
   acute hemolytic transfusion r.
   acute phase r.
   addition r.
   alkaline r.
   allergic transfusion r.
   alloxan-Schiff r.
   amphoteric r.
   anamnestic r.
   anaphylactic transfusion r.
   anaphylactoid r.
   anoxia r.
   antibody-dependent cell-mediated cytotoxicity r. (ADCC reaction)

antigen-antibody r.
antigen-antiglobulin r.
argentaffin r.
Arias-Stella r. (ASR)
Arthus r.
Ascoli r.
associative r.
autoimmune r.
azo coupling r.
bacterial transfusion r.
Bauer r.
Bence Jones r.
Berthelot r.
biuret r.
Bloch r.
blocking antibody r.
Bordet-Gengou r.
Burchard-Liebermann r.
Cannizzaro r.
capsular precipitation r.
Carr-Price r.
cell-mediated r.
r. center (RC)
chain r.
Chantemesse r.
chemical r.
chill-fever r.
chloroacetate esterase r.
cholera-red r.
CHR r.
Christeller r.
chromaffin r.
clot r.
cocarde r.
colloidal gold r.
competitive reverse transcription polymerase chain r. (cRT-PCR)
complement-fixation r.
constitutional r.
contrast media r.
cross r.
cutaneous r.
cytokeratin antigen-antibody r.
cytotoxic hypersensitivity r.
DAB r.
Dale r.
dark r.
decidual r.
degenerate oligonucleotide primed polymerase chain r. (DOP-PCR)
delayed hemolytic transfusion r.
delayed hypersensitivity r.
depot r.
dermotuberculin r.
diaminobenzidine r.
diazo r.
digitonin r.
diphtheria toxin immunization r.
Dold r.

R

dopa r.
early r.
Edman r.
Ehrlich benzaldehyde r.
Ehrlich diazo r.
elimination r.
endergonic r.
endogenous antigen cell-bound antibody r.
endogenous antigen-circulating antibody r.
endogenous antigen-transferred
  cell-bound antibody r.
enthalpy of r.
exergonic r.
exogenous antigen cell-bound
  antibody r.
exogenous antigen-circulating
  antibody r.
false-negative r.
false-positive r.
febrile nonhemolytic transfusion r.
Felix-Weil r. (FWR)
Fenton r.
Fernandez r.
Feulgen r.
first-order r.
fixation r.
flocculation r. (FR)
focal r.
foreign body r.
Forssman antigen-antibody r.
Frei-Hoffmann r.
fuchsinophil r.
Fujiwara r.
furfural r.
galactose oxidase Schiff r.
gapped ligase chain r.
gel diffusion r.
Gell and Coombs r.
generalized Sanarelli-Shwartzman r. (GSSR)
generalized Shwartzman r. (GSR)
Gerhardt r.
giant cell r.
glycine-arginine r.
graft versus host r. (GVHR)
Grimelius argyrophil r.
group r.
Gruber-Widal r.
Haber-Weiss r.
heat of r.
hemoclastic r.
hemolytic r.
hemolytic transfusion r.
Henle r.
Herxheimer r.
heterophil antigen r.
highly complex series of r.
hypersensitivity r. type I
idiosyncratic r.
immediate hypersensitivity r.

immune complex-mediated
  hypersensitivity r.
immune inflammatory r.
incompatible blood transfusion r.
inflammatory r.
intense inflammatory r.
r. intermediate
intracutaneous r.
intradermal r. (IDR)
irreversible r.
Jaffe r.
Jarisch-Herxheimer r.
Jones-Mote r.
Klebanoff r.
Langhans type of giant cell r.
late r.
Leder r.
lepromin r.
leukemoid r.
leukoerythroblastic r.
Liebermann-Burchard r.
ligase chain r. (LCR)
ligase detection r.
light r. (LR)
local r.
localized Schwartzman r.
Loewenthal r.
lymphocytic leukemoid r.
Marchi r.
Meinicke turbidity r. (MTR)
miostagmin r.
Mitsuda r.
mixed agglutination r.
mixed lymphocyte r. (MLR)
mixed lymphocyte culture r.
monocytic leukemoid r.
myelocytic leukemoid r.
Nadi r.
Nagler r.
Nessler r.
Neufeld r.
Nickerson-Kveim test r.
ninhydrin r.
ninhydrin-Schiff r.
nitritoid r.
r. of degeneration
r. of identity
r. of partial identity
osteoclastic r.
oxidase r.
oxidation-reduction r.
Pirquet r.
PK r.
plasmal r.
plasmocytic leukemoid r.
polymerase chain r. (PCR)
Porter-Silber r.
Prausnitz-Kustner r.
precipitin r.

reaction (*continued*)

Price precipitation r. (PPR)
primary r.
propagating nuclear r.
prozone r.
quanti-Pirquet r. (QP)
quellung r.
r. quotient
r. rate
reagin r.
redox r.
repair chain r.
reversed Prausnitz-Küstner r.
reverse transcriptase polymerase chain r. (RT-PCR)
reverse transcription polymerase chain r.
rheumatoid factor r.
Sakaguchi r.
Sanarelli-Shwartzman r.
Schmorl r.
Schultz r.
Schultz-Charlton r.
Schultz-Dale r.
second-order r.
sedimentation r.
Selivanoff r.
serum r.
Shwartzman r.
sigma r. (SR)
skin r.
so-called false-positive r.
specific r.
streptococcal toxin immunization r.
substitution r.
symptomatic r.
Szent-Györgyi r.
tetanus toxin immunization r.
thermoprecipitin r.
r. time (RT)
transcription-based chain r.
transferred antigen-cell-bound antibody r.
transferred antigen-transferred antibody r.
transfusion r.
Treponema pallidum immobilization r.
triketohydrindene r.
Trinder r.
tuberculin r.
tuberculin-type r.
type I–IV delayed-type r.
type I–IV hypersensitivity r.
typhoid immunization r.
unpredictable hypersensitivity-like r.
vaccinoid r.
Voges-Proskauer r.
von Kossa r.

Wassermann r.
Weidel r.
Weil-Felix r. (WFR)
Weinberg r.
wheal-and-erythema r.
wheal-and-flare r.
Widal r.
Yorke autolytic r.
zero-order r.
Zimmermann r.

reactivate

reactivation

dark r.

reactive

r. airways dysfunction syndrome (RADS)
r. astrocyte
atypical favor r.
r. cell
r. change
r. ductal proliferation
r. eosinophilic pleuritis (REP)
r. follicular hyperplasia
r. hyperemia (RH)
r. hyperemia blood flow (RHBF)
r. lymphocytes
r. lymphoid tissue (RLT)
r. material
r. oxygen metabolite (ROM)
r. oxygen species (ROS)
r. perforating collagenosis (RPC)
r. protein (RP)
r. spindle cell nodule (RSCN)
r. thrombocytosis
weakly r. (WR)

reactivity

CK20 r.
r. hazard rating
juxtanuclear Golgi r.
nonspecific bronchial r. (NSBR)

reactone red test

reactor

biologic false-positive r. (BFR)

readability

reader

Affinity multimode plate r.
Bio-Tek EIx800 plate r.
Cardiac R.
mark sense r.

reading

albumin r.
r. frame

Readit SNP genotyping system

readout

readthrough

re-aerosolization

reagent

Advia Centaur anti-HBs r.
Advia Centaur HBc IgM r.

analyte-specific r. (ASR)
analytical r. (AR)
Benedict-Hopkins-Cole r.
Bial r.
CellProbe cytoenzymology r.
chlorous acid r.
Cleland r.
Coleman-Schiff r.
CRPH high-sensitivity C-reactive
 protein r.
diazo r.
DNA synthesis r.
Drabkin r.
Edlefsen r.
Ehrlich diazo r.
Elecsys RBC folate
 hemolyzing r.
Eosinofix r.
Esbach r.
Folin-Ciocalteu r.
Fouchet r.
FPN r.
Frohn r.
furfural r.
Girard r.
gold chloride r.
r. grade
Gram-Sure r.
Griess r.
Günzberg r.
Hahn oxine r.
Hammarsten r.
Hanker-Yates r.
Horm collagen r.
Ilosvay r.
immunoassay r.
immunochemistry r.
immunohistochemistry r.
IntraPrep permeabilization r.
IOPath immunohistochemistry r.
Kasten fluorescent Schiff r.
KP1 immunohistochemical r.
Life Technologies TRIzol r.
LipoClear Plus lipemia
 clearing r.
Lloyd r.
lysing r.
MAK6 immunohistochemical r.
Mandelin r.
Marme r.
Marquis r.
maximum impurities r.
Mecke r.
Millon r.
Nanoprobes GoldEnhance r.
Nanoprobes Nanogold r.
Nichols r.
OptiLyse lysing r.
PTT-LA r.

r. red blood cell
Rosenthaler-Turk r.
Sanger r.
Schaer r.
Scheibler r.
Schiff r.
Selivanoff r.
Sickledex r.
Stravigen immunohistochemical r.
streptavidin-Nanogold r.
r. strip
Sulkowitch r.
test r.
TRIzol r.
Vectabond r.
Vectastain immunohistochemical r.
Vector Elite r.
reagin
 atopic r.
 automated r.
 rapid plasma r. (RPR)
 r. reaction
 unheated serum r. (USR)
reaginic antibody
REAL
 Revised European-American Lymphoma
 REAL classification
real number
real-time
 r.-t. clock
 r.-t. reverse-transcriptase PCR
reanneal
rearrangement
 bcl-2 gene r.
 breakpoint cluster region r.
 clonal gene r.
 gene r.
 immunoglobulin gene r.
 promiscuous antigen receptor
 gene r.
reassignment
 gender r.
reassociation
 DNA r.
Réaumur
 R. scale (R)
 R. thermometer
rebiopsy
rebound thrombocytosis
Rebuck skin window technique
recalcification time
**receiver operating characteristic
 (ROC)**
recent
 r. embolus
 r. infarct
 r. thrombus
receptogram pattern
receptoma

R

receptor

r. activator of nuclear factor kappa B ligand (RANKL)
alpha adrenergic r.
androgen r. (AR)
antiasialoglycoprotein r.
antiestrogen r.
antiprogesterone r.
asialoglycoprotein r. (ASGPR)
r. assay
autocrine motility factor r. (AMFR)
B-cell antigen r.
beta adrenergic r.
bombesin r.
calcitonin receptor-like r.
calcium-sensing r.
cell surface r.
c-kit r.
c-mp1 r.
complement r. (CR)
complement r. 3 (CR3)
dihydropyridine r.
discoidin domain r. (DDR)
endothelin-A, -B r.
epidermal growth factor r. (EGFR)
estradiol r.
estrogen r. (ER)
Fas r. (FasR)
Fc r. (FcR)
fibroblast growth factor r. (FGFR)
fMLP r.
folic acid r.
GABA r.
glucocorticoid r. (GR)
glycoprotein r.
GPC-R5b r.
GPC-R5c r.
GPC-R5d r.
G protein-coupled r. (GPCR)
G protein-linked r.
hormonal r.
hormone r.
human epidermal growth r. 2
hyperactive glutamate r.
importin r.
J r.
juxtapulmonary-capillary r.
kainate r.
kappa opioid r. (KOR)
killer immunoglobulin-like r. (KIR)
laminin r.
low-affinity nerve growth factor r. (LNGFR)
low density lipoprotein r.
lymphatic endothelial hyaluronan r. (LYVE1)
lymphocyte homing r.
mineralocorticoid r.
M3 muscarinic acetylcholine r.
muscarinic r.
neurotransporter r.
neurotrophic factor r.
Notch r.
opsonin r.
progesterone r. (PgR, PR)
prolactin r.
protease-activated r. (PAR)
PTCH r.
RAIG1 family r.
retinoic acid r. (RARS)
retinoid X r. (RXR)
ryanodine r.
scavenger r.
sensory r.
serotonergic r.
serum soluble transferrin r.
r. site
soluble interleukin-2 r.
soluble NSF-attachment protein r. (SNARE)
soluble transferrin r. (sTfR)
somatostatin r.
specific cell r.
steroid hormone r.
stretch r.
T-cell r. (TCR)
T-cell antigen r.
T-cell/E-rosette r.
thrombopoietin r.
toll-like r. 4 (TLR4)
transferrin r.
tumor necrosis factor r. (TNFR)
tyrosine kinase r.
r. tyrosine kinase
urokinase plasminogen activator r. (uPAR)
vascular endothelial growth factor r. 3 (VEGFR3)
vitronectin r.

receptor-destroying enzyme (RDE)
receptor-mediated endocytosis
recessive

autosomal r.
r. character
r. gene
r. inheritance

recidivans

leishmaniasis r. (LR)

recipient
reciprocal

r. transfusion
r. translocation

Recklinghausen

R. disease
R. tumor

Recklinghausen-Applebaum syndrome

reclotting phenomenon
reclusa
    Loxosceles r.
Reclus disease
recognition
    antigen r.
    r. factor
    r. of antigen
recombinant
    r. DNA (rDNA)
    r. erythropoietin
    r. human insulin-like growth factor (rhIGF)
    r. immunoblot assay (RIBA)
    r. platelet-derived growth factor (rPDGF)
    r. strain
    r. vaccine
    r. vector
recombination
    r. frequency
    genetic r.
    high-frequency r. (Hfr)
    homologous r.
    meiotic r.
    r. signal sequence (RSS)
RecombiPlasTin thromboplastin
reconditum
    Dipetalonema r.
reconfigurable
reconstruction
    Born method of wax plate r.
record
    dental identification r.
    logical r.
    medical r.
recorded
    not r. (NR)
recorder
recording
    r. electrode
    r. thermometer
recovery
    detect, incident command, scene safety and security, assess hazard, support required, triage and treatment, evacuation, r. (DISASTER)
    granulocyte r.
    r. time
recrudescent
    r. typhus
    r. typhus fever
recruitment
    leukocyte r.
recta (*pl. of* rectum)
rectae
    arteriolae r.
    venae r.

rectal
    r. bleeding
    r. column
    r. corticosteroid
    r. shelf tumor
rectale
    Eubacterium r.
recti
    Alcaligenes r.
    folliculi lymphatici r.
    stratum circulare tunicae muscularis r.
    stratum longitudinale tunicae muscularis r.
    tubuli seminiferi r.
    tunica muscularis r.
rectification
rectifier
    bridge r.
    full-wave r.
    half-wave r.
    silicon-controlled r.
rectitis
rectivirgula
    Saccharopolyspora r.
rectocele
rectocolitis
rectolabial fistula
rectostenosis
rectourethral fistula
rectovaginal fistula
rectovesical fistula
rectovestibular fistula
rectovulvar fistula
rectum, *pl.* **rectums, recta**
    benign lymphoma of r.
    vasa recta
rectums (*pl. of* rectum)
rectus
    Campylobacter r.
    tubulus r.
recumbinant interferon-9
recurrence
    local r.
    r. risk
recurrent
    r. albuminuria
    r. bacterial infection
    r. bouts of nephrotic syndrome
    r. carcinoma
    r. encephalopathy
    r. fetal loss (RFL)
    r. hepatitis C virus infection
    r. inflammation
    r. respiratory papillomatosis (RRP)
    r. sinus and pulmonary infection
    r. upper respiratory tract infection (RURTI)
    r. vasospasm

R

recurrentis
  Borrelia r.
recurring digital fibroma of childhood
recursion
recursive
  r. definition
  r. subroutine
recurvatum
  Echinoparyphium r.
  genu r.
red
  acid r. 87, 91
  alizarin r.
  alizarin r. S
  amidonaphthol r.
  r. atrophy
  Biebrich scarlet r.
  r. blood cell (RBC)
  r. blood cell cast
  r. blood cell cholinesterase
    (RBC-ChE)
  r. blood cell count
  r. blood cell enzyme deficiency
  r. blood cell injury
  r. blood cell mass (RBCM)
  r. blood cell morphology
  r. blood cells per high-power field
    (RBC/hpf)
  r. blood cell survival
  r. blood cell survival time
  r. blood cell volume (RBCV)
  r. bone marrow
  brilliant vital r.
  calcium r.
  r. cell adherence phenomenon
  r. cell adherence test
  r. cell aplasia
  r. cell count (RCC)
  r. cell destruction
  r. cell diameter width
  r. cell distribution width
    (RDW)
  r. cell folate (RCF)
  r. cell fragility
  r. cell fragmentation syndrome
  r. cell indices
  r. cell iron turnover rate
  r. cell lake
  r. cell mass (RCM)
  r. cell membrane protein defect
  r. cell survival test
  r. cell volume (RCV)
  chlorophenol r.
  chrome r.
  Congo r.
  r. corpuscle
  cresol r.
  Darrow r.
  r. degeneration

  r. eye syndrome
  r. fiber
  r. half-moon
  r. hepatization
  r. induration
  r. infarct
  r. litmus paper
  medicinal scarlet r.
  methyl r. (MR)
  r. mite
  r. muscle
  r. neuron
  neutral r.
  r. nucleus of midbrain
  r. oil
  r. phosphorus (RP)
  r. pulp
  r. pulp cord
  quinaldine r.
  ruthenium r.
  scarlet r.
  scharlach r.
  Sirius r.
  r. squill
  Sudan r. I
  r. thrombus
  toluylene r.
  trypan r.
  turkey r.
  r. venous blood (RVB)
  vital r.
reddish-blue mottling
reddish-brown infarct
redia
Redlich-Fisher miliary plaques
redox
  r. couple
  r. indicator
  r. potential
  r. reaction
Redquant kit
reduce
reduced
  r. enamel epithelium
  r. Fhit protein expression
  r. glutathione
  r. hematin
  r. hemoglobin (HHb)
  r. nicotinamide-adenine dinucleotide
  r. penetrance
reducing
  r. agent
  r. substances in urine
  r. sugar
reductant
reductase
  acetoacetyl-CoA r.
  cytochrome b5 r.
  dihydrofolate r. (DHFR)

dihydropteridine r.
epoxide r.
folate r.
glutathione r. (GR)
glyoxylate r.
l-xylulose r.
lysine ketoglutarate r.
lysine-2-oxoglutaryl r.
methemoglobin r.
methylenetetrahydrofolate r. (MTHFR)
NADH methemoglobin r.
4-oxoproline r.
oxosteroid r.
pyrroline-5-carboxylate r.
thioredoxin r. (TrxR)
reduction
r. division
r. potential
tetrazolium r. (TR)
reduplication of meiotic chromosome
reduvid, reduviid
reduviid (*var. of* reduvid)
Reduviidae
Reduvius
redux
chancre r.
redwater disease
Reed cell
Reed-Hodgkin disease
Reed-Sternberg
R.-S. cell (RS)
Hodgkin and R.-S. (HRS)
Reed-variant
R.-v. cell
mononuclear R.-v. (MRV)
reentrant pathway
Rees culture medium
Rees-Ecker
R.-E. fluid
R.-E. method
Reeve rest
REF
renal erythropoietic factor
refect
refeeding syndrom
reference
common r.
r. distribution
r. electrode
r. interval (RI)
r. laboratory
laboratory r. (LR)
r. material
r. method
r. strain
r. value (RV)
Refetoff syndrome

reflectance spectrophotometry
reflecting microscope
reflection
angle of r.
diffuse r.
specular r.
total internal r.
reflective testing
reflex
esophagosalivary r.
gag r.
Magnus and de Kleijn neck r.
Roger r.
r. sympathetic dystrophy
viscerotrophic r.
reflexa
tunica r.
reflexus
Argas r.
reflux
biliary r.
esophageal r.
r. esophagitis
r. gastritis
gastroesophageal r.
hepatojugular r.
r. nephropathy
ureteral r.
vesicoureteral r.
refluxate
refracting medium
refraction
angle of r.
double r.
index of r.
refractionometer (*var. of* refractometer)
refractive index (RI)
refractometer, refractionometer
refractometry
refractory
r. anemia with excess blasts in transformation
r. anemia with excess blasts in transition (RAEBT)
r. anemia with excess of blasts (RAEB)
r. anemia with ringed sideroblasts (RARS)
r. period (RP)
r. sideroblastic anemia
refringens
Borrelia r.
Treponema r.
Refsum disease
Regan isoenzyme
Regaud
R. fixative
R. pattern of growth
residual body of R.

R

regeneration
    atypical r.
    r. cell
    compensatory r.
    epimorphic r.
    incomplete r.
    morphallactic r.
regeneration-associated muscle protease (RAMP)
regenerative
    r. blood shift
    r. crypt
    r. endometrium
    r. medicine field of research
    r. micronodularity
    r. polyp
regia
    aqua r.
regina
regio
    r. olfactoria tunicae
    r. respiratoria tunicae mucosae
region
    abnormal banding r.
    antigen-binding r.
    argyrophilic nucleolar organizer r. (AgNOR)
    breakpoint r.
    C r.
    cell-cell contact r.
    centromeric r.
    complementarity determining r. (CDR)
    constant r.
    critical r.
    C-terminus r.
    D-loop r.
    hinge r.
    homogeneous staining r. (HSR)
    homology r.
    hypervariable r.
    hypochondriac r.
    I r.
    major breakpoint r. (MBR)
    midcervical r.
    midthoracic r.
    minor cluster r. (MCR)
    mutation cluster r. (MCR)
    nucleolar organizing r. (NOR)
    nucleolus organizing r. (NOR)
    promotor r.
    ringworm of genitocrural r.
    silver-stained nucleolar organizer r. (AgNOR)
    silver-stained nucleolar organizing r. (AgNOR)
    variable r.
regional
    r. cerebral blood volume (RCBV)

    r. colitis
    r. enteritis (RE)
    r. enterocolitis
    r. granulomatous lymphadenitis
    r. ileitis (RI)
    r. lymph node
register
    index r.
    shift r.
registry
    Agency for Toxic Substances Disease R. (ATSDR)
    Ovarian Tumor R. (OTR)
    tumor r.
Regitine
regressing atypical histiocytosis (RAH)
regression
    absent r.
    r. coefficient (R)
    r. curve
    extensive r.
    focal r.
regressive staining
regulated
    r. area
    r. on activation, normal T expressed and secreted (RANTES)
regulation
    genetic r.
    lipolysis r.
regulator
    autocrine-paracrine growth r.
    autoimmune r. (Aire)
    cell-cycle r.
    current r.
    cystic fibrosis transmembrane conductance r. (CFTR)
    r. gene
    humoral r.
    r. of G protein signaling protein 5 (RGS5)
    r. of invasion
    voltage r.
regulatory
    r. albuminuria
    r. gene
    r. hormone
    myogenic r. (MyoD)
    r. sequence
regurgitation
    aortic r. (Ao regurg, aor regurg)
    cardiac valvular r.
    r. jaundice
    mitral r.
    tricuspid r.
rehydration
Reibachia agariperforans

Reichmann
>R. disease
>R. syndrome

Reid
>R. base line (RBL)
>R. index

Reifenstein syndrome
Reinekea marinisedimentorum
reinfection tuberculosis
Reinke
>R. crystal
>R. crystalloid

reinnervation
reinoculation
Reinsch test
Reis-Bücklers corneal lattice dystrophy
Reisseisen muscle
Reissner membrane
Reiter
>R. disease
>R. protein complement-fixation
>(RPCF)
>R. syndrome

Reitland-Franklin (RF)
>R.-F. unit

rejection
>accelerated r.
>acute cellular r.
>acute humoral r.
>acute vascular r.
>allograft r.
>antibody-mediated r.
>chronic allograft r.
>first-set graft r.
>graft r.
>homograft r.
>hyperacute r.
>kidney transplant r.
>primary r.
>second-set graft r.
>transplant r.

rejuvenescence
relapsing
>r. disease
>r. febrile nodular panniculitis
>r. fever
>r. pancreatitis
>r. perichondritis
>r. polychondritis

relation
>Duane-Hunt r.
>equivalence r.

relationship
>host-parasite r.

relative
>r. biological effectiveness (RBE)
>r. centrifugal force (RCF)
>r. erythrocytosis
>r. fluorescence (RF)

>r. hepatic dullness (RHD)
>r. immunity
>r. leukocytosis
>r. polycythemia
>r. refractory period (RRP)
>r. retention time
>r. risk
>r. sagittal depth
>r. sensitivity
>r. specific activity (RSA)
>r. specificity
>r. standard deviation (RSD)
>r. value index (RVI)

relaxin
relay
>mercury-wetted r.

release
>clandestine aerosol r.
>renin r. (RR)

releasing
>r. factor (RF)
>r. hormone (RH)

REM
>reticular erythematous mucinosis

remains
>commingled r.
>human r.

Remak
>R. fiber
>R. paralysis

remanantlike lipoprotein particle (RLP)
remission
>spontaneous r.

remittent
>r. malaria
>r. malarial fever

remnant
>allantoic duct r.
>Cloquet canal r.
>mesonephric r.
>omphalomesenteric duct r.
>sinus venosus r.

**remnantlike lipoprotein
particles-cholesterol (RLP-C)**
remodeling
removal
>adduct r.
>wax r.

renal
>r. adenocarcinoma
>r. agenesis
>r. amyloidosis
>r. angiomyolipoma
>r. artery stenosis (RAS)
>r. atheroembolic disease
>r. azotemia
>r. blockade
>r. calculus
>r. capsule

renal (*continued*)
r. carbuncle
r. carcinosarcoma
r. cast
r. cell carcinoma (RCC)
r. clear cell carcinoma
r. colic
r. column
r. corpuscle
r. cortex
r. cortical adenoma
r. cortical lobule
r. cortical necrosis
r. cyst
r. cystic disease
r. diabetes
r. dysplasia complex
r. epithelioid oxyphilic neoplasm
r. erythropoietic factor (REF)
r. failure
r. fascia
r. function study (RFS)
r. function test
r. glycosuria
r. hamartoma
r. hemangioma
r. hematuria
r. hemorrhage
r. hypertension
r. hypoplasia
r. infarction
r. insufficiency
r. labyrinth
r. medullary necrosis
r. obstruction
r. oncocytoma
r. osteodystrophy
r. papillae
r. papillary necrosis
r. plasma flow (RPF)
r. pressor substance (RPS)
r. rickets
r. schwannoma
r. shutdown
r. synovial sarcoma
r. threshold
r. transplant
r. tuberculosis
r. tubular acidosis (RTA)
r. tubular dysgenesis
r. tubular epithelial (RTE)
r. tubular epithelial cell
r. tumor
r. uriniferous tubule
r. vascular resistance (RVR)
r. vein renin activity (RVRA)
r. vein renin concentration (RVRC)
r. vein thrombosis (RVT)
r. venous renin assay (RVRA)

renale
Corynebacterium r.
Dioctophyma r.

renales
columnae r.

renalis
area cribrosa papillae r.
cortex r.
fascia r.
hilum r.
lobulus corticalis r.

renal-retinal dysplasia
renaturation
DNA r.
Renaut body (RB)
Rendu-Osler-Weber
R.-O.-W. disease
R.-O.-W. syndrome
reniculi (*pl. of* reniculus)
reniculus, *pl.* **reniculi**
reniform nucleus
renin
r. assay
r. release (RR)
r. secreting tumor
r. stimulation test
renin-aldosterone axis
renin-angiotensin-aldosterone system
renin-release rate (RRR)
renis
arteriae arcuatae r.
capsula adiposa r.
corpusculum r.
ectopia r.
foramina papillaria r.
porta r.
tunica fibrosa r.
venulae rectae r.
venulae stellatae r.
rennin
renomedullary interstitial cell tumor
renomegaly
renovascular hypertension
Renpenning syndrome
Renshaw cell
REON
renal epithelioid oxyphilic neoplasm
Reoviridae
reovirus-like agent
reovirus type 1, 2, 3
REP
reactive eosinophilic pleuritis
repair
r. chain reaction
density-dependent r.

R

DNA r.
fibrous r.
mismatch r. (MMR)
postoperative r.
primary r.
secondary r.
tendon r.
reparative giant cell granuloma
repeat
dinucleotide r.
interspersed r.'s
inverted r.
mononucleotide r.
tandem trinucleotide r.
trinucleotide r.
triplet r.
variable number of tandem r.'s
(VNTR)
repeatability
wavelength r.
repeated DNA sequence
repens
Aspergillus r.
dermatitis r.
Dirofilaria r.
erythema gyratum r.
repere
point de r. (point of reference)
reperfusion injury
repertoire
HLA sequence in NK r.
KIR sequence in NK r.
repetitive stimulation
replacement
aortic valve r. (AVR)
r. bone
r. fibrosis
fibrous r.
replenisher
replica
freeze-fracture r.
r. grating
replicase
Q beta r.
replicate punch
replication
r. and transfer (RTF)
r. bubble
r. cycle
r. fork
local r.
normal r.
self-sustained sequence r. (3SR)
replicative
r. form
r. state
replicator
replicon
repolarization

repression
catabolite r.
end-product r.
enzyme r.
negative control r.
positive control r.
repressor gene
reproducibility
reproduction
asexual r.
sexual r.
reproductive cell
reptilase
r. fibrin
r. time
reptilase-R time
Reptilia
repullulation
repulsion
ReQ helicase
RER
rough endoplasmic reticulum
RER⁺ phenotype
RES
reticuloendothelial system
resazurin
rescue
marker r.
research
histocytologic r.
regenerative medicine field of r.
resection
laparoscopic renal r.
surgical r.
total gastric r.
resequencing microarray
reserve
r. cell
r. cell carcinoma
r. cell hyperplasia
reservoir
chromatin r.
r. host
r. of infection
r. of virus
rodent r.
resident cell
residua (*pl. of* residuum)
residual
r. abscess
r. air
r. body
r. body of Regaud
r. carcinoma
r. cleft
r. lumen
r. lung capacity (RLC)
r. urine
r. volume (RV)

residue
 amino acid r.
 gunshot r. (GSR)
 methanol-extruded r. (MER)
 nucleotide r. (NR)
 organized old thrombotic r.
 punctate nitrate r.
 spill r.
residuum, *pl.* **residua**
 gastric residua
resin
 anion-exchange r.
 cation exchange r.
 Chelex r.
 cholestyramine r.
 Effapoxy r.
 Epon-Araldite r.
 epoxy r.
 Harleco synthetic r.
 ion-exchange r.
 methacrylate r.
 podophyllin r.
 polyamine-methylene r.
 polyester r.
 quinine carbarcylic r.
 Spurr r.
 r. uptake
Resinicium
resin-uptake ratio (RUR)
resistance
 activated protein C r. (APCR)
 airway r.
 APC r.
 bacteriophage r.
 cerebrovascular r. (CVR)
 chemotherapy r.
 r. determinant (RD)
 r. factor
 r. inducing factor (RIF)
 insulin r.
 internal r. (IR)
 main site of airway r.
 multidrug r. (MDR)
 multidrug r. 1
 multiple drug r. (MDR)
 r. plasmid
 pulmonary r. (Rp)
 renal vascular r. (RVR)
 systemic vascular r. (SVR)
 r. thermometer
 total peripheral r. (TPR)
 total pulmonary vascular r.
  (TPVR)
 r. to venous return
 r. transfer factor (RTF)
 r. transferring episome
 r. unit (RU)
 vascular r. (VR)
resistivity

resistor
 r. capacitor (RC)
 carbon r.
 carbon-film r.
 r. color code
 composition r.
 power r.
 precision r.
 trimming r.
 variable r.
 wire-wound r.
resolution
 energy r.
 limit of r.
 radius of r.
 spectral r.
resolved
 not r. (NR)
resolvent
resolving
 r. power
 r. time
resonance
 electron paramagnetic r.
 electron spin r. (ESR)
 r. fluorescence
 r. line
resorcin
resorcin-fuchsin
resorcinol
 r. phthalic anhydride
 r. test
resorcinolphthalein sodium
resorption
 alveolar bone r.
 bone r.
 dissection r.
 r. lacunae
 lacunar r.
 osteoclastic r.
resource
 R. Conservation and Recovery Act
 death investigation r.'s
respiraculi
 Ralstonia r.
 Wautersia r.
respiration
 aerobic r.
 anaerobic r.
 Biot r.
 cellular r.
 Kussmaul r.
 Kussmaul-Kien r.
respirator
 air-purifying r. (APR)
 r. brain
 supplied air r. (SAR)
respiratorii
 bronchioli r.

respiratory
    r. acid-base disorder
    r. acidosis
    r. alkalosis
    r. angiocentric lymphoma
    r. bronchiole
    r. bronchiolitis
    r. burst
    r. chain
    r. depression
    r. distress syndrome (RDS)
    r. distress syndrome of newborn
    r. enteric orphan virus
    r. epithelial adenomatoid
      hamartoma
    r. epithelium
    r. exanthematous virus
    r. failure
    r. function
    r. illness (RI)
    r. infection virus
    r. inflammation
    r. insufficiency
    r. lobule
    r. mucosa
    r. pigment
    r. protein
    r. quotient
    r. scleroma
    r. syncytial (RS)
    r. syncytial virus (RSV)
    r. syncytial virus antibody test
    r. syncytial virus antigen
    r. syncytial virus antigen test
    r. syncytial virus infection
    r. syncytial virus nucleic acid
    r. syncytial virus serology
    r. system neoplasm
    Taiwan acute r. (TWAR)
    r. tract
    r. tract fluid (RTF)
    r. tuberculosis
    r. viral disease
Respirovirus
responder
    r. cell
    first r.
response
    anamnestic r.
    biphasic r.
    booster r.
    clinical r.
    concentration-dependent nanomolar r.
    delayed-phase skin r.
    dramatic r.
    early-phase r.
    galvanic skin r. (GSR)
    heat shock r.
    host r.

    humoral immune r.
    immediate-phase skin r.
    immune r. (Ir)
    isomorphic r.
    late-phase r.
    lymphoplasmacytic r.
    osteoblastic r.
    primary immune r.
    reticulocyte r.
    secondary immune r.
    sensitization r. (SR)
    spectral r.
    stringent r.
    total r. (TR)
    visual evoked r.
responsibility
    safety r.
rest
    aberrant r.
    adrenal r.
    cartilaginous r.
    congenital r.
    embryonal r.
    epithelial r.
    Erdheim r.
    intralobar nephrogenic r. (ILNR)
    Marchand r.
    mesonephric r.
    Müllerian r.
    nephrogenic r. (NR)
    Reeve r.
    Walthard cell r.
    wolffian r.
restiform
resting
    r. B cell
    r. membrane potential
    r. stage
    r. wandering cell
restitope
restless legs syndrome
restricted
    r. access laboratory
    r. light chain
restriction
    r. endonuclease
    r. endonuclease analysis (REA)
    r. enzyme
    r. fragment length polymorphism
      (RFLP)
    r. map
    MHC r.
restrictive
    r. cardiomyopathy
    r. lung disease
restrictus
    Azovibrio r.
    Dehalobacter r.
restructured cell

R

restuans
Culex r.
result
macrophage presented antigen r.
r. of severe fracture
Surveillance, Epidemiology, and End
R.'s (SEER)
retained
r. foreign body (RFB)
r. placental fragment
r. products of conception
r. testis
retardation
familial mental r. (FMR)
growth r.
Wilms tumor, aniridia, genital
anomalies, mental r. (WAGR)
ret detach
rete, *pl.* **retia**
r. cell tumor
r. cord
r. cutaneum corii
r. cyst of ovary
malpighian r.
r. peg
r. ridge
r. subpapillare
r. testis
retention
r. cyst
fluid r.
gas r.
increased sodium r.
r. index
r. jaundice
mucus r.
r. polyp
r. time
urinary r.
r. volume
retia (*pl. of* rete)
retial
Retic-Chex linearity assay
reticle
ocular r.
reticONE system
reticula (*pl. of* reticulum)
reticular, reticulated
r. activating system (RAS)
r. cartilage
r. cell
r. degeneration
r. dermis
r. dysgenesis (RD)
r. erythematous mucinosis
(REM)
r. fiber
r. fibers in wall of central
vein

r. formation
r. growth pattern
r. keratitis
r. lamina
r. layer of corium
r. membrane of spinal organ
r. substance
r. tissue
reticularis
angiitis livedo r.
r. cell
dermatopathia pigmentosa r.
fetal r.
formatio r.
livedo r.
substantia r.
zona r.
reticulata
folliculitis ulerythematosa r.
reticulate body
reticulated (*var. of* reticular)
r. bone
r. corpuscle
r. erythrocyte
reticulating colliquation
reticulation
intralobar r.
reticulatum
atrophoderma r.
reticulatus
Dermacentor r.
reticulin
r. fiber
marrow r.
r. stain
r. staining
reticuliscabiei
Streptomyces r.
reticulocyte (retic)
r. count
r. distribution width (RDWr)
hemoglobin content of r.'s
r. mean corpuscular volume (MCVr)
r. response
shift r.
r. staining
stress r.
reticulocytic
r. marrow
r. production index (RPI)
reticulocytopenia
reticulocytosis
reticuloendothelial (RE)
r. cell
r. cell hyperplasia
r. iron stores
r. sarcoma
r. system (RES)
reticuloendothelioma

reticuloendotheliosis
    avian r.
    leukemic r.
    systemic r.
reticuloendothelium
reticulofilamentosa
    substantia r.
reticulohistiocytic granuloma
reticulohistiocytoma
reticulohistiocytosis
    multicentric r.
reticuloid
    actinic r.
reticulopenia
reticulosis
    benign inoculation r.
    histiocytic medullary r.
    Ketron-Goodman pagetoid r.
    leukemic r.
    lipomelanic r.
    lipomelanotic r.
    medullary histiocytic r.
    myeloid r.
    polymorphic r. (PMR)
    Sézary r.
    Woringer-Kolopp pagetoid r.
reticulum, *pl.* **reticula**
    agranular endoplasmic r.
    r. cell
    r. cell hyperplasia
    r. cell lymphosarcoma
    r. cell sarcoma (RCS, RSA)
    cistern of cytoplasmic r.
    Ebner r.
    endoplasmic r. (ER)
    Golgi internal r.
    granular endoplasmic r.
    Kölliker r.
    rough endoplasmic r. (RER)
    rough-surfaced endoplasmic r.
    sarcoplasmic r.
    smooth endoplasmic r. (SER)
    smooth-surfaced endoplasmic r.
    r. stain
    stellate r.
    trabecular r.
    r. trabeculare sclerae
    Wilder stain for r.
retiform
    r. hemangioendothelioma
    r. Sertoli-Leydig cell tumor
retina, *pl.* **retinae**
    ablatio retinae
    cerebral layer of r.
    cone cell of r.
    ganglion cell of r.
    ischemia retinae
    layer of r.
    limiting membrane of r.

    macula retinae
    neural layer of r.
    ora serrata retinae
    strata nuclearia externa et interna
      retinae
    stratum cerebrale retinae
    stratum moleculare retinae
    stratum neuroepitheliale retinae
    stratum pigmenti retinae
retinacula (*pl. of* retinaculum)
retinaculum, *pl.* **retinacula**
retinae (*pl. of* retina)
retinal
    r. anlage tumor
    r. aplasia
    r. artery occlusion
    r. cone
    r. detachment
    r. disorder
    r. embolism
    r. microaneurysm
retinalis
    lipemia r.
retinitis
    r. pigmentosa
    r. proliferans
retinoblastoma
    r. gene (RB1)
    r. protein
retinochoroiditis
    r. juxtapapillaris
    toxoplasmic r.
retinoic
    r. acid
    r. acid binding protein 1 gene
    r. acid receptor (RARS)
retinoid
    r. X receptor (RXR)
    r. X receptor alpha
retinol
retinol-binding protein (RBP)
retinopathy
    circinate r.
    diabetic r. (DR)
    r. of prematurity (ROP)
retoperithelium
retort
Retortamonas intestinalis
retothelioma
retractile testis
retraction
    r. artifact
    clot r.
    impaired clot r.
    massive vitreous r. (MVR)
retrieval
    antigen r.
    epitope r.
    heat-induced epitope r. (HIER)

retrieval (*continued*)
    heat-mediated antigen r.
    information r.
    low-temperature antigen r. (LTAR)
    low-temperature, heat-mediated
      antigen r. (LTHMAR)
    sonication-induced epitope r. (SIER)
retrobulbar
    r. neuropathy
retrocardiac tumor
retrocolic hernia
retroflection (*var. of* retroflexion)
retroflexion, retroflection
retrograde
    r. chromatolysis
    r. degeneration
    r. embolism
    r. intussusception
    r. metamorphosis
    r. pyelography
retrogression
retrolental fibroplasia (RLF)
retromammary mastitis
retromorphosis
retroperitoneal
    r. fibromatosis
    r. fibrosis
    r. gas insufflation
    r. lymph node dissection
retroperitoneum
retroperitonitis
    idiopathic fibrous r.
retroplacental hematoma
retroplasia
retrospective study
retrosternal
    r. hernia
    r. tumor
retroversion
retroviral oncogene
Retroviridae
retrovirus
    AKT8 r.
    jaagsiekte sheep r.
    zoonotic r.
RETRX
    retraction
Retsch MM200 mixer mill
Rettgerella rettgeri
rettgeri
    Proteus r.
    Providencia r.
    Rettgerella r.
Rett syndrome
return
    resistance to venous r. (RVR)
Retzius
    calcification line of R.
    R. fiber

    R. line
    line of R.
    R. parallel striae
    sheath of Key and R.
reuniens
    canaliculus r.
    canalis r.
    ductus r.
Reuss
    R. formula
    R. test
revaccination
reverse
    r. agglutination
    r. banding
    r. bias
    r. blood typing
    r. dot-blot
    r. genetics
    r. grouping
    r. hemolytic plaque assay
    r. immunoelectrophoresis
    r. line probe
    r. mutation
    r. passive hemagglutination
    r. passive latex agglutination
      (RPLA)
    r. T_3
    r. transcriptase
    r. transcriptase polymerase chain
      reaction (RT-PCR)
    r. transcription
    r. transcription polymerase chain
      reaction
    r. triiodothyronine (rT_3)
reversed
    r. albumin-globulin ratio
    r. passive anaphylaxis
    r. Prausnitz-Küstner reaction
reversible
    r. calcinosis
    r. change
    r. injury
reversion
revertant
review
    drug utilization r.
revised
    R. European-American Classification
      of Lymphoid Neoplasms
    R. European-American Lymphoma
      (REAL)
    R. European-American Lymphoma
      classification
revision
    fusiform skin r. (FSR)
Revival Menopause Home Test
revivescence
revolutions per minute (rpm)

revolutum
    Echinostoma r.
revolver
Rexed
    lamina of R.
Reye syndrome
Reynolds
    R. lead citrate
    R. number
    R. pentad
RF
    Reitland-Franklin
    relative fluorescence
    releasing factor
    rheumatic fever
    rheumatoid factor
RFB
    retained foreign body
RFL
    recurrent fetal loss
RFLA
    rheumatoid factor-like activity
RFLP
    restriction fragment length
     polymorphism
      RFLP Southern hybridization analysis
RFS
    renal function study
rgp120 protein
RGS5
    regulator of G protein signaling
     protein 5
RH
    reactive hyperemia
    releasing hormone
rh
    rheumatic
Rh
    rhesus
      Rh agglutinin
      Rh antibody
      Rh antigen
      Rh blocking test
      Rh blood group
      Rh factor
      Rh immunization
      Rh incompatibility
      Rh isoantigen
      Rh isoimmunization syndrome
      Rh negative
      Rh null syndrome
      Rh positive
      Rh type
      Rh typing
Rhabdiasoidea
Rhabditida
rhabditiform
Rhabditis hominis
rhabdocyte

rhabdoid
    r. cell
    r. phenotype
    r. phenotype of large-cell carcinoma
    r. predisposition
    r. tumor of the kidney
Rhabdomonas
rhabdomyoblast
rhabdomyoblastic differentiation
rhabdomyolysis
    acute recurrent r.
    familial paroxysmal r.
    idiopathic paroxysmal r.
rhabdomyoma
rhabdomyosarcoma (RM, RMS),
  rhabdosarcoma
    alveolar r. (ARMS)
    botryoid r.
    embryonal r. (ERMS)
    r. marker
    pleomorphic r.
rhabdosarcoma (*var. of* rhabdomyosarcoma)
Rhabdoviridae
rhabdovirus
Rhadinovirus
rhagades
rhagadiform
rhagiocrine
    r. cell
    r. vacuole
RHBF
    reactive hyperemia blood flow
RHD
    relative hepatic dullness
    rheumatic heart disease
Rheinberg microscope
Rheinheimera
    R. baltica
    R. pacifica
rhenobacensis
    Rhodopseudomonas r.
rheobase
Rheolog device
rheostat
rheostosis
rheotaxis
rheotropism
rhestocythemia
rhesus (Rh)
    r. monkey kidney (RMK)
rheum
    rheumatic
rheumatic (rh, rheum)
    r. arteritis
    r. arthralgia
    r. carditis
    r. endocarditis
    r. fever (RF)
    r. heart disease (RHD)

R

rheumatic (*continued*)
    r. lung disease
    r. myocarditis
    r. nodule
    r. pericarditis
    r. pneumonia
    r. pneumonitis
    r. valvulitis
rheumatica
    polymyalgia r.
    scarlatina r.
rheumaticum
    erythema marginatum r.
rheumatid
rheumatism
    articular r.
    chronic r.
    gonorrheal r.
    inflammatory r.
    Macleod r.
    muscular r.
    nodose r.
    tuberculous r.
rheumatismal
rheumatoid
    r. agglutinator
    r. ankylosing spondylitis
    r. aortitis
    r. arteritis
    r. arthritis (RA)
    r. arthritis factor (RAF)
    r. episcleritis
    r. factor (RF)
    r. factor-like activity (RFLA)
    r. factor reaction
    r. factor test
    r. heart disease
    r. lung
    r. neutrophilic dermatosis
    r. nodule
    r. pneumoconiosis
    r. synovitis
rhIGF
    recombinant human insulin-like growth factor
rhinaria
    Linguatula r.
rhinitis
    acute r.
    allergic r.
    atrophic r.
    fetid r.
    r. nervosa
    nonallergic r.
    seasonal r.
    vasomotor r. (VMR)
rhinoantritis
rhinocerebral
    r. aspergillosis

    r. disease
    r. zygomycosis
Rhinocladiella
Rhinocladium
rhinocleisis
rhinoentomophthoromycosis
rhinoestrosis
Rhinoestrus purpureus
rhinolaryngitis
rhinomucormycosis
rhinomycosis
rhinonecrosis
rhinopharyngitis mutilans
rhinophycomycosis
rhinophyma
rhinopneumonitis
    equine r. (ERP)
rhinoscleroma bacillus
rhinoscleromatis
    Klebsiella pneumonia r.
rhinosporidiosis
Rhinosporidium seeberi
rhinotracheitis
    feline viral r.
    infectious bovine r. (IBR)
Rhinotrichum
rhinovirus
    bovine r.
    equine r.
Rhipicentor
rhipicephali
    Rickettsia r.
Rhipicephalus sanguineus
Rhizidiomyces
Rhizidiovirus
Rhizobiaceae
Rhizobieae
Rhizobium
    R. indigoferae
    R. japonicum
    R. larrymoorei
    R. loessense
    R. radiobacter
    R. rhizogenes
    R. rubi
    R. sullae
    R. undicola
    R. vitis
    R. yanglingense
Rhizoctonia
rhizogenes
    Rhizobium r.
Rhizoglyphus parasiticus
rhizoid
rhizomelia
Rhizomucor
rhizophila
    Kocuria r.
    Stenotrophomonas r.

rhizoplast
rhizopod
Rhizopoda
Rhizopodasida
Rhizopodea
rhizopodoformis
    Rhizopus r.
Rhizopus
    R. arrhizus
    R. equinus
    R. niger
    R. nigricans
    R. oryzae
    R. rhizopodoformis
Rhizosphaera
rhizosphaerae
    Pseudomonas r.
rhizosphaericus
    Streptomyces r.
rhizospherae
    Agromyces r.
Rh_{null} disease
rhodamine
    lissamine r. B 200
    r. B
    r. stain
rhodanate
rhodanic acid
rhodanile blue
Rhodanobacter lindaniclasticus
Rhodesian trypanosomiasis
rhodesianum
    Methylobacterium r.
rhodesiense
    Trypanosoma brucei r.
rhodina
    Botryosphaeria r.
rhodinum
    Methylobacterium r.
Rhodnius prolixus
Rhodobaca bogoriensis
Rhodobacteria
Rhodoblastus acidophilus
Rhodocista pekingensis
Rhodococcus
    R. aetherivorans
    R. baikonurensis
    R. equi
    R. gordoniae
    R. jostii
    R. koreensis
    R. maanshanensis
    R. pyridinivorans
Rhodoferax
    R. antarcticus
    R. ferrireducens
Rhodoglobus vestalii
Rhodomyces
rhodophylactic

rhodophylaxis
Rhodophyllus sinuatus
Rhodopirellula baltica
Rhodopseudomonas
    R. faecalis
    R. rhenobacensis
rhodopsin
Rhodospirillaceae
Rhodospirillales
Rhodosporidium
Rhodotorula
    R. mucilaginosa
    R. rubra
rhodotorulosis
rho factor
RhoGAM vaccine
rhombencephalitis
rhombic lip
rhombocele
rhomboidalis
rhomboidal sinus, sinus rhomboidalis
Rhombomys
rhopheocytosis
rhoptry protein
RHPA
    reverse hemolytic plaque
    assay
Rhus
    R. toxicodendron antigen
    R. venenata antigen
rhusiopathiae
    Actinomyces r.
    Erysipelothrix r.
rhypophagy
rhysodes
    Acanthamoeba r.
rhythm
    circadian r.
    infradian r.
    isochronal r.
    metachronal r.
    ultradian r.
rhytidosis
RI
    reference interval
    refractive index
    regional ileitis
    respiratory illness
RIA
    radioimmunoassay
        CA15-3 RIA
        triiodothyronine by RIA
RIBA
    recombinant immunoblot assay
        RIBA 1, 2, 3
Ribas-Torres disease
ribavirin
Ribbert theory
ribbon stool

R

riboflavin, riboflavine
  r. assay
  r. loading test
  r. unit
riboflavine (*var. of* riboflavin)
riboflavin-5′-phosphate
ribonuclear protein (RNP)
ribonuclease (RNase, RNAse)
  r. (pancreatic)
  r. protection assay
  r. solution
ribonucleic acid (RNA)
ribonucleoprotein (RNP)
  r. antibody test
  r. complex
  small nuclear r.'s (SNRPs)
ribonucleoside
  thymine r.
ribonucleoside-5′-phosphate
  thymine r.-5.-p.
ribonucleotide
riboprobe
  digoxigenin-labeled r.
  EBER1 r.
  U6 r.
ribose
ribose-1-phosphate
ribose-5-phosphate
ribosomal
  r. ambiguity
  r. DNA (rDNA)
  r. RNA (rRNA)
ribosome
  disaggregated r.
  free r.
ribosome-lamella complex
ribosuria
ribothymidylic acid
ribotyping
ribovirus
ribulose
ribulose-5-phosphate
rice
  r. blast
  r. body
  r. starch
rice-flour breath test
rice-Tween agar
rice-water stools
Richard-Allan Scientific Ultrafast Papanicolaou stain
richardsiae
Richards-Rundle syndrome
Richet aneurysm
Richter
  R. hernia
  R. syndrome
ricin A, B chain
ricinoleic acid

ricinus
  R. communis
  Ixodes r.
rickets
  acute r.
  adult r.
  celiac r.
  hemorrhagic r.
  hypophosphatemic r.
  renal r.
  vitamin-D-dependent r.
  vitamin-D-resistant r.
rickettsi
  Dermacentroxenus r.
rickettsia
  R. aeschlimannii
  R. africae
  R. akari
  R. australis
  R. conorii
  R. felis
  R. honei
  R. japonica
  R. massiliae
  R. montana
  R. pediculi
  R. prowazekii
  R. rhipicephali
  R. rickettsii
  R. sennetsu
  R. sibirica
  R. slovaca
  R. tsutsugamushi
  R. typhi
  r. vaccine, attenuated
Rickettsiaceae
rickettsiae
Rickettsiales
rickettsial infection
rickettsialpox
Rickettsieae
rickettsii
  Rickettsia r.
rickettsiosis
rickettsiostatic
Ricketts organism
RID
  radial immunodiffusion
  RID assay
Rida virus
Rideal-Walker
  R.-W. coefficient
  R.-W. method
ridge
  epidermal r.
  gonadal r.
  interpapillary r.
  mucosal r.
  r. of intramembranous particle

R

rete r.
skin r.
riding embolism
Riechert-Mundiger stereotactic
device
Riedel
R. disease
R. struma
R. thyroiditis
Rieder
R. cell
R. cell leukemia
R. lymphocyte
Rieger syndrome
Riehl melanosis
RIF
resistance inducing factor
RIFA
radioiodinated fatty acid
rifamycinica
Amycolatopsis r.
rifietoensis
Planococcus r.
rifling impression
Rift
R. Valley fever
R. Valley fever virus
Riga-Fede disease
Rigg disease
right
r. anterior measurement (RAM)
r. atrial enlargement (RAE)
r. atrial hypertrophy (RAH)
r. axis deviation (RAD)
deviation to the r.
r. lower quadrant
r. ovarian vein syndrome
shield to the r.
r. ventricle double outlet
r. ventricular dysplasia
r. ventricular enlargement (RVE)
r. ventricular failure
r. ventricular hypertrophy (RVH)
r. ventricular hypoplasia
right-handed alpha helix
right-to-know law
rigidity
decerebrate r.
lead-pipe r.
muscular r.
nuchal r.
postmortem r.
rigor mortis
rigorous
RIHSA
radioactive iodinated human serum
albumin
Riley-Day syndrome
Riley-Smith syndrome

rim
abrasion r.
R. A.R.C. Mono test
r. pattern
Rimini
R. test
R. testRimini test
rinderpest virus
Rindfleisch cell
ring
abrasion r.
aromatic r.
Balbiani r.
Bandl r.
Biondi r.
r. chromosome
connecting r.
contractile r.
corrin r.
r. counter
esophageal r.
F-actin r.
Fleischer r.
r. form
r. granuloma
Kayser-Fleischer r.
Liesegang r.
lower r.
mesangial r.
r. mosaic
nipple arranged in a r.
r. precipitin test
Schatzki r.
signet r.
vascular r.
Waldeyer r.
ring-chain tautomer
ringed sideroblast
Ringer
R. injection
R. irrigation
R. lactate solution (RLS)
R. mixture
ringeri
ring-wall lesion
ringworm
black-dot r.
crusted r.
gray-patch r.
honeycomb r.
r. of beard
r. of body
r. of genitocrural region
r. of nails
r. of scalp
Oriental r.
scaly r.
Tokelau r.
Rinkel test

Rinne test (R)
riot
>r. control
>r. control agent

RIP
>radioimmunoprecipitation

RIPA
>radioimmunoprecipitation assay

ripening
ripple
>r. counter
>r. factor
>r. voltage

RISA
>radioactive iodinated serum albumin
>radioiodinated serum albumin
>RISA test

RISHN
>radiation-induced sarcoma of the head and neck

risk
>r. factor
>Gail index of breast cancer r.
>r. group stratification
>recurrence r.
>relative r.

risk-adapted therapy
RIST
>radioimmunosorbent test

risticii
>*Ehrlichia r.*
>*Neorickettsia r.*

ristocetin cofactor (RcoF)
Ritter disease
Ritter-Oleson (RO)
>R.-O. technique

rittmannii
>*Alicyclobacillus acidocaldarius*
>subsp. *r.*

ritual ligature strangulation (incaprettamento)
RIU
>radioactive iodine uptake

river blindness
Rivinus
>R. duct
>R. gland

rivolta
>*Isospora r.*

riziform
RLC
>residual lung capacity

RLF
>retrolental fibroplasia

RLP
>remanantlike lipoprotein particle

RLP-C
>remnantlike lipoprotein
>particles-cholesterol

RLP-Cholesterol Immunoseparation Assay kit
RLS
>Ringer lactate solution

RLT
>reactive lymphoid tissue

RM
>rhabdomyosarcoma

R-meter
>rate meter

RMK
>rhesus monkey kidney

RMP
>rapidly miscible pool

RMS
>rhabdomyosarcoma

RMSF
>Rocky Mountain spotted fever

RNA
>ribonucleic acid
>>chromosomal RNA (cRNA)
>>Epstein-Barr encoded RNA (EBER)
>>expressed RNA
>>hMAM RNA
>>RNA nucleotidyltransferase
>>RNA polymerase
>>RNA processing
>>ribosomal RNA (rRNA)
>>short-interference RNA (siRNA)
>>RNA splicing
>>transfer RNA (tRNA)
>>translation control RNA (tcRNA)
>>RNA tumor virus

RNA-driven hybridization
RNA-RNA hybridization
RNase, RNAse
>ribonuclease
>RNase A
>alkaline RNase
>RNase I

RNase-free condition
RNAzol
>RNAzol B RNA extraction method
>RNAzol Reagent Extractor

RNP
>ribonuclear protein
>ribonucleoprotein
>RNP complex

RO
>Ritter-Oleson

Roaf
>R. syndrome
>R. syndrome

robertsiae
>*Wingea r.*

robertsonian translocation
Roberts syndrome
Robiginitalea biformata

Robin
>R. sequence
>R. syndrome

Robinow syndrome

Robinson disease

Roble disease

robot
>ORCA R.

Robson
>R. point
>R. stage I, II renal carcinoma

robustum
>*Ketogulonicigenium r.*

robustus
>*Atrax r.*
>*Gordius r.*

ROC
>receiver operating characteristic
>ROC curve

roccellin

Rochalimaea
>*R. henselae*
>*R. quintana*

Roche
>R. Septi-Chek blood culture system
>R. Sysmex hematology system

rocker microtome

rocket immunoelectrophoresis

rocking microtome

Rocky
>R. Mountain spotted fever (RMSF)
>R. Mountain spotted fever antibody test
>R. Mountain spotted fever serology
>R. Mountain spotted fever vaccine

rod
>anaerobic r.
>Auer r.
>Corti r.
>r. disc
>enamel r.
>r. fiber
>r. granule
>motile r.
>r. myopathy
>nemaline r.
>r. neutrophil
>r. nuclear cell
>r. photoreceptor cell
>policeman glass stirring r.
>r. shaped bacterium
>slightly curved r.
>spore-forming r.
>straight r.

rodent
>r. reservoir
>r. ulcer

rodenticide

rodentium
>*Veillonella parvula* subsp. *r.*

Rodrigues aneurysm

rod-shaped
>r.-s. polymer
>r.-s. structure

roetheln

Roger
>R. disease
>maladie de R.
>R. reflex
>R. syndrome

Rohr stria

Rohypnol

Rokitansky
>R. disease
>R. pelvis
>R. protuberance

Rokitansky-Aschoff sinus

Rokitansky-Küster-Hauser syndrome

rolandic epilepsy

Rolando
>R. cell
>R. fissure
>R. gelatinous substance

role
>prognostic r.

roll
>iliac r.
>scleral r.
>r. tube
>r. tube technique

rolled sample

Rollet stroma

rolling hernia

ROM
>range of motion
>reactive oxygen metabolite
>rupture of membranes

Romaña
>R. sign
>R. sign/trill

Roman bridge formation

Romanovsky (*var. of* Romanowsky)

Romano-Ward syndrome

Romanowsky, Romanovsky
>R. blood stain
>R. type stain

Romanowsky-Giemsa stain

Romberg
>R. disease
>R. syndrome
>R. trophoneurosis

rombergism

romeroi
>*Pyrenochaeta r.*

Römer test

Rommelaere sign

ronds
> corps r.

ronnel

room
> cold r.
> decontaminating r.
> negative-pressure r.
> r. temperature (RT)

root
> hair r.
> mandrake r.
> nerve r.
> r. sheath

root-mean-square

ROP
> retinopathy of prematurity

ropalocytosis

Ropes test

ropey collagen

ROS
> reactive oxygen species

rosa
> *Novosphingobium r.*

rosacea
> acne r.

rosacea-like tuberculid

rosaceum
> *Trichophyton r.*

Rosai-Dorfman disease (RDD)

rosanilin dye

rosaniline

rosary
> rachitic r.
> scorbutic r.

rosati

rosatii
> *Neotestudina r.*

rose
> r. bengal
> r. bengal antigen (RBA)
> r. bengal radioactive ^{131}I test
> r. bengal sodium
> r. cold
> R. test

rosea
> pityriasis r.

Rose-Bradford kidney

Roseburia intestinalis

Roseibium
> *R. denhamense*
> *R. hamelinense*

roseiflava
> *Sphingomonas r.*

Roseiflexus castenholzii

Roseinatronobacter thiooxidans

Roseivivax
> *R. halodurans*
> *R. halotolerans*

Rosellinia

Rosenbach
> R. disease
> R. syndrome
> R. test

Rosenbach-Gmelin test

rosenbergii
> *Hyphomonas r.*

Rosen criteria for lymphovascular invasion

Rosenmüller
> R. gland
> R. node

Rosenow veal-brain broth

Rosenthal
> R. fiber
> R. fiber
> R. syndrome

Rosenthaler-Turk reagent

Rosenthal-Kloepfer syndrome

Roseococcus thiosulfatophilus

roseola
> epidemic r.
> r. infantilis
> r. infantum virus
> r. vaccine

Roseolovirus

Roseomonas
> *R. gilardii*
> *R. mucosa*

roseosalivarius
> *Hymenobacter r.*

Roseospira
> *R. marina*
> *R. navarrensis*

Roseospirillum parvum

Roseovarius nubinhibens

rosette
> erythrocyte r.
> Flexner-Wintersteiner r.
> Homer-Wright r.
> hyalinizing spindle cell tumor with giant r.'s
> malarial r.
> neural r.
> pineocytomatous r.
> r. test
> T-lymphocyte r.

rosette-forming cell

rosetting

roseum
> *Trichothecium r.*

roseus
> *Arthrobacter r.*
> *Muricoccus r.*

Rose-Waaler test

Rosewater syndrome

Ross
> R. River fever
> R. River virus

Rossbach disease
Ross-Jones test
rostellum
rostrate pelvis
Rosys Plato Gene
  Machine
rot
>Barcoo r.
>liver r.
>r. value
rotamer
rotary microtome
rotation
>axis of r.
>optical r.
>specific r.
rotator
>r. cuff injury
>r. cuff tear
rotavirus serology
Rotazyme test
rotenone
Roth
>R. disease
>R. spot
>R. syndrome
Roth-Bernhardt
>R.-B. disease
>R.-B. syndrome
Rothera nitroprusside test
Rothia
>*R. aeria*
>*R. amarae*
>*R. dentocariosa*
>*R. mucilaginosa*
>*R. nasimurium*
Rothmann-Makai syndrome
Rothmund syndrome
Rothmund-Thomson syndrome
rotiferianus
>*Vibrio r.*
Rotor syndrome
Rotter
>R. node
>R. syndrome
>R. test
rotunda
>fenestra r.
rouge
>homme r.
Rouget
>R. cell
>R. muscle
>R. pericyte
Rouget-Neumann sheath
rough
>r. bacterium
>r. colony
>r. determinant

>r. endoplasmic reticulum
>(RER)
>r. factor
>r. plasmid
rough-smooth variation
rough-surfaced endoplasmic
  reticulum
Roughton-Scholander
>R.-S. apparatus
>R.-S. syringe
Rougnon-Heberden disease
rouleau formation
round
>r. atelectasis
>r. cell
>r. cell sarcoma
>high-velocity steel-core r.
>jacketed high-velocity r.
>lead core high-velocity r.
>r. secretory granule
>r. window
rounded
>r. atelectasis
>r. mononuclear cell
rounding
roundworm
Rourke-Ernstein sedimentation
  rate
Rous
>R. sarcoma
>R. sarcoma virus
>R. test
>R. tumor
Rous-associated virus (RAV)
Roussy-Dejerine syndrome
Roussy-Lévy
>R.-L. disease
>R.-L. syndrome
routine
>r. test dilution (RTD)
>trace r.
Roux
>R. bottle
>R. spatula
>R. stain
Rovsing syndrome
rowbothamii
>*Legionella r.*
Rowntree and Geraghty test
RP
>reactive protein
>red phosphorus
>refractory period
Rp
>pulmonary resistance
RPA
>ribonuclease protection assay
RPC
>reactive perforating collagenosis

RPCF
Reiter protein complement-fixation
RPCF test
rPDGF
recombinant platelet-derived growth
factor
RPF
renal plasma flow
RPGN
rapidly progressive glomerulonephritis
RPI
reticulocytic production index
RPLA
reverse passive latex agglutination
RPLND
retroperitoneal lymph node dissection
rpm
revolutions per minute
RPMI-1640 contrast medium
RPO
radiation protection officer
RPR
rapid plasma reagin
RPR test
RPR-CT
rapid plasma reagin circle card
test
RPS
renal pressor substance
RR
renin release
RRA
radioreceptor assay
RR-HPO
rapid recompression-high pressure
oxygen
rRNA
ribosomal RNA
RRP
recurrent respiratory papillomatosis
relative refractory period
RRR
renin-release rate
RRT
relative retention time
RRV
Ross River virus
RS
Reed-Sternberg cell
respiratory syncytial
RSA
rapid susceptibility assay
relative specific activity
reticulum cell sarcoma
RSCN
reactive spindle cell nodule
RSD
relative sagittal depth
relative standard deviation

RSS
recombination signal sequence
RST
radiosensitivity test
RSV
respiratory syncytial virus
RSV culture
Rs virus
rank correlation coefficient
RT
reaction time
room temperature
RTA
renal tubular acidosis
classic RTA
distal RTA
RTD
renal tubular dysgenesis
routine test dilution
RTE
renal tubular epithelial
RTE cell
RTE cell cast
RTF
replication and transfer
resistance transfer factor
respiratory tract fluid
RTK
rhabdoid tumor of the kidney
rTMP
ribothymidylic acid
RT-PCR
reverse transcriptase polymerase chain
reaction
RU
rat unit
resistance unit
rub
pleural friction r.
Rubarth
R. disease
R. disease virus
rubber
r. pelvis
r. policeman
rubeanic acid
rubella
r. antibody test
r. HI test
measles, mumps, and r. (MMR)
r. serology
r. virus (RV)
r. virus culture
r. virus vaccine, live
rubeola
r. serology
r. virus
ruber
Salinibacter r.

Thermovibrio r.
Vibrio r.
rubescens
Amanita r.
rubescent
rubi
Rhizobium r.
rubida
Amycolatopsis r.
rubidaea
Serratia r.
rubidomycin
rubidus
Hyostrongylus r.
Rubinstein syndrome
Rubinstein-Taybi syndrome
Rubin test
Rubivirus
Rubner test
rubor
rubra
Basipetospora r.
Leifsonia r.
medulla ossium r.
miliaria r.
pityriasis r.
polycythemia r.
Rhodotorula r.
trichomycosis r.
rubratoxin
rubredoxin
rubriblast
rubricyte
polychromatophilic r.
rubrifaciens
Acidisphaera r.
Rubrimonas cliftonensis
Rubritepida flocculans
Rubrobacteraceae
Rubrobacterales
Rubrobacteridae
Rubrobacter taiwanensis
rubropertincta
Gordonia r.
rubrum
r. Congo
Epidermophyton r.
r. scarlatinum
Trichophyton r.
Rubulavirus
ruby spot
rucksack paralysis
rudimentary
r. finger
r. lung
r. structure
r. testis syndrome
rudis
Ornithodoros r.

Rudivirus
rudongensis
Ancylobacter r.
Rud syndrome
Ruegeria
R. algicola
R. atlantica
R. gelatinovorans
ruestringensis
Muricauda r.
rufescens
Protostrongylus r.
Ruffini
R. corpuscle
flower-spray organ of R.
ruficornis
Sarcophaga r.
Ruge solution
rugglesi
Simulium r.
rugosa
Prauserella r.
rule
Clark r.
Goriaew r.
two-cell type r.
rulerule
Rumack-Matthew nomogram
ruminantium
Cowdria r.
ruminant
ruminicola
Bacteroides r.
ruminis
Pseudobutyrivibrio r.
Ruminococcus luti
Rummo disease
rump
crown r. (CR)
Rumpel-Leede test
Rundles-Falls syndrome
Runeberg formula
Runella zeae
runt disease
runting syndrome
Runyon
R. classification
R. mycobacteria group I–IV
ruoffiae
Ignavigranum r.
rupial syphilis
rupioides psoriasis
rupture
esophageal r.
focal plaque r.
inflammatory r.
r. of membranes (ROM)
plaque r.
premature r.

R

rupture (*continued*)
  prosthesis r.
  tendon r.
  traumatic r.
ruptured
  r. aneurysm
  r. ectopic pregnancy
  r. myocardial infarct
  r. viscera
rupture-delivery interval (RDI)
RUR
  resin-uptake ratio
RURTI
  recurrent upper respiratory tract
  infection
Rushton body
Russell
  R. body
  R. corpuscle
  R. double-sugar agar
  R. syndrome
  R. unit
  R. viper venom (RVV)
  R. viper venom time (RVVT)
Russell-Crooke cell
russellii
  Zobellia r.
Russell-Movat pentachrome stain
russensis
  Dethiosulfovibrio r.
Russian
  R. autumn encephalitis
  R. autumn encephalitis virus
  R. spring-summer encephalitis virus
  R. tick-borne encephalitis
russicus
  Arthrobacter r.
russii
  Fusobacterium r.
Russula emetica
Rust
  R. disease
  R. syndrome
rusty sputum
RUT
  rapid urease test
ruthenica
  Pseudoalteromonas r.
ruthenium
  r. red
  r. red labeling

rutherford (Rd)
  r. scattering
rutidosis
Rutstroemia
Ruysch
  R. disease
  R. glomerulus
  R. membrane
RV
  rat virus
  reference value
  residual volume
  rubella virus
RVB
  red venous blood
RVE
  right ventricular enlargement
RVH
  right ventricular hypertrophy
RVI
  relative value index
RVR
  renal vascular resistance
  resistance to venous return
RVRA
  renal vein renin activity
  renal venous renin assay
RVRC
  renal vein renin
  concentration
RVT
  renal vein thrombosis
RVV
  Russell viper venom
RVVT
  Russell viper venom time
RXR
  retinoid X receptor
  RXR alpha
ryanodine receptor
ryanodine-sensitive calcium transient
Ryan stain
Rye
  R. classification of Hodgkin
  disease
  R. histopathologic Hodgkin disease
  classification
  R. modification
Rymovirus
Ryparobius
ryukyuensis

S
　serum
　sulfur
　supravergence
　Svedberg unit of sedimentation
　　coefficient
　　S and s antigen
　　S antigen
　　S cell
　　S colony
　　S phase
　　S unit of streptomycin
s
　second
S-100
　　S-100 antibody
　　S-100 immunostain
　　S-100 marker
　　S-100 protein
　　S-100 protein antigen
　　S-100 protein
　　　immunopositivity
SA
　NATO code for arsine
　sarcoma
　secondary amenorrhea
　serum albumin
　sinoatrial
　Stokes-Adams
　　SA node
　　SA 3100 surface area and pore
　　　size analyzer
SAA
　serum amyloid A
　　SAA protein
SAAG
　serum ascites albumin
　　gradient
saalensis
　　Sedimentibacter s.
SAB
　significant asymptomatic
　　bacteriuria
　streptavidin-biotin
s-ABC peroxidase
saber
　　s. shin
　　s. tibia
Sabethes
Sabhi agar
Sabia virus
Sabin-Feldman
　　S.-F. dye test
　　S.-F. syndrome
Sabin vaccine

sabot
　　coeur en s.
　　s. heart
saboteur
Sabouraud
　　S. dextrose and brain heart infusion
　　　agar
　　S. medium
sabouraudi
　　Trichophyton s.
Sabouraudites
sabulous
sac
　　air s.
　　alveolar s.
　　aneurysmal s.
　　dental s.
　　hydrocele s.
　　tooth s.
sacbrood
saccate
saccharase
saccharephidrosis
sacchari
　　Amycolatopsis s.
　　Burkholderia s.
　　Thermoactinomyces s.
saccharic acid
saccharin
saccharobutylicum
　　Clostridium s.
saccharogenic assay
saccharoid
saccharolytica
　　Soehngenia s.
saccharolyticum
　　Thermoanaerobacterium s.
saccharometer
Saccharomonospora
　　S. halophila
　　S. paurometabolica
　　S. viridis
saccharomyces
　　S. albicans
　　S. anginae
　　S. apiculatus
　　Busse s.
　　S. capillitii
　　S. carlsbergensis
　　S. cerevisiae
　　S. coprogenus
　　S. epidermica
　　S. galacticolus
　　S. glutinis
　　S. hominis

saccharomyces (*continued*)
    S. lemonnieri
    S. mellis
    S. mycoderma
    S. neoformans
    S. pastorianus
Saccharomycetaceae
Saccharomycetales
Saccharomycodes
Saccharomycopsis
saccharomycosis
saccharophilum
    Halonatronum s.
saccharopine dehydrogenase
saccharopinuria
Saccharopolyspora
    S. flava
    S. rectivirgula
    S. thermophila
saccharorrhea
saccharose-mannitol agar
Saccharospirillum impatiens
saccharosuria
Saccharothrix
    S. albidocapillata
    S. algeriensis
    S. tangerinus
    S. violacea
Saccomanno
    S. collection fluid
    S. fixative
saccular
    s. aneurysm
    s. bronchiectasis
    s. gland
    s. spot
sacculated
    s. aneurysm
    s. pleurisy
saccule
sacculi (*pl. of* sacculus)
sacculotubular element
sacculus, *pl.* **sacculi**
    s. alveolaris
    s. communis
    macula sacculi
    s. proprius
    s. vestibuli
SACD
    subacute combined degeneration
sacelli
    Brachybacterium s.
Sachs disease
Sachs-Georgi (S-G)
    S.-G. test
sacrococcygeal
    s. chordoma
    s. teratoma
sacroiliitis

sacroplasmic cisternae
saddle embolism
S-adenosyl-l-homocysteine
S-adenosyl-l-methionine
Saemisch ulcer
Saenger macula
saerimneri
    Lactobacillus s.
Saethre-Chotzen syndrome
SafeCrit microhematocrit tube
Safetex tube
Safe-T Lance Plus lancet
safety
    s. program
    s. responsibility
    s. shower
SAF fixative
safflower oil
safranin
    s. O
    s. stain
safranophil, safranophile
safranophile (*var. of* safranophil)
sagamiensis
    Pseudoalteromonas s.
SAGE
    serial analysis of gene expression
S100A gene
Sagian
    S. automated assay optimization
    S. 180 CO2 incubator
saginata
    Taenia s.
sagitta
    Dipus s.
sago spleen
Sagrahamala
SAH
    subarachnoid hemorrhage
saheli
    Ensifer s.
Sahli method
sailor's skin
Saint Anthony's fire
sairae
    Shewanella s.
Sakaguchi reaction
Sakamoto
    S. classification
    S. poorly differentiated carcinoma
sakazakii
    Enterobacter s.
Saksenaea vasiformis
sakuensis
    Serratia marcescens subsp. *s.*
Sakura
    S. Finetek Tissue-Tek VIP 300E automatic tissue processor

S. Seiki Autosmear automatic smear machine

SAL
synchronous airway lesion

salaam spasm

Sala cell

Salana multivorans

salegens
Salegentibacter s.

Salegentibacter
S. *holothuriorum*
S. *salegens*

SalEst
S. system
S. test

salexigens
Aestuariibacter s.
Chromohalobacter s.
Salibacillus s.
Virgibacillus s.

Salibacillus
S. *marismortui*
S. *salexigens*

salicampi
Lentibacillus s.

salicin fermentation

salicylamide

salicylate
s. assay
s. intoxication
s. level
sodium s.
s. toxicity

salicylatoxidans
Pseudaminobacter s.

salicylic
s. acid
s. acid test

salicylism

salicylsalicylic acid

salicylsulfonic acid

salicyluric acid

salimeter

salina
Enhygromyxa s.
Nocardiopsis s.
Streptomonospora s.

salinaria
Orenia s.

salinarius
Culex s.
Halanaerobacter s.

saline
s. agglutination test
s. agglutinin
citrate-buffered s. (CBS)
s. infusion primary
hyperaldosteronism test
s. solution

s. technique
Tris-buffered s.

saline-agglutinating antibody

Salinibacterium amurskyense

Salinibacter ruber

Salinicoccus alkaliphilus

Salinisphaera shabanensis

Salinivibrio costicola subsp. *vallismortis*

salinus
Halobacillus s.

Salipiger mucescens

Salisbury common cold virus

salitolerans
Swaminathania s.

salivae
Prevotella s.

saliva ovulation test

salivaria
glandula s.

salivarium
Mycoplasma s.

salivarius
Lactobacillus s.
Streptococcus s.

salivary
s. amylase
s. calculus
s. corpuscle
s. duct
s. duct obstruction
s. fistula
s. gland (SG)
s. gland angiosarcoma
s. gland anlage tumor (SGAT)
s. gland carcinoma
s. gland tumor
s. gland virus (SGV)
s. gland virus disease
s. urate test

Salk vaccine

salmincola
Nanophyetus s.
Troglotrema s.

salmonella, *pl.* **salmonellae**
s. agglutinin
S. *arizonae*
S. *bongori*
S. *cholerae suis kuzendorf*
S. *choleraesuis* subsp. *arizona*
Enteritidis s.
S. *enteritidis*
S. *enteritidis* serotype *agona*
S. *enteritidis* serotype *heidelberg*
S. *enteritidis* serotype *hirschfeldii*
S. *enteritidis* serotype *infantis*
S. *enteritidis* serotype *montevideo*
S. *enteritidis* serotype *newport*
S. *enteritidis* serotype *paratyphi A*
S. *enteritidis* serotype *schottmulleri*

S

salmonella (*continued*)
   S. enteritidis serotype
    typhimurium
   s. group
   S. paratyphi
   s. poisoning
   S. titer
salmonellae (*pl. of* salmonella)
Salmonella-Shigella (**SS**)
   S.-S. agar
Salmonelleae
salmonellosis
salmoneum
   Acrodontium s.
salmonicida
   Aeromonas s.
salmonis
   Piscirickettsia s.
salmon patch
salmositica
   Cryptobia s.
salomonii
   Pseudomonas s.
salpinges (*pl. of*
  salpinx)
salpingioma
salpingitis
   chronic interstitial s.
   follicular s.
   foreign body s.
   gonorrheal s.
   s. isthmica nodosa
   pyogenic s.
salpingo-oophoritis
salpingoperitonitis
salpinx, *pl.* **salpinges**
salsalate
salsilacus
   Loktanella s.
salt
   s. agglutination
   s. antagonism
   bile s.'s
   s. bridge
   diazonium s.
   s. dye
   hexazonium s.
   insoluble s.
   s. loading
   s. sensitivity (SS)
   tetrazonium s.
   trisodium foscarnet s.
   s. wasting
   water-soluble s.
saltans
   Bodo s.
   thrombophlebitis s.
saltation
Saltatoria

saltatory
   s. conduction
   s. spasm
salted
   s. plasma
   s. serum
Salter-Harris 1–5 fracture
salting-in
salting-out procedure
salt-losing
   s.-l. crisis
   s.-l. nephritis
   s.-l. syndrome
salts-sucrose
   thiosulfate citrate-bile s.-s. (TCBS)
Saltzstein pseudolymphoma
saluresis
saluretic
salvage
   blood s.
   cell s.
   intraoperative cell s.
   s. therapy
salvarsanized serum
Salvia
   S. horminium
   S. sclarea
Salzer-Kuntschik grading system
Salzman method
SAM
   salicylamide
   sulfated acid mucopolysaccharide
samarium (Sm)
sample
   clinical s.
   s. distribution
   environmental s.
   formalin-fixed paraffin-embedded s.
   s. interaction
   multiple stage random s.
   population s. (PS)
   proficiency s.
   random s.
   rolled s.
   simple random s.
   s. steady state
   stratified random s.
sampler
   air s.
sampling
   chorionic villus s. (CVS)
   inferior petrosal sinus s.
   inferior petrosal vein s.
   transabdominal chorionic villus s.
   transcervical chorionic villus s.
Samsonia erythrinae
San
   S. Joaquin Valley fever
   S. Miguel sea lion virus

Sanarelli phenomenon
Sanarelli-Shwartzman
    S.-S. phenomenon (SSP)
    S.-S. reaction
Sanchez Salorio syndrome
sand
    s. body
    brain s.
    s. granule
    intestinal s.
    s. tumor
    urinary s.
sandal foot
sandalwood oil
Sanders disease
Sanderson polster
sandfly
    s. fever
    s. fever virus
Sandhoff disease
Sandison-Clark chamber
sandpaper gallbladder
sandramycini
    Kribbella s.
Sandström body
sandwich
    s. hybridization
    s. nucleic acid hybridization assay
    s. radioimmunoassay
sandworm
Sanfilippo syndrome
Sanford test
Sanger
    S. DNA sequencing method
    S. reagent
Sanguibacteraceae
sanguifacient
sanguiferous
sanguification
sanguinegens
    Sneathia s.
sanguineous
    s. cyst
    s. infiltration
sanguineus
    Allodermanyssus s.
    Porphyrobacter s.
    Rhipicephalus s.
    sudor s.
sanguinis
    Brevibacterium s.
    Filaria s.
    fragilitas s.
    Gemella s.
    Luteococcus s.
    Turicibacter s.
sanguinolent
sanguinolentis
    fetus s.

sanguinopurulent
sanguis
    Streptococcus s.
Sanguisuga
sanguivorous myiasis
sanies
saniopurulent
sanioserous
sanious pus
sanitary bacteriology
sanitization
santal oil
santonin
Santorini
    S. canal
    S. duct
    S. fissure
    S. major caruncle
    S. minor caruncle
SAP
    serum alkaline phosphatase
    sporadic adenomatous polyp
    systemic arterial pressure
sap
    cell s.
    nuclear s.
saponifiable fraction
saponification
saponify
saponin
    hemolysin s.
    s. lysing reagent stock solution
    steroid s.
    triterpenoid s.
Sapovirus
Sappinea diploidea
sapremia
saprobe
saprobic
saprogen
saprogenic, saprogenous
saprogenous (*var. of* saprogenic)
Saprolegnia
sapronosis
saprophilous
saprophilus
    Mycetocola s.
saprophyte
saprophytic infestation
saprophyticus
    Staphylococcus s.
Saprospira
saprozoic
saprozoonosis
SAR
    supplied air respirator
saramycetin
Sarcina ventriculi
Sarcinomyces phaeomuriformis

S

Sarcinosporon inkin
sarcoblast
sarcocele
sarcocyst
sarcocystin
Sarcocystis
    S. bovihominis
    S. fusiformis
    S. hominis
    S. lindemanni
    S. miescheriana
    S. suihominis
    S. tenella
sarcocystosis
sarcocyte
sarcode
Sarcodina
Sarcodontia
sarcoendoplasmic
    s. reticulum calcium-ATPase (SERCA)
    s. reticulum calcium-ATPase enzyme
sarcogenic cell
sarcoglia
sarcoglycan
sarcoid
    Boeck s.
    Darier-Roussy s.
    granuloma s.
    s. granuloma
    Schaumann s.
    Spiegler-Fendt s.
    verrucous s.
sarcoidal granuloma
sarcoidosis
    HHV 8 DNA in s.
    hypercalcemic s.
    mycobacterial DNA in s.
    propionibacterial DNA in s.
    pulmonary s.
sarcolemma
sarcolemmal, sarcolemmic, sarcolemmous
    s. folding
    s. integrity
sarcolemmic (*var. of* sarcolemmal)
sarcolemmous (*var. of* sarcolemmal)
sarcoma
    AIDS-related Kaposi s. (AIDS-KS)
    alveolar soft-part s. (ASPS)
    ameloblastic s.
    angiolithic s.
    avian s.
    biphasic synovial s.
    botryoid s.
    s. botryoid
    cerebellar s.
    clear cell s.
    endometrial stromal s. (ESS)
    endothelial s.
    epithelioid s. (ES)

    Ewing s. (ES)
    fascicular s.
    fibromyxoid s.
    follicular dendritic cell s.
    granulocytic s. (GS)
    hemangioendothelial s.
    Hodgkin s.
    immunoblastic s.
    interdigitating cell s.
    interdigitating dendritic cell s.
      (IDCS)
    Jensen s.
    juxtacortical osteogenic s.
    Kaposi s.
    Kupffer cell s.
    leukocytic s.
    low-grade endometrial stromal s.
      (LGESS)
    low-grade fibromyxoid s.
    lymphangioendothelial s.
    lymphatic s.
    lymphosarcoma-reticulum cell s.
      (LSA/RCS)
    mast cell s.
    medullary s.
    meningeal s.
    mesothelial s.
    monophasic synovial s. (MSS)
    multiple idiopathic hemorrhagic s.
    myelogenic s.
    myeloid s. (MS)
    myxoid synovial s.
    neurogenic s.
    osteogenic s.
    pleomorphic s.
    pulmonary intimal s. (PIS)
    renal synovial s.
    reticuloendothelial s.
    reticulum cell s. (RCS, RSA)
    round cell s.
    Rous s.
    small cell s.
    spindle cell s.
    stromal s.
    synovial s. (SS, SYS)
    telangiectatic osteogenic s.
    undifferentiated s.
sarcoma-like mural nodule (SLMN)
Sarcomastigophora
sarcomatodes
    lipoma s.
sarcomatoid
    s. carcinoma
    s. mesothelioma
    s. thymic carcinoma (STC)
    s. tumor
    s. urothelial carcinoma
sarcomatosis
    meningeal s.

sarcomatosum
    lipoma s.
    myxoma s.
sarcomatous component
sarcomere
sarcomeric actin
sarconeme
Sarcophaga
    S. carnaria
    S. dux
    S. fuscicauda
    S. haemorrhoidalis
    S. ruficornis
Sarcophagidae
sarcoplasm
sarcoplasmic reticulum
sarcoplast
Sarcopsylla penetrans
Sarcopsyllidae
Sarcoptes scabiei
sarcoptic mange
sarcoptid
Sarcoptidae
sarcoptidosis
sarcosine dehydrogenase
sarcosinemia
sarcosis
sarcosome
Sarcosporidia
sarcosporidiosis
sarcostosis
sarcotic
sarcotubule
sarcous
sardinae
    Eimeria s.
sarin
    NATO code for s. (GB)
SARS
    severe acute respiratory syndrome
SARS-CoV
    severe acute respiratory syndrome
      coronavirus
        antibody to S.-C.
SART
    standard acid reflux test
SAS
    supravalvular aortic stenosis
      SAS Rota test
saskatchewanense
    Mycobacterium s.
Sassone score
SAT
    subacute thyroiditis
sat
    saturated
    saturation
satelles
    Shuttleworthia s.

satellite
    s. abscess
    s. cell
    s. cell necrosis
    s. colony
    s. metastasis
    s. nodule
    s. phenomenon
    s. vesicular lesion
satellite-rich heterochromatin
satellitism
    platelet s.
satellitosis
Sattler elastic layer
saturated (sat)
    ambient temperature and pressure, s.
     (ATPS)
    body temperature, ambient pressure,
     s. (BTPS)
    s. fatty acid
    s. hydrocarbon
    s. solution (SS)
    s. solution of potassium iodide
     (SSKI)
saturation (sat)
    s. analysis
    s. and displacement assay
    arterial oxygen s.
    s. current
    s. hybridization
    s. index (SI)
    s. limit
    oxygen s.
    transferrin s.
Saturday night palsy
saturnina
    arthralgia s.
saturnine
    s. encephalopathy
    s. gout
saturnus
    Williopsis s.
saucerize
Saundby test
Saunders disease
sauriasis
sauriderma
sauriosis
sauroderma
    ichthyosis s.
sausage finger
saved
    years of life s. (YLS)
savigni
    Ornithodoros s.
Savill disease
sawing
    bone s.
sawtooth wave

S

saxitoxin
saxobsidens
   Blastococcus s.
Sayeed stain
SB
  serum bilirubin
  Southern blot
  stillbirth
SBB
  Sudan black B
SBE
  subacute bacterial endocarditis
SBF
  splanchnic blood flow
SBH
  sequencing by hybridization
SBI
  silicone breast implant
SBP
  selenium binding protein
  spontaneous bacterial peritonitis
SBR
  Scarf-Bloom-Richardson
    SBR tumor grading system
SBS
  shaken baby syndrome
SBT
  sequenced-based typing
  serous borderline tumor
  serum bactericidal test
SBTI
  soybean trypsin inhibitor
SC
  sickle cell
  subcutaneous
Sc
  scandium
SCA
  single-chain antigen-binding
    SCA protein
scabby mouth
scabiei
   Acarus s.
   Sarcoptes s.
scabies
scabrisporus
   Streptomyces s.
SCAD
  segmental colitis associated with
    diverticulosis
  spontaneous coronary artery dissection
scaffolding protein
scala
   Löwenberg s.
   s. media
   s. vestibuli
scalaris
   Fannia s.
scalar product

S100 calcium binding protein A1 gene
scalded skin syndrome (SSS)
scale
  absolute temperature s.
  Bauermeister s.
  Baumé s. (B)
  Benoist s. (B)
  Bethesda Pap smear rating s.
  Bloom-Richardson s.
  Celsius temperature s. (C)
  centigrade temperature s. (C)
  s. crust
  customary temperature s.
  full s.
  Gaffky s.
  gray s.
  Hamilton Rating S. (HRS)
  hydrometer s.
  interval s.
  kelvin temperature s. (k)
  positive and negative symptom s.
   (PANSS)
  Rankine temperature s. (Rank)
  ratio s.
  Réaumur s. (R)
scalene node biopsy (SNB)
scalenus anticus syndrome (SAS)
scaler
scaler-timer
scallop
  flail s.
scalloped pattern
scalloping
  endosteal s.
scalp
  s. contusion
  s. pH
  pilar tumor of s.
  ringworm of s.
scaly ringworm
scan
  biliary s.
  bilirubin s.
  bone marrow s.
  dot s.
  duplex s.
  indium leukocyte s.
  s. information density
  tomographic s.
scandium (Sc)
scanning
  s. electron micrograph (SEM)
  s. electron microscope (SEM)
  s. electron microscopy (SEM)
  s. probe microscopy (SPM)
  s. sequence
  s. transmission electron microscopy
  s. tunneling microscopy (STM)
scaphohydrocephalus, scaphohydrocephaly

scaphohydrocephaly (*var. of* scaphohydrocephalus)
scaphoid
s. facies
s. fracture
scapularis
Ixodes s.
scar
s. cancer
s. carcinoma
cigarette-paper s.
hypertrophic s.
radial s.
scleroelastotic s.
scarabiasis
Scardovia inopinata
scardovii
Bifidobacterium s.
Scarf-Bloom-Richardson (SBR)
scarification test
scarlatina
s. anginosa
anginose s.
s. hemorrhagica
s. latens
s. maligna
s. rheumatica
s. simplex
scarlatinal nephritis
scarlatinella
scarlatiniform
scarlatinoid
scarlatinum
rubrum s.
scarless healing
scarlet
Biebrich s.
s. fever (SF)
s. fever antitoxin
s. fever erythrogenic toxin
s. red
s. red stain
s. red sulfonate
water-soluble s.
scarring
myocardial s.
SCAT
sheep cell agglutination test
sickle cell anemia test
Scatchard
S. equation
S. plot
scatemia
scatologic
scatology
scatoma
scatophagy
scatophila
scatoscopy

scatter
s. diagram
forward s. (FSC)
optical light s.
scattergram
scattering
elastic s.
inelastic s.
rutherford s.
scatterplot
Scaurus
scavenger
s. cell
radical s.
s. receptor
SCBA
self-contained breathing apparatus
pressure-demand SCBA
SCC
small cell cancer
squamous cell carcinoma
SCCA, SCC-Ag
squamous-cell carcinoma antigen
SCD
subacute combined degeneration
sudden cardiac death
sudden coronary death
Scedosporium
S. apiospermum
S. inflatum
S. prolificans
SCF
stem cell factor
SCG
serum chemistry graft
Schaedler blood agar
Schaeffer-Fulton stain
Schaer reagent
Schafer syndrome
Schaffer test
Schales and Schales method for chloride
Schallibaum solution
Schamberg
S. dermatitis
S. disease
Schanz
S. disease
S. syndrome
scharlach red
Schatzki ring
Schaudinn fixative
Schaumann
S. body
S. disease
S. lymphogranuloma
S. sarcoid
S. syndrome

S

811

Scheibler reagent
Scheie syndrome
Scheloribates
schematic
scheme
    classification s.
    decay s.
    Facklam classification s.
    Van Nuys s.
Schenck disease
schenckii
    Sporothrix s.
    Sporotrichum s.
Scheuermann disease
Schick
    S. method
    S. test
    S. test toxin
Schiff
    S. base
    S. reagent
    S. stain
Schilder disease
Schiller-Duval body
Schiller test
Schilling
    S. band cell
    S. blood count
    S. classification
    S. index
    S. test
    S. type of monocytic leukemia
Schimmelbusch disease
schindleri
    Acinetobacter s.
Schirmer
    S. syndrome
    S. test
schistocelia
schistocystis
schistocyte, schizocyte
schistocytosis
schistorrhachis
Schistosoma
    S. haematobium
    S. hematobium
    S. intercalatum
    S. japonicum
    S. malayensis
    S. mansoni
    S. mattheei
    S. mekongi
schistosomal cystitis
Schistosomatidae
Schistosomatoidea
schistosome granuloma
schistosomiasis serological test
schistosomicidal
schistosomicide

schistosomule
schistosomulum
Schistotaenia srivastavai
schizaxon
schizencephalic microcephaly
schizencephaly
Schizoblastosporion
schizocyte (*var. of* schistocyte)
schizocytosis
schizogenesis
schizogonic cycle
schizogony
schizogyria
schizomycete
Schizomycetes
Schizonella
schizont
schizonticide
Schizophora
Schizophyllum commune
Schizopora
Schizosaccharomyces pombe
schizotonia
Schizotrypanum cruzi
schizozoite
Schlatter disease, Schlatter-Osgood
    disease
Schlatter-Osgood disease
Schlegelella thermodepolymerans
schlegeliana
    Shewanella s.
Schlemm
    canal of S.
schlieren microscope
Schmid-Fraccaro syndrome
Schmidt
    S. syndrome
    S. test
Schmidt-Lanterman
    S.-L. cleft
    S.-L. incisure
Schmincke
    S. pattern
    S. pattern of growth
Schmitz bacillus
Schmorl
    S. bacillus
    S. body
    S. disease
    S. ferric-ferricyanide reduction
        stain
    S. mosaic
    S. nodule
    S. picrothionin stain
    S. reaction
Schnabel cavernous degeneration
Schneider carmine
schneideri
    Elaeophora s.

schneiderian
> s. carcinoma
> s. membrane
> s. papilloma

schoenbuchensis
> *Bartonella s.*

schoenleinii
> *Trichophyton s.*

Scholz disease
Schönbein test
Schönlein
> S. disease
> S. purpura

Schottmuller disease
schottmulleri
> *Salmonella enteritidis*
> serotype *s.*

Schreger line
Schridde
> S. cancer hair
> S. syndrome

Schroeder
> S. disease
> S. syndrome

schroeteri
> *Kytococcus s.*

Schüffner
> S. dot
> S. granule

Schüller
> S. disease
> S. duct
> S. syndrome

Schüller-Christian
> S.-C. disease
> S.-C. syndrome

Schultz
> S. disease
> S. reaction
> S. stain
> S. syndrome

Schultz-Charlton
> S.-C. phenomenon
> S.-C. reaction

Schultz-Dale
> S.-D. reaction
> S.-D. test

Schultze
> S. cell
> S. membrane
> S. test

Schultze-Chvostek sign
Schumm test
Schwalbe
> S. corpuscle
> S. space

Schwann
> S. cell
> S. nucleus

> sheath of S.
> S. white substance
> white substance of S.

schwannian
Schwanniomyces
schwannoma
> acoustic s.
> ancient s.
> cellular s.
> glandular s.
> granular cell s.
> malignant s.
> melanotic s.
> plexiform s.
> psammomatous-melanotic s.
> renal s.

schwannosis
Schwartz-Bartter syndrome
Schwartz syndrome
Schwarz test
Schweigger-Seidel
> sheath of S.-S.

Schweninger-Buzzi
> S.-B. anetoderma
> S.-B. disease

SCI
> Sertoli cell index

Scianna blood group system
sciatica
SCID
> severe combined immunodeficiency

science
> mortuary s.
> National Accrediting Agency for
> Clinical Laboratory S.'s

scientific notation
scientist
> biomedical s.

scimitar sign
scintigraph
> octreotide s.

scintigraphy
scintillation
> s. camera
> s. count
> s. counter
> s. crystal
> s. technique

scintillator
> liquid s.

scirrhoid
scirrhosity
scirrhous
> s. adenocarcinoma
> s. carcinoma

scirrhus
SCIS
> surface carcinoma in situ

scissiparity

S

scissors
    mini s.
SCJ
    squamocolumnar junction
SCK
    serum creatine kinase
SCL
    scleroderma
sclarea
    Salvia s.
SCLC
    small-cell lung carcinoma
sclera, *pl.* sclerae
    corneoscleral part of trabecular
      tissue of s.
    lamina cribrosa sclerae
    lamina fusca sclerae
    reticulum trabeculare sclerae
    substantia propria sclerae
scleradenitis
sclerae (*pl. of* sclera)
scleral roll
scleratogenous
scleredema
    s. adultorum
    Buschke s.
sclerema
    s. adiposum
    s. neonatorum
sclerencephalia (*var. of* sclerencephaly)
sclerencephaly, sclerencephalia
scleriasis
scleroatrophy, sclerotylosis
sclerocornea
sclerocorneal junction
sclerodactylia (*var. of* sclerodactyly)
sclerodactyly, sclerodactylia
scleroderma
    s. antibody
    limited s.
    localized s.
    s. renal crisis
    systemic s.
sclerodermatitis
sclerodermatous
scleroelastotic scar
sclerogenic (*var. of* sclerogenous)
sclerogenous, sclerogenic
scleroid
scleroma
    respiratory s.
scleromalacia
scleromyxedema
sclero-oophoritis
Sclerophoma
sclerosal
sclerose
sclerosing
    s. bronchioloalveolar carcinoma

s. cholangitis
s. epithelioid fibrosarcoma
s. hemangioma
s. hyaline necrosis
s. inflammation
s. keratitis
s. mediastinitis
s. mucoepidermoid carcinoma with
  eosinophilia (SMECE)
s. osteitis
s. paraganglioma
s. polycystic adenosis
s. sarcomatoid transitional cell
  carcinoma
s. Sertoli cell tumor
s. sialadenitis
s. sinusitis
sclerosis
    s. adenosis
    Alzheimer s.
    amyotrophic lateral s. (ALC, ALS)
    arterial s.
    arteriocapillary s.
    arteriolar s.
    bone s.
    Canavan s.
    cardiac s.
    central hyaline s.
    combined s.
    s. corii
    s. cutanea
    cutaneous systemic s.
    diffuse infantile familial s.
    disseminated s.
    endocardial s.
    endomyocardial s.
    focal segmental glomerular s.
     (FSGS)
    glomerular s.
    hippocampal s. (HS)
    hyaline s.
    insular s.
    laminar cortical s.
    lobar s.
    mantle s.
    menstrual s.
    Mönckeberg medial calcific s.
    multiple s. (MS)
    nodular s. (NS)
    s. of white matter
    ovulational s.
    posterior spinal s.
    primary endocardial s.
    primary mediastinal large cell
     lymphoma with s. (PMLS)
    progressive systemic s. (PSS)
    subacute combined s.
    systemic s.
    tuberous s.

tumor-induced stromal s.
unicellular s.
vascular s.
sclerostenosis
Sclerostoma
sclerosus
lupus s.
sclerotic
s. body
s. coat
s. gastritis
s. kidney
s. margin
s. stomach
s. stroma
sclerotica
otitis s.
tunica s.
Sclerotinia
sclerotium
S.
sclerotylosis (*var. of* scleroatrophy)
sclerous
SCML
small cell malignant lymphoma
SCNB
stereotactic core-needle biopsy
SCNC
small cell neuroendocrine carcinoma
scoleces (*pl. of* scolex)
scoleciasis
scoleciform
Scolecobasidium
scolecoid
scolecology
scolex, *pl.* **scoleces, scolices**
scolices (*pl. of* scolex)
scoliodontum
Treponema s.
scoliosis series
scoliotic pelvis
Scolopendra
scomber
Cystoopsis s.
scombroid poisoning
scop
scopolamine
scopiformis
Streptomyces s.
scopolamine (scop)
Scopulariopsis
S. americana
S. aureus
S. blochi
S. brevicaulis
S. cinereus
S. koningi
S. minimus
scopulariopsosis

scorbutic
s. dysentery
s. gingivitis
s. rosary
score
CD44v6 s.
Child-Turcotte-Pugh s.
Gleason prostate carcinoma s.
initial prognostic s. (IPS)
International Prostate Symptom S.
(IPPS)
LAP s.
leukocyte alkaline phosphatase s.
LOD s.
MSTS s.
Sassone s.
standard s.
Z s.
scoring
Barr body s.
specific IgE antibody s.
Scorpiones
Scorpionida
Scotch tape method
scoticum
Diphyllobothrium s.
Scotobacteria
scotochromogen
scotochromogenic mycobacteria
scotoma, *pl.* **scotomata**
scotomata (*pl. of* scotoma)
scotopic
scotopsin
Scott
S. syndrome
S. tap water substitute
SCPK
serum creatine phosphokinase
Scr
concentration of creatinine in serum
scraper
cervical s.
scrapie
scraping
balloon s.
scratch-pad memory
scratch test
screen
amino acid s.
Ashkenazi s.
s. burn
cold agglutinin s.
cord blood s.
drug abuse s.
s. filtration pressure (SFP)
fungal antibody s.
glucose-6-phosphate dehydrogenase s.
heavy metal s.
hypercoagulable state coagulation s.

S

screen (*continued*)
  infertility s.
  intravascular coagulation s.
  latex s.
  multiple marker s.
  newborn s.
  stool s.
  substance abuse s.
  sugar water test s.
  T_4 newborn s.
  Triage Tox drug s.
  triple s.
  urine drug s. (UDS)
  volatile s.
screening
  amino acid s.
  antibody s.
  automated multiphasic s. (AMS)
  cytologic s.
  s. dipstick
  genetic s.
  multiphasic s.
  neonatal s.
  plasma amino acid s.
  prenatal s.
  rapid drug screen on-site
   drug s.
  s. test
screw artery
screw-cup container
screwworm, screw worm
  New World s.
  Old World s.
scrobiculate
scrofula
scrofulaceum
  Mycobacterium s.
scrofuloderma, scrofulodermia
  s. gummosa
  tuberculous s.
  ulcerative s.
  verrucous s.
scrofulodermia (*var. of* scrofuloderma)
scrofulosorum
  lichen s.
scrofulotuberculosis
scrofulous
scroll ear
scrota (*pl. of* scrotum)
scroti
  elephantiasis s.
scrotitis
scrotum, *pl.* **scrota, scrotums**
  lymph s.
  watering-can s.
scrotums (*pl. of* scrotum)
scrub typhus
SCT
  sex chromatin test

  squamous cell carcinoma of the
   thyroid
  staphylococcal clumping test
scum
SCUNC
  small cell undifferentiated
   neuroendocrine carcinoma
scurvy
  land s.
scute (*var. of* scutum)
scutellaris
  Trombicula s.
Scutigera
scutular
scutularis
scutulata
  ichthyosis s.
  porrigo s.
scutulum
scutum, scute
scybalous stool
Scytalidium
SD
  septal defect
  serologically defined
  serum defect
  solvent detergent treatment
  spontaneous delivery
  stable disease
  standard deviation
   SD antigen
   SD plasma
SDA
  strand displacement amplification
SDG
  sucrose density gradient
SDS
  sodium dodecyl sulfate
  sudden death syndrome
   SDS gel electrophoresis
   SDS gel filtration chromatography
SDS-PAGE
  sodium dodecyl sulfate-polyacrylamide
   gel electrophoresis
SE
  standard error
Se
  selenium
sea
  s. anemone ulcer
  s. urchin granuloma
sea-blue
  s.-b. histiocyte disease
  s.-b. histiocytosis
seal
  hermetic s.
  S. Rock hemoglobin
sealed
  s. beta gamma source

s. envelope technique
s. radioactive source

sealing

impulse s.

seared

s. skin
s. wound margin

seasonal rhinitis

Seattle graft-versus-host disease classification

seatworm

SEB

staphylococcal enterotoxin B

sebaceae

glandulae s.

sebaceous, sebaceus

s. adenocarcinoma
s. adenoma
s. carcinoma
s. cyst
s. epithelioma
s. follicle
s. gland
s. horn
lupus s.
s. miliaria
s. neoplasm
s. nevus
nevus s. (NS)
s. tubercle

sebaceum

adenoma s.
ichthyosis sebacea
tuberculum s.

sebaceus (*var. of* sebaceous)

Sebastian syndrome

sebi

Wallemia s.

sebiagogic

sebiferous

sebiparous

sebolith

seborrhea

seborrheic

s. dermatitis
s. keratosis
s. verruca
s. wart

seborrheica

acanthoma verrucosa s.
keratosis s.
verruca s.

Sebright bantam syndrome

sebum preputiale

SEC

sertoliform endometrioid carcinoma
subepidermal connective tissue

Secernentasida

Secernentia

Seckel syndrome

second (s)

cycle per s. (cps)
s. filial generation (F_2)
forced expiratory volume at 1 s. (FEV-1, FEV1)
forced expiratory time in s.'s (FETS)
kilocycles per s. (kcps)
vibration s. (vs)

secondary

s. active transport
s. aerosolization
s. agammaglobulinemia
s. amenorrhea (SA)
s. amine
s. amyloidosis
s. antibody deficiency
s. antiphospholipid syndrome
s. atelectasis
s. attack rate
s. bacterial peritonitis
s. blast injury
s. bleeding time
s. buffer
s. carcinoma
s. cementum
s. center of ossification
s. coccidioidomycosis
s. coil
s. cold agglutinin disease
s. constriction
s. contamination
s. culture
s. degeneration
s. dextrocardia
s. encephalitis
s. eosinophilic pneumonia
s. fixation
s. glaucoma
s. granule
s. hemochromatosis
s. hyperaldosteronism
s. hyperparathyroidism
s. hyperplasia
s. hypertrophic osteoarthropathy (SHO)
s. hypoadrenocorticism
s. hypogammaglobulinemia
s. immune response
s. immunodeficiency
s. infection
s. lymphoid follicle
s. lysosome
s. methemoglobinemia
s. mucinosis
s. myeloid metaplasia
s. nodule
s. ovarian follicle

S

secondary (*continued*)
s. point of ossification
s. polycythemia
s. pulmonary hemosiderosis (SPH)
s. pulmonary lobule
s. pyoderma
s. reference aterials
s. reference materials
s. refractory anemia
s. renal tubular acidosis
s. repair
s. sex character
s. spermatocyte
s. structure
s. thrombus
s. trisomy
s. tuberculosis
s. union
s. viremia
s. X zone
second-degree
s.-d. burn
s.-d. frostbite
s.-d. heart block
s.-d. radiation injury
second-order reaction
second-set
s.-s. graft rejection
s.-s. phenomenon
second-strain infection
Secrétan syndrome
secreted
regulated on activation, normal T expressed and s. (RANTES)
s. toxin
secretin pancreozymin test
secretin-cholecystokinin-pancreatozymin stimulation test
secreting hydrochloric
secretion
aldosterone s.
cervical s.
corrosive gastric s.'s
cytocrine s.
eccrine sweat gland s.
gland of internal s.
luteinizing hormone s.
s. rate (SR)
stimulate enzyme s.
transport and s.
tubular s.
secretogranin
secretor
s. factor
s. gene
s. phenotype
s. trait

secretory
s. acinar element
s. acinus
s. adenosis
s. canaliculus
s. carcinoma
s. cell
s. component
s. cyst
s. duct
s. endometrium
s. exhaustion
s. gland
s. granule
s. IgA (sIgA)
s. immunoglobulin
s. otitis media
s. pattern
s. portion
s. stage
section
attached cranial s.
capture cross s.
celloidin s.
coronal s.
cryostat s.
s. cutting
detached cranial s.
en face s.
eosin-stained microscopic s.
formalin-fixed tissue s.
s. freeze substitution technique
frozen s. (FS, FZ)
longitudinal s.
lung s.
microscopic s.
Pitres s.
pituitary stalk s.
semithin frozen s.
serial s.
thin s.
tuberculosis organisms in tissue s.
ultrathin s.
vibratome tissue s.
whole-mount s.
sectioning
Albert-Linder bone s.
lymph node s.
multiple level s.
step s.
tangential s.
secular equilibrium
secundarium
punctum ossificationis s.
Securline blood band
SED
spondyloepiphysial dysplasia
Sed-Chek 2 bilevel whole blood reference control

sediment
> spun urine s.
> stained urinary s.
> s. tube
> urinary s.

sedimentate

sedimentation
> s. coefficient
> s. equilibrium
> erythrocyte s.
> s. index
> s. rate (sed rate, SR)
> s. rate test (SRT)
> s. reaction
> s. technique
> s. time
> s. tube
> velocity-diffusion s.
> s. velocity-diffusion

sedimentator

sedimented red cell (SRC)

Sedimentibacter
> S. hydroxybenzoicus
> S. saalensis

sedimentometer

sedimentum lateritium

sedoheptulose 7-phosphate

sed rate
> sedimentation rate

SEE
> standard error of estimate

seeberi
> Rhinosporidium s.

seed
> s. agar
> prostate s.

seeding
> cell s.
> metachronous s.

SEER
> Surveillance, Epidemiology, and End Results

seg
> segmented neutrophil

SEGA
> subependymal giant cell astrocytoma

segbwema
> Prototheca s.

segment
> frame-scanning s.
> initial s.
> interannular s.
> internodal s.
> Lanterman s.
> s. long-spacing (SLS)
> Okazaki s.
> Ranvier s.

segmental

> s. colitis associated with diverticulosis (SCAD)
> s. glomerulonephritis

segmentation
> s. nucleus
> s. sphere

segmented
> s. cell
> s. granulocyte
> s. hyalinizing vasculitis
> s. leukocyte
> s. neutrophil (seg)

segmenter

Segmentina

Segmentininae

segmentum internodale

segnis
> Haemophilus s.
> Leptopsylla s.

segregation
> HLA haplotype s.

segregator
> Luys s.

Séguin sign

SeHCAT test

Seibert tuberculin

Seitelberger disease

Seitz filter

seizure
> psychogenic s.

selangorensis

Selas filter

Seldinger technique

Select-a-Fuge microcentrifuge machine

selected photomicrograph

selectin

selection
> s. against heterozygotes
> coefficient of s.
> directional s.
> natural s.
> s. pressure

selective
> s. affinity
> s. deficiency
> s. medium
> s. stain
> s. transport

selectivity ratio

Selenihalanaerobacter shriftii

selenite broth

selenite-cystine broth

selenitireducens
> Bacillus s.

selenium (Se)
> s. assay
> s. binding protein (SBP)

selenium-75

selenocyte

S

selenoid body
Selenomonas
selenoprotein P gene
Selenotila
self-absorption
self-complementary DNA
self-contained breathing apparatus (SCBA)
self-dose
self-immolation
self-infection
selfing
self-limited
    s.-l. colitis
    s.-l. disease
self-nucleate
self-reacting IgG
self-renewal
self-renewing cell
self-replication
self-sustained sequence replication (3SR)
self-testing
    INRatio PT/INR monitoring for patient s.-t.
Selivanoff
    S. reaction
    S. reagent
    S. test
sella
    empty s.
    s. turcica syndrome
Selter disease
Selye syndrome
SEM
    scanning electron micrograph
    scanning electron microscope
    scanning electron microscopy
    SEM freeze-fracture method
semelincident
semen
    acid phosphatase test for s.
    s. analysis
    s. examination
    hyaluronidase unit for s. (HUS)
semenuria, seminuria, spermaturia
semialdehyde
    glutamate s.
semiapochromatic objective
semiautomated susceptibility testing
semiautomatic handgun
semicanal
semicanalis
semicarbazide hydrochloride
semicircular
    s. canal
    s. duct
semicircularis
    ductus semicirculares
    epithelium ductus s.

    membrana basalis ductus s.
    membrana propria ductus s.
semiconductor
    s. device
    extrinsic s.
    intrinsic s.
semidominance
semiinterquartile range
semilethal mutation
semilunar
semilunatum
    planum s.
seminal
    s. coagulum
    s. colliculus
    s. fibrinolysin
    s. fluid
    s. granule
    s. vesical cyst
seminalis
    ductus excretorius vesiculae s.
semi-nester primer
seminiferous
    s. epithelium
    s. tubule
    s. tubule dysgenesis
seminis
    Allofustis s.
seminoma
    anaplastic s.
    immune rejection of s.
    spermacytic s.
    spermatocytic s.
    syncytiotrophoblastic cell of s.
seminomatous
seminuria (*var. of* semenuria)
semipermeable membrane
Semi-Q hCG combo test
semiquantitative
    s. analysis
    s. viral culture
semiquinone
Semisulcospina
semithin frozen section
Semliki Forest virus
Semple vaccine
senagalensis
    Curvularia s.
sendaiensis
    Alicyclobacillus s.
Sendai virus
Senear-Usher
    S.-U. disease
    S.-U. syndrome
seneciella
seneciosis
senescence
    cellular s.
    immune s.

senile
    s. amyloidosis
    s. arteriosclerosis
    s. atrophy
    s. degeneration
    s. dwarfism
    s. ectasia
    s. elastosis
    s. fibroma
    s. hemangioma
    s. hip disease
    s. involution
    s. keratoderma
    s. keratoma
    s. keratosis
    malum coxae s.
    s. nephrosclerosis
    s. osteomalacia
    s. plaques
    s. sebaceous
      hyperplasia
    s. wart

senilis
    arcus s.
    keratosis s.
    malum articulorum s.
    vaginitis s.
    verruca plana s.

sennetsu
    Ehrlichia s.
    Neorickettsia s.
    Rickettsia s.

sennoside

Sensa
    Hemoccult S.

sense
    s. organ
    s. strand

SensiCath system

Sensititre *Streptococcus pneumoniae* **HPB susceptibility plate**

sensitive membrane antigen rapid test (SMART)

sensitivity
    acquired s.
    analytical s.
    antibiotic s.
    antigen s.
    clinical s.
    contact s.
    culture and s. (C&S)
    diagnostic s.
    electrode s.
    idiosyncratic s.
    induced s.
    multiple chemical s.
    primaquine s.
    relative s.
    salt s. (SS)

sensitization
    active s.
    autoerythrocyte s.
    s. response (SR)

sensitize

sensitized
    s. antigen
    s. cell
    s. culture

sensitizer

sensitizing
    s. dose
    s. injection
    s. substance

sensor

sensorineural, sensory/neural

sensory
    s. crossway
    s. receptor

sensory/neural (*var. of* sensorineural)

sensuum
    organa s.

sentinel
    s. animal
    s. case
    s. event
    s. gland
    s. laboratory
    s. lymph node (SLN)
    s. lymph node biopsy
    s. pile
    s. tag

SEOC
    serous epithelial ovarian
    carcinoma

seoi
    Gymnophalloides s.

seoulensis
    Fibricola s.

Sepacell RZ-2000 device

separating medium

separation
    immunomagnetic cell s.
    multiangle polarized scatter s.
    (MAPSS)
    solid-phase s.

separator
    Amicus s.

separatory funnel

Sepedonium

Sepharose
    protein G S.

Sepsidae

sepsis
    Chlamydia s.
    intestinal s.
    s. lenta
    overwhelming postsplenectomy s.
    s. syndrome

S

sepsis (*continued*)
    tularemia s.
    tularemic s.
septa (*pl. of* septum)
septal
    s. bone
    s. cell
    s. defect (SD)
    s. fibrosis of liver
    s. panniculitis
    s. panniculitis without vasculitis
Septata intestinalis
septate mycelium
septectomy
SEPT9 gene
septic
    s. abortion
    s. arthritis
    s. disease
    s. embolus
    s. endocarditis
    s. fever
    s. infarct
    s. intoxication
    s. knee
    s. necrosis
    s. peritonitis
    s. phlebitis
    s. pneumonia
    s. shock
septica
    iridocyclitis s.
septicemia
    acute fulminating meningococcal s.
    anthrax s.
    cryptogenic s.
    puerperal s.
    Staphylococcus s.
    typhoid s.
septicemic
    s. abscess
    s. anthrax
    s. plague
Septi-Chek culture system
septicopyemia
septicopyemic
septicum
    Clostridium s.
    Mycobacterium s.
septin gene family
septique
    Vibrion s.
Septobasidium cokeri
Septomyxa
septooptic dysplasia
septulum testis
septum, *pl.* **septa**
    alveolar s.
    atrial s.

    connective tissue septa
    deviated s.
    fibrovascular s.
    interalveolar s.
    s. interalveolare
    interlobular connective tissue s.
    transverse s.
sequela, *pl.* **sequelae**
sequelae (*pl. of* sequela)
sequence
    insertion s.
    intervening s.
    s. ladder
    long terminal repeat s. (LTR)
    recombination signal s. (RSS)
    regulatory s.
    repeated DNA s.
    Robin s.
    scanning s.
    s. specific oligonucleotide probe (SSOP)
    termination s.
    unstable trinucleotide repeat s.'s
sequenced-based typing (SBT)
sequencer
    amino acid s.
sequencing
    s. by hybridization (SBH)
    direct s.
    DNA s.
    genome s.
    nucleic acid s.
    nucleotide s.
sequential
    s. access
    s. analysis
    s. multichannel autoanalyzer (SMA)
    s. multiple analyzer (SMA)
    s. multiple analyzer computer (SMAC)
Sequenza immunostaining system
sequester
sequestered antigen
sequestral
sequestrant
sequestration
    biochemical s.
    s. bronchopneumonia
    bronchopulmonary s.
    s. crisis
    s. cyst
    s. dermoid
    extralobar s.
    intralobar s.
Sequestrene iron chelate
sequestrum
    primary s.
Sequivirus
sequoiosis
SER
    smooth endoplasmic reticulum

sera (*pl. of* serum)
seralbumin
SERCA
    sarcoendoplasmic reticulum
      calcium-ATPase
      SERCA enzyme
Sereny test
SEREX
    serological expression of cDNA
      expression
      SEREX method
sergenti
serial
    s. analysis of gene expression (SAGE)
    s. cardiac isoenzyme assay
    s. data transmission
    s. dilution
    s. operation
    s. passage
    s. section
    s. thrombin time (STT)
serialis
    Coenurus s.
    Multiceps s.
sericata
    Lucilia s.
Sericopelma communis
series, *pl.* series
    Accurin 515 drug resistant mutant
      control s.
    s. circuit
    erythrocytic s.
    granulocytic s.
    homologous s.
    lymphocytic s.
    lymphoid s.
    monohistiocytic s.
    myeloid s.
    scoliosis s.
    thrombocytic s.
serine
    transmembrane protease s. 3
      (TMPRSS3)
serine/threonine
    s. protein kinase ATR
    s. protein phosphatase
Serinicoccus marinus
seriniphilus
serocolitis
seroconversion
serocystic
serodiagnosis
    Leptospira s.
serodiagnostic test
seroenteritis
seroepidemiology
serofast
serofibrinous
    s. effusion

    s. inflammation
    s. pericarditis
    s. pleurisy
serogroup
serologic
    s. pipette
    s. test for syphilis (STS)
serological expression of cDNA
  expression (SEREX)
serologically
    s. defined (SD)
    s. defined antigen
serology
    AIDS s.
    Aspergillus s.
    bacterial s.
    blastomycosis s.
    diagnostic s.
    Epstein-Barr virus s.
    fungal s.
    Helicobacter pylori s.
    hepatitis C s.
    hepatitis D s.
    histoplasmosis s.
    HIV-1 s.
    hypersensitivity pneumonitis s.
    Lyme disease s.
    mumps s.
    Mycoplasma s.
    respiratory syncytial virus s.
    Rocky Mountain spotted fever s.
    rotavirus s.
    rubella s.
    rubeola s.
    SLEV s.
    sporotrichosis s.
    s. test
    s. test for syphilis (STS)
    toxoplasmosis s.
    trichinosis s.
    varicella-zoster virus s.
seroma
seromucoid
    acid s.
    alpha s.
    alpha-1 s.
seromucosa
    glandula s.
seromucous
    s. cell
    s. gland
seronegative
    s. spondyloarthropathy (SNSA)
seropedicae
    Herbaspirillum s.
serophilic
seropositive
seropurulent
seropus

seroreversion
serosa
    glandula s.
    membrana s.
    polyemia s.
    tunica s.
serosal surface
serosamucin
serosanguineous effusion
serositis
    multiple s.
serosity
serosum
serosynovial
serosynovitis
serotherapy
serothorax
serotonergic receptor
serotonin
    s. assay
    s. release assay (SRA)
serotype
    heterologous s.
    homologous s.
serous
    s. acinus
    s. acute inflammation
    s. acute synovitis
    s. atrophy
    s. borderline tumor (SBT)
    s. carcinoma
    s. cell
    s. coat
    s. cyst
    s. cystadenocarcinoma
    s. cystadenofibroma
    s. cystadenoma
    s. cystoma
    s. demilune
    s. effusion
    s. epithelial ovarian carcinoma
    (SEOC)
    s. fluid
    s. gland
    s. membrane
    s. meningitis
    s. otitis media (SOM)
    s. pleurisy
    s. psammocarcinoma
    s. tunic
serovaccination
serovar
    Mycobacterium avium s. 1–29
serozyme
serpens
    Bacteroides s.
serpent
    s. infection
    s. worm

serpentine
    s. aneurysm
    s. blastema
serpiginosa
    elastosis perforans s. (EPS)
    zona s.
serpiginosum
    angioma s.
serpiginosus
    lupus s.
serpiginous
    s. configuration
    s. keratitis
    s. ulcer
serpigo
Serpula
serrata
    Linguatula s.
    ora s.
serrate
serrated
    s. adenoma
    s. colorectal polyp
Serratia
    S. liquefaciens
    S. marcescens
    S. marcescens subsp. *sakuensis*
    S. plymuthica
    S. proteamaculans
    S. quinivorans
    S. rubidaea
    S. urinary tract infection
serraticeps
    Pulex s.
Serratieae
serration
Serres gland
serrulate, serrulated
serrulated (*var. of* serrulate)
serrulatus
    Tityus s.
Ser-Thr kinase
Sertoli
    S. cell
    S. cell index (SCI)
    S. cell only syndrome
    S. cell tumor
    S. column
    S. stromal cell tumor
sertoliform
    s. component
    s. endometrioid carcinoma (SEC)
Sertoli-Leydig cell tumor
Sertoli-like pattern
serum, *pl.* **serums, sera**
    s. accelerator globulin
    s. accident
    acid phosphatase s.
    s. agar

aged s.
s. agglutinin
s. albumin (SA)
s. alkaline phosphatase (SAP)
s. alkaline phosphatase test
s. amylase
s. amylase test
s. amyloid A (SAA)
anallergenic s.
anticholera s.
anticolibacillary s.
anticomplementary s.
antidiphtheric s.
antiepithelial s.
antihepatic s.
antihuman lymphocyte s. (AHLS)
antilymphocyte s. (ALS)
antimacrophage s. (AMS)
antimeningococcus s.
antimouse lymphocyte s. (AMLS)
antineutrophilic s. (ANS)
antinsulin s. (AIS)
antipertussis s.
antiplague s.
antiplatelet s.
antipneumococcus s.
antirabies s. (ARS)
antireticular cytotoxic s. (ACS)
antiscarlatinal s.
antistaphylococcus s.
antistreptococcus s.
antitetanic s. (ATS)
antithymocyte s. (ATS)
antitoxic s.
antityphoid s.
antivenomous s.
s. ascites albumin gradient (SAAG)
s. bacterial test
s. bactericidal test (SBT)
bacteriolytic s.
s. beta-2 microglobulin
s. bicarbonate
s. bilirubin (SB)
s. bilirubin test
blood grouping s.
s. broth
s. calcium test
s. chemistry graft (SCG)
concentration of creatinine in s.
 (Scr)
concentration of sodium in s. (SNa)
convalescent s.
Coombs s.
s. creatine kinase (SCK)
s. creatine kinase test
s. creatine phosphokinase (SCPK)
s. creatinine clearance
s. creatinine test
s. defect (SD)

s. diagnosis
s. disease
dried human s.
s. drug level
s. electrolyte
endotheliolytic s.
s. enzyme
s. enzyme test
equine antihuman lymphoblast s.
 (EAHLS)
s. estriol
fetal bovine s. (FBS)
Flexner s.
foreign s.
s. globulin test
s. glutamic oxaloacetic transaminase
 (SGOT)
s. glutamic pyruvic transaminase
 (SGPT)
guinea pig s. (GPS)
guinea pig antiinsulin s. (GPAIS)
s. hepatitis (SH)
s. hepatitis virus
hereditary erythrocytic multinuclearity
 with positive acidified s.
 (HEMPAS)
s. HER-2/neu
heterologous s.
hog cholera s.
homologous s.
horse s. (HS)
human measles immune s.
human pertussis immune s.
human scarlet fever immune s.
s. hydroxybutyrate dehydrogenase
 (SHBD)
hyperimmune s.
immune s.
s. immunofixation electrophoresis
inactivated leukocytolytic s.
s. intoxication
s. iron (SI)
s. isocitric dehydrogenase (SICD)
s. lactate dehydrogenase (SLD,
 SLDH)
liquid human s.
Löffler blood s.
measles convalescent s.
motile s.
muscle s.
s. nephritis
nephrotoxic s.
nonimmune s.
normal blood s. (NBS)
normal horse s. (NHS)
normal human s. (NHS)
normal rabbit s. (NRS)
normal reference s. (NRS)
s. p24 antigen concentration

S

serum (*continued*)
   s. phenylalanine
   s. phosphorus test
   plague s.
   polyvalent s.
   pooled blood s.
   s. precipitable iodine (SPI)
   pregnant mare s. (PMS)
   prophylactic s.
   s. protein-bound iodine (SPBI)
   s. protein electrophoresis (SPE, SPEP)
   s. protein electrophoresis test
   s. protein immunofixation electrophoresis (SPIFE)
   s. prothrombin conversion
   s. prothrombin conversion acceleration (SPCA)
   s. prothrombin conversion accelerator (SPCA)
   s. prothrombin conversion accelerator factor
   s. prothrombin time
   quality control s.
   s. rash
   s. reaction
   salted s.
   salvarsanized s.
   s. shock
   s. sickness
   silver-acidified s. (Ag-AS)
   s. soluble transferrin receptor
   specific s.
   streptococcus s.
   s. therapy
   s. thrombotic accelerator (STA)
   thyrotoxic s.
   s. thyroxine measured by column chromatography ($T_4(C)$)
   s. urea nitrogen (SUN)
   s. uric acid (SUA)
   veronal-buffered saline/fetal bovine s.
serumal
serum-fast
serum-neutralizing (SN)
serums (*pl. of* serum)
service
   Department of Health and Human S.'s (DHHS)
   morgue s.
   National Council of Health Laboratory S.'s (NCHLS)
servomechanism
servomotor
seryl
sesame oil
sesquiterpene
sessile
   s. hydatid

   s. phagocyte
   s. polyp
   s. serrated adenoma
set
   medical equipment s. (MES)
   NAPP tablet s.
   s. of idiotopes
   s. point
   Shamrock Safety Winged S.
seta, *pl.* **setae**
setaceous
setae (*pl. of* seta)
Setaria
   S. cervi
   S. equina
setariasis
setiferous, setigerous
setigerous (*var. of* setiferous)
Setosphaeria
SETTLE
   spindle cell epithelial tumor with thymus-like differentiation
settled particulate
seven-segment display
severe
   s. acute respiratory syndrome (SARS)
   s. acute respiratory syndrome coronavirus (SARS-CoV)
   s. atypical pneumonia
   s. combined immunodeficiency (SCID)
   s. hemolytic anemia
   s. protein deprivation
severely
   s. malnourished alcoholic
   s. subnormal (SSN)
Severinghaus electrode
severity of illness
Sever syndrome
Sevier-Munger stain
sex
   s. cell
   s. chromatin
   s. chromatin study
   s. chromatin test (SCT)
   s. chromosome
   s. chromosome abnormality
   s. cord
   s. cord-stromal tumor
   s. cord tumor with annular tubule
   s. determination
   s. differentiation
   s. factor
   heterogametic s.
   homogametic s.
   s. hormone (SH)
   s. hormone-binding globulin
   s. pili
sexalatus

sex-conditioned character
sexivalent
sex-limited character
sex-linked
    s.-l. character
    s.-l. gene
    s.-l. heredity
    s.-l. inheritance
sex-reversed mutation
sextant
    s. biopsy
    s. site
sexual
    s. gland
    s. reproduction
sexually transmitted disease (STD)
Sézary
    S. cell
    S. count
    S. erythroderma
    S. reticulosis
    S. syndrome (SS)
SF
    scarlet fever
SFG
    spotted fever group
SFP
    screen filtration pressure
SFT
    solitary fibrous tumor
S-G
    Sachs-Georgi
SG
    skin graft
    specific gravity
SGAT
    salivary gland anlage tumor
SGC
    sweat gland carcinoma
SGD
    single gene disorder
14-3-3s gene
SGF2
    fog oil
SGOT
    serum glutamic oxaloacetic
    transaminase
SGPT
    serum glutamic pyruvic transaminase
SGV
    salivary gland virus
SH
    serum hepatitis
    sex hormone
    sinus histiocytosis
shabanensis
    Salinisphaera s.
shackletonii
    Bacillus s.

shadow
    s. cell
    s. corpuscle
    Gumprecht s.
    mediastinal s.
    s. nucleus
    Ponfick s.
shadow-casting
Shaffer-Hartmann method
shaft
    cortex of hair s.
    medulla of hair s.
shaggy pericardium
shagreen
    s. lesion
    s. patch
    s. skin
shahii
    Leptotrichia s.
    Prevotella s.
shake
    s. culture
    s. test
shaken
    s. adult syndrome
    s. baby syndrome (SBS)
    s. impact syndrome
    s. infant syndrome
Shamrock Safety Winged Set
Shandon
    S. Cadenza immunostainer
    S. Cytospin chamber
    S. fixative
shape
    flattened s.
    plurilobulated s.
shaped
    racquet s.
shared hallucination
Sharpey fiber
shave biopsy
Shaver disease
SHb
    sulfhemoglobin
SHBD
    serum hydroxybutyrate dehydrogenase
SHBG
    steroid hormone binding globulin
sheath
    archnoid s.
    caudal s.
    dentinal s.
    dural s.
    enamel rod s.
    external root s.
    fibrous tendon s.
    giant cell tumor of tendon s. (GCTTS)
    glissonian s.
    Henle s.

S

sheath (*continued*)
    Huxley s.
    internal root s.
    Mauthner s.
    medullary s.
    mitochondrial s.
    myelin s.
    nerve s. (NS)
    Neumann s.
    notochordal s.
    s. of Key and Retzius
    s. of Schwann
    s. of Schweigger-Seidel
    s.'s of vessels
    root s.
    Rouget-Neumann s.
    synovial s.
    tail s.
sheathed
Sheather
    S. sugar flotation method
    S. sugar flotation procedure
shedding
    syncytial s.
    virus s.
Sheehan syndrome
sheep
    s. blood agar
    s. cell agglutination test (SCAT)
    contagious ecthyma (pustular
      dermatitis) virus of s.
    s. liver fluke
    s. pox
    s. pox virus
    s. red blood cell (SRBC)
sheet
    beta-pleated s.
    material safety data s. (MSDS)
    pleated s.
sheeting
    architectural s.
sheetlike aggregate
Shelf-Life Extension Program (SLEP)
shell
    diffusion s.
    s. nail
    staining s.
Sherman-Bourquin unit of vitamin B$_2$
Sherman-Munsell unit
Sherman unit
Shewanella
    S. *affinis*
    S. *denitrificans*
    S. *fidelis*
    S. *gaetbuli*
    S. *japonica*
    S. *livingstonensis*
    S. *marinintestina*
    S. *olleyana*

    S. *pacifica*
    S. *pealeana*
    S. *sairae*
    S. *schlegeliana*
    S. *waksmanii*
Shewanellaceae
SHH
    sonic hedgehog
    SHH gene
    SHH protein
Shichito disease
shield
    chloride s.
    face s.
    gonadal s.
    syringe s.
    tabletop s.
    s. to the left
    s. to the right
shielding
shift
    antigenic s.
    bathochromic s.
    chemical s.
    chloride s.
    colloid s.
    s. counter
    hyperchromic s.
    hypochromic s.
    hypsochromic s.
    isohydric s.
    left s.
    left s. (increased band forms on
      WBC differential)
    midline s.
    regenerative blood s.
    s. register
    s. reticulocyte
    Stokes s.
Shiga
    S. bacillus
    S. toxin (Stx)
Shigalike toxin
Shigella
    S. *arabinotarda*
    S. *boydii*
    S. *dysenteriae*
    S. *flexneri*
    S. rapid latex test
    S. *sonnei*
shigelloides
    Aeromonas (*Plesiomonas*) s.
    Plesiomonas s.
shigellosis
Shiiki
    method of S.
Shikimate dehydrogenase
shilonii
    Vibrio s.

Shimada classification
Shimadzu hemoglobin determination
shimamushi disease
Shimoda blood group system
Shimosato-Mukai classification
shin
> saber s.
> s. splint

shingles
Shinowara-Jones-Reinhard (SJR)
> S.-J.-R. unit

shinshuensis
> *Leifsonia s.*

shiny surface colony
ship
> s. fever
> s. rat

shipping fever virus
shirt-stud abscess
shivering thermogenesis
sHLA
> soluble human leukocyte antigen
> sHLA protein

SHML
> sinus histiocytosis with massive
> lymphadenopathy

SHO
> secondary hypertrophic osteoarthropathy

shock
> anaphylactic s.
> anaphylactoid s.
> s. antigen
> s. artifact
> cardiogenic s.
> colloid s.
> endotoxic s.
> endotoxin s.
> faradic s.
> Forssman s.
> hemoclastic s.
> hemorrhagic s.
> histamine s.
> hypoglycemic s.
> hypovolemic s.
> insulin s.
> s. lung
> neurogenic s.
> osmotic s.
> protein s.
> pseudoanaphylactic s.
> septic s.
> serum s.
> thyrotoxin s.
> toxic s.
> vasogenic s.

shocking dose
Shone anomaly
Shope
> S. fibroma

S. fibroma virus
> S. papilloma
> S. papilloma virus

shored-exit wound
Shorr trichrome stain
short
> s. bowel syndrome
> s. circuit
> s. fascicular growth pattern
> s. increment sensitivity index (SISI)
> s. incubation hepatitis
> s. stature

shortened
> s. bleeding time
> s. coagulation time

shortening
> abnormal s.
> telomere s.

short-interference RNA (siRNA)
short-lived evidence
short-strip pouchitis
shottsii
> *Mycobacterium s.*

shotty
> s. breast
> s. lymphadenopathy
> s. pustule

showae
> *Campylobacter s.*

shower
> safety s.

showing
> fenestrated capillary s.

Shprintzen syndrome
shrapnel
shriftii
> *Selenihalanaerobacter s.*

shrinkage
> postremoval and postfixation s.

shuffle pit
Shulman syndrome
shunt, shunting
> s. determination
> hexose monophosphate s.
> (HMPS)
> Le Veen s.
> s. nephritis

shunting (*var. of* shunt)
shutdown
> renal s.

Shuttleworthia satelles
Shwachman-Diamond syndrome
Shwachman syndrome
Shwartzman reaction
Shy-Drager syndrome
SI
> International System of Units
> saturation index
> serum iron

S

SI (*continued*)
    soluble insulin
    syncytium inducing
        SI variant
        SI variant of HIV
SIA
    slide immunoenzymatic assay
Siadenovirus
SIADH
    syndrome of inappropriate secretion of
      antidiuretic hormone
sialadenitis, sialoadenitis
    HIV s.
    myoepithelial s. (MESA)
    sclerosing s.
sialadenoncus
sialadenosis
sialectasis
sialic acid
sialidase digestion
sialoadenitis (*var. of* sialadenitis)
sialoblastoma
sialocele
sialoglycoprotein
    homologous single-pass membrane s.
sialolithiasis
sialometaplasia
    necrotizing s.
sialomucin
sialoprotein
    bone s.
sialorrhea
Sialosyl-Tn antigen
sialyl
    s. Lewis X (SLex)
    s. moiety
siamense
    Gnathostoma s.
siamensis
    Asaia s.
Siamese twins
Siberian tick fever
sibericus
    Dermacentroxenus s.
Sibine
sibirica
    Rickettsia s.
sibiricum
    Anoxynatronum s.
    Thialkalimicrobium s.
sibiricus
    Thermococcus s.
Sibirina
Sibley-Lehninger (SL)
    S.-L. unit
sibling species
sibship
Sicard syndrome
Sicariidae

sicca
    bronchiectasia s.
    cholera s.
    s. complex
    keratoconjunctivitis s.
    Neisseria s.
    s. syndrome
siccant
siccative
siccolabile
siccostabile, siccostable
siccostable (*var. of* siccostabile)
siccus
SICD
    serum isocitric dehydrogenase
sick
    s. building syndrome
    s. sinus syndrome (SSS)
sickle
    s. cell (SC)
    s. cell anemia
    s. cell anemia test (SCAT)
    s. cell beta thalassemia
    s. cell crisis
    s. cell hemoglobin (HbS)
    s. cell hemoglobin C, D disease
    s. cell nephropathy
    s. cell test
    s. cell thalassemia disease
    s. cell trait
Sickle-Chex
sickled
    s. cell
    s. erythrocyte
Sickledex
    S. reagent
    S. test
sicklemia
Sicklequik test
sickling
    s. disorder
    s. hemoglobin
    s. test
sickness
    African horse s.
    African sleeping s.
    altitude s.
    decompensation s.
    decompression s.
    green s.
    Jamaican vomiting s.
    radiation s.
    serum s.
    sleeping s.
siculi
    Thermococcus s.
side-chain theory
sidedness
    membrane s.

side effect (SE)
sideramine
sideroachrestic anemia (*var. of* sideroblastic anemia)
sideroblast
    refractory anemia with ringed s.'s (RARS)
    ringed s.
sideroblastica
    anemia refractoria s.
sideroblastic anemia, sideroachrestic anemia
Siderocapsa
Siderocapsaceae
siderochrome
Siderococcus
siderocyte stain
siderocytic granule
sideroderma
siderofibrosis
siderogenous
sideromycin
sideropenia
sideropenic
    s. anemia
    s. dysphagia
siderophage
siderophagocytosis
siderophil, siderophile
siderophile (*var. of* siderophil)
siderophilin
siderophilous
siderophore
siderosilicosis
siderosis
    Bantu s.
siderosome
siderotic
    s. granule
    s. nodule
siderotica
    granulomatosis s.
    pneumoconiosis s.
SIDS
    sudden infant death syndrome
Siemens Advia Centaur immunoassay system
sienata
    Nocardia s.
SIER
    sonication-induced epitope retrieval
sieve
    s. bone
    molecular s.
sievert (Sv)
sIg
    surface immunoglobulin
Siggaard-Andersen alignment nomogram

sigma, σ
    s. bond
    S. Glycergel
    s. isoform
    s. reaction (SR)
    S. Tween proteinase
sigmoid
    s. colon
    s. shape of the curve
sigmoiditis
sigmoidovesical fistula
Sigmund gland
sign
    Amoss s.
    André Thomas s.
    Argyll Robertson pupil s.
    Arroyo s.
    Auspitz s.
    Azzopardi s.
    Brudzinski meningeal s.
    Chvostek s.
    Chvostek-Weiss s.
    Coopernail s.
    Courvoisier s.
    crescent s.
    Crichton-Browne s.
    Cullen s.
    dimple s.
    Fajersztajn crossed sciatic s.
    filarial dance s.
    Froment paper s.
    Grey Turner s.
    groove s.
    Hawkins s.
    Higoumenakia s.
    Kernig meningeal s.
    Krisovski s.
    lemon s.
    Leser-Trélat s.
    long tract s.
    Mendel-Bekhterev s.
    Mirchamp s.
    Nikolsky s.
    Ortolani s.
    pseudo-Graefe s.
    pulvinar s.
    Romaña s.
    Rommelaere s.
    Schultze-Chvostek s.
    scimitar s.
    Séguin s.
    sonographic Murphy s.
    string s.
    Vierra s.
    vital s.'s (VS)
signal
    s. amplification
    analog s.
    s. averaging

S

signal (*continued*)
　　common mode s.
　　deflection s.
　　insufficient s. (IS)
　　s. level
　　s. node
　　nuclear s.
　　proinflammatory s.
　　ras s.
　　spatial syndromic s.
　　s. to noise ratio (S:N)
　　s. transducer and activator of
　　　transcription (STAT)
　　trophic s.
signaling
　　s. molecule
　　suppressor of cytokine s.
　　　(SOCS)
signature
　　gene expression s.
　　immunophenotypic s.
　　microRNA s.
　　tumor s.
signed
　　s. magnitude
　　s. rank test
signet
　　s. ring
　　s. ring adenocarcinoma
　　s. ring cell
　　s. ring cell carcinoma
　　s. ring cell ductal carcinoma in
　　　situ
signet-ring configuration
significance
　　atypical glandular cell of
　　　undetermined s. (AGUS)
　　atypical glandular cell of unknown
　　　s. (AGUS)
　　atypical squamous cells of
　　　undetermined s. (ASCUS)
　　s. level
　　monoclonal gammopathy of
　　　undetermined s. (MGUS)
　　monoclonal gammopathy of
　　　unknown s. (MGUS)
　　s. probability
　　test of s. (t)
significant (sig)
　　s. asymptomatic bacteriuria (SAB)
　　s. digit
　　not s. (NS)
　　not statistically s. (NSS)
　　statistically s. (SS)
Signify
　　S. DOA test
　　S. ER drug screen test
sign/trill
　　Romaña s.

SiHa cell
sihwensis
　　Gordonia s.
SIL
　　squamous intraepithelial lesion
silacea
　　Chrysops s.
silanated slide
silane
silanization
silastic
silencing
　　epigenetic s.
　　gene s.
silent
　　s. gene
　　s. mutation
　　s. myocardial infarction (SMI)
　　s. thalassemia
　　s. thyroiditis
Silferskiöld syndrome
silhouette
　　cardiac s.
silica (SiO$_2$)
　　s. gel
　　s. granuloma
silicate
silicatosis
Silicibacter
　　S. lacuscaerulensis
　　S. pomeroyi
silicic acid
silicofluoride
　　sodium s.
silicon-controlled
　　s.-c. rectifier
　　s.-c. switch
silicone
　　s. breast implant (SBI)
　　s. dioxide
　　s. granuloma
　　s. lymphadenopathy
　　s. oil
siliconoma
silicon-oxygen (Si-O)
silicoproteinosis
silicosis
　　complication of s.
silicotic nodule
silo-filler's
　　s.-f. disease
　　s.-f. lung
silver (Ag)
　　s. ammoniacal silver stain
　　s. cell
　　Grocott methenamine s. (GMS)
　　s. impregnation
　　methenamine s.
　　s. nitrate

s. nitrate stain
s. nitrate with hematoxylin
s. nitroprusside test
s. protein stain
S. syndrome
silver-acidified serum (Ag-AS)
silver-ammoniac silver stain
Silver-Russell
S.-R. dwarfism
S.-R. syndrome
silver/silver chloride electrode
silver-stained
s.-s. nucleolar organizer region (AgNOR)
s.-s. nucleolar organizing region (AgNOR)
Silvestrini-Corda syndrome
Silvex
silylation
Simbu
S. hepatitis
S. virus
simiae
Aeromonas s.
Herpesvirus s.
Mycobacterium s.
Trypanosoma s.
simian
s. crease
s. immunodeficiency virus (SIV)
s. sarcoma virus (SSV)
s. vacuolating virus No. 40
s. virus (SV)
simicola
Pneumonyssus s.
simii
Trichophyton s.
similarity
antigenic s.
Simkaniaceae
Simkania negevensis
simkin
simulation kinetics
simkin analysis
Simmonds disease
Simmons citrate agar
Simonea folliculorum
Simons disease
Simon septic factor
Simonsiella
Simonsiellaceae
Simplate heterotrophic plate count method
simple
s. adenosis
s. asphyxiant
s. atrophy
s. bone cyst
s. ciliated cuboidal

s. fracture
s. goiter
s. hypertrophy
s. lymphangiectasis
s. microscope
s. necrosis
s. protein
s. pulmonary eosinophilia
s. radiological device
s. random sample
s. renal cyst
s. solitary cyst
s. ulcer
s. urethritis
simplex
adiposis tuberosa s.
carcinoma s.
epidermolysis bullosa s.
hemangioma s.
herpes s. (HS)
ichthyosis s.
lymphangioma superficium s.
prurigo s.
scarlatina s.
toxoplasmosis, rubella, cytomegalovirus, and herpes s. (TORCH)
verruca s.
xanthoma tuberosum s.
Simplexvirus
simplicissima
Spicaria s.
Simplify D-dimer assay
Sims-Huhner test
simulans
Corynebacterium s.
Staphylococcus s.
simulated
s. hypertrophy
s. matrix reference materials
simulation kinetics (simkin)
Simuliidae
Simulium
S. damnosum
S. neavei
S. ochraceum
S. rugglesi
simultaneous multiple analyzer (SMA)
sincalide
Sindbis
S. fever
S. virus
sinensis
Knoellia s.
Opisthorchis s.
Streptococcus s.
sinesedis
Gordonia s.

S

sine wave
singaporensis
    Actinopolymorpha s.
    Desulforhopalus s.
singer's
    s. node
    s. nodule
single
    s. breath carbon monoxide diffusing capacity
    s. breath nitrogen elimination
    s. copy gene
    s. copy gene marker
    s. diffusion
    s. (gel) diffusion precipitin test in one dimension
    s. (gel) diffusion precipitin test in two dimensions
    s. gene disorder (SGD)
    s. human leukocyte antigen
    s. immunodiffusion
    s. nucleotide change
    s. nucleotide polymorphism (SNP)
    s. nucleotide polymorphism scoring technology
    S. Use Diagnostic System (SUDS)
    s. vial fixative
single-agent kinetic enzyme assay
single-analyte
    s.-a. immunologic assay
    s.-a. molecular assay
single-chain antigen-binding (SCA)
single-diffusion radial immunodiffusion
single-donor
    s.-d. plasma
    s.-d. platelets
single-dot pattern
single-phase
single-stranded
    s.-s. conformation polymorphism (SSCP)
    s.-s. DNA (SS-DNA)
single-to-multiple layers of follicular cell
Singleton-Merten syndrome
sinica
    Borrelia s.
sinistra
sinistrocardia
    isolated s.
sink
    heat s.
sinoatrial (SA), sinuatrial
sinonasal
    s. carcinoma
    s. myxoma
    s. smooth muscle cell tumor
    s. undifferentiated carcinoma (SNUC)

Sinorhizobium
    S. kummerowiae
    S. morelense
sinuatrial (*var. of* sinoatrial)
sinuatum
    Entoloma s.
sinuatus
    Rhodophyllus s.
sinus, *pl.* **sinus, sinuses**
    anal s.
    Aschoff-Rokitansky s.
    cavernous s.
    coronary s.
    s. cyst
    dermal s.
    ethmoidal s.
    s. ethmoidales
    s. histiocytosis (SH)
    s. histiocytosis with massive lymphadenopathy (SHML)
    s. intercavernosi anterior et posterior
    lactiferous s.
    s. lienis
    lymph s.
    lymphatic s.
    medullary s.
    s. mucocele
    s. node dysfunction syndrome
    s. of nail
    s. of Valsalva aneurysm
    Oribacterium s.
    s. phlebitis
    pilonidal s.
    rhomboidal s.
    Rokitansky-Aschoff s.
    splenic s.
    superior sagittal s.
    s. unguis
    s. venosus remnant
    venous s.
sinusarabici
    Flexistipes s.
sinusitis
    allergic fungal s.
    sclerosing s.
sinusoid
    blood s.
    hepatic s.
sinusoidal
    s. capillary
    s. dilatation
    s. endothelial cell
    s. foam cell cluster
    s. inflammation
Si-O
    silicon-oxygen
SiO_2
    silica
    silicone dioxide

Siphona irritans
Siphonaptera
siphonis
> *Aquicella s.*

Siphoviridae
Siphunculina
Sipple syndrome
siralis
> *Bacillus s.*

sirenomelia
Sirius red
siRNA
> short-interference RNA

siro
> *Acarus s.*
> *Tyroglyphus s.*

Sirobasidium
SIRS
> soluble immune response suppressor

SISI
> short increment sensitivity index
> SISI test

sister
> s. chromatid
> S. Mary Joseph nodule

Sistotrema
Sisyrosea
site
> allosteric s.
> antibody combining s.
> antigen-binding s.
> antigen-combining s.
> combining s.
> extravascular s.
> immunologically privileged s.
> implantation s.
> ligand-induced binding s. (LIBS)
> s. of venous obstruction
> privileged s.
> receptor s.
> sextant s.
> small discrete s.

site-specific biopsy mapping
sitophila
> *Chrysonilia s.*

sitosterolemia
> beta s.

situ
> adenocarcinoma in s. (AIS)
> apocrine ductal carcinoma in s.
> argyrophilic ductal carcinoma in s.
> carcinoma in s. (CIS)
> clinging ductal carcinoma in s.
> comedo ductal carcinoma in s.
> cystic hypersecretory ductal
>   carcinoma in s.
> ductal carcinoma in s. (DCIS)
> endocrine ductal carcinoma in s.
>   (E-DCIS)

> endometrial carcinoma in s. (ECIS)
> epidermoid carcinoma in s.
> in s.
> isolated gland carcinoma in s.
>   (GCIS)
> lobular carcinoma in s. (LCIS)
> malignant melanoma in s.
> melanoma in s.
> neuroendocrine ductal carcinoma in
>   s.
> signet ring cell ductal carcinoma in
>   s.
> squamous cell carcinoma in s.
> surface carcinoma in s. (SCIS)
> tumor in s. (TIS)

situs inversus
SIUD
> sudden intrauterine unexplained
> death

SIV
> simian immunodeficiency virus

sivashensis
> *Orenia s.*

Siwe-Letterer disease
sixth venereal disease
size
> laser diffraction particle s.
> mean follicle s.

size-exclusion chromatography
sizing
> platelet s.

Sjögren
> S. antibody
> S. disease
> S. syndrome

Sjögren-Larsson syndrome
SJR
> Shinowara-Jones-Reinhard
> SJR unit

skagerrakense
> *Tenacibaculum s.*

skatole
skatoxyl
skein cell
skeinoid fiber
skeletal
> s. disease
> s. fluorosis
> s. muscle
> s. muscle antibody
> s. muscle component of cardiac
>   isoenzymes (MM)
> s. muscle fiber
> s. muscle tissue
> s. myxoid chondrosarcoma (SMC)
> s. survey

skeletal-muscle myosin
skeleti
> musculus s.

S

skeleton
> gel-embedded GA-fixed s.
> gill-arch s.
> s. hand
> membrane s.

Skene
> Bartholin, urethral, S. (BUS)
> S. gland

skeneitis, skenitis
skenitis (*var. of* skeneitis)
Skermanella parooensis
Skevas-Zerfus disease
skew
skewed distribution
skewness
skin
> alligator s.
> s. biopsy
> s. carcinoma
> congenital localized absence of s.
> (CLAS)
> deciduous s.
> elastic s.
> farmer's s.
> fish s.
> s. fungus culture
> glabrous s.
> s. graft (SG)
> s. groove
> hyperextensible s.
> layer of s.
> loose s.
> mixed tumor of s.
> s. mycobacteria culture
> porcupine s.
> s. puncture
> s. reaction
> s. reaction pattern
> s. ridge
> sailor's s.
> seared s.
> shagreen s.
> s. shave biopsy
> stippling of s.
> s. stone
> stretchable s.
> s. tag
> s. test dose (STD)
> s. test unit (STU)
> thick s.
> thin s.
> s. tumor
> washerwoman's s.
> s. window test

skinbound disease
Skinner partially edentulous classification
skin-puncture test
skin-reactive factor (SRF)
Skinsense gloves

skin-sensitizing antibody (SSA)
skin-specific histocompatibility antigen
skin-to-tumor distance (STD)
skip
> s. areae
> s. lesion
> s. metastasis

skip-segment Hirschsprung disease
skull
> cloverleaf s.
> maplike s.
> steeple s.
> tower s.

sky blue
skyensis
sl
> slyke

SL
> Sibley-Lehninger
> small lymphocyte
> SL unit

SLA
> slide latex agglutination
> soluble liver antigen

Slackia
> *S. exigua*
> *S. heliotrinireducens*

slant culture
slaty anemia
SLD
> serum lactate dehydrogenase

SLDH
> serum lactate dehydrogenase

SLE
> St. Louis encephalitis
> systemic lupus erythematosus

sleep
> s. apnea syndrome
> s. disorder

sleeping sickness
sleeve lobectomy
SLEP
> Shelf-Life Extension Program

SLEV
> St. Louis encephalitis virus
> SLEV serology

SLex
> sialyl Lewis X
> blood group antigen SLex

SLFIA
> substrate-labeled fluorescence
> immunoassay
> substrate-labeled fluorescent immunoassay

SLI
> somatostatin-like immunoreactivity

slide
> s. agglutination test
> aminopropyltriethyoxysilane-coated
> glass s.

s. bile solubility test
ChemMate capillary gap s.
Colorfrost disposable microscope s.
Colormark s.
s. flocculation test
Genta s.
hydrogel coated s.
s. immunoenzymatic assay (SIA)
s. latex agglutination (SLA)
s. micrometer
s. platelet aggregation test (SPAT)
silanated s.
Superfrost Plus glass s.
triethylenethiophosphoramide
  precoated s.
Ventana silanized capillary gap s.
SlidePro slide heater
slide-wire potentiometer
sliding microtome
slightly curved rod
sling fiber
slippage
polymerase s.
slit
filtration s.
s. lamp
s. pore
slitlike
s. margin
s. space
SLKC
superior limbic keratoconjunctivitis
SLL
small lymphocytic lymphoma
SLMN
sarcoma-like mural nodule
SLN
sentinel lymph node
SLO
streptolysin O
slope culture
slot-blot
slot exhaust
slough
sloughing ulcer
slovaca
Rickettsia s.
slow
s. fever
s. hemoglobin
s. neutron
s. reacting factor of anaphylaxis
  (SRF-A)
s. reacting substance of anaphylaxis
  (SRS-A)
s. virus
s. virus disease
s. vital capacity (SVC)
slow-moving protease (SMP)

slow-reacting
s.-r. substance (SRS)
SLS
segment long-spacing
SLS collagen
Sluder syndrome
sludge
sludged blood
sluggish layer
slurry
SLVL
splenic lymphoma with villous
  lymphocyte
Sly
S. disease
S. syndrome
slyke (sl)
SM
splenomegaly
Sm
samarium
Sm antigen
SMA
sequential multichannel autoanalyzer
sequential multiple analyzer
simultaneous multiple analyzer
smooth muscle actin
smooth muscle antibody
infantile SMA
juvenile SMA
SMAC
sequential multiple analyzer computer
SMAC 6, 7, 10, 12, 20
SMAC test
SMAF
specific macrophage-arming factor
small
s. bowel ischemia
s. calorie (c, cal)
s. cell cancer (SCC)
s. cell malignant lymphoma (SCML)
s. cell neuroendocrine carcinoma
  (SCNC)
s. cell sarcoma
s. cell undifferentiated
  neuroendocrine carcinoma (SCUNC)
s. cleaved cell
s. discrete site
s. glandular pattern
s. intestine polyp
s. intestine tumor
s. lymphocyte (SL, T, T cell)
s. lymphocytic lymphoma (SLL)
s. noncleaved cell (SNCC)
s. noncleaved cell, non-Burkitt
  lymphoma
s. nuclear ribonucleoproteins (SNRPs)
s. peptide
s. round cell tumor (SRCT)

S

small-bowel biopsy
small-cell
    s.-c. lung carcinoma (SCLC)
    s.-c. tumor
small-intestine bacterial overgrowth
smallpox
    s. as biological weapon
    coherent s.
    confluent s.
    discrete s.
    flat s.
    fulminating s.
    hemorrhagic s.
    s. immunization
    inoculation s.
    malignant s.
    modified s.
    ordinary s.
    s. vaccine
    s. vaccine
    s. virus
    West Indian s.
SMA-12 profile test
SMART
    sensitive membrane antigen rapid test
SmartCycler realtime PCR system
smart terminal
SMC
    skeletal myxoid chondrosarcoma
    somatomedin C
SMCD
    systemic mast cell disease
smear
    acid-fast s.
    AFB s.
    air-dried s.
    alcohol fixed s.
    alimentary tract s.
    auramine-stained buffy coat s.
    s. background
    Bethesda Pap s.
    blood s.
    Breed s.
    broad s.
    bronchoscopic s.
    buccal s.
    buffy coat s.
    cervical s.
    colonic s.
    cul-de-sac s.
    s. culture
    cytologic s.
    cytopuncture s.
    cytospin slide centrifuge gram-stained s.
    Diff-Quik s.
    dried s.
    duodenal s.
    ectocervical s.
    endocervical s.

    endometrial s.
    eosinophil s.
    esophageal s.
    fast s.
    FGT cytologic s.
    fungus s.
    gastric s.
    Legionella pneumophila direct fA s.
    malaria s.
    nasal s.
    Neisseria gonorrhoeae s.
    Nickerson medium s.
    oral s.
    s. preparation and staining for
      blood parasites
    sputum s.
    sputum tuberculosis acid-fast s.
    TB s.
    s. test
    Tzanck s.
    urinary s.
    vaginal irrigation s. (VIS)
    VCE s.
    VEE s.
SMECE
    sclerosing mucoepidermoid carcinoma
    with eosinophilia
smegma
    s. bacillus
    s. clitoridis
    s. embryonum
    s. preputii
smegmalith
smegmatis
    Mycobacterium s.
smell
    organ of s.
***S*-methylmalonyl-CoA mutase**
Smith
    S. disease
    S. silver stain
Smithella propionica
Smith-Lemli-Opitz syndrome
Smith-Magenis syndrome
Smith-Riley syndrome
Smith-Strang disease
SMN
    survival motor neuron
      SMN telomeric gene
SMO
    smoothened
      SMO gene
smog
SMOH
    smoothened homolog
smoke
    NATO code for military obscurant s.
      (zinc oxide and hexachloroethane,
      grained aluminum)

smoke-producing munition
smoker's
    s. granule
    s. polycythemia
smoky
    s. melanin
    s. urine
smoldering
    s. form of ATLL
    s. leukemia
SMON
    subacute myelooptic neuropathy
S-Monovette blood collection system
smooth
    s. bacterium
    s. colony
    s. endoplasmic reticulum
    (SER)
    s. leprosy
    s. muscle
    s. muscle actin (SMA)
    s. muscle antibody (SMA)
    s. muscle cell
    s. muscle marker
    s. muscle metaplasia
    s. muscle tissue
    s. muscle tumor (SMT)
    s. muscle tumor of uncertain
    malignant potential (SMTUMP)
smoothened (SMO)
    s. homolog (SMOH)
smoothing
smooth-rough variation
smooth-surfaced endoplasmic
  reticulum
smooth-walled cyst
SMP
    slow-moving protease
SMR
    somnolent metabolic rate
    standard morbidity ratio
    standard mortality ratio
SMT
    smooth muscle tumor
SMTUMP
    smooth muscle tumor of uncertain
    malignant potential
smudge cell
smudged
    s. cell
    s. nucleus
smut
    wheat s.
SMZL
    splenic marginal zone lymphoma
S:N
    signal to noise ratio
SN
    serum-neutralizing

SNa
    concentration of sodium in serum
snakebite
snake venom (SV)
SNAP
    soluble NSF attachment protein
snap-freezing of tissue
snap-frozen specimen
SNARE
    soluble NSF-attachment protein
    receptor
snatching
    body s.
SNB
    scalene node biopsy
SNCC
    small noncleaved cell
        SNCC Burkitt lymphoma
        SNCC lymphoma
        SNCC non-Burkitt lymphoma
Sneathia sanguinegens
Sneddon syndrome
Sneddon-Wilkinson disease
sneeze gas
Snell law
S-nitrosohemoglobin
SNOMED
    systematized nomenclature of
    medicine
Snook reticulum stain
SNOP
    Systematized Nomenclature of
    Pathology
snout
    cytoplasmic s.
snowshoe hare virus
snowstorm
    lead s.
SNP
    single nucleotide polymorphism
      SNP scoring technology
SNPstream genotyping system
SNRPs
    small nuclear ribonucleoproteins
snub-nose dwarfism
SNUC
    sinonasal undifferentiated carcinoma
soap
        SoftCIDE-EC antimicrobial hand s.
        SoftCIDE hand s.
        SoftCIDE-NA plain hand s.
soap-bubble radiolucency
Sobel
    gravimetric method of S.
Sobemovirus
sobria
    Aeromonas s.
so-called false-positive reaction
socia parotidis

S

society
 American Chemical S. (ACS)
 S. for Pediatric Pathology (SPP)
 Musculoskeletal Tumor S. (MSTS)
socket
 tooth s.
socks and gloves petechial rash
SOCS
 suppressor of cytokine signaling
SOD
 superoxide dismutase
soda-lime glassware
Sodalis glossinidius
sodium
 s. acetarsol
 s. acetate
 s. acetazolamide
 s. acid citrate
 s. acid phosphate
 s. alginate
 s. alizarinsulfonate
 s. amobarbital
 s. and potassium assays
 s. antimonyltartrate
 s. arsenate
 s. ascorbate
 s. aurothiomalate
 s. aurothiosuccinate
 s. aurothiosulfate
 s. azide
 s. benzoate
 s. benzosulfimide
 s. bicarbonate
 s. biphosphate
 s. bisulfite stain
 s. borate
 s. bromide
 s. butabarbital
 s. cacodylate
 s. calcium edetate
 s. caprylate
 carbenicillin indanyl s.
 s. carbonate
 s. caseinate
 s. cellulose phosphate
 s. chloride (NaCl)
 s. chloride broth
 s. chloride culture medium
 s. chloride-sodium citrate solution
 (SSC)
 s. chromate
 s. clearance
 colistimethate s.
 s. cyanide (NaCN)
 s. cyclamate
 danaparoid s.
 dextrothyroxine s.
 s. diphenylhydantoin (SDPH)
 s. dithionate

 s. dodecyl sulfate (SDS)
 s. dodecyl sulfate-polyacrylamide gel
 electrophoresis (SDS-PAGE)
 exchangeable s.
 fecal s.
 fluorescein s.
 s. fluoride
 s. fluoroacetate
 s. fluorosilicate
 s. folate
 fractional excretion of s.
 (FENa)
 s. fusidate
 s. glutamate
 s. glycolate
 s. hexafluorosilicate
 s. hydrate
 s. hydroxide stain
 s. hypochlorite
 s. hyposulfite
 s. imbalance
 s. indigotin disulfonate
 s. iodide
 s. lactate
 s. lauryl sulfate
 mercaptomerin s.
 s. metabisulfite sickle hemoglobin
 test
 s. monofluorophosphate
 s. morrhuate
 s. nitrate
 s. nitrite
 s. nitroferricyanide
 s. nitroprusside
 s. orthovanadate
 s. oxybate
 s. *p*-aminohippurate
 s. *p*-aminohippuric acid
 s. *para*-aminosalicylate
 s. pentobarbital
 s. perborate
 s. phenobarbital
 s. phenylethylbarbiturate
 s. phenytoin
 s. phytate
 plasma s. (P_{Na})
 s. polyethylene sulfonate
 s. potassium sodium
 tartrate
 s. propionate
 s. pyroborate
 s. pyrophosphate
 s. pyrosulfite
 resorcinolphthalein s.
 s. rhodizonate stain
 rose bengal s.
 s. salicylate
 s. silicofluoride
 s. stearate

s. stibocaptate
stool s.
s. succinate
s. sulfite
sulfobromophthalein s.
s. sulfoxone
s. taurocholate
s. test
s. tetraborate
s. tetradecyl sulfate
s. thiamylal
s. thiocyanate (NaSCN)
s. thiopental
s. thiosulfate stain
s. tolbutamide
s. trimetaphosphate
s. tungstoborate
tyropanoate s.
urine s.
s. warfarin
Yb-169 pentetate s.
sodium-iodide transport protein
sodium-iodine symporter (NIS)
Soehngenia saccharolytica
Soemmerring
S. ganglion
S. spot
soft
s. chancre
s. papilloma
s. parts giant cell tumor (SP-GCT)
s. sore
s. tissue calcification (STC)
s. tissue lipoma
s. tissue tumor
s. tubercle
s. ulcer
s. wart
Sof-Tact
S.-T. diabetes management system
S.-T. glucose monitor
SoftCIDE-EC antimicrobial hand soap
SoftCIDE hand soap
SoftCIDE-NA plain hand soap
SoftGrip pipette
SoftGUARD hand cream
soft-spin technique
software
CellQuest Pro 4.0 flow cytometry s.
Expo 32 flow cytometry s.
Sohval-Soffer syndrome
SOL
solution
space-occupying lesion
sol
metal s.
solid s.
solanae
Fusarium s.

solani
Kribbella s.
solanine
Solanum carolinense
solar
s. elastosis
s. fever
s. keratosis
s. lentigo
s. urticaria
solder spot
soldier's patch
solenocyte
solenoid
Solenopotes capillatus
Solenopsis
sole nucleus
sole-plate ending
solfataricum
Desulfotomaculum s.
soli
Bacillus s.
Fulvimonas s.
Nocardia s.
Weissella s.
solid
s. adenocarcinoma
s. ameloblastoma
s. angle
s. carbon dioxide
s. carcinoma
s. edema
s. growth pattern
s. masses of epithelial cell
s. pattern
s. phase fluorescence immunoassay (SPFIA)
s. phase immunoassay
s. pseudopapillary tumor
s. sol
s. state
s. teratoma
total s.'s (TS)
solidistic pathology
solid-phase
s.-p. hybridization
s.-p. radioimmunoassay
s.-p. separation
Solirubrobacter pauli
solitarii
folliculi lymphatici s.
tractus s.
solitary
s. bone cyst
s. fibrous tumor (SFT)
s. follicle
s. gland
s. rectal ulcer syndrome

S

solium
    Taenia s.
sollicitans
    Aedes s.
Solobacterium moorei
solochrome
    s. azurine staining method
    s. cyanine stain
solubility
    s. coefficient
    s. product
    s. test
solubilization defect
solubilize
solubilized hemoglobin
solubilizer
soluble
    s. HLA
    s. HLA protein
    s. human leukocyte antigen (sHLA)
    s. immune response suppressor
    (SIRS)
    s. insulin (SI)
    s. interleukin-2 receptor
    s. liver antigen (SLA)
    s. NSF attachment protein (SNAP)
    s. NSF-attachment protein receptor
    (SNARE)
    s. ribonucleic acid (sRNA)
    s. specific substance
    s. transferrin receptor (sTfR)
solute
    total body s. (TBS)
solution (SOL)
    ammoniacal silver s.
    anticoagulant heparin s.
    aqueous s.
    Atroxin s.
    azeotropic s.
    Balamuth buffer s.
    balanced salt s. (BSS)
    Belzer s.
    Benedict s.
    blocking s.
    Bouin s.
    buffered saline s. (BSS)
    Burow s.
    Cajal formol ammonium bromide s.
    carrageenin s.
    Celsior s.
    cleaning s.
    Coleman Feulgen s.
    CryoStor cell freezing s.
    Cytyc CytoLyt preservative s.
    Cytyc PreservCyt preservative s.
    Dakin s.
    Dako target retrieval s.
    Delafield fixative s.
    Denhardt s.

    Diaphane s.
    disclosing s.
    Dragendorff s.
    Earle s.
    Fehling s.
    Fonio s.
    formaldehyde s.
    formalin s.
    Fowler s.
    FU-48 Zenker fixative s.
    Gallego differentiating s.
    Gowers s.
    Gram s.
    Hartmann s.
    Hayem s.
    heat of s.
    Hinfl s.
    Histoclear slide processing s.
    Hollande s.
    Hucker-Conn crystal violet s.
    s. hybridization
    hydrogen peroxide s.
    ideal s.
    iodine s.
    isotonic sodium chloride s.
    Kaiserling s.
    Karnovsky II s.
    Krebs-Ringer s.
    lactated Ringer s. (LRS)
    Lange s.
    Locke s.
    Locke-Ringer s.
    Lugol iodine s.
    Lumi-Phos s.
    Monsel s.
    mordant s.
    nonideal s.
    NoTox formalin substitute s.
    Oncor antifade mounting s.
    Orth s.
    Progen antibiotic s.
    propidium iodide s.
    pyridoxalated stroma-free hemoglobin
    s.
    ribonuclease s.
    Ringer lactate s. (RLS)
    Ruge s.
    saline s.
    saponin lysing reagent stock s.
    saturated s. (SS)
    Schallibaum s.
    sodium chloride-sodium citrate s.
    (SSC)
    standard s.
    TAC s.
    Tellyesnicky fixative s.
    test s. (TS)
    tetrazolium salt s.
    Toison s.

volumetric s. (VS)
Weigert iodine s.
Zamboni s.
Zenker s.
solvate
solvation
solvent
    aprotic s.
    s. detergent treatment (SD)
    s. extraction
    organic s.
    protic s.
solvolysis
soma
somaliensis
    Streptomyces s.
soman
    NATO code for s. (GD)
somat
    somatic
somatic (somat)
    s. agglutinin
    s. antigen
    s. cell
    s. cell deoxyribonucleic acid
      (somatic cell DNA)
    s. cell genetics
    s. chromosome
    s. death
    s. fibromatosis
    s. motor neuron
    s. mutation theory of cancer
    s. pairing
    s. point mutation
somatochrome
somatomammotropin
    chorionic s. (CS)
    human chorionic s. (hCSM)
    immunoradioassayable human
      chorionic s. (IRHCS)
somatomedin C (SMC)
somatoplasm
somatosexual ambiguity
somatostatin-like immunoreactivity (SLI)
somatostatinoma
somatostatin-producing small cell
somatostatin receptor
somatotrope (*var. of* somatotroph)
somatotroph, somatotrope
    s. adenoma
    s. release inhibiting factor
somatotrophic (*var. of* somatotropic)
somatotropic, somatotrophic
    s. adenoma
    s. hormone (STH)
somatotropin
somatotropin-releasing
    s.-r. factor (SRF)
    s.-r. hormone (SRH)

somerae
    Cetobacterium s.
somni
    Histophilus s.
somniferum
somnolent metabolic rate (SMR)
Somogyi
    S. effect
    S. method
    S. unit
sonicate
sonication
sonication-induced epitope retrieval
    (SIER)
sonic hedgehog (SHH)
sonification
sonifier
sonify
Sonne-Duval bacillus
Sonne dysentery
sonnei
    Shigella s.
sonographic Murphy sign
sonorensis
    Bacillus s.
soot wart
sooty capsule
SOP
    standard operating procedure
sorbate
    potassium s.
sorbefacient
sorbent
sorbic acid
sorbitol dehydrogenase
sorbitol-MacConkey medium
Sordaria
sordellii
    Clostridium s.
sordidicola
    Burkholderia s.
sore
    canker s.
    Ceylon mouth s.
    cold s.
    fungating s.
    hard s.
    s. mouth
    Oriental s.
    soft s.
    venereal s.
sorehead
soremouth virus
soremuzzle
Soret
    S. band
    S. effect
    S. phenomenon
sorption

S

Sorsby syndrome
sorter
      fluorescence-activated cell s. (FACS)
SOS bacterial DNA repair system
Sotos syndrome of cerebral gigantism
soudanense
      Trichophyton s.
souniana
      Vulcanisaeta s.
source
      alpha s.
      flood s.
      hidden radiation s.
      neutron s.
      sealed beta gamma s.
      sealed radioactive s.
      s. statement
      unsealed beta gamma s.
      unsealed radioactive s.
sourekii
      Facklamia s.
South
      S. African-type porphyria
      S. American blastomycosis
Southern
      S. blot (SB)
      S. blot analysis
      S. blot technique
      S. blot test
souvenir knife
soybean
      s. test
      s. trypsin inhibitor (SBTI)
Soymovirus
s/p
      status post
sp
      species
space
      air-filled tubular s.
      anterior incisural s.
      Blessig s.
      Bowman s.
      canalicular s.
      capillary-like s.
      capsomer capsular s.
      capsular s.
      cartilage s.
      cavernous s.
      s. charge
      corneal s.
      Czermak s.
      Disse s.
      extravascular s.
      filtration s.
      Fontana s.
      haversian s.
      His perivascular s.
      honeycomb-like s.

      intercristal s.
      interglobular s.
      intervillous s.
      intracisternal s.
      intracristal s.
      intramembranous s.
      intravascular s.
      Kiernan s.
      labyrinthine s.
      lymph s.
      Max-Joseph s.
      medium incisural s.
      Nuel s.
      s. of iridocorneal angle
      Poiseuille s.
      posterior incisural s.
      Schwalbe s.
      slitlike s.
      subarachnoid s.
      subchorial s.
      Virchow-Robin s.
      vitreous s.
      zonular s.
space-occupying lesion (SOL)
spacer
spacing
      third s.
spade
      s. finger
      s. hand
SPAI
      steroid protein activity index
spallation product
spalling
Spanish influenza
spanius
      Achromobacter s.
Sparassis
sparganoma
sparganosis
Sparganum proliferum
sparing
      orthokeratotic s.
sparteine
spasm
      bladder s.
      cadaveric s.
      diffuse esophageal s.
      esophageal s.
      infantile s. (IS)
      s. of accommodation
      salaam s.
      saltatory s.
spasmogen
spastic
      s. anemia
      s. colitis
      s. colon
      s. ileus

SPAT
    slide platelet aggregation test
spatia (*pl. of* spatium)
spatial
    s. isomerism
    s. scan statistic
    s. syndromic signal
spatium, *pl.* **spatia**
    spatia anguli iridocornealis
    s. interglobulare
    s. intervaginale subarachnoidale nervi
      optici
    spatia zonularia
spatula
    Ayre s.
    Roux s.
spatulata
    Cooperia s.
SPBI
    serum protein-bound iodine
SPCA
    serum prothrombin conversion
      acceleration
    serum prothrombin conversion
      accelerator
    SPCA deficiency
    SPCA factor
SPE
    serum protein electrophoresis
Spearman rank correlation coefficient
special
    s. pathology
    s. reference method
specialist dissection technique
specialization
    globose s.
specialized
    s. epithelium
    s. transduction
speciation
species (sp)
    reactive oxygen s. (ROS)
    sibling s.
    type s.
species-specific antigen
specific
    s. absorptivity
    s. active immunity
    s. anergy
    s. antibody deficiency
    s. antigen
    s. antiserum
    s. autoantibody
    s. bactericide
    s. capsular substance
    s. cell receptor
    s. coagulation factor deficiency
    s. disease

    s. dynamic action
    s. gene
    s. granule
    s. gravity (SG, sp gr)
    s. gravity test
    s. heat
    s. heat capacity
    s. hemolysin
    s. IgE
    s. IgE antibody scoring
    s. IgE antibody testing
    s. immune globulin (human)
    s. ionization
    s. macrophage-arming factor
      (SMAF)
    s. opsonin
    s. passive immunity
    s. pathogen-free (SPF)
    s. rate
    s. reaction
    s. rotation
    s. serum
    s. soluble polysaccharide
    s. soluble substance (SSS)
    s. soluble sugar
    s. transduction
specificity
    analytical s.
    anti-P blood group s.
    diagnostic s.
    HLA-C locus s.
    kappa chain s.
    lambda chain s.
    relative s.
    tumor s.
specified
    not otherwise s. (NOS)
Speci-Gard specimen transport bag
specimen
    bacteriologic s.
    biopsy s.
    brush s.
    clean-catch urine s.
    clean-voided s. (CVS)
    cytologic s.
    double-voided urine s.
    EDTA contamination of s.
    first morning urine s.
    grab urine s.
    mammary aspiration s. (MAS)
    normocellular bone marrow s.
    postmortem s.
    s. radiography
    random urine s.
    snap-frozen s.
    surgical s.
    swab s.
    touch-smear s.
    trimmed s.

S

speckled pattern
spectral
   s. color
   s. interference
   s. karyotype
   s. karyotyping
   s. overlap
   s. resolution
   s. response
spectrin
spectrofluorometer
spectrograph
   mass s.
spectrometer
   energy dispersive s. (EDS)
   gamma s.
   mass s.
spectrometry
   clinical s.
   gamma s.
   gas chromatography-mass s.
    (GC-MS)
   isotope dilution-mass s.
   MALDI-TOF mass s.
   mass s. (MS)
   matrix-assisted laser desorption and
    ionization mass s. (MALDIMS)
   surface-enhanced laser desorption
    ionization time-of-flight mass s.
    (SELDI-TOF-MS)
   tandem mass s.
spectrophotometer
   atomic absorption s. (AAS)
   Cary 100 UV-Vis s.
   DU Series 500, DU 800 UV/Vis s.
spectrophotometric assay
spectrophotometry
   atomic absorption s. (AAS)
   flame emission s.
   infrared s. (IRS)
   reflectance s.
   ultraviolet/visible s.
spectroscope
   direct vision s.
spectroscopic test
spectroscopy
   atomic absorption s.
   clinical s.
   emission s.
   energy dispersive x-ray s. (EDS)
   flame emission s. (FES)
   fluorescence correlation s. (FCS)
   infrared s.
   mass s.
   microabsorption s.
   nuclear magnetic resonance s.
   proton s.
   Raman s.
   vibrational s.

spectrum
   absorption s.
   s. action
   action s.
   s. analyzer
   antimicrobial s.
   atomic s.
   band s.
   broad s.
   chemical s.
   clinical s.
   continuous s.
   emission s.
   excitation s.
   fiber s.
   fluorescence s.
   gamma-ray s.
   gaseous s.
   line s.
   toxin s.
   wide s.
specular reflection
speed vacuum concentrator
Spegazzinia
speibonae
   Streptomyces s.
spelencephaly
Spelotrema nicolli
Spencer disease
spencerii
   Aedes s.
Spencer-Wells forceps
Spen syndrome
spent platelet
SPEP
   serum protein electrophoresis
sperm, spermatozoon
   s. agglutinating antibody
   s. cell
   s. crystal
   muzzled s.
   s. nucleus
   s. penetration assay
spermacytic seminoma
spermagglutination
spermatic
   s. duct
   s. filament
   s. fistula
spermatici
   tunicae funiculi s.
spermatid
   nuclear envelope of s.
spermatin
spermatoblast
spermatocele, spermatocyst
spermatocyst (*var. of*
 spermatocele)
spermatocytal

spermatocyte
  primary s.
  secondary s.
spermatocytic
  s. granuloma
  s. seminoma
spermatocytogenesis, spermatogeny, spermatogenesis
spermatogenetic
spermatogenic, spermatogenous, spermatopoietic
  s. granuloma
  s. maturation arrest
spermatogeny
spermatogone
spermatogonium, spermatogone
spermatoid
spermatology
spermatolysin
spermatolysis, spermolysis
spermatolytic, spermolytic
spermatophore
spermatopoietic (*var. of* spermatogenic)
spermatotoxin (*var. of* spermatoxin)
spermatoxin, spermatotoxin, spermotoxin
spermatozoa
spermatozoal, spermatozoan
spermatozoan (*var. of* spermatozoal)
spermatozoon (*var. of* sperm)
  mature s.
spermaturia (*var. of* semenuria)
spermia (*pl. of* spermium)
spermiation
spermidine
spermiduct
spermin crystal
spermine crystal
spermiogenesis
spermium, *pl.* **spermia**
spermolith
spermolysis (*var. of* spermatolysis)
spermolytic (*var. of* spermatolytic)
Spermophilus
Spermospora
spermotoxin
sperm-ubiquitin tag immunoassay (SUTI)
SPF
  specific pathogen-free
SPFIA
  solid phase fluorescence immunoassay
SP-GCT
  soft parts giant cell tumor
sp gr
  specific gravity
SPH
  secondary pulmonary hemosiderosis

sphacelate
sphacelation
sphacelism
sphaceloderma
sphacelous
sphacelus
Sphaerella
Sphaeria
sphaerica
  Nigrospora s.
sphaericus
  Bacillus s.
Sphaerobacteraceae
Sphaerobacterales
Sphaerobacteridae
Sphaerobolus
Sphaerophorus
  necrophorus
Sphaeropsis subglobosa
sphaerospora
  Xylogone s.
Sphaerotilus natans
S-phase fraction
sphenisci
  Corynebacterium s.
spheniscorum
  Corynebacterium s.
sphenoides
  Clostridium s.
sphenoiditis
sphenooccipital synchondrosis
sphenopetrosal synchondrosis, sphenopetrous synchondrosis
sphere
  attraction s.
  embryonic s.
  Morgagni s.
  prelytic s.
  segmentation s.
  vitelline s.
spherical polar coordinates
spherocytic
  s. anemia
  s. hereditary elliptocytosis
  s. jaundice
spherocytosis
  congenital s.
  hereditary s. (HS)
spherophakia-brachymorphia syndrome
spheroplast
spherospermia
spherule
spherulin
spherulosis
  collagenous s.
sphincter
  urinary tract s.
sphincteral achalasia

S

sphincteric structure
sphincteritis
sphinganine
sphingenine
Sphingobacteria
Sphingobacteriaceae
Sphingobium
    S. amiense
    S. chlorophenolicum
    S. herbicidovorans
    S. yanoikuyae
sphingolipidoses (*pl. of* sphingolipidosis)
sphingolipidosis, sphingolipodystrophy, *pl.*
  sphingolipidoses
    cerebral s.
sphingolipid storage disease
sphingolipodystrophy (*var. of* sphingolipidosis)
Sphingomonadaceae
Sphingomonas
    S. aerolata
    S. alaskensis
    S. aquatilis
    S. aurantiaca
    S. chungbukensis
    S. cloacae
    S. faeni
    S. koreensis
    S. melonis
    S. pituitosa
    S. roseiflava
    S. taejonensis
    S. wittichii
    S. xenophaga
    S. yanoikuyae
sphingomyelin
    s. lipidosis
    s. phosphodiesterase
sphingomyelinase
sphingomyelinosis
Sphingopyxis
    S. alaskensis
    S. chilensis
    S. macrogoltabida
    S. terrae
    S. witflariensis
sphingosine
SPI
    serum precipitable iodine
Spicaria simplicissima
spicheri
    Lactobacillus s.
spicifera
    Bipolaris s.
spicular
spiculated
    s. body
    s. edge
spicule of bone
spiculum

spider
    s. angioma
    arterial s.
    black widow s.
    brown recluse s.
    s. burst
    s. cancer
    s. cell
    s. mole
    s. nevus
    s. pelvis
    s. telangiectasia
    vascular s.
spidery
Spiegler-Fendt
    S.-F. pseudolymphoma
    pseudolymphoma of S.-F.
    S.-F. sarcoid
Spielmeyer acute swelling
Spielmeyer-Stock disease
Spielmeyer-Vogt disease
SPIFE
    serum protein immunofixation
    electrophoresis
        SPIFE acid hemoglobin assay
        SPIFE alkaline hemoglobin assay
spike
    s. and dome appearance
    M s.
    monoclonal M s.
spill
    cellular s.
    s. control
    s. control kit
    s. residue
spiloma
Spilopsyllus cuniculi
spilus
    nevus s.
spina, *pl.* spinae
    s. bifida
    s. bifida aperta
    s. bifida cystica
    s. bifida manifesta
    s. bifida occulta
    s. ventosa
spinae (*pl. of* spina)
spinal
    s. cord compression (SCC)
    s. cord concussion
    s. cord demyelination
    s. cord disease
    s. cord infection
    s. cord inflammation
    s. cord injury
    s. cord tumor
    s. cord vascular malformation
    s. embolism
    s. fluid

s. fluid culture
s. fluid leak
s. fluid leukocyte count
s. meningioma
s. muscular atrophy (SMA)
s. neoplasm
s. stenosis

spinalis

hydrocele s.

Spinchron DLX, 15 series centrifuge

spindle

achromatic s.
s. attachment
barbiturate s.
bipolar s.
s. cell
s. cell carcinoma
s. cell component
s. cell epithelial tumor with
thymus-like differentiation (SETTLE)
s. cell fascicular pattern
s. cell lipoma
s. cell melanoma
s. cell nevus
s. cell nodule
s. cell pseudotumor
s. cell sarcoma
s. cell thymoma
s. cell tumor
central s.
cleavage s.
s. fiber
Krukenberg s.
Kühne s.
mitotic s.
multipolar s.
muscle s.
neuromuscular s.
neurotendinous s.
nuclear s.

spindle-celled layer
spindle-shaped neoplastic stromal cell
spindling
spindly squamoid cell
spine

s. cell
cleft s.
dendritic s.
poker s.

spiniger

S.
Heterodoxus s.

spinigera

Haemaphysalis s.

spinigerum

Gnathostoma s.

spinipalpis

Ixodes s.

spinnbarkeit

spinner

DiffSpin slide s.

spinosa

ichthyosis s.

spinosispora

Pseudonocardia s.

spinosum

stratum s.

spinous layer
spinulosum
spiracle
spiradenitis
spiradenoma

eccrine s.

spiral

s. artery
s. crest
Curschmann s.
s. foraminous tract
s. fracture
Herxheimer s.
s. hypha
s. lamina
s. ligament of cochlea
s. membrane
s. organ
s. plate
s. plica
s. tubule
s. visual field
s. wound (SW)

spirale

organum s.

spiralis

Acuaria s.
crista s.
membrana reticularis organi s.
Trichinella s.
Trichurus s.

spiramycin
Spirillaceae
Spirillales
spirillar dysentery
Spirilleae
spirillosis
spirillum

S.
S. minus
Obermeier s.
S. volutans

spirit lamp
Spirocerca lupi
Spirochaeta

S. americana
S. bajacaliforniensis
S. eurystrepta
S. pallida
S. plicatilis
S. stenostrepta

S

Spirochaetaceae
Spirochaetae
Spirochaetales
Spirochaetes
spirochetal
spirochete
    Dutton s.
spirochetemia
spirochetes
    Becker stain for s.
spirochetolysis
spirochetosis
    icterogenic s.
spirogram
    forced expiratory s. (FES)
Spirolate broth
Spirometra
    S. mansoni
    S. mansonoides
Spiromicrovirus
spironolactone test
Spiroplasmataceae
Spirosomaceae
Spirotrichum
Spirurata
Spirurida
Spiruridae
Spiruroidea
spiruroid larva migrans
Spitz-like melanoma
Spitz nevus
spitzoid melanocytic lesion
SPL
    spontaneous lesion
splanchnic
    s. blood flow (SBF)
    s. mesenchyme
splanchnicus
    Bacteroides s.
splanchnocystica
    dysencephalia s.
splanchnoptosia (*var. of* splanchnoptosis)
splanchnoptosis, splanchnoptosia
splanchnosclerosis
splatter
    back s.
    impact s.
splatter-borne agent
spleen
    accessory s.
    Banti s.
    diffuse waxy s.
    Gandy-Gamna s.
    hilum of s.
    lardaceous s.
    malpighian body of s.
    sago s.
    sugar-coated s.
    waxy s.

splen accessorius
splenauxe
splendens
    linea s.
Splendore-Hoeppli phenomenon
splenectopia, splenectopy
splenectopy (*var. of* splenectopia)
splenelcosis
splenemphraxis
splenic
    s. anemia
    s. cell
    s. cord
    s. corpuscle
    s. flexure
    s. hemangiosarcoma
    s. index
    s. leukemia
    s. lymph follicle
    s. lymph nodule
    s. lymphoma with villous
        lymphocyte (SLVL)
    s. marginal zone lymphoma (SMZL)
    s. pulp
    s. red pulp
    s. sequestration of platelets
    s. sinus
    s. tumor
splenica
    pulpa s.
splenicum
    hilum s.
splenis
    tunica fibrosa s.
splenitis
    acute s.
splenocele
splenogonadal fusion
splenohepatomegalia (*var. of*
  splenohepatomegaly)
splenohepatomegaly, splenohepatomegalia
splenoma
splenomalacia
splenomedullary
splenomegalia (*var. of* splenomegaly)
splenomegalic polycythemia
splenomegaly (SM), splenomegalia
    congestive s.
    Egyptian s.
    fibrocongestive s.
    hemolytic s.
splenomyelogenous
splenomyelomalacia
splenoncus
splenosis
splenotoxin
spliceosome
    major GU-AG s.
    minor AU-AC s.

splicing
  gene s.
  RNA s.
splint
  shin s.
split
  s. collection urine test
  s. gene
  s. pelvis
  s. renal function (SRF)
  s. renal function study
    (SRFS)
  s. renal function test
  s. tolerance
split-thickness skin graft (STSG)
splitting
  beam s.
split-virus vaccine
SPM
  scanning probe microscopy
spodogenous
spodogram
spodography
spodophorous
SPO1-like viruses
Spondweni virus
spondylitis
  ankylosing s.
  rheumatoid ankylosing s.
  tuberculous s.
spondyloarthropathy
  seronegative s. (SNSA)
spondylocace
Spondylocladium
spondyloepiphyseal (*var. of*
  spondyloepiphysial)
spondyloepiphysial, spondyloepiphyseal
  s. dysplasia (SED)
spondylolisthesis
spondylolisthetic pelvis
spondylolysis
spondylomalacia
spondylopathy
spondyloptosis
spondylopyosis
spondyloschisis
spondylosis
  cervical s.
  hyperostotic s.
  lumbar s.
spondylosyndesis
sponge disease
spongiform
  s. degeneration
  s. encephalopathy
  s. pustule of Kogoj
spongioblast
spongioblastoma
spongiocyte

spongioid
spongiosa
  substantia s.
spongiosi
  trabecula corporis s.
  trabeculae corporis s.
  tunica albuginea corporis s.
spongiosis
spongiositis
spongiosum
  corpus s.
  osteoma s.
  stratum s.
spongiosus
  status s.
spongiotic dermatitis
Spongipellis
Spongiporus
spongy
  s. bone
  s. degenerative-type leukodystrophy
  s. nevus
spontanea
  dactylolysis s.
spontaneous
  s. abortion
  s. agglutination
  s. amputation
  s. bacterial peritonitis (SBP)
  s. coagulation
  s. coronary artery dissection
    (SCAD)
  s. delivery (SD)
  s. generation
  s. lesion (SPL)
  s. mutation
  s. phagocytosis
  s. pneumothorax
  s. remission
sporadic
  s. adenomatous polyp (SAP)
  Alzheimer disease familial and s.
  s. diffuse goiter
  s. dysentery
  s. nodular goiter
  s. papillary renal cell carcinoma
sporadin
Sporanaerobacter acetigenes
sporangiophore
sporangiospore
sporangium
spore
  anthrax s.
  bacterial s.
  central s.
  drumstick s.
  s. form
  fungal s.
  midterminal s.

S

spore (*continued*)
    oval subterminal s.
    s. strip
spore-forming rod
Sporendonema
Sporichthyaceae
sporicidal
sporicide
Sporidesmium
Sporidiobolus
sporidium
sporoagglutination
Sporobacterium olearium
sporoblast
Sporobolomyces
Sporocybe
sporocyst
Sporocystinea
sporodochium
sporogenes
    Caminicella s.
    Clostridium s.
sporogenesis
sporogenous
sporogeny (*var. of* sporogony)
sporogony, sporogeny
Sporomusa aerivorans
sporont
sporophore
sporoplasm
Sporormiella
Sporosarcina
    S. aquimarina
    S. globispora
    S. macmurdoensis
    S. pasteurii
    S. psychrophila
sporotheca
Sporothrix schenckii
Sporotomaculum syntrophicum
sporotrichosis
    lymphocutaneous s.
    s. serology
sporotrichositic chancre
Sporotrichum
    S. beurmanni
    S. gougerotii
    S. pruinosum
    S. schenckii
sporozoan
Sporozoasida
Sporozoea
sporozoite
sporozooid
sporozoon
sports-related sudden death
sporular
sporulate
sporulation

sporule
spot
    acoustic s.
    ash-leaf s.
    Bitot s.
    blood s.
    blue s.
    Brushfield s.
    café au lait s.
    cayenne pepper s.
    cherry red s.
    Christopher s.
    chromatin s.
    cold s.
    de Morgan s.
    dried blood s.
    electronic focal s.
    embryonic s.
    eye s.
    s. film
    Fordyce s.
    germinal s.
    hot s.
    intranuclear s.
    Koplik s.
    lance-ovate s.
    milk s.
    milky s.
    mongolian s.
    Roth s.
    S. RT Monochrome Kodak
      KAI-2000 CCD digital camera
    ruby s.
    saccular s.
    Soemmerring s.
    solder s.
    Stephen s.
    Tardieu s.
    telomere s.
    tendinous s.
    s. test
    s. test for infectious mononucleosis
    utricular s.
    white s.
    Wischnewsky s.'s
    yellow s. (YS)
spot-blot
spotted
    s. fever
    s. fever group (SFG)
spotty lobular necrosis
SPOV
    Spondweni virus
SPP
    Society for Pediatric Pathology
spray
    cryogenic s.
    Fisher Scientific Histo-freeze 2000
      freezing s.

Spray-Cyte slide fixative
spreading factor
spread plate
spring
    s. catarrhal conjunctivitis
    hemoglobin Constant S.
    s. ophthalmia
Sprinz-Nelson syndrome
sprue
    celiac s.
    collagenous s.
    nontropical s.
    tropical s. (TS)
spruelike syndrome
spumae
    Tsukamurella s.
Spumavirinae
spumicola
    Friedmanniella s.
spun urine sediment
spur
    s. cell
    s. cell anemia
spuria
    hemospermia s.
    placenta s.
spurious
    s. cast
    s. parasite
spurium
Spurr resin
Spurway syndrome
sputa (*pl. of* sputum)
sputi
    Gordonia s.
Sputolysin
sputorum
    Campylobacter s.
    Vibrio s.
sputum, *pl.* **sputa**
    s. aerogenosum
    s. cytology
    s. examination
    s. fungus culture
    globular s.
    green s.
    s. induction
    s. mycobacteria culture
    nummular s.
    prune juice s.
    rusty s.
    s. smear
    s. tube
    s. tuberculosis acid-fast smear
SQ
    squalene
    subcutaneous
squalene
squama, squame, *pl.* **squamae**

squamae (*pl. of* squama)
squamate
squamatization
squame (*var. of* squama)
squamocellular
squamocolumnar junction (SCJ)
squamoid pattern
squamous
    s. alveolar cell
    s. cell carcinoma (SCC)
    s. cell carcinoma in situ
    s. cell carcinoma of the thyroid
        (SCT)
    s. cell index
    s. cell papilloma
    s. dysplasia
    s. eddy
    s. epithelial cell
    s. epithelium
    s. intraepithelial lesion (SIL)
    s. metaplasia
    s. metaplasia of amnion
    s. morule
    s. odontogenic tumor
    s. pearl
    s. syringometaplasia
squamous-cell carcinoma antigen (SCCA, SCC-Ag)
square wave
squarrose
squill
    red s.
3SR
    self-sustained sequence replication
^{90}Sr
    strontium
    strontium-90
SR
    screen
    secretion rate
    sedimentation rate
    sensitization response
    sigma reaction
    stimulation ratio
Sr
    strontium
sr
    steradian
SRA
    serotonin release assay
SRBC
    sheep red blood cell
SRC
    sedimented red cell
SRCT
    small round cell tumor
SRF
    skin-reactive factor
    somatotropin-releasing factor

S

SRF (*continued*)
    split renal function
    subretinal fluid
SRF-A
    slow reacting factor of anaphylaxis
SRFS
    split renal function study
SRH
    somatotropin-releasing hormone
srivastavai
      Schistotaenia s.
sRNA
    soluble ribonucleic acid
SRS
    slow-reacting substance
SRS-A
    slow reacting substance of anaphylaxis
SRT
    sedimentation rate test
SS
    Salmonella-Shigella
    saturated solution
    Sézary syndrome
    statistically significant
    subaortic stenosis
    supersaturated
    synovial sarcoma
    systemic sclerosis
SSA
    skin-sensitizing antibody
    sulfosalicylic acid
SS-A/Ro antigen
SS-B/La antigen
SSC
    sodium chloride-sodium citrate solution
    standard saline citrate
SSCP
    single-stranded conformation
     polymorphism
      SSCP assay
SSD
    sum of square deviations
SS-DNA
    single-stranded DNA
SSKI
    saturated solution of potassium iodide
SSN
    severely subnormal
SSOP
    sequence specific oligonucleotide probe
SSP
    Sanarelli-Shwartzman phenomenon
SSPE
    subacute sclerosing panencephalitis
ssRNA virus
SSS
    scalded skin syndrome
    specific soluble substance
S-sulfoglutathione

SSV
    simian sarcoma virus
ST
    surface tension
St.
    Saint
      St. Anthony dance
      St. Guy dance
      St. John dance
      St. Jude pediatric oncology staging
       system
      St. Louis encephalitis (SLE)
      St. Louis encephalitis virus
       (SLEV)
STA
    serum thrombotic accelerator
    STA hemostasis system
    STA Liatest control N+P
    STA Liatest D-DI
     coagulation/inflammation test kit
stab
    s. cell
    s. culture
    s. neutrophil (stab)
    s. wound
stabilate
stabile
stabilis
    Burkholderia s.
stability
    genome s.
stable
    s. cell
    s. disease (SD)
    s. factor
    s. factor deficiency
    s. fly
stachybotryotoxicosis
Stachybotrys
Stachylidium
stachyose
Staclot
    S. LA
    S. Protein S test kit
STA-Compact hemostasis system
Stadie-Riggs microtome
staff cell
stage
    algid s.
    Arneth s.
    cold s.
    defervescent s.
    Dukes A, B, C tumor s.
    end s.
    imperfect s.
    incubative s.
    latent s.
    menstrual s.
    s. of invasion

s.'s of labor
prodromal s.
proliferative s.
resting s.
secretory s.
Tanner s.
tumor s.
vegetative s.

staghorn calculus

staging

American Joint Committee on
Cancer S. (AJCCS)
Braak neurofibrillary tangle s.
Butchart tumor s.
cancer s.
Clark malignant melanoma s.
Dukes s.
Durie and Salmon multiple
myeloma clinical s.
FAB tumor s.
FIGO classification of tumor s.
Jewett and Strong s.
malignant melanoma s.
molecular s.
Rai s.
TNM s.
tumor s.

stagnant

s. anoxia
s. hypoxia
s. loop syndrome

Stagnicola

stagnora

Prototheca s.

stain

acetoorcein s.
Achucarro s.
acid-fast s.
acid phosphatase s.
acid-Schiff s.
acridine orange s.
AE1 immunoperoxidase s.
AFB s.
Ag-AS s.
Albert diphtheria s.
Alcian blue s.
alizarin red s.
alkaline phosphatase s.
alpha 3, 4, 5 chain collagen s.
Altmann anilin-acid fuchsin s.
Alzheimer s.
3-amino-9-ethylcarbazole s.
ammonium silver carbonate s.
amyloid s.
aniline blue modified
trichrome s.
antibody s.
anticytokeratin s.
antimony s.

argentaffin s.
argyrophil s.
arsenic s.
astrocyte s.
ATPase s.
Attwood S.
auramine O fluorescent s.
auramine-rhodamine s.
azan s.
azure-eosin s.
azure II-methylene blue s.
B72.3 s.
bacterial s.
basic fuchsin-methylene blue s.
Bauer chromic acid leucofuchsin s.
Bennhold Congo red s.
Ber-EP4 immunoperoxidase s.
Berg s.
Best carmine s.
beta amyloid precursor protein
immunohistochemical s.
Betke s.
Betke-Kleihauer s.
Bielschowsky s.
Biondi-Heidenhain s.
bipolar s.
Birch-Hirschfeld s.
Bodian copper-protargol s.
Bodian histochemical s.
Borrel blue s.
Bowie s.
Brown-Brenn s.
Brown-Hopp tissue Gram s.
butyrate esterase s.
Cajal astrocyte s.
Cajal gold sublimate s.
calcofluor white s.
carbol fuchsin s.
carbol-thionin s.
C-banding s.
CD10 s.
CEA Gold-5 s.
CEA immunoperoxidase s.
centromere banding s.
certified s.
cervical Gram s.
chloracetate esterase histochemical s.
chlorazol black E s.
chondroitin sulfate s.
ChrA immunoperoxidase s.
chrome alum hematoxylin-phloxine s.
Churukian-Schenck s.
chymotrypsin s.
Ciaccio s.
CK5 s.
colloidal iron s.
Congo red s.
contrast s.
cresyl blue brilliant s.

S

stain (*continued*)

cresyl violet s.
crystal violet s.
cyclin D s.
Da Fano s.
Dane and Herman
  keratin s.
DAPI s.
Darrow red s.
Delafield hematoxylin s.
del Rio Hortega s.
deoxyribonucleic acid s.
diaminobenzidine s.
diastase-periodic acid-Schiff s.
Dieterle s.
differential s.
Diff-Quik histochemical s.
direct fluorescent antibody s.
DOPA s.
Dorner s.
double s.
D-PAS s.
E-cadherin s.
Ehrlich acid hematoxylin s.
Ehrlich aniline crystal
  violet s.
Ehrlich triacid s.
Ehrlich triple s.
Einarson gallocyanin-chrome
  alum s.
elastica van Gieson s.
elastic fiber s.
elastin s.
en-bloc s.
eosin Y derivative of fluorescein s.
Eranko fluorescence s.
ethidium bromide s.
fast green FCF s.
fecal fat s.
ferric ammonium sulfate s.
Feulgen s.
fibrin histochemical s.
Field rapid s.
Fink-Heimer s.
Fite s.
Fite-Faraco s.
Flemming triple s.
fluorescence plus Giemsa s.
Fontana-Masson silver s.
Fontana methenamine silver s.
Foot reticulin impregnation s.
Fouchet s.
fuchsin s.
fungal s.
Fungalase-F s.
ganglioside GD2 s.
G-banding s.
Genta s.
gentian orange s.

gentian violet s.
Giemsa chromosome banding s.
Gill #2 hematoxylin blue s.
Gimenez s.
glycogen s.
glycolipid s.
glycoprotein s.
Goldner trichrome s.
Golgi s.
Gomori aldehyde fuchsin s.
Gomori chrome alum
  hematoxylin-phloxine s.
Gomori-Jones periodic
  acid-methenamine silver s.
Gomori methenamine silver s.
  (GMS stain)
Gomori nonspecific acid
  phosphatase s.
Gomori nonspecific alkaline
  phosphatase s.
Gomori one-step trichrome s.
Gomori silver impregnation s.
Gomori-Takamatsu s.
Goodpasture s.
Gordon and Sweets s.
Gram s.
Gram-chromotrope s.
Gram-Weigert s.
Gridley s.
Grimelius s.
Grocott-Gomori methenamine
  silver s.
Hale colloidal iron s.
Hansel s.
H&E s.
Heidenhain azan s.
Heidenhain iron hematoxylin s.
Heinz body s.
hematoxylin s.
hematoxylin-malachite green-basic
  fuchsin s.
hematoxylin-phloxine B s.
hemosiderin s.
heparan sulfate PG s.
heparan sulfate proteoglycan s.
HHF 35 s.
Hirsch-Peiffer s.
Hiss capsule s.
histochemical s.
Holmes s.
Hortega neuroglia s.
Hucker-Conn s.
immunoalkaline phosphatase s.
immunofluorescent s.
immunohistochemical s.
immunoperoxidase s.
India ink capsule s.
indigo-carmine s.
intravital s.

iodine s.
iron s.
iron hematoxylin s.
Jenner s.
Jenner-Giemsa s.
Jones methenamine silver s.
Kasten fluorescent Feulgen s.
Kasten fluorescent PAS s.
keratin s.
Kinyoun carbolfuchsin s.
Kittrich s.
Kleihauer s.
Kleihauer-Betke s.
Klüver-Barrera Luxol fast blue s.
Kokoskin s.
Kossa s.
Kronecker s.
lactophenol cotton blue s.
LAP s.
Lawless s.
lead citrate s.
lead hydroxide s.
Leder s.
Leishman s.
Lendrum inclusion body s.
Lendrum phloxine-tartrazine s.
Lepehne-Pickworth s.
leukocyte acid phosphatase s.
Leukostat s.
LeuM1 immunoperoxidase s.
Leung s.
Levaditi s.
Levine alkaline Congo red s.
Lillie allochrome connective
  tissue s.
Lillie azure-eosin s.
Lillie ferrous iron s.
Lillie sulfuric acid Nile blue s.
lipase 105 s.
lipid s.
Liquichek reticulocyte control and s.
Lison-Dunn s.
Löffler caustic s.
Lugol s.
Luna-Ishak s.
Luxol fast blue s.
Macchiavello s.
MacNeal tetrachrome blood s.
malachite green s.
malarial pigment s.
Maldonado-San Jose s.
Mallory aniline blue s.
Mallory collagen s.
Mallory iodine s.
Mallory phloxine s.
Mallory phosphotungstic acid
  hematoxylin s.
Mallory trichrome s.
Mallory triple s.

Mancini iodine s.
Mann methyl blue-eosin s.
Marchi s.
maspin s.
Masson argentaffin s.
Masson-Fontana ammoniacal silver s.
Masson-Fontana ammoniac silver s.
Masson trichrome s.
Mayer acid alum hematoxylin s.
Mayer hemalum s.
Mayer hematoxylin s.
Mayer mucicarmine s.
Mayer mucihematein s.
May-Grünwald s.
May-Grünwald-Giemsa s.
meconium s.
Meissel s.
Merck new fuchsin s.
metachromatic s.
methenamine silver s.
methylene blue s.
methyl green-pyronin s.
M'Fadyean s.
Milligan trichrome s.
modified acid-fast s.
modified Steiner s.
Movat pentachrome s.
Mowry colloidal iron s.
MSB trichrome s.
mucicarmine s.
mucopolysaccharide s.
multiple s.
Musto s.
MY-10 clone s.
myeloperoxidase s.
myoglobin s.
myosin s.
Nakanishi s.
naphthol ASBI phosphate s.
NASDCE s.
Nauta s.
negative s.
Neisser s.
neutral s.
nicotinamide adenine dinucleotide
  diaphorase s. (NADH diaphorase
  stain)
Nile blue fat s.
Nissl s.
nitroblue tetrazolium s.
Noble s.
Novelli s.
NSE s.
nuclear fast red s.
oil red O s.
oligodendroglia s.
orcein s.
Orth s.
osmium tetroxide s.

stain (*continued*)
oxalic acid s.
oxytalan fiber s.
plasma s.
plasmatic s.
plasmic s.
plastic section s.
polychrome methylene blue s.
Pontamine sky blue s.
port-wine s.
positive s.
potassium metabisulfate s.
potassium permanganate s.
propidium iodine s.
Protargol s.
Prussian blue iron s.
PTA s.
PTAH s.
Puchtler-Sweat s.
pyrrol blue s.
Q-banding s.
quinacrine chromosome banding s.
Rambourg chromic
acid-phosphotungstic acid s.
Rambourg periodic acid-chromic
methenamine-silver s.
Ranson pyridine silver s.
R-banding s.
reticulin s.
reticulum s.
rhodamine s.
Richard-Allan Scientific Ultrafast
Papanicolaou s.
Romanowsky blood s.
Romanowsky-Giemsa s.
Romanowsky type s.
Roux s.
Russell-Movat pentachrome s.
Ryan s.
safranin s.
Sayeed s.
scarlet red s.
Schaeffer-Fulton s.
Schiff s.
Schmorl ferric-ferricyanide
reduction s.
Schmorl picrothionin s.
Schultz s.
selective s.
Sevier-Munger s.
Shorr trichrome s.
siderocyte s.
silver ammoniacal silver s.
silver-ammoniac silver s.
silver nitrate s.
silver protein s.
Smith silver s.
Snook reticulum s.
sodium bisulfite s.

sodium hydroxide s.
sodium rhodizonate s.
sodium thiosulfate s.
solochrome cyanine s.
Steiner s.
Stirling modification of Gram s.
stool fecal fat s.
Sudan black B fat s.
supravital s.
synaptophysin s.
Taenzer s.
Taenzer-Unna s.
Takayama s.
telomeric R-banding s.
tetrachrome s.
Tetragonolobus purpureas lectin s.
tetramethylbenzidine s.
thiazin s.
thioflavin T s.
thionin s.
thyroglobulin s.
Tilden s.
Tizzoni s.
T method s.
Toison s.
toluidine blue s.
TRAP s.
trichrome s.
Truant auramine-rhodamine s.
trypsin G-banding s.
Turnbull blue s.
TWAR s.
ultrafast Pap s.
Unna s.
Unna-Pappenheim s.
Unna-Taenzer s.
uranyl acetate s.
urate crystal s.
van Ermengen s.
van Gieson s.
Ventana ES s.
Verhoeff elastic tissue s.
Verhoeff-van Gieson elastin s.
Victoria blue s.
vimentin immunoperoxidase s.
vital s.
von Kossa calcium s.
VVG s.
Wade-Fite-Faraco s.
Warthin-Starry silver s.
Wayson s.
Weber s.
Weber-modified trichome s.
Weigert-Gram s.
Weigert iron hematoxylin s.
Weigert-Pal s.
Weil myelin sheath s.
Williams s.
Wright s.

Wright-Giemsa s.
Ziehl s.
Ziehl-Neelsen s.

stainable
s. hemosiderin
s. iron

stained
s. cortex
s. urinary sediment (SUS)

stainer
Code-On Immunoslide s.
Hematek 2000 slide s.
Midas II automated s.
Quick Slide automated s.
Ventana Medical Systems Techmate
  500 automated s.

stainer/cytocentrifuge
Aerospray acid-fast bacteria slide s.
Aerospray hematology slide s.

staining
acid phosphatase s.
alkaline phosphatase s.
amyloid s.
anti-GFAP s.
astrocyte s.
automated slide s.
bacterial s.
bipolar s.
card-amplified nanogold-gold s.
card-amplified nanogold-silver s.
CD34 s.
chondroitin sulfate s.
cytokeratin s.
cytoplasmic s.
deoxyribonucleic acid s.
enterochromaffin s.
fat s.
fibrin s.
fluorescent s.
fluoro jade s.
fungus s.
glycogen s.
glycolipid s.
glycophorin A s.
glycoprotein s.
Gordon-Sweet s.
H and E s.
hemosiderin s.
histologic s.
immunoenzymometric s.
immunofluorescent s.
immunogold-silver s. (IGSS)
immunohistochemical s.
iodine s.
keratin s.
maspin nuclear s.
mast cell s.
mucopolysaccharide s.
nuclear s.

oligodendroglia s.
podoplanin s.
progressive s.
regressive s.
reticulin s.
reticulocyte s.
s. shell
Steiner s.
supravital s.
surface marker s.
thioflavin S s.
vital s.

Stains-All
Staleya guttiformis
stalk
infundibular s.
pituitary s.
s. to basilar artery ratio
Staller
S. kit
S. point
Stamey test
Stamnosoma
Stamper-Woodruff assay
stand
standard
s. acid reflux test (SART)
air quality s.
s. bicarbonate
certified s.
s. curve
s. deviation (SD)
s. electrode potential
s. enthalpy of formation
s. error (SE)
s. error of estimate (SEE)
S.'s for Reporting of Diagnostic
  Accuracy (STARD)
s. free energy
gold s.
s. hydrogen electrode
internal s.
internal telomerase s. (ITAS)
s. method agar
s. morbidity ratio (SMR)
s. mortality ratio (SMR)
National Committee for Clinical
  Laboratory S.'s (NCCLS)
s. operating procedure (SOP)
Prader bead s.
primary s.
quantitation s. (QS)
s. reduction potential
s. saline citrate (SSC)
s. score
s. serologic test for syphilis
s. solution
s. state
s. temperature and pressure

S

standard (*continued*)
 s. temperature and pressure, dry (STPD)
 s. test for syphilis (STS)
 s. urea clearance
standardization
standardize
standardized
 s. protocol
 s. rate
standing plasma test
standstill
 cardiac s.
stannic
stannous
Stanton disease
staph
 staphylococcus
Staph-Ident test
Staph-Trac test
staphyline
staphylococcal
 s. clumping test (SCT)
 s. enteritis
 s. enterotoxin
 s. enterotoxin B (SEB)
 s. pneumonia
 s. protein A binding assay
 s. scalded skin syndrome
Staphylococceae
staphylococcemia
staphylococcin
staphylococcolysin
staphylococcolysis
Staphylococcus
 S. albus
 S. aureus nasopharyngeal culture
 S. aureus neutral proteinase
 S. aureus urinary tract infection
 S. citreus
 S. epidermidis
 S. equorum subsp. *linens*
 S. fleurettii
 S. haemolyticus
 S. hominis
 S. hominis novobiosepticus
 methicillin-resistant coagulase-negative *S.* (MRCNS)
 methicillin-susceptible coagulase-negative *S.* (MSCNS)
 S. nepalensis
 S. pyogenes
 S. pyogenes albus
 S. pyogenes aureus
 S. saprophyticus
 S. septicemia
 S. simulans
 S. succinus subsp. *casei*

 S. viridans
 S. warneri
staphylococcus (staph)
 s. antitoxin
 s. vaccine
staphylohemia
staphylohemolysin
staphylokinase
staphylolysin
 alpha s.
 beta s.
 delta s.
 epsilon s.
 gamma s.
staphyloma
staphyloopsonic index
Staphylothermus hellenicus
staphylotoxin
star
 lens s.
 macular s.
 venous s.
 Verheyen s.
 Winslow s.
starburst pattern
starch
 s. hydrolysis test
 hydroxyethyl s.
 rice s.
 s. tolerance test
STARD
 Standards for Reporting of Diagnostic Accuracy
Stargardt disease
Starkeya novella
Starkeyomyces
Starling law
starrii
 Bacteriovorax s.
starry
starry-sky
 s.-s. appearance
 s.-s. macrophage
 s.-s. pattern
 s.-s. phenomenon
start
 S. 8 clot detection system
 s. codon
starter pistol
StarTox 5 drugs of abuse screening test
starvation-induced protein breakdown
starvation ketoacidosis
stases (*pl. of* stasis)
stasis, *pl.* **stases**
 bile s.
 s. cirrhosis
 s. dermatitis
 s. syndrome

s. ulcer (SU)
venous s.
Stasisia
STAT
signal transducer and activator of transcription
stat
S. Profile pHOx blood gas analyzer
s. test
Stat-60 centrifuge
state
absorptive s.
carrier s.
central excitatory s. (CES)
central inhibitory s. (CIS)
chronic carrier s.
complement deficiency s.
euthyroid sick s.
excited s.
fasted s.
ground s.
hypercoagulable s. (HCS)
immunity deficiency s. (IDS)
imperfect s.
metastable s.
nonreplicative s.
oxidation s.
platelet-refractory s.
postabsorptive s.
pseudo-Cushing s.
replicative s.
sample steady s.
solid s.
standard s.
steady s.
transition s.
statement
assignment s.
source s.
static
s. balance receptor cell
s. gangrene
s. pulmonary compliance
s. storage allocation
s. telepathology
statin
stationary phase
statistic
Mann-Whitney rank sum s.
Office of National S.'s (ONS)
spatial scan s.
test s.
Wilcoxon signed rank s.
statistically significant (SS)
statistical symbol
statoconia
statoconial membrane
statoconiorum
membrana s.

statolith
statosphere
STAT-Site M Hgb test system
StatSpin
S. Express 2 centrifuge
S. MP centrifuge
stature
short s.
status
s. asthmaticus
s. choreicus
s. cribrosus
s. criticus
S. Cup Plus drug testing device
s. dysmyelinisatus
s. dysraphicus
s. epilepticus
s. hemicranicus
hormone receptor s.
Karnofsky s.
s. lacunaris
s. lymphaticus
s. marmoratus
s. nervosus
s. post (s/p)
s. raptus
s. spongiosus
s. thymicolymphaticus
s. thymicus
Staub-Traugott effect
Staurophoma
staurosporine
STC
sarcomatoid thymic carcinoma
soft tissue calcification
STD
sexually transmitted disease
skin test dose
skin-to-tumor distance
steady state
steady-state condition
steam-fitter's asthma
steapsin
stearate
polyoxyethylene s. (POES)
sodium s.
stearic acid
stearin
stearothermophilus
Bacillus s.
Geobacillus s.
stearrhea (*var. of* steatorrhea)
steatitis
steatocystoma multiplex
steatohepatitis
nonalcoholic s. (NASH)
steatolytic enzyme
steatomatosis
steatonecrosis

S

steatopyga, steatopygia
steatopygia (*var. of* steatopyga)
steatopygous
steatorrhea, stearrhea
steatosis
    centrilobar s.
    s. cordis
    hepatic s.
    macrovesicular s.
steatozoon
Steele-Richardson-Olszewski syndrome
Steenbock unit
steeple skull, tower skull
Stefan-Boltzmann law
stege
stegnosis
Stegobium
Stegomyia
stegomyiae
    Myxococcidium s.
Steinbrocker syndrome
Steiner
    S. stain
    S. staining
    S. syndrome
Steinert disease
Stein-Leventhal syndrome
steinstrasse (cobbled street ureteric lumen)
Stelangium
stella
    s. lentis hyaloidea
    s. lentis iridica
Stellantchasmus falcatus
stellata
    Hemispora s.
stellatae
    venae s.
stellate
    s. abscess
    s. cell
    s. density
    s. fracture
    s. reticulum
    s. vein
    s. venule
stellate-cell lipidosis
stellatoidea
    Candida s.
stellifer
stellipolaris
    Alteromonas s.
stelliscabiei
    Streptomyces s.
stellulae
    s. vasculosae
    s. verheyenii
    s. winslowii

stem
    s. cell
    s. cell assay
    s. cell factor (SCF)
    s. cell leukemia
    s. cell lymphoma
    s. cell renewal factor
    gliosis of brain s.
    infundibular s.
    s. kit CD34+HPC enumeration system
stemline
stemonitis
    Doratomyces s.
    S. flavogenita
Stemphylium macrosporoidium
Stem-Trol control cell
Stender dish
Stenella araguata
Stenoglossa
stenosal
stenosed (sten)
stenoses (*pl. of* stenosis)
stenosing odditis
stenosis, *pl.* **stenoses**
    aortic valvular s.
    buttonhole s.
    calcific bicuspid aortic valve s.
    calcific nodular aortic s.
    carotid artery s.
    cervical canal s.
    congenital pyloric s.
    coronary ostial s.
    discrete subaortic s.
    Dittrich s.
    hypertrophic muscular subaortic s. (HMSAS)
    hypertrophic pyloric s. (HPS)
    idiopathic hypertrophic subaortic s. (IHSS)
    infundibular s.
    internal carotid s.
    lumbar canal s.
    mitral incompetency and s.
    muscular subaortic s.
    nodular calcific aortic s.
    pulmonary artery s. (PAS)
    pulmonary infundibular s.
    pyloric s. (PS)
    renal artery s. (RAS)
    spinal s.
    subaortic s. (SS)
    subvalvar s.
    supravalvular aortic s. (SAS, SVAS)
    tricuspid s.
    valvular s.
    vascular s.
stenostrepta
    Spirochaeta s.

stenothermal
stenotic
Stenotrophomonas
    S. acidaminiphila
    S. maltophilia
    S. nitritireducens
    S. rhizophila
stenoxenous
Stensen duct, Steno
  duct
step
    s. function
    s. sectioning
step-down transformer
Stephanoascus ciferii
Stephanofilaria stilesi
Stephanosporium
stephanostomum
    Oesophagostomum s.
Stephanurus dentatus
stephensi
    Anopheles s.
Stephen spot
step-up transformer
steradian (sr)
stercobilin
stercobilinogen
stercolith
stercoraceous ulcer
stercoral
    s. abscess
    s. appendicitis
    s. fistula
    s. ulcer
stercoralis
    Strongyloides s.
stercoricanis
    Sutterella s.
stercorihominis
    Anaerofustis s.
stercoris
    Collinsella s.
stercorisuis
    Hespellia s.
stercoroma
Sterculia
stereochemical isomerism
stereochemistry
stereocilium
stereognosis
stereoisomer
stereoisomerism
stereology
stereometer
stereometry
stereomicroscopic
stereophotomicrograph
stereoscope
stereoscopic

    s. microscope
    s. radiography
stereospecific numbering
stereotactic, stereotaxic
    s. brain biopsy
    s. breast biopsy
    s. core-needle biopsy (SCNB)
stereotaxic (*var. of* stereotactic)
    s. instrument
stereotaxis, stereotaxy
stereotaxy (*var. of* stereotaxis)
Stereum
steric
    s. exclusion
    s. hindrance
sterigma
Sterigmatocystis
Sterigmatomyces
sterile
    s. abscess
    s. cyst
    s. pyuria
    s. stick
sterilisans
    therapia magna s.
sterility
    s. culture
    s. test broth
sterilization
    discontinuous s.
    fractional s.
    intermittent s.
sterilize
sterilizer
    gas s.
    Sterrad 100 s.
    Sterrad 50 s.
sternal synchondrosis
Sternberg
    S. disease
    S. giant cell
Sternberg-Reed cell
Sterneedle tuberculin test
Sternheimer-Malbin positive cell
sterni
    mucro s.
sternocostale
    trigonum s.
sternocostal triangle
sternoglossal
steroid
    anabolic s.
    s. cell tumor
    s. fever
    s. hormone
    s. hormone binding globulin
      (SHBG)
    s. hormone receptor
    17-ketogenic s.

S

steroid (*continued*)
    ketogenic s. (KGS)
    s. protein activity index (SPAI)
    s. saponin
    s. sulfatase (STS)
    s. sulfatase gene
steroid-binding betaglobulin
steroid-21-hydroxylase
steroid-21-monooxygenase
steroidogenesis
steroidogenic hormone
steroid-receptor complex
sterol
    s. carrier protein
    s. glycoside
Sterolibacterium denitrificans
Sterrad
    S. 50, 100, and 200 acid
      sterilization system
    S. 50, 100 sterilizer
stetharteritis
stethomyositis
Stevens-Johnson syndrome
Stewart-Bluefarb syndrome
Stewart-Morel syndrome
Stewart-Treves syndrome
sTfR
    soluble transferrin receptor
STH
    somatotropic hormone
STI
    systolic time interval
stibine
stibocaptate
    sodium s.
stichochrome cell
stick
    sterile s.
stick-and-ball-shaped virion
  particle
Sticker disease
sticklandii
    Clostridium s.
Stickler syndrome
Stictis
Stieda disease
stigma, *pl.* **stigmas, stigmata**
    follicular s.
    s. ventriculi
stigmas (*pl. of* stigma)
stigmata (*pl. of* stigma)
stigmataophilia
Stigonematales
stilbene dye
stilbestrol
stilbospora
    Taeniolella s.
stilesi
    Stephanofilaria s.

still
    S. disease
    S. layer
stillbirth (SB)
    macerated s.
Still-Chauffard syndrome
Stilling
    S. canal
    S. gelatinous substance
    S. syndrome
Stilling-Turk-Duane syndrome
stimulate enzyme secretion
stimulation
    prolonged estrogen s.
    s. ratio (SR)
    repetitive s.
stimulator
    B lymphocyte s. (BLyS)
    s. cell
    long-acting thyroid s.
      (LATS)
stipple cell
stippled epiphysis
stippling
    basophilic s.
    gunpowder s.
    s. of skin
    pseudo-gunpowder s.
    Ziemann s.
Stirling modification of Gram stain
stitch abscess
STKS automated cell counting
  instrument
STM
    scanning tunneling microscopy
Stobo antigen
stochastic
stock
    s. culture
    s. strain
    s. vaccine
stockpile
    National Pharmaceutical S.
      (NPS)
stoichiology
stoichiometry
Stokes
    S. law
    S. shift
Stokes-Adams (SA)
    S.-A. disease
    S.-A. syndrome
Stokvis-Talma syndrome
Stokvis test
Stoll dilution egg count technique
stolon
stolpii
    Bacteriovorax s.
stoma, *pl.* **stomas, stomata**

stomach
    bilocular s.
    s. cancer
    s. carcinoma
    chief cell of s.
    drain-trap s.
    hourglass s.
    leather-bottle s.
    sclerotic s.
    theca cell of s.
    trifid s.
    s. tumor
    wallet s.
    watermelon s.
    water-trap s.
stomal ulcer
stomas (*pl. of* stoma)
stomata (*pl. of* stoma)
stomatitis
    angular s.
    aphthous s.
    bovine papular s.
    gangrenous s.
    herpetic s.
    lead s.
    primary herpetic s.
    vesicular s.
    Vincent s.
Stomatococcus mucilaginosus
stomatocyte
stomatocytic hereditary elliptocytosis
stomatocytosis
    hereditary s.
stomodeal ectoderm
stomodeum
Stomoxys calcitrans
stone
    ammonium magnesium phosphate s.
    cystine s.
    s. heart
    skin s.
    vein s.
stonelike debris
stone-stripper's asthma
stool
    acholic s.
    s. analysis
    bloody s.
    s. carbohydrate
    s. chloride
    s. collection
    s. color
    s. consistency
    s. electrolytes
    s. examination
    fat in s.
    s. fecal fat stain
    s. fungus culture
    s. guaiac

    s. guaiac test
    s. leukocyte
    s. leukocyte count
    s. lipids
    melanotic s.
    s. mucus
    s. muscle fiber
    s. mycobacteria culture
    s. nitrogen
    s. occult blood
    s. osmolality
    s. pH
    s. porphyrin
    s. potassium
    s. reducing substances test
    ribbon s.
    rice-water s.'s
    s. screen
    scybalous s.
    s. sodium
    tarry s.
    s. toxin assay
    s. trypsin
    s. urobilinogen
stopcock
stop codon
storage
    s. allocation
    autologous leukapheresis, processing, and s. (ALPS)
    bone marrow iron s.'s
    s. capacity
    common s.
    compressed gas s.
    ether s.
    external s.
    glycogen s.
    internal s.
    s. limit
    s. location
    mass s.
    s. oscilloscope
    s. phosphor autoradiography
    s. pool disease
    reticuloendothelial iron s.'s
    transport and s.
storiform
    s. neurofibroma
    s. pattern
storm
    thyroid s.
Stormer viscosimeter
Stormorken syndrome
Stovall-Black method
STPD
    standard temperature and pressure, dry
    STPD conditions of gas
Strachan syndrome
straddling embolism

S

straight
    s. rod
    s. tubule
strain
    attenuated s.
    avirulent s.
    s. birefringence
    carrier s.
    cell s.
    clostridial s.
    HFR s.
    hypothetical mean s. (HMS)
    lysogenic s.
    McKrae herpes simplex virus s.
    Mycobacterium bovis BCG s.
    pseudolysogenic s.
    recombinant s.
    reference s.
    stock s.
    type s.
    virulent Schu S4 tularemia s.
stramonium
    Datura s.
strand
    complementary s.
    s. displacement amplification (SDA)
    homology of s.'s
    leading s.
    minus s.
    plus s.
    sense s.
    viral s.
strandjordii
    Tsukamurella s.
strangling
strangulated hernia
strangulation
    ritual ligature s. (incaprettamento)
strap cell
Strassburg test
Strasseria
strata (*pl. of* stratum)
Stratagene CastAway sequencing device
stratification
    s. index
    risk group s.
stratified
    s. random sample
    s. thrombus
stratiform
Stratiomyidae
stratum, *pl.* **strata**
    s. aculeatum
    s. basale
    s. basale epidermidis
    s. basalis
    s. cerebrale retinae
    s. circulare membranae tympani
    s. circulare tunicae muscularis recti

    s. circulare tunicae muscularis ventriculi
    s. compactum
    s. corneum
    s. corneum epidermidis
    s. corneum unguis
    s. cutaneum membranae tympani
    s. cylindricum
    s. disjunctum
    s. fibrosum capsulae articularis
    s. functionale
    s. ganglionare nervi optici
    s. germinativum
    s. germinativum unguis
    s. granulosum
    s. granulosum corticis cerebelli
    s. granulosum epidermidis
    s. granulosum folliculi ovarici vesiculosi
    s. granulosum ovarii
    s. longitudinale tunicae muscularis coli
    s. longitudinale tunicae muscularis intestini tenuis
    s. longitudinale tunicae muscularis recti
    s. longitudinale tunicae muscularis ventriculi
    s. lucidum
    malpighian s.
    s. malpighii
    s. moleculare
    s. moleculare corticis cerebelli
    s. moleculare retinae
    s. neuroepitheliale retinae
    strata nuclearia externa et interna retinae
    s. papillare corii
    s. pigmenti bulbi
    s. pigmenti corporis ciliaris
    s. pigmenti iridis
    s. pigmenti retinae
    s. radiatum membranae tympani
    s. reticulare corii
    s. reticulare cutis
    s. spinosum
    s. spinosum epidermidis
    s. spongiosum
    s. subcutaneum
    s. synoviale
Stratus II automatic analyzer
Strauss
    allergic granulomatosis of Churg and S.
Stravigen immunohistochemical reagent
strawberry
    s. birthmark
    s. gallbladder
    s. gums

s. mark
s. nevus
strawberry-cream blood
stray light
streak
angioid s.
s. culture
fibrous s.
s. gonad
gonadal s.
s. hyperostosis
meningitic s.
s. plate
streaming movement
street virus
Strengeria
strength
dielectric s.
ionic s.
magnetic field s.
tensile s.
strep
streptococcus
Streptococcus
Acceava Strep A
Strep A OIA Max
Strep B OIA
strep throat
Streptacidiphilus
S. albus
S. carbonis
S. neutrinimicus
streptavidin
streptavidin-biotin (SAB)
s.-b. peroxidase method
streptavidin-biotin-based detection
system
streptavidin-biotin-complex technique
streptavidin-Nanogold reagent
strepticemia
Streptobacillus
S. moniliformis
S. pseudotuberculosis
streptocerca
Acanthocheilonema s.
Dipetalonema s.
Mansonella s.
streptocerciasis
Streptococcaceae
streptococcal
s. antigen test
s. carditis
s. cellulitis
s. fibrinolysin
s. infection
s. pneumonia
s. toxic shock syndrome
s. toxin immunization reaction
streptococcemia

streptococci (*pl. of* streptococcus)
Streptococcus
S. agalactiae
S. anaerobius
S. anginosus
S. anginosus-constellatus
S. australis
S. bovis
S. canis
S. caprinus
S. constellatus
S. cremoris
S. devriesei
S. didelphis
S. durans
S. endocarditis
S. entericus
S. equi
S. evolutus
S. faecalis
S. faecium
S. gallinaceus
S. gallolyticus subsp. *macedonicus*
S. gallolyticus subsp. *pasteurianus*
S. garvieae
S. gordonii
group A *S.*
group B *S.*
group D *S.*
group N *S.*
S. halichoeri
S. infantarius
S. infantarius subsp. *coli*
S. infantarius subsp. *infantarius*
S. intermedius
S. lutetiensis
S. M antigen
S. minor
S. mitis
S. morbillorum
S. mutans
S. oligofermentans
S. orisratti
S. ovis
S. pasteurianus
S. pneumoniae
S. pyogenes
S. salivarius
S. sanguis
S. sinensis
S. uberis
S. urinalis
streptococcus (strep), *pl.* **streptococci**
alpha s.
anaerobic s.
anhemolytic s.
Bargen s.
beta s.
beta hemolytic s. (BHS)

S

streptococcus (*continued*)
    s. erythrogenic toxin
    Fehleisen s.
    gamma s.
    hemolytic s.
    microaerophilic s.
    nonhemolytic s.
    s. serum
streptolysin
    s. O (SLO)
    s. O test
Streptomonospora
    S. alba
    S. salina
Streptomyces
    S. africanus
    S. albus
    S. annulatus
    S. asiaticus
    S. aureus
    S. avermectinius
    S. avermitilis
    S. beijiangensis
    S. cangkringensis
    S. drozdowiczii
    S. europaeiscabiei
    S. gibsonii
    S. hebeiensis
    S. indonesiensis
    S. javensis
    S. laceyi
    S. luridiscabiei
    S. luteireticuli
    S. madurae
    S. mexicanus
    S. niveiscabiei
    S. pelletieri
    S. puniciscabiei
    S. reticuliscabiei
    S. rhizosphaericus
    S. scabrisporus
    S. scopiformis
    S. somaliensis
    S. speibonae
    S. stelliscabiei
    S. thermocoprophilus
    S. thermospinosisporus
    S. yatensis
    S. yeochonensis
    S. yunnanensis
Streptomycetaceae
Streptomycetales
Streptomycetes
streptomycin
    s. assay agar with yeast extract
    G unit of s.
    L unit of s.
    S unit of s.
    s. unit

Streptomycineae
streptomycosis
streptosepticemia
Streptosporangiaceae
Streptosporangineae
Streptosporangium subroseum
Streptothrix
streptotrichosis
streptozyme test
stress
    environmental s.
    s. erythrocytosis
    s. fiber
    fluid shear s.
    s. fracture
    oxidant s.
    oxidative s.
    s. protein
    s. reticulocyte
    s. ulcer
stretch
    carbon-hydrogen s.
    C-H s.
    s. device
    myocyte s.
    s. receptor
stretchable skin
stria, *pl.* **striae**
    Amici s.
    striae atrophicae
    Baillarger s.
    brown striae
    striae cutis distensae
    striae gravidarum
    Langhans s.
    Monakow s.
    Nitabuch s.
    striae of Zahn
    Retzius parallel
     striae
    Rohr s.
    s. vascularis ductus
     cochlearis
    Wickham striae
striae (*pl. of* stria)
striata
    area s.
    osteopathia s.
striate body
striated
    s. brush border
    s. duct
    s. muscle
striation
    basal s.
    cross s.
    cytoplasmic s.
    tabby cat s.
    tigroid s.

striatonigral
- s. degeneration
- s. fiber

striatum
- corpus s.
- *Corynebacterium s.*

striatus
- lichen s.
- limbus s.

stricto
- *Borrelia burgdorferi sensu s.*

stricture
- biliary s.
- esophageal s.
- Hunner s.
- urethral s.

stridor

Strigeata

strigiphila
- *Tetrameres s.*

string
- auditory s.
- s. sign
- s. test for duodenal parasite

stringency

stringent response

strip
- Albustix reagent s.
- Cardiac Reader IQC test s.
- reagent s.
- spore s.
- Titan III H cellulose acetate s.
- UrinChek 10+ urine test s.'s

stripe
- Baillarger s.
- Hensen s.
- Kaes-Bekhterev s.
- vascular s.

striped form of interstitial fibrosis

stripped nucleus

stripping
- electrolytic s.

strobe light

strobila

strobilocercus

strobiloid

stroboscopic microscope

stroke

stroma, *pl.* **stromata**
- s. cell
- cellular s.
- collagenous s.
- connective tissue s.
- desmoplastic s.
- fibrocollagenous s.
- fibrovascular s.
- s. glandulae thyroideae
- host s.
- hyalinized s.

- hypocellular s.
- s. iridis
- juxtatumoral s.
- lymphatic s.
- mesenchymal s.
- mucinous s.
- mucohyaline s.
- myxoid s.
- s. of ovary
- s. of vitreous
- s. ovarii
- papillary s.
- periductal s.
- pseudosarcomatous s.
- Rollet s.
- sclerotic s.
- tumor s.
- vascular s.
- vascularized s.
- s. vitreum

stroma-free
- s.-f. hemoglobin
- s.-f. methemoglobin

stromal
- s. cell neoplasm
- s. collagen band
- s. component
- s. desmoplasia
- s. edema
- s. endometriosis
- s. hyperplasia
- s. hyperthecosis
- s. invasion
- s. luteoma
- s. mucopolysaccharide
- s. myofibroblast
- s. sarcoma

stromal-epithelial neoplasm

stromata (*pl. of* stroma)

stromatin

Stromatinia

stromatolysis

stromatosis
- endometrial s.

stromelysin

stromic

stromomyoma

stromovascular hyperplasia

Strong bacillus

Strongylata

strongyle

Strongylidae

strongylina
- *Ascarops s.*

Strongyloidea

Strongyloides
- *S. fuelleborni*
- *S. stercoralis*

strongyloidiasis, strongyloidosis

S

Strongyloididae
strongyloidosis (*var. of* strongyloidiasis)
strongylosis
Strongylus
    S. *asini*
    S. *edentatus*
    S. *equinus*
    S. *radiatus*
    S. *ventricosus*
    S. *vulgaris*
strontium (Sr)
strontium-90 (^{90}Sr)
Stropharia
structural
    s. collapse
    s. correlation
    s. gene
    s. isomerism
    s. lesion
    s. protein
structure
    analogous s.
    s. collapse
    dimorphic s.
    dipolar s.
    fine s.
    glandular s.
    homologous s.
    lentiginous melanocytic s.
    list s.
    maturation of gonadal s.
    neuroid melanocytic s.
    primary s.
    quaternary s.
    rod-shaped s.
    rudimentary s.
    secondary s.
    sphincteric s.
    tertiary s.
    tuboreticular s.
struma, *pl.* **strumae**
    s. aberrata
    s. colloides
    cystic s.
    Hashimoto s.
    ligneous s.
    s. lymphomatosa
    s. maligna
    s. medicamentosa
    s. ovarii
    Riedel s.
strumae (*pl. of* struma)
strumal carcinoid
strumatosis
strumiform
strumipriva
    cachexia s.
strumitis
strumosis

strumous
Strümpell disease
Strümpell-Leichtenstern disease
Strümpell-Lorrain disease
Strümpell-Marie disease
Strümpell-Westphal disease
struvite calculus
strychnine assay
Stryker-Halbeisen syndrome
STS
    serologic test for syphilis
    serology test for syphilis
    standard test for syphilis
    steroid sulfatase
        STS gene
STS-7 continuous glucose monitoring system
STSG
    split-thickness skin graft
^{90}**St**
    strontium-90
STT
    serial thrombin time
STU
    skin test unit
Stuart
    S. broth
    S. factor
stuartii
    Proteus s.
    Providencia s.
Stuart-Prower factor
stubby microvillus
Student-Newman-Keuls test
Student test
studeri
    Bertiella s.
study
    blood chemistry s.
    buffy coat smear s.
    cardiopulmonary sleep s.
    case-control s.
    clinicopathologic s.
    clonality s.
    cohort s.
    cytogenetic s.
    double-blind s.
    double-contrast s.
    dual-contrast s.
    electrophysiology s.
    enzyme s.
    erythrokinetic s.
    esophageal motility s.
    fat absorption s.
    ferrokinetics s.
    gastrointestinal bleed
      localization s.
    gene arrangement s.
    haplotype association s.

immunophenotypic s.
Johns Hopkins Center for Civilian Biodefense Studies
National Wilms Tumor S.
Ostor s.
prospective s.
renal function s. (RFS)
retrospective s.
sex chromatin s.
split renal function s. (SRFS)
ultrastructural s.

stump
    s. cancer
    s. carcinoma

stunned myocardium

stunted
    s. embryo
    s. fetus

Sturge-Kalischer-Weber syndrome
Sturge syndrome
Sturge-Weber syndrome
stutzeri
    Pseudomonas s.

STVA
    subtotal villous atrophy

stye
    meibomian s.
    zeisian s.

stygium
    Novosphingobium s.

stylet, stylette
    Liberator universal locking s.

stylette (*var. of* stylet)
styloiditis
styloid process
stylosteophyte
Styloviridae
styptic
    chemical s.
    mechanical s.
    vascular s.

Stypven
    S. time
    S. time test

styrene
styrone
Stysanus
SUA
    serum uric acid

subacute
    s. abscess
    s. bacterial endocarditis (SBE)
    s. bronchopneumonia
    s. combined degeneration (SACD, SCD)
    s. combined sclerosis
    s. cutaneous lupus
    s. glomerulonephritis
    s. granulomatous thyroiditis

s. hepatitis
s. inclusion body encephalitis
s. infective endocarditis
s. inflammation
s. meningitis
s. myelomonocytic leukemia
s. myelooptic neuropathy (SMON)
s. necrotizing encephalopathy
s. necrotizing myelitis
s. nephritis
s. sclerosing leukoencephalitis
s. sclerosing panencephalitis (SSPE)
s. spongiform encephalopathy
s. thyroiditis (SAT)

subadventitial fibrosis
subaortic stenosis (SAS, SS)
subarachnoid
    s. hemorrhage (SAH)
    s. space

subarcticum
    Novosphingobium s.

subareolar duct papillomatosis
subcapsular
subcartilaginous
subcellular
subchondral
subchorial
    s. lake
    s. space

subchorionic
    s. fibrin
    fibrin, s.

subchoroidal
subclass
    immunoglobulin s.

subclassification
    Lukes-Butler histologic s.

subclavian steal syndrome
subclinical coccidioidomycosis
subcommissural organ
subconjunctival
subcorneal
    s. bulla
    s. pustular dermatitis
    s. pustular dermatosis

subcortical
    s. arteriosclerotic encephalopathy
    s. arteriosclerotic leukoencephalopathy

subculture
subcutanea
    tela s.

subcutaneous (SC, SQ, subcu, subq)
    s. emphysema
    s. fat
    s. fat necrosis of newborn
    s. nodule
    s. tissue

subcutaneous/sublingual provocation

S

subcutaneum
  stratum s.
subcuticular
subcutis
  superficial s.
subdermal
subdermic
subdural
  s. empyema
  s. hematoma
  s. hematorrhachis
  s. hygroma
subendocardial
  s. connective tissue
  s. layer
  s. myocardial infarction
subendothelial
  s. immune complex deposition
  s. layer
subendothelium
subependymal
  s. giant cell astrocytoma
  s. glioma
subependymoma
subepidermal, subepidermic
  s. blister
  s. connective tissue
    (SEC)
  s. fibrosis
subepidermic (*var. of*
  subepidermal)
  s. bulla
subepithelial
  s. collagen
  s. collagen band
subepithelium
suberosis
suberyl arginine
subfamily
subflava
  Neisseria s.
subfolium
subgemmal
subgenus
subglobosa
  Sphaeropsis s.
subgranular
subgroup
  mucopolysaccharidosis s.
subicteric
subinfection
subinflammatory
subintegumental
subintimal
subinvolution
subitum
  exanthema s.
subkingdom
sublabial adhesion

subleukemia
subleukemic
  s. granulocytic
    leukemia
  s. lymphocytic
    leukemia
  s. monocytic leukemia
  s. myelosis
sublimation
  heat of s.
sublingual
  s. cyst
  s. gland
sublingualis
  glandula s.
sublithincola
  Aequorivita s.
sublobular
subluxation
  atlantoaxial s.
sublymphemia
submammary mastitis
submandibular duct
submandibularis
  ductus s.
  glandula s.
submarinus
  Desulfonauticus s.
  Psychrobacter s.
submassive confluent
  necrosis
submaxillaris
  ductus s.
submaxillary
  s. duct
  s. gland
  s. glycoprotein
submembranous
submetacentric
submicrometastasis
submicronic
submicroscopic
submorphous
submucosa
  tela s.
  tunica s.
submucosal
submucous
subneural apparatus
subnitrate
  bismuth s.
subnormal
  severely s. (SSN)
  s. temperature
subnuclear vacuolated cell
subnucleus
suborder
subpapillare
  rete s.

subpapillary
s. layer
s. network
subpapular
subparta
ileus s.
subperitoneal appendicitis
subphylum
subplacental
subplasmalemmal
s. dense zone
s. density
s. microfilament
subpleural bleb
subq
subcutaneous
subretinal fluid (SRF)
subroseum
Streptosporangium s.
subrostratus
Felicola s.
subroutine
recursive s.
subsclerotic
subscripted variable
subserosal (*var. of* subserous)
subserous, subserosal
subset
lymphocyte s.
subsinusoidal fibrosis
subspecies
substage
substance
s. abuse screen
alpha s.
antidiuretic s. (ADS)
bacteriotropic s.
basophil s.
beta s.
blood group s.
blood group-specific s. A, B
cement s.
cementing s.
chromidial s.
chromophil s.
s. concentration
controlled s.
cortical s.
erythrocyte-sensitizing s. (ESS)
exophthalmos-producing s. (EPS)
extracellular ground s.
fat-mobilizing s. (FMS)
filar s.
gelatinous s.
ground s.
H s.
hazardous s.
hemolytic s.

immunity s.
interspongioplastic s.
medullary s.
methylene blue active s. (MBAS)
neurosecretory s.
Nissl s.
s. P (SP)
s. P neuropeptide
pressor s.
proper s.
prostaglandin-like s. (PLS)
rabbit aorta-contracting s.
renal pressor s. (RPS)
reticular s.
Rolando gelatinous s.
Schwann white s.
sensitizing s.
slow-reacting s. (SRS)
soluble specific s.
specific capsular s.
specific soluble s. (SSS)
Stilling gelatinous s.
threshold s.
thromboplastic s.
tigroid s.
tumor polysaccharide s. (TPS)
white s.
zymoplastic s.
substantia
s. adamantina
s. alba
s. basophilia
s. compacta
s. compacta ossium
s. corticalis
s. eburnea
s. fundamentalis
s. gelatinosa
s. gelatinosa centralis
s. glandularis prostatae
s. intermedia centralis
s. lentis
s. medullaris
s. metachromaticogranularis
s. muscularis prostatae
s. nigra
s. ossea dentis
s. propria corneae
s. propria membranae tympani
s. propria of cornea
s. propria sclerae
s. reticularis
s. reticulofilamentosa
s. spongiosa
s. trabecularis
s. vitrea
substernal goiter
substituent

S

substitute
> blood s.
> plasma s.
> PolyHeme blood s.
> Scott tap water s.
> volume s.

substitution
> generic s.
> s. product
> s. reaction

substrate
> defined s. (DS)
> s. level phosphorylation

substrate-labeled
> s.-l. fluorescence immunoassay (SLFIA)
> s.-l. fluorescent immunoassay (SLFIA)

substratum

substructure

subsurface
> s. basement membrane
> s. cisterna

subsynchronous vibration

subtegumental

subtelocentric

Subtercola
> *S. boreus*
> *S. frigoramans*
> *S. pratensis*

subterranea
> *Knoellia s.*
> *Thermotoga s.*

subterraneum
> *Novosphingobium s.*
> *Sulfurihydrogenibium s.*

subterraneus
> *Bacillus s.*
> *Caldanaerobacter s.*
> *Caldanaerobacter subterraneus* subsp. *s.*
> *Geobacillus s.*
> *Hydrogenobacter s.*
> *Thermaerobacter s.*
> *Thermoanaerobacter s.*

subtilis
> *Bacillus s.*
> *Copromonas s.*

subtotal villous atrophy (STVA)

subtraction
> immunofixation by s.

subtribe

subtype
> chondroblastic s.
> desmoplastic s.

subungual, subunguial
> s. melanoma

subunguial (*var. of* subungual)

subunit
> chorionic gonadotropin-alpha s.
> chorionic gonadotropin-beta s.
> four s.
> HCG alpha s.
> HCG beta s.
> s. vaccine

subvalvar stenosis

subvibrioides
> *Brevundimonas s.*

subvital mutation

succentorius
> lien s.

succenturiata
> placenta s.

succenturiate lobe

successional lamina

succi (*pl. of* succus)

succinate
> s. dehydrogenase
> sodium s.

succinate-ubiquinone-oxidoreductase

succinatimandens

succinic acid

succiniciproducens
> *Anaerobiospirillum s.*

succinifaciens
> *Treponema s.*

Succinivibrio dextrinosolvens

Succinivibrionaceae

succinylcoenzyme A

succus, *pl.* **succi**

sucking louse

Sucquet canal

Sucquet-Hoyer canal

sucrase

sucrase-isomaltase

sucrose
> s. alpha-d-glucohydrolase
> s. density gradient (SDG)
> s. density gradient analysis
> s. density gradient ultracentrifugation
> s. hemolysis test
> s. intolerance
> s. pad nuclear exchange assay

sucrosemia

sucrosuria

suction method

suction-type biopsy

Suctoria

suctorial

SUD
> sudden unexpected death
> sudden unexplained death

Sudan
> S. black
> S. black B (SBB)
> S. black B fat stain
> S. black Bizzozero

black Bizzozero, S.
S. brown
S. red III
S. yellow
S. yellow G
sudanophil
sudanophilia
sudanophilic leukodystrophy
sudanophobic
s. unit
s. zone
sudden
s. cardiac death (SCD)
s. coronary death (SCD)
s. death syndrome (SDS)
s. infant death syndrome (SIDS)
s. intrauterine unexplained death (SIUD)
s. unexpected death (SUD)
s. unexpected death in infancy (SUDI)
s. unexpected, unexplained death (SUUD)
s. unexplained death (SUD)
s. unexplained death in epilepsy (SUDEP)
s. unexplained infant death (SUID)
Sudeck
S. atrophy
S. disease
S. point
Sudeck-Leriche syndrome
SUDEP
sudden unexplained death in epilepsy
SUDI
sudden unexpected death in infancy
sudomotor fiber
sudor
s. sanguineus
s. urinosus
sudoriferae
corpus glandulae s.
glandulae s.
sudoriferous
s. abscess
s. duct
s. gland
sudoriferus
ductus s.
porus s.
sudorikeratosis
sudoriparous abscess
SUDS
Single Use Diagnostic System
SUDS HIV-1 test
sueciensis
Helcococcus s.
sufentanil

sufficient
s. condition
not s. (NS)
quantity not s. (QNS)
suffocation
indirect s.
suffocative goiter
suffodiens
folliculitis abscedens et s.
suffusion
suffusus
Centruroides s.
sufrartyfex
sugar
s. acid
s. assimilation assay
blood s. (BS)
s. broth
capillary blood s. (CBS)
fasting blood s. (FBS)
s. fermentation assay
invert s.
postprandial blood s. (PPBS)
reducing s.
specific soluble s.
s. tumor
s. water test screen
Sugar-Chex II glucose control
sugar-coated spleen
sugar-icing liver
suggillation
postmortem s.
suicide
s. gene
hot antigen s.
s. machine
suicloacalis
Atopostipes s.
suicordis
Corynebacterium s.
SUID
sudden unexplained infant death
suid herpesvirus
suihominis
Sarcocystis s.
suillum
Dechlorosoma s.
Suillus
suimastitidis
Actinomyces s.
suipestifer
Bacillus s.
Suipoxvirus
suis
Balantidium s.
Brucella s.
Haemophilus s.
Isospora s.
Mycoplasma s.

S

suis (*continued*)
    Trichomonas s.
    Trichuris s.
    Trypanosoma s.
suit
    chemical splash s.
sulcatum
    keratoderma plantare s.
    keratoma plantare s.
sulci (*pl. of* sulcus)
sulcular
    s. epithelium
    s. fluid
sulcus, *pl.* sulci
    sulci cutis
    external spiral s.
    s. matricis unguis
    s. spiralis externus
sulfa
    sulfa drug
    sulfa film
sulfabenzamide
sulfacetamide
sulfadiazine
sulfaguanidine
sulfamerazine
sulfameter
sulfamethazine
sulfamethizole
sulfamethoxazole
sulfanilamide
sulfanilic acid
sulfapyridine
sulfatase
    iduronic s.
    l-sulfoiduronate s.
    steroid s. (STS)
    sulfatide s.
sulfate, sulphate
    1-adamantanamine s.
    ammonium s.
    chondroitin s.
    colistin s.
    copper s.
    dehydroepiandrosterone s. (DHEAS)
    dermatan s.
    diethyl s.
    dimethyl s.
    heparan s.
    indoxyl s.
    keratan s.
    polymyxin B s.
    potassium s.
    protamine s.
    sodium dodecyl s. (SDS)
    sodium lauryl s.
    sodium tetradecyl s.
    thallium s.
sulfated acid mucopolysaccharide (SAM)

sulfatemia
sulfatiazole
sulfatidase
sulfatide
    cerebroside s.
    s. lipidosis
    s. sulfatase
sulfation factor
sulfexigens
    Desulfocapsa s.
sulfhemoglobin (HbS, SHb)
sulfhemoglobinemia
sulfhemoglobinuria
sulfhydryl group
sulfidaeris
    Halomonas s.
sulfide
    dichlorodiethyl s.
    hydrogen s.
    Timm silver s.
sulfidifaciens
    Globicatella s.
sulfidophilum
    Heliobacterium s.
sulfindigotic acid
sulfinic acid
sulfinpyrazone
sulfinyl
sulfisoxazole
sulfite
    s. agar
    anhydrous sodium s.
    s. challenge
    exsiccated sodium s.
    s. oxidase
    s. oxidase deficiency
    sodium s.
Sulfitobacter
    S. brevis
    S. delicatus
    S. dubius
    S. mediterraneus
    S. pontiacus
sulfmethemoglobin
sulfobromophthalein sodium
sulfolipid
Sulfolobaceae
Sulfolobales
sulfolobus
    S. SNDV-like viruses
    S. tokodaii
sulfomucin
sulfonamide
    s. antagonist
    s. assay
sulfonate
    alkylbenzene s. (ABS)
    scarlet red s.
    sodium polyethylene s.

sulfonation
sulfone
sulfonic acid
sulfonivorans
    Arthrobacter s.
    Hyphomicrobium s.
sulfonmethane
sulfonyl
sulfonylurea assay
sulfoprotein
sulforhodamine B
sulfosalicylic
    s. acid (SSA)
    s. acid turbidity test
sulfotransferase
sulfoxide
    dimethyl s.
sulfoxone
    sodium s.
sulfur (S), sulphur
    s. bacterium
    s. dioxide
    s. dye
    s. granule
    s. oxide
    s. pearl of Namibia
    s. trioxide
sulfur-containing amino acid
sulfuric acid
Sulfurihydrogenibium
    S. azorense
    S. subterraneum
Sulfurimonas autotrophica
Sulfurospirillum
    S. arsenophilum
    S. halorespirans
    S. multivorans
sulfurous acid
Sulfurovum lithotrophicum
sulfurreducens
    Geobacter s.
Sulkowitch
    S. reagent
    S. test
sullae
    Rhizobium s.
sulphate (*var. of* sulfate)
sulphur (*var. of* sulfur)
sulphureum
    Trichophyton s.
    Trichophyton tonsurans s.
sulphureus
    Laetiporus s.
Sulzberger-Garbe syndrome
summa
    Pygidiopsis s.
summer
    s. asthma
    s. prurigo of Hutchinson

sum of square deviations (SSD)
SUN
    serum urea nitrogen
sunburst form
sundaicus
    Anopheles s.
sun stroke (*var. of* sunstroke)
sunstroke, sun stroke
sup
    superficial
superacidity
superantigen
supercooled
superdistention
superdominance
superfamily
superfemale
superficial (sup)
    s. burn
    s. cell
    s. implantation
    s. malignant fibrous histiocytoma
    s. multicentric basal cell carcinoma
    s. mycosis
    s. spreading melanoma
    s. subcutis
    s. ulcerating rheumatoid necrobiosis
    s. wound
superficialis
    colitis cystica s.
    lupus s.
    nodi lymphoidei inguinales
        superficiales
Superfrost Plus glass slide
supergene
    immunoglobulin s.
superheated
superinduce
superinfection
superior
    ductulus aberrans s.
    s. limbic keratoconjunctivitis (SLKC)
    lipodystrophia progessiva s.
    s. pulmonary sulcus tumor
    s. sagittal sinus
    s. sulcus tumor
    tarsus s.
    tela choroidea s.
    s. vena caval syndrome
    s. vena cava syndrome
Supermount slide fixative
supernatant
    culture fluid s.
    hybridoma s.
    postmitochondrial s. (PMS)
supernate
supernumerary
    s. kidney
    s. marker

S

supernumerary (*continued*)
    s. organ
    s. segmental artery
superoxide
    s. anion
    s. assay
    s. dismutase
    s. dismutase gene
superparasite
superparasitism
superpictus
    Anopheles s.
superpigmentation
supersaturated
**Super Sensitive kit multistep detection
system**
Superstitionia donensis
supervoltage
superwarfarin
sulphureum
    Trichphyton s.
supplemental inheritance
supplementary gene
supplied air respirator (SAR)
supply
    double blood s.
    endometrial blood s.
    power s.
support
    granulocyte transfusion s.
    Joint Task Force for Civil S. (of
    the Defense Department)
    s. medium
    s. zone
supporting cell
suppressibility
suppression
    bone marrow s.
    bystander s.
    s. of cell cycle
    s. subtractive hybridization
suppressor
    s. cell
    s. gene
    s. mutation
    s. of cytokine signaling (SOCS)
    p53 tumor s.
    soluble immune response s. (SIRS)
    s. T lymphocyte
    tRNA s.
suppressor-sensitive mutant
suppurant
suppurate
suppuration
suppurativa
    hidradenitis s.
suppurative
    s. acute appendicitis
    s. acute inflammation

    s. arthritis
    s. cerebritis
    s. cholangitis
    s. chronic inflammation
    s. chronic otitis media
    s. encephalitis
    s. granulomatous inflammation
    s. hepatitis
    s. infection
    s. keratitis
    s. mastitis
    s. necrosis
    s. nephritis
    s. pericarditis
    s. pleurisy
    s. pneumonia
    s. synovitis
suprabasal
    s. cell layer
    s. clefting
suprabasilar bulla
suprahyoid gland
supranormal venous oxygen content
supranuclear
supraoptic nucleus
supraopticohypophysialis
    tractus s.
supraopticohypophysial tract
suprapapillary
suprapubic
    s. needle aspiration
    s. puncture
suprarenal
    s. body
    s. capsule
    s. cortex
    s. gland
suprarenalis
    cortex glandulae s.
    glandula s.
    macrogenitosomia praecox s.
    medulla glandulae s.
suprasellar
    s. cyst
    s. meningioma
supravalvular aortic stenosis (SAS, SVAS)
supraventricular tachycardia
supravergence (S)
supravital
    s. stain
    s. staining
Supre-Heme buffer
suramin
Sure Blot membrane
Surecut needle
SureStep
    S. Flexx professional blood glucose
    management system
    S. Pro glucose analyzer

surf
  surfactant
surface
  abluminal s.
  s. absorptive cell
  s. antigen
  apical s.
  s. carcinoma in situ
    (SCIS)
  CellBIND cell culture s.
  cut s.
  s. denudation
  s. epithelial-stromal tumor
  s. epithelium
  s. expression
  s. immunoglobulin
  intimal s.
  s. marker
  s. marker staining
  s. mucous cell
  serosal s.
  s. tension (ST)
surface-active agent
surface-barrier detector
surface-enhanced laser desorption
  ionization time-of-flight mass
  spectrometry (SELDI-TOF-MS)
surface-oriented pinocytic activity
surfactant
  amniotic fluid s.
  amniotic fluid pulmonary s.
  s. nanoemulsion
  s. protein A, B, C
  pulmonary s.
surgery
  bariatric s.
  video-assisted transthoracic s.
    (VATS)
surgical
  s. ciliated cyst
  s. defect
  s. emphysema
  s. pathology
  s. resection
  s. specimen
  s. wound
Surgicutt device
Surgipath Decalcifier I, II
surivivin protein
surnumerary chromosome
surra
surrogate
  biofidelic human s.
surveillance
  Surveillance, Epidemiology, and End
    Results (SEER)
  immune s.
  immunological s.
  syndromic s.

survey
  cross-sectional s.
  iodine-131 thyroid
    metastatic s.
  metastatic bone s.
  s. meter
  proficiency s.
  s. program
  radiation s.
  skeletal s.
survival
  chromium-51 red cell s.
  disease-free s. (DFS)
  disease-specific s.
  metastasis-free s.
  s. motor neuron (SMN)
  s. motor neuron telomeric
    gene
  s. of cancer cell
  overall s. (OS)
  predictor of patient s.
  red blood cell s.
  s. time
survivin
  s. expression
  s. protein
SUS
  stained urinary sediment
susceptibility
  disease s.
  electric s.
  genetic s.
  magnetic s.
  s. test
  s. testing
suspended particulate
suspension
  DNAzole cell s.
  extended insulin zinc s.
suspicious cell
sustentacular cell
SUTI
  sperm-ubiquitin tag immunoassay
Sutterella
  S. stercoricanis
  S. wadsworthensis
Sutton
  S. disease
  S. nevus
  S. ulcer
Suttonella indologenes
suture
  s. granuloma
  localization s.
SUUD
  sudden unexpected, unexplained death
suum
  Ascaris s.
Suzanne gland

S

SV
   simian virus
   snake venom
      SV 40 T antigen
Sv
   sievert
SV40-adenovirus hybrid
SVAS
   supravalvular aortic stenosis
SVC
   slow vital capacity
Svedberg
      S. equation
      S. unit of sedimentation
        coefficient (S)
SVR
   systemic vascular resistance
SW
   spiral wound
Sw^a antigen
swab
      nasopharyngeal s.
      s. specimen
Swachman-Diamond syndrome
Swaminathania salitolerans
swamp
      s. fever
      s. fever virus
Swann antigen
swan-neck deformity
swarming
sweat
      s. chloride level
      s. duct
      s. duct adenoma
      excretory duct of s.
      s. gland
      s. gland adenocarcinoma
      s. gland adenoma
      s. gland carcinoma
       (SGC)
      s. gland tumor
      s. pore
      s. test
Sweat-Chek conductivity analyzer
Swediaur disease
Sweet
      S. disease
      S. method
      S. syndrome
swelling
      albuminous s.
      brain s.
      Calabar s.
      cellular s.
      cloudy s.
      fugitive s.
      high amplitude s.
      hydropic s.

      Neufeld capsular s.
      Spielmeyer acute s.
Swift disease
Swift-Feer disease
swimmer's itch
swimming
      s. pool conjunctivitis
      s. pool granuloma
swine
      atrophic rhinitis of s.
      s. encephalitis virus
      s. fever
      s. fever virus
      s. influenza
      s. influenza virus
      s. pest
      s. rotlauf bacillus
      transmissible gastroenteritis virus
       of s.
      s. vesicular disease
swinepox virus
swirling comet tail colony
SWI/SNF complex
Swiss
      S. cheese endometrium
      S. cheese hyperplasia
      S. mouse leukemia virus
Swiss-type
      S.-t. agammaglobulinemia
      S.-t. hypogammaglobulinemia
switch
      angiogenic s.
      class s.
      double-pole double-throw s.
      double-pole single-throw s.
      silicon-controlled s.
switching
      class s.
      isotype s.
swollen crista
Sx
   symptoms
sycoma
sycosis
      tinea s.
Sydenham
      S. chorea
      S. disease
Sydney
      S. classification
      S. classification for gastritis
      S. classification system
Sydowia
sylvatic plague
Sylvest disease
Symbiobacterium thermophilum
symbion, symbiont
symbiont (*var. of* symbion)
symbiosis

symbiosum
　　Fusobacterium s.
symbiote
symbiotic
symblepharon
symbol
　　hazard s.
　　statistical s.
sym-**dichloroethylene**
Symmers
　　S. clay pipestem fibrosis
　　S. disease
symmetric
　　s. adenolipomatosis
　　s. distribution
symmetrica
　　keratoderma s.
symmetrical gangrene
symmetry
　　axis of s.
　　bilateral s.
　　s. element
　　s. group
　　icosahedral s.
　　s. operation
　　s. plane
　　radial s.
sympathetic
　　s. chain
　　s. formative cell
　　s. imbalance
　　s. neuroblast
　　s. ophthalmia
　　s. ophthalmitis
　　s. pharmacology
sympathetoblast
sympathetoblastoma
sympathicectomy
sympathicoblast
sympathicoblastoma
sympathicogonioma
sympathiconeuritis
sympathicopathy
sympathicotonia
sympathicotripsy
sympathicotropic cell
sympathoblast
sympathoblastoma
sympathochromaffin cell
sympathogonia
sympathogonioma
sympathomimetic
sympathotropic cell
sympexis
symphyses (*pl. and gen. of* symphysis)
symphysis, *pl.* **symphyses**
symplasmatic
Sympodiophora
symport

symporter
　　human sodium/iodide s.
　　　(hNIS)
　　sodium-iodine s. (NIS)
symptomatic
　　s. fever
　　s. myeloid metaplasia
　　s. porphyria
　　s. reaction
　　s. ulcer
　　s. varicocele
symptomatica
　　livedo reticularis s.
symptomatology
symptomatolytic, symptomolytic
symptomolytic (*var. of* symptomatolytic)
symptoms (Sx)
SYN
　　synaptophysin
synapse
　　axoaxonic s.
　　axodendritic s.
　　axosomatic s.
　　electrotonic s.
synapsing
　　nerves s.
synapsis
synaptic
　　s. bouton
　　s. cleft
　　s. ending
　　s. phase
　　s. terminal
　　s. trough
　　s. vesicle
synaptinemal complex
synaptobrevin
synaptology
synaptonemal complex
synaptophysin (SYN)
　　s. antibody
　　s. stain
synaptopodin
　　s. gene
　　s. protein
synaptosomal protein of 25 kDa
synaptosome
synaptotagmin
Syncephalastrum racemosum
syncephalus
synchondrosis
　　sphenooccipital s.
　　sphenopetrosal s.
　　sternal s.
Synchron
　　S. CX9 ALX clinical system
　　S. CX clinical chemistry system
　　S. CX4, CX5, CX9, CX500,
　　　CX1000 PRO clinical system

S

Synchron (*continued*)
   S. CX3, CX4, CX5 Delta clinical
      system
   S. CX4, CX5, CX7 Super clinical
      system
   S. LX clinical chemistry system
   S. LX20 clinical system
   S. LX4201 clinical system
   S. LXi 725 clinical system
   S. LX20, LX2000 PRO clinical
      system
synchronism
   developmental s.
synchronized culture
synchronous
   s. airway lesion (SAL)
   s. cancer
   s. counter
   s. data transmission
   s. mass lesion
   s. neoplasm
Synchytrium endobioticum
Syncleistostroma
syncope
   vasovagal s.
syncyanea
   Pseudomonas s.
syncyanin
synctia (*pl. of* synctium)
syncytial
   s. alteration
   s. endometritis
   s. knot
   s. knotting
   s. morphology
   respiratory s. (RS)
   s. shedding
   s. trophoblast
syncytiotrophoblast
syncytiotrophoblastic
   s. cell
   s. cell of seminoma
syncytium, *pl.* **synctia**
   s. inducing (SI)
syndactyly
syndecan
syndecan-1
syndesmitis
syndesmophyte
syndromal dysplasia
syndrome
   Aarskog s.
   Aarskog-Scott s.
   abdominal muscle
      deficiency s.
   Abercrombie s.
   Achard s.
   Achard-Thiers s.
   Achenbach s.

acquired immunodeficiency s.
   (AIDS)
acrofacial s.
acute coronary s. (ACS)
acute radiation s. (ARS)
acute respiratory distress s. (ARDS)
acute urethral s.
Adair-Dighton s.
addisonian s.
Adie s.
adrenal feminizing s.
adrenal gland virilizing s.
adrenogenital s. (AGS)
adult respiratory distress s. (ARDS)
Ahumada-Del Castillo s.
Aicardi s.
Alagille s.
Albright s.
Albright-McCune-Sternberg s.
Aldrich s.
Alezzandrini s.
Allen-Masters s.
Alport s.
Alström s.
amenorrhea-galactorrhea s.
amniotic band s.
Amsterdam s.
Andersen s.
Andrade s.
androgen insensitivity s. (AIS)
Angelman s.
Angelucci s.
angioosteohypertrophy s.
antibody deficiency s. (ADS)
antiphospholipid s. (APS)
antiphospholipid antibody s.
antisynthetase s.
Anton s.
apallic s.
aplastic anemia s.
Argonz-Del Castillo s.
Arias s.
Arndt-Gottron s.
Arnold-Chiari s.
Arnold nerve reflex cough s.
arthritis-dermatitis s.
Ascher s.
Asherman s.
ataxia telangiectasia s.
autoerythrocyte sensitization s.
autoimmune lymphoproliferative s.
   (ALPS)
Avellis s.
Axenfeld s.
Ayerza s.
Baastrup s.
Babinski s.
Babinski-Fröhlich s.
Babinski-Nageotte s.

Babinski-Vaquez s.
bacterial overgrowth s.
Bäfverstedt s.
Balint s.
Baller-Gerold s.
Bamberger-Marie s.
Bannayan-Riley-Ruvalcaba s. (BRRS)
Bannayan-Zonana s. (BZS)
Banti s.
Bardet-Biedl s.
bare lymphocyte s. type 1
base lymphocyte s. (BLS)
Barlow s.
Barré-Guillain s.
Barrett s.
Bart s.
Bart s.
Bartter s.
basal cell nevus s.
base lymphocyte s. (BLS)
Bassen-Kornzweig s.
Bateman s.
Batten-Mayou s.
Bazex s.
Beau s.
Beckwith s.
Beckwith-Wiedemann s.
Behçet s.
Benedikt s.
Beradinelli s.
Berlin breakage s.
Bernard s.
Bernard-Horner s.
Bernard-Sergent s.
Bernard-Soulier s. (BSS)
Bernhardt-Roth s.
Bernheim s.
Bertolotti s.
Besnier-Boeck-Schaumann s.
Bianchi s.
Biemond s.
bile salt deficiency s.
Birt-Hogg-Dube s.
Björnstad s.
Blackfan-Diamond s.
black thyroid s.
Blatin s.
blind loop s.
Bloch-Sulzberger s.
Bloom s.
blue diaper s.
Blum s.
body of Luys s.
bodypacker s.
Boerhaave s.
Bonnet-Dechaume-Blanc s.
Bonnevie-Ullrich s.
Bonnier s.
Böök s.

Börjeson s.
Börjeson-Forssman-Lehmann s.
Bouillaud s.
Bouveret s.
bowel bypass s.
Brachmann-de Lange s.
brachymesomelia-renal s.
brain death s.
Brennemann s.
Briquet s.
Brissaud-Marie s.
Brissaud-Sicard s.
Bristowe s.
Brock s.
bronchiolitis obliterans s.
brown bowel s.
Brown-Séquard s.
Brugsch s.
Brugsch s.
Bruns s.
Brunsting s.
Buckley s.
Budd s.
Budd-Chiari s.
Bürger-Grütz s.
Burnett s.
Buschke-Ollendorf s.
Byler s.
Bywaters s.
Cacchi-Ricci s.
Caffey s.
Caffey-Silverman s.
Canada-Cronkhite s.
Capgras s.
Caplan s.
carcinoid s.
cardiolipin antibody s.
Carney s.
carotid sinus s.
carpal tunnel s.
Carpenter s.
Castleman s.
cat's cry s.
cat's eye s.
Ceelen-Gellerstedt s.
cellular immunity deficiency s.
  (CIDS)
cerebellomedullary malformation s.
cerebral salt-washing s.
cerebrohepatorenal s.
cervical disk s.
cervical rib s.
Cestan s.
Cestan-Chenais s.
Cestan-Raymond s.
chancriform s.
Charcot s.
Charcot-Weiss-Baker s.
CHARGE s.

S

syndrome (*continued*)

Charlin s.
Chauffard s.
Chauffard-Still s.
Chédiak-Higashi s.
Chédiak-Steinbrinck-Higashi s.
Cheney s.
Chiari-Arnold s.
Chiari-Budd s.
Chiari-Frommel s.
Chiari II s.
Chilaiditi s.
CHILD s.
childhood hemolytic uremic s.
Chinese restaurant s.
   (CRS)
choriodecidual inflammatory
   response s.
Chotzen s.
Christian s.
Christ-Siemens s.
Christ-Siemens-Touraine s.
chromosomal breakage s.
chromosomal deletion s.
chromosomal malformation s.
chromosome breakage s.
chronic brain s. (CBS)
chronic fatigue immune dysfunction
   s. (CFIDS)
chronic intestinal pseudoobstructive
   s. (CIPS)
Churg-Strauss s.
Citelli s.
Clarke-Hadfield s.
Claude Bernard-Horner s.
Clough-Richter s.
Clouston s.
Cockayne s.
Coffin-Lowry s.
Coffin-Siris s.
Cogan s.
cold agglutinin s. (CAS)
Collet s.
Collet-Sicard s.
coloboma s.
combined immunodeficiency s.
   (CIDS)
common variable
   immunodeficiency s.
compartment s.
compartmental s.
complete androgen insensitivity s.
   (CAIS)
congenital rubella s.
Conn s.
Cornelia de Lange s.
coronary insufficiency s.
Costello s.
Costen s.

Cotard s.
Courvoisier-Terrier s.
Cowden s.
Crandall s.
CREST s.
cri du chat s.
Crigler-Najjar s.
Cronkhite-Canada s.
Crouzon s.
Crow-Fukase s.
CRST s.
crush s.
Cruveilhier-Baumgarten s.
cryopathic hemolytic s.
cryptophthalmus s.
Curtis-Fitz-Hugh s.
Curtius s.
Cushing s.
cutaneomucouveal s.
CVID s.
Cyriax s.
DaCosta s.
Danbolt-Closs s.
Dandy-Walker s.
Danlos s.
Debré-Semelaigne s.
de Clerambault s.
defibrination s.
Degos s.
Dejerine s.
Dejerine-Klumpke s.
Dejerine-Roussy s.
Dejerine-Sottas s.
de Lange s.
del Castillo s.
dengue shock s.
Dennie-Marfan s.
de novo myelodysplastic s.
Denys-Drash s.
de Sanctis-Cacchione s.
de Toni-Fanconi s.
Devon polyposis s.
dialysis dysequilibrium s.
Diamond-Blackfan s.
DiGeorge s.
Di Guglielmo s.
Donath-Landsteiner s.
Donohue s.
Down s. (DS)
Dresbach s.
Dressler s.
Duane s.
Dubin-Johnson s.
Dubin-Sprinz s.
Dubreuil-Chambardel s.
Duchenne s.
Duchenne-Erb s.
dumping s.
Duncan s.

Duplay s.
Dupré s.
Dyggve-Melchior-Clausen s.
Dyke-Davidoff-Masson s.
dysmyelopoietic s.
dysplastic nevus s.
dyspoietic s.
dystrophy-dystocia s. (DDS)
dysuria-pyuria s.
Eagle s.
Eaton-Lambert s.
economy class s.
ectopic ACTH s.
Eddowes s.
Edwards s.
Edwards-Patau s.
Ehlers-Danlos s. (EDS)
Eisenlohr s.
Eisenmenger s.
Ekbom s.
Ellis-van Creveld s.
EMG s.
empty sella s.
endocrine polyglandular s.
eosinophilia-myalgia s. (EMS)
Epstein s.
Erb s.
erythrodysesthesia s.
Evans s.
excited skin s.
Faber s.
facet s.
Fallot s.
Fanconi s.
Fanconi-Zinsser s.
Farber s.
Farber-Uzman s.
fat embolism s.
Fechtner s.
Felty s.
fertile eunuch s.
fetal alcohol s.
fetal face s.
fetal hydantoin s.
fetal trimethadione s.
Feuerstein-Mims s.
fibrinogen-fibrin conversion s.
Fiessinger-Leroy-Reiter s.
Figueira s.
first arch s.
Fisher s.
Fitz s.
Fitz-Hugh and Curtis s.
Fleischner s.
Flynn-Aird s.
focal dermal hypoplasia s.
Foix s.
folded-lung s.
Forbes-Albright s.

Forney s.
Foster Kennedy s.
Foville s.
fragile X s.
Fraley s.
Franceschetti s.
Franceschetti-Jadassohn s.
François s.
Fraser s.
Freeman-Sheldon s.
Frenkel anterior ocular traumatic s.
Frey s.
Friderichsen-Waterhouse s.
Friedmann vasomotor s.
Fröhlich s.
Froin s.
Frommel-Chiari s.
Fryn s.
Fuchs s.
Furst-Ostrum s.
G s.
Gaisböck s.
Gamstorp s.
Ganser s.
Gardner s.
Gardner-Diamond s.
Gasser s.
gay lymph node s.
Gélineau s.
Gerhardt s.
Gerstmann s.
Gianotti-Crosti s.
giant platelet s.
Gilbert s.
Gilles de la Tourette s.
Gitelman s.
Glanzmann-Riniker s.
glomangiomatous osseous
  malformation s.
glutaric aciduria type 2 s.
Goldberg-Maxwell s.
Goldenhar s.
Goldz-Gorlin s.
Goltz s.
gonococcal arthritis-dermatitis s.
Good s.
Goodpasture s.
Gopalan s.
Gordon s.
Gorlin s.
Gorlin-Chaudhry-Moss s.
Gorlin-Goltz s.
Gorlin-Psaume s.
Gorman s.
Gougerot-Blum s.
Gougerot-Carteaud s.
Gowers s.
gracilis s.
Gradenigo s.

S

syndrome (*continued*)
Graham Little s.
gray platelet s. (GPS)
Greig s.
Griscelli s.
Grönblad-Strandberg s.
Gruber s.
Gubler s.
Guillain-Barré s.
Gulf War s.
Gull-Sutton s.
Gunn s.
gustatory sweating s.
Haber s.
Haddad s.
Hadfield-Clarke s.
Hakim s.
Hallermann-Streiff s.
Hallermann-Streiff-François s.
Hallervorden s.
Hallervorden-Spatz s.
Hallgren s.
Hallopeau-Siemens s.
Hamman s.
Hamman-Rich s.
hand-foot s.
hand-foot-uterus s.
Hanhart s.
Hanot-Chauffard s.
hantavirus pulmonary s.
happy puppet s.
Harada s.
Hare s.
Harris s.
Hartnup s.
Hassin s.
Hayem-Widal s.
heart-hand s.
Heerfordt s.
Hegglin s.
Heidenhain s.
HELLP s.
Helweg-Larssen s.
hemangioma-thrombocytopenia s.
hemolytic-uremic s. (HUS)
hemophagocytic s. (HPS)
hemorrhagic colitis s.
hemorrhagic fever with renal s.
Hench-Rosenberg s.
Henoch-Schönlein s.
hepatorenal s. (HRS)
hereditary flat adenoma s. (HFAS)
hereditary mixed polyposis s.
Herlitz s.
Hermansky-Pudlak s.
herniated disc s. (HDS)
Herrmann s.
Hines-Bannick s.
Hirschowitz s.

Hoffmann-Werdnig s.
Holmes-Adie s.
Holt-Oram s.
Homén s.
Horner s.
Horton s.
Houssay s.
Hünermann s.
hungry bone s.
Hunt s.
Hunter s.
Hunter-Hurler s.
Hurler s. (HS)
Hutchinson s.
Hutchinson-Gilford s.
Hutchison s.
hypereosinophilic s.
hyper-IgE s.
hyper-IgM s.
hyperventilation s.
hyperviscosity s.
hypophysial s.
idiopathic nephrotic s. (INS)
idiopathic respiratory distress s.
 (IRDS)
Imerslund-Grasbeck s.
immersion s.
immotile cilia s.
immune dysfunction s.
immunodeficiency s.
impingement s.
inappropriate antidiuretic hormone s.
India rubber man s.
infantile respiratory distress s.
infection-associated hemophagocytic
 s. (IAHS)
intersex s.
iridocorneal endothelial s.
 (ICE)
irradiation CVS/CNS s.
irradiation hematopoietic s.
irritable bowel s. (IBS)
Irvine s.
Ivemark s.
Jaccoud s.
Jackson s.
Jacod s.
Jadassohn-Lewandowski s.
Jaffe-Campanacci s.
Jahnke s.
Jeghers-Peutz s.
Jervell and Lange-Nielsen s.
Jeune s.
Job s.
Johnson-Dubin s.
Joseph s.
juvenile polyposis s.
Kallmann s.
Kandinskii-Clerambault s.

Kanner s.
Kartagener s.
Kasabach-Merritt s.
Kast s.
Kearns s.
Kearns-Sayre s.
Kennedy s.
Kiloh-Nevin s.
Kimmelstiel-Wilson s.
Kinsbourne s.
Klauder s.
Kleine-Levin s.
Klinefelter s. (KS)
Klippel-Feil s. (KFS)
Klippel-Trenaunay s.
Klippel-Trenaunay-Weber s.
Klumpke-Dejerine s.
Klüver-Bucy s.
Kniest s.
Kocher-Debré-Semelaigne s.
Koenig s.
Koerber-Salus-Elschnig s.
Korsakoff s.
Kostmann s.
Krabbe s.
Krause s.
Kunkel s.
Kuskokwim s.
kwashiorkor-marasmus s.
Laband s.
Labbé neurocirculatory s.
Ladd s.
LAMB s.
Lambert-Eaton s.
Lambert-Eaton myasthenic s.
  (LEMS)
Landry s.
Landry-Guillain-Barré s.
Larsen s.
Launois s.
Launois-Bensaude s.
Launois-Cléret s.
Laurence-Biedl s.
Laurence-Moon s.
Laurence-Moon-Bardet-Biedl s.
Laurence-Moon-Biedl s.
Lawford s.
Lawrence-Seip s.
lazy leukocyte s.
Lennox s.
Lenz s.
LEOPARD s.
Leriche s.
Leri-Weill s.
Lermoyez s.
Lesch-Nyhan s.
Lévy-Roussy s.
Leyden-Mobius s.
Lhermitte-McAlpine s.

Libman-Sacks s.
Lichtheim s.
Liddle s.
Li-Fraumeni cancer s.
light chain Fanconi s.
Lightwood s.
Lignac s.
Lignac-Fanconi s.
linear sebaceous nevus s.
Lobstein s.
Looser-Milkman s.
Lorain-Lévi s.
Louis-Bar s.
Lowe s.
Lowe-Terrey-MacLachlan s.
Lown-Ganong-Levine s.
Lucey-Driscoll s.
Lutembacher s.
Luys body s.
Lyell s.
lymphadenopathy s.
lymphoproliferative s.
Lynch II s.
MacKenzie s.
Macleod s.
Maffucci s.
malabsorption s.
male Turner s.
malformation s.
Mali s.
malignant carcinoid s.
Malin s.
Mallory-Weiss s.
mandibulofacial dysotosis s.
mandibulooculofacial s.
Marañón s.
Marchesani s.
Marchiafava-Micheli s.
Marcus Gunn s.
Marfan s.
Margolis s.
Marie s.
Marie-Bamberger s.
Marie-Robinson s.
Marinesco-Garland s.
Marinesco-Sjögren s.
Maroteaux-Lamy s.
Marshall s.
Martorell s.
Mauriac s.
Mayer-Rokitansky-Küster s.
McCune-Albright s. (MAS)
Meckel s.
Meckel-Gruber s.
megacystic s.
Meigs s.
MELAS s.
Melchior s.
Melkersson s.

S

syndrome (*continued*)

Melkersson-Rosenthal s.
Melnick-Needles s.
Ménétrier s.
Mengert shock s.
Ménière s.
Menkes s.
menopausal s.
metabolic s.
metastatic carcinoid s.
methionine malabsorption s.
Meyenburg-Altherr-Uehlinger s.
Meyer-Betz s.
Meyer-Schwickerath and Weyers s.
microdeletion s.
middle lobe s.
Miescher s.
Mikulicz s.
milk-alkali s.
Milkman s.
Millard-Gubler s.
Miller-Dieker s.
minimal-change nephrotic s.
Minkowski-Chauffard s.
Minot-von Willebrand s.
Mirizzi s.
mixed cryoglobulin s.
Möbius s.
Monakow s.
Montreal platelet s. (MPS)
Moore s.
Morel s.
Morgagni s.
Morgagni-Adams-Stokes s.
Morgagni-Stewart-Morel s.
Morquio s.
Morquio-Brailsford s.
Morquio-Ullrich s.
Morris s.
Morton s.
Morvan s.
Mosse s.
Mounier-Kuhn s.
Mucha-Habermann s.
Muckle-Wells s.
mucocutaneous lymph node s.
mucosal neuroma s.
mucosal prolapse s.
Muir-Torre s.
multiple hamartoma s.
multiple lentigines s.
multiple mucosal neuroma s.
multiple organ dysfunction s.
Murchison-Sanderson s.
mycosis fungoides/Sézary s. (MF/SS)
myelodysplastic s. (MDS)
myeloproliferative s.
Myhre s.
myofascial s.

Naffziger s.
Nägeli s.
nail-patella s.
NAME s.
Nelson s.
Nelson-Salassa s.
neonatal respiratory distress s.
nephritic s.
nephrotic s. (NS)
Netherton s.
neurocutaneous phacomatosis s.
neuroleptic malignant s.
nevoid basal cell carcinoma s. (NBCCS)
newborn respiratory s.
Nezelof s.
Nijmegen breakage s. (NBS)
Noack s.
nonketotic hyperosmolar s.
Nonne-Milroy-Meige s.
nonspecific viral s.
Noonan s.
nutritional recovery s.
OAV s.
ocular-mucous membrane s.
oculobuccogenital s.
oculocerebral s.
oculocerebrorenal s.
oculodentodigital s.
oculovertebral s.
ODD s.
OFD s. 1–8
s. of inappropriate secretion of antidiuretic hormone (SIADH)
Ogilvie s.
Omenn s.
OMM s.
Opitz GBBB s.
Oppenheim s.
opsoclonus-myoclonus s.
organic brain s. (OBS)
organic dust toxic s.
Osler-Weber-Rendu s.
osteomyelofibrotic s.
Ostrum-Furst s.
otomandibular s.
ovarian hyperstimulation s. (OHS)
overlap s.
pacemaker twiddler's s.
4p deletion s.
Pitt-Rogers-Danks s.
Plummer-Vinson s.
POEMS s.
Poland s.
Polhemus-Schafer-Ivemark s.
polycystic ovary s.
polysplenia s.
polytoxicomaniac s.
postgastrectomy dumping s.

postmenopausal s.
postpump s. (PPS)
postrubella s.
postvagotomy s.
Potter s.
pouch s.
Prader-Willi s.
premature senility s.
primary fibrinogenolysis s.
primary fibromyalgia s.
Profichet s.
Proteus s. (PS)
prune belly s. (PBS)
pseudo-Felty s.
pseudomyasthenic s.
pseudothalidomide s.
pseudo-Turner s.
pterygium s.
pulmonary dysmaturity s.
pulmonary-renal s.
Putnam-Dana s.
radial aplasia-thrombocytopenia s.
Raeder paratrigeminal s.
Ramsay Hunt s.
Rapp-Hodgkin s.
Raymond-Cestan s.
reactive airways dysfunction s.
 (RADS)
Recklinghausen-Applebaum s.
recurrent bouts of nephrotic s.
red cell fragmentation s.
red eye s.
refeeding s.
Refetoff s.
Reichmann s.
Reifenstein s.
Reiter s.
REM s.
Rendu-Osler-Weber s.
Renpenning s.
respiratory distress s.
 (RDS)
restless legs s. (RLS)
Rett s.
Reye s.
Rh isoimmunization s.
Rh null s.
Richards-Rundle s.
Richter s.
Rieger s.
right ovarian vein s.
Riley-Day s.
Riley-Smith s.
Roaf s.
Roberts s.
Robin s.
Robinow s.
Roger s.
Rokitansky-Küster-Hauser s.

Romano-Ward s.
Romberg s.
Rosenbach s.
Rosenthal s.
Rosenthal-Kloepfer s.
Rosewater s.
Roth s.
Roth-Bernhardt s.
Rothmann-Makai s.
Rothmund s.
Rothmund-Thomson s.
Rotor s.
Rotter s.
Roussy-Dejerine s.
Roussy-Lévy s.
Rovsing s.
Rubinstein s.
Rubinstein-Taybi s.
Rud s.
rudimentary testis s.
Rundles-Falls s.
runting s.
Russell s.
Rust s.
Sabin-Feldman s.
Saethre-Chotzen s.
salt-losing s.
Sanchez Salorio s.
Sanfilippo s.
scalded skin s. (SSS)
scalenus anticus s.
Schafer s.
Schanz s.
Schaumann s.
Scheie s.
Schirmer s.
Schmid-Fraccaro s.
Schmidt s.
Schridde s.
Schroeder s.
Schüller s.
Schüller-Christian s.
Schultz s.
Schwartz s.
Schwartz-Bartter s.
Scott s.
Sebastian s.
Sebright bantam s.
Seckel s.
secondary antiphospholipid s.
Secrétan s.
sella turcica s.
Selye s.
Senear-Usher s.
sepsis s.
Sertoli cell only s.
Sever s.
severe acute respiratory s. (SARS)
Sézary s. (SS)

S

syndrome (*continued*)
shaken adult s.
shaken baby s. (SBS)
shaken impact s.
shaken infant s.
Sheehan s.
short bowel s.
Shprintzen s.
Shulman s.
Shwachman s.
Shwachman-Diamond s.
Shy-Drager s.
Sicard s.
sicca s.
sick building s.
sick sinus s. (SSS)
Silferskiöld s.
Silver s.
Silver-Russell s.
Silvestrini-Corda s.
Singleton-Merten s.
sinus node dysfunction s.
Sipple s.
Sjögren s.
Sjögren-Larsson s.
sleep apnea s.
Sluder s.
Sly s.
Smith-Lemli-Opitz s.
Smith-Magenis s.
Smith-Riley s.
Sneddon s.
Sohval-Soffer s.
solitary rectal ulcer s.
Sorsby s.
Spen s.
spherophakia-brachymorphia s.
Sprinz-Nelson s.
spruelike s.
Spurway s.
stagnant loop s.
staphylococcal scalded skin s.
stasis s.
Steele-Richardson-Olszewski s.
Steinbrocker s.
Steiner s.
Stein-Leventhal s.
Stevens-Johnson s.
Stewart-Bluefarb s.
Stewart-Morel s.
Stewart-Treves s.
Stickler s.
Still-Chauffard s.
Stilling s.
Stilling-Turk-Duane s.
Stokes-Adams s.
Stokvis-Talma s.
Stormorken s.
Strachan s.

streptococcal toxic shock s.
Stryker-Halbeisen s.
Sturge s.
Sturge-Kalischer-Weber s.
Sturge-Weber s.
subclavian steal s.
sudden death s. (SDS)
sudden infant death s. (SIDS)
Sudeck-Leriche s.
Sulzberger-Garbe s.
superior vena cava s.
superior vena caval s.
Swachman-Diamond s.
Sweet s.
Takayasu s.
Tapia s.
TAR s.
tarsal tunnel s. (TTS)
Taussig-Bing s.
Terry s.
Terson s.
testicular feminization s. (Tfm, TFS)
testicular regression s.
thalassemia s.
Thibierge-Weissenbach s.
third and fourth pharyngeal
pouch s.
thoracic outlet s. (TOS)
Thorn s.
thrombocytopenia with absent
radii s.
thrombopathic s.
thrombotic thrombocytopenic purpura
and hemolytic uremic s.
(TTP-HUS)
Tietze s.
Timme s.
Tolosa-Hunt s.
TORCH s.
Torkelson s.
Tornwaldt s.
Torre s.
Torsten Sjögren s.
Touraine-Solente-Goĺe s.
toxic shock s. (TSS)
Treacher Collins s.
triad s.
trichorhinophalangeal s.
triple X s.
trisomy 8,13,18,20,21,22 s.
Troisier s.
tropical splenomegaly s. (TSS)
Trousseau s.
tryptophan malabsorption s.
tumor lysis s. (TLS)
Turcot s.
Turner s.
twiddler's s.
twin-to-twin transfusion s. (TTTS)

twin-twin transfusion s. (TTTS)
Uehlinger s.
Ullrich-Feichtiger s.
Ullrich-Turner s.
Ulysses s.
undifferentiated connective tissue s.
urogenital s.
Usher s.
uveoencephalitic s.
van Buchem s.
van der Hoeve s.
Van der Woude s.
velocardiofacial s. (VCFS)
Verner-Morrison s.
Vernet s.
vertebral basilar artery s.
vertebral crush-fracture s.
Villaret s.
Vinson s.
virilizing s.
virus-associated hemophagocytic s.
  (VAHS)
Vogt s.
Vogt-Koyanagi s.
Vohwinkel s.
Volkmann s.
von Hippel-Lindau s. (vHL)
von Willebrand s.
Waardenburg s.
WAGR s.
Waldenström s.
Wallenberg s.
Ward-Romano s.
Warkany s.
wasting s.
Waterhouse-Friderichsen s.
WDHA s.
Weber s.
Weber-Cockayne s.
Weber-Dubler s.
Wegener s.
Weil s.
Weill-Marchesani s.
Wells s.
Wermer s.
Werner s.
Wernicke s.
Wernicke-Korsakoff s.
West s.
Weyers oligodactyly s.
Weyers-Thier s.
whistling face s.
white clot s.
Widal s.
Wiedemann-Beckwith s.
Wildervanck s.
Willebrand s.
Williams s.
Williams-Campbell s.

Wilson s.
Wilson-Mikity s.
Winter s.
Wiskott-Aldrich s. (WAS)
Witkop-Von Sallmann s.
Wolf s.
Wolff-Parkinson-White s.
Wolf-Hirschhorn s.
Wolfram s.
Wright s.
s. X
XLP s.
XO s.
XXY s.
XYZ s.
yellow nail s.
Young s.
Zellweger s.
Zieve s.
Zinsser-Cole-Engman s.
Zollinger-Ellison s. (ZES)
syndromic
  s. surveillance
  s. surveillance system
synechia, *pl.* **synechiae**
  s. pericardii
  posterior iridolenticular synechiae
synechiae (*pl. of* synechia)
synencephalocele
syneresis
synergism
  agent, state, body site, effects,
  severity, time course, other
  (diagnoses), s. (ASBESTOS)
synergist
synergistic
synergy
Syngamidae
Syngamus
  S. laryngeus
  S. trachea
syngamy
syngeneic
  s. graft
  s. transplant
syngenesioplastic transplant
syngenesioplasty
syngenesiotransplantation
syngenic
syngraft
synkaryon
synophthalmia, synophthalmus,
  synophthalmos
synophthalmos (*var. of* synophthalmia)
synophthalmus (*var. of* synophthalmia)
synorchidism, synorchism
synorchism (*var. of* synorchidism)
synosteosis (*var. of* synostosis)
Synosternus pallidus

S

synostosis, synosteosis
 tribasilar s.
synotus
synovial
 s. cancer
 s. cavity
 s. cell
 s. chondromatosis
 s. crypt
 s. cyst
 s. fluid
 s. fluid analysis
 s. fluid examination
 s. fringe
 s. membrane
 s. membrane biopsy
 s. osteochondromatosis
 s. sarcoma (SS, SYS)
 s. sheath
 s. tuft
 s. tumor
 s. villi
 s. villus protrusion
synoviale
 stratum s.
synoviales
 villi s.
synovialis
 membrana s.
synoviocyte
 knee s.
synovioma
 malignant s.
synovitis
 acute serous s.
 dendritic s.
 lymphoplasmacytic s.
 proliferative s.
 purulent s.
 rheumatoid s.
 serous acute s.
 suppurative s.
 tendinous s.
 vaginal s.
 villonodular pigmented s.
synovium
syntaxin
syntectic
syntenic
synteny
syntexis
synthase
 fatty acid s. (FAS)
 glycogen (starch) s.
 methionine s.
 nitric oxide s. (NOS)
 porphobilinogen s.
 thymidylate s.
 uroporphyrinogen I s.

syntheses (*pl. of* synthesis)
synthesis, *pl.* **syntheses**
 ATP s.
 collagenase s.
 DNA s.
 eicosanoid s.
 endogenous s.
 fatty acid s.
 globin-chain s.
 glycogen s.
 lipid s.
 s. period
 s. phase
 porphyrin s.
 protein s.
 triacylglyceride s.
 urea s.
synthesize oxytocin
synthetase
 acetyl-CoA s.
 acyl-CoA s.
 alanyl-ribonucleic acid s.
 alanyl-RNA s.
 argininosuccinate s.
 carbamoyl phosphate s. (CPS)
 carbamyl phosphate s. (CPS)
 glutamine s.
 glutathione s.
 heme s. (HS)
 inducible nitric oxide s.
  (iNOS)
 isoleucyl-RNA s.
 leucyl-RNA s.
 methionyl-RNA s.
 oligoadenylate s.
 polydeoxyribonucleotide s.
 tyrosyl-RNA s.
 valyl-RNA s.
synthetic
 s. antigen
 s. dye
 s. lethal
syntrophicum
 Sporotomaculum s.
syntrophism
Syntrophomonadaceae
Syntrophomonas curvata
Syntrophothermus lipocalidus
Syntrophus aciditrophicus
syntropic
synuclein
 alpha s.
Syphacia obvelata
syphilemia
syphilid
 bullous s.
 gummatous s.
 nodular s.
syphilimetry

syphilis
- endemic s.
- hemagglutination treponemal test for s.
- quaternary s.
- rupial s.
- serologic test for s. (STS)
- serology test for s. (STS)
- standard serologic test for s.
- standard test for s. (STS)
- tertiary s.
- s. test

syphilitic
- s. abscess
- s. aneurysm
- s. aortitis
- s. fever
- s. gumma
- s. lymphadenopathy
- s. meningitis
- s. meningoencephalitis
- s. nephritis
- s. node
- s. osteochondritis
- s. periarteritis
- s. ulcer

syphiliticum
- tuberculum s.

syphiloma of Fournier

syphilomatous

syringadenoma

syringe
- Luer lock glass s.
- Roughton-Scholander s.
- s. shield

syringeal

syringitis

syringoadenoma

syringobulbia

syringocarcinoma

syringocele

syringocystadenoma papilliferum

syringocystoma

syringoencephalomyelia

syringoid

syringoma
- chondroid s.

syringomatous
- s. adenoma
- s. growth pattern
- s. metamorphosis

syringomeningocele

syringometaplasia
- squamous s.

syringomyelia

syringomyelocele

syringopontia

Syringospora albicans

syrinx

Syrphidae

SYS
- synovial sarcoma

Sysmex
- S. CA-6000 coagulation instrument
- S. HS-330 robotic hematology system
- S. NE-8000 CBC analyzer
- S. R-1000 reticulocyte counter
- S. XE-2100 hematology analyzer
- S. XT-2000i automated hematology analyzer

system
- 10-20 s.
- ABC immunodetection s.
- Access 2 immunoassay s.
- ACIT s.
- ACL Advance coagulation testing s.
- ACL 1000 coagulation testing s.
- ACL Elite coagulation testing s.
- ACL Top coagulation testing s.
- ACS 180 SE automated chemiluminescent immunoassay s.
- Adeza TLi fetal fibronectin analysis s.
- Advia 120 hematology s.
- AEC detection s.
- Aeroset clinical chemistry s.
- Affymetrix GeneChip s.
- Aldefluor reagent s.
- Alpha Dx point-of-need test s.
- Amersham International ECL gene detection s.
- A2 MicroArray s.
- Ann Arbor staging s.
- API 20 Strep S.
- Array 360, 360CE/CE-AL protein/drug/serology s.
- ASAP biopsy s.
- association s.
- AutoCyte PREP s.
- automated cellular imaging s. (ACIS)
- autonomous detection s. (ADS)
- avidin-biotin based detection s.
- avidin-biotin complex immunodetection s.
- BacT/Alert automated microbial detection s.
- Bactec blood culture s.
- Bactec 9000 MB s.
- Batson s.
- Bayer AG II chemistry analyzer s.
- BD BBL CultureSwab Plus collection and transport s.
- BD Phoenix automated microbiology s.
- Bethesda s.
- bicarbonate buffer s.

system (*continued*)

biohazard detection s. (BDS)
blood group systems (ABO)
buffer s.
cardiovascular system and central nervous s. (CVS/CNS)
CAS 200 Image Analysis s.
catalyzed signal amplification s.
CellaVision DM96 s.
cell-free s.
CellPrep sample preparation s.
CenSlide 2000 urinalysis s.
centimeter-gram-second s.
central nervous s. (CNS)
Ceprate SC stem cell concentration s.
CEQ 8000, 8800 genetic analysis s.
CGS s.
ChemMate multistep detection s.
CHEMXpress s.
Christopherson nuclear grading s.
chromaffin s.
CipherGen Express software biomarker analysis s.
CoaguChek Pro/DM s.
Colormate Tlc.BiliTest s.
combined DNA index s. (CODIS)
complement s.
Coulter reticONE s.
Coulter tetraONE s.
countercurrent multiplier s.
Crit-Line III TQA s.
Cryo-Vac-A cryostat vacuum s.
CX9 ALX clinical s.
CX4, CX5, CX9, CX500, CX1000 PRO clinical s.
CX3, CX4, CX5 Delta clinical s.
CX4, CX5, CX7 super clinical s.
Cymbal blood collection s.
CytoLite luminescence assay s.
Cytomics FC 500 series flow cytometry s.
CytoRich cervical cytology monolayer s.
Dako Artisan Staining S.
Dako Fast Red Substrate S.
DexCom STS continuous glucose monitoring s.
dichroic filter s.
Diego blood group s.
Difco ESP testing s.
diffuse neuroendocrine s.
DL2000 data management s.
DNA-Prep workstation reagent s.
DSX automated ELISA s.
Duffy blood group s.
DxI 800 immunoassay s.
Early Aberration Reporting S. (EARS)

Edmondson tumor grading s.
Ehrenreich and Churg membranous nephropathy staging s.
Elecsys troponin T immunoassay s.
Electra 1400C, 1800C coagulation s.
enteric nervous s. (ENS)
EnVision non-avidin-biotin detection s.
Epics Altra cell sorting s.
Epics XL, XLMCL flow cytometer s.
ES300-Cardiac T ELISA troponin T immunoassay s.
ESP II s.
excurrent duct s.
extrinsic s.
FastPack blood analyzer s.
fibrinolytic s.
FiltraCheck-UTI colorimetric filtration s.
FiltraCheck-UTI disposable colorimetric bacteriuria detection s.
First Warning S.
FreeStyle blood glucose monitoring s.
Fuhrman s.
gamma motor s.
GenomeLab GeXP genetic analysis s.
GenomeLab SNPstream genotyping s.
Gerbich blood group s.
glandular s.
S. Gold HPLC
Halon s.
haversian s.
hematopoietic s.
HemoCue hemoglobin test s.
heparan sulfate-antithrombin III s.
His-Tawara s.
HmX H20 hematology s.
Huvos grading s.
Hybrid Capture s.
Hybritech PSA determination s.
hypophyseoportal s.
hypothalamohypophysial portal s.
hypothalamoneurohypophysial s.
ID-Micro typing s.
Immage immunochemistry s.
Immulite 1000, 2000, 2500 immunoassay s.
Immulite 2500 SMS immunoassay s.
immune s.
ImmunoPrep reagent s.
Impact on-site drug and alcohol test s.
In Charge diabetes control s.
indicator s.

Infectious Disease Surveillance Information S. (ISIS)
Integrated Core s.
integumentary s.
Intercept platelet s.
intermediary s.
International Neuroblastoma Staging S. (INSS)
intrinsic s.
Isolator blood culture s.
Isolex 300i magnetic cell selection s.
I-TRAC Plus transfusion s.
Jass staging s.
kallikrein s.
Kell blood group s.
Kidd blood group s.
kinin s.
LaChrom HPLC s.
Leitz image analysis s.
LightCycler s.
Lipoprint cholesterol subfraction test s.
LSAB2 multistep detection s.
LS 6500 liquid scintillation counting s.
Lutheran blood group s.
LX4201 clinical s.
LXi 725 clinical s.
LX20, LX200, LX2000 PRO clinical s.
lymphoreticular s.
Macroduct collecting s.
male reproductive s.
Mammotome biopsy s.
Masaoka thymic cancer staging s.
MB-Redox s.
MDS s.
mesolimbic dopaminergic s.
meter-kilogram-second s.
metric s.
metropolitan medical response s. (MMRS)
MFO s.
microbiology identification s.
microsomal enzyme s.
mixed function oxidase s.
MKS s.
modified Masaoka thymic cancer staging s.
monocyte-macrophage s.
mononuclear phagocyte s. (MPS)
MSTS staging s.
Munich tumor classification s.
myeloperoxidase s.
myeloperoxidase H_2O_2 halide s.
Nanoduct neonatal sweat analysis s.
National Electronic Disease Surveillance S. (NEDSS)

National Notifiable Diseases Surveillance S. (NNDSS)
NIOX nitric oxide monitoring s.
nonisotopic gel detection s.
nonspecific s.
s. of macrophages
s. of macrophases
Oncor Inform HER2/neu gene amplification detection s.
on-demand s.
operating s.
OptiMax immunostaining s.
Ortho Summit donor screening s.
P/ACE MDQ series capillary electrophoresis s.
plasminogen-plasmin activator s.
PlateTrak automated microplate processing s.
POG surgicopathologic staging s.
Poly-Chem automated chemistry-immunoassay s.
Polytech 2000 laboratory information s.
portal s.
properdin s.
protein characterization s.
ProteinChip Biomarker DU, PA s.
ProteinChip System Series 4000 biomarker/assay s.
ProteomeLab DU, PA 800 protein characterization s.
ProteomeLab PF 2D protein fractionation s.
ProteomeLab XL-A, XL-I protein characterization s.
ProTime microcoagulation s.
ProTime prothrombin time test s.
PSI chromosome analysis s.
Purkinje s.
Q-beta replicase s.
RAG-1, -2 recombinase enzyme s.
RAMP biological test s.
random access immunoassay s.
Rapid One single dipstick s.
Readit SNP genotyping s.
renin-angiotensin-aldosterone s.
reticONE s.
reticular activating s. (RAS)
reticuloendothelial s. (RES)
Roche Septi-Chek blood culture s.
Roche Sysmex hematology s.
SalEst s.
Salzer-Kuntschik grading s.
SBR tumor grading s.
Scianna blood group s.
SensiCath s.
Septi-Chek culture s.
Sequenza immunostaining s.
Shimoda blood group s.

S

system (*continued*)
Siemens Advia Centaur
immunoassay s.
Single Use Diagnostic S. (SUDS)
SmartCycler realtime PCR s.
S-Monovette blood collection s.
SNPstream genotyping s.
Sof-Tact diabetes management s.
SOS bacterial DNA repair s.
STA-Compact hemostasis s.
STA hemostasis s.
STart 8 clot detection s.
STAT-Site M Hgb test s.
stem kit CD34+HPC enumeration s.
Sterrad 100, 200 and 50 acid
sterilization s.
St. Jude pediatric oncology
staging s.
streptavidin-biotin-based detection s.
STS-7 continuous glucose
monitoring s.
Super Sensitive kit multistep
detection s.
SureStep Flexx professional blood
glucose management s.
Sydney classification s.
Synchron CX9 ALX clinical s.
Synchron CX clinical chemistry s.
Synchron CX4, CX5, CX9, CX500,
CX1000 PRO clinical s.
Synchron CX3, CX4, CX5 Delta
clinical s.
Synchron CX4, CX5, CX7 Super
clinical s.
Synchron LX20 clinical s.
Synchron LX4201 clinical s.
Synchron LX clinical chemistry s.
Synchron LXi 725 clinical s.
Synchron LX20, LX2000 PRO
clinical s.
syndromic surveillance s.
Sysmex HS-330 robotic hematology s.
T s.
TD glucose monitoring s.
TechMate 500 automated
immunohistochemical s.
tetraONE s.
The Bethesda S. (TBS)
TheraTest Laboratories EL-RF test
kit s.
ThinPrep Imaging s.
thrombin-thrombomodulin-protein
C s.
TNM staging s.
T-tubular s.
Typenex blood-recipient
identification s.
ubiquitin-proteasome s. (UPS)
Ultima II refrigerator s.

UniCel Dxl 800 immunoassay s.
Unopette s.
UP*link* point of care sample testing
s.
Uriscreen bacteriuria detection s.
Vectastain Elite ABC s.
ViraType In Situ S.
ViroSeq HIV-1 genotyping s.
Wampole Isolater blood culture s.
Whitmore-Jewett tumor staging s.
Xga blood group s.

10-20 system
systema
systematic
s. bacteriology
s. error
systematized
s. nevus
s. nomenclature of medicine
(SNOMED)
S. Nomenclature of Pathology
(SNOP)
Système International d'Unités
systemic
s. air embolism
s. anaphylaxis
s. arterial pressure (SAP)
s. autoimmune disease
s. calciphylaxis
s. chondromalacia
s. familial primary amyloidosis
s. febrile disease
s. histiocytosis
s. hyalinosis
s. l-carnitine deficiency
s. lesion
s. lupus erythematosus (SLE)
s. mast cell disease (SMCD)
s. mycosis
s. myelitis
s. poisoning
s. reticuloendotheliosis
s. scleroderma
s. sclerosis
s. vascular resistance (SVR)
systemoid
systolic
s. hypertension
s. time interval (STI)
Syva EMIT-II assay
syzygial
syzygii
Acetobacter s.
Ralstonia s.
syzygium
syzygy
Szent-Györgyi reaction
szulgai
Mycobacterium \ s.

t

test of significance

t distribution

t test

T

temperature

tesla

T agglutination

T agglutinogen

T and B lymphocyte subset assay

T antibody

T antigen

T banding

T (cell) cytolytic

T (cell) cytotoxic (Tc)

T cytotoxic cell (Tc)

T factor

T helper cell

T lymphocyte

T method stain

T system

T tubule

T1/2

terminal half-life

T0

no evidence of primary tumor

T2

T2 mycotoxin

T2 toxin

T₃

triiodothyronine

reverse T₃

T₃ uptake

T₃ uptake test

T₄

levothyroxine

free T₄

T₄ newborn screen

TA

alkaline tuberculin

therapeutic abortion

titratable acid

toxin-antitoxin

tube agglutination

TA-4

tumor-antigen 4

TAB

typhoid, paratyphoid A, and paratyphoid B

TAB 250 antibody

TAB vaccine

tabacinasalis

Facklamia t.

tabanid

Tabanidae

Tabanus

tabby

t. cat heart

t. cat striation

tabescence

tabescent

tabes dorsalis

tabetic

tabetiform

table

anthropomorphic t.

contingency t.

decision t.

Gaffky t.

life t.

thickened subepithelial collagen t.

truth t.

tablet

graph t.

Ictotest reagent t.

tabletop shield

tabun

NATO code for t. (GA)

TAC

tetracaine, Adrenalin (epinephrine), and cocaine

TAC antigen

TAC solution

Tacaribe complex of viruses

tache

t. blanche

t. laiteuse

tachetic

tachycardia

supraventricular t. (SVT)

ventricular t. (V-TACH, V tach)

tachyphylaxis

tachypnea

tachyzoite

extracellular t.

tacrolimus

tactile

t. cell

t. corpuscle

t. disc

t. meniscus

t. papilla

tactoid body

tactor

tactus

meniscus t.

organum t.

corpusculum t.

TAD

thoracic asphyxiant dystrophy

tadpole cell

T

taejonensis
> *Sphingomonas* t.

taenia (*var. of* tenia)
> T. *africana*
> T. *armata*
> T. *bremneri*
> T. *canina*
> T. *confusa*
> T. *crassicollis*
> T. *cucurbitina*
> T. *demerariensis*
> T. *dentata*
> T. *diminuta*
> T. *echinococcus*
> T. *equina*
> T. *hominis*
> T. *hydatigena*
> T. *lata*
> T. *madagascariensis*
> T. *mediocanellata*
> T. *minima*
> T. *multiceps*
> T. *murina*
> T. *nana*
> T. *ovis*
> T. *philippina*
> T. *pisiformis*
> T. *quadrilobata*
> T. *saginata*
> T. *solium*
> T. *taeniaeformis*

taeniacide (*var. of* teniacide)

taeniaeformis
> *Hydatigera* t.
> *Taenia* t.

taenial (*var. of* tenial)

Taeniarhynchus

taeniasis (*var. of* teniasis)

taeniform (*var. of* teniform)

taeniid

Taeniidae

taenioid (*var. of* tenioid)

taenioides
> *Diphyllobothrium* t.

Taeniolella stilbospora

taeniorhynchus
> *Aedes* t.

Taenzer stain

Taenzer-Unna stain

TAF
  albumose-free tuberculin
  toxoid-antitoxoid floccule
  trypsin-aldehyde-fuchsin
  tumor angiogenic factor

tag
> anal skin t.
> hymenal t.
> sentinel t.
> skin t.

TAG
  tumor-associated glycoprotein

TAG-72 antigen

tagging
> COOH-terminal t.

T-agglutination

TAGVHD
  transfusion-associated graft-versus-host
  disease

Tahyna virus

tail
> cytoplasmic t.
> t. poikilocyte
> polyA t.
> polyadenylate t.
> t. sheath

tailed red cell

tailing

tainanensis
> *Chitinibacter* t.

Taiwan acute respiratory (TWAR)

taiwanensis
> *Chitinimonas* t.
> *Natrialba* t.
> *Pseudoxanthomonas* t.
> *Ralstonia* t.
> *Rubrobacter* t.
> *Wautersia* t.

Takahara disease

Takara
> T. Biomedicals One-Step RNA PCR
> kit
> T. Biomedicals Suprec tube

Takata-Ara test

Takayama stain

Takayasu
> T. arteritis
> T. disease
> T. syndrome

TAL
  thymic alymphoplasia

talaje
> *Alectorobius* t.
> *Ornithodoros* t.

Talaromyces

talc
> t. crystal
> t. plaques
> t. pneumoconiosis

talcosis

Talerman classification

Talfan disease

talgut cyst

T-ALL
> T-cell acute lymphoblastic leukemia

tall cell variant (TCV)

Talma disease

TALP
> tumor-assisted lymphoid proliferation

TAM
 toxoid-antitoxoid mixture
Tamm-Horsfall
 T.-H. mucoprotein (THM)
 T.-H. protein
tamponade, tamponage
 cardiac t.
tamponage (*var. of* tamponade)
Tamulus
TAN
 tropical ataxic neuropathy
tandem
 t. mass spectrometry
 t. repeat analysis
 t. trinucleotide repeat
tandoii
 Acinetobacter t.
tangent
tangential
 t. plane
 t. sectioning
tangerinus
 Saccharothrix t.
Tangier disease
tangle
 neurofibrillary t.
 t. only dementia
tangle-bearing neuron
tangle-free neuron
tannate
 albumin t.
tanned
 t. red cell (TRC)
 t. red cell hemagglutination
 inhibition test
tannerae
 Prevotella t.
Tannerella forsythensis
Tanner stage
tannic acid
tannophilus
 Pachysolen t.
tanycyte
TAO
 thromboangiitis obliterans
tap
 dry t.
tapasin
tape
 Dissolve-A-Way t.
 magnetic t.
 t. mark
 t. transport
tapetal cell
tapeticola
 Halospirulina t.
tapetum
 t. nigrum
 t. oculi

tapeworm
 beef t.
 broad fish t.
 dwarf t.
 fish t.
 pork t.
 rat t.
Taphrina
Tapia syndrome
Tapinella
tapir mouth
TAP1/TAP2 heterodimer
Taq
 T. deoxyribonucleic acid polymerase
 (taq DNA polymerase)
 T. DyeDeoxy Terminator Cycle
 Sequencing kit
 T. Master Mix kit
TaqI restriction digest
TaqMan real-time PCR
tar
 coal t.
 t. keratosis
 T. syndrome
TAR
 thrombocytopenia-absent radius
TARA
 tumor-associated rejection
 antigen
tarantula
tarda
 Edwardsiella t.
 osteogenesis imperfecta t.
 porphyria cutanea t. (PCT)
tardaugens
 Novosphingobium t.
Tardieu
 T. ecchymoses
 T. petechiae
 T. spot
 T. test
tardive
 forme t.
tare
target
 t. amplification
 t. cell
 t. cell anemia
 t. fiber
 t. gland
 t. lesion
 t. organ
targetoid
 t. hemosiderotic hemangioma
 t. pattern
Tarlov cyst
tarry
 t. cyst
 t. stool

899

tarsal
t. coalition
t. cyst
t. gland
t. plates
t. tunnel syndrome
tarsalis
Culex t.
glandulae tarsales
tarsi (*pl. of* tarsus)
tarsitis
tarsoepiphyseal aclasis
tarsomegaly
tarsophyma
tarsus, *pl.* **tarsi**
t. inferior
t. superior
tartaric acid
tart cell
tartrate
t. inhibited acid phosphatase
potassium acid t.
potassium sodium t.
sodium potassium sodium t.
tartrate-resistant
t.-r. acid phosphatase (TRAcP, TRAP)
t.-r. acid phosphate
t.-r. leukocyte acid phosphatase
tartrazine
TARU
technical advisory response unit
Tarui disease
tasmaniensis
Vibrio t.
taste
t. bud
t. bulb
t. cell
t. corpuscle
t. hair
organ of t.
t. pore
TAT
tetanus antitoxin
thromboplastin activation test
total antitryptic activity
toxin-antitoxin
treponemal antibody test
turn-around time
TATA
tumor-associated transplantation antigen
tataouinensis
Ramlibacter t.
Tatlockia micdadei
tattoo
dental amalgam t.
tattooing abrasion
tau
neurofibrillary degeneration

t. gene
t. molecular marker
t. pathology class I–IV
t. protein
t. protein pathology
tauopathy class I–IV
taurine
taurinensis
Legionella t.
taurochenodeoxycholate
taurochenodeoxycholic acid
taurocholate
sodium t.
taurocholemia
taurocholic acid
taurodeoxycholic acid
taurolithocholic acid
Taussig-Bing
T.-B. disease
T.-B. syndrome
tautomer
keto-enol t.
proton t.
ring-chain t.
valence t.
tautomeric fiber
taxis
taxon
taxonomic
taxonomy
numerical t.
Tay disease
Taylor disease
Taylorella asinigenitalis
Tay-Sachs disease (TSD)
TB
toluidine blue
tubercle bacillus
tuberculosis
TB smear
TBA
testosterone-binding affinity
thiobarbituric acid test
thyroxine-binding albumin
TBBx
transbronchial lung biopsy
TBC
tuberculous
TBD
total body density
TBF
total body fat
TBG
thyroid-binding globulin
thyroxine-binding globulin
TBG assay
TBG cap
TBGP
total blood granulocyte pool

TBH
total body hematocrit
TBI
thyroxine-binding index
traumatic brain injury
TBII
TSH binding inhibitory
immunoglobulin
TBK
total body potassium
TBLB
transbronchial lung biopsy
T/B lymphocyte assay
TBM
tuberculous meningitis
tubular basement membrane
TBNA
transbronchial needle aspiration
TBP
thyroxine-binding protein
TBPA
thyroxine-binding prealbumin
TB-RD
tuberculosis-respiratory disease
TBS
The Bethesda System
total body solute
TBSAH
traumatic basal subarachnoid
hemorrhage
TBT
tolbutamide test
TBV
total blood volume
TBW
total body water
total body weight
T$_4$(C)
serum thyroxine measured by column
chromatography
TC
temperature compensation
thermal conductivity
tissue culture
to contain
total cholesterol
TC detector
TC pipette
Tc
T (cell) cytotoxic
TCA
total colonic aganglionosis
tricarboxylic acid
TCA cycle
TCBS
thiosulfate citrate-bile salts-sucrose
TCBS agar
TCC
transitional cell carcinoma

high-grade TCC
low-grade TCC
TCC of renal pelvis
TCCA
tissue culture cytotoxin assay
TCD
tissue culture dose
TCD$_{50}$
median tissue culture dose
TCDD
2,3,7,8-tetrachlorodibenzo-p-dioxin
TCDD intoxication
T-cell
T-c. acute lymphoblastic leukemia
T-c. ALL
T-c. antibody labeling
T-c. antigen
T-c. antigen receptor
T-c. chronic lymphocytic leukemia
T-c. disorder
T-c. growth factor (TGF)
T-c. growth factor-1
T-c. growth factor-2
T-c. immunodeficiency
T-c. lymphoma
T-c. marker
T-c. mediated disease
T-c. priming
T-c. proliferation
T-c. prolymphocytic leukemia (T-PLL)
T-c. receptor (TCR)
T-c. receptor complex
T-c. replacing factor (TRF)
T-c. restricted intracellular antigen
(TIA)
T-c. rich B-cell lymphoma
(TCRBCL)
T-c. turnover
T-cell/E-rosette receptor
TCF
tissue-coding factor
TCH
thiophen-2-carboxylic acid hydrazide
total circulating hemoglobin
TCI
transient cerebral ischemia
TCID
tissue culture infective dose
TCID$_{50}$
median tissue culture infective dose
TCIE
transient cerebral ischemic episode
TCM
tissue culture medium
TCPI Rapid HIV test
TCR
T-cell receptor
TCR complex
TCR Vgamma9 test

TCRBCL
  T-cell rich B-cell lymphoma
tcRNA
  translation control RNA
TCT
  thrombin clotting time
  thymic carcinoid tumor
  thyrocalcitonin
TCV
  tall cell variant
TD
  teratoma differentiated
  tetanus-diphtheria
  thymus-dependent
  to deliver
    TD glucose monitoring
    system
    TD pipette
T2D
  Type 2 diabetes
TDA
  TSH displacing antibody
TDE
  tetrachlorodiphenylethane
T-dependent antigen
TDF
  testis-determining factor
  thoracic duct fistula
TDI
  total-dose infusion
TDLU
  terminal duct lobular unit
TDM
  therapeutic drug monitoring
TDP
  thiamine diphosphate
TDT
  thermal death time
    TDT immunostain
TdT
  terminal deoxynucleotidyltransferase
TDTH cell
**TdT-mediated dUTP nick-end labeling
  (TUNEL)**
TDxFlx analyzer
TE
  tissue-equivalent
  total estrogen (excretion)
Te
  tellurium
  tetanus
team
    Disaster Medical Assistance T.
      (DMAT)
    Disaster Mortuary T. (DMORT)
    Infectious Disease Death Review T.
      (IDDRT)
    National Medical Response T.
      (NMRT)

tear
  cruciate ligament t.
  t. gas
  Mallory-Weiss t.
  meniscal t.
  rotator cuff t.
  tendon t.
  triangular fibrocartilage complex t.
  triangular-shaped skin t.
teardrop red cell
teargas (*var. of* tear gas)
teasing
tebenquichense
    Halorubrum t.
TeBG
  testosterone-estradiol binding globulin
TEC
  transient erythroblastopenia of
  childhood
TechMate
  T. 500 automated
    immunohistochemical system
  T. 1000 immunostainer
technetium (Tc)
technetium-99m (^{99m}Tc)
technic (*var. of* technique)
**technical advisory response unit
  (TARU)**
technician
  histologic t. (HT)
  medical laboratory t.
technique
  ABC t.
  alkaline phosphatase antialkaline
    phosphatase t.
  antibody-coated microprobe t.
  antibody panning t.
  antigen-retrieval t.
  APAAP t.
  avidin-biotin immunoperoxidase t.
  Brecher new methylene blue t.
  Brown-Brenn t.
  Carey Ranvier t.
  Cattoretti t.
  cellulose tape t.
  Corbin rhinoplasty t.
  counterstaining t.
  Crocker silver impregnation t.
  crypt isolation t.
  cumulative-summation t.
    (cusum)
  cytoblock t.
  Dennis left atrium cannulation t.
  DGGE t.
  dilution-filtration t.
  direct fluorescent antibody t.
  DNA slot blot t.
  double antibody t.
  double-layer fluorescent antibody t.

double staining t.
Duhamel t.
enzyme-assisted immunoassay t.
enzyme-dependent colorimetric t.
enzyme-multiplied immunoassay t.
(EMIT)
extracorporeal photophoresis t.
FA t.
Ficoll-Hypaque t.
Florescent Amplification Catalyzed
by T7-polymerase T. (FACTT)
flotation t.
fluorescent antibody t.
freeze-fracture t.
Gallyas silver staining t.
general dissection t.
glove juice t.
Highman Congo red t.
Hotchkiss-McManus PAS t.
hybridoma t.
immunofluorescence t.
immunohistochemical t.
immunoperoxidase t.
Jerne t.
Kato thick smear t.
Knott t.
Kohn one-step staining t.
Laurell t.
McMaster t.
membrane filter t.
micropore filter t.
modified zinc sulfate centrifugal
flotation t.
multiblock t.
Northern blot t.
Ouchterlony t.
PACONA t.
plaque t.
pop-off t.
program evaluation and review t.
(PERT)
protein A gold complex t.
Q-band t.
rapid frozen section t.
Rebuck skin window t.
Ritter-Oleson t.
roll tube t.
saline t.
scintillation t.
sealed envelope t.
section freeze substitution t.
sedimentation t.
Seldinger t.
soft-spin t.
Southern blot t.
specialist dissection t.
Stoll dilution egg count t.
streptavidin-biotin-complex t.
thin-layer cervical cytology t.

time diffusion t.
titration t.
trypsin digest t.
Western blot t.
wet scanning t.
whole blood lysis t.
zinc sulfate centrifugal flotation t.
technologic life
technologist
medical t. (MT)
technology
automated cell-counter t.
Biobarcode t.
bioelectronic sensor t.
c-mycERTAM stem cell
expansion t.
DNA microarray t.
ExpressDetect t.
FFF t.
gene chip t.
nucleic acid chip t.
single nucleotide polymorphism
scoring t.
SNP scoring t.
tissue microarray t. (TMA)
Up-Converting Phosphor t. (UPT)
tecta
zona t.
Tectiviridae
Tectivirus
tectorium
TED
threshold erythema dose
thromboembolic disease
TEF
tracheoesophageal fistula
TEG
thromboelastographic monitor device
TEG trace
Teichobacteria
Teichococcus ludipueritiae
teichoic
t. acid
t. acid antibody
tela, *pl.* **telae**
t. choroidea
t. choroidea inferior
t. choroidea of fourth ventricle
t. choroidea of third ventricle
t. choroidea superior
t. choroidea ventriculi quarti
t. choroidea ventriculi tertii
t. conjunctiva
t. elastica
in t.
t. subcutanea
t. submucosa
Teladorsagia davtiani
telae (*pl. of* tela)

telangiectases (*pl. of* telangiectasis)
telangiectasia
    ataxia t.
    calcinosis cutis, Raynaud
      phenomenon, sclerodactyly, and t.
      (CRST)
    calcinosis, Raynaud phenomenon,
      esophageal motility disorders,
      sclerodactyly, and t. (CREST)
    cephalooculocutaneous t.
    essential t.
    hereditary hemorrhagic t. (HHT)
    t. lymphatica
    t. macularis eruptiva perstans
    spider t.
    t. verrucosa
telangiectasis, *pl.* **telangiectases**
telangiectatic
    t. angioma
    t. angiomatosis
    t. cancer
    t. fibroma
    t. glioma
    t. lipoma
    t. osteogenic sarcoma
    t. osteosarcoma
    t. wart
telangiectatica
    livedo t.
telangiectaticum
    granuloma t.
telangiectodes
    elephantiasis t.
    neuroma t.
    purpura annularis t.
telangioma
telangion
telecytology
telehealth journal
telemedicine
telencephalization
teleomorph
teleonomy
telepathology
    dynamic real-time t.
    static t.
television microscope
tellurate
tellurite
    t. glycine agar
    t. medium
tellurium (Te)
    t. assay
Tellyesnicky fixative solution
telocentric
telodendron
telogen hair
teloglia
telolysosome

telomerase
    t. activity
    t. enzyme
    t. function
    t. repeat amplification protocol
      (TRAP)
telomere
    t. banding
    t. shortening
    t. spot
telomeric
    t. R-banding stain
    t. repeat amplification protocol
      (TRAP)
    t. repeat amplification protocol
      assay
    t. restriction fragment (TRF)
telopeptide
telophase
Telosporea
Telosporidia
TEM
    transmission electron microscope
    transmission electron microscopy
temperate
    t. bacteriophage
    t. phage
    t. virus
temperature (T)
    ambient t.
    annealing t.
    body t.
    t. coefficient (Q_{10})
    t. compensation (TC)
    corpse t.
    critical t.
    effective t. (ET)
    eutectic t.
    flash-point t.
    ignition t.
    increased t.
    maximal growth t.
    maximum t. (T-MAX, T-max, T_{max})
    melting t. (Tm)
    minimal growth t.
    minimum t.
    normal body t.
    optimal growth t.
    optimum t.
    t. programming
    room t. (RT)
    subnormal t.
    ultra low t. (ULT)
    wet bulb globe t.
temperature-gradient gel electrophoresis
  (TGGE)
temperature-sensitive
    t.-s. mutant
    t.-s. mutation

template
> t. bleeding time
> t. bleeding time method
> DNA t.

temporal
> t. arteritis
> t. cluster
> t. lobe epilepsy
> t. temperature gradient gel electrophoresis (TTGE)

temporary
> t. cartilage
> t. cavitation
> t. parasite

TEMT
> tubular epithelial-myofibroblast transdifferentiation

TEN
> toxic epidermal necrolysis

Tenacibaculum
> *T. amylolyticum*
> *T. maritimum*
> *T. mesophilum*
> *T. ovolyticum*
> *T. skagerrakense*

tenacity
> cellular t.

tenaculum

tenascin

tenascin-C

tenascin-X deficiency

tenase complex

tenax
> *Trichomonas t.*

tendency
> central t.

Tenderlett Plus finger-stick blood collection device

tender line

tendinea
> inscriptio t.
> intersectio t.
> macula t.

tendinis
> theca t.
> vagina mucosa t.
> vagina synovialis t.

tendinitis, tendonitis
> hypertrophic infiltrative t. (HIT)

tendinopathy

tendinous
> t. inscription
> t. intersection
> t. spot
> t. synovitis

tendomucin, tendomucoid

tendomucoid (*var. of* tendomucin)

tendon
> t. bundle

> t. cell
> coronary t.
> t. entrapment
> t. injury
> mucous sheath of t.
> t. organ
> t. repair
> t. rupture
> t. tear

tendonitis (*var. of* tendinitis)

tendosynovitis (*var. of* tenosynovitis)

tendovaginitis (*var. of* tenosynovitis)
> radial styloid t.

Tenebrio

tenella
> *Sarcocystis t.*

Tenericutes

tenerifensis
> *Nocardia t.*

tenesmus

tengcongensis
> *Caldanaerobacter subterraneus* subsp. *t.*
> *Thermoanaerobacter t.*

tenia, taenia, *pl.* **teniae**
> teniae coli

teniacide, taeniacide

teniae (*pl. of* tenia)

teniafuge

tenial, taenial

teniasis, taeniasis

teniform, taeniform

tenioid, taenioid

teniposide

Tenney change

tennis
> t. elbow
> t. racket cell

tenofibril

tenonitis

tenontolemmitis

tenontothecitis

tenophyte

tenoreceptor

tenositis

tenostosis

tenosynovial giant cell tumor

tenosynovitis, tendosynovitis tendovaginitis, tenovaginitis
> t. crepitans
> de Quervain t.
> localized nodular t.
> villonodular pigmented t.
> villous t.

tenovaginitis (*var. of* tenosynovitis)

tensile strength

Tensilon test

tensin gene

tension
>carbon dioxide t.
>t. cyst
>end-tidal CO_2 t.
>t. headache
>oxygen t.
>surface t. (ST)

tension-type headache
tenue
>*Eubacterium t.*

tenuicollis
>*Cysticercus t.*

tenuis
>*Alternaria t.*
>*Dirofilaria t.*
>plicae circulares intestini t.
>stratum longitudinale tunicae
> muscularis intestini t.
>*Trichostrongylus t.*
>tunica mucosa intestini t.
>tunica muscularis intestini t.
>tunica serosa intestini t.

Tenuivirus
Tephrocybe
tephromalacia
tepidarius
>*Thermithiobacillus t.*

Tepidibacter
>*T. formicigenes*
>*T. thalassicus*

Tepidimonas
>*T. aquatica*
>*T. ignava*

Tepidiphilus margaritifer
tepidum
>*Chlorobaculum t.*
>*Haliangium t.*

terahertz (THz)
terangae
>*Ensifer t.*

Terasakiella pusilla
teratoblastoma
teratocarcinoma
teratogen
teratogenesis
teratogenetic (*var. of*
  teratogenic)
teratogenic, teratogenetic
teratogenicity
teratoid tumor
teratology
teratoma
>adult cystic t.
>anaplastic malignant t.
>benign cystic t.
>cystic dermoid t.
>t. differentiated (TD)
>differentiated t.
>embryonal t.

>immature t.
>malignant trophoblastic t.
> (MTT)
>mature t.
>monodermal t.
>ovarian t.
>sacrococcygeal t.
>solid t.
>triphyllomatous t.
>trophoblastic malignant t.
>undifferentiated malignant t.

teratomatous cyst
teratospermia
terebrans
>ulcus t.

Teredinibacter turnerae
terephthalate
>polyethylene t. (PETG)

terminal
>t. addition enzyme
>amino t. (Nt)
>t. axolysis
>axon t.
>t. banding
>t. bar
>t. bouton
>t. bronchiole
>carboxyl t.
>t. cisterna
>t. deletion
>t. deoxynucleotidyltransferase
> (TdT)
>t. deoxyribonucleotidyl
> transferase
>t. differentiation
>t. duct adenocarcinoma
>t. duct carcinoma
>t. duct lobular unit (TDLU)
>t. endocarditis
>graphic t.
>t. half-life (T $\frac{1}{2}$)
>t. hematuria
>t. ileitis
>t. ileum
>t. latency
>t. leukocytosis
>t. nerve corpuscle
>smart t.
>synaptic t.
>t. web

terminale
>filum t.

terminalia
>corpuscula nervosa t.

terminalis
>crista t.

terminalization
terminally truncated variant
terminatio

termination
    t. codon
    t. factor
    t. sequence
terminator
    dideoxy t.
terminaux
terminus
Termitomyces
termone
ternary acid
Ternidens deminutus
terpene
terphase cell
terrae
    Gordonia t.
    Janibacter t.
    Mycobacterium t.
    Opitutus t.
    Sphingopyxis t.
terragena
    Demetria t.
Terranova decipiens
terrenus
    Ureibacillus t.
terrestre
    Halorubrum t.
    Trichophyton t.
terrestris
terreus
    Aspergillus t.
terricola
    Burkholderia t.
terrigena
    Raoultella t.
territorial matrix
terrorism
    agricultural t.
    biological t.
    emergency response to t. (ERT)
Terry syndrome
Terson
    T. gland
    T. syndrome
tertian
    t. fever
    t. malaria
tertiarism, tertiarismus
tertiarismus (*var. of* tertiarism)
tertiary
    t. amine
    t. blast injury
    t. cortex
    t. hyperparathyroidism
    t. structure
    t. syphilis
    t. trisomy
tertii
    tela choroidea ventriculi t.

tertium
    Clostridium t.
Teschen
    T. disease
    T. virus
TESE
    testicular sperm extraction
tesla (T)
tessellated
test
    AAN t.
    Abrams t.
    ACB t.
    Access AccuTnI t.
    Access Hybritech PSA t.
    Access Ostase t.
    AccuDx t.
    AccuTnI t.
    acetic acid and potassium
      ferrocyanide t.
    acetic acid-induced writhing t.
    acetoacetic acid t.
    acetoin t.
    acetone t.
    acetowhite t.
    acid challenge t.
    acid clearance t. (ACT)
    acid elution t.
    acid hemolysin t.
    acid hemolysis t.
    acidified serum lysis t.
    acidity reduction t.
    acid lability t.
    acidosis t.
    acid perfusion t.
    acid phosphatase t.
    acid reflux t.
    ACPA t.
    Actalyke t.
    ACTH stimulation t.
    activated partial thromboplastin
      substitution t.
    active rosette t.
    Activin AB free beta-HCG ELISA
      t.
    Adamkiewicz t.
    AD7C Alzheimer t.
    Addis t.
    adhesion t.
    Adler t.
    adrenal ascorbic acid depletion t.
    adrenal function t.
    adrenaline t.
    adrenocortical inhibition t.
    adrenocorticotropic hormone
      suppression t.
    Aeroset abused drugs/toxicology t.
    AFP t.
    agglutination t.

T

test (*continued*)
ALA t.
AlaSTAT latex allergy t.
albumin cobalt binding t.
albumin suspension t.
aldolase t.
aldosterone stimulation t.
aldosterone suppression t.
alizarin t.
alkali denaturation t.
alkaline denaturation t.
alkaline phosphatase antialkaline
    phosphatase antibody t.
alkali tolerance t.
alkaloid t.
alkaptonuria t.
Allen t.
Allen-Doisy t.
allergen challenge t.
alpha amino nitrogen t.
ALT t.
Ames t.
aminopyrine breath t. (ABT)
ammoniacal silver nitrate t.
ammonium chloride loading t.
amniotic fluid fern t.
amniotic fluid foam stability t.
amniotic fluid shake t.
AmpliChip CYP450 genotyping t.
Amplicor CT/NG t.
Amplicor HIV-1 monitor t.
amylase t.
Anderson and Goldberger t.
Anderson-Collip t.
androstenedione t.
AnemiaPro self-screening t.
AneuVysion prenatal t.
angiotensin I, II t.
anion gap t.
antibiotic sensitivity t.
antibody screening t.
anti-*Chlamydia* antibody t.
antichymotrypsin t.
antideoxyribonuclease B titer t.
antiendomysial antibody t.
antiglobulin t. (AGT)
antihuman globulin t.
anti-LA/SS-B t.
anti-Rho-D titer t.
anti-Ro/SS-A t.
anti-Sm t.
antithrombin III t.
antitrypsin t.
Anton t.
APAAP t.
APC gene stool t.
Apt t.
APTT t.
arabitol t.

arginine insulin tolerance t. (AITT)
arginine stimulation t.
arginine tolerance t. (ATT)
Argo corn starch t.
arylsulfatase t.
ascariasis serological t.
Aschheim-Zondek pregnancy t.
Ascoli t.
ascorbate-cyanide t.
ascorbic acid t.
ASO t.
Aspergillus antibody t.
ASPIRINcheck urine t.
aspirin tolerance t.
AspirinWorks diagnostic urine t.
AST t.
Astwood t.
atropine suppression t.
augmented histamine t. (AHT)
autohemolysis t.
Autolet blood glucose t.
automated reagin t. (ART)
Autopath QC t.
Aware HIV-1/2 oral fluid rapid t.
AxSYM free PSA t.
A-Z pregnancy t.
babesiosis serological t.
Babystart ovulation t.
Bachman t.
Bachman-Pettit t.
bacitracin disc t.
Baker acid hematein t.
Baker pyridine extraction t.
Bang t.
Barany caloric t.
barium t.
Barr body t.
basal gastric secretion t.
basal secretory flow rate t.
basophil degranulation t.
Bauer-Kirby t.
BCR-ABL protein t.
BD BeAware t.
Beard t.
bedtime salivary cortisol t.
BEI t.
Bence Jones protein t.
Benedict t.
bentiromide t.
bentonite flocculation t. (BFT)
benzidine t.
Bernstein t.
Berson t.
beta galactosidase t.
beta-hCG t.
beta-lactamase t.
beta quick strep t.
Betke-Kleihauer t.
Bettendorff t.

Beutler t.
BG t.
Bial t.
bicarbonate titration t.
bicolor guaiac t. (BCG)
bile acid tolerance t.
bile esculin hydrolysis t.
bile pigment t.
bile salt breath t.
bile solubility t.
bilirubin tolerance t.
Binax Now *Legionella* urine antigen t.
Binax Now Malaria T.
Binax Now *Streptococcus pneumoniae* antigen t.
Binax Now urinary antigen t.
Binz t.
Biosafe TSH t.
BioStar *Strep A* OIA MAX *Streptococcus A* t.
biuret t.
bleeding time t.
blind t.
blood urea nitrogen t.
Bloor t.
blot t.
Blount t.
Bloxam t.
Boas t.
Bonanno t.
borderline glucose tolerance t. (BGTT)
Bordet-Gengou t.
Bouchardat t.
BRACAnalysis genetic susceptibility breast and ovarian cancer t.
Bradshaw t.
breath analysis t.
BreathTek UBT *H. pylori* t.
bromocriptine suppression t.
bromphenol t.
bromsulphalein t.
bronchial challenge t.
Brucella agglutination t.
BSFR t.
BSP excretion t.
buffy coat smear t.
butanol-extractable iodine t.
calcium oxalate t.
Calmette t.
Cambridge Biotech HIV-1 urine Western blot t.
CAMP t.
CanDia5 candida rapid t.
Candida precipitin t.
candidiasis serologic t.
capillary fragility t.
capon-comb-growth t.

carbohydrate fermentation t.
carbohydrate identification t.
carbohydrate tolerance t.
carbohydrate utilization t.
carbon dioxide challenge t.
carbon dioxide combining power t.
carbon 13-labeled ketoisocaproate breath t.
carbon monoxide t.
carcinoembryonic antigen t.
Cardiac Reader D-Dimer t.
Cardiac Reader M myoglobin t.
Cardiac Reader T quantitative troponin-T t.
Cardiac STATus CK-MB t.
Cardiac STATus CK-MB/myoglobin panel t.
Cardiac STATus myoglobin/troponin I t.
Cardiac STATus rapid format troponin I panel t.
cardiolipin t.
cardiopulmonary stress t.
Carrell t.
Carr-Price t.
Casoni intradermal t.
Castellani t.
catatorulin t.
catecholamine t.
14C-cholylglycine breath excretion t.
CDC t.
CEA t.
CEDIA drug of abuse t.
cephalin-cholesterol flocculation t.
cephalin flocculation t.
cercaria-hullen reaction schistosomiasis t.
cercarien-hullen-reaktion t.
ceruloplasmin t.
cervical mucus sperm penetration t.
cetylpyridium chloride t.
CF t.
CFF t.
C-glycocholic acid breath t.
7C gold urine protein t.
Chagas disease serological t.
checkerboard microdilution t.
Chédiak t.
chemical inhibition isoamylase t.
chemiluminescence t.
Chemstrip BG t.
Chen t.
chenodeoxycholic acid t.
Cherry-Crandall serum lipase t.
Chick-Martin t.
Chlamydia trachomatis direct FA t.
Chlamydiazyme t.
chlormerodrin accumulation t. (CAT)
cholecystokinin t.

T

test (*continued*)

cholesterol t.
cholesterol-lecithin flocculation t.
cholinesterase blood t.
chorionic gonadotropin t.
chromaffin reaction t.
chromogenic cephalosporin t.
chromogenic enzyme substrate t.
cis/trans t.
citrate t.
CK-MB tandem t.
C lactose t.
Clark t.
Clauberg t.
ClearCourse solution drug screening t.
ClearView C. Diff A t.
Clinitest stool t.
CLO t.
clomiphene t.
clonidine suppression t.
coagulase t.
coagulation time t.
Cobas Amplicor HIV-1 monitor t.
$^{14}CO_2$-cholyl-glycine breath t.
cold agglutinin t.
cold hemolysin t.
collagen gel droplet-embedded drug sensitivity t. (CD-DST)
colloidal gold t.
ColorPAC toxin A t.
Coloscreen Self t.
comb-growth t.
combined pituitary function t.
compatibility t.
competitive protein-binding t.
complement direct Coombs t.
complement-fixation t. (CFT)
complement lysis sensitivity t.
concentration and dilution t.
confirmatory t.
conglutinating complement absorption t. (CCAT)
Congo red t.
contraction stress t.
Coombs t. (CT)
copper-binding protein t.
copper reduction t.
copper sulfate t.
coproporphyrin t.
corneal impression t. (CIT)
Corner-Allen t.
cortisone-glucose tolerance t. (CGTT)
cortisone-primed oral glucose tolerance t. (COGTT)
cosyntropin t.
C-peptide t.

C-reactive protein t.
creatine kinase t.
creatinine clearance t.
cresol-ammonia spot t.
critical flicker fusion t.
^{51}Cr red cell survival t.
CRSFungal Profile diagnostic t.
C&S t.
CSF glutamine t.
cutaneous tuberculin t.
cutireaction t.
^{14}C-xylose breath t.
cyanide-ascorbate t.
cyanide-nitroprusside t.
cyclic AMP t.
CYP2D6 drug screen t.
cysteine t.
cystic fibrosis t.
cystinuria t.
cytochrome oxidase t.
cytotropic antibody t.
Davidsohn differential absorption t.
Davidsohn modification of Paul-Bunnell heterophile antibody t.
Day t.
D-dimer t.
deferoxamine challenge t.
deferoxamine mesylate infusion t.
deoxycorticosterone t.
deoxycortisol t.
deoxyribonuclease t.
deoxyuridine suppression t.
dexamethasone suppression t. (DST)
dextrose t.
DFA t.
DFA-TP t.
DHEA t.
DHT t.
Diagnex Blue t.
Diatest diabetes breath t.
diazepam breath t.
Dick t.
differential renal function t.
differential ureteral catheterization t.
Digene hc2 high-risk HPV DNA t.
diluted whole blood clot lysis t.
dilution t.
dinitrophenylhydrazine t.
diphtheria t.
direct agglutination t. (DAT)
direct agglutination pregnancy t. (DAPT)
direct antiglobulin t. (DAGT, DAT)
direct bilirubin t.
direct Coombs t. (DCT)
direct fluorescent antibody t.
direct fluorescent antibody-*Treponema pallidum* t. (DFA-TP)

disaccharide tolerance t.
disc approximation synergy t.
disc diffusion t.
dithionite t.
Dixon t.
DNA-FluHunter t.
DNase t.
DNPH t.
Dold t.
Donath-Landsteiner t.
Donné t.
dot blot t.
double diffusion t.
Dragendorff t.
DR-70 tumor marker t.
DRx quantitative hCG patient
  monitor t.
Ducrey t.
Duke bleeding time t.
Duncan multiple-range t.
Dunnett multiple component t.
d-xylose absorption t.
d-xylose tolerance t.
dye exclusion t.
dye excretion t.
E t.
echinococcosis serological t.
edrophonium chloride t.
Ehrlich t.
Elecsys total PSA t.
electrophoresis t.
electrotransfer t.
Elek t.
Ellsworth-Howard t.
Emmens S/L t.
Entamoeba histolytica serological t.
EnteroScreen 4 single-tube
  pathogen t.
enzyme-linked antibody t.
enzyme-linked antiglobulin t. (ELAT)
EP t.
EPCA-2 prostate cancer t.
ergonovine provocation t.
E-rosette t.
erythrocyte adherence t.
erythrocyte fragility t.
erythrocyte protoporphyrin t.
erythropoietin t.
esculin hydrolysis t.
esophageal acid infusion t.
esterase t.
estradiol t.
estrogen stimulation t.
ethanol gelation t.
euglobulin clot t. (ECT)
euglobulin lysis t.
ExacTech blood glucose meter t.
exoantigen t.
EZ-HP *Helicobacter pylori* t.

factor V Leiden mutation t.
FANA t.
Farber t.
Farr t.
fastFISH amnio t.
fat absorption t.
febrile agglutination t.
fecal fat t.
fecal occult blood t. (FOBT)
fecal reducing substances t.
Fehling t.
fermentation t.
fern t.
ferric chloride t.
ferric ferricyanide reduction t.
FertilMARQ fertility screening t.
fetal antigen t.
fetal hemoglobin t.
Feulgen t.
FFN t.
fibrinogen titer t.
fibrinopeptide t.
fibrin stabilizing factor t.
fibrin titer t.
FIBROSpec t.
FiF t.
FIGLU excretion t.
filariasis serological t.
filter paper microscopic t.
FiltraCheck-UTI t.
Finn chamber patch t.
First Check 12 Drug t.
First Check home-screening t.
Fischer exact t.
Fishberg concentration t.
Fisher exact t.
fixation t.
Fleitmann t.
flocculation t.
flotation t.
FLU OIA A/B rapid t.
fluorescent allergosorbent t. (FAST)
fluorescent antibody t. (FAT)
fluorescent antinuclear antibody t.
fluorescent treponemal
  antibody-absorption t.
fluoroscopic diaphragmatic paralysis
  sniff t.
foam/shake t.
foam stability t.
Folin t.
Folin-Ciocalteu t.
Folin-Looney t.
foodSCAN food allergy t.
formol-gel t.
Forsure One Step Dip Read drug
  screen t.
Foshay t.
Fouchet t.

T

test (*continued*)
    fragility t.
    Francis skin t.
    free beta t.
    free protein S t.
    free/total PSA ratio t.
    free urinary cortisol t.
    Frei t.
    Friedman t.
    frog t.
    fructose t.
    FTA-ABS t.
    Gaddum and Schild t.
    galactose breath t.
    galactose tolerance t.
    GASDirect t.
    gastric acid stimulation t.
    gastric function t.
    gastrin-calcium infusion
      stimulation t.
    gastrin-protein stimulation t.
    gastrin-secretin stimulation t.
    Gastroccult t.
    gastrointestinal blood loss t.
    gastrointestinal protein loss t.
    gel diffusion precipitin t.
    Genetic Systems HIV-1 Western
      blot t.
    Geraghty t.
    Gerhardt ferric chloride t.
    germination tube t.
    germ tube t.
    Gibson-Cooke sweat t.
    globulin t.
    glucagon response t.
    glucose fingerstick t.
    glucose insulin tolerance t. (GITT)
    glucose oxidase t.
    glucose oxidase paper strip t.
    glucose-6-phosphate dehydrogenase t.
    glucose suppression t.
    glucose tolerance t. (GTT)
    glutathione instability t.
    glutathione stability t.
    glycogen storage t.
    glycolic acid t.
    glycosylated hemoglobin t.
    glycyltryptophan t.
    glyoxylic acid t.
    Gmelin t.
    Gofman t.
    gold sol t.
    gonadotropin t.
    gonadotropin-releasing hormone
      stimulation t.
    Gordon t.
    Göthlin capillary fragility t.
    Graham-Cole t.
    Gravindex pregnancy t.

    growth hormone suppression t.
    GSR t.
    guaiac t.
    guaiac-based fecal occult blood t.
    Gunning-Lieben t.
    Günzberg t.
    Guthrie t.
    Gutzeit t.
    Haagensen t.
    Haenszel t.
    HAIRscreen drug t.
    Hamel t.
    Hammarsten t.
    Ham paroxysmal nocturnal
      hemoglobinuria t.
    hamster egg penetration t.
    Hanger t.
    haptoglobin t.
    Harris and Ray t.
    Harrison t.
    hatching t.
    hc2 CMV DNA t.
    hc2 HPV DNA t.
    HealthCheck HDL home-screening t.
    HealthCheck One-Step One Minute
      pregnancy t.
    HealthCheck total cholesterol
      home-screening t.
    HealthEssist urine-based t.
    heat coagulation t.
    heat instability t.
    heat labile t.
    heat precipitation t.
    heat stability t.
    heavy metal screening t.
    Heinz body t.
    Helicobacter pylori breath t.
    Helicobacter pylori gII t.
    Helisal rapid blood t.
    hemadsorption inhibition t.
    hemadsorption virus t.
    hemagglutination t.
    hemagglutination-inhibition t. (HIT)
    hematein t.
    Hematest reagent tablet t.
    heme t.
    heme-porphyrin fecal occult blood t.
    Hemoccult fecal occult blood t.
    Hemoccult II Sensa fecal occult
      blood t.
    hemodilution t.
    hemoglobin S t.
    HemoQuant fecal blood t.
    hemosiderin t.
    hemosiderinuria t.
    Henry fructose t.
    hepatic function t.
    hepatitis B surface antigen t.
    HercepTest immunohistochemical t.

HER-2/neu serum t.
Herter t.
heterophil antibody t.
Hickey-Hare t.
Hicks-Pitney thromboplastin
  generation t.
Hinton t.
hippuric acid excretion t.
Histalog t.
histamine flare t.
histamine stimulation t.
histidine loading t.
histoplasmin-latex t.
Hivagen t.
HIV antibody t.
Hoesch t.
Hoffman t.
Hofmeister t.
Hogben t.
Hollander t.
Home Access hepatitis C Check t.
homocystinuria t.
homogentisic acid t.
homovanillic acid t.
Hooker-Forbes t.
Hopkins-Cole t.
Hoppe-Seyler t.
2-hour postprandial blood sugar t.
2-hour postprandial plasma
  glucose t.
Howard t.
Howell prothrombin t.
Huddleston agglutination t.
Huhner t.
human chorionic gonadotropin
  injection t.
human erythrocyte agglutination t.
  (HEAT)
human growth hormone
  stimulation t.
human papillomavirus DNA probe t.
HVA t.
Hybrid Capture 2 Chlamydia t.
Hybrid Capture 2 HPV DNA t.
Hybritech free PSA t.
Hybritech PSA blood t.
hydrostatic t.
hydroxybutyric t.
17-hydroxycorticosteroid t.
5-hydroxyindoleacetic t.
17-hydroxyprogesterone t.
IBD First Step t.
ice water calorics t.
ICG excretion t.
Icon 25 hCG t.
icterus index t.
Ide t.
IDI-Strep B t.
Immulite 1000 free PSA t.

Immulite 2000 free PSA t.
Immulite free PSA t.
immune adhesion t.
immunoassay fecal occult blood t.
  (iFOBT)
immunoblot t.
ImmunoCard STAT! rotavirus t.
immunochemical fecal occult
  blood t.
ImmunoCyt cytopathology recurrent
  bladder cancer t.
ImmunoDip urinary albumin t.
immunofluorescence t. (IFT)
immunoglobulin A, D, E,G, M t.
immunologic pregnancy t.
immunoperoxidase t.
implantation t. (IT)
indican t.
indigo-carmine t.
indirect antiglobulin t.
indirect bilirubin t.
indirect Coombs t.
indirect fluorescent antibody t.
indirect hemagglutination t.
indirect immunofluorescence t.
indocyanine green t.
indophenol t.
infectious mononucleosis screening t.
influenza t.
ingestion challenge t.
inhibition t.
In-Line Strep A t.
inosithin neutralization t.
Instant-View fecal occult blood t.
INSTI HIV-1 rapid antibody t.
insulin clearance t.
insulin-glucose tolerance t.
insulin hypoglycemia t.
insulin sensitivity t. (IST)
insulin tolerance t. (ITT)
InSure fecal immunochemical t.
interference t.
intracavernous injection t.
intradermal t. (IT)
intraesophageal pH t.
intravenous glucose tolerance t.
  (IVGTT)
intravenous tolbutamide tolerance t.
  (IVTTT)
invasive activity t. (IAT)
in vivo compatibility t.
iodine t.
iodine-azide t. (IAT)
iodine-131 uptake t.
iron-binding capacity t.
islet cell antibody screening t.
isocitrate dehydrogenase t.
isoniazid phenotype t.
isopropanol precipitation t.

T

test (*continued*)

Ito-Reenstierna t.
[131]I uptake t.
Ivy bleeding time t.
Jacquemin t.
Jaffe t.
Jaworski t.
Jolles t.
Jones-Cantarow t.
Kahn t.
Katayama t.
Keto-Diastix urine ketone and glucose t.
ketogenic corticoid t.
ketone body t.
KidneyScreen At·Home mail-in t.
Kirby-Bauer t.
Kleihauer t.
Kleihauer-Betke t.
Kober t.
KOH t.
Kolmer t.
Kowarsky t.
Krokiewicz t.
Kruskal-Wallis t.
Kunkel t.
Kurzrok-Ratner t.
Kveim t.
Kveim-Stilzbach t.
lactate dehydrogenase t.
lactic dehydrogenase t.
lactose tolerance t.
Ladendorff t.
LAL gram-negative bacteria t.
Lancefield precipitation t.
Landsteiner-Donath t.
Lang t.
Lange colloidal gold t.
LAP t.
latex agglutination t.
latex agglutination-inhibition t. (LAIT)
latex fixation t.
latex flocculation t. (LFT)
latex particle agglutination t.
latex slide agglutination t.
LATS t.
LE cell t.
Lee-White clotting t.
Legal t.
leishmaniasis serological t.
lepromin skin t.
leucine aminopeptidase t.
leucine tolerance t.
leukoagglutinin t.
leukocyte adherence assay t.
leukocyte bactericidal assay t.
leukocyte esterase t. (LET)
leukocyte histamine release t.

Levinson t.
levulose tolerance t.
LHMT t.
Liebermann-Burchard t.
limulus lysate t.
line t.
lipase t.
lipid t.
Lipoprint LDL subfraction t.
lipoprotein electrophoresis t.
liver flocculation t.
liver function t.'s (LFT)
Lowenthal t.
Lücke t.
lupus band t.
lymphocyte transfer t.
lymphocyte transformation t.
lysozyme t.
Machado-Guerreiro t.
macrophage migration inhibition t.
magnesium t.
malaria film t.
male frog t.
male toad t.
mallein t.
Malmejde t.
mammary aspiration specimen cytology t. (MASCT)
Mantoux skin t.
mast cell degranulation t.
Master 2-step t.
mastic t.
maximal Histalog t.
Mazzotti t.
McNemar t.
McPhail t.
t. meal
Meinicke t.
melanin t.
melanogen t.
menopause home t.
metabisulfite t.
metachromatic stain t.
metanephrine t.
methanol t.
methionine t.
methoxy-4-hydroxymandelic acid t.
methylene blue t.
methyl red t.
Metopirone t.
Metra DPD t.
metrotrophic t.
metyrapone stimulation t.
Micral urine dipstick t.
microalbumin t.
microbore t.
Microflow t.
microhemagglutination-*Treponema pallidum* t.

microimmunofluorescence t.
microlymphocytotoxicity t.
microprecipitation t.
microsomal thyroid antibody t.
Middlebrook-Dubos
  hemagglutination t.
MIF t.
migration inhibition t.
migration-inhibitory factor t.
Millon-Nasse t.
minimum bactericidal
  concentration t.
mixed agglutination t.
mixed lymphocyte culture t.
MLC t.
mobilization t.
Molisch t.
Moloney t.
monocyte function t.
Mono-Diff t.
MonoPrep Pap t. (MPPT)
Monoscreen t.
monospecific direct Coombs t.
Monospot t.
Monosticon Dri-Dot t.
Mono-Vacc t.
Montenegro skin t.
Mörner t.
Mosenthal t.
motility t.
Motulsky dye reduction t.
mucin clot t.
mucopolysaccharide t.
mucoprotein t.
Mulder t.
multiple antigen stimulation t.
  (MAST)
multiple puncture tuberculin t.
multipuncture tuberculin skin t.
multithread allergosorbent t. (MAST)
mumps sensitivity t.
Murex *Candida albicans* CA50 t.
Murphy-Pattee t.
mutagenicity t.
MycoAKT latex bead
  agglutination t.
myoglobin cardiac diagnostic t.
myoglobin clearance t.
NAP bacteria differentiation t.
Napier formol-gel t.
nares swab anthrax spore t.
neonatal thyroid-stimulating
  hormone t.
neoprecipitin t. (NPT)
neutralization t. (NT)
niacin t.
Nickerson-Kveim t.
Nicklès t.
nicotine t.

nighttime salivary cortisol t.
nitrate reduction t.
nitrate utilization t.
nitric acid t.
nitrite t.
nitroblue tetrazolium t.
nitropropiol t.
nitroprusside t.
nitroso-indole-nitrate t.
N-MID osteocalcin ELISA t.
NMP22 BladderChek t.
nocturnal penile tumescence t.
Nonne t.
nonprotein nitrogen t.
nonstress t. (NST)
nontreponemal antibody t.
normal lymphocyte transfer t. (NLT)
Northern blot t.
novel microbiology t.
novel toxicology t.
nucleic acid t.
nucleic acid amplification t. (NAT)
OAAD t.
Obermayer t.
Obermüller t.
OBIS albicans rapid colorimetric t.
t. object
occult blood t. (OBT)
t. of significance (t)
17-OH corticoid t.
oleic acid uptake t.
one-stage prothrombin time t.
One-Step hCG combo t.
one-tailed t.
ONPG t.
O&P t.
Optochin susceptibility t.
oral glucose tolerance t. (OGTT)
oral lactose tolerance t.
OralScreen 3-panel oral fluids t.
OralScreen 4 substance abuse t.
OraQuick rapid HIV-1 antibody t.
OraTest oral cancer t.
orcinol t.
osazone t.
osmotic fragility t.
OsteoGram bone density t.
Osteosal osteoporosis t.
Ouchterlony t.
ovarian tumor triage t.
ovulation t.
oxidase t.
oxidation-fermentation t.
oxytocin challenge t. (OCT)
p-aminohippurate clearance t.
t. paper
pineapple t.
pine wood t.
Pirquet cutaneous tuberculin t.

T

test (*continued*)
 pituitary function t.
 PKU t.
 PLAC coronary heart disease t.
 placental and fetoplacental function t.'s
 plant protease t. (PPT)
 plasma cortisol t.
 plasmacrit t.
 plasma hemoglobin t.
 platelet adhesion t.
 platelet adhesiveness t.
 platelet aggregation t.
 platelet function t.
 platelet retention t.
 platelet survival t.
 Porges-Meier t.
 Porges-Salomon t.
 porphobilinogen t.
 porphyrin t.
 Porter-Silber chromogen t.
 Porteus maze t.
 positive-pressure t.
 positive whiff t.
 potassium hydroxide t.
 P&P t.
 PP-CAP IgA enzyme immunoassay t.
 PPD skin t.
 Prausnitz-Küstner t.
 prealbumin t.
 precipitation t.
 precipitin t.
 Precision-G handheld blood glucose t.
 Precision QI-D handheld blood glucose t.
 Pre-Gen 26 colorectal cancer t.
 pregnancy t.
 presumptive heterophil t.
 prick t.
 t. profile
 Profile-ER one-step qualitative drug t.
 prolactin t.
 Pro-PredictRx diagnostic t.
 prostaglandin t.
 protamine sulfate t.
 protamine titration t.
 protection t.
 protein t.
 protein-bound iodine t.
 protein-bound iodine-131 t.
 ProteinChip t.
 protein truncation t.
 prothrombin and proconvertin t.
 prothrombin consumption t.
 prothrombin time t.
 Protocult t.

 protoporphyrin t.
 provocative chelation t.
 provocative Wassermann t.
 pulmonary capacity t.
 pulmonary function t.'s (PFT)
 purified protein derivative skin t.
 purine bodies t.
 qualitative fecal fat t.
 qualitative urine myoglobin dipstick t.
 QuantiFERON-TB t.
 quantitation t.
 Queckenstedt t.
 quellung t.
 Quick tourniquet t.
 QuickVue Advance *Gardnerella vaginalis* t.
 QuickVue Advance pH and amines t.
 QuickVue *Chlamydia* t.
 QuickVue *H. pylori* gII t.
 QuickVue iFOB t.
 QuickVue+ infectious mononucleosis t.
 QuickVue influenza t.
 QuickVue 1 step *Helicobacter pylori* t.
 QuickVue UrinChek 10+ urine t.
 quinine carbacrylic resin t.
 Quinlan t.
 QuPID pregnancy t.
 rabbit t.
 radioactive fibrinogen uptake t.
 radioactive iodide uptake t.
 radioactive iodine uptake t.
 radioallergosorbent assay t. (RAST)
 radioimmunosorbent t. (RIST)
 radioisotope renal excretion t.
 radiosensitivity t. (RST)
 RAI t.
 RA latex fixation t.
 RAMP anthrax t.
 RAMP botulinum toxin t.
 RAMP heart attack t.
 RAMP myoglobin t.
 RAMP ricin t.
 RAMP smallpox t.
 RAMP West Nile Virus t.
 random plasma glucose t.
 rank sum t.
 rapid ACTH t.
 RapID ANA II t.
 rapid corticotropin t.
 Rapid flu A&B t.
 Rapid One lateral flow immunoassay t.
 rapid plasma reagin circle card t. (RPR-CT)

rapid serum amylase t.
rapid urease t. (RUT)
RapiTex ASO latex
  agglutination t.
RapiTex Hp t.
Rapoport t.
reactone red t.
t. reagent
red cell adherence t.
red cell survival t.
Reinsch t.
renal function t.
renin stimulation t.
resorcinol t.
respiratory syncytial virus
  antibody t.
respiratory syncytial virus
  antigen t.
Reuss t.
Revival Menopause Home T.
Rh blocking t.
rheumatoid factor t.
riboflavin loading t.
ribonucleoprotein antibody t.
rice-flour breath t.
RIM A.R.C. Mono t.
Rimini t.
ring precipitin t.
Rinkel t.
Rinne t. (R)
RISA t.
Rocky Mountain spotted fever
  antibody t.
Römer t.
Ropes t.
Rose t.
rose bengal radioactive ^{131}I t.
Rosenbach t.
Rosenbach-Gmelin t.
rosette t.
Rose-Waaler t.
Ross-Jones t.
Rotazyme t.
Rothera nitroprusside t.
Rotter t.
Rous t.
Rowntree and Geraghty t.
RPCF t.
RPR t.
rubella antibody t.
rubella HI t.
Rubin t.
Rubner t.
Rumpel-Leede t.
Sabin-Feldman dye t.
Sachs-Georgi t.
SalEst t.
salicylic acid t.
saline agglutination t.

saline infusion primary
  hyperaldosteronism t.
saliva ovulation t.
salivary urate t.
Sanford t.
SAS Rota t.
Saundby t.
scarification t.
Schaffer t.
Schick t.
Schiller t.
Schilling t.
Schirmer t.
schistosomiasis serological t.
Schmidt t.
Schönbein t.
Schultz-Dale t.
Schultze t.
Schumm t.
Schwarz t.
scratch t.
screening t.
secretin-cholecystokinin-
  pancreatozymin
  stimulation t.
secretin pancreozymin t.
sedimentation rate t. (SRT)
SeHCAT t.
Selivanoff t.
Semi-Q hCG combo t.
sensitive membrane antigen rapid t.
  (SMART)
Sereny t.
serodiagnostic t.
serology t.
serum alkaline phosphatase t.
serum amylase t.
serum bacterial t.
serum bactericidal t. (SBT)
serum bilirubin t.
serum calcium t.
serum creatine kinase t.
serum creatinine t.
serum enzyme t.
serum globulin t.
serum phosphorus t.
serum protein electrophoresis t.
sex chromatin t. (SCT)
shake t.
sheep cell agglutination t. (SCAT)
Shigella rapid latex t.
sickle cell t.
sickle cell anemia t. (SCAT)
Sickledex t.
Sicklequik t.
sickling t.
signed rank t.
Signify DOA t.
Signify ER drug screen t.

T

test (*continued*)
  silver nitroprusside t.
  Sims-Huhner t.
  SISI t.
  skin-puncture t.
  skin window t.
  slide agglutination t.
  slide bile solubility t.
  slide flocculation t.
  slide platelet aggregation t.
    (SPAT)
  SMAC t.
  SMA-12 profile t.
  smear t.
  sodium t.
  sodium metabisulfite sickle
    hemoglobin t.
  solubility t.
  t. solution (TS)
  Southern blot t.
  soybean t.
  specific gravity t.
  spectroscopic t.
  spironolactone t.
  split collection urine t.
  split renal function t.
  spot t.
  Stamey t.
  standard acid reflux t. (SART)
  standing plasma t.
  Staph-Ident t.
  Staph-Trac t.
  staphylococcal clumping t. (SCT)
  starch hydrolysis t.
  starch tolerance t.
  StarTox 5 drugs of abuse
    screening t.
  stat t.
  t. statistic
  Sterneedle tuberculin t.
  Stokvis t.
  stool guaiac t.
  stool reducing substances t.
  Strassburg t.
  streptococcal antigen t.
  streptolysin O t.
  streptozyme t.
  Student t.
  Student-Newman-Keuls t.
  Stypven time t.
  sucrose hemolysis t.
  SUDS HIV-1 t.
  sulfosalicylic acid turbidity t.
  Sulkowitch t.
  susceptibility t.
  sweat t.
  syphilis t.
  t t.
  Takata-Ara t.

  tanned red cell hemagglutination
    inhibition t.
  Tardieu t.
  TCPI Rapid HIV t.
  TCR Vgamma9 t.
  Tensilon t.
  tetrazolium t.
  Thayer-Martin t.
  thermostable opsonin t.
  thiamine t.
  thiobarbituric acid t. (TBA)
  Thompson t.
  Thormählen t.
  Thorn t.
  three-glass t.
  thrombin time t.
  thromboplastin activation t. (TAT)
  thromboplastin generation t. (TGT)
  thromboplastin substitution t.
  Thrombo-Wellcotest t.
  Thudichum t.
  thymol turbidity t.
  thyroid antibody t.
  thyroid function t. (TFT)
  thyroid-stimulating hormone
    stimulation t.
  thyroid suppression t.
  thyroid uptake t.
  thyrotropin-releasing hormone
    challenge t.
  thyrotropin-releasing hormone
    stimulation t.
  thyroxine-binding index t.
  TIBC t.
  time-kill kinetics t.
  tine t.
  tissue oxidase t.
  tissue thromboplastin inhibition t.
    (TTIT)
  titratable acidity t.
  toad t.
  tolbutamide t. (TBT)
  tolbutamide tolerance t. (TTT)
  Töpfer t.
  total catecholamine t.
  TPH t.
  TPI t.
  transaminase t.
  transferrin t.
  treponemal antibody t. (TAT)
  treponemal immobilization t.
  Treponema pallidum complement
    fixation t.
  TRH stimulation t.
  Triage BNP t.
  triiodothyronine resin uptake t.
  triiodothyronine suppression t.
  Trinder t.
  triple t.

Trousseau t.
trypsin t.
tryptophan challenge t.
tryptophan load t.
TSH stimulating t.
TSH stimulation t.
T_3U t.
t. tube
tube dilution t.
tubeless gastric analysis t.
tuberculin skin t.
tuberculosis skin t.
tubular reabsorption of phosphate t.
tumor marker t.
tumor skin t. (TST)
T_3 uptake t.
two-glass t.
two-stage PT t.
two-tail t.
typhus antibody t.
tyramine t.
tyrosine t.
Tzanck t.
Uffelmann t.
unheated serum reagin t.
Uni-Gold *H. pylori* t.
Uni-Gold Recombigen HIV t.
Uni-Gold Recombigen rapid HIV antibody t.
urea breath t. (UBT)
urea clearance t.
urea concentration t.
urea nitrogen t.
urease t.
urecholine supersensitivity t.
uric acid t.
Uricult dipslide t.
urinary concentration t.
urine acetone t.
urine amylase excretion t.
urine myoglobin t.
urine spot t.
Uriscreen t.
UriSite microalbumin/creatinine urine t.
Uri-Test protein in urine t.
urobilinogen t.
uroporphyrin t.
UroVysion bladder cancer recurrence t.
UroVysion FISH t.
Valentine t.
van Deen t.
van den Bergh t.
van der Velden t.
vanillylmandelic acid t.
Van Slyke t.
VAP cholesterol t.
varicella-zoster antibody t.

VDRL t.
Verdict-II drug screening t.
Vgamma9 t.
ViraPap t.
virus neutralization t.
visual fluorescent screening t.
vitamin A clearance t.
vitamin B_{12} absorption t.
VMA t.
Voges-Proskauer t.
Volhard t.
Vollmer t.
t. volume
VP t.
Wagner t.
Waldenström t.
Wang t.
Wassén t.
Wassermann t.
water deprivation diabetes insipidus differentiation t.
water gurgle t.
water loading t.
Watson-Schwartz t.
Weber t.
Webster t.
Weil-Felix t.
Welcozyme HIV 12 ELISA antibody t.
Werner t.
Westergren sedimentation rate t.
Western blot electrotransfer t.
Western immunoblot t.
West Nile virus IgM capture t.
Wetzel t.
wheal-and-erythema skin t.
Wheeler-Johnson t.
whiff t.
Whipple t.
Widal serum t.
wire-loop t.
Wormley t.
Wurster t.
Xenopus laevis t.
Xpert EV meningitis t.
Xpert EV rapid viral meningitis t.
Xpert MRSA t.
xylose absorption t.
xylose concentration t.
Yvon t.
Zimmermann t.
zinc flocculation t.
zinc sulfate turbidity t.
Zollinger-Ellison t.
zona-free hamster egg penetration t.
Zsigmondy t.

testacea
  Nocardia t.
Testacealobosia

testcross
tester
    Novapath HIV-1 immunoblot t.
testes (*pl. of* testis)
testi
    tubuli seminiferi recti t.
testibumin
testicular
    t. agenesis
    t. cancer
    t. duct
    t. dysgenesis
    t. failure
    t. feminization
    t. feminization syndrome (Tfm, TFS)
    t. germ cell tumor (TGCT)
    t. hormone
    t. regression syndrome
    t. Sertoli cell tumor
    t. sperm extraction (TESE)
    t. torsion
    t. tubular adenoma
testicular-splenic fusion
testing
    antibacterial agent susceptibility t.
    avidity t.
    bacterial susceptibility t.
    biochemical t.
    calcitonin t.
    cardiopulmonary exercise t.
    confirmatory t.
    Crithidia immunofluorescence t.
    direct immunofluorescence t.
    epicutaneous t.
    evocative t.
    forensic urine drug t. (FUDT)
    fungal skin t.
    histocompatibility t.
    homocysteine t.
    homocystine t.
    human genetic identity t.
    hypothesis t.
    Intercept oral fluid drug t.
    intracutaneous allergy t.
    intracutaneous tuberculin skin t.
    intradermal allergy t.
    minipool nucleic acid t.
    molecular resistance t.
    multiple puncture tuberculin skin t.
    neonatal t.
    neuromuscular junction t.
    nucleic acid amplification t.
    point-of-care t. (POCT)
    point of care INR t.
    polymerase chain reaction-based identity t.

presumptive t.
proficiency t.
reflective t.
semiautomated susceptibility t.
specific IgE antibody t.
susceptibility t.
thallium stress t.
testis, *pl.* **testes**
    t. carcinoma
    cryptorchid t.
    ductuli efferentes t.
    dysgenetic testes
    ectopia t.
    ectopic t.
    t. inflammation
    interstitial cell tumor of t.
    inverted t.
    lobule of t.
    lobuli t.
    movable t.
    obstructed t.
    retained t.
    rete t.
    retractile t.
    septulum t.
    torsion of t.
    trabecula t.
    tubule of t.
    tunica albuginea t.
    tunica vaginalis t.
    tunica vasculosa t.
    undescended t.
testis-determining factor (TDF)
testitis (*var. of* orchitis)
testoid hyperthecosis
testos
    testosterone
testosterone production rate (TPR)
testosterone-binding affinity (TBA)
testosterone-estradiol binding globulin (TeBG)
testosteroni
    Pseudomonas t.
TestPackChlamydia
testudineum
    Mycoplasma t.
testudinoris
    Corynebacterium t.
tet
    tetralogy of Fallot
tetani
    Bacillus t.
    Clostridium t.
tetanizing
tetanolysin
tetanomorphum
    Clostridium t.
tetanospasmin

tetanotoxin
tetanus
- t. antibody
- t. antitoxin (TAT)
- t. antitoxin unit
- t. bacillus
- t. immune globulin
- t. immunoglobulin
- t. toxin
- t. toxin immunization reaction
- t. vaccine

tetanus-diphtheria (TD)
tetanus-perfringens antitoxin
tetany
Tete virus
Tetko nylon mesh filter
tetraborate
- sodium t.

tetrabrachius
- dicephalus dipus t.

tetracaine, Adrenalin (epinephrine), and cocaine
tetracarcinoma cell
tetrachloride
- carbon t. (CCl4)

2,3,7,8-tetrachlorodibenzo-p-dioxin (TCDD)
tetrachlorodiphenylethane (TDE)
tetrachloroethane poisoning
tetrachloroethylene
tetrachrome stain
tetracycline
tetrad
tetradecapeptide
tetradius
- Anaerococcus t.

tetraethylammonium
tetragena
- Entamoeba t.
- Gaffkya t.

Tetragonolobus purpureas lectin stain
tetrahedron chest
tetrahydrobiopterin
tetrahydrocannabinol (THC)
tetrahydrochloride
- diaminobenzidine t.

tetrahydrocortisol (THC)
tetrahydrocortisone (THE)
tetrahydrodeoxycorticosterone (THDOC)
tetrahydro-11-deoxycortisol
tetrahydrofolate dehydrogenase
tetrahydrofolic acid
tetrahydrofuran
tetrahydropteroylglutamate methyltransferase
6-tetrahydropyridine (var. of 1-methyl-4-phenyl-1,2,3,6-tetrahydropyridine)

Tetrahymena pyriformis
tetralogy
- t. of Eisenmenger
- t. of Fallot (tet, TF)

tetramastigote
tetramer analysis
Tetrameres strigiphila
tetramethyl acridine
tetramethylbenzidine
- t. chromogen
- t. stain

tetramethylcarbazole
tetra-methylrhodamine ethyl ester (TMRE)
tetramethylrhodamine isothiocyanate (XRITC)
Tetramitidae
tetranectin
tetranitrate
tetranucleotide
tetraodonis
- Pseudoalteromonas t.

tetraONE system
tetraparesis
Tetrapetalonema
tetraplegia
Tetraploa aristata
tetraploidization
tetraploid tumor
tetraploidy
tetraptera
- Aspiculuris t.

tetrasomic
tetrasomy
Tetrasphaera
- T. australiensis
- T. elongata
- T. japonica

tetrathionate enrichment broth
Tetratrichomonas
- T. buccalis
- T. hominis
- T. ovis

tetravalent
tetra-X chromosomal aberration
tetrazole
tetrazolium
- nitroblue t. (NBT)
- t. reduction (TR)
- t. reduction inhibition (TRI)
- t. salt solution
- t. test

tetrazonium salt
tetrin macrolide antibiotic
tetrodotoxin
tetrose
tetroxide
- dinitrogen t.
- osmium t. (OsO4)

T

tetter
    honeycomb t.
textiform
textiloma
textural
texture
    fractal t.
    markovian t.
textus
TF
    tetralogy of Fallot
    thymol flocculation
    tissue-damaging factor
    tissue factor
    transfer factor
    tuberculin filtrate
    tubular fluid
TFA
    total fatty acid
TFAA
    trifluoroacetic anhydride
TFF [1–3]
    trefoil family factor
TFI
    tubular-fertility index
TFL
    tumefactive fibroinflammatory lesion
        TFL of head and neck
TFPI
    tissue factor pathway inhibitor
TFS
    testicular feminization syndrome
TFT
    thyroid function test
TG
    thyroglobulin
    toxic goiter
    triglyceride
TGA
    transposition of great arteries
TGase
    transglutaminase
Tg cell
TGCT
    testicular germ cell tumor
TGE
    transmissible gastroenteritis
        TGE virus
TGF
    T-cell growth factor
TGGE
    temperature-gradient gel
        electrophoresis
TGT
    thromboplastin generation test
    thromboplastin generation time
TGV
    thoracic gas volume
    transposition of great vessels

TH
    thermite
    tyrosine hydroxylase
Th
    thorium
thailandensis
        Weissella t.
thalamic hyperesthetic anesthesia
thalassanemia (*var. of* thalassemia)
thalassemia, thalassanemia
    alpha t.
    beta-delta t.
    delta t.
    F t.
    gamma t.
    hemoglobin SC-alpha t.
    heterozygous t.
    heterozygous alpha t. 1
    homozygous t.
    homozygous alpha t. 1, 2
    t. intermedia
    Lepore t.
    t. major
    t. minor
    mixed t.
    sickle cell beta t.
    silent t.
    t. syndrome
    t. trait
thalassemia-sickle cell disease
thalassicus
        Tepidibacter t.
Thalassolituus oleivorans
Thalassomonas
        T. ganghwensis
        T. viridans
Thalassospira lucentensis
thalidomide
thallasanemia (*var. of* thalassemia)
thallic
thallitoxicosis
thallium (Tl)
    t. assay
    t. poisoning
    t. stress testing
    t. sulfate
Thallophyta
thallophyte
thallospore
thallus
Thamnidium
Thamnostylum
Thanatephorus
thanatophoric dwarfism
thanatopsia (*var. of* thanatopsy)
thanatopsy, thanatopsia
thapsigargin
Thauera
        T. aminoaromatica

T. chlorobenzoica
T. phenylacetica
thaumatropy
Thaumetopoea
Thaumetopoeidae
Thayer-Martin
    T.-M. agar
    T.-M. medium
    T.-M. test
Thaysen disease
THBR
    thyroid hormone binding ratio
THC
    tetrahydrocannabinol
    tetrahydrocortisol
THDOC
    tetrahydrodeoxycorticosterone
THE
    tetrahydrocortisone
thebaine
The Bethesda System (TBS)
theca
    t. cell-granuloma cell tumor
    t. cell of stomach
    t. cordis
    t. externa
    t. folliculi
    t. interna
    t. interna cell
    t. interna cone
    t. lutein cell
    t. lutein cyst
    t. lutein tumor
    t. tendinis
thecitis
thecoma
thecomatosis
Theile gland
Theiler
    T. disease
    T. mouse encephalomyelitis
     virus
    T. original virus
theileri
    Trypanosoma t.
Theileria
theileriasis
Theileriidae
theileriosis
Thelazia
    T. californiensis
    T. callipaeda
thelaziasis
Thelebolus
thelia (*pl. of* thelium)
theliolymphocyte
thelium, *pl.* **thelia**
theloncus
T-helper/inducer subset marker

Theobald Smith phenomenon
theobromae
    Botryodiplodia t.
theophylline
    AccuMeter t.
    t. assay
theorem
    Bayes t.
    Bernoulli t.
    central limit t.
theoretical plate
theory
    Altmann t.
    Arrhenius t.
    Arrhenius-Madsen t.
    cellular immune t.
    clonal deletion t.
    clonal selection t.
    Cohnheim t.
    deletion t.
    Ehrlich side-chain t.
    emigration t.
    fitter cell t.
    Frerichs t.
    gametoid t.
    germ t.
    information t.
    instructive t.
    kern-plasma relation t.
    Metchnikoff t.
    monophyletic t.
    myelostimulatory t.
    neoplastic t.
    polyphyletic t.
    Ribbert t.
    side-chain t.
    Warburg t.
thèque
therapeutic
    t. abortion (TA, TAb, TAB)
    t. cloning
    t. cytapheresis
    t. drug level
    t. drug monitoring (TDM)
    t. malaria
    t. phlebotomy
    t. plasma exchange
    t. pneumothorax
    t. ratio
therapia (*var. of* therapy)
therapy, therapia
    allogeneic cellular immune t.
    (ACIT)
    alpha interferon t.
    anticoagulant t. (ACT)
    antimicrobial t.
    autoserum t.
    cancer management t.
    chelation t.

T

therapy (*continued*)
    corticosteroid t.
    cytoreductive t.
    desensitization t.
    eradication t.
    fibrinolytic t.
    foreign protein t.
    gene t.
    glucocorticoid t.
    gold t.
    heterovaccine t.
    hormonal t.
    induction t.
    insulin coma t. (ICT)
    insulin shock t. (IST)
    L-asparaginase t.
    t. magna sterilisans
    methylprednisdone pulse t.
        (MPPT)
    molecularly targeted t.
    myeloablative t.
    nonspecific t.
    obidoxime t.
    plasma t.
    protein shock t.
    radiation t.
    risk-adapted t.
    salvage t.
    serum t.
    thrombolytic t.
    warfarin t.
**TheraTest Laboratories EL-RF test kit
  system**
Thermaceae
thermacidophilum
    Bifidobacterium thermacidophilum
    subsp. *t.*
Thermaerobacter
    T. nagasakiensis
    T. subterraneus
thermal
    t. conductivity (λ, TC)
    t. conductivity detector
    t. death point
    t. death time
    t. equilibrium
    t. neutron
Thermales
Thermanaeromonas toyohensis
Thermanaerovibrio
    T. acidaminovorans
    T. velox
thermantarcticus
    Bacillus t.
thermautotrophica
    Carboxydocella t.
thermelometer
Thermicanus aegyptius
thermionic emission

thermistor
thermite (TH)
Thermithiobacillus tepidarius
Thermoactinomyces
    T. candidus
    T. sacchari
    T. vulgaris
thermo agent
Thermoanaerobacter
    T. subterraneus
    T. tengcongensis
    T. yonseiensis
Thermoanaerobacterium
    T. polysaccharolyticum
    T. saccharolyticum
    T. zeae
Thermoascus aurantiacus
Thermobacillus xylanilyticus
thermocatenulatus
    Geobacillus t.
Thermococcaceae
Thermococcales
Thermococci
Thermococcus
    T. acidaminovorans
    T. aegaeus
    T. alcaliphilus
    T. atlanticus
    T. barophilus
    T. gammatolerans
    T. sibiricus
    T. siculi
    T. waiotapuensis
thermocoprophilus
    Streptomyces t.
thermocouple thermometer
Thermocrinis albus
thermocycler
    GeneAmp PCR System 9600
    t.
thermodenitrificans
    Bacillus t.
    Geobacillus t.
thermodepolymerans
    Schlegelella t.
Thermodesulfatator indicus
Thermodesulfobacteria
Thermodesulfobacteriaceae
Thermodesulfobacteriales
Thermodesulfobacterium
    T. hveragerdense
    T. hydrogeniphilum
Thermodesulfobiaceae
Thermodesulfobium narugense
Thermodesulfovibrio islandicus
thermodilution method
Thermodiscus maritimus
thermoduric
thermodynamic equilibrium

thermodynamics
thermoferrooxidans
    Leptospirillum t.
Thermofilaceae
thermogenesis
    shivering t.
thermogenic action
thermoglucosidasius
    Geobacillus t.
thermograph
Thermohalobacter berrensis
thermohalophila
    Anaerophaga t.
thermolabile opsonin
thermolacticum
    Clostridium stercorarium
    subsp. *t.*
thermoleovorans
    Geobacillus t.
Thermolospora viridis
thermoluminescence
thermoluminescent
    t. detector
    t. dosimeter (TLD)
thermolysis
thermometer
    air t.
    alcohol t.
    Beckmann t.
    bimetal t.
    Celsius t.
    centigrade t.
    differential t.
    Fahrenheit t.
    gas t.
    kelvin t.
    liquid-in-glass t.
    maximum t.
    mercurial t.
    metallic t.
    metastatic t.
    minimum t.
    Rankine t.
    Réaumur t.
    recording t.
    resistance t.
    thermocouple t.
thermometry
Thermomicrobia
Thermomicrobiaceae
Thermomicrobiales
Thermomonas
    T. brevis
    T. fusca
    T. haemolytica
    T. hydrothermalis
Thermomonosporaceae
Thermomyces lanuginosus
thermophil (*var. of* thermophile)

thermophila
    Anaerolinea t.
    Hydrogenimonas t.
    Saccharopolyspora t.
thermophile, thermophil
thermophilic
    t. actinomycete
    t. bacterium
thermophilum
    Caenibacterium t.
    Symbiobacterium t.
thermophilus
    Deferribacter t.
Thermoplasma acidophilum
Thermoplasmata
Thermoplasmataceae
Thermoplasmatales
thermoprecipitin reaction
thermopropionicum
Thermoproteaceae
Thermoproteales
Thermoprotei
Thermoproteus uzoniensis
thermoregulation
thermoresistant
thermosaccharolyticum
    Clostridium t.
Thermosipho
    T. geolei
    T. japonicus
thermosphaericus
    Ureibacillus t.
thermospinosisporus
    Streptomyces t.
thermostable
    t. alkaline phosphatase
    t. body
    t. opsonin
    t. opsonin test
thermosyntrophicum
    Desulfotomaculum thermobenzoicum
    subsp. *t.*
thermotaxis
thermoterrenum
    Anaerobaculum t.
Thermotoga
    T. lettingae
    T. naphthophila
    T. petrophila
    T. subterranea
Thermotogaceae
Thermotogae
Thermotogales
thermotolerans
    Haloterrigena t.
    Lactobacillus t.
    Pseudomonas t.
thermotropism
Thermovenabulum ferriorganovorum

T

Thermovibrio
    T. ammonificans
    T. ruber
Thermus
    T. antranikianii
    T. aquaticus
    T. igniterrae
thesaurismosis
    lipoid t.
thesaurocyte
theta
    t. antigen
    t. band
thetaiotamicron
    Bacteroides t.
THF
    thymic humoral factor
Thialkalicoccus limnaeus
Thialkalimicrobium
    T. aerophilum
    T. cyclicum
    T. sibiricum
Thialkalivibrio
    T. denitrificans
    T. jannaschii
    T. nitratireducens
    T. nitratis
    T. paradoxus
    T. thiocyanoxidans
    T. versutus
thiamin (*var. of* thiamine)
thiamine, thiamin
    t. assay
    t. chloride unit
    t. deficiency
    t. diphosphate (TDP)
    t. hydrochloride unit
    t. test
thiamphenicol assay
thiamylal
    sodium t.
Thiara
Thiaridae
thiazide diuretic
thiazin
    t. dye
    t. stain
thiazole dye
Thibierge-Weissenbach syndrome
thick
    t. fibrous band
    t. myofilament
    t. skin
thickened subepithelial collagen table
thickening
    concentric intimal t.
    fibrointimal t.
    hyaline t.
    trophoblast basement membrane t.

thickness
    Breslow t.
    mean corpuscular t. (MCT)
thiel
Thielavia
Thielaviopsis
Thiel-Behnke corneal lattice dystrophy
Thiemann disease
thiemia
Thiersch canaliculus
thimerosal
thin
    t. basement membrane disease
    t. basement membrane nephropathy
    t. elastic fiber
    t. myofilament
    t. section
    t. skin
thin-layer
    t.-l. cervical cytology technique
    t.-l. chromatography (TLC)
    t.-l. cytology
    t.-l. electrophoresis (TLE)
    t.-l. immunoassay
thin-needle biopsy
ThinPrep
    T. cytologic preparation
    T. cytology
    T. Imaging system
    T. processor
    T. slide process
thioacetamide
thioaldehyde
Thioalkalispira microaerophila
Thiobaca trueperi
Thiobacilleae
Thiobacteria
thiobarbiturate
thiobarbituric acid test (TBA)
Thiocapsa
    T. litoralis
    T. marina
Thiocapsaceae
thiocarbonyl group
thiochrome
thioctic acid
thiocyanate
    potassium t.
    sodium t. (NaSCN)
thiocyanoxidans
    Thialkalivibrio t.
thiodismutans
    Desulfonatronum t.
thioester
thioethanolamine
thioether
thioflavin, thioflavine
    t. S staining
    t. T stain

thioflavine (*var. of* thioflavin)
thiogenes
    Trichlorobacter t.
thioglycolate, thioglycollate
    t. broth
    t. medium
thioglycolic acid
thioglycollate (*var. of* thioglycolate)
thioketone
thiol
thiolaminopropionic acid
thiolase
    acetoacetyl-CoA t.
    alpha-methylacetoacetyl CoA t.
thiolysis
Thiomargarita namibiensis
thionine
thionin stain
thiooxidans
    Acidithiobacillus t.
    Limnobacter t.
    Roseinatronobacter t.
thiooxydans
    Ottowia t.
thiopental
    sodium t.
thiophen-2-carboxylic acid hydrazide (TCH)
thiophilus
    Geovibrio t.
thioredoxin
    t. reductase (TrxR)
    t. reductase gene
thioridazine assay
thiosulfate
    amyl nitrite, sodium nitrite, and sodium t.
    t. citrate-bile salts-sucrose (TCBS)
thiosulfatigenes
    Desulfonispora t.
thiosulfatiphilum
    Chlorobaculum t.
thiosulfatireducens
    Clostridium t.
thiosulfatophilus
    Roseococcus t.
thiothixene
Thiothrix
    T. disciformis
    T. flexilis
thiourea
    alpha-naphthol t.
thioxanthene tranquilizer
third
    t. and fourth pharyngeal pouch syndrome
    t. corpuscle
    t. disease

    t. spacing
    t. tonsil
third-degree
    t.-d. burn
    t.-d. frostbite
    t.-d. heart block
    t.-d. radiation injury
third-space fluid loss
thistle seed agar
thivervalensis
    Pseudomonas t.
thixotropic
thixotropy
THM
    Tamm-Horsfall mucoprotein
Thogotovirus
tholozani
    Ornithodoros t.
Thoma
    T. counting chamber
    T. fixative
Thomas antigen
thomasii
    Anaerobiospirillum t.
Thominx aerophilus
Thompson test
Thomsen
    T. antibody
    T. disease
Thomsen-Friedenreich antigen
Thoms method
thoracentesis
thoracic
    t. actinomycosis
    t. aneurysm
    t. asphyxiant dystrophy (TAD)
    t. duct fistula (TDF)
    t. gas volume (TGV)
    t. goiter
    t. index (TI)
    t. outlet syndrome (TOS)
thoracic-pelvic-phalangeal dystrophy
thorium (Th)
    t. dioxide
Thormählen test
thorn
    t. apple crystal
    dendritic t.
    T. syndrome
    T. test
Thornwaldt (*var. of* Tornwaldt)
Thorotrast
Thr
    threonine
thracensis
thread
    mucous t.
threadworm

threatened abortion
three-day
  t.-d. fever
  t.-d. measles
three dimensional composition
three-glass test
three-part mitosis
three-phase current
three-point cross
threonine (Thr)
threonyl
threose
thresher's lung
threshold
  t. body
  t. erythema dose (TED)
  t. limit value (TLV)
  mean cell t.
  median detection t. (MDT)
  renal t.
  t. substance
thrive
  failure to t.
throat
  t. culture
  putrid t.
  strep t.
thrombase
thrombasthenia
  Glanzmann t.
  Glanzmann-Naegeli t.
  hereditary hemorrhagic t.
thrombi (pl. of thrombus)
thrombin
  t. clotting time (TCT)
  t. time (TT)
  t. time test
thrombinogen
thrombinogenesis
thrombin-thrombomodulin-protein C
  system
thromboagglutinin
thromboangiitis obliterans (TAO)
thromboarteritis purulenta
thromboasthenia
thromboblast
thromboclasis
thrombocyst, thrombocystis
thrombocystis (var. of thrombocyst)
thrombocytapheresis
thrombocytasthenia
thrombocyte
thrombocythemia
  essential t. (ET)
  hemorrhagic t.
  primary t.
thrombocytic
  t. leukemia
  t. series

thrombocytin
thrombocytopathy
thrombocytopenia
  alloimmune t.
  amegakaryocytic t.
  autoimmune neonatal t.
  dilutional t.
  drug-induced t. (DIT)
  essential t.
  heparin-associated t. (HAT)
  heparin-induced t. (HIT)
  idiopathic t.
  immune t.
  isoimmune neonatal t.
  neonatal alloimmune t. (NAIT)
  neonatal autoimmune t.
  t. with absent radii syndrome
  X-linked t. (XLT)
thrombocytopenia-absent radius (TAR)
thrombocytopenia-thrombosis
  heparin-induced t.-t. (HITT)
thrombocytopenic purpura (TP)
thrombocytopoiesis
thrombocytopoietic
thrombocytosis
  clonal t.
  essential t.
  reactive t.
  rebound t.
thromboelastogram
thromboelastograph
thromboelastographic monitor device
  (TEG)
thromboembolic disease (TED)
thromboembolism
  pulmonary t. (PTE)
thromboendarteritis
thromboendocarditis
thrombogen
thrombogene
thrombogenic hypothesis
thrombogenicity
thromboglobulin
  beta t.
thromboid
thrombokatilysin
thrombokinase
thrombolic
thrombolus
thrombolymphangitis
thrombolysis
thrombolytic
  t. agent
  t. therapy
thrombometer
thrombomodulin glycoprotein (TM)
thrombon
thrombonecrosis
  arteriolar t.

thrombopathic syndrome
thrombopathy
    constitutional t.
thrombopenia
thrombopenic anemia
thrombophilia
    hereditary t.
thrombophlebitis
    t. migrans
    migrating t.
    t. saltans
thromboplastic
    t. plasma component (TPC)
    t. substance
thromboplastid
thromboplastin
    t. activation test (TAT)
    t. antecedent deficiency
    automated activated partial t.
    cofactor of t.
    t. generation accelerator
    t. generation test (TGT)
    t. generation time (TGT)
    RecombiPlasTin t.
    t. substitution test
    tissue t.
thromboplastinogen
thromboplastinogenase
thromboplastinogenemia
thrombopoiesis
thrombopoietin (TPO)
    t. receptor
thromboresistance
    endothelial t.
thrombosed
    t. arteriosclerotic aneurysm
    t. hemorrhoid
thromboses (*pl. of* thrombosis)
thrombosin
thrombosis, *pl.* **thromboses**
    agonal t.
    arterial t.
    atrophic t.
    cardiac t.
    cavernous sinus t.
    cerebral t. (CT)
    coronary t. (CT)
    deep vein t. (DVT)
    dilatation t.
    fetal stem artery t.
    generalized activation of t.
    hepatic vein t.
    intracellular t.
    marantic t.
    marasmic t.
    mesenteric t.
    placental t.
    plate t.
    platelet t.

    portal vein t. (PVT)
    propagating t.
    puerperal t.
    renal vein t. (RVT)
    traumatic t.
    venous t.
thrombospondin
thrombostasis
thrombosthenin
Thrombotest
thrombotic
    t. gangrene
    t. infarct
    t. microangiopathy (TMA)
    t. nonbacterial endocarditis
    t. occlusion
    t. phlegmasia
    t. pulmonary hypertension
    t. thrombocytopenic purpura
        (TTP)
    t. thrombocytopenic purpura and
        hemolytic uremic syndrome
        (TTP-HUS)
    t. thrombocytopenic purpura assay
thrombotonin
Thrombo-Wellcotest test
thromboxane A_2, B_2
thrombozyme
thrombus, *pl.* **thrombi**
    agglutinative t.
    agonal t.
    antemortem t.
    ball t.
    ball-valve t.
    bile t.
    canalized t.
    fibrin t.
    globular t.
    hyaline t.
    infective t.
    laminated t.
    marantic t.
    marasmic t.
    mixed t.
    mural t.
    old t.
    organized t.
    platelet t.
    postmortem t.
    t. precursor protein
    recent t.
    red t.
    secondary t.
    stratified t.
    t. tumor
    tumor t.
    valvular t.
    vascular t.
    white t.

T

through-and-through myocardial infarction
through-the-eyepiece photomicrography
thrush
    t. breast heart
    t. fungus
    vaginal t.
thrust culture
thryotroph cell
Thudichum test
thulium (Tm)
thumb
    cortical t.
    hitchhiker t.
thumbprinting
thuringiensis
    Bacillus t.
Thy-1 antigen
Thygeson disease
thylacitis
thymectomy
    adult t.
    neonatal t.
thymi (*pl. of* thymus)
thymic
    t. agenesis
    t. alymphoplasia (TAL)
    t. carcinoid tumor (TCT)
    t. carcinoma
    t. cell emperipolesis
    t. corpuscle
    t. cortex
    t. dysplasia
    t. epithelial cell
    t. epitheliocyte
    t. humoral factor
    t. hypoplasia
    t. leukemia
    t. lymphopoietic factor
    t. replacing factor
    t. reticulum cell
thymica
    mors t.
thymicolymphaticus
    status t.
thymic-parathyroid aplasia
thymicus
    status t.
thymidine
    t. diphosphate (dTDP)
    t. kinase
    t. monophosphate
    t. triphosphate
    tritiated t. (TTH)
thymidine-5′-phosphate
thymidylate synthase
thymidylic acid
thymidylyl
thymin

thymine
    t. dimer
    t. ribonucleoside
    t. ribonucleoside-5′-phosphate
thymine-2-deoxyriboside
thymitis
thymocyte
    antimouse t.
thymocytotoxic autoantibody
thymofibrolipoma
thymol
    t. blue
    t. flocculation (TF)
    t. turbidity (TT)
    t. turbidity test
thymolipoma
    proliferating t.
thymoliposarcoma
thymolphthalein
thymoma
    cortical t.
    epithelial t.
    intrapulmonary spindle cell t.
    lymphocyte-predominant t. (LPT)
    lymphocytic t.
    malignant t.
    medullary t.
    microscopic t.
    organoid t.
    predominantly epithelial t. (PET)
    spindle cell t.
thymopathy
thymopoietin
thymosin
thymus, *pl.* **thymi, thymuses**
    congenital aplasia of t.
    cortex of t.
    t. gland
    t. leukemia (TL)
    lobule of t.
    lobuli thymi
    normal t.
    t. nurse cell
thymus-dependent (TD)
    t.-d. antigen
    t.-d. cell
    t.-d. zone
thymus-derived cell
thymuses (*pl. of* thymus)
thymus-independent antigen
thymus-leukemia antigen
Thynnascaris
thyristor
thyroadenitis
thyrocalcitonin (TCT)
thyrocardiac disease
thyrocele
thyrocolloid

thyroglobulin (TG)
    t. antibody
    iodinated t.
    t. stain
thyroglossal
    t. duct cyst
    t. fistula
thyroid
    accessory t.
    t. adenoma
    t. antibody test
    t. antimicrosomal antibody
    t. antithyroglobulin antibody
    t. biopsy
    t. body
    t. cachexia
    t. carcinoma
    t. colloid
    t. crisis
    t. cyst
    t. endocrine disorder
    t. follicle
    t. function test (TFT)
    t. gland
    t. hormone binding ratio (THBR)
    light cell of t.
    t. lobule
    medullary carcinoma of t.
    t. microsomal antibody (TMAb)
    t. ophthalmopathy
    t. orbitopathy
    squamous cell carcinoma of the t. (SCT)
    t. storm
    t. suppression test
    t. transcription factor-1 (TTF-1)
    t. transcription factor 1 immunostain (TTF-1)
    t. tumor
    t. uptake test
thyroidal clearance
thyroid-binding globulin (TBG)
thyroidea
    t. accessoria
    glandula t.
thyroideae
    folliculi glandulae t.
    lobuli glandulae t.
    stroma glandulae t.
thyroiditis
    acute t.
    autoimmune t.
    chronic atrophic t.
    de Quervain t.
    fibrous t.
    focal lymphocytic t.
    giant cell t.
    granulomatous t.
    Hashimoto t.

    induced t.
    invasive fibrous t.
    ligneous t.
    lymphocytic t.
    postpartum t.
    Riedel t.
    silent t.
    subacute t. (SAT)
    subacute granulomatous t.
thyroid-stimulating
    t.-s. hormone (TSH)
    t.-s. hormone assay
    t.-s. hormone-releasing factor (TSH-RF)
    t.-s. hormone stimulation test
    t.-s. immunoglobulin (TSI)
thyroid-to-serum ratio (TSR)
thyrolingual cyst
thyrolytic
thyromegaly
thyroptosis
thyrosis
thyrotoxic
    t. complement-fixation factor
    t. encephalopathy
    t. heart disease
    t. myopathy
    t. serum
thyrotoxicosis factitia
thyrotoxin shock
thyrotrope adenoma
thyrotroph
    t. cell adenoma
    t. hyperplasia
thyrotropic hormone (TTH)
thyrotropin-producing adenoma
thyrotropin-receptor antibody (TSHR)
thyrotropin-releasing
    t.-r. factor (TRF)
    t.-r. hormone (TRH)
    t.-r. hormone challenge test
    t.-r. hormone stimulation test
thyroxin (*var. of* thyroxine)
thyroxine, thyroxin
    t. and cortisol treatment
    t. assay
    free (unbound) t. (FT_4)
    protein-bound t. (PBT4)
    total t. (TT)
thyroxine-binding
    t.-b. albumin (TBA)
    t.-b. globulin (TBG)
    t.-b. globulin assay
    t.-b. index (TBI)
    t.-b. index test
    t.-b. prealbumin (TBPA)
    t.-b. protein (TBP)
    t.-b. protein electrophoresis

T

thyroxine-specific activity (T₄SA)
thyrse
    en t.
Thysanophora
Thysanosoma actinoides
Thysanotaenia congolensis
THz
    terahertz
TI
    thoracic index
    time interval
    tricuspid incompetence
    tricuspid insufficiency
TIA
    T-cell restricted intracellular antigen
    transient ischemic attack
TIA-1 antibody
Tiarosporella
TIBC
    total iron-binding capacity
    TIBC test
tibetense
    Halorubrum t.
tibia, *pl.* tibiae
    saber t.
tibiae (*pl. of* tibia)
tibial
    t. cortical bone
    t. tuberosity
tibialis
    apophysitis t.
TIC
    trypsin-inhibitory capacity
ticarcillin
tic disorder
    diverticulum
tick
    t. fever
    t. paralysis
tick-borne
    t.-b. encephalitis (Central European
      subtype)
    t.-b. encephalitis (Eastern subtype)
    t.-b. encephalitis virus
ticket
    antibody-based lateral flow
      economical recognition t. (ALERT)
TID
    titrated initial dose
tidal
    t. air
    t. volume
tide
    acid t.
    alkaline t.
    fat t.
    t. mark
TIE
    transient ischemic episode

Tiedemann gland
tiedjei
    Desulfomonile t.
Tieghemella
Tieghemiomyces
Tierfellnaevus
tiering
Tietze syndrome
Tietz-Fiereck method
tiger
    t. heart
    t. lily heart
tight
    t. contact wound
    t. junction (TJ)
tigroid
    t. body
    t. striation
    t. substance
TIL
    tumor-infiltrating lymphocyte
Tilachlidium
Tilden stain
Tillaux disease
Tilletia
Tilletiopsis
tilorone
tilt table evaluation
time
    absolute retention t. (ART)
    access t.
    activated clotting t. (ACT)
    activated coagulation t. (ACT)
    activated partial thromboplastin t.
      (aPTT, APTT)
    automated coagulation t.
    bleeding t. (BT)
    blood-clot lysis t. (BLT)
    calcium t.
    cell cycle t.
    circulation t. (CT)
    clot lysis t. (CLT)
    clot retraction t.
    clotting t. (CT)
    coagulation t. (CT)
    compile t.
    corrected retention t.
    dead t.
    decimal reduction t.
    t. diffusion technique
    dilute Russell viper venom t.
      (DRVVT)
    doubling t.
    Duke method of bleeding t.
    electrode response t.
    euglobin lysis t.
    euglobulin clot lysis t. (ECLT)
    euglobulin lysis t. (ELT)
    execution t.

fast turnaround t.
filter bleeding t.
forced expiratory t. (FET)
gastric emptying t. (GET)
gastric emptying half t. (GET1/2)
generation t.
grain count halving t.
half t.
helium equilibration t. (HET)
t. interval (TI)
Ivy method of bleeding t.
Ivy template bleeding t.
kaolin-clotting t.
kaolin partial thromboplastin t. (KPTT)
lag t.
mean circulation t. (MCT)
mean generation t.
Mielke bleeding t.
occlusion t. (OT)
t. of flight (TOF)
t. of maximum concentration (T_{max})
one-stage prothrombin t.
operating t.
plasma clotting t.
plasma iron disappearance t. (PIDT)
plasma thrombin t.
prolonged bleeding t.
prolonged coagulation t.
prothrombin t. (PT)
prothrombin consumption t. (PCT)
reaction t. (RT)
recalcification t.
recovery t.
red blood cell survival t.
relative retention t.
reptilase t.
reptilase-R t.
resolving t.
retention t.
Russell viper venom t. (RVVT)
secondary bleeding t.
sedimentation t.
serial thrombin t. (STT)
serum prothrombin t.
shortened bleeding t.
shortened coagulation t.
Stypven t.
survival t.
template bleeding t.
thermal death t.
thrombin t. (TT)
thrombin clotting t. (TCT)
thromboplastin generation t. (TGT)
tissue thromboplastin inhibition t.
turn-around t. (TAT)
wash t.
wheal reaction t.
whole-blood clotting t.

timed
    t. 2-hour volume
    t. 24-hour volume
time-domain
time-kill kinetics test
time-of-flight
    matrix-assisted laser desorption
    ionization t.-o.-f. (MALDI-TOF)
time-resolved
    t.-r. fluorescence (TRF)
    t.-r. fluorescence immunoassay
    t.-r. fluorometry (TRF)
time-series plot
time-tension index (TTI)
timidum
    Mogibacterium t.
Timme syndrome
Timm silver sulfide
timonensis
timothy bacillus
TIMP-1
    tissue inhibitors of metalloproteinase-1
TIMP-2
    tissue inhibitors of metalloproteinase-2
TIMP-3
    tissue inhibitors of metalloproteinase-3
TIN
    tubulointerstitial nephropathy
Tinca
tinctable
tinction
tinctorial
tincture of iodine
Tindallia
    T. californiensis
    T. magadiensis
tinea
    t. amiantacea
    t. barbae
    t. capitis
    t. ciliorum
    t. circinata
    t. corporis
    t. cruris
    t. faciale
    t. favosa
    t. glabrosa
    t. imbricata
    t. inguinalis
    t. kerion
    t. manus
    t. manuum
    t. nigra
    t. pedis
    t. sycosis
    t. tonsurans
    t. tropicalis
    t. unguium
    t. versicolor

T

tine test
tingibility
tingible
    t. body
    t. body macrophage
tinnitus
tip
    Aerosol Resistant T.'s (ART)
    policeman t.
TIS
    tumor in situ
Tiselius
    T. electrophoresis cell
    T. procedure
Tissierella praeacuta
tissue
    aberrant t.
    adenoid t.
    adipose t.
    archival brain t.
    areolar connective t.
    t. artifact
    t. basophil
    bone t.
    bronchus-associated lymphoid t. (BALT)
    brown adipose t.
    bursa-equivalent t.
    cancellous t.
    capsular t.
    cardiac muscle t.
    cartilaginous t.
    cavernous t.
    chondroid t.
    chromaffin t.
    colon glandular t.
    compression of t.
    connective t.
    crushing of t.
    t. culture (TC)
    t. culture cytotoxin assay (TCCA)
    t. culture dose (TCD)
    t. culture infective dose (TCID)
    t. culture medium (TCM)
    cutaneous t.
    dartoic t.
    diffuse lymphatic t.
    t. displaceability
    t. displacement
    donor t.
    ectopic pancreatic t.
    ectopic thyroid t.
    elastic t.
    epithelial t.
    t. equivalent
    erectile t.
    extrathymic t.
    t. factor
    t. factor pathway inhibitor (TFPI)
    fatty intraosseous t.

fibroadipose t.
fibrohyaline t.
t. fibronectin
fibrous t. (FT)
t. fluid
formalin-fixed t.
gastrointestinal associated lymphoid t. (GALT)
gelatinous t.
gingival t.
t. glycogen
granulation t.
gut-associated lymphoid t. (GALT)
Haller vascular t.
hard t.
hematopoietic t.
t. hypoperfusion
t. hypoxia
inflammation of connective t. (ICT)
t. inhibitor of metalloproteinase-1 (TIMP-1)
interfascicular connective t.
interstitial t.
investing t.
islet t.
t. lymph
lymphatic t.
malignant rhabdoid tumor of soft t. (MRTS)
mesenchymal t.
mesonephric t.
metanephrogenic t.
t. microarray (TMA)
t. microarray technology (TMA)
mucosa-associated lymphoid t. (MALT)
mucous connective t.
t. multiblock
multilocular adipose t.
muscular t.
myeloid t.
t. necrosis
neoplastic hematopoietic t.
nervous t.
nodal t.
nonmucosa-associated lymphoid t. (non-MALT)
odontoblastic t.
osseous t.
osteogenic t.
osteoid t.
t. oxidase test
oxygenation of t.
t. pellet
peripancreatic adipose t.
t. plasminogen factor
t. processing
reactive lymphoid t. (RLT)
reticular t.
skeletal muscle t.

smooth muscle t.
snap-freezing of t.
subcutaneous t.
subendocardial connective t.
subepidermal connective t. (SEC)
t. thromboplastin
t. thromboplastin inhibition
t. thromboplastin inhibition test (TTIT)
t. thromboplastin inhibition time
t. tolerance dose (TTD)
tuberculosis granulation t.
t. typing
venous blood and t.
white adipose t.
WHO classification of tumors of the lymphoid t.

tissue-coding factor (TCF, TSF)
tissue-compatible plastic phantom
tissue-damaging factor (TF)
tissue-equivalent (TE)
tissue-nonspecific alkaline phosphatase (TNAP)
tissue-specific antigen
tissular
Tistrella mobilis
Titan

T. III H cellulose acetate strip
T. yellow

titanium dioxide pneumoconiosis
titer

agglutination t.
AH t.
antibody t.
anti-F1 antigen t.
antihyaluronidase t. (AHT)
anti-Rh t.
antistreptolysin-O t.
California encephalitis virus t.
CF antibody t.
Chlamydia group t.
cold agglutinin t.
cryptococcal antigen t.
Cryptococcus antibody t.
cysticercosis t.
differential agglutination t. (DAT)
Eastern equine encephalitis virus t.
fibrin t.
HAI t.
hemagglutination inhibition t.
Image T.
influenza A, B t.
lymphogranuloma venereum t.
mumps antibody t.
poliomyelitis I–III t.
psittacosis t.
Q fever t.
Salmonella t.

titin protein
titrant

titratable

t. acid (TA)
t. acidity test

titrated initial dose (TID)
titration

amperometric-coulometric t.
coulometric t.
potentiometric t.
t. technique

titrator

Cotlove t.

titrimetric
Tityus serrulatus
Tizzoni stain
TJ

tight junction

tjernbergiae

Acinetobacter t.

TL

thymus leukemia
TL antigen

Tl

thallium

TLA

total laboratory automation

TLC

thin-layer chromatography
total L-chain concentration
total lung capacity

TLD

thermoluminescent dosimeter
tumor lethal dose

T/LD$_{100}$

minimum dose causing death or malformation of 100% of fetuses

TLE

thin-layer electrophoresis

T1-like viruses
T4-like viruses
T5-like viruses
T7-like viruses
T-lineage
TLR4

toll-like receptor 4

TLS

tumor lysis syndrome

TLV

threshold limit value

T-lymphocyte rosette
TM

thrombomodulin glycoprotein

Tm

melting temperature
thulium
Tm cell

TMA

thrombotic microangiopathy
tissue microarray technology
transcription-mediated amplification

TMAb
thyroid microsomal antibody
T-MAX, T-max, T$_{max}$
maximum temperature
TMH-1 antibody
TMIF
tumor-cell migration-inhibition
factor
TMPRSS3
transmembrane protease serine 3
TMPRSS2-ERG gene fusion
TMRE
tetra-methylrhodamine ethyl
ester
TMV
tobacco mosaic virus
Tn
transposon
troponin
Tn antigen
T-natural
T-n. killer (TNK)
T-n. killer cell (TNK)
T-n. killer cell lymphoma
TnC
troponin C
TnC polypeptide
TNF
tumor necrosis factor
TNF alpha
TNF beta
TNFR
tumor necrosis factor receptor
TnI
troponin I
TnI polypeptide
TNK
T-natural killer
T-natural killer cell
TNM
(primary) tumor, (regional lymph)
nodes, (remote) metastasis
tumor-node-metastasis
TNM staging
TNM staging system
T-nodule
TnT
troponin T
TnT polypeptide
TNTC
too numerous to count
to
t. contain (TC)
t. deliver (TD)
TOA
tuboovarian abscess
toad
t. test
t. toxin

tobacco
t. amblyopia
t. mosaic virus (TMV)
Tobamovirus
Tobie, von Brand, and Mehlman diphasic medium
tobramycin
Tobravirus
tocainide
tocodynagraph
tocodynamometer
tocolytic agent
Todd
T. body
T. paralysis
T. unit (TU)
Todd-Hewitt broth
toe
clubbed t.
Hong Kong t.
webbed t.
toebii
Geobacillus t.
toenail
ingrown t. (IGTN)
Togaviridae
togavirus
Togobacteria
Toison
T. solution
T. stain
Tokelau ringworm
Toker clear cell
tokodaii
Sulfolobus t.
tolaasinivorans
Mycetocola t.
tolbutamide
sodium t.
t. test (TBT)
t. tolerance test
(TTT)
tolerance
aspirin t.
drug t.
glucose t. (GT)
high-dose t.
immune t.
immunological t.
t. interval
t. limit
nonresponder t.
split t.
tolerogen
tolerogenic
toll-like receptor 4 (TLR4)
Tolosa-Hunt syndrome
toluene 2,4-diisocyanate
toluic acid

toluidine
    t. blue (TB)
    t. blue O
    t. blue stain
toluol
toluolica
    Desulfobacula t.
toluvorans
    Azoarcus t.
toluylene red
Tolypocladium
tolypomycina
    Amycolatopsis t.
tomato
    Macrosporium t.
tombstone-like dermis
Tombusvirus
Tomes
    T. fiber
    T. granular layer
    T. process
Tommaselli disease
tomographic scan
tongue
    bifid t.
    black hairy t.
    t. blanching
    cleft t.
    geographic t.
    t. worm
tonicity
toning
    gold t.
tonofibril
tonofilament
tonometer
tonoplast
tonsil
    eustachian t.
    faucial t.
    Gerlach t.
    laryngeal t.
    lingual t.
    Luschka t.
    third t.
    tubal t.
tonsilla
    t. intestinalis
    t. lingualis
    t. palatina
    t. pharyngealis
    t. tubaria
tonsillar crypt
tonsillaris
    crypta t.
    cynanche t.
tonsillitis
    acute necrotizing ulcerative t.
tonsurans

    tinea t.
    Trichophyton t.
tool
    policeman transfer t.
too numerous to count (TNTC)
tooth
    auditory teeth
    t. cement
    Corti auditory teeth
    T. disease
    Huschke auditory teeth
    Hutchinson teeth
    impacted t.
    t. pulp
    t. sac
    t. socket
Töpfer test
tophaceous gout
tophus
    gouty t.
topical
    t. calciphylaxis
    t. corticosteroid
Topocuvirus
topo-II-alpha
    topoisomerase II-alpha
    topoisomerase II-alpha index
topoisomerase
    anti-DNA t.
    t. II-alpha (topo-II-alpha)
    t. II enzyme
topopathogenesis
TOPV
    trivalent oral poliovirus vaccine
Tor
    Vibrio cholerae biotype El T. (El Tor vibrio)
TORCH
    toxoplasmosis, rubella, cytomegalovirus, and herpes simplex
    TORCH syndrome
torcular herophili
Torkelson syndrome
Tornwaldt, Thornwaldt
    T. abscess
    T. disease
    T. syndrome
torocyte membrane
torose, torous
torous (*var. of* torose)
Torovirus
torque
torquis
    Psychroflexus t.
torr
Torre syndrome
torsade de pointes
torsion
    t. injury

T

torsion (*continued*)
    t. of testis
    ovarian t.
    testicular t.
Torsten Sjögren syndrome
torticollis
    congenital t.
tortuosum
    Eubacterium t.
tortuous
Torula
    T. capsulatus
    T. histolytica
torular meningitis
Torulaspora
toruloidea
    Hendersonula t.
toruloma
Torulomyces lagena
Torulopsis glabrata
torulopsosis
torulosis
TOS
    thoracic outlet syndrome
Tospovirus
tosylate
total
    t. acidity
    t. antitryptic activity (TAT)
    t. blood granulocyte pool (TBGP)
    t. blood volume (TBV)
    t. body clearance (Q_B)
    t. body density (TBD)
    t. body fat (TBF)
    t. body hematocrit (TBH)
    t. body potassium (TBK)
    t. body solute (TBS)
    t. body water (TBW)
    t. body weight (TBW)
    t. calcium assay
    t. carbon dioxide content
    t. catecholamine test
    t. cell count
    t. cholesterol (TC)
    t. circulating hemoglobin (TCH)
    t. colonic aganglionosis (TCA)
    complement t.
    t. estriol
    t. estrogen (excretion) (TE)
    t. exchangeable potassium measurement
    t. fatty acid (TFA)
    t. gastric resection
    t. hematuria
    t. hemoglobin
    t. hexosaminidase
    t. internal reflection
    t. iron-binding capacity (TIBC)
    t. laboratory automation (TLA)
    t. L-chain concentration (TLC)

    t. lesion
    t. lung capacity (TLC)
    t. necrosis
    t. oxidant
    t. parenteral nutrition (TPN)
    t. peripheral resistance (TPR)
    t. protein (TP)
    t. protein expression
    t. pulmonary vascular resistance (TPVR)
    t. response (TR)
    t. ridge count (TRC)
    t. serum bilirubin (TSB)
    t. serum IgE
    t. serum prostatic acid phosphatase (TSPAP)
    t. serum protein (TSP)
    t. solids (TS)
    t. thyroxine (TT)
    t. urinary gonadotropin (TUG)
    t. urine estrogen
total-dose infusion (TDI)
totalis
totipotence (*var. of* totipotency)
totipotency, totipotence
totipotent, totipotential
    t. cell
    t. HSC
    t. stem cell
totipotential (*var. of* totipotent)
    t. protoplasm
Totivirus
touch
    t. cell
    t. corpuscle
    t. imprint
    t. imprint cytology
    t. preparation
touch-smear specimen
Touraine-Solente-Golé syndrome
Tourette disease
Touton giant cell
towelette
    mini Hype-Wipe bleach t.
tower skull
Towne CMV low passage clinical isolate
towneri
    Acinetobacter t.
tox
    toxic
    toxicology
    toxin
toxalbumin
toxanemia
toxaphene
Toxascaris leonina
toxemia, toxicemia
    t. of pregnancy
    preeclamptic t. (PET)

toxemic jaundice
toxic (tox)
    t. adenoma
    t. anemia
    t. chemical agent
    t. chemical handling
    t. cirrhosis
    t. colitis
    t. cyanosis
    t. dermatitis
    t. epidermal necrolysis (TEN)
    t. equivalent
    t. erythema
    t. glycosuria
    t. goiter (TG)
    t. granulation
    t. granule
    t. hemoglobinuria
    t. idiopathy
    t. megacolon
    t. methemoglobinemia
    t. myocarditis
    t. nephrosis
    t. organophosphorous
    t. shock
    t. shock syndrome
    t. shock syndrome toxin (TSST1)
    t. soluble oligomer
    t. unit (TU)
    t. waste
toxicant
toxicemia (*var. of* toxemia)
toxicity
    acetaminophen hepatic t.
    aspirin t.
    delayed radiation t.
    EP t.
    immediate radiation t.
    manganese t.
    salicylate t.
toxicogenic conjunctivitis
toxicogenomics
toxicologic
toxicologist
toxicology (tox)
    analytical t.
    clinical t.
    environmental t.
    forensic t.
    free t.
    industrial t.
toxicopathic
toxicosis
    triiodothyronine t.
toxicum
    erythema t.
toxidrome
toxigenic bacterium
toxigenicity

toxin (tox)
    animal t.
    anthrax t.
    Bacillus anthracis t.
    bacterial t.
    bee venom t.
    botulinum t. (Botox)
    botulinus t.
    cagA t.
    cholera t. (CTX)
    Clostridium difficile t.
    Clostridium perfringens alpha t.
    Clostridium perfringens beta t.
    Clostridium perfringens epsilon t.
    Clostridium perfringens iota t.
    Coley t.
    diagnostic diphtheria t.
    Dick test t.
    dinoflagellate t.
    diphtheria t.
    disease-associated bacterial t.
    epsilon clostridial t.
    erythrogenic t.
    extracellular t.
    intracellular t.
    mitochondrial t.
    normal t.
    plant t.
    pyrogenic t.
    scarlet fever erythrogenic t.
    Schick test t.
    secreted t.
    Shiga t. (Stx)
    Shigalike t.
    t. spectrum
    streptococcus erythrogenic t.
    T2 t.
    tetanus t.
    toad t.
    toxic shock syndrome t. (TSST1)
    t. unit (TU)
toxin-antitoxin (TA, TAT)
toxinic
toxinogenic
toxinogenicity
toxinology
toxinosis, toxonosis
toxipathic
toxipathy
Toxocara
    T. canis
    T. cati
    T. mystax
toxocariasis
toxoid
    alum-precipitated t. (APT)
toxoid-antitoxoid
    t.-a. floccule (TAF)
    t.-a. mixture (TAM)

T

toxon, toxone
toxone (*var. of* toxon)
toxoneme
toxonosis
toxophil, toxophile
toxophile (*var. of* toxophil)
toxophore
toxophorous
Toxoplasma
    T. gondii
    T. pyrogenes
Toxoplasmatidae
Toxoplasmea
toxoplasmic retinochoroiditis
toxoplasmin
toxoplasmosis
    congenital t.
    toxoplasmosis, rubella, cytomegalovirus,
      and herpes simplex (TORCH)
    t. serology
Toynbee corpuscle
toyohensis
    Thermanaeromonas t.
TP
    thrombocytopenic purpura
    total protein
    tryptophan
    tube precipitin
    tuberculin precipitation
TPA
    Treponema pallidum agglutination
TPC
    thromboplastic plasma component
TPCF
    Treponema pallidum complement
      fixation
TPH
    transplacental hemorrhage
    treponemal hemagglutination
    Treponema pallidum hemagglutination
      TPH test
TPHA
    Treponema pallidum hemagglutination
      assay
TPI
    triosephosphate isomerase
      TPI assay
      TPI test
TPIA
    Treponema pallidum immobilization
      (immune) adherence
T-PLL
    T-cell prolymphocytic leukemia
TPMT
      Pro-PredictRx TPMT
TPN
    total parenteral nutrition
TPO
    thrombopoietin

TPR
    testosterone production rate
    total peripheral resistance
TPS
    tumor polysaccharide substance
TPVR
    total pulmonary vascular resistance
TQA Sensor Pad blood-flow rate
  device
TQ-Prep workstation
TR
    tetrazolium reduction
    total response
    tuberculin R (new tuberculin)
Tr
    trace
TRA
    transaldolase
      TRA antigen
tra operon
trabecula, *pl.* **trabeculae**
    arachnoid trabeculae
    arachnoid t.
    trabeculae carneae
    connective tissue t.
    trabeculae corporis spongiosi
    t. corporis spongiosi
    trabeculae corporum cavernosorum
    t. corporum cavernosorum
    t. of bone
    t. testis
trabeculae (*pl. of* trabecula)
trabecular
    t. adenocarcinoma
    t. adenoma
    t. blood vessel
    t. bone
    t. carcinoma
    t. meshwork
    t. network
    t. pattern
    t. reticulum
    t. zone
trabecularis
    substantia t.
trabeculate
trabeculation
trace (Tr)
    t. alternant
    t. element
    t. routine
    TEG t.
tracer
    radiocolloid t.
trachea, *pl.* **tracheae**
    Syngamus t.
    tunica mucosa tracheae
    tunica muscularis tracheae
tracheae (*pl. of* trachea)

tracheal
  t. aspiration
  t. gland
tracheales
  glandulae t.
tracheitis
trachelematoma
trachelocystitis
trachelomyitis
trachelopanus
trachelophyma
tracheoaerocele
tracheobiliary fistula
tracheobronchial
  t. amyloidosis
  t. dyskinesia
  t. tree
tracheobronchitis
tracheobronchomegaly
tracheoesophageal fistula (TEF)
tracheomalacia
tracheomegaly
tracheopathia osteoplastica
tracheopathy
Tracheophilus cucumerinum
tracheostenosis
Trachipleistophora
trachitis
trachoma
  t. body
  t. gland
  psittacosis-lymphogranuloma
    venereum t. (PLT)
  t. virus
trachoma-inclusion conjunctivitis (TRIC)
trachomatis
  Chlamydia t.
trachomatosus
Trachybdella bistriata
trachychromatic
tracking
  lymphatic t.
TRAcP
  tartrate resistant acid phosphatase
tract
  alimentary t.
  Arnold t.
  association t.
  benign mesothelioma of genital t.
  Bürdach t.
  census t. (CT)
  digestive t.
  female genital t. (FGT)
  geniculocalcarine t.
  geniculotemporal t.
  hypothalamohypophysial t.
  inflammatory sinus t.
  long t.
  portal t.

  respiratory t.
  spiral foraminous t.
  supraopticohypophysial t.
  upper aerodigestive t. (UADT)
  uveal t.
tractellum
traction
  t. aneurysm
  t. atrophy
  t. diverticulum
tractus, *pl.* **tractus**
  t. solitarii
  t. spiralis foraminosus
  t. supraopticohypophysialis
TRAF
  tumor receptor-associated factor
traffic
  cell t.
trafficking
  membrane t.
**TRA-1-60 human embryonal carcinoma
  marker antigen**
trait
  hemoglobin E t.
  hemoglobin G Philadelphia t.
  hemoglobin Lepore t.
  quantitative t.
  secretor t.
  sickle cell t.
  thalassemia t.
trajectory
TRALI
  transfusion-related acute lung injury
Trametes
tram-track appearance
tram-tracking
trance
  death t.
tranquilizer
  major t.
  minor t.
  thioxanthene t.
trans
  t. activation
  t. face
transabdominal
  t. chorionic villus sampling
  t. CVS
transaldolase
transaminase
  aspartate t.
  erythrocyte glutamic oxaloacetic t.
    (EGOT)
  glutamate-pyruvate t.
  glutamic-oxaloacetic t. (GOT)
  glutamic-pyruvic t. (GPT)
  hepatic t.
  serum glutamic oxaloacetic t.
    (SGOT)

transaminase (*continued*)
    serum glutamic pyruvic t. (SGPT)
    t. test
    valine t.
transamination
transbronchial
    t. lung biopsy (TBBx, TBLB)
    t. needle aspiration (TBNA)
transcapsidation
transcarbamoylase
    ornithine t. (OTC)
transcellular
    t. fluid
    t. pathway
transcervical
    t. chorionic villus sampling
    t. CVS
transcobalamin (Tc)
transconfiguration
transcortin
transcript
    BCR-ABL t.
    EWS-WT1 chimeric t.
    primary t.
transcriptase
    avian myeloblastosis leukemia virus
      reverse t. (AMLV-RT)
    human telomerase reverse t.
    reverse t.
transcription
    t. factor
    t. factor beta
    t. factor Cbfa1/Runx2
    t. factor neuroD
    gene t.
    inhibitor of t.
    metalloproteinase t.
    reverse t.
    signal transducer and activator of t.
      (STAT)
    t. unit
transcriptional
    t. profiling
    t. promoter
transcription-based chain reaction
transcription-dependent amplification
transcription-mediated amplification
  (TMA)
transcription/translation
    in vitro t. (IVTT)
transcriptome analysis
transdifferentiation
    tubular epithelial-myofibroblast t.
      (TEMT)
transduce
transducer cell
transductant
transduction
    abortive t.

    adenoviral t.
    complete t.
    general t.
    generalized t.
    high-frequency t.
    insulin receptor and signal t.
    low-frequency t.
    specialized t.
    specific t.
transepidermal water loss
  (TWL)
transethmoidal puncture
transfection
transfer
    DNA t.
    t. factor (TF)
    fluorescence resonance energy t.
      (FRET)
    fluorescent resonance energy t.
      (FRET)
    t. function
    t. gene
    group t.
    t. host
    linear energy t. (LET)
    t. pipette
    plasmid t.
    replication and t. (RTF)
    t. RNA (tRNA)
transferase
    adenylyl t.
    catechol-O-methyl t. (COMT)
    glucuronosyl t.
    terminal deoxyribonucleotidyl t.
    UDP-glucuronyl t.
transferred
    t. antigen-cell-bound antibody
      reaction
    t. antigen-transferred antibody
      reaction
transferrin
    t. assay
    t. receptor
    t. saturation
    t. test
transformant
transformation
    asbestos t.
    bacterial t.
    blastic t.
    cell t.
    globular-fibrous t.
    human lymphocyte t. (hLT)
    logit t.
    lymphocyte t.
    lymphocytic t.
    malignant t.
    oncocytic t.
    probit t.

pseudoxanthomatous t.
refractory anemia with excess blasts in t.

transformation-sensitive
large external t.-s. (LETS)

transformed lymphocyte

transformer
high-voltage t.
step-down t.
step-up t.
voltage-regulating t.

transforming
t. agent
t. gene
t. growth factor X
t. virus

transfusion
t. adult committee
autologous t.
coagulation factor t.
cryoprecipitate t.
directed donor t.
exchange t. (ET)
granulocyte t.
t. hepatitis
incompatible blood t.
intrauterine fetal t. (IVT)
leukocyte t.
massive t.
t. nephritis
platelet t.
predeposit autologous t.
t. reaction
reciprocal t.
t. transmitted virus (TTV)

transfusion-associated graft-versus-host disease (TAGVHD)

transfusion-mediated viral hepatitis

transfusion-related
t.-r. acute lung injury (TRALI)
t.-r. alloimmunization

transgene

transgenic mice

transglutaminase (TGase)

trans-Golgi

transheterozygosity

transient
t. acantholytic dermatosis
t. agammaglobulinemia
t. albuminuria
t. cerebral ischemia (TCI)
t. cerebral ischemic episode (TCIE)
t. derepression
t. enzyme abnormality
t. equilibrium
t. erythroblastopenia of childhood (TEC)
t. hypogammaglobulinemia

t. hypogammaglobulinemia of infancy
t. ischemic attack (TIA)
t. ischemic episode (TIE)
t. myeloproliferative disorder
ryanodine-sensitive calcium t.

transistor
field effect t.
insulated gate field effect t.
junction field effect t.
metal oxide semiconductor field effect t.
unijunction t.

transition
G to A stage tumor t.
isomeric t. (IT)
t. mutation
refractory anemia with excess blasts in t. (RAEBT)
t. state
t. zone (TZ)
t. zone biopsy

transitional
t. cell
t. cell carcinoma (TCC)
t. cell papilloma
t. cell tumor
t. epithelium
t. leukocyte
t. zone

transketolase
t. assay
erythrocyte t.

translation control RNA (tcRNA)

translator

translocation
autosome t.
balance t.
chromosome t.
t. factor
insertional t.
reciprocal t.
robertsonian t.
t. trisomy
XPII t.

translucency
fetal nuchal t.

translucent

translucida
Pseudoalteromonas t.

transmandibular projection

transmembrane
t. protease serine 3 (TMPRSS3)
t. protein

transmethylase

transmethylation

transmigration
leukocyte t.

transmigration (*continued*)
    t. macrophage
    t. neutrophil
transmissible
    t. dementia
    t. disease
    t. enteritis
    t. gastroenteritis
    t. gastroenteritis virus of swine
    t. mink encephalopathy
    t. plasmid
    t. spongiform encephalopathy
      (TSE)
    t. turkey enteritis virus
transmission
    asynchronous data t.
    t. electron microscope (TEM)
    t. electron microscopy (TEM)
    fecal-oral t.
    glutamatergic t.
    horizontal t.
    serial data t.
    synchronous data t.
    vertical t.
transmittance
    percent t.
transmitter-gated ion channel
transmogrification
    placental t.
transmogrify
transmural
    t. gradient
    t. lymphoid aggregate
    t. lymphoid hyperplasia
    t. myocardial infarction
transmutation
transnexus channel
transparent
transpeptidase
    gamma glutamyl t. (GGTP)
    glutamyl t. (GT)
transphosphorylase
transplacental hemorrhage (TPH)
transplant
    bone marrow t.
    canalicular organic anion t.
    orthotopic liver t. (Olt, OLT,
      OLTx)
    t. rejection
    renal t.
    syngeneic t.
    syngenesioplastic t.
    umbilical cord blood t.
    t. vascular disease
transplantation
    allogeneic t.
    allogeneic bone marrow t.
      (allo-BMT)
    t. antigen

    autologous blood and marrow t.
      (ABMT)
    autologous bone marrow t. (ABMT)
    autologous peripheral blood stem
      cell bone marrow t.
    bone marrow t. (BMT)
    hematopoietic progenitor cell t.
    heterotopic t.
    homotopic t.
    t. immunology
    International Society for Heart and
      Lung T. (ISHLT)
    orthoptic t.
    t. workup
transport
    active t.
    t. and secretion
    t. and storage
    axoplasmic t.
    carrier-mediated t.
    direct t.
    t. disease
    effective oxygen t. (EOT)
    indirect t.
    t. medium
    membrane t.
    t. of cancer cell
    primary active t.
    t. protein defect
    secondary active t.
    selective t.
    tape t.
transportation
    lysis, storage, and t. (LST)
transporter
    biliary acid t. (BAT)
    canicular multispecific organic anion
      t. (CMOAT)
    Dura-Temp specimen t.
    GLUT5 t.
    MDR1 t.
transposable element
transpose
transposition
    corrected t. (CT)
    incomplete t.
    t. of great arteries (TGA)
    t. of great vessels (TGV)
transposon
transrectal
    t. ultrasonography
    t. ultrasound-guided sextant biopsy
      (TRUS)
transseptal fiber
transsynaptic
    t. chromatolysis
    t. degeneration
transthyretin (TTR)
transubstantiation

transudate
  acute inflammatory t.
  inflammatory t.
transudation
  generalized t.
transudative
  t. inflammation
  t. pleural effusion
transuranic radionuclide
transurethral resection of prostate (TURP)
transvaalensis
  Alkaliphilus t.
transvalensis
  Nocardia t.
transvector
transverse
  t. disc
  t. ductules of epoophoron
  t. fracture
  t. myelitis
  t. myelopathy
  t. septum
transversion mutation
transversus
  tubulus t.
TRAP
  tartrate resistant acid phosphatase
  telomerase repeat amplification protocol
  telomeric repeat amplification protocol
  TRAP assay
  TRAP stain
Trapp formula
Trapp-Häser formula
trastuzumab
Traube
  T. corpuscle
  T. plug
trauma
  blunt t.
  blunt force t. (BFT)
  laryngeal intubation t.
  t. MCI
  orbital t.
traumatic
  t. abnormality
  t. anemia
  t. aneurysm
  t. atrophy
  t. basal subarachnoid hemorrhage (TBSAH)
  t. bone cyst
  t. brain injury (TBI)
  t. chylothorax
  t. fever
  t. hemolysis
  t. herpes
  t. neuroma
  t. osteoporosis

  t. progressive encephalopathy
  t. rupture
  t. subarachnoid hemorrhage (TSAH)
  t. thrombosis
traveler's diarrhea
TRC
  tanned red cell
  total ridge count
Treacher Collins syndrome
treatment (Tx)
  antiretroviral t. (ART)
  immunomodulatory t.
  isoserum t.
  preventive t.
  prophylactic t.
  PUVA t.
  solvent detergent t. (SD)
  thyroxine and cortisol t.
tree
  tracheobronchial t.
trefoil
  T. Factor Family (TFF [1–3])
  t. family factor (TFF)
  t. peptide
trehala
trehalose
trehalosi
  Nocardiopsis t.
Trematoda
trematode, trematoid
  blood t.
trematoid (*var. of* trematode)
Tremella
tremelloid, tremellose
tremellose (*var. of* tremelloid)
tremens
  delirium t. (DT)
tremor
  epidemic t.
trench
  t. fever
  t. foot
  t. mouth
trephine biopsy
trephocyte
Treponema
  T. azotonutricium
  T. buccale
  T. calligyrum
  T. carateum
  T. cuniculi
  T. denticola
  T. genitalis
  T. hyodysenteriae
  T. macrodentium
  T. microdentium
  T. mucosum
  T. orale
  T. pallidum

T

Treponema (*continued*)
>T. *pallidum* agglutination (TPA)
>T. *pallidum* complement fixation (TPCF)
>T. *pallidum* complement fixation test
>T. *pallidum* hemagglutination (TPH)
>T. *pallidum* hemagglutination assay (TPHA)
>T. *pallidum* immobilization (TPI)
>T. *pallidum* immobilization assay
>T. *pallidum* immobilization (immune) adherence (TPIA)
>T. *pallidum* immobilization reaction
>T. *parvum*
>T. *pectinovorum*
>T. *pertenue*
>T. *pintae*
>T. *primitia*
>T. *putidum*
>T. *refringens*
>T. *scoliodontum*
>T. *succinifaciens*
>T. *vincentii*

treponema-immobilizing antibody
treponemal
>t. antibody
>t. antibody test (TAT)
>t. hemagglutination (TPH)
>t. immobilization test

Treponemataceae
treponematosis
tresis
trevisanii
>*Leptotrichia* t.

Trevor disease
TRF
>T-cell replacing factor
>telomeric restriction fragment
>thyrotropin-releasing factor
>time-resolved fluorescence
>time-resolved fluorometry

TRH
>thyrotropin-releasing hormone
>TRH stimulation test

TRH-stimulation test
TRI
>tetrazolium reduction inhibition

triac
triacetate
>glyceryl t.

triacetin
triacetylglycerol
triacetyloleandomycin
triacsin C
triacylglyceride synthesis
triacylglycerol lipase
triad
>acute compression t.
>adrenomedullary t.

>Andersen t.
>Beck t.
>Charcot t.
>fragile histidine t. (FHIT)
>Hutchinson t.
>portal t.
>t. syndrome
>Virchow t.
>Whipple t.

triage
>T. BNP test
>T. Cardiac panel
>t. delayed
>HPV t.
>t. immediate
>T. MeterPlus
>t. minimal
>T. Tox drug screen

trial
>clinical t.

triamcinolone
triangle
>Alsberg t.
>gastrinoma t.
>sternocostal t.

triangular
>t. fibrocartilage complex tear
>t. lamella
>t. wave

triangular-shaped skin tear
triarylmethane dye
Triatoma
triatomae
>*Trypanosoma* t.

triatomic
triatomid
Triatominae
triatriatum
>cor t.

tribasic
>t. acid
>t. potassium phosphate

tribasilar synostosis
tribrachius
>dicephalus dipus t.
>dicephalus tripus t.

TRIC
>trachoma-inclusion conjunctivitis

tricarboxylic
>t. acid (TCA)
>t. acid cycle

Tricercomonas
trichangion
Trichaptum
trichatrophia
trichilemmal
>t. cyst
>t. cystic squamous cell carcinoma

trichilemmoma

trichina
  t.
Trichinella
  T. pseudospiralis
  T. spiralis
trichinelliasis
Trichinellicae
Trichinelloidea
trichinellosis
trichiniasis
trichiniferous
trichinization
trichinoscope
trichinosis serology
trichinous embolism
trichite
trichitis
trichiura
  Trichocephalus t.
  Trichuris t.
trichlorfon
trichloride
  acetylene t.
  antimony t.
  indium 111 t.
  vinyl t.
trichloroacetic acid
Trichlorobacter thiogenes
1,1,1-trichloroethane
1,1,2-trichloroethane
trichloroethylene
trichlorophenoxy acetic acid
Trichobilharzia physellae
trichoblastoma
  desmoplastic t.
trichocephaliasis
Trichocephalus trichiura
trichochrome
Trichocladium asperum
Trichococcus
  T. collinsii
  T. palustris
  T. pasteurii
Trichoconis padwickii
trichocyst
Trichodectes
trichodectis
  Cryptocystis t.
Trichoderma
trichodes
  Lactobacillus t.
trichodiscoma
trichoepithelioma
  desmoplastic t.
  hereditary multiple t.
  t. papillosum multiplex
trichofolliculoma
trichohyalin
trichoid

trichoides
  Cladosporium t.
tricholemmoma
Tricholoma
  T. magnivelare
  T. pardinum
trichomanas vaginitis
Trichomaris invadens
Trichometasphaeria
trichomonacide
trichomonad
Trichomonadidae
trichomonas
  T. buccalis
  T. foetus
  T. gallinarum
  T. hominis
  t. infestation
  T. intestinalis
  T. ovis
  T. preparation
  T. pulmonalis
  T. suis
  T. tenax
  T. urethritis
  T. vaginalis
trichomoniasis
trichomycosis
  t. axillaris
  t. chromatica
  t. favosa
  t. rubra
trichonodosis
trichophytic
trichophytid
trichophytin
Trichophyton, Trichophytum
  T. agar
  T. ajelloi
  T. asteroides
  T. concentricum
  T. cruris
  T. dankaliense
  T. epilans
  T. equinum
  T. equinum autotrophicum
  T. equinum equinum
  T. erinacei
  T. ferrugineum
  T. fischeri
  T. flavescens
  T. floccosum
  T. gallinae
  T. glabrum
  T. gloriae
  T. gourvilii
  T. granulare
  T. granulosum
  T. gypseum

T

Trichophyton (*continued*)
    T. inguinale
    T. interdigitale
    T. intertriginis
    T. kanei
    T. krajdenii
    T. longifusum
    T. megninii
    T. mentagrophytes
    T. mentagrophytes erinacei
    T. mentagrophytes interdigitale
    T. mentagrophytes mentagrophytes
    T. mentagrophytes nodulare
    T. mentagrophytes quinckeanum
    T. niveum
    T. nodulare
    T. pedis
    T. persicolor
    T. phaseoliforme
    T. proliferans
    T. purpureum
    T. radiolatum
    T. raubitschekii
    T. rosaceum
    T. rubrum
    T. sabouraudi
    T. schoenleinii
    T. simii
    T. soudanense
    T. sulphureum
    T. terrestre
    T. tonsurans
    T. tonsurans perforans
    T. vanbreuseghemii
    T. verrucosum
    T. violaceum
    T. yaoundei
trichophytosis
    t. barbae
    t. capitis
    t. corporis
    t. cruris
    t. unguium
Trichophytum (*var. of* Trichophyton)
Trichopleuris
Trichoprosopon
Trichoptera
trichorhinophalangeal syndrome
trichorrhexis nodosa
Trichosanthes cucumerina
trichosomatous
Trichosporon
    T. asahii
    T. asteroides
    T. beigelii
    T. cutaneum
    T. faecale

    T. fuscans
    T. giganteum
    T. gracile
    T. granulosum
    T. inkin
    T. loboi
    T. mucoides
    T. ovoides
    T. pedrosianum
    T. penicillatum
    T. proteolyticum
    T. pullulans
    T. variabile
Trichosporonoides
trichosporosis
trichostrongyle
trichostrongyliasis
Trichostrongylidae
Trichostrongyloidea
trichostrongylosis
Trichostrongylus
    T. axei
    T. brevis
    T. capricola
    T. colubriformis
    T. instabilis
    T. longispicularis
    T. orientalis
    T. probolurus
    T. tenuis
    T. vitrinus
trichothecene mycotoxin
Trichothecium roseum
trichotomy
trichotoxin
Trichovirus
trichrome stain
trichuriasis
Trichuris
    T. suis
    T. trichiura
    T. vulpis
Trichuroidea
Trichurus spiralis
tricorn protease
tricresol
tricresyl phosphate
Tricula
tricuspid, tricuspidal, tricuspidate
    t. atresia
    t. incompetence (TI)
    t. insufficiency (TI)
    t. regurgitation
    t. stenosis
    t. valve
    t. valve cleft leaflet
tricuspidal (*var. of* tricuspid)
tricuspidate (*var. of* tricuspid)

tricuspidatus
tricuspis
    Ollulanus t.
trident hand
tridermoma
triethanolamine
triethylenethiophosphoramide precoated slide
trifid stomach
trifluoride-methanol
    boron t.-m.
trifluoroacetic anhydride (TFAA)
trifluorocarbonylcyanide phenylhydrazone (FCCP)
trigeminal dermatome
triglyceride (TG)
    t. assay
    long-chain t. (LCT)
    medium-chain t. (MCT)
    plasma t.
trigona (*pl. of* trigonum)
trigonitis
trigonocephalum
    Bunostomum t.
Trigonopsis
trigonosporus
    Microascus t.
trigonum, *pl.* **trigona**
    t. sternocostale
trihexosidase
    ceramide t.
trihexoside
    ceramide t. (CTH)
trihydride
    arsenic t.
triiodide
    bismuth t.
triiodothyronine (T_3)
    t. assay
    t. by RIA
    free t. (FT_3)
    t. resin uptake (T_3RU)
    t. resin uptake test
    reverse t. (rT_3)
    t. suppression test
    t. toxicosis (T_3-toxicosis)
    t. uptake (T_3U)
triketohydrindene reaction
trilaminar
trilineage dysplasia
trilinear maturation
triloba
    placenta t.
trilobate placenta
trilocular heart
trilogy
Trilone
trimastigote
trimer

trimetaphosphate
    sodium t.
trimethoprim
trimethoxyamphetamine
trimethylacetate
    desoxycorticosterone t. (DCTMA)
trimethylamine
trimethylaminuria
trimmed specimen
trimming resistor
trimorphic
trimorphism
trimorphous
Trinder
    T. reaction
    T. test
trinitrotoluene
trinocular microscope
trinucleotide
    t. CAG
    t. repeat
    t. repeat disorder
tri-*o*-cresyl phosphate
Triodontophorus diminutus
triol
triolein I-131
triose
triosephosphate
    t. dehydrogenase
    t. isomerase
    t. isomerase assay
    t. isomerase deficiency
trioxide
    arsenic t. (As_2O_3)
    sulfur t.
2,6,8-trioxypurine
tripartita
    placenta t.
triphasic wave
triphenylacetate
    desoxycorticosterone t. (DCTPA)
triphenyl albumin
triphenylmethane dye
Triphleps insidiosus
triphosphatase
    adenosine t. (ATPase)
triphosphate (TP)
    adenosine t. (ATP)
    adenosine 5′-diphosphate/adenosine t.
    cytidine t. (CTP)
    cytosine t. (CTP)
    deoxythymidine t. (dTTP)
    deoxyuridine t. (DUTP)
    guanosine t. (GTP)
    inosine t.
    thymidine t.
    uridine t. (UTP)
5′-triphosphate
    2-deoxyguanosine 5.-t. (dGTP)

T

triphyllomatous teratoma
triple
- t. bond
- t. phosphate
- t. phosphate crystal
- t. point
- t. screen
- t. sugar iron (TSI)
- t. sugar iron agar
- t. symptom complex
- t. test
- t. X syndrome

triple-blind
triplet
- t. code
- coding t.
- nonsense t.
- t. repeat

triple-X chromosomal aberration
triploblastic
triploid mosaicism
triploidy
triradiate
trisacryl gelatin microsphere
Tris-buffered saline
triseriatus
- *Aedes t.*

Tris-HCl buffer
tris(hydroxymethyl) **aminomethane**
trisimilitubis
- *Isoparorchis t.*

trisodium foscarnet salt
trisomic cell
trisomy
- t. 12
- chromosome t.
- complete t.
- double t.
- t. 8 mosaicism
- primary t.
- primary t. 18
- secondary t.
- t. 8, 13, 18, 20, 21, 22 syndrome
- tertiary t.
- translocation t.
- t. XXY

tristearin
trisymptome
trit
- triturate

triterpene
triterpenoid saponin
tritiated
- t. gas
- t. thymidine (TTH)
- t. water

triticeous
tritici

Ochrobactrum t.
Pyemotes t.
Tritimovirus
Tritirachium
tritium (H3)
triton tumor
Triton-X 100
Tritrichomonas
triturate (trit)
Triturus automated ELISA immunoassay analyzer
trivalent oral poliovirus vaccine (TOPV)
triviale
- *Mycobacterium t.*

trivialis
- *Pseudomonas t.*

trivittatus
- *Aedes t.*

Trizma buffer concentrate
TRIzol reagent
trizonal
TRK-A gene expression
tRNA
- transfer RNA
- tRNA suppressor

Troglotrema salmincola
Troglotrematidae
Troisier
- T. ganglion
- T. node
- T. syndrome

troitsensis
- *Arenibacter t.*

Trojan horse inhibitor
troleandomycin
Tröltsch corpuscle
Trombicula
- T. akamushi
- T. alfreddugesi
- T. autumnalis
- T. deliensis
- T. pallida
- T. scutellaris
- T. tsalsahuatl

trombiculiasis
Trombiculidae
trombiculid mite
Trombidiidae
Trombidoidea
tromethamine
tropeolin
trophedema
Tropheryma whipplei
trophic
- t. gangrene
- t. lesion
- t. nucleus
- t. signal
- t. ulcer

trophoblast
- t. basement membrane thickening
- t. cell
- syncytial t.

trophoblastic
- t. cell membrane
- t. disease
- t. embolization
- malignant teratoma, t. (MTT)
- t. malignant teratoma
- t. neoplasia
- t. neoplasm
- t. tumor

trophoblastoma
trophochromatin
trophochromidia
trophocyte
trophoderm
trophodermatoneurosis
trophoneurosis
- facial t.
- Romberg t.

trophoneurotic leprosy
trophonucleus
trophoplasm
trophoplast
trophospongium
trophotaxis
trophozoite
tropica
- *Herpetomonas t.*
- *Leishmania t.*
- *Nocardiopsis t.*

tropical
- t. abscess
- t. anemia
- t. ataxic neuropathy (TAN)
- t. bubo
- t. diarrhea
- t. disease
- t. eosinophilia
- t. mask
- t. measles
- t. splenomegaly syndrome (TSS)
- t. sprue (TS)
- t. typhus

tropicalis
- *Acetobacter t.*
- adenitis t.
- *Candida t.*
- *Entamoeba t.*
- tinea t.

Tropicorbis
tropicum
- granuloma inguinale t.

tropicus
- *Amphibacillus t.*
- *Psychroflexus t.*

tropism
- negative t.
- positive t.
- viral t.

tropocollagen
tropoelastin
tropomodulin-1
- t.-1 antibody (TMOD1)
- t.-1 antigen

tropomyosin
- alpha t.

tropomyosin-binding protein
troponin
- Cardiac STATus controls for t. I
- Cardiac T rapid assay for t. T
- t. C (TnC)
- t. I (TnI)
- t. T (TnT)

trough
- synaptic t.

Trousseau
- T. syndrome
- T. test

Trousseau-Lallemand body
TRPC6 gene
T₃RU
- triiodothyronine resin uptake

TRU
- turbidity-reducing unit

Truant auramine-rhodamine stain
Tru-cut, Trucut
- T.-C. biopsy
- T.-C. needle

Trucut (*var. of* Tru-Cut)
true
- t. aneurysm
- t. diverticulum
- t. hypertrophy
- t. mucosal margin
- T. test kit

trueperi
- *Thiobaca t.*

TruGene HIV-1 genotyping kit
Trump fixative
truncate
Truncatella
truncation
truncatum
- *Pseudamphistomum t.*

trunci (*pl. of* truncus)
truncus, *pl.* **trunci**
- t. arteriosus (TA)
- t. fascicularis atrioventricularis

trunk
- t. abscess
- t. duplication
- t. of atrioventricular bundle
- pulmonary t. (PT)

951

TRUS
transrectal ultrasound-guided sextant biopsy
truth table
TrxR
thioredoxin reductase
tryosine kinase inhibitor
trypan
t. blue
t. red
trypanicidal
trypanicide
trypanid
trypanocidal
trypanocide
Trypanoplasma
Trypanosoma
T. ariarii
T. avium
T. brucei brucei
T. brucei gambiense
T. brucei rhodesiense
T. castellani
T. congolense
T. cruzi
T. dimorphon
T. equinum
T. equiperdum
T. escomelis
T. evansi
T. hominis
T. lewisi
T. melophagium
T. nigeriense
T. rangeli
T. simiae
T. suis
T. theileri
T. triatomae
T. ugandense
T. vivax
trypanosomatid
Trypanosomatidae
trypanosome
trypanosomiasis
African t.
American t.
Brazilian t.
East African (Rhodesian) t.
Gambian t.
Rhodesian t.
trypanosomic
trypanosomicidal
trypanosomicide
trypanosomid
tryparsamide
Trypetidae
trypomastigote

trypsin
t. assay
t. digest technique
fecal t.
t. G-banding stain
t. inhibitor
stool t.
t. test
trypsin-aldehyde-fuchsin (TAF)
trypsin-inhibitory capacity (TIC)
trypsinization
trypsinogen, trypsogen
trypsogen (*var. of* trypsinogen)
tryptamine
tryptase
t. immunostain
mast cell t.
tryptic
t. activity
t. soy agar
trypticase
t. soy agar (TSA)
t. soy with agar broth
t. soy yeast (TSY)
tryptone
tryptonemia
tryptophan (TP)
t. challenge test
t. load test
t. malabsorption syndrome
tryptophanemia
tryptophanuria
tryptophyl
TS
test solution
total solids
tropical sprue
T₄SA
thyroxine-specific activity
TSA
trypticase soy agar
tyramide signal amplification
TSAH
traumatic subarachnoid hemorrhage
tsalsahuatl
Trombicula t.
TSB
total serum bilirubin
TSC
tuberous sclerosis complex
TSC1 gene
TSC2 gene
TSD
Tay-Sachs disease
TSE
transmissible spongiform encephalopathy
tsetse fly

TSF
>tissue-coding factor

TSH
>thyroid-stimulating hormone
>>TSH assay
>>TSH binding inhibitory
>>immunoglobulin (TBII)
>>TSH displacing antibody (TDA)
>>TSH releasing hormone
>>TSH stimulating test
>>TSH stimulation test

TSHR
>thyrotropin-receptor antibody

TSH-RF
>thyroid-stimulating hormone-releasing
>factor

TSH-stimulating test
TSI
>thyroid-stimulating immunoglobulin
>triple sugar iron
>>TSI agar

TSIA
>triple sugar iron agar

TSLC1 gene
t-s mutation
TSNP
>two-step nested PCR

TSP
>total serum protein

TSPAP
>total serum prostatic acid phosphatase

TSR
>thyroid-to-serum ratio

TSS
>tropical splenomegaly syndrome

TSST1
>toxic shock syndrome toxin

TST
>tumor skin test

TSTA
>tumor-specific transplantation
>antigen

T-strain mycoplasma
Tsukamurella
>>*T. inchonensis*
>>*T. paurometabola*
>>*T. pulmonis*
>>*T. spumae*
>>*T. strandjordii*
>>*T. tyrosinosolvens*
>>*T. wratislaviensis*

Tsukamurellaceae
Tsunami laser
T-suppressor cell
T-suppressor/cytotoxic subset marker
tsuruhatensis
>>*Delftia t.*

tsutsugamushi
>t. disease

>t. fever
>>*Orientia t.*
>>*Rickettsia t.*

TSY
>trypticase soy yeast

TT
>thrombin time
>thymol turbidity
>total thyroxine

T$_4$/TBG ratio
TTD
>tissue tolerance dose

TTF-1
>thyroid transcription factor-1
>thyroid transcription factor-1
>immunostain

TTGE
>temporal temperature gradient gel
>electrophoresis

TTH
>thyrotropic hormone
>tritiated thymidine

TTI
>time-tension index
>>TTI procedure

TTIT
>tissue thromboplastin inhibition test

T/T Mega advanced multifunction microwave labstation
T$_3$-toxicosis
>triiodothyronine toxicosis

TTP
>thrombotic thrombocytopenic purpura
>>TTP assay

TTP-HUS
>thrombotic thrombocytopenic purpura
>and hemolytic uremic syndrome

TTR
>transthyretin

TTT
>tolbutamide tolerance test

TTTS
>twin-to-twin transfusion syndrome
>twin-twin transfusion syndrome

T-tubular system
TTV
>transfusion transmitted virus

TU
>Todd unit
>toxic unit
>toxin unit
>tuberculin unit

tuba, *pl.* **tubae**
>t. acustica
>t. auditiva
>t. auditoria
>t. eustachiana
>laciniae tubae

tub1 adenocarcinoma

T

tub2 adenocarcinoma
tubae (*pl. of* tuba)
tubaeforme
 Ancylostoma t.
tubal
 t. abortion
 t. air cell of pharyngotympanic tube
 t. infantilism
 t. pregnancy
 t. tonsil
tubaria
 tonsilla t.
tubariae
 glandulae t.
tube, tubing
 t. agglutination (TA)
 ampulla of uterine t.
 auditory t.
 Babcock t.
 capillary t.
 t. cast
 cathode ray t.
 t. cell
 ClearCRIT microhematocrit t.
 Corvac integrated serum separator t.
 Craigie t.
 t. culture
 digestive t.
 t. dilution test
 discharge t.
 Durham t.
 electron multiplier t.
 Eppendorf t.
 eustachian t.
 fermentation t.
 Ferrein t.
 fimbriae of uterine t.
 germ t.
 glow modulator t.
 Greiner Vacuette coagulation
  plastic t.
 Hamamatzu high-sensitivity
  photomultiplier t.
 Hemochron P214 glass-activated
  ACT t.
 indicator t.
 Isolator lysis-centrifugation t.
 lateral plate of cartilaginous
  auditory t.
 LipoClear reagent t.
 Luki aspirating t.
 medial plate of cartilaginous
  auditory t.
 Mett test t.
 microfuge t.
 mucous gland of auditory t.
 mycobacteria growth indicator t.
  (MGIT)
 NIXIE t.

otopharyngeal t.
t. precipitin (TP)
pus t.
roll t.
SafeCrit microhematocrit t.
Safetex t.
sediment t.
sedimentation t.
sputum t.
Takara Biomedicals Suprec t.
test t.
tubal air cell of pharyngotympanic
 t.
Unopette t.
Vacuette blood sample t.
vacuum t.
Veillon t.
voltage-regulator t.
Wintrobe hematocrit t.
tubeless
 t. gastric analysis
 t. gastric analysis test
tuber
tuberalis
tubercle
 anatomic t.
 anatomic t.
 Babès t.
 t. bacillus (TB)
 caseous t.
 dissection t.
 fibrous t.
 genital t.
 Ghon t.
 Ghon-Sachs t.
 hard t.
 hyaline t.
 Montgomery t.
 mycobacteria other than t.
  (MOTT)
 postmortem t.
 prosector's t.
 sebaceous t.
 soft t.
tubercular, tuberculated
tuberculated (*var. of* tubercular)
tuberculation
tuberculid
 nodular t.
 rosacea-like t.
tuberculin
 albumose-free t. (TAF)
 alkaline t. (TA)
 Büchner t.
 t. filtrate (TF)
 Koch old t.
 old t. (OT)
 t. precipitation (TP)
 purified protein derivative of t.

t. reaction
t. R (new tuberculin) (TR)
Seibert t.
t. skin test
t. unit (TU)
vacuum t. (VT)
tuberculin-type
t.-t. hypersensitivity
t.-t. reaction
tuberculitis
tuberculization
tuberculochemotherapeutic
tuberculocidal
tuberculoderma
tuberculofibroid
tuberculoid
t. granuloma
t. leprosy
tuberculoid-type granuloma
tuberculoma
tuberculoopsonic index
tuberculoprotein
tuberculosis (TB, TBC)
acute miliary t.
adult t.
anthracotic t.
arrested t.
attenuated t.
Bacillus t.
basal t.
central nervous system t.
cerebral t.
cutaneous t.
t. cutis
t. cutis luposa
t. cutis orificialis
t. cutis verrucosa
dermal t.
disseminated t.
endobronchial t.
extrapulmonary t.
gastrointestinal t.
general t.
generalized t.
t. granulation tissue
healed t.
inactive t.
laryngeal t.
t. lymphadenitis
miliary t.
Mycobacterium t. (MTB)
open t.
t. organisms in tissue section
placental t.
pleural t.
postprimary t.
primary t.
pulmonary t.
reinfection t.

renal t.
respiratory t.
secondary t.
t. skin test
t. ulcerosa
urinary t.
t. vaccine
tuberculosis-respiratory disease (TB-RD)
tuberculostat
tuberculostatic
tuberculostearic acid
tuberculostearicum
Corynebacterium t.
tuberculosus
lupus t.
tuberculous
t. abscess
t. bronchopneumonia
t. cystitis
t. gumma
t. infiltration
t. lymphadenitis
t. meningitis (TBM)
t. nephritis
t. osteomyelitis
t. pericarditis
t. peritonitis
t. prostatitis
t. rheumatism
t. scrofuloderma
t. spondylitis
t. wart
tuberculum
t. arthriticum
tubercula dolorosa
t. sebaceum
t. syphiliticum
tuberiferous
tuberin
tuberoeruptive xanthoma
tuberosa
urticaria t.
tuberosity
ischial t.
pubic t.
tibial t.
tuberosum
xanthoma t.
tuberous
t. sclerosis
t. sclerosis complex (TSC)
tuberum
Burkholderia t.
tubi (*pl. of* tubus)
Tubifera ferruginosa
tubing (*var. of* tube)
Tygon t.
tubocurarine

T

tuboendometrioid
    t. metaplasia
    t. type
tubo-ovarian (*var. of* tuboovarian)
tuboovarian, tubo-ovarian
    t. abscess (TOA)
    t. varicocele
tuboovaritis
tuboreticular structure
tubovesicular network
tubovillous adenoma
tubular
    t. adenocarcinoma
    t. adenoma
    t. adenosis
    t. aggregate
    t. aneurysm
    t. basement membrane (TBM)
    t. carcinoma
    t. cristae
    t. cyst
    t. epithelial-myofibroblast transdifferentiation (TEMT)
    t. fluid (TF)
    t. gland
    t. infiltration
    t. nephrosis
    t. pit
    t. reabsorption
    t. reabsorption of phosphate test
    t. secretion
    t. visual field
tubular-fertility index (TFI)
tubule
    Albarían y Dominguez t.
    aluminal t.
    connecting t.
    convoluted seminiferous t.
    dental t.
    dentin t.
    dentinal t.
    discharging t.
    t. formation
    Henle t.
    mesonephric t.
    metanephric t.
    t. of testis
    renal uriniferous t.
    seminiferous t.
    sex cord tumor with annular t.
    spiral t.
    straight t.
    T t.
    typical seminiferous t.
    uriniferous t.
tubuli (*pl. of* tubulus)
tubuliform
tubulin
    beta t.

tubulitis
tubuloacinar gland
tubuloalveolar mucous gland
tubulocyst
tubulocystic growth pattern
tubulodermoid
tubulointerstitial
    t. lesion
    t. nephritis
    t. nephropathy (TIN)
tubulonecrosis
tubuloneogenesis
tubulopapillary
    t. architectural pattern
    t. carcinoma
tubuloracemose
tubuloreticular aggregate
tubulorrhexis
tubulose (*var. of* tubulous)
tubulous, tubulose
tubulovesicle
tubulovesicular
tubulus, *pl.* **tubuli**
    tubuli biliferi
    tubuli contorti
    tubuli dentales
    tubuli epoophori
    tubuli galactophori
    tubuli lactiferi
    tubuli paroophori
    t. rectus
    t. renalis contortus
    tubuli seminiferi recti
    tubuli seminiferi recti testi
    t. transversus
tubus, *pl.* **tubi**
    t. digestorius
tucumana
    Filaria t.
    Mansonella t.
tuffstone body
tuft
    enamel t.
    glomerular t.
    malpighian t.
    synovial t.
tufted
    t. cell
    t. phalanx
tufting enteropathy
tuftsin deficiency
TUG
    total urinary gonadotropin
tularemia
    t. agglutinin
    enteric t.
    oculoglandular t.
    oropharyngeal t.
    t. pneumonia

pneumonia t.
pneumonic t.
t. sepsis
typhoidal t.
ulceroglandular t.
tularemic
    t. chancre
    t. conjunctivitis
    t. pneumonia
    t. sepsis
tularense
    Bacillus t.
tularensis
    Francisella t.
tumefacient
tumefaction
tumefactive fibroinflammatory lesion (TFL)
tumefy
tumentia
tumescence, turgescence
tumescent
tumeur d'emblée
tumid
tumidus
    lupus t.
tumor
    Abrikosov t.
    acellular t.
    acinar cell t.
    acinic cell t.
    acute splenic t.
    adenoid t.
    adenomatoid odontogenic t.
    adipose t.
    adrenal t.
    adrenocortical rest t.
    adult granulosa cell t. (AGCT)
    ameloblastic adenomatoid t.
    ampullary t.
    amyloid t.
    aneuploid t.
    t. aneuploidy
    t. angiogenesis
    t. angiogenic factor (TAF)
    angiomatoid t.
    t. antigen
    aortic body t.
    apocrine t.
    Askin t.
    astrocytic t.
    atypical carcinoid t.
    atypical teratoid t. (ATT)
    atypical teratoid/rhabdoid t. (AT/RT)
    basaloid t.
    Bednar t.
    benign epithelial breast t.
    biphasic t.
    bladder t. (BT)

blood t.
blue cell t.
t. blush
Bolande t.
bone t.
borderline ovarian t.
brain t. (BT)
brainstem t.
breast t.
Brenner t.
bronchogenic t.
Brooke t.
brown t.
Brown-Pearce t.
t. burden
Burkitt t.
burnt-out germ cell t.
Buschke-Löwenstein t.
calcifying epithelial odontogenic t. (CEOT)
t. capsule
carcinoid t.
carotid body t.
t. cell
t. cell kinetics
t. cell motility
t. cell population
cellular t.
central nervous system t.
cerebellar t.
cerebellopontine angle t.
chemoreceptor t.
chiasmal t.
chondromatous giant cell t.
chromaffin t.
chromophobe t.
clear cell borderline t.
clear cell sugar t.
Codman t.
collision t.
colon t.
compound t.
connective t.
cutaneous neural t. (CNT)
Dabska t.
dendritic cell t.
dentigerous mixed t.
dermal duct t.
dermoid t.
desmoid t.
desmoplastic small round cell t. (DSRCT)
diploid t.
ductectatic-type mucinous cystic t.
ductus deferens t.
dysembryoplastic neuroepithelial t.
dysplastic neuroepithelial t. (DNET)
eccrine t.

T

tumor (*continued*)
ectomesenchymal chondromyxoid t.
(ECT)
Ehrlich t.
eighth nerve t.
t. embolism
t. embolus
embryonal t.
embryonic t.
endobronchial t.
endocervical mucinous borderline t.
(EMBLT, EMBT)
endodermal sinus t.
endometrioid t.
epiphysial giant cell t.
epithelial t. (ET)
epithelial-stromal t.
Erdheim t.
esophageal t.
Ewing sarcoma family of t.'s
(ESFT)
Ewing sarcoma/peripheral
neuroectodermal t.
Ewing sarcoma/primitive
neuroectodermal t.
extracapsular t.
extragonadal germ cell t.
extrarenal rhabdoid t. (ERRT)
extrauterine-extraovarian endometrioid
stromal t.
exuberant t.
eye t.
fallopian tube t.
fecal t.
Fechner t.
feminizing t.
fibroblastic t.
fibroepithelial t.
fibroid t.
fibromyxoid t.
Fuhrman grade t.
functional t.
gastric t.
gastrointestinal autonomic nerve t.
(GANT)
gastrointestinal pacemaker cell t.
(GIPACT)
gastrointestinal smooth muscle t.
gastrointestinal stromal t. (GIST)
G-cell t.
gemistocytic t.
germ cell t.
giant cell t.
globoid encapsulated t.
glomus jugulare t.
Godwin t.
gonadal stromal t.
t. grading
granular cell t.

granulosa cell t.
granulosa-stromal cell t.
granulosa-theca cell t.
Grawitz t.
Gruber-Frantz t.
Gubler t.
hamartomatous t.
heart t.
hematopoietic t.
hepatic t.
heterologous t.
histoid t.
t. histology
homologous t.
Hürthle cell t.
hyalinizing trabecular t.
hylic t.
inflammatory fibromyxoid t.
inflammatory myofibroblastic t.
(IMT)
innocent t.
t. in situ (TIS)
interdigitating dendritic cell t.
intestinal mucinous borderline t.
(IMBT)
intracranial t.
intraductal papillary mucinous t.
(IPMT)
intratesticular t.
intravascular sclerosing
bronchioloalveolar t. (IVBAT)
islet cell t.
juvenile granulosa cell t.
(JGCT)
juxtaglomerular cell t. (JGCT)
Koenen t.
Krukenberg t.
lacrimal gland t.
lacrimal sac t.
Landschutz t.
large-cell calcifying Sertoli cell t.
(LCCSCT)
t. lethal dose (TLD)
Lewis lung t.
Leydig cell t.
Leydig-Sertoli cell t.
Lindau t.
lipophyllodes t.
localized fibrous t.
low-risk t. (LRT)
lung t.
luteinizing t.
lymphoid t.
Lynch syndrome t.
t. lysis syndrome (TLS)
malignant breast t.
malignant cartilaginous t.
malignant giant cell t. (MGCT)
malignant mixed t. (MMT)

malignant mixed mesodermal t. (MMMT)
malignant mixed müllerian t. (MMMT)
malignant peripheral nerve sheath t. (MPNST)
malignant plasma cell t.
malignant rhabdoid t. (MRT)
malignant triton t. (MTT)
malignant vascular t.
t. map
t. marker
t. marker test
Masson t.
mast cell t.
mediastinal yolk sac t. (MYST)
melanotic neuroectodermal t.
Merkel cell t.
mesenchymal t.
mesonephroid t.
metanephric stromal t.
metastatic t.
t. mitotic rate
mixed epithelial t.
mixed epithelial-mesenchymal t.
mixed germ cell t. (MGCT)
mixed mesodermal t.
monoclonal t.
mucinous borderline t. (MBT)
mucinous cystic t. (MCT)
mucoepidermoid t.
müllerian t.
multiple t.
myofibroblastic mammary stromal t.
napkin ring t.
necrosis t.
t. necrosis
t. necrosis factor (TNF)
t. necrosis factor alpha (TNF-alpha)
t. necrosis factor beta
t. necrosis factor receptor (TNFR)
Nelson t.
nerve sheath t.
t. nest
neuroectodermal t.
neuroendocrine t. (NET)
no evidence of primary t. (T0)
nomenclature of t.
nonmyogenous t.
nonseminomatous germ cell t. (NSGCT)
odontogenic ghost cell t.
t. of Capella
t. of germ cell origin
t. of thymic epitheliocyte
oil t.
oligodendroglial t.
oncocytic hepatocellular t.
orbital t.

organoid t.
ovarian borderline t.
ovarian granulosa cell t.
ovarian mucinous t. (OMT)
ovarian serous borderline t. (OSBT)
ovarian sex-cord t.
Pindborg t.
pituitary t.
placental site trophoblastic t. (PSTT)
plasmacytic t.
pleomorphic hyalinizing angiectatic t. (PHAT)
polyclonal t.
t. polysaccharide substance (TPS)
polyvesicular vitelline t.
pontine angle t.
primary bone t.
primitive neuroectodermal t. (PNET)
primitive peripheral neuroectodermal t. (pPNET)
primitive small-cell thoracopulmonary t.
t. progression marker
proliferating pillar t.
t. promoter
prostatic t.
pseudosarcomatous fibromyxoid t.
pseudosarcomatous myofibroblastic t. (PMT)
pulmonary endodermal t. (PET)
pure t.
Rathke pouch t.
t. receptor-associated factor (TRAF)
Recklinghausen t.
rectal shelf t.
t. registry
renal t.
renin secreting t.
renomedullary interstitial cell t.
rete cell t.
retiform Sertoli-Leydig cell t.
retinal anlage t.
retrocardiac t.
retrosternal t.
Rous t.
salivary gland t.
salivary gland anlage t. (SGAT)
sand t.
sarcomatoid t.
sclerosing Sertoli cell t.
serous borderline t. (SBT)
Sertoli cell t.
Sertoli-Leydig cell t.
Sertoli stromal cell t.
sex cord-stromal t.
t. signature
sinonasal smooth muscle cell t.
skin t.
t. skin test

tumor (*continued*)
    small-cell t.
    small intestine t.
    small round cell t. (SRCT)
    smooth muscle t. (SMT)
    soft parts giant cell t. (SP-GCT)
    soft tissue t.
    solid pseudopapillary t.
    solitary fibrous t. (SFT)
    t. specificity
    spinal cord t.
    spindle cell t.
    splenic t.
    squamous odontogenic t.
    t. stage
    t. stage at diagnosis
    t. staging
    steroid cell t.
    stomach t.
    t. stroma
    sugar t.
    superior pulmonary sulcus t.
    superior sulcus t.
    t. suppressor gene
    t. suppressor pathway
    surface epithelial-stromal t.
    sweat gland t.
    synovial t.
    tenosynovial giant cell t.
    teratoid t.
    testicular germ cell t. (TGCT)
    testicular Sertoli cell t.
    tetraploid t.
    theca cell-granuloma cell t.
    theca lutein t.
    thrombus t.
    t. thrombus
    thymic carcinoid t. (TCT)
    thyroid t.
    transitional cell t.
    triton t.
    trophoblastic t.
    turban t.
    ulcerogenic t.
    urethral t.
    uterine tumor resembling an ovarian sex-cord t. (UTROSCT)
    vaginal t.
    villous t.
    t. virus
    vulvar t.
    Warthin t.
    Wharton t.
    WHO histologic classification of ovarian t.'s
    Wilms t.
    xenograft t.
    xenografted t.
    Yaba t.
    yolk sac t.
    Zollinger-Ellison t.

tumoraffin
tumoral calcinosis
tumor-antigen 4 (TA-4)
tumor-assisted lymphoid proliferation (TALP)
tumor-associated
    t.-a. glycoprotein (TAG)
    t.-a. rejection antigen (TARA)
    t.-a. transplantation antigen (TATA)
tumor-cell migration-inhibition factor (TMIF)
tumorigenesis
    foreign body t.
tumorigenic
tumorigenicity
tumor-induced stromal sclerosis
tumor-infiltrating lymphocyte (TIL)
tumorlet
tumor-like lesion
tumor-node-metastasis (TNM)
tumorous
tumor-specific transplantation antigen (TSTA)
tumor-suppressor protein
tundrae
    Acetobacterium t.
TUNEL
    TdT-mediated dUTP nick-end labeling
    TUNEL assay
Tunga penetrans
tungiasis
Tungidae
Tungrovirus
tungstate
    lithium t.
tungsten
    t. arc lamp
    t. carbide pneumoconiosis
    t. halogen lamp
tungstic acid
tungstoborate
    sodium t.
tunic, tunica
    Bichat t.
    Brücke t.
    circular layer of muscular t.
    corneoscleral t.
    longitudinal layer of muscular t.
    mucosal t.
    muscular t.
    serous t.
tunica (*var. of* tunic)
    t. adventitia
    t. albuginea
    t. albuginea corporis spongiosi

t. albuginea corporum cavernosorum
t. albuginea oculi
t. albuginea testis
t. carnea
t. conjunctiva
t. conjunctiva bulbi
t. conjunctiva palpebrarum
t. dartos
t. elastica
t. externa
t. externa oculi
t. externa thecae folliculi
t. extima
t. fibrosa
t. fibrosa bulbi
t. fibrosa hepatis
t. fibrosa lienis
t. fibrosa renis
t. fibrosa splenis
t. interna thecae folliculi
t. intima
t. media
t. media of arteriole
t. mucosa
t. mucosa bronchi
t. mucosa cavitatis tympani
t. mucosa coli
t. mucosa ductus deferentis
t. mucosa esophagi
t. mucosa gastrica
t. mucosa intestini tenuis
t. mucosa laryngis
t. mucosa linguae
t. mucosa nasi
t. mucosa oris
t. mucosa pharyngis
t. mucosa tracheae
t. mucosa tubae auditivae
t. mucosa tubae uterinae
t. mucosa ureteris
t. mucosa urethrae femininae
t. mucosa uteri
t. mucosa vaginae
t. mucosa vesicae biliaris
t. mucosa vesicae felleae
t. mucosa vesicae urinariae
t. muscularis
t. muscularis bronchiorum
t. muscularis coli
t. muscularis ductus deferentis
t. muscularis esophagi
t. muscularis intestini tenuis
t. muscularis recti
t. muscularis tracheae
t. muscularis tubae uterinae
t. muscularis ureteris
t. muscularis urethrae femininae
t. muscularis uteri
t. muscularis vaginae

t. muscularis ventriculi
t. muscularis vesicae biliaris
t. muscularis vesicae felleae
t. muscularis vesicae urinariae
t. nervea
t. propria
t. propria corii
t. propria lienis
t. reflexa
t. sclerotica
t. serosa
t. serosa coli
t. serosa hepatis
t. serosa intestini tenuis
t. serosa peritonei
t. serosa tubae uterinae
t. serosa uteri
t. serosa ventriculi
t. serosa vesicae biliaris
t. serosa vesicae felleae
t. serosa vesicae urinariae
t. submucosa
t. vaginalis
t. vaginalis testis
t. vasculosa
t. vasculosa bulbi
t. vasculosa lentis
t. vasculosa oculi
t. vasculosa testis
t. vitrea

tunicae
    t. funiculi spermatici
    regio olfactoria t.

tunnel
    t. cell
    Corti t.

turban
    t. growth
    t. tumor

Turbatrix aceti
turbid
turbidimeter
turbidimetric
    t. aggregometry
    t. immunoassay
turbidimetry
turbidity
    increased t.
    thymol t. (TT)
turbidity-reducing unit (TRU)
turbinal varix
turcica
    Borrelia t.
Türck degeneration
Turcot
    T. syndrome
    T. syndrome
turgescence (*var. of* tumescence)
turgescent

T

turgid
turicata
    Ornithodoros t.
turicatae
    Borrelia t.
turicensis
Turicibacter sanguinis
Türk
    T. cell
    T. irritation leukocyte
turkey
    t. meningoencephalitis virus
    t. red
turkmenica
    Haloterrigena t.
Turlock virus
turn-around time (TAT)
Turnbull
    T. blue
    T. blue stain
turnerae
    Teredinibacter t.
Turner syndrome
turnover
    bone t.
    t. number
    plasma iron t. (PIT)
    protein t.
    T-cell t.
TURP
    transurethral resection of prostate
    TURP chip
turpentine oil
turricephaly
T₃U test
TV
    tidal volume
TWAR
    Taiwan acute respiratory
    TWAR stain
twiddler's syndrome
twig
    motor axon t.
twin
    t. cone
    conjoined t.'s
    corpora lutea t.'s
    t. crystal
    dichorionic placenta t.'s
    dizygotic t.'s
    fraternal t.'s
    heterokaryotic t.'s
    identical t.'s
    incomplete conjoined t.'s
    monoamniotic placenta t.'s
    monochorionic diamniotic placenta
      t.'s
    monozygotic t.'s
    t. placenta

    placenta t.'s
    Siamese t.'s
twin-to-twin transfusion syndrome (TTTS)
twin-twin transfusion syndrome (TTTS)
TWL
    transepidermal water loss
two-cell
    t.-c. type rule
    t.-c. wide vertical cord
two-dimensional (2D)
    t.-d. chromatography
    t.-d. gel electrophoresis
    t.-d. immunoelectrophoresis
    t.-d. polyacrylamide gel
      electrophoresis
two-glass test
two-parameter histogram
Twort-d'Herelle phenomenon
Twort phenomenon
two's complement
two-sided alternative
two-site immunoenzymometric assay
two-slide method
two-stage PT test
two-step nested PCR (TSNP)
two-tail test
two-tube nested PCR
Tx
    treatment
Ty
    typhoid
Tygon tubing
tylosis palmaris et plantaris
Tymovirus
tympana (*pl. of* tympanum)
tympani
    membrana t.
    stratum circulare membranae t.
    stratum cutaneum membranae t.
    stratum radiatum membranae t.
    substantia propria membranae t.
    tunica mucosa cavitatis t.
tympanic
    t. body
    t. cell
    t. gland
    t. membrane
tympanicae
    cellulae t.
tympanosclerosis
tympanum, *pl.* **tympana, tympanums**
    membrane of t.
tympanums (*pl. of* tympanum)
Tyndall effect
tyndallization
type
    t. A intercalated cell
    atypical melanocytic nevi of genital
      t. (AMNGT)

autoimmune polyendocrine syndrome t. 1 (APS1)
autosomal dominant osteopetrosis t. 2 (ADO2)
B cell lymphoma of MALT t.
t. B intercalated cell
blood t.
t. C nevus cell
t. culture
dengue virus, t. 1–4
t. 1–4 dextrocardia
T. 1 diabetes
T. 2 diabetes (T2D)
Duffy blood antibody t.
enterovirus t. 71 (EV 71)
familial multiple endocrine adenomatosis, t. 1, 2
hemadsorption virus t. 1, 2
hyperplasia of usual t. (HUT)
hypertyrosinemia, Oregon t.
t. I cell
t. I collagen gene
t. II alveolar epithelial cell
t. II alveolar epithelial cell adenocarcinoma
t. I, II dysgammaglobulinemia
t. I, II error
t. II membranoproliferative glomerulonephritis
t. I–IV delayed-type reaction
t. I–IV hypersensitivity reaction
t. I–IV pili
intraepidermal basal cell epithelioma, Borst-Jadassohn t.
intratubular germ cell neoplasia, unclassified t. (IGCNU)
t. I–XX collagen
Kell body antibody t.
Kidd blood antibody t.
Lutheran blood antibody t.
membrane t. 1–6
mixed epithelial papillary cystadenoma of borderline malignancy of müllerian t. (MEBMM)
neurotrophic tyrosine kinase receptor, t. 1 (NTRK1)
no specific t. (NST)
t. 1 pneumocyte
t. 2 pneumocyte
primary hyperoxaluria, t. 1 (PH1)
reovirus t. 1, 2, 3
Rh t.
t. species
t. strain
tuboendometrioid t.
t. V glycogenosis
wild t.

Typenex blood-recipient identification system
typhi
    Bacillus t.
    Eberthella t.
    Rickettsia t.
typhimurium
    Salmonella enteritidis serotype *t.*
typhinia
typhlectasis
typhlenteritis (*var. of* typhlitis)
typhlitis, typhlenteritis
Typhlocoelum cucumerinum
typhlomegaly
typhlonius
    Helicobacter t.
typhoid (Ty)
    t. bacillus
    t. bacteriophage
    t. cholera
    t. enteritis
    t. fever (TF)
    t. immunization reaction
    t., paratyphoid A, and paratyphoid B (TAB)
    provocation t.
    t. septicemia
typhoidal tularemia
typhoid-paratyphoid A and B vaccine
typholysin
typhosepsis
typhosus
    Bacillus t.
typhous
typhus
    t. antibody test
    endemic t.
    endemic murine t.
    t. epidemic
    epidemic louse-borne t.
    louse-borne t.
    mite t.
    murine t.
    recrudescent t.
    scrub t.
    tropical t.
    t. vaccine
typical
    t. seminiferous tubule
    t. smooth muscle cell
typing
    ABO t.
    ABO-Rh t.
    bacteriophage t.
    blood t.
    forward blood t.
    HLA t.
    molecular t.
    primed lymphocyte t.

T

typing (*continued*)
    reverse blood t.
    Rh t.
    $Rh_o(D)$ t.
    sequenced-based t. (SBT)
    tissue t.
tyramide signal amplification (TSA)
tyramine test
Tyroglyphidae
Tyroglyphus
    T. longior
    T. siro
tyroid
tyroketonuria
tyroma
Tyromyces
tyropanoate sodium
Tyrophagus putrescentiae
tyrosinase deficiency
tyrosine
    t. assay
    t. crystal
    t. hydroxylase (TH)
    kinase t. (KIT)
    t. kinase receptor
    t. phosphorylation
    t. test
tyrosinemia
    hereditary t.
tyrosinosis
tyrosinosolvens
    Tsukamurella t.
tyrosinuria
tyrosis
tyrosyl
tyrosyl-RNA synthetase
tyrosyluria
tyrothricin
TYSGM-9 medium
TY1-S-33 medium
Tyson gland
Tyzzer disease
Tyzzeria
TZ
    transition zone
Tzanck
    T. cell
    T. smear
    T. test
T-zone dysplasia

U
  unit
U6
  U6 riboprobe
  U6 snRNA molecule
UA
  uric acid
  urinalysis
  uterine aspiration
    PocketChem UA
UACL
  ulcer associated cell lineage
UADT
  upper aerodigestive tract
UBBC
  unsaturated vitamin B_{12}-binding
  capacity
uberis
    Streptococcus u.
UBF
  uterine blood flow
UBG
  urobilinogen
UBI
  ultraviolet blood irradiation
ubiq
  ubiquitin
ubiquinol
ubiquinone
ubiquitin (ubiq)
    u. C-terminal hydrolase
    u. ligase
ubiquitinated inclusion
ubiquitination
ubiquitin-protease pathway
ubiquitin-proteasome system
  (UPS)
ubisemiquinone
ubonensis
    Burkholderia u.
UBT
  urea breath test
UC
  ulcerative colitis
  ultracentrifugal
UcA
  urothelial carcinoma
U-cell lymphoma
UCG
  urinary chorionic gonadotropin
UCHL1 antibody
UCHL1^a antibody
UCL3D3 antibody
UCP
  urinary coproporphyrin

Ucr
  concentration of creatinine in urine
UD
  urethral discharge
UDCA
  ursodeoxycholic acid
Udeniomyces
UDG
  uracil DNA glycosylase
UDP
  uridine diphosphate
  urine drug panel
UDP-galactose
UDP-glucose
UDP-glucose-hexose-1-phosphate
    U.-g.-h.-1-p. uridylyltransferase
    U.-g.-h.-1-p. uridylyltransferase assay
UDP-glucuronate
UDP-glucuronic acid
UDP-glucuronyl transferase
UDP-iduronic acid
UDP-l-iduronate
UDP-*N*-acetyl-d-galactosamine
UDP-*N*-acetyl-d-glucosamine
UDP-xylose
UDS
  urine drug screen
UE
    Ulex europaeus
UEC
  uterine endometrial carcinoma
Uehlinger syndrome
UF
  ulcerating form
UFA
  unesterified fatty acid
Uffelmann test
U fiber
U-fiber
    cortical U-f.
Uganda S virus
ugandense
    Trypanosoma u.
UGI
  upper gastrointestinal
Uhl anomaly
UIBC
  unsaturated iron-binding capacity
UIF
  undegraded insulin factor
UIP
  usual interstitial pneumonia
  usual interstitial pneumonitis
UJ13A monoclonal antibody
UJ127.11 antibody

UL
   undifferentiated lymphoma
ulcer
   amebic u.
   amputating u.
   aphthous ileal u.
   u. associated cell lineage (UACL)
   Bairnsdale u.
   Barrett u.
   Buruli u.
   chancroidal u.
   chiclero u.
   chronic u.
   cockscomb u.
   cold u.
   constitutional u.
   corneal u.
   creeping u.
   Cruveilhier u.
   Curling u.
   Cushing u.
   decubitus u.
   diabetic u.
   diphtheritic u.
   discoid u.
   distention u.
   duodenal u.
   Fenwick-Hunner u.
   focal u.
   gastric u. (GU)
   groin u.
   gummatous u.
   hard u.
   healed u.
   hemorrhagic u.
   herpetic u.
   Hunner u.
   indolent u.
   inflamed u.
   Kocher dilation u.
   linear u.
   Lipschütz u.
   lupoid u.
   marginal u.
   Marjolin u.
   Meleney u.
   rodent u.
   Saemisch u.
   sea anemone u.
   serpiginous u.
   simple u.
   sloughing u.
   soft u.
   stasis u.
   stercoraceous u.
   stercoral u.
   stomal u.
   stress u.
   Sutton u.

   symptomatic u.
   syphilitic u.
   trophic u.
   varicose u.
   venereal u.
   warty u.
   Zambesi u.
ulcera (*pl. of* ulcus)
ulcerans
   Corynebacterium u.
   Mycobacterium u.
ulcerate
ulcerating form (UF)
ulceration
   acute hemorrhagic u.
   aphthous u.
   crateriform u.
   diffuse u.
ulcerative
   u. colitis (UC)
   u. cystitis
   u. dermatosis
   u. inflammation
   u. scrofuloderma
ulcerogenic tumor
ulceroglandular tularemia
ulceromembranous
ulcerosa
   blepharitis u.
   tuberculosis u.
ulcerous
ULCL4D12 antibody
ulcus, *pl.* **ulcera**
   u. ambulans
   u. terebrans
   u. venereum
   u. vulvae acutum
ulegyria
ulerythema ophryogenes
Ulex
   U. europaeus (UE)
   U. europaeus agglutinin
   U. lectin
uli
   Olsenella u.
uliginosa
   Cellulophaga u.
   Zobellia u.
uliginosum
   Clostridium u.
Ullmann line
Ullrich-Feichtiger syndrome
Ullrich-Turner syndrome
ulmi
   Xylanibacterium u.
ULMS
   uterine leiomyosarcoma
ULN
   upper limits of normal

ulnar nerve entrapment
Ulocladium chartarum
ulodermatitis
uloid
ULT
ultra low temperature
Ultima II refrigerator system
ultimate principle
ultimobranchial body
ultimum moriens
ultracentrifugal (UC)
ultracentrifugation
preparative u.
sucrose density gradient u.
ultracentrifuge
Airfuge u.
analytic u.
Discovery SE u.
Optima L-XP, L-90 K, LE-80 K
preparative u.
Optima Max, Max-E, TLX personal
benchtop u.
ultracytostome
ultradian rhythm
ultrafast Pap stain
ultrafilter
ultrafiltration hemodialyzer
ultrahigh vacuum
ultra low temperature (ULT)
ultramicroanalysis
ultramicroscope
ultramicroscopic
ultramicrotome
ultramicrotomy
**ultrashort-segment Hirschsprung
disease**
ultrasonic
u. cell disrupter
u. microscope
u. nebulizer (USN)
ultrasonication
ultrasonography
endoscopic u.
transrectal u.
ultrasound
intravascular coronary u.
ultrastructural
u. anatomy
u. characteristic
u. difference
u. immunochemistry
u. morphology of bone mineral
u. study
ultrastructure
ultrathin section
ultra-trace element
ultraviolet (UV)
u. blood irradiation (UBI)
u. burn

u. fluorescent dosimeter
u. irradiation
u. light
u. light-induced mutation
u. microscope
u. radiation
ultraviolet/visible spectrophotometry
ultravirus
ultropaque method
ulvae
Pseudoalteromonas u.
Ulvibacter litoralis
Ulysses syndrome
umbilical
u. cord blood transplant
u. cyst
u. fistula
u. hernia
u. polyp
Umbravirus
umbrella cell
Umbre virus
umidischolae
Nocardiopsis u.
UMP
undetermined malignant
potential
umsongensis
Pseudomonas u.
UN
urea nitrogen
UNa
concentration of sodium in urine
unaggregated
unamae
Burkholderia u.
unbiased estimate
**unbound thyroxine-binding globulin
(UTBG)**
uncal herniation
uncertainty principle
uncia
Uncinaria
U. americana
U. duodenalis
uncinariasis
uncinate epilepsy
Uncinocarpus
unclassified
arbovirus group u.
carcinoma in situ/intratubular germ
cell neoplasia u. (CIS/ITGCNU)
uncoded amino acid
uncommon developmental disorder
uncompensated
u. acidosis
u. alkalosis
uncomplemented
unconditional jump

U

unconjugated
    u. bilirubin
    u. estriol
    u. hyperbilirubinemia
uncontained criticality
uncontrolled fission
uncoossified
uncoupler
    oxidative phosphorylation u.
unctuous
undae
    Exiguobacterium u.
undecaprenol phosphate
undegraded insulin factor (UIF)
underflow
underlying cause of death
underphosphorylated protein expression
understain
Underwood disease
undescended testis
undetermined
    u. malignant potential (UMP)
    u. nitrogen
undicola
    Rhizobium u.
undifferentiated
    u. adenocarcinoma
    u. cell
    u. cell adenoma
    u. connective tissue syndrome
    u. epidermoid carcinoma
    u. lymphoma (UL)
    malignant teratoma, u. (MTU)
    u. malignant teratoma
    u. osteosarcoma (UOS)
    u. sarcoma
    u. squamous cell carcinoma
    u. type fever
undifferentiation
undosum
    Heliobacterium u.
Undritz anomaly
undulans
    Entamoeba u.
undulant fever
undulate
undulating membrane, undulatory membrane
undulipodium
unequal
    u. crossing over
    u. crossing over model
unesterified fatty acid (UFA)
unexplained death
UNG
    uracil-N-glycosylase
unglycosylated
ungues (*pl. of* unguis)

unguis, *pl.* **ungues**
    sinus u.
    stratum corneum u.
    stratum germinativum u.
    sulcus matricis u.
    vallecula u.
unguium
    achromia u.
    dystrophia u.
    tinea u.
    trichophytosis u.
unheated
    u. serum reagin (USR)
    u. serum reagin test
uniaxial
Unibacteria
Uniblue A
unicameral bone cyst
UniCel Dxl 800 immunoassay system
unicellular
    u. gland
    u. sclerosis
unicentral
unicentric blastoma
unicornis uterus
unicystic ameloblastoma
unidirectional
uniflagellate
UniFluidics
unifocal eosinophilic granuloma
uniforate
uniform
uniformly positive (UP)
unigene database
uniglandular
uni-gold
    U.-G. *H. pylori* test
    U.-G. Recombigen HIV test
    U.-G. Recombigen rapid HIV antibody test
unijunction transistor
unilaminar primary follicle
unilateral renal agenesis
unilobar
unilocular
    u. echinococcosis
    u. fat
    u. hydatid cyst
unimodal peak
uninuclear, uninucleate
uninucleate (*var. of* uninuclear)
union
    faulty u.
    fibrous u.
    primary u.
    secondary u.
    vicious u.
unionized hemoglobin (HHb)
uniovular

unipapillary
uniparental disomy (UPD)
unipolar
    u. cell
    u. neuron
uniport
unipotential
unirenicular
uniseptate
Unistat bilirubinometer
unit (U)
    absolute system of u.'s
    acinar u.
    alexin u.
    Allen-Doisy u.
    alpha u.
    amboceptor u.
    androgen u.
    antigen u.
    antitoxin u. (AU)
    atomic mass u. (amu)
    atomic weight u. (awu)
    base u.
    Behnken u. (R)
    Bessey-Lowry u. (BLU)
    Bethesda u. (BU)
    biological standard u.
    bird u.
    BLB u.
    Bodansky u. (BU)
    Bowers-McComb u.
    British thermal u. (BTU)
    cat u.
    u. cell
    central processing u.
    CGS u.
    chlorophyll u.
    chorionic gonadotropin u.
    Clauberg u.
    colony-forming u. (CFU)
    complement u.
    Corner-Allen u.
    corpus luteum hormone u.
    Dam u.
    dial u.
    digitalis u.
    diphtheria antitoxin u.
    dog u.
    Ehrlich u. (EU)
    electromagnetic u. (emu)
    electrostatic u. (ESU)
    enzyme u. (EU)
    epidermal-melanin u.
    equine gonadotropin u.
    estradiol benzoate u.
    estrone u.
    Fishman-Lerner u.
    Florey u.
    flotation u.

Gutman u.
Hazardous Materials Response U. (HMRU)
heat u. (HU)
hemagglutinating u. (HU)
hemolysin u.
hemolytic u.
hemorrhagin u.
heparin u.
Holzknecht u. (H)
Hounsfield u. (H)
Howell u.
hyperemia u. (HU)
immunizing u. (IU)
u. inheritance
insulin u.
international u. (IU)
International benzoate u. (IBU)
International System of U.'s (SI)
Jenner-Kay u.
kallikrein-inhibiting u. (KIU)
Karmen u. (KU)
King u.
King-Armstrong u. (KAU)
lung u.
Mache u. (MU)
map u.
u. membrane
meter-kilogram-second u. (MKS)
Mett u.
minimal hemolytic u.
mobile chilling u.
Montevideo u. (MU)
mouse u. (MU)
mouse uterine u. (MUU)
u. of intermedin
u. of luteinizing activity
u. of mass
u. of oxytocin
u. of penicillin
u. of progestational activity
u. of thyrotrophic activity
u. of vasopressin
u. of wavelength
u. of weight
Oxford u.
plaque-forming u. (PFU)
progesterone u.
prolactin u.
protein nitrogen u. (PNU)
radiation measuring u.
rat u. (RU)
RcoF u.
Reitland-Franklin u.
resistance u. (RU)
riboflavin u.
Russell u.
Sherman u.
Sherman-Munsell u.

U

unit (*continued*)
    Shinowara-Jones-Reinhard u.
    Sibley-Lehninger u.
    SJR u.
    skin test u. (STU)
    SL u.
    Somogyi u.
    Steenbock u.
    streptomycin u.
    sudanophobic u.
    technical advisory response u.
      (TARU)
    terminal duct lobular u.
      (TDLU)
    tetanus antitoxin u.
    thiamine chloride u.
    thiamine hydrochloride u.
    Todd u. (TU)
    toxic u. (TU)
    toxin u. (TU)
    transcription u.
    tuberculin u. (TU)
    turbidity-reducing u. (TRU)
    vitamin A u.
    vitamin B_2 u.
    vitamin B_6 u.
    vitamin B_1 hydrochloride u.
    vitamin C u.
    vitamin D u.
    vitamin E u.
    vitamin K u.
    Wohlgemuth u.
unitarian hypothesis
unit-culture
    colony-forming u.-c. (CFUC,
      CFU-C)
United States Army Medical Research Institute of Infectious Disease (USAMRIID)
unit-erythroid
    burst-forming u.-e. (BFU-E)
    colony-forming u.-e. (CFU-E)
uniting
    u. canal
    u. cartilage
    u. duct
unit-megakaryocyte
    colony-forming u.-m. (CFU-Meg)
units/mL
    colony-forming u. (CFU/mL)
unit-spleen
    colony-forming u.-s. (CFU-S)
univalent antibody
univariate analysis
universal
    u. donor
    U. ISH detection kit
    u. leukoreduction
    u. precautions

universale
    melasma u.
universalis
    adiposis u.
    alopecia u.
    calcinosis u.
univitelline
unknown
    u. etiology
    u. radioactivity
unmasking
    enzymatic antigen u.
    epitope u.
unmedullated
unmyelinated
    u. axon
    u. fiber
Unna
    U. cell
    U. disease
    U. mark
    U. stain
Unna-Pappenheim stain
Unna-Taenzer stain
Unopette
    U. system
    U. tube
unorganized virus
unpredictable hypersensitivity-like reaction
unrearranged germline
unresolved
    u. hepatitis
    u. lobar pneumonia
unresponsiveness
    immunologic u.
unrest
    nuclear u.
unsaturated
    u. hydrocarbon
    u. iron-binding capacity (UIBC)
    u. vitamin B_{12}-binding capacity
      (UBBC)
unsealed
    u. beta gamma source
    u. radioactive source
unspun peripheral blood
unstable
    u. hemoglobin
    u. hemoglobin disease
    u. hemoglobin hemolytic anemia
    u. trinucleotide repeat sequences
unstriated muscle, unstriped muscle
unstriped muscle (*var of* unstriated muscle)
ununited fracture
unusual isolates/fastidious organisms
Unverricht disease
unwinding protein

UOS
    undifferentiated osteosarcoma
up
    colony stands u.
U:P
    urine-plasma ratio
UP
    uniformly positive
    uroporphyrin
uPA
    urokinase plasminogen activator
uPAR
    urokinase plasminogen activator
    receptor
UP1a uroplakin gene
UP1b uroplakin gene
Up-Converting Phosphor technology
(UPT)
UPD
    uniparental disomy
UPEP
    urine protein electrophoresis
UPG
    uroporphyrinogen
UPI
    uteroplacental insufficiency
UPII
    uroplakin II
    UPII gene
UPIII
    uroplakin III
    UPIII gene
UP*link* point of care sample testing
system
upper
    u. aerodigestive tract (UADT)
    u. anal canal
    u. gastrointestinal (UGI)
    u. limits of normal (ULN)
    u. motor neuron
    u. respiratory disease (URD)
    u. respiratory infection (URI)
    u. respiratory tract infection
        (URTI)
up-regulation
UPS
    ubiquitin-proteasome system
upsilon
upstream binding factor
UPT
    Up-Converting Phosphor technology
uptake
    absolute iodine u. (AIU)
    bipolar u.
    oxygen u.
    radioactive iodine u. (RAIU, RIU)
    radiocalcium u.
    resin u.
    T_3 u.

triiodothyronine u. (T_3U)
triiodothyronine resin u. (T_3RU)
uptime
urachal
    u. carcinoma
    u. cyst
    u. fistula
urachus
uracil DNA glycosylase (UDG)
uracil-N-glycosylase (UNG)
uracrasia
uranin
uranium
    depleted u. (DU)
    u. nephritis
uranyl acetate stain
uraroma
urarthritis
UrAssist pum-assisted urine
collection
urate
    u. calculus
    u. crystal
    u. crystal stain
    de Galantha method for u.'s
    monosodium u. (MSU)
uratemia
uratica
    arthritis u.
uratohistechia
uratoma
uratosis
uraturia
Urbach-Oppenheim disease
Urbach-Wiethe disease
urban plague
URD
    upper respiratory disease
urea
    u. agar
    u. breath test (UBT)
    u. clearance
    u. clearance test
    u. concentration test
    u. cycle
    u. nitrogen (UN)
    u. nitrogen assay
    u. nitrogen or plasma
    u. nitrogen test
    u. synthesis
ureae
    Nitrosomonas u.
urealyticum
    Ureaplasma u.
Ureaplasma
    U. parvum
    U. urealyticum
    U. urealyticum genital culture
ureapoiesis

U

urease
u. enzyme
Helicobacter pylori u.
u. test
u. test broth
urea-splitting bacterial infection
urecchysis
urecholine supersensitivity test
uredema, uroedema
Ureibacillus
U. terrenus
U. thermosphaericus
urelcosis
uremia, urinemia
hypercalcemic u.
uremic
u. cachexia
u. cardiomyopathy
u. colitis
u. coma
u. eclampsia
u. encephalopathy
u. inflammation
u. lung
u. pericarditis
u. pneumonia
u. pneumonitis
uremigenic
ureolyticus
Bacteroides u.
ureotelic
ureter
bifid u.
ureteral, ureteric
u. atresia
u. calculus
u. carcinoma
u. hyperperistalsis
u. ileus
u. peristalsis disorder
u. reflux
ureterectasia
ureteric (*var. of* ureteral)
ureteris
tunica mucosa u.
tunica muscularis u.
ureteritis
u. cystica
u. glandularis
ureterocele
ureterocutaneous fistula
ureterohydronephrosis
ureterolith
ureterolithiasis
ureterolysis
ureteropelvic
u. junction
u. junction obstruction
ureteropyelitis

ureteropyelonephritis
ureteropyosis
ureterostegnosis (*var. of* ureterostenosis)
ureterostenoma (*var. of* ureterostenosis)
ureterostenosis, ureterostegnosis, ureterostenoma
ureterostoma
ureterovaginal fistula
ureterovesical obstruction
urethrae
corpus cavernosum u.
urethral
u. caruncle
u. discharge (UD)
u. diverticulum
u. hematuria
u. obstruction
u. stricture
u. tumor
urethralis
Oligella u.
urethratresia
urethrism, urethrismus, urethrospasm
urethrismus (*var. of* urethrism)
urethritis
follicular u.
granular u.
nongonococcal u. (NGU)
nonspecific u. (NSU)
u. petrificans
posterior u.
postgonococcal u.
simple u.
Trichomonas u.
urethrocele
urethrocystitis
urethrophyma
urethrospasm (*var. of* urethrism)
urethrostenosis
urethrovaginal fistula
URF
uterine-relaxing factor
urhidrosis
URI
upper respiratory infection
uric
u. acid (UA)
u. acid assay
u. acid calculus
u. acid crystal
u. acid infarct
u. acid test
uricacidemia
uricemia
uricolytic index
uricosuria
uricosuric
Uricult dipslide test

uridine
  u. diphosphate (UDP)
  u. monophosphate
  u. triphosphate (UTP)
uridine-5′-phosphate
uridrosis
uridylic acid
uridyltransferase
  galactose-1-phosphate u. (GALT)
  galactose phosphate u. (GPUT)
  hexose-1-phosphate u.
uridylyl
uridylyltransferase
  UDP-glucose-hexose-1-phosphate u.
urinae
  ardor u.
urinaehominis
  Aerococcus u.
urinale
  Actinobaculum u.
urinalis
  Streptococcus u.
urinalysis (UA)
  fractional u. (FU)
  midstream u.
urinaria
  Bodo u.
urinariae
  tunica mucosa vesicae u.
  tunica muscularis vesicae u.
  tunica serosa vesicae u.
urinarius
  Bodo u.
urinary
  u. amylase
  u. bladder fistula
  u. bladder hernia
  u. calculus
  u. cast
  u. catecholamine
  u. chorionic gonadotropin
    (UCG)
  u. concentration test
  u. coproporphyrin (UCP)
  u. cyst
  u. estriol
  u. free cortisol
  u. frequency
  u. hydroxyproline
  u. incontinence
  u. nitrogen
  u. obstruction
  u. retention
  u. sand
  u. sediment
  u. smear
  u. tract brush biopsy
  u. tract disease
  u. tract infection (UTI)

  u. tract sphincter
  u. tuberculosis
UrinChek 10+ urine test strips
urine
  u. acetone test
  alkalinization of u.
  u. alpha hydroxybutyric acid
  u. amino acid
  ammoniacal u.
  u. amylase
  u. amylase excretion test
  u. argininosuccinic acid
  black u.
  u. blood pigment
  u. calcium
  u. chloride
  chylous u.
  u. citrulline
  cloudy u.
  concentration of creatinine in u.
    (Ucr)
  concentration of sodium in u.
    (UNa)
  u. copper
  u. coproporphyrin
  u. creatinine
  crude u.
  u. crystals
  u. cystathionine
  u. cystine
  u. cytology
  diabetic u.
  u. 2,5-dihydroxyphenylacetic acid
  u. dopamine
  u. drug panel (UDP)
  u. drug screen (UDS)
  u. epinephrine
  u. estradiol fraction
  u. estriol fraction
  febrile u.
  feverish u.
  u. fungus culture
  Gerhardt test for urobilin in the u.
  u. glucose
  u. glycine
  gouty u.
  u. heptacarboxyporphyrin
  u. hexacarboxyporphyrin
  u. histidine
  u. homocystine
  u. homogentisic acid
  honey u.
  u. 5-hydroxyindoleacetic acid
  u. hydroxyproline
  u. isoleucine
  u. leucine
  u. leukocyte esterase
  u. lysozyme
  u. magnesium

U

urine (*continued*)
   u. metanephrine
   u. microscopy
   milky u.
   u. mycobacteria culture
   u. myoglobin test
   nebulous u.
   u. norepinephrine
   u. normetanephrine
   u. osmolality
   u. oxalate
   u. pentacarboxyporphyrin
   u. phenylalanine
   u. phosphoethanolamine
   u. placental estriol
   u. porphobilinogen
   u. porphyrin
   u. potassium
   pregnancy u. (PU)
   u. pregnanediol
   u. pregnanetriol
   u. proline
   u. protein electrophoresis (UPEP)
   u. pyridinoline cross-link
   reducing substances in u.
   residual u.
   u. sediment crystal
   smoky u.
   u. sodium
   u. specimen collection
   u. spot test
   u. total estrogen
   u. urea nitrogen (UUN)
   u. uric acid
   u. urobilinogen (UU)
   u. uroporphyrin
   u. valine
   u. vanillylmandelic acid
urinemia (*var. of* uremia)
urine-plasma ratio (U:P)
uriniferous tubule
urinific
uriniparous
urinoma
urinometer, urometer
urinometry
urinoscopy
urinosus
   sudor u.
urinothorax
urinous
Uriscreen
   U. bacteriuria detection system
   U. test
UriSite microalbumin/creatinine urine
  test
Urisys 2400 urine analyzer
Uri-Test protein in urine test
uroammoniac

urobenzoic acid
urobilin assay
urobilinemia
urobilinogen (UBG)
   u. assay
   fecal u. (FU)
   increased urine u.
   stool u.
   u. test
   urine u. (UU)
urobilinogenuria (*var. of* urobilinuria)
urobilinuria, urobilinogenuria
urocanic acid
urocele, uroscheocele
urocheras (*var. of* uropsammus)
urochrome
urocortisol
urocrisia, urocrisis
urocrisis (*var. of* urocrisia)
urocyanin
urocyanogen
urocyanosis
Urocystis
urocystitis
UROD
   uroporphyrinogen decarboxylase
uroedema (*var. of* uredema)
uroerythrin
urofuscohematin
urogastrone
urogenital
   u. disorder
   u. fistula
   u. syndrome
urogenitalis
   Actinomyces u.
   Amoeba u.
uroglaucin
urogram
   excretory u. (XU)
urography
urogravimeter
urohemolytic coefficient
urokinase
   u. plasminogen activator (uPA)
   u. plasminogen activator receptor
   (uPAR)
urolith
urolithiasis
urolithic
urometer (*var. of* urinometer)
uromucoid assay
uroncus
Uronema caudatum
uronephrosis
uronic acid
uronophile
uronoscopy (*var. of* uroscopy)
uropathogen

uropathy
    obstructive u.
uropepsin
uropepsinogen assay
urophanic
urophein
urophilia
uroplakin
    u. I
    u. II (UPII)
    u. III (UPIII)
uroporphyria
uroporphyrin (UP)
    u. assay
    u. test
    urine u.
uroporphyrinogen (UPG)
    u. decarboxylase (UROD)
    u. decarboxylase deficiency
    u. III cosynthase
    u. III cosynthase deficiency
    u. I synthase
    u. synthase deficiency
uroporphyrinuria
uropsammus, urocheras
urorosein
urorubin
urorubrohematin
uroscheocele (*var. of* urocele)
uroschesis
uroscopic
uroscopy, uronoscopy
urosemiology
urosepsin
urosepsis
uroseptic
urothelial
    u. carcinoma (UcA)
    u. leiomyomatous hamartoma
    u. neoplasm
    u. papilloma
urothelium
urotoxic coefficient
uroureter
UroVysion
    U. bladder cancer recurrence test
    U. FISH test
uroxanthin
ursincola
    Blastomonas u.
ursingii
    Acinetobacter u.
ursodeoxycholic acid (UDCA)
URTI
    upper respiratory tract infection
urticaria
    aquagenic u.
    cholinergic u.
    cold u.

    congelation u.
    factitious u.
    giant u.
    u. gigantea
    u. perstans
    u. pigmentosa
    pressure u.
    solar u.
    u. tuberosa
urticate
urticating
    u. agent
    u. caterpillar
Uruma virus
usage
    Working Formulation for Clinical U. (WF)
USAMRIID
    United States Army Medical Research Institute of Infectious Disease
USC
    uterine serous carcinoma
useful life
Usher syndrome
US-licensed formaldehyde-killed whole bacilli vaccine
USN
    ultrasonic nebulizer
U1 snRNA molecule
U2 snRNA molecule
U4 snRNA molecule
U5 snRNA molecule
USR
    unheated serum reagin
ustilaginism
Ustilago
    U. maydis
    U. zeae
usual
    u. interstitial pneumonia (UIP)
    u. interstitial pneumonitis (UIP)
    u. type papillary carcinoma (UTPC)
uta
utahensis
    Halorhabdus u.
UTBG
    unbound thyroxine-binding globulin
uteri (*pl. of* uterus)
uterina
    rachitis u.
uterinae
    ampulla tubae u.
    fimbriae tubae u.
    glandulae u.
    tunica mucosa tubae u.
    tunica muscularis tubae u.
    tunica serosa tubae u.

uterine
  u. aspiration (UA)
  u. blood flow (UBF)
  u. calculus
  u. cancer
  u. colic
  u. descensus
  u. endometrial carcinoma (UEC)
  u. endometriosis
  u. gland
  u. granuloma
  u. leiomyoma
  u. leiomyosarcoma (ULMS)
  u. serous carcinoma (USC)
  u. surface carcinoma
  u. tumor resembling an ovarian
    sex-cord tumor (UTROSCT)
uterine-relaxing factor (URF)
uteritis
utero
  dead fetus in u. (DFU)
  in u.
uterolith
uteroovarian varicocele
uteroperitoneal fistula
uteroplacental
  u. fibrinoid layer
  u. insufficiency (UPI)
uterus, *pl.* **uteri**
  adenomyosis uteri
  arcuatus u.
  asymmetric u.
  bicornuate u.
  bifid u.
  cervical gland of u.
  coiled artery of the u.
  fibroid u.
  glandulae cervicales uteri
  gliosis uteri
  ichthyosis uteri
  infantile u.
  inversion of u.
  male rudimentary u.
  tunica mucosa uteri
  tunica muscularis uteri
  tunica serosa uteri
  unicornis u.
UTI
  urinary tract infection
utilization
  ketone body u.
  net protein u. (NPU)

UTP
  uridine
    triphosphate
UTPC
  usual type papillary
    carcinoma
utricle
utricular
  u. cyst
  u. spot
utricularis
  Badhamia u.
utriculi (*pl. of* utriculus)
utriculitis
utriculosaccular duct
utriculosaccularis
  ductus u.
utriculus, *pl.* **utriculi**
  macula utriculi
utrophin marker
UTROSCT
  uterine tumor resembling an ovarian
    sex-cord tumor
UU
  urine urobilinogen
UUN
  urine urea nitrogen
UV
  ultraviolet
uvea
uveal
  u. melanoma
  u. tract
uveitides (*pl. of* uveitis)
uveitis, *pl.* **uveitides**
  induced u.
  lens-induced u.
uveoencephalitic
  syndrome
uveomeningitis
uveoparotid fever
uviform
uviofast
uvioresistant
uviosensitive
UV-irradiated nevus
Uvitex 2B
uvulitis
uzenensis
  Geobacillus u.
uzoniensis
  Thermoproteus u.

V

valine
vanadium
volt
   V agent
   V antigen

VA

vacuum aspiration
volt-ampere
   phenotype VA

VACB

vacuum-assisted core biopsy

vaccenic acid

vaccimaxillae

   Actinomyces v.

vaccinal

vaccinate

vaccinated

   distantly v.

vaccinator

vaccinatum

   eczema v.

vaccine

   adjuvant v.
   aqueous v.
   attenuated v.
   autogenous v.
   BCG v.
   Brucella strain 19 v.
   Calmette-Gúerin v.
   cholera v.
   Cox v.
   crystal violet v.
   diphtheria, tetanus, and pertussis v.
    (DTP)
   diphtheria toxoid, tetanus toxoid,
    and pertussis v.
   duck embryo origin v.
   Flury strain v.
   foot-and-mouth disease virus v.
   Haemophilus pertussis v. (HPV)
   Haffkine v.
   hepatitis B v.
   heterogenous v.
   high egg-passage Flury strain rabies
    v.
   hog cholera v.
   human diploid cell rabies v.
    (HDCV)
   inactivated poliovirus v. (IPV)
   inactivated ricin toxoid v.
   influenza virus v.
   killed v. (KV)
   killed measles virus v. (KMV)
   live oral poliovirus v.

   low egg-passage v.
   v. lymph
   measles, mumps, and rubella v.
   measles virus v.
   multivalent v.
   mumps virus v.
   oil v.
   oral poliovirus v.
   plague v.
   pneumococcal v.
   poliomyelitis v.
   poliovirus v.
   polyvalent v.
   rabies v.
   recombinant v.
   RhoGAM v.
   Rocky Mountain spotted fever v.
   roseola v.
   Sabin v.
   Salk v.
   Semple v.
   smallpox v.
   smallpox v.
   split-virus v.
   staphylococcus v.
   stock v.
   subunit v.
   TAB v.
   tetanus v.
   trivalent oral poliovirus v. (TOPV)
   tuberculosis v.
   typhoid-paratyphoid A and B v.
   typhus v.
   US-licensed formaldehyde-killed
    whole bacilli v.
   variola v.
   v. virus
   whooping cough v.
   yellow fever v.

vaccinia

   fetal v.
   v. gangrenosa
   generalized v.
   v. immune globulin (VIG)
   v. nervosum
   progressive v.
   variola v.
   v. virus

vaccinial

vacciniform

vaccinist

vaccinization

vaccinogen

vaccinogenous

vaccinoid reaction

V

vaccinostyle
Vacuette blood sample tube
vacuo
  in v.
vacuolar
  v. degeneration
  v. interface dermatitis
  v. nephrosis
vacuolate, vacuolated
vacuolated (*var. of* vacuolate)
  v. cell
  v. cytoplasm
  v. lymphocyte
  v. platelet
vacuolating
  v. agent
  v. virus
vacuolation, vacuolization
  cytoplasmic v.
vacuolatus
  Desulforhopalus v.
vacuole
  v. alteration phagocytosis
  autophagic v.
  condensing v.
  contractile v.
  cytoplasmic v.
  digestion v.
  extracellular v.
  heterophagic v.
  intracytoplasmic v.
  paranuclear v.
  plasmocrine v.
  rhagiocrine v.
vacuolization (*var. of* vacuolation)
vacuome
Vacutainer
vacuum
  v. aspiration (VA)
  v. breaker
  v. distillation
  v. flask
  v. gauge
  high v.
  v. tube
  v. tuberculin (VT)
  v. tube voltmeter (VTVM)
  ultrahigh v.
vacuum-assisted core biopsy (VACB)
VAD
  venous access device
  phenotype VAD
vadensis
  Victivallis v.
vagabond's
  v. disease
  v. melanosis
vagale
  glomus v.

vagina, *pl.* **vaginae**
  v. cellulosa
  congenital absence of v. (CAV)
  v., ectocervix, endocervix
    (VCE)
  v. mucosa tendinis
  v. synovialis tendinis
  tunica mucosa vaginae
  tunica muscularis vaginae
  vaginae vasorum
vaginae (*pl. of* vagina)
vaginal
  v. adenosis
  v. atresia
  v. cancer
  v. carcinoma
  v. clear cell adenocarcinoma
  v. epithelium
  v. gland
  v. intraepithelial neoplasia
  v. irrigation smear
    (VIS)
  v. leukocyte
  v. pool
  v. synovial membrane
  v. synovitis
  v. thrush
  v. tumor
vaginalis
  Anaerococcus v.
  Gardnerella v.
  Haemophilus v.
  processus v.
  Trichomonas v.
  tunica v.
vaginalitis
vaginate
vaginism (*var. of* vaginismus)
vaginismus, vaginism
vaginitis
  adhesive v.
  bacterial v.
  v. cystica
  desquamative inflammatory v.
  v. emphysematosa
  emphysematous v.
  granular v.
  v. senilis
  trichomanas v.
vaginomycosis
Vaginulus plebeius
Vagitest
Vagococcus carniphilus
Vahlkampfia
VAHS
  virus-associated hemophagocytic
    syndrome
Val
  valine

valence, valency
 v. electron
 v. tautomer
valency (*var. of* valence)
Valentin corpuscle
Valentine test
valerianellae
 Acidovorax v.
valeric acid
valgum
 genu v.
valgus deformity
validation
valine (V, Val)
 v. aminotransferase
 v. transaminase
 urine v.
valinemia
valinuria
vallatae
vallate papilla
vallecula unguis
valley fever
vallismortis
 Salinivibrio costicola
 subsp. *v.*
vallum
valproic acid
Valsa
Valsalva maneuver
value
 absolute v.
 acetyl v.
 acid v.
 buffer v.
 cot v.
 crisis v.
 D v.
 GC v.
 globular v.
 iodine v.
 negative predictive v. (NPV)
 normal v.
 P v.
 positive predictive v. (PPV)
 predictive v.
 reference v. (RV)
 rot v.
 threshold limit v. (TLV)
valva, *pl.* **valvae**
valvae (*pl. of* valva)
valvarum
 Cardiobacterium v.
valvate
valve
 Amussat v.
 atrioventricular v.
 Bianchi v.
 congenital v.

 damaged fibrotic v.
 incompetent aortic v.
 incompetent foramen ovale v.
 incompetent mitral v.
 incompetent pulmonic v.
 incompetent tricuspid v.
 Kerckring v.
 mitral v.
 v. of coronary vein
 tricuspid v.
valvotomy, valvulotomy
valvula (*var. of* valvule)
 Amussat v.
 Gerlach v.
valvulae conniventes
valvular
 v. atresia
 v. disease of heart (VDH)
 v. endocarditis
 v. incompetence
 v. stenosis
 v. thrombus
 v. tissue embolus
valvule, valvula
valvulitis
 rheumatic v.
valvulotomy (*var. of* valvotomy)
valyl
valyl-RNA synthetase
Vampirolepis
van
 v. Bogaert disease
 v. Buchem syndrome
 v. Buren disease
 v. Deen test
 v. den Bergh test
 v. der Hoeve syndrome
 v. der Velden test
 v. der Waals equation
 v. der Waals forces
 V. der Woude syndrome
 V. Diest criteria
 v. Ermengen stain
 v. Gieson stain
 v. Hansemann cell
 V. Nuys scheme
 V. Slyke and Cullen method
 V. Slyke apparatus
 V. Slyke formula
 V. Slyke test
vanadium (V)
vanbaalenii
 Mycobacterium v.
vanbreuseghemi
 Microsporum v.
vanbreuseghemii
 Microsporum v.
 Trichophyton v.
vancomycin

vancomycin-insensitive *Staphylococcus aureus* (**VISA**)
vancomycin-resistant
    v.-r. *Enterococcus* (VRE)
    v.-r. enterococcus assay (VRE)
vancoresmycina
    Amycolatopsis v.
vanillic acid
vanillism
vanillylmandelic
    v. acid (VMA)
    v. acid test
VAP cholesterol test
vapor
    combustible v.
    v. pressure
    v. pressure depression osmometer
vaporization
    heat of v.
vaporize
vapor-phase chromatography (VPC)
VaporTrode Vaporization Electrode
Vapro vapor pressure osmometer
Vaquez disease
Vaquez-Osler disease
var
    variant
variabile
    Cellulosimicrobium v.
    Trichosporon v.
variabilis
    Brevundimonas v.
    Dermacentor v.
    erythrokeratodermia v.
    Isoptericola v.
    Mesocestoides v.
variability
    interobserver v.
    intraobserver v.
variable
    v. autotransformer
    v. capacitor
    common v.
    dependent v.
    dichotomous v.
    double-precision v.
    dummy v.
    endogenous v.
    exogenous v.
    fixed-point v.
    floating-point v.
    independent v.
    label v.
    v. number of tandem repeats (VNTR)
    ordinal v.
    pointer v.
    random v.
    v. region

    v. resistor
    subscripted v.
variably positive (VP)
variance
    analysis of v. (ANOVA)
    multivariate analysis of v. (MANOVA)
varians
    Micrococcus v.
variant (var)
    aggressive follicular v.
    blastoid v.
    columnar cell v. (CCV)
    cribriform-morular v.
    diffuse follicular v.
    floral v.
    germline v.
    v. hemoglobin
    inherited albumin v.
    L-phase v.
    macrofollicular v.
    v. pattern
    Pittsburgh v.
    SI v.
    v. sickling hemoglobin anemia
    tall cell v. (TCV)
    terminally truncated v.
variate
    binary v.
variation
    alpha-beta v.
    coefficient of v. (CV)
    contingent negative v. (CNV)
    meristic v.
    microbial v.
    negative v. (NV)
    rough-smooth v.
    smooth-rough v.
Varibaculum cambriense
varication
variceal
varicella
    v. encephalitis
    v. virus
varicellation
varicella-zoster (VZ, V-Z)
    v.-z. antibody test
    v.-z. virus (VZV)
    v.-z. virus serology
varicelliform eruption
varicelloid smallpox
varicellosus
    herpes zoster v.
Varicellovirus
varices (*pl. of* varix)
variciform
varicocele
    ovarian v.
    symptomatic v.

tuboovarian v.
uteroovarian v.
varicoid
varicole
varicophlebitis
Varicosavirus
varicose
v. aneurysm
v. ulcer
v. vein
varicosis
varicosity
varicosum
lymphangioma capillare v.
varicule
variegata
variegate porphyria
variegatum
Amblyomma v.
Hyalomma v.
variegatus
Aedes v.
variglandis
Austrobilharzia v.
Microbilharzia v.
variicola
Klebsiella v.
variola
v. benigna
v. hemorrhagica
v. major
v. maligna
v. miliaris
v. minor
v. pemphigosa
v. sine eruptione
v. vaccine
v. vaccinia
v. vera
v. verrucosa
v. virus
variolar
variolate
variolation, variolization
variolic
varioliform gastritis
varioliformis
variolization (*var. of* variolation)
varioloid
variolous
variolovaccine
varium
Fusobacterium v.
Procerovum v.
varius
varix, *pl.* **varices**
v. anastomoticus
aneurysmal v.
cirsoid v.

esophageal varices
lymph v.
v. lymphaticus
turbinal v.
varum
genu v.
varus deformity
vas, *pl.* **vasa, vasorum**
vasa aberrantia
v. afferens
v. capillare
v. deferens
v. efferens
vasa previa
vasa recta
vaginae vasorum
vasa vasorum
vasa (*pl. of* vas)
vascular
v. addressin
v. anomaly
v. birthmark
v. bud
v. cell adhesion molecule-1
(VCAM-1)
v. cone
v. corrosion cast
v. dementia
v. density
v. disorder
v. dissection
v. ectasia
v. endothelial cadherin (VE-cadherin)
v. endothelial growth factor (VEGF)
v. endothelial growth factor receptor
3 (VEGFR3)
v. gland
v. hemophilia
v. invasion (VI)
v. keratitis
v. lacune
v. lake
v. layer
v. leakage
v. leiomyoma
v. malformation
v. morphology
v. myelopathy
v. myxoma
v. neoplasia
v. nevus
v. papilla
v. permeability
v. permeability factor
v. polyp
v. resistance (VR)
v. ring
v. sclerosis
v. smooth muscle cell (VSMC)

V

vascular (*continued*)
　v. spider
　v. stenosis
　v. stripe
　v. stroma
　v. styptic
　v. thrombus
vasculare
　poikiloderma atrophicans v.
vascularization
　corneal v.
vascularize
vascularized stroma
vasculature
　lesion of v.
vasculitide
　immune-mediated v.
vasculitis
　Churg-Strauss v.
　cryoglobulinemic v.
　cutaneous v.
　hypersensitivity v.
　leukocytoclastic v.
　livedo v.
　lymphocytic v.
　lymphohistiocytic v.
　necrotizing v.
　nodular v.
　pustular v.
　segmented hyalinizing v.
　septal panniculitis without v.
vasculocardiac syndrome of hyperserotonemia
vasculomyelinopathy
vasculoocclusive process
vasculopathic
vasculosa
　Haller tunica v.
　tunica v.
vasculosae
　stellulae v.
vasculosi
　coni v.
vasculosum
　punctum v.
vasculosyncytial membrane
vasculotoxic
vasiformis
　Saksenaea v.
vasitis nodosa
vasoactive
　v. amine
　v. intestinal peptide (VIP)
　v. intestinal polypeptide (VIP)
　v. mediator
vasoconstriction
　hypoxic v.
vasodepressor material (VDM)
vasoexcitor material (VEM)

vasoformative cell
vasoganglion
vasogenic shock
vasomotor
　v. hypotonia
　v. instability
　v. paralysis
　v. rhinitis (VMR)
vasoocclusive crisis
vasoparalysis
vasoparesis
vasopressin (VP)
　arginine v. (AVP)
　unit of v.
vasorum (*pl. of* vas)
vasospasm
　recurrent v.
vasospastic
vasovagal
　v. attack
　v. syncope
Vater corpuscle
VATER
　vertebral defects, anal atresia, tracheoesophageal fistula with esophageal atresia, and radial and renal anomalies
　VATER complex
Vaterian carcinoma
Vater-Pacini corpuscle
VATS
　video-assisted transthoracic surgery
Vav1 signal transducer protein
VCA
　viral capsid antigen
　VCA IgM
VCAM-1
　vascular cell adhesion molecule-1
VCE
　vagina, ectocervix, endocervix
　VCE smear
VCFS
　velocardiofacial syndrome
VD
　venereal disease
　phenotype VD
VDBR
　volume of distribution of bilirubin
VDEL
　venereal disease experimental laboratory
VDG
　venereal disease gonorrhea
VDH
　valvular disease of heart
VDM
　vasodepressor material

VDRL
  Venereal Disease Research Laboratory
    VDRL test
VDS
  venereal disease-syphilis
VE
  NATO code for nerve agent O-ethyl
  S-[2-(diethylamino)ethyl]
  ethylphosphonothioate
VE-cadherin
  vascular endothelial cadherin
Vectabond reagent
Vectastain
    V. ABC Elit kit
    V. Elite ABC system
    V. immunohistochemical reagent
    V. Universal Elite ABC kit
    V. Universal Quick kit
vection
vector
    biological v.
    cloning v.
    electric field v.
    V. Elite reagent
    expression v.
    V. Laboratories VectaShield
      antifading buffer
    mechanical v.
    V. MOM kit
    plasmid v.
    v. product
    recombinant v.
vectorial
VEE
  Venezuelan equine encephalomyelitis
    VEE smear
    VEE virus
VEFG
  vascular endothelial growth
  factor
vegetans
    keratosis v.
    pyoderma v.
    pyostomatitis v.
vegetation
    bacterial v.
    verrucous v.
vegetative
    v. anthrax bacilli
    v. bacillus
    v. bacteriophage
    v. cell
    v. endocarditis
    v. multiplication
    v. stage
VEGF
  vascular endothelial growth
  factor
VEGF-A gene

VEGFR3
  vascular endothelial growth factor
  receptor 3
    VEGFR3 marker
VEGF-related protein
vehiculated nutrient
veil
    aqueduct v.
    v. cell
veiled cell
Veillonaceae
Veillonella
    V. alcalescens subsp. *alcalescens*
    V. alcalescens subsp. *dispar*
    V. montpellierensis
    V. parvula
    V. parvula subsp. *atypica*
    V. parvula subsp. *rodentium*
Veillonellaceae
Veillon tube
vein, vena
    arterialization of v.
    capillary v.
    external pudendal v.
    hemorrhoidal v.
    key v.
    Krukenberg v.
    large v.
    medium v.
    obturator v.
    portal v.
    reticular fibers in wall of
      central v.
    stellate v.
    v. stone
    valve of coronary v.
    varicose v.
veined
veinlet
vein-to-vein anastomosis
Vejovis
vela (*pl. of* velum)
velamentous
    v. cord
    v. insertion
    v. vessel
velamentum
velamen vulva
Vel antigen
velar
veliform
vellicate
vellication
vellus
    v. anagen follicle
    v. hair
    v. hair cyst
    v. telogen follicle
velocardiofacial syndrome (VCFS)

velocity
    v. coefficient
    wave v.
velocity-diffusion
    v.-d. sedimentation
    sedimentation v.-d.
velogenic Newcastle disease
velopharyngeal insufficiency
velox
    Thermanaerovibrio v.
velum, *pl.* **vela**
VEM
    vasoexcitor material
vena (*var. of* vein), *pl.* **venae**
    v. cava obstruction
    venae centrales hepatis
    venae rectae
    venae stellatae
venae (*pl. of* vena)
Ven antigen
venenata
    dermatitis v.
veneniferous
venenous
venereal
    v. disease (VD)
    v. disease experimental laboratory (VDEL)
    v. disease gonorrhea (VDG)
    V. Disease Research Laboratory (VDRL)
    v. disease-syphilis (VDS)
    v. lymphogranuloma
    v. sore
    v. ulcer
    v. wart
venerealis
    Campylobacter fetus subsp. *v.*
venereology
venereum
    lymphogranuloma v. (LGV)
    lymphopathia v.
    ulcus v.
veneris
    corona v.
venesect
Venezuelan
    V. equine A encephalomyelitis virus
    V. equine encephalitis
    V. equine encephalomyelitis (VEE)
    V. equine encephalomyelitis virus
venezuelensis
    Borrelia v.
    Leishmania mexicana v.
    Ornithodoros v.
venin
venipuncture
venofibrosis
venogram

venolymphatic
venom
    antisnake v. (ASV)
    cobra v.
    hymenoptera v.
    kokoi v.
    Malayan pit viper v.
    Protac v.
    Russell viper v. (RVV)
    snake v. (SV)
    viper v. (VV)
venosclerosis
venostasis
venosus
    nevus v.
venous
    v. access device (VAD)
    v. blood and tissue
    v. capillary
    v. claudication
    v. congestion
    v. embolism
    v. gangrene
    v. hematocrit (VH)
    v. insufficiency
    v. lake
    mixed v.
    v. occlusion
    v. pressure
    v. sinus
    v. star
    v. stasis
    v. thrombosis
Ventana
    V. alkaline phosphatase blue detection kit
    V. automated immunostainer
    V. ES slide processor machine
    V. ES stain
    V. Inform HPV
    V. Medical Systems Techmate 500 automated stainer
    V. NexES immunostainer
    V. silanized capillary gap slide
    V. TechMate 100 immunostainer
ventilation
    v. defect
    local exhaust v.
    maximum voluntary v. (MVV)
    mechanical v.
ventilation-perfusion ratio
ventilator (*var. of* respirator)
ventilator-associated pneumonia
ventilatory failure
ventosa
    spina v.
ventosae
    Halomonas v.
ventral respiratory group

ventricle
    tela choroidea of fourth v.
    tela choroidea of third v.
ventricose
ventricosus
    Haemodipsus v.
    Strongylus v.
ventricular
    v. aneurysm
    v. bigeminy
    v. diverticulum
    v. dysfunction
    v. hypertrophy
    v. layer
    v. septal defect (VSD)
    v. tachycardia
ventriculi (*pl. of* ventriculus)
ventriculography
    radionucleotide v.
ventriculonector
ventriculoradial dysplasia
ventriculus, *pl.* **ventriculi**
    anadenia ventriculi
    descensus ventriculi
    Sarcina ventriculi
    stigma ventriculi
    stratum circulare tunicae muscularis
      ventriculi
    stratum longitudinale tunicae
      muscularis ventriculi
    tunica muscularis ventriculi
    tunica serosa ventriculi
ventriosum
    Eubacterium v.
ventroptosia (*var. of* ventroptosis)
ventroptosis, ventroptosia
Venturia
venula, venule, *pl.* **venulae**
    venulae rectae renis
    venulae stellatae renis
venulae (*pl. of* venula)
venular
venule (*var. of* venula)
    high-endothelial v. (HEV)
    postcapillary v.
    stellate v.
venulitis
    cutaneous necrotizing v.
venulosum
    Oesophagostomum v.
venulous
venustensis
    Alcanivorax v.
vera
    cutis v.
    decidua v.
    hemospermia v.
    myeloid metaplasia with
      polycythemia v. (PCV-M)

    polycythemia v. (PCV, PV)
    polycythemia rubra v.
      (PRV)
    variola v.
verapamil
verbascose
Verdict-II
    V.-I. drug screening device
    V.-I. drug screening test
verdoglobin
verdohemochrome
verdohemoglobin
verdoperoxidase
verge
    anal v.
vergeture
verheyenii
    stellulae v.
Verheyen star
Verhoeff elastic tissue stain
Verhoeff-van
    V.-v. Gieson (VVG)
    V.-v. Gieson elastin stain
veriformis
    Hartmannella v.
vermicidal
vermicide
vermicular
Vermicularia
vermicularis
    Enterobius v.
    Oxyuris v.
vermicule
vermiculous
vermiculus
vermiform
vermiformis
    appendix v.
    folliculi lymphatici aggregati
      appendicis v.
vermifugal
vermifuge
vermilion
    v. border
    v. zone
vermin
verminal
vermination
verminous
    v. abscess
    v. colic
vermis
verna
    Amanita v.
vernal
    v. conjunctivitis
    v. encephalitis
Verner-Morrison syndrome
Vernet syndrome

V

Verneuil
V. disease
hidradenitis axillaris of V.
V. neuroma
vernier dial caliper
vernix caseosa
vero
V. cell
v. cytotoxin
Verocay body
Veronaea botryosa
veronal buffer
veronal-buffered saline/fetal bovine serum
verotoxin
Verpa bohemica
verruca
v. acuminata
v. digitata
v. filiformis
v. glabra
v. mollusciformis
v. necrogenica
v. palmaris
v. peruana
v. plana
v. plana juvenilis
v. plana senilis
v. plantaris
seborrheic v.
v. seborrheica
v. simplex
v. virus
v. vulgaris
verrucal
v. atypical endocarditis
v. nonbacterial endocarditis
verrucarum
verruciform
verruciformis
acrokeratosis v.
epidermodysplasia v.
Verrucomicrobiaceae
Verrucomicrobiae
Verrucomicrobiales
verrucopapillary
v. alteration
v. external genital lesion
verrucosa
Amoeba v.
dermatitis v.
pachyderma v.
telangiectasia v.
tuberculosis cutis v.
variola v.
verrucose (*var. of* verrucous)
verrucosis
lymphostatic v.
verrucosum
eczema v.

molluscum v.
Trichophyton v.
verrucosus
lupus v.
Ornithodoros v.
verrucous, verrucose
v. acanthosis
v. angiosarcoma
v. carcinoma
v. carditis
v. endocarditis
v. hyperplasia
v. melanoma
v. nevus
v. papilloma
v. sarcoid
v. scrofuloderma
v. vegetation
v. xanthoma
verruculosa
Curvularia v.
verruga peruana
Versant HCV RNA 3.0 assay
Verse disease
Versene
versican
versicolor
Aspergillus v.
membrana v.
pityriasis v.
Pityrosporum v.
tinea v.
versiforme
Natrinema v.
version
HD allele v.
versmoldensis
Lactobacillus v.
versutus
Thialkalivibrio v.
vertebral
v. arthritis
v. basilar artery syndrome
v. crush-fracture syndrome
v. defects, anal atresia,
tracheoesophageal fistula with
esophageal atresia, and radial and
renal anomalies (VATER)
v. polyarthritis
vertical
v. melanoma growth
phase
v. transmission
verticil
verticillate
Verticillium
V. alboatrum
V. graphii
vertigo

verumontanitis
very
    v. large scale integration (VLSI)
    v. late activation (VLA)
very-high-density lipoprotein (VHDL)
very-high frequency
very-low birth weight (VLBW)
very-low-density lipoprotein (VLDL)
vesica, *pl.* **vesicae**
    bullous edema vesicae
    ectopia vesicae
    malacoplakia vesicae
    pachyderma vesicae
vesicae (*pl. of* vesica)
vesical
    v. blood fluke
    v. calculus
    v. diverticulum
    v. dysplasia
    v. endometriosis
    v. fistula
    v. gland
    v. hematuria
vesicalis
    anus v.
vesicant
vesicating agent
vesicle
    acrosomal v.
    air v.
    Baer v.
    clathrin-coated v.
    coated electron-lucent v.
    electron-lucent v.
    excretory duct of seminal v.
    germinal v.
    matrix v.
    micropinocytotic v.
    nonmelanosomal v.
    pinocytotic v.
    presynaptic v.
    synaptic v.
    villous v.
vesicobullous
vesicocolic fistula
vesicocutaneous fistula
vesicointestinal fistula
vesicolithiasis
vesicopustular
vesicopustule
vesico-sphincter dyssynergia
vesicoureteral reflux
vesicouterine fistula
vesicovaginal fistula
vesicovaginorectal fistula
vesicula, *pl.* **vesiculae**
vesiculae (*pl. of* vesicula)
vesicular
    v. acute inflammation

    v. chromatin pattern
    v. emphysema
    v. exanthema
    v. exanthema of swine virus
    v. granulomatous inflammation
    v. keratitis
    v. mole
    v. nucleus
    v. ovarian follicle
    v. stomatitis
    v. stomatitis virus (VSV)
vesicularis
    Brevundimonas v.
    Pseudomonas v.
vesiculate
vesiculated
vesiculation
vesiculiform
vesiculin
vesiculitis
vesiculocavernous
vesiculopapular
vesiculoprostatitis
vesiculopustular
vesiculose
vesiculosi
    stratum granulosum folliculi ovarici
    v.
vesiculosum
    eczema v.
    hydroa v.
vesiculosus
    folliculus ovaricus v.
vesiculous
Vesiculovirus
Vesivirus
vessel
    aberrant renal v.
    blood v.
    capillary v.
    chyle v.
    efferent lymphatic v.
    endothelial lining of v.
    great v.
    lacteal v.
    newly formed v.
    pinocytotic v.
    trabecular blood v.
    transposition of great v.'s (TGV)
    velamentous v.
vestalii
    Rhodoglobus v.
vestfoldensis
    Loktanella v.
vestibular
    v. anus
    v. canal
    v. gland
    v. hair cell

V

vestibular (*continued*)
    v. membrane
    v. organ
    v. window
vestibule
    fenestra of the v.
vestibuli
    aqueductus v.
    fenestra v.
    sacculus v.
    scala v.
vestigial
vestimenti
vestimentorum
vestrisii
    Bosea v.
vesuvin
veterana
    Nocardia v.
veterinary vaccine Stern strain *Bacillus anthracis*
vexans
    Aedes v.
vexator
VG
    NATO code for nerve agent O,O-diethyl S-[2-(diethylamino)ethyl] phosphonothioate
VGA
    villoglandular adenocarcinoma
Vgamma9 test
VH
    venous hematocrit
VHD
    viral hematodepressive disease
VHDL
    very-high-density lipoprotein
VHF
    viral hemorrhagic fever
VHL
    von Hippel-Lindau
      VHL gene
Vi
    Vi agglutination
    Vi antibody
    Vi antigen
VI
    vascular invasion
VIA
    virus-inactivating agent
viability
viable cell count
vial
vibration
    v. second (vs)
    subsynchronous v.
vibrational spectroscopy
vibratome tissue section

Vibrio
    V. aerogenes
    V. aestuarianus
    V. agarivorans
    V. alginolyticus
    V. brasiliensis
    V. calviensis
    V. chagasii
    V. cholerae
    V. cholerae biotype El Tor (El Tor vibrio)
    V. coralliilyticus
    V. cyclitrophicus
    V. fluvialis
    V. fortis
    V. furnissii
    V. gallicus
    V. group F (EF-6)
    V. hepatarius
    V. hispanicus
    V. hollisae
    V. kanaloae
    V. lentus
    V. metschnikovii
    V. mimicus
    V. neptunius
    V. pacinii
    V. parahaemolyticus
    V. pomeroyi
    V. proteolyticus
    V. proteus
    V. rotiferianus
    V. ruber
    V. shilonii
    V. sputorum
    V. tasmaniensis
    V. viscosus
    V. vulnificus
    V. wodanis
    V. xuii
vibrio
    Celebes v.
    cholera v.
    Nasik v.
    nonagglutinating v.
vibrioides
    Propionispora v.
Vibrionaceae
Vibrion septique
vibriosis
vicarious
    v. hemoptysis
    v. hypertrophy
Vi-CELL series cell viability analyzer
Vicia graminea
vicinal neuron
vicine
vicious union
victim identification

Victivallales
Victivallis vadensis
Victoria
    V. blue
    V. blue stain
    V. orange
Vidal disease
vidarabine
Vidas
    V. probe
    V. total PSA assay kit
vide infra
video-assisted transthoracic surgery (VATS)
video time-lapse microscopy
Vidiera
    V. NsD nucleic sample detection
    V. NsP nucleic sample preparation
Vielle menopause home test kit
Vierra sign
vietnamensis
    Desulfovibrio v.
view
    field of v.
    radius of v.
VIG
    vaccinia immune globulin
vigil
    Wohlfahrtia v.
Vignal cell
Villaret syndrome
villi (*pl. of* villus)
villiform configuration
villin
villitis of unknown etiology (VUE)
villoglandular adenocarcinoma (VGA)
villoma
villonodular
    v. pigmented synovitis
    v. pigmented tenosynovitis
villorum
    Enterococcus v.
villosa
    polyarthritis chronica v.
villose (*var. of* villous)
villositis
villosity
villous, villose
    v. adenoma
    v. atrophy
    v. capillary hypervascularity
    v. carcinoma
    v. ischemic necrosis
    v. papilloma
    v. polyp
    v. tenosynovitis
    v. tumor
    v. vesicle

villus, *pl.* **villi**
    abnormal chorionic v.
    arachnoid v.
    chorionic v.
    intestinal v.
    villi intestinales
    molar villi
    villi pericardiaci
    villi peritoneales
    pleural villi
    villi pleurales
    synovial villi
    villi synoviales
vimentin
    v. antibody
    v. immunoperoxidase stain
    v. protein
VIN
    vulvar intraepithelial neoplasia
    warty VIN
vinacea
    Nocardia v.
vinaceus
    Actinomyces v.
Vincent
    V. angina
    V. bacillus
    V. disease
    V. organism
    V. stomatitis
    V. white mycetoma
vincentii
    Borrelia v.
    Treponema v.
vincristine neuropathy
vinculin protein
Vindelov procedure
vindobonensis
    Promicromonospora v.
vinegar acid
vinsonii
    Bartonella v.
Vinson syndrome
vinyl
    v. chloride
    v. chloride disease
    v. polymer
    v. trichloride
violacea
    Lentzea v.
    Saccharothrix v.
violaceinigra
    Duganella v.
violaceous
violaceum
    Cardiobacterium v.
    Chromobacterium v.
    Trichophyton v.

V

violet
    amethyst v.
    ammonium oxalate crystal v.
    aniline gentian v. (AGV)
    Bensley safranin acid v.
    Bernthsen methylene v.
    chrome v.
    cresyl v. (CV)
    cresylecht v.
    cresyl fast v.
    crystal v.
    gentian v. (GV)
    hexamethyl v.
    Hoffman v.
    Lauth v.
    methyl v.
    methylene v.
viomycin
viosterol
VIP
    vasoactive intestinal peptide
    vasoactive intestinal polypeptide
    voluntary interruption of pregnancy
viper venom (VV)
VIPoma
viral
    v. capsid antigen (VCA)
    v. carcinogenesis
    v. culture
    v. dysentery
    v. encephalomyelitis
    v. envelope
    v. gastroenteritis
    v. genome
    v. genomic diversity
    v. hemagglutination
    v. hematodepressive disease (VHD)
    v. hemorrhagic fever (VHF)
    v. hemorrhagic fever virus
    v. hepatitis, type A–E
    v. hybrid capture
    v. inclusion
    v. load
    v. meningitis
    v. myocarditis
    v. neutralization
    v. nucleic acid
    v. pericarditis
    v. pneumonia
    v. probe
    v. respiratory infection (VRI)
    v. strand
    v. tropism
    v. wart
ViraPap test
ViraType In Situ System
Virchow
    V. cell
    V. corpuscle
    V. crystal
    V. disease
    V. hydatid
    V. law
    V. node
    V. psammoma
    V. triad
Virchow-Hassall body
Virchow-Robin space
viremia
    asymptomatic v.
    secondary v.
vireti
    Bacillus v.
Virgibacillus
    V. carmonensis
    V. marismortui
    V. necropolis
    V. picturae
    V. salexigens
virginal hypertrophy
virgin B cell
virginity
Virgisporangium
    V. aurantiacum
    V. ochraceum
viricidal (*var. of* virucidal)
viricide (*var. of* virucide)
viridans
    Aerococcus v.
    Carnobacterium v.
    Staphylococcus v.
    Thalassomonas v.
viridilutea
    Actinomadura v.
viridis
    Euglena v.
    Saccharomonospora v.
    Thermolospora v.
virilism
    adrenal v.
    congenital adrenal v. (CAV)
virilization
    adrenal v.
virilizing syndrome
virion
virogene
viroid
virologist
virology laboratory
viropexis
virosa
    Amanita v.
ViroSeq HIV-1 genotyping system
Virotrol syphilis total control
virtual autopsy
virtually diagnostic
virucidal, viricidal
virucide, viricide

virucopria
virulence factor
virulent
    v. bacteriophage
    v. Schu S4 tularemia strain
viruliferous
viruria
2060 virus
virus
    2060 v.
    Abelson murine leukemia v.
    adeno-associated v. (AAV)
    adenosatellite v.
    African horse sickness v.
    African swine fever v.
    AIDS-related v. (ARV)
    Akabane v.
    AKT1 v.
    Aleutian mink disease v.
    amphotropic v.
    animal v.
    v. animatum
    APC v.
    apeu v.
    Argentine hemorrhagic fever v.
    attenuated v.
    Aujeszky disease v.
    Australian X disease v.
    Australian X encephalitis v.
    avian encephalomyelitis v.
    avian erythroblastosis v.
    avian infectious laryngotracheitis v.
    avian influenza v.
    avian leukosis-sarcoma v.
    avian lymphomatosis v.
    avian myeloblastosis v.
    avian myelocytomatosis v. (AMV2)
    avian neurolymphomatosis v.
    avian pneumoencephalitis v.
    avian sarcoma v.
    avian viral arthritis v.
    bacterial v.
    Bittner v.
    biundulant milk fever v.
    BK v.
    v. blockade
    bluecomb v.
    bluetongue v.
    Borna disease v.
    Bornholm disease v.
    bovine leukemia v. (BLV)
    bovine leukosis v.
    bovine papular stomatitis v.
    breakpoint cluster region-Abelson
      murine leukemia v. (BCR-ABL)
    brick-shaped v.
    v. bronchopneumonia
    Brunhilde v.
    Bunyamwera v.

    Bwamba fever v.
    C v.
    CA v.
    Cache Valley v.
    California encephalitis v.
    California myxoma v.
    canarypox v.
    canine distemper v.
    Capim v.
    Caraparu v.
    cat distemper v.
    cattle plague v.
    Catu v.
    CELO v.
    Central European encephalitis v.
      (CEEV)
    Central European tick-borne
      encephalitis v.
    C group v.
    Chagres v.
    chicken embryo lethal orphan v.
    chickenpox v.
    chikungunya fever v.
    c2-like v.
    Coe v.
    cold v.
    Colorado tick fever v.
    Columbia SK v.
    common cold v.
    contagious pustular stomatitis v.
    coryza v.
    cowpox v.
    Crimean-Congo hemorrhagic fever v.
    Crimean hemorrhagic fever v.
    croup-associated v.
    cytomegalic inclusion disease v.
    cytopathogenic v.
    defective v.
    delta v.
    diphasic meningoencephalitis v.
    diphasic milk fever v.
    distemper v.
    DNA v.
    dog distemper v.
    double-stranded DNA v.
    duck hepatitis v.
    duck influenza v.
    duck plague v.
    Eastern equine encephalomyelitis v.
    EB v.
    Ebola v.
    Ebola-like v.
    ECBO v.
    ECDO v.
    ECHO v.
    ECMO v.
    ecotropic v.
    ECSO v.
    ecthyma infectiosum v.

V

virus (*continued*)

ectromelia v.
EEE v.
EMC v.
emerging v.
encephalitis v.
encephalomyocarditis v.
enteric orphan v.
entomopox v.
enzootic encephalomyelitis v.
ephemeral fever v.
epidemic gastroenteritis v.
epidemic keratoconjunctivitis v.
epidemic myalgia v.
epidemic parotitis v.
epidemic pleurodynia v.
Epstein-Barr v. (EBV)
equine abortion v.
equine arteritis v.
equine coital exanthema v.
equine encephalomyelitis v.
equine infectious anemia v.
equine influenza v.
equine rhinopneumonitis v.
feline ataxia v. (FAV)
feline leukemia v. (FeLV)
feline panleukopenia v.
feline rhinotracheitis v.
fibrous bacterial v.
fifth disease v.
filamentous bacterial v.
filterable v.
fixed v.
Flury strain rabies v.
FMD v.
foamy v.
foot-and-mouth disease v.
fowl erythroblastosis v.
fowl lymphomatosis v.
fowl myeloblastosis v.
fowl neurolymphomatosis v.
fowl plague v.
fowlpox v.
fox encephalitis v.
Friend leukemia v.
GAL v.
gallus adenolike v.
gastroenteritis v. type A, B
Gauma v.
German measles v.
Germiston v.
gibbon ape lymphosarcoma v.
 (GaLV)
Graffi v.
green monkey v.
Gross leukemia v.
group B arbor v.
Guama v.
Guanarito v.

Guaroa v.
hand-foot-and-mouth disease v.
Hantaan v.
hard pad v.
helper v.
hepatitis v.
hepatitis A v. (HAV)
hepatitis B v. (HBV)
hepatitis C v. (HCV)
hepatitis D v. (HDV)
hepatitis delta v. (HDV)
hepatitis E v. (HEV)
hepatitis E-like viruses
hepatitis G v. (HGV)
hepatitis GB v. (HGBV)
herpangina v.
herpes v.
herpeslike v. (HLV)
herpes simplex v. (HSV)
herpes simplex v. I (HSV I)
herpes-type v. (HTV)
herpes zoster v.
hog cholera v.
horsepox v.
human B lymphotropic v. (HBLV)
human immunodeficiency v.
 (HIV)
human T-cell leukemia-lymphoma v.
 (HTLV)
human T-cell lymphotropic v. type I
 (HTLV-I)
human T-cell lymphotropic v. type
 II (HTLV-II)
human T-cell lymphotropic v. type
 III (HTLV-III)
Ibaraki v.
IBR v.
Ictalurid herpes-like viruses
IgM anti-hepatitis A v.
Ilhéus v.
inadvertent inoculation of vaccinia
 v.
inclusion conjunctivitis v.
infantile gastroenteritis v.
infectious bovine rhinotracheitis v.
infectious bronchitis v. (IBV)
infectious ectromelia v.
infectious hepatitis v.
infectious laryngo-tracheitis-like v.
infectious papilloma v.
infectious porcine encephalomyelitis
 v.
influenza v.
insect v.
iridescent v.
Itaqui v.
Jamestown Canyon v.
Japanese B encephalitis v.
JC v.

JH v.
Junin v.
K v.
Kelev strain rabies v.
v. keratoconjunctivitis
Kilham rat v.
Kisenyi sheep disease v.
Koongol v.
Korean hemorrhagic fever v.
Kumba v.
Kyasanur Forest disease v.
La Crosse v.
lactate dehydrogenase v.
lactic dehydrogenase v. (LDV)
Lansing v.
Lassa v.
latent rat v.
LCM v.
Leon v.
louping ill v.
Lucké v.
Lunyo v.
lymphadenopathy-associated v. (LAV)
lymphocytic choriomeningitis v.
lymphogranuloma venereum v.
Machupo v.
maedi v.
Maloney leukemia v.
mammary tumor v. (MTV)
Marburg v.
Marburg-like v.
Marek disease v.
Marek disease-like v.
Marituba v.
marmoset v.
masked v.
Mason-Pfizer monkey v.
Mayaro v.
measles v.
Mengo v.
milker's nodule v.
mink enteritis v.
MM v.
Mokola v.
molluscum contagiosum v. (MCV)
molluscum sebaceum v.
Moloney leukemogenic v. (MLV)
Moloney sarcoma v. (MSV)
monkey B v.
monkeypox v.
mouse encephalomyelitis v.
mouse hepatitis v.
mouse leukemia v. (MLV)
mouse mammary tumor v. (MMTV)
mouse parotid tumor v.
mouse poliomyelitis v.
mousepox v.
mouse thymic v.

mucosal disease v.
mu-like v.
mumps v.
murine sarcoma v. (MSV)
Murutucu v.
MVE v.
myxomatosis v.
Nairobi sheep disease v.
naked v.
ND v.
Nebraska calf scours v.
Neethling v.
negative strand v.
Negishi v.
neonatal calf diarrhea v.
neurotropic v.
v. neutralization test
newborn pneumonitis v.
Newcastle disease v. (NDV)
nonbacterial gastroenteritis v.
nonenveloped RNA v.
nonoccluded v.
Norwalk v. *(Norovirus)*
Ntaya v.
occluded v.
Omsk hemorrhagic fever v.
oncogenic v.
O'nyong-nyong fever v.
orf v.
Oriboca v.
ornithosis v.
Oropouche v.
orphan v.
Pacheco parrot disease v.
plant v.
P1-like v.
P2-like v.
P4-like v.
P22-like v.
PLT group v.
v. pneumonia of pigs
pneumonitis v.
poliomyelitis v.
v. poliomyelitis
polyoma v.
porcine hemagglutinating encephalomyelitis v.
Powassan v.
progressive pneumonia v.
pseudocowpox v.
pseudolymphocytic choriomeningitis v.
pseudorabies v.
psittacosis v.
PVM v.
quail bronchitis v.
Quaranfil v.
rabbit fibroma v.
rabbitpox v.

V

virus (*continued*)
 rabies v.
 rat v. (RV)
 Rauscher leukemia v.
 reservoir of v.
 respiratory enteric orphan v.
 respiratory exanthematous v.
 respiratory infection v.
 respiratory syncytial v. (RSV)
 Rida v.
 Rift Valley fever v.
 rinderpest v.
 RNA tumor v.
 roseola infantum v.
 Ross River v.
 Rous-associated v. (RAV)
 Rous sarcoma v.
 Rs v.
 Rubarth disease v.
 rubella v. (RV)
 rubeola v.
 Russian autumn encephalitis v.
 Russian spring-summer
  encephalitis v.
 Sabia v.
 Salisbury common cold v.
 salivary gland v. (SGV)
 sandfly fever v.
 San Miguel sea lion v.
 Semliki Forest v.
 Sendai v.
 serum hepatitis v.
 v. shedding
 sheep pox v.
 shipping fever v.
 Shope fibroma v.
 Shope papilloma v.
 Simbu v.
 simian v. (SV)
 simian immunodeficiency v. (SIV)
 simian sarcoma v. (SSV)
 s. vacuolating v. No. 40
 Sindbis v.
 slow v.
 smallpox v.
 snowshoe hare v.
 soremouth v.
 SPO1-like viruses
 Spondweni v.
 ssRNA v.
 St. Louis encephalitis v.
 street v.
 Sulfolobus SNDV-like v.
 swamp fever v.
 swine encephalitis v.
 swine fever v.
 swine influenza v.
 swinepox v.
 Swiss mouse leukemia v.

Tacaribe complex of v.'s
Tahyna v.
temperate v.
Teschen v.
Tete v.
TGE v.
Theiler mouse encephalomyelitis v.
Theiler original v.
tick-borne encephalitis v.
T1-like v.
T4-like v.
T5-like v.
T7-like v.
tobacco mosaic v. (TMV)
trachoma v.
transforming v.
transfusion transmitted v. (TTV)
transmissible turkey enteritis v.
TT v.
tumor v.
turkey meningoencephalitis v.
Turlock v.
Uganda S v.
Umbre v.
unorganized v.
Uruma v.
vaccine v.
vaccinia v.
vacuolating v.
varicella v.
varicella-zoster v. (VZV)
variola v.
VEE v.
Venezuelan equine A
 encephalomyelitis v.
Venezuelan equine
 encephalomyelitis v. (VEE)
verruca v.
vesicular exanthema of swine v.
vesicular stomatitis v. (VSV)
viral hemorrhagic fever v.
visceral disease v.
visna v.
v. VP1 capsid protein
VS v.
WEE v.
Wesselsbron disease v.
Western equine encephalomyelitis v.
 (WEE)
West Nile encephalitis v.
Willowbrook v.
v. X disease
xenotropic v.
Yaba monkey v.
yellow fever v.
Zika v.
virus-associated hemophagocytic
 syndrome (VAHS)
virus-inactivating agent (VIA)

virus-neutralizing (VN)
virusoid
virus-transformed cell
VIS
  vaginal irrigation smear
VISA
  vancomycin-insensitive *Staphylococcus aureus*
viscera (*pl. of* viscus)
visceral
  v. disease virus
  v. inversion
  v. larva migrans
  v. leishmaniasis
  v. lymphomatosis
  v. motor neuron
  v. pleurisy
viscerale
visceromegaly
visceroptosia (*var. of* visceroptosis)
visceroptosis, visceroptosia
viscerotomy
viscerotrophic reflex
viscid
viscidity
viscidosis
viscometer
viscosa
  Moritella v.
viscose
viscosimeter
  Ostwald v.
  Stormer v.
viscosimetry
viscosity
  absolute v.
  dynamic v.
  increased v.
  kinematic v.
viscosus
  Actinomyces v.
  Vibrio v.
  Xanthobacter v.
viscous
viscus, *pl.* **viscera**
  abdominal viscera
  ruptured viscera
visible light
vision
  cribriform field of v.
VisionSaver lab lamp
Visiprep solid-phase extraction vacuum manifold
visna virus
visual
  v. evoked potential
  v. evoked response
  v. fluorescent screening test
  v. receptor cell

vital
  v. dye
  v. red
  v. signs (VS)
  v. stain
  v. staining
vitamin
  v. A
  v. A_1
  v. A_1 aldehyde
  v. A_2
  v. A and carotene assays
  v. A clearance test
  v. A, D intoxication
  v. A unit (international)
  v. B complex
  v. B_1
  v. B_1 hydrochloride unit
  v. B_2
  v. B_2 unit
  v. B_3
  v. B_6
  v. B_6 assay
  v. B_6 unit
  v. B_7
  v. B_{12}
  v. B_{12a}
  v. B_{12} absorption test
  v. B_{12} assay
  v. B_{12} deficiency
  v. B_{12} neuropathy
  v. B_{12} unsaturated binding capacity
  v. B_c
  v. B_x
  v. C unit
  v. D_3
  v. D assay
  v. deficiency anemia
  v. D unit
  v. E assay
  v. E unit
  v. K_1
  v. K_1 oxide
  v. K_2 (MK-6)
  v. K_3
  v. K assay
  v. K deficiency
  v. K dependent plasma protein
  v. K unit
  microbial v.
  water-soluble v.
vitamin-D-dependent rickets
vitamin-D-resistant rickets
vitaminoid action
Vitek GPI
vitellarium
Vitellibacter vladivostokensis
vitellin

V

vitellina
    membrana v.
vitelline
    polyvesicular v.
    v. sphere
vitellointestinal cyst
viterbiensis
    Caloramator v.
vitiation
vitiliginous
vitiligo
    circumnevic v.
vitiligoidea
vitis
    Rhizobium v.
Vitivirus
vitrea
    lamina v.
    membrana v.
    substantia v.
    tunica v.
Vitreoscillaceae
vitreous
    v. body
    v. cavity
    v. cell
    v. humor
    v. lamella
    v. membrane
    v. space
    stroma of v.
vitreum
    corpus v.
    stroma v.
vitreus
    humor v.
vitrinus
    Trichostrongylus v.
vitro
    in v.
vitronectin receptor
Vitros
    V. analyzer
    V. anti-HBs assay
    V. HBsAg assay
    V. HBsAg confirmatory kit
    V. Immunodiagnostic Products
    anti-HBc calibrator
    V. Immunodiagnostic Products
    anti-HBc reagent pack
Vittaforma
vituli
    Acholeplasma v.
vitulorum
    Neoascaris v.
Viva-E drug testing analyzer
vivax
    v. fever
    v. malaria

    Plasmodium v.
    Trypanosoma v.
viverrini
    Opisthorchis v.
vivipara
    Probstymayria v.
Viviparidae
viviparus
    Dictyocaulus v.
vivo
    ex v.
    in v.
vivum
    contagium v.
VLA
    very late activation
    VLA antigen
vladivostokensis
    Vitellibacter v.
VLBW
    very-low birth weight
VLDL
    very-low-density lipoprotein
VLSI
    very large scale integration
VM
    NATO code for nerve agent O-ethyl
    S-[2-(diethylamino)ethyl]
    methylphosphonothioate
VMA
    vanillylmandelic acid
    VMA test
VMC
    von Meyenburg complex
VMR
    vasomotor rhinitis
VN
    virus-neutralizing
VNTR
    variable number of tandem
    repeats
VOC
    volatile organic compound
vocal
    v. cord disease
    v. cord paralysis
    v. fold nodule
    v. fold polyp
vogeli
    Echinococcus v.
Voges-Proskauer (VP)
    V.-P. broth
    methyl red, V.-P. (MR-VP)
    V.-P. reaction
    V.-P. test
Vogt-Koyanagi syndrome
Vogt-Spielmeyer disease
Vogt syndrome
Vohwinkel syndrome

voinovskiensis
  Anoxybacillus v.
volatile
  v. nerve agent
  v. oil
  v. organic compound (VOC)
  v. organic substances assay
  v. screen
  v. substance inhalation
volatility
volatilization
vole
  v. bacillus
  field v.
Volhard test
Volkmann
  V. canal
  V. contracture
  V. disease
  V. ischemic paralysis
  V. membrane
  V. syndrome
Vollmer test
volt (V)
  ampere-second per v. (As/V)
  electron v. (eV)
  giga electron v. (geV)
  kiloelectron v. (keV)
  megaelectron v. (MeV)
  million electron v.'s (MeV)
voltage
  anode v.
  v. divider
  v. drop
  high v.
  v. regulator
  ripple v.
voltage-gated channel
voltage-regulating transformer
voltage-regulator tube
voltage-to-frequency converter
voltammetry
volt-ampere (VA)
voltmeter
  digital v.
  vacuum tube v. (VTVM)
volt-ohm-milliammeter
Voltolini disease
Volucribacter
  V. amazonae
  V. psittacicida
volume
  amniotic fluid total v.
  blood v. (BV)
  cell v. (CV)
  central blood v. (CBV)
  circulating blood v. (CBV)
  v. coefficient
  v. conduction

conductivity cell v. (CCV)
corpuscular v. (CV)
corrected blood v. (CBV)
v. depletion
effective circulating v. (ECV)
effective circulating blood v. (ECBV)
euvolemic v.
v. expansion
extracellular v. (ECV)
extracellular fluid v. (ECFV, EFV)
fluid v. (FV)
increased v.
v. index (VI)
inspiratory reserve v. (IRV)
intracellular fluid v. (IFV)
intrathoracic gas v. (IGV)
maximum expiratory flow v. (MEFV)
mean cell v. (MCV)
mean corpuscular v. (MCV)
mean platelet v. (MVP)
minute v. (MV)
v. of distribution of bilirubin (VDBR)
v. of isoflow
v. of packed cells (VPC)
v. of packed red cells (VPRC)
packed cell v. (PCV)
placental residual blood v. (PRBV)
plasma v. (PV)
pulmonary capillary blood v.
red blood cell v. (RBCV, VRBC)
red cell v. (RCV)
regional cerebral blood v. (RCBV)
residual v. (RV)
retention v.
reticulocyte mean corpuscular v. (MCVr)
v. substitute
test v.
thoracic gas v. (TGV)
tidal v. (TV, VT)
timed 2-hour v.
timed 24-hour v.
total blood v. (TBV)
weight per v. (w/v)
volumetric
  v. flask
  v. pipette
  v. solution (VS)
voluntary interruption of pregnancy
volutans
  Spirillum v.
Volutella cinerescens
volutin
Volvariella
Volvox
volvulosis

V

volvulus
    Filaria v.
    gastric v.
    Onchocerca v.
vomica
vomicose
vomiting, vomition
    v. agent
    epidemic v.
vomition (*var. of* vomiting)
vomitoria
    Calliphora v.
vomitoxin
vomitus
    colonic v.
    fecal v.
von
    v. Apathy gum syrup medium
    v. Bechterew disease
    v. Brunn nest
    v. Clauss method
    v. Economo disease
    v. Economo encephalitis
    v. Gierke disease
    v. Hansemann histiocyte
    v. Hansemann macrophage
    v. Hippel disease
    v. Hippel-Lindau (VHL)
    v. Hippel-Lindau disease
    v. Hippel-Lindau gene
    v. Hippel-Lindau syndrome
    v. Jaksch disease
    v. Kossa calcium assay
    v. Kossa calcium stain
    v. Kossa method
    v. Kossa reaction
    v. Meyenburg complex (VMC)
    v. Meyenburg disease
    v. Recklinghausen disease
    v. Willebrand disease (VW)
    v. Willebrand factor
    v. Willebrand factor antigen
    v. Willebrand factor assay
    v. Willebrand factor multimer assay
    v. Willebrand syndrome
    v. Zumbusch psoriasis
Voorhoeve disease
vortex
vortexing
Vorticella
vorticose
VP
    variably positive
    vasopressin
    Voges-Proskauer
    VP test
VPC
    vapor-phase chromatography
    volume of packed cells

VPRC
    volume of packed red cells
V/Q mismatch
VR
    vascular resistance
VRE
    vancomycin-resistant *Enterococcus*
    vancomycin-resistant *Enterococcus*
      assay
VRI
    viral respiratory infection
Vrolik disease
VS
    vital signs
    volumetric solution
      VS virus
vs
    vibration second
VSD
    ventricular septal defect
VSMC
    vascular smooth muscle cell
      VSMC infolding
VSV
    vesicular stomatitis virus
VT
    tidal volume
    vacuum tuberculin
VTVM
    vacuum tube voltmeter
V-Twin drug testing analyzer
VUE
    villitis of unknown
      etiology
Vuilleminia
vulcanalis
    Alicyclobacillus v.
vulcani
    Bacillus v.
Vulcanisaeta
    V. distributa
    V. souniana
vulgare
    Ketogulonicigenium v.
vulgaris
    acne v.
    Cellvibrio v.
    ichthyosis v.
    impetigo v.
    lupus v.
    Nitrobacter v.
    Proteus v.
    psoriasis v.
    Strongylus v.
    Thermoactinomyces v.
      (TV)
    verruca v.
vulneris
    Escherichia v.

vulnificus
    Vibrio v.
vulpis
    Crenosoma v.
    Trichuris v.
vulva, *pl.* **vulvae**
    elephantiasis v.
    kraurosis vulvae
    leukoplakia v.
    lichen sclerosus of v.
    multinucleated atypia of the v.
      (MAV)
    velamen v.
vulvae (*pl. of* vulva)
vulval (*var. of* vulvar)
vulvar, vulval
    v. cancer
    v. dystrophy
    v. intraepithelial neoplasia (VIN)
    v. squamous hyperplasia
    v. tumor
vulvitis
    chronic atrophic v.
    chronic hypertrophic v.

    hypertrophic chronic v.
    leukoplakic v.
    plasma cell v.
vulvovaginal
    v. anus
    v. candidiasis
    v. gland
vulvovaginitis
    Candida v.
VV
    viper venom
VVG
    Verhoeff-van Gieson
      VVG stain
VW
    von Willebrand disease
Vw antigen
Vycor glassware
Vysis probe
VZ, V-Z
    varicella-zoster
VZV
    varicella-zoster virus
      VZV culture

V

W
watt
W factor
Waardenburg syndrome
Wachstein-Meissel stain for
calcium-magnesium-ATPase
Waddliaceae
Waddlia chondrophila
Wade-Fite-Faraco stain
wadei
Leptotrichia w.
wadsworthensis
Sutterella w.
wadsworthia
Bilophila w.
wadsworthii
Legionella w.
Wagner
W. disease
W. test
Wagner-Meissner corpuscle
WAGR
Wilms tumor, aniridia, genital
anomalies, mental retardation
WAGR syndrome
WAIHA
warm autoimmune hemolytic anemia
Waikavirus
waiotapuensis
Thermococcus w.
Wako
W. 1% crude papain
W. NEFA test kit
waksmanii
Shewanella w.
Waldenström
W. disease
W. macroglobulinemia (WM)
W. purpura
W. syndrome
W. test
Waldermaria
Waldeyer
W. gland
W. ring
W. ring lymphoma
Walker
W. carcinoma
W. carcinosarcoma
wall
anterior w.
cell w.
cross w.
hypertrophy of chamber w.
Wallemia sebi

Wallenberg syndrome
wallerian degeneration (WD)
wallet stomach
Walsh average
Walthard
W. cell
W. cell rest
Walther
W. canal
W. duct
Waltomyces
Wampole
W. *Clostridium difficile* Tox A/B II
W. Isolater blood culture system
wandering
w. abscess
w. cell
w. goiter
w. liver
w. nucleolonema
w. organ
w. pacemaker
w. pneumonia
Wang
W. needle
W. test
Wangiella dermatitidis
warble fly
Warburg theory
Wardomyces inflatus
Wardomycopsis
Ward-Romano syndrome
Wardrop disease
warfare
biological w. (BW)
chemical w. (CW)
chemical and biological w.
(CBW)
warfarin
w. assay
w. dosing decision
sodium w.
w. therapy
Warkany syndrome
warm
w. agglutination
w. agglutinin
w. autoantibody
w. autoimmune hemolytic anemia
(WAIHA)
w. hemagglutinin
w. reactive antibody
warm-and-cold-type autoimmune
hemolytic anemia
warm-cold hemolysin

W

warming
  blood w.
warneri
  Staphylococcus w.
wart
  anatomic w.
  anatomical w.
  anogenital w.
  cattle w.
  common w.
  digitate w.
  fig w.
  filiform w.
  flat w.
  genital w.
  Hassall-Henle w.
  infectious w.
  moist w.
  mosaic w.
  necrogenic w.
  pitch w.
  plane w.
  plantar w.
  pointed w.
  postmortem w.
  prosector's w.
  seborrheic w.
  senile w.
  soft w.
  soot w.
  telangiectatic w.
  tuberculous w.
  venereal w.
  viral w.
Wartenberg disease
Warthin-Finkeldey multinucleate giant cell
Warthin-Finkeldey-type polykaryocyte
Warthin-Starry
  W.-S. method
  W.-S. silver stain
Warthin tumor
wartpox
warty
  w. carcinoma
  w. dyskeratoma
  w. horn
  w. ulcer
  w. VIN
WAS
  Wiskott-Aldrich syndrome
wasabiae
wash
  Gravlee jet w.
  w. time
  xylene w.
  Zila Pro-Wash antiseptic hand w.

washed
  w. out deposit
  w. platelet activation
  w. red blood cell
  w. red cell (WRC)
washerwoman's skin
washing
  bronchial w.
  w. cytology
washout pipette
Wasmann gland
WASP
  Wiskott-Aldrich syndrome protein
  World Association of Societies of Pathology
Wassén test
wasserhelle
  w. cell
  w. hyperplasia
Wassermann
  W. antibody
  W. antigen
  W. reaction
  W. test
Wassermann-fast
Wassilieff disease
waste
  chemical w.
  infectious w.
  w. product
  radioactive w.
  toxic w.
wasting
  w. disease
  salt w.
  w. syndrome
Watanabe silver impregnation
water
  w. aspirator
  w. bacterium
  w. balance
  w. bath
  w. clear cytoplasm
  w. conductivity
  DEPC-treated w.
  w. deprivation diabetes insipidus differentiation test
  dextrose in w. (percent)
  extracellular w. (ECW)
  w. gas
  gentian aniline w.
  w. gurgle test
  heavy w.
  HPLC w.
  w. immersion
  w. in oil (W/O)
  interstitial w. (ISW)
  w. intoxication

intracellular w. (ICW)
light w.
w. loading test
oil in w. (O/W)
5 percent dextrose in w. (D_5W, D5W)
radiostable w.
ratio of number of ATPs produced to number of atmospheric oxygen molecules converted to w. (P:O)
total body w. (TBW)
tritiated w.

waterborne pathogen
water-clear
    w.-c. cell
    w.-c. cell hyperplasia
    w.-c. cell of parathyroid
Waterhouse-Friderichsen syndrome
watering-can
    w.-c. perineum
    w.-c. scrotum
Waterman blue ink
watermelon stomach
waterpox
water-soluble
    w.-s. salt
    w.-s. scarlet
    w.-s. vitamin
water-trap stomach
watery diarrhea, hypokalemia, achlorhydria (WDHA)
watsoni
    Cladorchis w.
    Watsonius w.
Watsonius watsoni
Watson-Schwartz test
watt (W)
Wautersia
    W. basilensis
    W. campinensis
    W. eutropha
    W. gilardii
    W. metallidurans
    W. oxalatica
    W. paucula
    W. respiraculi
    W. taiwanensis
wave
    acid w.
    alkaline w.
    w. amplitude
    w. analyzer
    diphasic w.
    monophasic w.
    polyphasic w.
    sawtooth w.
    sine w.
    square w.

triangular w.
triphasic w.
w. velocity
waveform
wavefront phenomenon
waveguide
wavelength
    w. accuracy
    w. repeatability
    unit of w.
wavenumber, wave number
wavy
    w. border colony
    w. fiber
wax
    embedding w.
    grave w.
    w. removal
waxy
    w. degeneration
    w. finger
    w. kidney
    w. liver
    w. spleen
    w. urinary cast
Wayson stain
waywayandensis
    Lentzea w.
WB
    whole blood
Wb
    weber
WBC
    white blood cell
        WBC urinary cast
WBC/hpf
    white blood cells per high-power field
WBF
    whole-blood folate
WBGT
    wet bulb globe temperature
WBH
    whole-blood hematocrit
WC
    whole complement
WCC
    white cell count
WCD
    Weber-Christian disease
WD
    wallerian degeneration
    well-differentiated
    Wilson disease
WDCA
    well-differentiated carcinoma
WDFA
    well-differentiated fetal adenocarcinoma

W

WDHA
watery diarrhea, hypokalemia, achlorhydria
WDHA syndrome
WDLL
well-differentiated lymphocytic lymphoma
WE
Western encephalitis
Western encephalomyelitis
weakly
w. positive (WP)
w. reactive (WR)
weakness
congenital vascular w.
excessive w.
weapon
aerosolized plague w.
anthrax as biological w.
biological w.
bone w.
CBRN w.
w. grade
mass-casualty w. (MCW)
w. of mass destruction (WMD)
smallpox as biological w.
weaponized T2 mycotoxin
weapons-grade nuclear material
wear-and-tear
w.-a.-t. pigment
w.-a.-t. pigmentation
web
actin-myosin w.
cell w.
esophageal w.
laryngeal w.
terminal w.
Webb antigen
webbed
w. finger
w. neck
w. toe
webbing
weber (Wb)
W. gland
W. paralysis
W. stain
W. syndrome
W. test
Weber-Christian disease
Weber-Cockayne syndrome
Weber-Dubler syndrome
Weber-modified trichome stain
Weber-Rendu-Osler disease
Webster test
weddellite calculus
WEE
Western equine encephalomyelitis
WEE virus

weed
Jimson w.
Weeks bacillus
Weeksella zoohelcum
Wegener
W. granulomatosis
W. syndrome
Wegner
W. disease
W. line
Weibel-Palade body
Weichselbaum diplococcus
Weidel reaction
weigert
W. iodine solution
W. iron hematoxylin
W. iron hematoxylin stain
W. stain for *Actinomyces*
W. stain for elastin
W. stain for fibrin
W. stain for myelin
W. stain for neuroglia
Weigert-Gram stain
Weigert-Pal stain
weighing
weight (wt)
atomic w.
fat-free dry w. (FFDW)
fat-free wet w. (FFWW)
gram molecular w. (GMW)
high birth w. (HBW)
high molecular w. (HMW)
ideal body w. (IBW)
low birth w. (LBW)
low molecular w. (LMW)
molar w.
molecular w. (MW)
w. per volume (w/v)
total body w. (TBW)
unit of w.
very-low birth w. (VLBW)
weighted average
weihenstephanensis
Bacillus w.
Weil
W. basal layer
W. basal zone
W. disease
W. myelin sheath stain
W. syndrome
Weil-Felix
W.-F. agglutinin
W.-F. reaction (WFR)
W.-F. test
Weill-Marchesani syndrome
Weinberg reaction
Weinman medium
Weir Mitchell disease
Weiss criteria

Weissella
> *W. cibaria*
> *W. kimchii*
> *W. koreensis*
> *W. minor*
> *W. soli*
> *W. thailandensis*

Welch bacillus
welchii
> *Bacillus w.*
> *Clostridium w.*

Welcozyme HIV 1&2 ELISA antibody test
welder's
> w. conjunctivitis
> w. lung

Welker method
well
> alive and w. (A&W)
> w. differentiated
> worried w.

well-differentiated (WD)
> w.-d. carcinoma (WDCA)
> w.-d. fetal adenocarcinoma (WDFA)
> w.-d. lymphocytic lymphoma (WDLL)

Wells syndrome
welt
wen
Wenckebach disease
wenyonii
> *Mycoplasma w.*

Wepfer gland
Werdnig-Hoffmann disease
Werlhof disease
Wermer syndrome
werneckii
> *Cladosporium w.*
> *Exophiala w.*
> *Hortaea w.*

Werner
> W. syndrome
> W. test

Werner-His disease
Werner-Schultz disease
Wernicke
> W. encephalopathy
> W. syndrome

Wernicke-Korsakoff (WK)
> W.-K. encephalopathy
> W.-K. syndrome

Wescor Sweat-Chek conductivity analyzer
Wesenberg-Hamazaki body
Wesselsbron
> W. disease
> W. disease virus
> W. fever

West
> W. African fever
> W. Indian smallpox
> W. Nile encephalitis virus
> W. Nile fever
> W. Nile virus IgM capture test
> W. syndrome

Westerdykella
Westergren
> W. sedimentation rate
> W. sedimentation rate test

westermani
Western
> W. blot
> W. blot analysis
> W. blot electrotransfer test
> W. blot technique
> W. encephalitis (WE)
> W. encephalomyelitis (WE)
> W. equine encephalitis
> W. equine encephalomyelitis (WEE)
> W. equine encephalomyelitis virus
> W. immunoblot test
> W. subtype Russian spring-summer encephalitis

western-type intestinal lymphoma
westfalica
> *Gordonia w.*

Westgard
> W. multirule procedure
> W. selection grid

Westphal disease
Westphal-Strümpell
> W.-S. disease
> W.-S. pseudosclerosis

wet
> w. beriberi
> w. bulb globe temperature (WBGT)
> w. gangrene
> w. mount
> w. pleurisy
> w. prep
> w. preparation
> w. scanning technique

wetting agent
Wetzel test
Weyers oligodactyly syndrome
Weyers-Thier syndrome
WF
> Working Formulation for Clinical Usage

WFR
> Weil-Felix reaction

WGA
> wheat germ agglutinin
> whole genome amplification
> MDA in WGA

W

Wharton
>   W. duct
>   W. jelly
>   W. tumor

whartonitis
Whatman paper
wheal-and-erythema
>   w.-a.-e. reaction
>   w.-a.-e. skin test

wheal-and-flare reaction
wheal reaction time
wheat
>   w. broth
>   w. germ agglutinin (WGA)
>   w. smut

Wheatstone bridge
Wheeler-Johnson test
whetstone crystal
whewellite calculus
whey
>   w. acidic protein
>   litmus w.

whiff test
whiplash
Whipple
>   W. disease
>   W. method
>   W. test
>   W. triad

whipplei
>   *Tropheryma w.*

whipworm infection
Whispovirus
whistling face syndrome
white
>   w. adipose tissue
>   w. bile
>   w. blood cell (WBC)
>   w. blood cell antibody
>   w. blood cell cast
>   w. blood cell count
>   w. blood cells per high-power field
>   (WBC/hpf)
>   w. cell count (WCC)
>   w. clot syndrome
>   w. corpuscle
>   W. disease
>   w. fat
>   w. fiber
>   w. gangrene
>   w. graft
>   w. infarct
>   w. leg
>   w. matter
>   methylene w.
>   w. muscle
>   w. muscle disease
>   w. of eye
>   w. patch

>   w. phosphorus (WP)
>   w. piedra
>   w. pneumonia
>   w. pulp
>   w. spot
>   w. spot disease
>   w. substance
>   w. substance of Schwann
>   w. thrombus

whitehead
whitepox
whitlow
>   herpes w.
>   herpetic w.
>   melanotic w.

Whitmore
>   W. bacillus
>   W. disease
>   W. fever
>   W. melioidosis

Whitmore-Jewett tumor staging system
whitmori
>   *Bacillus w.*
>   *Malleomyces w.*

Whitten effect
WHO
>   World Health Organization
>   WHO classification of tumors of
>   the lymphoid tissue
>   WHO histologic classification of
>   ovarian tumors

WHO/ISUP
>   World Health Organization/International
>   Society of Urologic Pathologists
>   WHO/ISUP classification

whole
>   w. blood (B, WB)
>   w. blood lysis technique
>   w. complement (WC)
>   w. genome amplification (WGA)
>   w. ragweed extract (WRE)

whole-arm fusion
whole-blood
>   w.-b. clotting time
>   w.-b. folate (WBF)
>   w.-b. hematocrit (WBH)
>   w.-b. mercury level

whole-body titration curve
whole-mount section
whooping
>   w. cough
>   w. cough vaccine

whorl
>   bone w.
>   keratin w.

whorled
>   w. appearance
>   w. mass
>   w. storiform pattern

whorling cell
whorl-like array
Whytt disease
WI-38 cell
Wickerhamia
Wickerhamiella
wickerhamii
    Prototheca w.
Wickersheimer medium
wick fixative
Wickham striae
Widal
    W. reaction
    W. serum test
    W. syndrome
wide
    w. rete peg
    w. spectrum
widefield
    w. capillary microscopy
    w. eyepiece
    w. ocular
wide-spectrum keratin
WiDr human colorectal cancer cell line
width
    hemoglobin distribution w. (HDW)
    platelet distribution w. (PDW)
    red cell diameter w.
    red cell distribution w. (RDW)
    reticulocyte distribution w. (RDWr)
Wiedemann-Beckwith syndrome
WIF
    wnt inhibitory factor
Wilcoxon signed rank statistic
wild
    w. type
    w. yeast
Wilder stain for reticulum
Wildervanck syndrome
wild-type
    w.-t. allele
    w.-t. gene
Wilkie disease
Wilkins-Chilgren agar
Willebrand syndrome
Willemze type A lymphocyte
Williams
    W. factor
    W. stain
    W. syndrome
Williams-Campbell syndrome
williamsi
    Iodamoeba w.
Williamsia maris
Williopsis saturnus
Willis
    W. cord
    W. disease

willisii
    chordae w.
Willowbrook virus
Wilms
    W. tumor
    W. tumor, aniridia, genital anomalies, mental retardation (WAGR)
Wilson
    W. disease (WD)
    W. method
    W. syndrome
wilsonian fulminant hepatitis
Wilson-Mikity syndrome
Winckel disease
wind
    blast w.
    w. contusion
windage
Windelmann granuloma
window
    cochlear w.
    w. frame appearance
    oval w.
    round w.
    vestibular w.
windpipe
Windscheid disease
wing cell
Wingea robertsiae
wingless
    w. gene
    w. signaling pathway in *Drosophila*
Winiwarter-Buerger disease
Winkler disease
winogradskyi
    Algoriphagus w.
winslowii
    stellulae w.
Winslow star
winter
    w. itch
    W. syndrome
winthemi
    Margaropus w.
Winton disease
Wintrobe
    W. and Landsberg method
    W. hematocrit tube
    macromethod of W.
    W. sedimentation rate
    W. sedimentation rate method
wipe
    bullet w.
    decontamination w.
wire-like collagen
wire-loop
    w.-l. abnormality

W

wire-loop (*continued*)
    w.-l. lesion
    w.-l. test
wire-wound resistor
Wirsung
    W. canal
    W. duct
wiry
Wischnewsky spots
Wiskott-Aldrich
    W.-A. syndrome (WAS)
    W.-A. syndrome protein (WASP)
WISP1
    wnt-1-induced secreted protein 1
wispy adhesion
Wistar rat
witflariensis
    Sphingopyxis w.
withering crypt appearance
within normal limits (WNL)
Witkop disease
Witkop-Von Sallmann syndrome
wittichii
    Sphingomonas w.
Wizard
    W. MagneSil PCR cleanup
    W. MagneSil plasmid purification
    W. MagneSil sequencing cleanup
    W. SV 96 plasmid purification
WK
    Wernicke-Korsakoff
WM
    Waldenström macroglobulinemia
WMD
    weapon of mass destruction
    biologic WMD
    chemical WMD
WMR
    work metabolic rate
WNL
    within normal limits
wnt
    wnt inhibitory factor (WIF)
    wnt signaling transduction pathway
wnt9b gene
wnt11 gene
wnt-1-induced secreted protein 1 (WISP1)
W/O
    water in oil
wobble hypothesis
wodanis
    Vibrio w.
woesei
    Conexibacter w.
wohlfahrtia
    W. magnifica
    W. opaca
    W. vigil

wohlfahrtiosis
Wohlfart-Kugelberg-Welander disease
Wohlgemuth unit
Wojnowicia
Wolbachieae
Wolfe breast carcinoma
Wolff-Chaikoff effect
wolffian
    w. cyst
    w. duct
    w. duct carcinoma
    w. rest
Wolff-Parkinson-White (WPW)
    W.-P.-W. syndrome
Wolf-Hirschhorn syndrome
wolfii
    Mortierella w.
Wolfiporia
Wölfler gland
Wolf-Orton body
Wolfram syndrome
Wolfring gland
Wolf syndrome
Wolhynia fever
Wolinella
Wolman
    W. disease
    W. xanthoma
woman
    PMP w.
Wood
    W. glass
    W. lamp
    W. light
woodcutter's encephalitis
Woodsholea maritima
woodworker's lung
Wookey skin flap
woolgathering
woolsorter's
    w. disease (anthrax)
    w. pneumonia
Woringer-Kolopp
    W.-K. disease
    W.-K. pagetoid reticulosis
Workcell
    LH 755 hematology W.
worker
    abattoir w.
working
    w. distance
    W. Formulation for Clinical Usage (WF)
    W. Group on Civilian Biodefense
work metabolic rate (WMR)
workstation
    Biomek 2000, 3000, FX, FX assay, NX laboratory automation w.

Coulter Gen-S Cell hematology w.
Coulter TQ-Prep w.
NanoChip molecular biology w.
PrepPlus series w.
Q-Prep w.
TQ-Prep w.

workup

neonatal cholestasis w.
transplantation w.

world

W. Association of Societies of
Pathology (WASP)
W. Health Organization (WHO)
W. Health Organization/International
Society of Urologic Pathologists
(WHO/ISUP)

worm

w. abscess
Bancroft filarial w.
dragon w.
Eustoma rotundatum parasitic w.
serpent w.
tongue w.

Wormley test
worried well
wort broth
wound

w. aspiration
w. botulism
bullet w.
center-fire rifle w.
close range entrance w.
contact entrance w.
cranial gunshot w.
w. culture
distant range entrance w.
w. elasticity
entrance w.
entry w.
exit w.
w. fever
forensic evaluation of handgun w.
gunshot w.
w. healing
hesitation w.
incised w.
indeterminate range entrance w.
intermediate range entrance w.
lacerated w.
long-range w.
loose contact w.
missile w.
mutilating w.
progressive contraction of w.
shored-exit w.

spiral w. (SW)
stab w.
superficial w.
surgical w.
tight contact w.
zone of antemortem w.

woven bone
WP

weakly positive
white phosphorus

WPW

Wolff-Parkinson-White

WR

weakly reactive

Wr^a antigen
wrap
wratislaviensis

Tsukamurella w.

Wratten filter
Wr^b antigen
WRC

washed red cell

WRE

whole ragweed extract

Wright

W. antigen
W. stain
W. syndrome

Wright-Giemsa

W.-G. stain
W.-G. stained touch imprint

wrinkled

w. nucleus
w. silk appearance

writer's paralysis
WRN

WRN gene
WRN protein

wt

weight

wt1 gene
WT-1 marker
Wu

Folin and W. (FW)

Wuchereria

W. bancrofti
W. malayi
W. pacifica

wuchereriasis
Wurster test
wurstgift (sausage poison)
w/v

weight per volume

Wyeomyia
Wyeth bifurcated needle

W

X
magnification
X chromatin
X chromatin body
X chromosome
X deletion
X karyotype
X zone
xanchromatic
xanthelasma
generalized x.
x. palpebrarum
xanthelasmoidea
xanthelasmoideum
lymphangioma x.
xanthematin
xanthemia
xanthene dye
xanthine oxidase (XO)
xanthinuria, xanthiuria, xanthuria
xanthiuria (*var. of* xanthinuria)
xanthoastrocytoma
pleomorphic x. (PXA)
Xanthobacter
X. *aminoxidans*
X. *viscosus*
xanthochromatic
xanthochromia
xanthochromic
xanthocyte
xanthoderma
xanthoerythrodermia perstans
xanthogranuloma
adult-type x.
juvenile x. (JXG)
necrobiotic x.
xanthogranulomatous
x. bursitis
x. cholecystitis
x. prostatitis
x. pyelonephritis (XPN)
xanthoma
x. cell
x. disseminatum (XD)
fibrous x.
x. generalisata ossium
juvenile x.
x. palpebrarum
x. planum
x. striatum plamare
tuberoeruptive x.
x. tuberosum
x. tuberosum simplex
verrucous x.
Wolman x.

xanthomatosis
biliary x.
cerebrotendinous x.
normal cholesteremic x.
xanthomatous
x. deposition
x. pseudotumor
Xanthomonas
X. *cynarae*
X. *maltophilia*
X. *oryzae*
Xanthophyllomyces
xanthopia (*var. of* xanthopsia)
xanthopsia, xanthopia
xanthopsydracia
xanthopterin
xanthosine monophosphate
xanthosine-5′-phosphate
xanthosis
xanthous
xanthum
Flavobacterium x.
xanthurenic
x. acid
x. aciduria
xanthuria (*var. of* xanthinuria)
xanthylic acid
XAP101 gene
x-axis
XD
xanthoma disseminatum
XDP
xeroderma pigmentosum
¹²⁷Xe
xenon-127
¹³³Xe
xenon-133
Xe
xenon
xenic culture
xenoantigen
xenobiotic
xenocytophilic antibody
xenodiagnosis
xenogeneic graft
xenogenic
xenogenous
xenografted tumor
xenograft tumor
xenology
Xenomeris
xenon (Xe)
xenon-127 (¹²⁷Xe)
xenon-133 (¹³³Xe)
xenon-arc discharge lamp

X

xenoparasite
xenophaga
    Sphingomonas x.
xenopi
    Mycobacterium x.
Xenopsylla
    X. *astia*
    X. *brasiliensis*
    X. *cheopis*
Xenopus
    X. *laevis*
    X. *laevis* test
xenotransplantation
    organ x.
xenotropic virus
xenovorans
    Burkholderia x.
xeransis
xerantic
Xerocomus
xerocytosis
xeroderma pigmentosum (XDP, XP)
xeronosus (*var. of* xerosis)
xerophthalmia
xerosis, xeronosus
    Corynebacterium x.
xerostomia
xerotic
Xerula
Xga blood group system
Xg antigen
xiligouense
    Myceligenerans x.
X-inactivation
xinjiangense
    Flavobacterium x.
    Halorubrum x.
xinjiangensis
    Ensifer x.
    Nocardiopsis x.
    Pseudonocardia x.
xinjisis
    Nesterenkonia x.
xiphoiditis
XLA
    X-linked agammaglobulinemia
    XLA gene
XLD
    xylose-lysine-deoxycholate
    XLD agar
X-linked
    X-l. agammaglobulinemia (XLA)
    X-l. agammaglobulinemia of Bruton
    X-l. character
    X-l. dominant inheritance
    X-l. familial hypophosphatemia
    X-l. gene
    X-l. heredity
    X-l. ichthyosis

X-l. infantile
    hypogammaglobulinemia
X-l. lymphoproliferative (XLP)
X-l. lymphoproliferative disease
X-l. microthrombocytopenia
X-l. recessive disorder
X-l. recessive inheritance
X-l. thrombocytopenia (XLT)
XLP
    X-linked lymphoproliferative
    XLP gene
    XLP syndrome
XLT
    X-linked thrombocytopenia
XM
    crossmatch
XO
    xanthine oxidase
    XO gonadal dysgenesis
    XO karyotype
    XO syndrome
X-Omat AR film
XP
    xeroderma pigmentosum
XPC gene
Xpert
    X. EV assay
    X. EV enterovirus assay
    X. EV meningitis test
    X. EV rapid viral meningitis test
    X. MRSA test
XPII translocation
XPN
    xanthogranulomatous pyelonephritis
X-PO4
    protein X-PO4
x-ray
    x-r. crystallography
    full-body x-r.
    x-r. microscope
    postmortem dental x-r.
XRITC
    tetramethylrhodamine isothiocyanate
x-scanning
    fast x-s.
XU
    excretory urogram
Xu
    x-unit
xuii
    Vibrio x.
x-unit (Xu)
XX
    XX gonadal dysgenesis
    XX karyotype
XXX
    XXX disorder
    XXX karyotype
XXXX disorder

XXXXY disorder
XXXY disorder
XX/XY sex chromosome pattern
XXY
    XXY karyotype
    XXY syndrome
    trisomy XXY
45,X/46,XY mosaicism
XXYY disorder
XY
    XY female
    XY gonadal dysgenesis
    XY karyotype
Xylanibacterium ulmi
xylanilytica
    Cellulomonas x.
xylanilyticus
    Thermobacillus x.
Xylanimicrobium pachnodae
Xylanimonas cellulosilytica
xylanivorans
    Pseudobutyrivibrio x.
xylanovorans
    Clostridium x.
Xylaria
xylene (*var. of* xylol)
xylene-soluble mounting medium
xyli
    Leifsonia x.
    Leifsonia xyli subsp. *x.*

xylidine
    ponceau de x.
xylinus
    Acetobacter x.
xylitol dehydrogenase
Xylogone sphaerospora
Xylohypha
xyloketose
xylol, xylene
    acetone, methylbenzoate, x.
    (AMeX)
    x. artifact
    modified acetone methylbenzoate x.
    (ModAMeX)
    x. wash
xylose
    x. absorption test
    x. concentration
    test
xylose-lysine-deoxycholate
  (XLD)
xylosuria
xylulose
xylulosuria
xysma
XYY karyotype
47,XYY male
X-Y-Z beam scanning method
  coordinates
XYZ syndrome

X

Y
Y body
Y cartilage
Y chromatin
Y chromosome
Yaba
Y. monkey virus
Y. tumor
YAC
yeast artificial chromosome
YAC probe
Yakima
hemoglobin Y.
yamanashiensis
Nocardia y.
yanglingense
Rhizobium y.
Yania halotolerans
yanoikuyae
Sphingobium y.
Sphingomonas y.
yaoundei
Trichophyton y.
Yarrowia
Yatapoxvirus
yatensis
Streptomyces y.
yawing projectile
yaws
crab y.
forest y.
y-axis
Yb
ytterbium
YB1
Y-box binding protein
Y-box binding protein (YB1)
Yb-169 pentetate sodium
years of life saved (YLS)
yeast
y. artificial chromosome (YAC)
baker's y.
dried y.
y. extract agar
y. fungus
imperfect y.
y. peptone dextrose
trypticase soy y. (TSY)
wild y.
yellow
acridine y.
alizarin y.
y. atrophy of liver
y. body

y. bone marrow
brilliant y.
butter y.
y. cartilage
chrome y.
y. corallin
corralin y.
fast y.
y. fat
y. fever
y. fever vaccine
y. fever virus
y. fiber
fuchsin, amido black, and naphthol y. (FAN)
y. hepatization
hydrazine y.
Leipzig y.
martius y.
metaniline y.
methyl y.
y. nail
y. nail syndrome
naphthol y. S
y. phosphorus
y. rain
y. spot (YS)
Sudan y.
Titan y.
yellow-brown wear and tear pigment
yellowish
eosin y.
light green SF y.
yeochonensis
Streptomyces y.
Yersinia
Y. enterocolitica
Y. enterocolitica antibody
Y. enterocolitica subsp. *palearctica*
Y. frederiksenii
Y. intermedia
Y. kristensenii
Y. pestis
Y. pestis antibody
Y. pestis F1 capsular antigen
Y. pseudotuberculosis
Yersinia-related enterocolitis
Yersinieae
yersiniosis
yield
quantum y.
y-intercept
YKL-40

Y-linked
> Y-l. character
> Y-l. gene

YLS
> years of life saved

YNS
> yellow nail syndrome

Yokogawa fluke

yokogawai
> *Metagonimus y.*

yolk
> y. cell
> y. membrane
> y. sac antigen
> y. sac carcinoma
> y. sac tumor

yonseiensis
> *Caldanaerobacter subterraneus*
> subsp. *y.*
> *Thermoanaerobacter y.*

Yorke autolytic reaction

young
> maturity onset diabetes of the y.
> (MODY)
> Y. syndrome

Yperite (mustard gas)

YS
> yellow spot

Y-shaped

YSI 2300 STAT glucose and lactate
analyzer

Yta antigen

ytterbium
(Yb)

yuanmingense
> *Bradyrhizobium y.*

yunnanensis
> *Pseudonocardia y.*
> *Streptomyces y.*

Yvon test

Z

    Z band
    Z disc
    Z filament
    Z line
    Z score

Zahn

    Z. infarct
    Z. line
    lines of Z.
    striae of Z.

Zahorsky disease

Zambesi ulcer

Zamboni

    Z. fluid
    Z. solution

Zambusch

    generalized pustular psoriasis of Z.

ZAP-70 deficiency

Zappert counting chamber

zatmanii

    Methylobacterium z.

Zavarzinia compransoris

z-axis

ZB4 antibody

Z2 Coulter Counter

Z/D

    zero defects

Z-dependent protease inhibitor (ZPI)

ZDV

    zidovudine

ZE

    Zollinger-Ellison

zeae

    Runella z.
    Thermoanaerobacterium z.
    Ustilago z.

zeaxanthinifaciens

zebra body

Zebrina

Zein agar

Zeis gland

zeisian stye

Zeiss

    Z. Axiophot fluorescent microscope
    Z. Axioplan microscope
    Z. Axioskop microscope
    Z. counting cell
    Z. LSM-10 laser microscope
    Z. transmission electron microscope

Zellballen pattern

zellen

    helle z. (pale cells)

Zellweger syndrome

Zenker

    Z. degeneration
    Z. diverticulum
    Z. dysplasia
    Z. fixative
    Z. fluid
    Z. necrosis
    Z. solution

zenkerize

zeolite

zero

    absolute z.
    z. defects (Z/D)
    limes z. (L_0)

zero-order

    z.-o. kinetics
    z.-o. reaction

ZES

    Zollinger-Ellison syndrome

zeta

    z. isoform
    z. potential
    z. sedimentation rate (ZSR)

zetacrit

zidovudine (ZDV)

Ziehen-Oppenheim disease

Ziehl-Neelsen

    Z.-N. carbolfuchsin
    Z.-N. method
    Z.-N. stain

Ziehl stain

Ziemann

    Z. dot
    Z. stippling

Zieve syndrome

ZIG

    zoster immune globulin

zijingensis

    Pseudonocardia z.

Zika

    Z. fever
    Z. virus

Zila

    Z. Pro-Scrub
    Z. Pro-Wash antiseptic hand wash

Zimmermann

    Z. corpuscle
    Z. elementary particle
    Z. granule
    Z. pericyte
    polkissen of Z.
    Z. reaction
    Z. test

Z

Zimmermannella
- Z. *alba*
- Z. *bifida*
- Z. *faecalis*
- Z. *helvola*

zinc
- z. assay
- z. deficiency
- z. finger gene
- z. finger protein
- z. flocculation test
- z. formalin
- z. oxide
- z. phosphide
- z. protoporphyrin (ZPP)
- z. sulfate centrifugal flotation technique
- z. sulfate flotation concentration
- z. sulfate turbidity test

zincalism
zinc-containing endopeptidase
Zinn zonule
Zinsser-Brill disease
Zinsser-Cole-Engman syndrome
ziram
zirconium granuloma
Z-line
Zobellia
- Z. *amurskyensis*
- Z. *galactanivorans*
- Z. *laminariae*
- Z. *russellii*
- Z. *uliginosa*

zobellii
- Idiomarina z.

zoite
Zollinger-Ellison (ZE)
- Z.-E. syndrome (ZE, ZES)
- Z.-E. test
- Z.-E. tumor

zombie cell
zona, *pl.* **zonae**
- z. arcuata
- z. ciliaris
- z. dermatica
- z. epithelioserosa
- z. facialis
- z. fasciculata
- z. glomerulosa
- z. ignea
- z. medullovasculosa
- z. ophthalmica
- z. pectinata
- z. pellucida
- z. perforata
- z. reticularis
- z. serpiginosa
- z. tecta

zonae (*pl. of* zona)
zona-free hamster egg penetration test
zonal
- z. aganglionosis
- z. centrifugation
- z. electrophoresis
- z. necrosis

zonary
zonate
zonation effect
zone
- androgenic z.
- antibody excess z.
- arcuate z.
- basement membrane z.
- centrilobular z.
- ciliary z.
- decontamination z.
- z. electrophoresis
- entry z.
- ependymal z.
- epileptogenic z.
- equivalence z.
- extranodal marginal z.
- fetal z.
- flame intensity z.
- focal z.
- Golgi z.
- grenz z.
- hemorrhoidal z.
- hot z.
- hyperesthetic z.
- mantle z.
- marginal z. (MZ)
- z. necrosis
- z. of antemortem wound
- z. of equivalence
- z. ossification
- Rappaport acinus z. 1
- Rappaport acinus z. 3
- secondary X z.
- subplasmalemmal dense z.
- sudanophobic z.
- support z.
- thymus-dependent z.
- trabecular z.
- transition z. (TZ)
- transitional z.
- vermilion z.
- Weil basal z.
- X z.

zoning
zonula, *pl.* **zonulae**
- z. adherens
- z. ciliaris
- z. occludens

zonulae (*pl. of* zonula)

zonular
 z. fiber
 z. keratitis
 z. space
zonulares
 fibrae z.
zonularia
 spatia z.
zonule
 ciliary z.
 Zinn z.
zooanthroponosis
zooblast
zoofulvin
Zoogloea
zoograft
zoohelcum
 Weeksella z.
zooid
Zoomastigina
Zoomastigophorasida
Zoomastigophorea
zoomylus
Zoon balanitis
zoonosis
 bacterial z.
 enteric helminthic z.
zoonotic
 z. disease
 z. infection
 z. potential
 z. retrovirus
zooparasite
zoophilic
zoophyte
zooprophylaxis
Zooshikella ganghwensis
zoospermia
zootoxin
Zopfia
zopfii
 Prototheca z.
ZO-1 protein
zoster
 z. encephalomyelitis
 herpes z. (HZ)
 z. immune globulin (ZIG)
zosterae
 Desulfovibrio z.
ZPI
 Z-dependent protease inhibitor
 ZPI deficiency
ZPP
 zinc protoporphyrin
Z-protein
Zsigmondy test

ZSR
 zeta sedimentation rate
ZSR method
ZstatFlu
 Z. rapid diagnostic test for influenza A and B
 Z. test kit
Zuberella
zuckergussleber
Zuckerkandl
 Z. body
 Z. organ
Zülch
 monstrocellular sarcoma of Z.
Zurich
 hemoglobin Z.
Zyderm collagen
ZYF gene
Zygoascus
Zygofabospora
Zygohansenula
Zygolipomyces
Zygomycetes
zygomycosis
 rhinocerebral z.
zygonema
Zygopichia
Zygorenospora
Zygorhynchus
Zygosaccharomyces
zygosperm
zygospore
Zygosporium mansonii
zygote
zygotene
zygotoblast
zygotomere
Zygowillia
Zymobacterium
Zymodebaryomyces
zymodeme
zymogen granule
zymogenic cell
zymogram
zymographic analysis
zymography
 gelatin z.
Zymomonas
Zymonema
Zymopichia
zymoplastic substance
zymosan
Zyplast implant
Zythia
Z1, Z2 series Coulter counter

Contents: The Appendices

Anatomical Illustrations

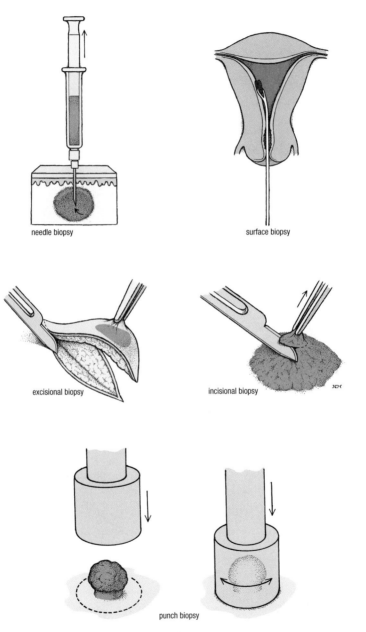

needle biopsy

surface biopsy

excisional biopsy

incisional biopsy

punch biopsy

biopsy techniques

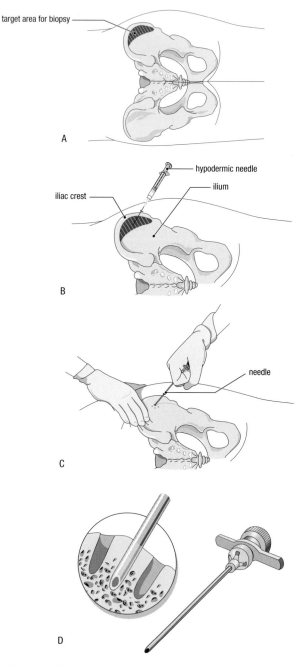

target area for biopsy

A

hypodermic needle

iliac crest

ilium

B

needle

C

D

bone marrow biopsy: (A) posterior view of pelvic region with target area for bone marrow biopsy highlighted; (B) hypodermic needle penetrating skin at an angle to reach the ilium just below the iliac crest; (C) procedure used to obtain a bone marrow sample for biopsy from ilium by aspiration through needle; (D) close-up of aspiration technique and needle used for procedure

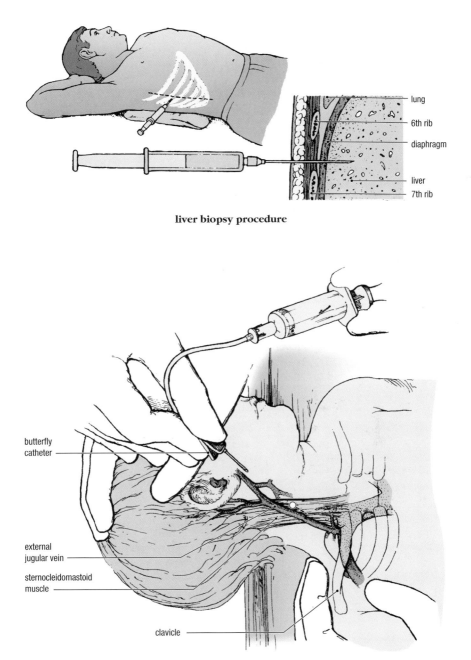

liver biopsy procedure

lung

6th rib

diaphragm

liver

7th rib

butterfly
catheter

external
jugular vein

sternocleidomastoid
muscle

clavicle

technique used in external jugular venipuncture: butterfly catheter is about to be inserted
into external jugular vein of supine infant

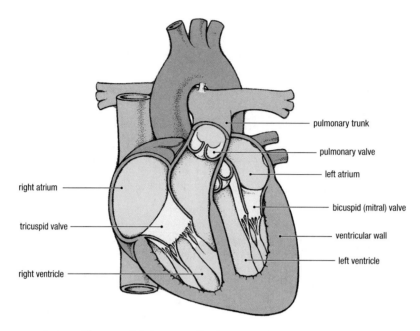

coronal view of heart with left ventricular hypertrophy: notice the thickened ventricular wall

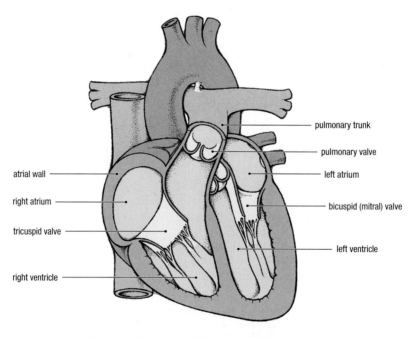

coronal view of heart with right atrial hypertrophy: notice the thickened atrial wall

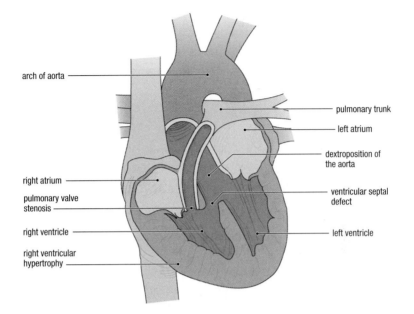

arch of aorta

pulmonary trunk

left atrium

dextroposition of the aorta

right atrium

ventricular septal defect

pulmonary valve stenosis

right ventricle

left ventricle

right ventricular hypertrophy

coronal view of heart in tetralogy of Fallot: characteristics include pulmonary valve stenosis, right ventricular hypertrophy, dextroposition of the aorta, and ventricular septal defect

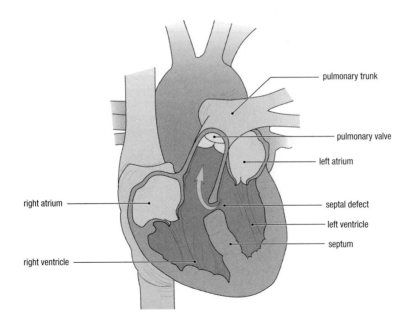

pulmonary trunk

pulmonary valve

left atrium

right atrium

septal defect

left ventricle

septum

right ventricle

coronal view of heart with a congenital ventricular septal defect: oxygenated blood is allowed to travel from the left to right ventricle into the pulmonary trunk

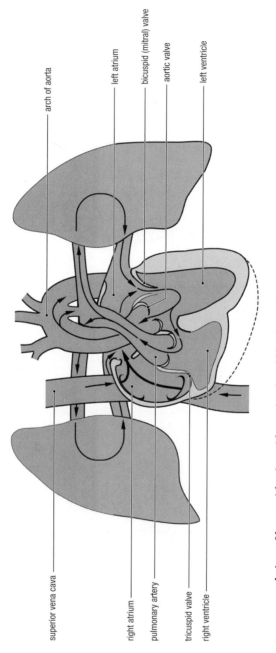

coronal view of heart with tricuspid atresia: altered blood circulation due to a congenital lack of the tricuspid valve depicted

arch of aorta

left atrium

bicuspid (mitral) valve

aortic valve

left ventricle

superior vena cava

right atrium

pulmonary artery

tricuspid valve

right ventricle

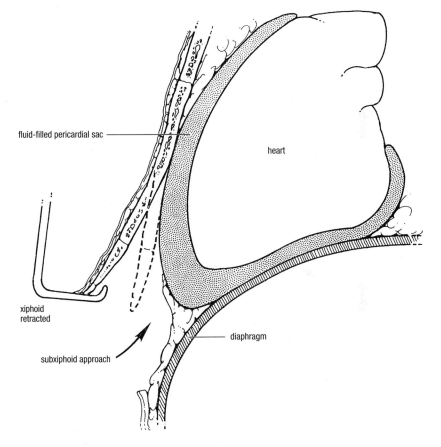

fluid-filled pericardial sac

heart

xiphoid
retracted

subxiphoid approach

diaphragm

cardiac tamponade: midsagittal view showing fluid-filled pericardial sac and subxiphoid
surgical approach

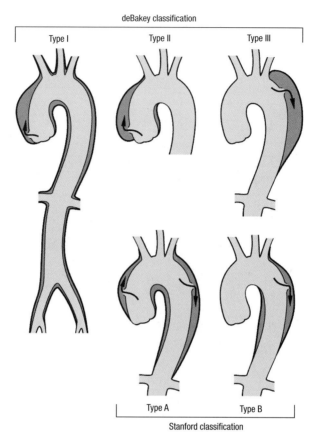

schematic illustration showing types of aneurysms affecting the aorta

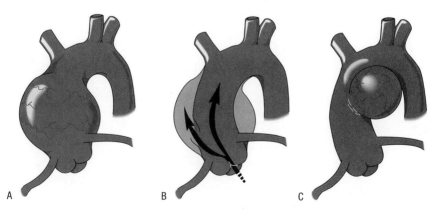

types of aortic aneurysms: (A) ascending aortic aneurysm; (B) aortic aneurysm; (C) aortic dissection

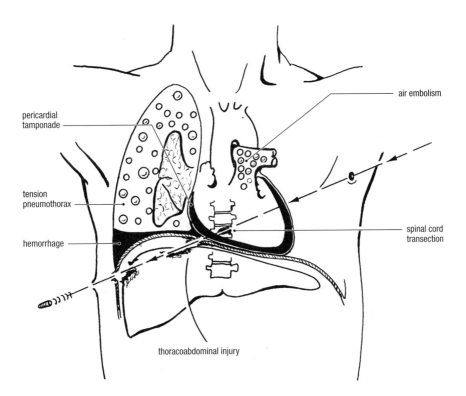

air embolism

pericardial
tamponade

tension
pneumothorax

hemorrhage

spinal cord
transection

thoracoabdominal injury

mechanisms of shock in penetrating thoracic trauma

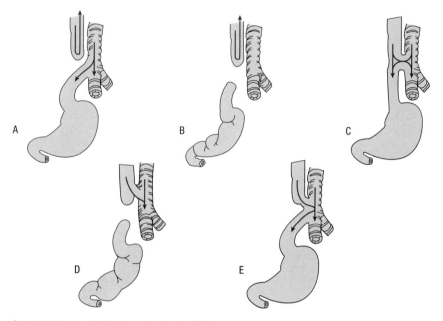

five variations of esophageal atresia: (A) the most common is when the esophagus ends in a blind pouch; (B) both upper and lower segments end in blind pouches; (C) both upper and lower segments communicate with trachea; (D) very rarely, the upper segment ends in a blind pouch and communicates by a fistula to the trachea; (E) fistula connects to both upper and lower segments of the esophagus

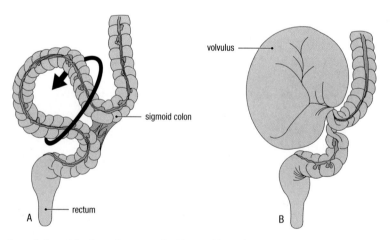

volvulus of sigmoid colon: the unattached loop of bowel twists (left), causing the bowel lumen to become obstructed (right), which leads to the inability of stool to pass and compression of the blood supply to the looped bowel segment

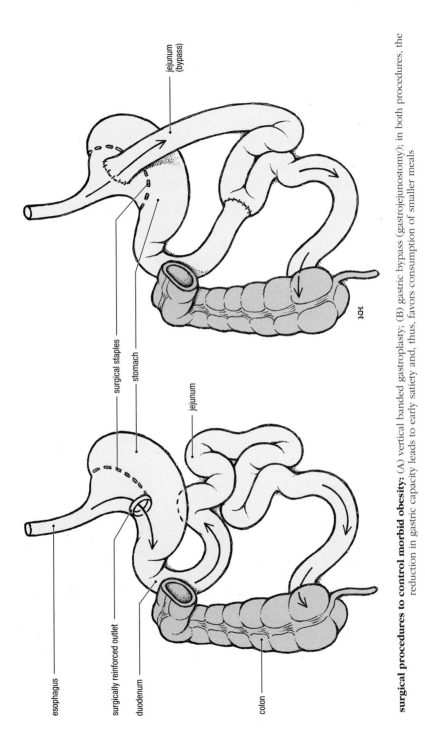

surgical procedures to control morbid obesity: (A) vertical banded gastroplasty; (B) gastric bypass (gastrojejunostomy); in both procedures, the reduction in gastric capacity leads to early satiety and, thus, favors consumption of smaller meals

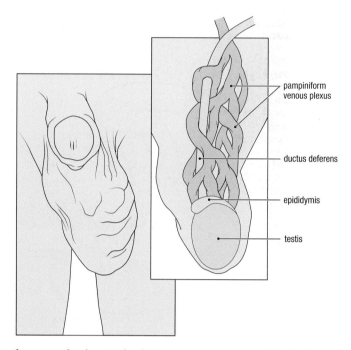

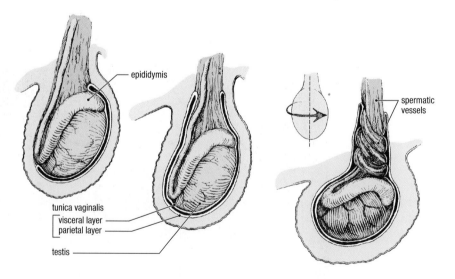

varicocele: image of male genitalia showing anatomical abnormality of left scrotum ("bag of worms" appearance); insert shows internal anatomy of scrotum with abnormal dilation of the cre-master and pampiniform venous plexuses surrounding the spermatic cord

torsion: normal testicular anatomy (left); a bell-clapper deformity in the tunica vaginalis (middle), which can permit torsion of spermatic cord vessels (right)

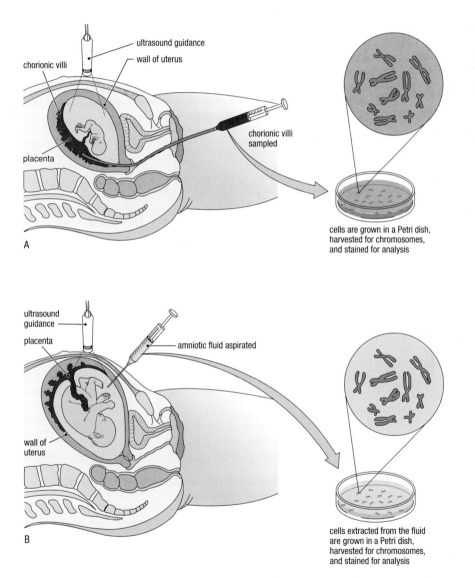

(A) chorionic villus sampling (9 to 11 weeks); (B) amniocentesis (15 to 18 weeks)

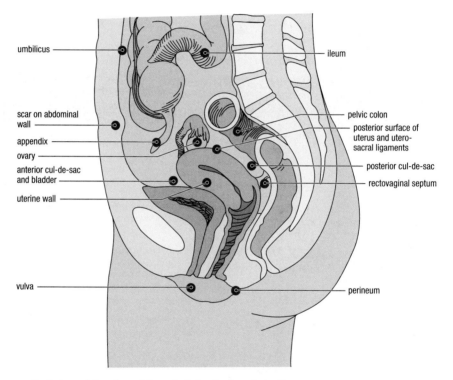

sagittal view of female pelvic and abdominal regions showing common sites (dots) of endometriosis formation)

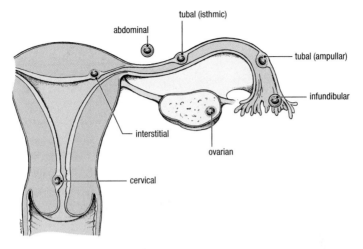

sites of ectopic pregnancy

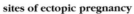

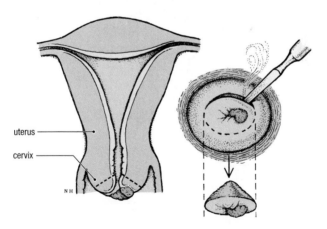

conization: neoplasm shown as darkest area, dashed line shows extent of resection

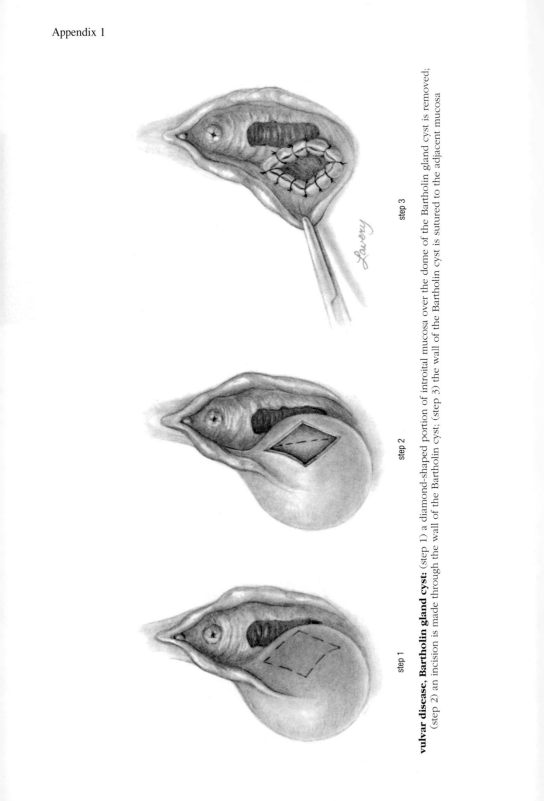

step 1   step 2   step 3

vulvar disease, Bartholin gland cyst: (step 1) a diamond-shaped portion of introital mucosa over the dome of the Bartholin gland cyst is removed; (step 2) an incision is made through the wall of the Bartholin cyst; (step 3) the wall of the Bartholin cyst is sutured to the adjacent mucosa

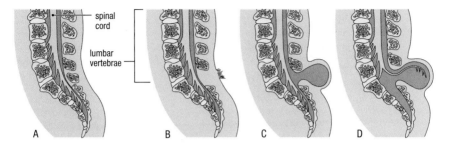

four degrees of spinal cord anomalies: (A) normal spinal cord; (B) spina bifida occulta; (C) meningocele; (D) myelomeningocele

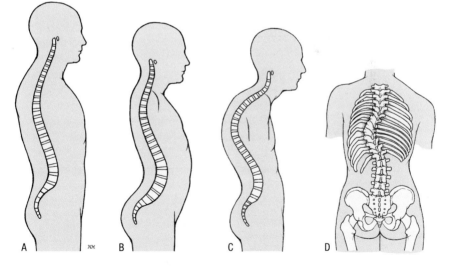

spinal curvatures: (A) normal; (B) lordosis; (C) kyphosis; (D) scoliosis

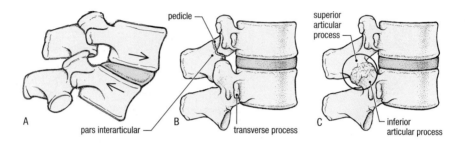

spondylolisthesis: (A) showing forward slippage of lumbar vertebra; spondylolysis: (B) showing fracture of pars interarticularis; spondylosis: (C) showing fixation of the articular processes

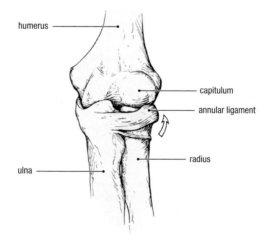

nursemaid's elbow: anatomy of injury to elbow joint; interposition of annular ligament between radial head and capitellum

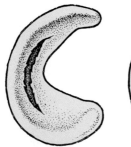
longitudinal tear

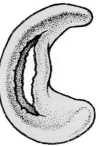
bucket-handle tear

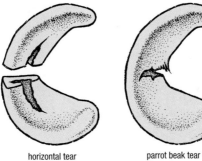
horizontal tear

parrot beak tear

meniscal tears

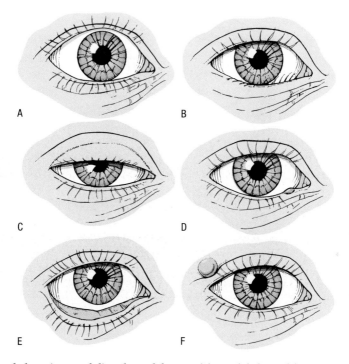

structural alterations and disorders of the eye: (A) exophthalmos; (B) entropion; (C) ptosis; (D) sty; (E) ectropion; (F) chalazion

Culture Media

(von) Apathy gum syrup medium
A1 broth, medium
acetamide nutrient broth
acetate agar
Acetobacter agar
acid broth
acriflavine-ceftazidime agar
actinomycete isolation agar
Aeromonas isolation agar base
agar No.1 bacteriological
agar No.2 bacteriological
agarose gel
algae culture agar, broth
Amies transport medium
Amies with charcoal
Amies without charcoal
AmnioMAX C-100 basal medium
anaerobe identification medium base
anaerobic agar, brewer's
anaerobic blood agar
anaerobic blood agar according to CDC
anaerobic egg agar base
antibiotic agar, broth
antibiotic broth
antibiotic medium 1 (See Penassay seed agar)
antibiotic medium 11 (See neomycin assay agar)
antibiotic medium 2 (See Penassay base agar)
antibiotic medium 3 (See Penassay broth)
antibiotic medium 5 (See streptomycin assay agar)
APT (all purpose Tween) agar
ascitic agar
aseptic commissioning broth
asparagine proline broth
Aspergillus differentiation agar base
ASS (antibiotic sulfonamide sensitivity) test agar

azide blood agar base
azide dextrose broth
azide glucose broth
Azotobacter agar glucose
Azotobacter agar mannitol

B12 assay broth USP
Bacillus cereus agar
Bacillus cereus egg yolk polymyxin agar base
Bacillus cereus selective agar
Bacillus medium
bacteriological peptone
Baird Parker agar, base, medium
Balamuth culture medium
Barnes agar
BBE (*Bacteroides* bile esculin) agar
BCYE (buffered charcoal yeast extract) agar
BDG (buffered deoxycholate glucose) broth
BDG (buffered deoxycholate glucose) broth, Hajna
beef extract dehydrated
beef heart infusion lactose agar
beef lactose agar
beta *Streptococcus* agar
BG (brilliant green)
BG (brilliant green) sulfa agar
BHI (brain-heart infusion) agar, broth
BHIS (brain heart infusion with fetal calf serum) broth
BiGGY (bismuth glycine glucose yeast) agar (See Nickerson agar)
bile broth
bile esculin agar
bile salt agar
bile salts brilliant green starch agar
biotin assay medium
biphasic broth medium

birdseed (*Guizotia abysinnica*) agar

BISC (bismuth iron sulfite cycloserine) medium

bismuth sulfite agar

bismuth sulphate sugar base A, base B

blood agar base

blood culture broth, medium

Boeck-Drbohlav-Locke egg-serum medium

Bordet-Gengou medium

Bordet-Gengou potato blood agar

boric acid broth

BPL (brilliant green, phenol red, lactose) agar according to Kauffmann

BPLS (brilliant green, phenol red, lactose, sucrose) agar

brain heart agar (See brain heart infusion agar)

Brazier CCEY (cefoxitin-cycloserine egg yolk) agar

Brettanomyces selective broth

brewer's anaerobic agar

BRILA (brilliant green bile lactose) broth

BRILA MUG (brilliant green bile, lactose, 4-methylumbelliferyl-B-D-glucuronide) broth

brilliant green 2%-bile broth

brilliant green agar modified

brilliant green agar with phosphates

brilliant green bile salt agar

BROLAC (bromothymol-blue, lactose) agar

BROLACIN (bromothymol-blue, lactose, cystine) agar

BROLACIN MUG(bromothymol-blue, lactose, cystine 4-methylumbelliferyl-B-D-glucuronide) agar

bromcresol purple lactose agar

bromocresol purple azide broth

Brucella agar

Brucella sheep blood agar

BSM (*Bifidus* selective medium) agar, broth, supplement

buffalo green monkey cells

buffered *Listeria* broth

buffered peptone water

buffered yeast agar (See yeast agar, buffered)

calcium caseinate agar

Campylobacter agar, broth

Campylobacter blood-free medium

Campylobacter selective agar according to Karmali (See Karmali *Campylobacter* agar)

Campylobacter selective supplement

CAN (colistin-nalidixic acid) agar

Candida Ident agar

carbohydrate broth

Cary Blair medium

casein agar

casein peptone lecithin polysorbate broth

casein peptone soybean flour peptone agar (See CASO agar or tryptic soy agar)

casein peptone soybean flour peptone broth (See CASO broth or tryptic soy broth)

casein soya broth (See tryptic soy broth or CASO broth)

casein-peptone dextrose yeast agar (See plate count agar)

casein-peptone dextrose yeast MUG(4-methylumbelliferyl-B-D-glucuronide) agar (See plate count MUG agar)

Casman broth

CASO (casein soy), salt broth (See tryptic soy salt broth)

CATC (citrate azide Tween carbonate) agar

cation-adjusted Mueller-Hinton broth

CB (chocolate blood) agar

CDC (Centers for Disease Control) anaerobic blood agar
CE (*Campylobacter* enrichment) broth
cetrimide agar
Chang complete medium
Chapman agar (*Staphylococcus* agar)
China Blue lactose agar
chlortetracycline selective supplement
chopped meat broth, medium
Christensen urea agar
CIN (cefsulodin-Irgasan-novobiocin) agar (See *Yersinia* agar)
citrate agar
citrate utilization test (See Simmons citrate agar)
citrate-citric acid buffer
clearing medium
CLED (cystine, lactose, electrolyte deficient) agar
CLED MUG (cystine, lactose, electrolyte deficient, 4-methylumbelliferyl-B-D-glucuronide) agar (See BROLACIN MUG agar)
clostridial differential broth
clostridial nutrient medium
Clostridium difficile agar base
Clostridium difficile supplement
coliform PA (presence absence) broth
Columbia agar base
Columbia blood agar
Columbia calcium nutrient agar
Columbia horse blood CAN (colistin-nalidixic acid) agar
Columbia medium
cooked meat broth, medium
cornmeal agar
Corynebacterium selective agar
CPC (cellobiose, polymyxin, colistin) agar, base
CPC (cellobiose, polymyxin, colistin) selective supplement
Cryo-Gel embedding medium

CTA (cystine trypticase agar)
culture medium
CVS (chorionic villi) medium
cycloserine-cefoxitin-fructose agar
Czapek solution agar
Czapek-Dox agar, medium

DCA (deoxycholate citrate agar)
DCA (deoxycholate citrate agar) Hynes modification
DCA (deoxycholate citrate agar) Leifson (See Leifson agar)
DCLS (deoxycholate, citrate, lactose, sucrose) agar
decarboxylase broth
deep agar
deoxycholate, desoxycholate agar
deoxycholate lactose agar
DEV Endo agar
DEV gelatin agar
DEV glucose broth
DEV glutamate broth
DEV lactose broth
DEV lactose peptone broth
DEV nutrient agar
DEV nutrient gelatin
DEV tryptophan broth
dextrose agar, broth
dextrose casein peptone agar
dextrose tryptone agar
DHL (deoxycholate hydrogen sulfide lactose) agar
DIASSALM (diagnostic semisolid *Salmonella*) agar
differential agar
differential medium
dispersive medium
DNase (deoxyribonuclease) agar, test agar
DRBC (dichloran rose bengal) agar
DRCM (See clostridial differential broth)
Drigalski LL (litmus lactose) agar

DTM (dermatophyte test medium)
DTM (dermatophyte test medium) agar
Duncan Strong broth, modified

Eagle basal medium
Easter and Gibson preenrichment broth
Easter and Gibson *Salmonella* medium
EC (*Escherichia coli*) broth, medium
ECD (*Escherichia coli* direct) agar
ECD MUG (*Escherichia coli* direct,
    4-methylumbelliferyl-B-D-
    glucuronide) agar
EE (Enterobacteriaceae enrichment)
    broth (See Mossel broth)
egg yolk agar
egg yolk emulsion
egg yolk tellurite emulsion
Eijkman lactose broth
Elliker broth
Ellinghausen-McCullough/Johnson-
    Harris medium
EMB (eosin methylene blue) agar, base
EMEM (Eagle minimum essential
    medium)
Emmon modification of Sabouraud
    dextrose agar
Endo agar, medium
enriched medium
enrichment medium
Enterococcus selective agar
Escherichia coli MUG
    (4-methylumbelliferyl-B-D-
    glucuronide) agar
EVA (ethyl violet azide) broth

FAA (fastidious anaerobe agar)
FAB (fastidious anaerobe broth)
Farrant medium
FIL-IDF (Fédération Internationale de
    Laiterie, International Dairy
    Federation)
FDA (Federal Drug Administration)
fluid Sabouraud medium
fluid thioglycolate medium, USP

fluorescence agar
folic acid assay medium
formate ricinoleate broth
Fraser broth
Fraser broth base
FTM (fluid thioglycolate medium)

Gassner agar
GC (gonococcus) agar base
gelatin phosphate buffer
gelatin phosphate salt agar
germ count agar for foodstuffs
germ count agar sugar-free
    FIL-IDF
Giolitti Cantoni broth
glucose azide broth
glucose broth
glucose casein-peptone agar
glucose salt Teepol broth
glucose-format broth
glycerin broth
glycerin-potato broth
glycerol gelatin medium
GN (gram-negative) broth
GN (gram-negative) broth Hajna
GN (gram-negative) enrichment broth
GPS (gelatin phosphate salt) agar
GSP (glutamate starch phenol red)
    agar

Haemophilus medium
Halobacterium agar
Ham F-10 complete medium
Hanahan broth (See SOB broth)
HAT (hypoxanthine, aminopterin, and
    thymidine) medium
HBT (human blood Tween) agar
heart infusion agar
Hektoen enteric agar
Helicobacter pylori agar base
hippurate broth
HITES (hydrocortisone, insulin,
    transferrin, estradiol, and selenium)
    medium

Hoyle medium, base

IMA (inhibitory mold agar)
indole-nitrate broth
inositol gelatin medium
iron broth
iron sulfite agar (See sulfite iron
  agar)

KAA (kanamycin aesculin azide) agar,
  broth
kanamycin agar for *Streptococcus*
kanamycin broth
Kaper agar
Karmali *Campylobacter* agar, base
KIA (Kligler iron agar)
King agar A, B
Kirchner TB (tuberculosis) medium
Koser citrate broth
KRANEP (potassium thiocyanate,
  actidione, sodium azide,egg-yolk,
  pyruvate) agar
Kundrat agar
KVLBA (kanamycin,vancomycin.laked
  blood agar)

Lactobacillus agar according to DeMan,
  Rogosa and Sharpe (See MRS agar)
Lactobacillus broth (See Elliker broth)
Lactobacillus broth according to
  DeMan, Rogosa and Sharpe (See
  MRS broth)
Lactobacillus bulgaricus agar, base
Lactobacillus selective agar (See
  Rogosa agar)
lactose broth
lactose fuchsin sulfite agar (See DEV
  Endo agar)
lactose gelatin broth
Lambda medium
Lash casein hydrolysate-serum medium
lauryl casein peptone broth (See lauryl
  sulfate broth)
lauryl sulfate broth

lauryl tryptose broth
LB (laked blood) agar, broth
LB (Luria Bertani) agar
LB top (Luria Bertani) agar
LDS (lysine decarboxylase sulfhydrase)
  test medium according to Costin
LE broth (*Listeria* enrichment)
LE/FDA broth (*Listeria* enrichment
  according to FDA/IDF-FIL)
lead broth
LEB (*Listeria* enrichment broth)
  according to FDA/IDF-FIL
Leifson agar (See DCA Leifson)
Letheen agar
Letheen agar base modified
Levine EMB (eosin methylene blue)
  agar
Lim broth
lipase-salt-mannitol agar
liquid Baird-Parker medium
Listeria broth
Listeria identification agar, PALCAM
  (See PALCAM *Listeria* selective
  agar)
Listeria identification broth, PALCAM
  (See L-PALCAM *Listeria* selective
  enrichment broth)
Listeria medium
Listeria Oxford medium (See Oxford
  agar)
Listeria selective agar
Listeria selective agar, Oxford (See
  Oxford agar)
Listeria selective enrichment
  supplement according to FDA
Listeria selective enrichment
  supplement according to IDF/FIL
litmus milk
liver broth
liver broth, starch
LL (lactose litmus) broth
LL (litmus lactose) agar according to
  Drigalski
Loeffler, Löffler agar

Culture Media

Loeffler, Löffler blood culture medium
Loeffler, Löffler coagulated serum
  medium
Loeffler, Löffler serum medium
Lowenstein-Jensen medium
L-PALCAM (*Listeria* polymixin,
  acriflavine, lithium chloride,
  ceftazidine, aesculin, mannitol)
  selective enrichment broth
LPM (lithium chloride phenyl ethanol
  moxalactam) plating agar
LS (*Lactobacillus Streptococcus*)
  differential agar
LST (lauryl sulfate tryptose)
LST-MUG (lauryl sulfate tryptose
  4-methylumbelliferyl-B-D-
  glucuronide) broth
lysine arginine iron agar
lysine decarboxylase salt broth
lysine-iron agar

M (membrane filter) azide broth
M (membrane filter) broth
M (membrane filter) *Enterococcus* agar
M (membrane filter) *Enterococcus* agar,
  modified
M (membrane filter) standard methods
  broth
M 17 agar, broth
M BCG (membrane filter bromcresol
  green) yeast and mold broth
M Endo (membrane filter Endo) broth
MacConkey agar
MacConkey agar No. 3
MacConkey agar, sorbitol
MacConkey agar, with salt
MacConkey agar, without salt
MacConkey broth
MacConkey broth purple
MacConkey sorbitol agar
magnesium chloride malachite green
  broth (See RVS broth, modified)
malachite green broth
malonate phenylalanine broth

malt agar
malt extract agar, broth, powder
mammalian cells
mannitol salt agar
mannitol salt phenol red agar
mannitol, lysine, crystal violet,
  brilliant
mannitol-egg yolk-Polymyxin agar (See
  c*ereus* selective agar)
Martin broth
Martin-Lester agar, medium
maximal recovery diluent
McBride agar
McClung Toabe agar base
McCoy cells
m-CP (membrane filter *Clostridium
  perfringens*) agar base
meat liver agar
MEM alpha (minimum essential
  medium with alpha modification)
membrane filter rinse fluid, USP
M-HD (membrane filter Hajna Damon)
  Endo broth with brilliant green
MF (membrane filter) Endo broth
m-FC (membrane focal coli) broth with
  rosolic acid
M-H (Mueller-Hinton) agar, broth
M-Hajna Damon Endo broth with
  brilliant green
M-HD (membrane filter Hajna Damon)
  Endo broth
Middlebrook agar, broth, medium
milk agar
milk agar with cetrimide
milk agar, modified according to Brown
  & Scott
milk plate count agar
mineral modified glutamate broth, base,
  medium
Mitchison medium
MLS (membrane lauryl sulfate) broth
modified Holt-Harris & Teague medium
modified NYC (New York city) medium
modified Stuart medium

modified Thayer-Martin agar
modified Tinsdale agar
modified TSB for E. coli 0157
Mossel broth
motility medium
motility nitrate agar
MOX (magnesium oxalate) agar
MRS (deMan, Rogosa, Sharpe) agar,
  broth
MR-VP (methyl red and Voges-
  Proskauer) broth, medium
MSA (mannitol salt agar)
MSRV (modified semisold
  Rappaport-Vassiliadis) medium
Mucate broth
Mueller-Hinton agar, broth
Mueller-Kauffman tetra broth
MUG (4-methylumbelliferyl-B-D-
  glucuronide) agar
MUG (4-methylumbelliferyl-B-D-
  glucuronide) tryptone soya agar
MY (malt extract yeast extract) glucose
  agar
mycobiotic agar

neomycin assay agar
Neussel-Linzenmeier agar
niacin assay medium
Nickerson BiGGY agar (See BiGGY
  agar)
NIH (National Institutes of Health)
  thioglycolate broth
nitrate agar, broth
nonselective medium
Novy- McNeal-Nicolle medium
Nu Sens agar
nutrient agar
nutrient agar for oxidase
nutrient agar with NaCl
nutrient broth
nutrient broth E
nutrient broth No 2
nutrient broth without NaCl
nutrient gelatin

nutrient medium
oatmeal-tomato paste agar

OF (oxidation fermentation) medium
OF (oxidation fermentation) basal
  medium
OF (oxidation fermentation) test
  nutrient agar
OGY (oxytetracycline glucose yeast)
  agar
OGYE (oxytetracycline, glucose, yeast
  extract) agar base
ÖNÖZ agar (*Salmonella* agar according
  to Önöz)
OPSP (oleandomycin, polymyxin,
  sulfadiazine *perfringens*) medium
orange serum agar, broth
Oxford agar base
Oxford *Listeria* selective agar
oxidative-fermentative-polymixin
  B-bacitracin-lactose agar

PA (presence absence) broth
Pai agar
PALCAM (polymixin, acriflavine,
  lithium chloride, ceftazidine,
  aesculin, mannitol) agar base
PALCAM (polymixin, acriflavine,
  lithium chloride, ceftazidine,
  aesculin, mannitol) *Listeria* selective
  supplement according to Van Netten
  et al.
pantothenate medium USP
Parietti broth
Park and Sanders enrichment broth
  (base)
Park and Sanders selective supplement
  I, II
passive medium
PBW (peptone water,
  phosphate-buffered)
PC (*Pseudomonas cepacia*) agar
PEA (phenylethyl alcohol) agar
PEA (phenylethyl alcohol) blood agar

Penassay base agar, broth
Penassay base agar, Grove and Randall antibiotic agar
Penassay broth, Grove and Randall antibiotic broth
Penassay seed agar
peptone proteose (See proteose-peptone)
peptone sorbitol bile broth
peptone water (See tryptone water)
peptone water tryptic digest (See tryptone water)
peptone water, phosphate-buffered
peptone yeast dextrose agar, broth (See YPD agar, broth)
peptone yeast extract agar (See YEPD agar)
peptone yeast extract iron citrate agar
peptonized milk agar
perfringens agar base (See OPSP)
perfringens selective agar according to Angelotti (See SPS agar)
perfringens supplement I, II
Petragnani medium
Pfeiffer blood agar
phenethyl alcohol agar
phenol red broth base
phenylalanine agar
phosphate gelatin buffer (See gelatin phosphate buffer)
Pike streptococcal broth
plant tissue culture media
plate count agar
plate count agar APHA
plate count agar with antibiotic free skim milk (See plate count skim milk agar)
plate count agar, special
plate count MUG (4-methylumbelliferyl-B-D-glucuronide) agar
plate count skim milk agar
PM (penicillin in milk) indicator agar
polysorbate 80 medium

potassium chlorate supplement
potassium tellurite solution
potassium thiocyanate actidione sodium azide egg-yolk pyruvate agar (See KRANEP agar)
potato dextrose (glucose) agar
potato flakes agar
potato glucose rose bengal agar, base
potato glucose sucrose agar
preenrichment broth
Preuss broth
Pril mannitol agar
Propionibacteria growth supplement
proteose-peptone
PRYES (pentachloro rose bengal yeast extract) agar
Pseudomonas agar (King agar B)
Pseudomonas agar base
Pseudomonas agar F
Pseudomonas agar F base
Pseudomonas agar P
Pseudomonas agar P base
Pseudomonas and *Aeromonas* selective agar according to Kielwein (See GSP agar)
Pseudomonas asparagine broth
Pseudomonas isolation agar
Pseudomonas selective agar base (See cetrimide agar)
purple carbohydrate fermentation broth (See bromocresol purple azide broth)

rabbit blood agar
Raka Ray broth
Rambach equivalent agar (See *Salmonella* Chromogen agar)
RBC (rose bengal chloramphenicol) agar, base
RC agar (*Clostridium* agar)
RCA (reinforced Clostridial agar)
RCM (reinforced clostridial medium) (See clostridial nutrient medium)
REA (rice extract agar)

Rees culture medium
refracting medium
Regan-Lowe charcoal agar
Regan-Lowe transport medium
rice-Tween agar
Rogosa agar
Rogosa agar, modified
Rogosa SL agar
Rosenow veal-brain broth
Roswell Park Memorial Institute
   medium
RVS (Rappaport Vassiliadis) broth,
   medium
RVS (Rappaport Vassiliadis) broth,
   modified
RVS (Rappaport Vassiliadis) enrichment
   broth
RVS (Rappaport Vassiliadis) semisolid
   medium

Sabhi agar, medium
Sabouraud 2% dextrose (glucose) agar
Sabouraud 4% dextrose (glucose)
   agar
Sabouraud agar modified
Sabouraud dextrose broth
Sabouraud glucose agar modified (See
   Sabouraud 2% glucose agar)
Sabouraud liquid medium USP
Sabouraud maltose agar, broth
Saccharomyces medium
salicin broth
Salmonella agar according to Önöz
Salmonella chromogen agar
Salmonella enrichment broth according
   to Rappaport and Vassiliadis (See
   RVS broth, modified)
salt meat broth
SBM (selenite brilliant green mannitol)
   enrichment broth
Schaedler blood agar
Schaedler medium
Schleifer-Kramer agar
SDA (Sabouraud dextrose agar)

selective agar for pathogenic fungi
selective blood agar
selective medium
selenite broth base
selenite cystine broth
selenite enrichment broth
sensitivity test agar
separating medium
serum agar, broth
SFP (sugar-free penicillin) agar
Shapton agar
sheep blood agar
Simmons citrate agar
single step *Staphylococcus* selective
   agar (4S medium)
skim milk agar
Slanetz and Bartley agar (See
   Enterococcus selective agar)
sodium biselenite
sodium chloride (6.5%) culture
   medium
sorbic acid agar, base
sorbitol-MacConkey agar
soy agar, broth
soybean casein digest agar (See CASO
   agar or tryptic soy agar)
soybean casein digest broth (See CASO
   broth or tryptic soy broth)
soybean casein digest MUG agar (See
   CASO MUG agar)
soybean casein digest salt broth (See
   tryptic soy salt broth)
SP4 medium
Spirolate broth
SPS (sulfite polymyxin sulfadiazine)
   agar, modified
SS (*Salmonella Shigella*) agar
standard II nutrient agar
standard methods agar (See plate count
   agar)
Staphylococcus agar, medium
Staphylococcus enrichment broth
   according to Giolitti and Cantoni (See
   Giolitti Cantoni broth)

Staphylococcus selective agar (See
    Baird Parker agar)
sterility test broth
Streptococcus agalactiae selective agar
    (See TKT agar)
Streptococcus selective agar
Streptococcus thermophilus isolation
    agar
Streptomyces medium
Streptomycin assay agar
Stuart broth
Stuart Ringertz agar
Stuart transport medium
sucrose broth
sucrose-phosphate-glutamate transport
    medium
sugar broth
sugar-free agar
sulfate reducing broth
sulfite iron agar
Superbroth agar
supplemented anaerobic blood agar
support medium
synthetic medium old tuberculin
    trichloroacetic acid (precipitated)

Tartoff-Hobbs broth, modified (See
    terrific broth, modified)
TAT broth base
TB (tetrathionate broth)
TB (tetrathionate broth) agar
TBG (tetrathionate, brilliant green, bile)
    enrichment broth
TBX (tryptone bile X-glucuronide) agar
TCBS (thiosulfate citrate bile salts
    sucrose) *cholerae* medium
TCBS (thiosulfate citrate bile sucrose)
    agar
tellurite glycine agar, base, medium
Tergitol-7 agar
terrific broth, modified (See Tartoff-
    Hobbs broth)
test agar for the residue test according to
    Kundrat (See Kundrat agar)

tetrathionate crystal violet enrichment
    broth according to Preuss (See Preuss
    broth)
tetrathionate enrichment broth
    according to Muller-Kauffmann
TG (thioglycolate) broth, medium
TG (thioglycolate) broth with
    Resazurine
TG (thioglycolate)-135C broth
Thermoacidurans agar
Ticarcillin supplement
tissue culture medium
TKT (thallium sulfate, crystal violet, B
    toxin blood) agar
TM (Thayer-Martin) agar, medium
TMAO (trimethylamine N-oxide) agar
Tobie, von Brand, and Mehlman
    diphasic medium
Todd-Hewitt agar, broth
tomato juice agar, broth
TPB (tryptone phosphate broth)
TPEY (tellurite polymyxin egg yolk)
    agar, base
transport medium
transport medium according to Stuart,
    modified by Ringertz (See Stuart
    Ringertz agar)
tributyrin agar
tryptic soy agar (See CASO agar)
tryptic soy broth (See CASO
    broth)
tryptic soy lecithin polysorbate broth
    (See casein peptone lecithin
    polysorbate broth)
tryptic soy MUG (4-methylumbelliferyl-
    B-D-glucuronide) agar (See CASO
    MUG agar)
tryptic soy salt broth
tryptic soy yeast extract broth
trypticase soy agar
trypticase soy with agar broth
tryptone agar
tryptone bile agar
tryptone bile glucuronide agar

tryptone glucose yeast extract agar (See plate count agar)

tryptone medium

tryptone phosphate water (See peptone water, phosphate-buffered)

tryptone soy agar USP

tryptone soy broth USP

tryptone soya agar (See tryptic soy agar or CASO agar)

tryptone soya broth (See tryptic soy broth or CASO broth)

tryptone soya lecithin polysorbate broth (See casein peptone lecithin polysorbate broth)

tryptone soya MUG (4-methylumbelliferyl-B-D-glucuronide) agar (See CASO MUG agar)

tryptone soya salt agar with magnesium sulfate

tryptone soya salt broth (See tryptic soy salt broth)

tryptone water (See also peptone water)

tryptone yeast extract agar

tryptose agar, broth

tryptose blood agar base

TSA (tryptic soy agar) (See CASO agar

TSA tryptic soy agar) blood agar base

TSAMS (See tryptone soya salt agar with magnesium sulfate)

TSB (trypticase soy broth)

TSC (tryptose sulfite cycloserine) agar (See *perfringens* agar)

TSI (triple sugar iron) agar

TT (tetrathionate) broth, base, enrichment broth

TTC (triphenyltetrazolium chloride) solution

TYC (trypticase, yeast extract, cystine) medium

Tyrobutyricum broth (base)

UB (universal beer) agar

urea agar base according to Christensen (See Christensen urea agar)

urea agar, base, broth

urea test agar (See Christensen urea agar)

urease test broth

USP (United States Pharmacopeia)

UVM (University of Vermont) broth base

UVM (University of Vermont) *Listeria* broth, medium

UVM (University of Vermont) *Listeria* selective enrichment broth, modified

V-8 agar for lactobacilli (See tomato juice agar, broth)

vaginalis agar

Vibrio selective agar (See TCBS agar)

vitamin B12 assay broth base, medium

vitamin biotin assay broth

vitamin folic acid assay broth base

vitamin nicotinic acid assay broth

vitamin pantothenic acid assay broth

VJ agar (Vogel-Johnson) agar

VP (Voges Proskauer) broth, modified

VP (Voges-Proskauer) broth

VPSA (*Vibrio parahaemolyticus* sucrose agar)

VRB (violet red bile) agar

VRB MUG (violet red bile 4-methylumbelliferyl-B-D-glucuronide) agar

VRBD (violet red bile dextrose) agar

VRBG (violet red bile glucose) agar

Wadsworth *Brucella* blood agar

Wagatsuma agar

water agar

water blue metachrome-yellow lactose agar according to Gassner (See Gassner agar)

Weinman medium

Wesley broth

West-Wilkins medium

wheat broth
Wilkins-Chalgren agar, broth
Wilson Blair selective media (See
   bismuth sulfite agar)
WL (Wallerstein Laboratory)
   differential agar
WL (Wallerstein Laboratory) nutrient
   agar, medium
wort agar, broth

XLD (xylose-lysine-deoxycholate) agar

yeast agar, buffered
yeast and mold broth
yeast carbon base
yeast extract agar
yeast extract powder

yeast nitrogen base
yeast nitrogen base without amino
   acids
yeast nitrogen base without amino acids
   and ammonium sulfate
YEPD (yeast extract peptone dextrose)
   agar, broth (See YPD)
YER (yeast extract rose bengal) broth,
   base
Yersinia enrichment broth base
Yersinia isolation agar
Yersinia selective agar (See CIN)
YGC (yeast extract glucose
   chloramphenicol) agar
YM (yeast malt) agar, broth
YPD (yeast peptone dextrose) agar,
   broth (See YEPD)

Stains, Dyes, and Fixatives

Abbott stain
aceto-orcein stain
acetic-lacmoid stain
Achúcarro stain
acid blue 45
acid dye
acid fuchsin stain
acid green 25
acid phosphatase stain
acid phosphatase stain with tartrate
acid phosphatase stain without tartrate
acid red 87
acid red 91
acid stain
acid-methenamine-silver stain
acid-Schiff stain
acridine dye
acridine orange stain
acridine yellow
acriflavine HCl
acriflavine neutral
acriflavine stain
ACS (amino-cupric-silver)
AFB (acid fast bacillus) stain
Ag-AS (silver-ammoniacal silver) stain
Albert diphtheria stain
Albert stain No. 1
Alcian blue 8GX
Alcian blue stain
Alcian yellow stain
alizarin
alizarin cyanin
alizarin cyanin BBS stain
alizarin purpurin
alizarin red
alizarin red S
alizarin red stain
alizarin yellow
alizarin yellow R
alizarin yellow R sodium salt
alkaline phosphatase stain

alkaline toluidine blue O
alpha-naphthyl esterase stain with or
    without fluoride
Altmann aniline-acid fuchsin stain
alum carmine
Alzheimer stain
amaranth
amethyst violet
amido black 10B stain
amidonaphthol red
aminoanthraquinone dye
3-amino-9-ethylcarbazole stain
ammonium oxalate crystal violet
ammonium silver carbonate stain
amphoteric dye
aniline blue
aniline blue modified trichrome stain
aniline blue water soluble
aniline gentian violet
aniline xylene
anionic dye
anthracene blue
antimony stain
Archibald stain
argentaffin stain
argyrophil stain
arsenic stain
auramine O fluorescent stain
auramine-rhodamine stain
azan stain
azocarmine B stain
azovan blue
azure I, II
azure A, B, C stain
azure-eosin stain
azure II-methylene blue stain
Baker Sudan black
basic fuchsin hydrochloride
basic fuchsin stain
basic fuchsin-methylene blue stain
Bauer chromic acid leucofuchsin stain

Becker stain
Belke-Kleihauer stain
Bennhold Congo red stain
Bensley aniline-acid fuchsin-methyl
  green
Bensley safranin acid violet
benzo fast pink 2BL
benzo sky blue method
benzopurpurin 4B
Berg stain
Berlin blue
Bernthsen methylene violet
Best carmine stain
beta-glucuronidase stain
Betke stain
Biebrich scarlet red
Biebrich scarlet water soluble
Biebrich scarlet-picroaniline blue
Bielschowsky stain
Biondi-Heidenhain stain
bipolar stain
Birch-Hirschfeld stain
Bismarck brown R
Bismarck brown stain
Bismarck brown Y stain
Bodian copper-Protargol stain
Borrel blue stain
Bowie stain
brilliant black BN
brilliant blue G250
brilliant blue R250
brilliant cresyl blue stain
brilliant crocein MOO
brilliant green
brilliant vital red
brilliant yellow
bromcresol purple
bromocresol green
bromocresol purple desoxycholate
bromphenol blue
bromthymol blue
Brown-Brenn stain
butyrate esterase stain
Cajal astrocyte stain

Cajal gold sublimate stain
calcium red
calcofluor white stain
carbolfuchsin stain
carbolfuchsin-methylene blue stain
carbol-thionin stain
carmine
carminic acid 50%
carminic acid 95%
C-banding stain
CEA gold-5 stain
CEA immunoperoxidase stain
celestine blue B
Chicago sky blue 6B
China blue
chlorazol black E stain
chlorophenol red
chocolate brown
chondroitin sulfate stain
ChrA (chromogranin A)
  immunoperoxidase stain
chromate stain
chrome alum carmine
chrome alum hematoxylin-phloxine
  stain
chrome azurol S
chrome red
chrome violet
chrome violet CG
chrome yellow
chromotrope 2B
chromotrope 2R
chromoxane cyanine R
chrysophenine
Churukian-Schenck stain
Ciaccio stain
Clayton yellow
cochineal red A
colloidal iron stain
colophonium alcohol
Congo Corinth
Congo red stain
contrast stain
Coomassie brilliant blue G-250

Coomassie brilliant blue R-250
cotton blue
cresol red
cresyl blue
cresyl blue brilliant
cresyl fast violet
cresyl violet
cresyl violet acetate
Cresylecht violet
crocein scarlet 3B
crystal violet stain
curcumin
cyclin D stain
Da Fano stain
Dane and Herman keratin stain
Dane stain
DAPI (46′-diamidino-2-phenylindole-2 HCl) dye, stain
Darrow red stain
del Rio-Hortega stain
Delafield hematoxylin stain
deoxyribonucleic acid stain
dextran blue
Diagnex Blue
diaminobenzidine stain
diazo blue B
diazo stain
dibromofluorescein
Dieterle stain
differential stain
Diff-Quik stain
diphenylmethane dye
direct fluorescent antibody stain
DOPA (dihydroxyphenylalanine) stain
Dorner stain
double stain
D-PAS (diastase-periodic acid-Schiff) stain
eau de Javelle
Ehrlich acid hematoxylin stain
Ehrlich aniline crystal violet stain
Ehrlich triacid stain
Ehrlich triple stain
Einarson gallocyanin-chrome alum stain

elastic fiber stain
elastica-van Gieson stain
endolymphatic dye
eosin B spirit soluble
eosin B stain
eosin B water soluble
eosin stain
eosin Y free acid
eosin Y sodium salt
eosin Y stain
eosin-methylene blue
Eranko fluorescence stain
eriochrome black A
eriochrome black T reagent ACS
eriochrome blue black R
eriochrome cyanine R
erioglaucine
erythrosine B
erythrosine B free acid
ethidium bromide stain
ethyl eosin
ethyl green
ethyl orange
ethyl violet
Evans blue
Farrant medium
fast blue B stain
fast garnet GBC base, salt
fast green FCF
fast green stain
fast red B stain
fast sulphon black F
fast yellow stain
ferric ammonium sulfate stain
Feulgen stain (Schiff reagent)
Feulgen sulfurous acid solution
Field rapid stain
Fink-Heimer stain
Fite stain
Fite-Faraco stain
Flemming triple stain
fluorescein alcohol soluble
fluorescein alcohol soluble USP
fluorescein stain

fluorescein water soluble
fluorescence plus Giemsa stain
fluorescent dye
fluorescent stain
fluorochrome stain
Fontana-Masson silver stain
Fontana methenamine silver stain
Fontana stain
Foot reticulin impregnation stain
Foot silver solution
formol-calcium
Fouchet stain
Fraser-Lendrum stain
fuchsin acid
fuchsin basic
fuchsin stain
fungal stain
Fungalase-F stain
gallamine blue
gallein
gallocyanine
ganglioside GD2 stain
G-banding stain
Genta stain
gentian orange stain
gentian violet stain
Giemsa chromosome banding
    stain
Giemsa stain
Gill #2 hematoxylin blue stain
Gill hematoxylin stain
Gimenez stain
Glenner-Lillie stain
glycogen stain
glycolipid stain
glycoprotein stain
GMS (Gomori methenamine-silver)
    stain
Golgi stain
Gomori aldehyde fuchsin stain
Gomori chrome alum
    hematoxylin-phloxine stain
Gomori-Jones periodic
    acid-methenamine-silver stain

Gomori nonspecific acid phosphatase
    stain
Gomori nonspecific alkaline
    phosphatase stain
Gomori one-step trichrome stain
Gomori silver impregnation stain
Gomori-Takamatsu stain
Gomori trichrome stain
Goodpasture stain
Gordon and Sweet stain
Gothard differentiator
Gram iodine stain
Gram stain
Gram-chromotrope stain
Gram-Weigert stain
Gridley stain
Grimelius argyrophil stain
Grimelius stain
Grocott-Gomori methenamine-silver
    stain
Grocott methenamine silver stain
guinea green B
Hale colloidal iron stain
Hansel stain
Harris hematoxylin
H&E (hematoxylin and eosin) stain
Heidenhain azan stain
Heidenhain iron hematoxylin stain
Heinz body stain
Helly fixative
hemalum
hematein
hematoxylin and eosin (H&E) stain
hematoxylin stain
hematoxylin, malachite green, basic
    fuchsin
hematoxylin-phloxine B stain
hematoxylin, phloxine, saffron
hemosiderin stain
heparan sulfate PG (proteoglycan) stain
hexamethyl violet
Highman Congo red
Hirsch-Peiffer stain
Hiss capsule stain

histochemical stain
Hoechst dye
Hoffman violet
Holmes stain
Hortega neuroglia stain
Hucker-Conn crystal violet solution
Hucker-Conn stain
hydrazine yellow
hydroxyketone dye
8-hydroxy-136-pyrenetrisulfonic acid trisodium salt
immunoalkaline phosphatase stain
immunofluorescent stain
immunogold-silver stain
immunohistochemical stain
immunoperoxidase stain
indamine dye
India ink capsule stain
India ink stain
indigo blue
indigo carmine
indigo synthetic
indigoid dye
indocyanine green
indophenol blue
indophenol dye
indulin water soluble
intravital stain
iodine stain
iodonitrotetrazolium
iron hematoxylin stain
iron stain
Isamine blue
isosulfan blue
Janus green B
Jenner-Giemsa stain
Jenner stain
Jones methenamine silver stain
Jones stain
Kaiserling fixative
Kasten fluorescent Feulgen staing
Kasten fluorescent PAS (periodic acid-Schiff) stain
Kermes dye

ketonimine dye
Kinyoun acid-fast stain
Kinyoun carbolfuchsin stain
Kinyoun stain
Kittrich stain
Kleihauer stain
Kleihauer-Betke stain
Klinger-Ludwig acid-thionin stain
Klüver-Barrera Luxol fast blue stain
Kokoskin stain
Kossa stain
Kronecker stain
Kühne methylene blue
laccaic acid
lacmoid
lactone dye
lactophenol cotton blue stain
LAP (leukocyte alkaline phosphatase) stain
Lauth violet
Lawless stain
lead citrate stain
lead hydroxide stain
Leder stain
Leipzig yellow
Leishman stain
Lendrum inclusion body stain
Lendrum phloxine-tartrazine stain
Lepehne-Pickworth stain
leuco crystal violet
leuco patent blue
leucomethylene blue
leukocyte acid phosphatase stain
Leukostat stain
Leung stain
Levaditi stain
Levine alkaline Congo red stain
light green SF
light green SF yellowish
Lillie allochrome connective tissue stain
Lillie azure-eosin stain
Lillie ferrous iron stain
Lillie sulfuric acid Nile blue stain
Liquichek reticulocyte control and stain

Lison-Dunn staing
lissamine green B
lithium carmine
Loeffler, Löffler caustic stain
Loeffler, Löffler methylene blue
Loeffler, Löffler stain
Lugol stain
Luna-Ishak staing
Luxol fast blue stain
Macchiavello staing
MacNeal tetrachrome blood stain
malachite green
malachite green oxalate
malarial pigment stain
Maldonado-San Jose stain
Mallory aniline blue stain
Mallory collagen stain
Mallory iodine stain
Mallory phloxine stain
Mallory phosphotungstic acid
   hematoxylin
Mallory trichrome stain
Mallory triple stain
Mancini iodine stain
Mann methyl blue-eosin stain
Marchi stain
martius scarlet blue
martius yellow
Masson argentaffin stain
Masson trichrome stain
Masson-Fontana ammoniacal silver
   stain
Maximow stain
Mayer acid alum hematoxylin stain
Mayer hemalum stain
Mayer hematoxylin stain
Mayer mucicarmine stain
Mayer mucihematein stain
May-Grünwald stain
May-Grünwald-Giemsa stain
Meissel stain
mercurochrome 220
metachromatic dye
metachromatic stain

metanil yellow stain
methenamine silver stain
methine dye
methyl blue
methyl green
methyl green-pyronin
methyl green zinc chloride salt
methyl green-pyronin stain
methyl orange
methyl orange reagent ACS
methyl red
methyl violet
methyl violet 2B
methyl yellow
methylene azure
methylene blue
methylene blue chloride
methylene blue dye
methylene blue stain
methylene green
methylene violet
methylene violet 3RAX
methylene white
methylthymol blue
Milligan trichrome stain
modified acid-fast stain
modified auramine-rhodamine stain
modified Kinyoun stain
modified Steiner stain
modified Ziehl-Nielsen stain
Morin (fluorescent) stain
Movat pentachrome stain
Mowry colloidal iron stain
MSB (martius scarlet blue) trichrome
   stain
mucicarmine stain
Musto stain
myeloperoxidase stain
n-propyl red
Nakanishi stain
naphthol-ASD chloroacetate esterase
   stain
naphthol green B
naphthol yellow S stain

natural dye
natural red Certistain
Nauta stain
NBT (nitroblue tetrazolium) dye, stain
negative stain
Neisser stain
neutral red
neutral stain
new coccine dye
new fuchsin
new methylene blue
new methylene blue N
Nicolle stain
night blue stain
nigrosin stain
nigrosin water soluble
nigrosin B alcohol soluble
Nile blue
Nile blue A
Nile blue A chloride
Nile blue A sulfateg
Nile red
ninhydrin-Schiff stain
Nissl stain
nitro dye
nitroso dye
Noble stain
Novelli stain
NSE (nonspecific esterase) stain
nuclear fast red stain
nuclear stain
oil red O stain
orange II, IV
orange IV
orange G stain
orcein stain
Orth lithium carmine stain
osmium tetroxide stain
oxalic acid stain
oxazin dye
oxytalan fiber stain
Padykula-Herman stain
Paget-Eccleston stain
Palmgren silver impregnation stain

panoptic stain
PAP (peroxidase-antiperoxidase) stain
Pap stain
paracarmine stain
Paragon blue stain
pararosaniline acetate
pararosaniline HCl
Paris green
Paris yellow
PAS (periodic acid-Schiff) stain
PAS-orange G stain
patent blue
patent blue A
patent blue V dye
patent blue VF
patent blue violet
Pearl iron stain
pentamethyl violet
periodic acid-silver methenamine stain
Perls Prussian blue stain
peroxidase stain
phenosafranin
4-(phenylazo)-1-naphthalenamine
    hydrochloride (Chrysoidin)
phloxine B stain
phloxine-tartrazine stain
phosphomolybdic acid stain
phthalocyanine dye
picric stain
picrocarmine stain
picroindigocarmine stain
picro-Mallory trichrome stain
picronigrosin stain
Pizzolato peroxide-silver
plasmocorinth B
polychrome methylene blue stain
polymethine dye
Ponceau 3R
Ponceau 4R
Ponceau 6R stain
Ponceau G R 2R
Ponceau S
Pontamine sky blue stain
potassium metabisulfate stain

potassium permanganate stain
Procion blue HB
p-rosaniline acetate stain
p-rosaniline acetate powder
Protargol stain
Prussian blue iron stain
Prussian blue stain
PTA (phosphotungstic acid) stain
PTAH (phosphotungstic acid
   hematoxylin) stain
Puchtler alkaline Congo red
Puchtler Sirius red
Puchtler-Sweat stain
pyronin B
pyronin Y
pyrrol blue stain
Q-banding stain
quinacrine chromosome banding stain
quinaldine red
quinoline dye
quinoline yellow
quinoline yellow SS
Rambourg periodic acid, chromic acid,
   methenamine silver stain
Ranson pyridine silver stain
reactive red 4
rhodamine 6G
rhodamine B
rhodamine B base alcohol soluble
rhodamine B O
rhodamine blue
rhodamine stain
Romanowsky blood stain
Romanowsky stain
Romanowsky-Giemsa stain
rosaniline dye
rose bengal stain
rosolic acid
Roux stain
ruthenium red
Ryan stain
Sabin-Feldman dye
saffron
safranin O

safranin stain
salt dye
Sayeed stain
SBB (Sudan black B) stain
scarlet red stain
scarlet red sulfonate
Schaeffer-Fulton stain
scharlach red
Schiff stain
Schmorl ferric-ferricyanide reduction
   stain
Schmorl picrothionin stain
Schneider carmine
Schultz stain
selective stain
Sevier-Munger stain
Shorr trichrome stain
silver impregnation
silver nitrate stain
silver nitroprusside
silver protein stain
silver stain
silver-ammoniacal silver stain
Sirius red
Sirius red F3B
Smith silver stain
Snook reticulum stain
sodium bisulfite stain
sodium hydroxide stain
sodium thiosulfate stain
Steiner stain
Sternheimer-Malbin Sedi-stain
Sternheimer-Malbin stain
stilbene dye
stilbene yellow
Stirling modification of Gram stain
Sudan I, II, III, IV
Sudan black stain
Sudan brown
Sudan orange G
Sudan red 7B
Sudan red III
Sudan yellow
Sudan yellow G

sulfur dye
supravital stain
Susa fixativeg
synthetic dye
Taenzer stain
Taenzer-Unna stain
Takayama stain
tartrazine stain
tetrachrome stain
tetramethylbenzidine stain
thiazin dye
thiazole dye
thioflavine S
thioflavine T, TG
thionin acetate
thionin stain
thymol blue
Tilden stain
Timm silver sulfide
titan yellow
Tizzoni stain
Toison stain
toluidine blue O
toluidine blue stain
toluylene red
TRAP (tartrate-resistant acid
   phosphatase) stain
triarylmethane dye
trichrome stain
triphenylmethane dye
tropaeolin O
Truant auramine-rhodamine stain
trypan blue
trypan red
Turk blood counting fluid
Turkey red
Turnbull blue stain
ultrafast Pap stain
ultramarine blue
Unna stain
Unna-Pappenheim stain
Unna-Taenzer stain

uranyl acetate stain
urate crystals stain
van Ermengen stain
van Gieson stain
Ventana ES stain
Verhoeff elastic tissue stain
Victoria blue B
Victoria blue R
Victoria blue stain
Victoria orange
vimentin immunoperoxidase
   stain
vital dye
vital red
vital stain
von Kossa stain
VVG (Verhoeff-van Gieson) stain
Wachstein-Meissel stain
Wade-Fite-Faraco stain
Warthin-Starry silver stain
water blue-orcein
Wayson stain
Weber-modified trichome stain
Weber stain
Weigert-Gram stain
Weigert-Pal stain
Weigert iron hematoxylin stain
Weigert stain
Weil myelin sheath stain
Wilder stain
Williams stain
Wright stain
Wright-Giemsa stain
xanthene dye
xylene cyanol FF
xylidine Ponceau 2 R
xylidine Ponceau stain
yellow corallin
Zenker formol
Ziehl stain
Ziehl-Neelsen stain
Zike flagella mordant

Appendix 4
Greek Alphabet

Lower case	Name	Upper case
α	alpha	A
β	beta	B
γ	gamma	Γ
δ	delta	Δ
ε	epsilon	E
ζ	zeta	Z
η	eta	H
θ	theta	Θ
ι	iota	I
κ	kappa	K
λ	lambda	Λ
μ	mu	M
ν	nu	N
ξ	xi	Ξ
ο	omicron	O
π	pi	Π
ρ	rho	P
ς, σ	sigma	Σ
τ	tau	T
υ	upsilon	Υ
φ	phi	Φ
χ	chi	X
ψ	psi	Ψ
ω	omega	Ω

Elements and Symbols

Symbol	Element	Symbol	Element
Ac	actinium	Hf	hafnium
Ag	silver	Hg	mercury
Al	aluminum	Ho	holmium
Am	americium	I	iodine
Ar	argon	In	indium
As	arsenic	Ir	iridium
At	astatine	K	potassium
Au	gold	Kr	krypton
B	boron	La	lanthanum
Ba	barium	Li	lithium
Be	beryllium	Lr	lawrencium
Bi	bismuth	Lu	lutetium
Bk	berkelium	Md	mendelevium
Br	bromine	Mg	magnesium
C	carbon	Mn	manganese
Ca	calcium	Mo	molybdenum
Cd	cadmium	N	nitrogen
Ce	cerium	Na	sodium
Cf	californium	Nb	niobium
Cl	chlorine	Nd	neodymium
Cm	curium	Ne	neon
Co	cobalt	Ni	nickel
Cr	chromium	No	nobelium
Cs	cesium	O	oxygen
Cu	copper	Os	osmium
Dy	dysprosium	P	phosphorus
Er	erbium	Pa	protactinium
Es	einsteinium	Pb	lead
Eu	europium	Pd	palladium
F	fluorine	Pm	promethium
Fe	fermium	Po	polonium
Fe	iron	Pr	praseodymium
Fr	francium	Pt	platinum
Ga	gallium	Pu	plutonium
Gd	gadolinium	Ra	radium
Ge	germanium	Rb	rubidium
H	hydrogen	Re	rhenium
He	helium	Rh	rhodium

Symbol	Element	Symbol	Element
Rn	radon	U	uranium
Ru	ruthenium	Une	unnilennium
S	sulfur	Unh	unnilhexium
Sb	antimony	Uno	unniloctium
Sc	scandium	Unp	unnilpentium
Se	selenium	Unq	unnilquadium
Si	silicon	Uns	unnilseptium
Sm	samarium	Uun	ununnilium
Sn	tin	Uup	ununpentium
Sr	strontium	Uut	ununtrium
Ta	tantalum	V	vanadium
Tb	terbium	W	tungsten
Tc	technetium	Xe	xenon
Te	tellurium	Y	yttrium
Th	thorium	Yb	ytterbium
Ti	titanium	Z	zirconium
Tl	thallium	Zn	zinc
Tm	thulium		

Element	Symbol	Element	Symbol
actinium	Ac	cesium	Cs
aluminum	Al	chlorine	Cl
americium	Am	chromium	Cr
antimony	Sb	cobalt	Co
argon	Ar	copper	Cu
arsenic	As	curium	Cm
astatine	At	dysprosium	Dy
barium	Ba	einsteinium	Es
berkelium	Bk	erbium	Er
beryllium	Be	europium	Eu
bismuth	Bi	fermium	Fe
boron	B	fluorine	F
bromine	Br	francium	Fr
cadmium	Cd	gadolinium	Gd
calcium	Ca	gallium	Ga
californium	Cf	germanium	Ge
carbon	C	gold	Au
cerium	Ce	hafnium	Hf

Element	Symbol	Element	Symbol
helium	He	rhodium	Rh
holmium	Ho	rubidium	Rb
hydrogen	H	ruthenium	Ru
indium	In	samarium	Sm
iodine	I	scandium	Sc
iridium	Ir	selenium	Se
iron	Fe	silicon	Si
krypton	Kr	silver	Ag
lanthanum	La	sodium	Na
lawrencium	Lr	strontium	Sr
lead	Pb	sulfur	S
lithium	Li	tantalum	Ta
lutetium	Lu	technetium	Tc
magnesium	Mg	tellurium	Te
manganese	Mn	terbium	Tb
mendelevium	Md	thallium	Tl
mercury	Hg	thorium	Th
molybdenum	Mo	thulium	Tm
neodymium	Nd	tin	Sn
neon	Ne	titanium	Ti
nickel	Ni	tungsten	W
niobium	Nb	unnilennium	Une
nitrogen	N	unnilhexium	Unh
nobelium	No	unniloctium	Uno
osmium	Os	unnilpentium	Unp
oxygen	O	unnilquadium	Unq
palladium	Pd	unnilseptium	Uns
phosphorus	P	ununnilium	Uun
platinum	Pt	ununpentium	Uup
plutonium	Pu	ununtrium	Uut
polonium	Po	uranium	U
potassium	K	vanadium	V
praseodymium	Pr	xenon	Xe
promethium	Pm	ytterbium	Yb
protactinium	Pa	yttrium	Y
radium	Ra	zinc	Zn
radon	Rn	zirconium	Z
rhenium	Re		

Appendix 6
Units of Measure for Pathology

Basic SI Units

Unit Name	SI Unit	Symbol
length	meter	m
mass	kilogram	kg
time	second	s
electric current	ampere	A
thermodynamic temperature	kelvin	K
amount of substance	mole	mol
luminous intensity	candela	cd

Derived SI Units

Unit Name	SI Unit	Symbol
frequency	hertz	Hz
force	newton	N
pressure	pascal	Pa
energy (all forms)	joule	J
power	watt	W
electric charge	coulomb	C
electric potential difference	volt	V
electrical capacitance	farad	F
electrical resistance	ohm	Ω
electrical conductance	siemens	S
magnetic flux	weber	Wb
magnetic induction	tesla	T
inductance	henry	H
luminous flux	lumen	lm
illumination	lux	lx
activity (of a radionuclide)	becquerel	Bq
absorbed dose	gray	Gy
dose equivalent	sievert	Sv
catalytic activity	katal	kat
Celsius temperature	degree Celsius	°C
plane angle	radian	rad
solid angle	steradian	sr

Sample Immunodiagnostic Panels

ARBOVIRUS COMPETITIVE ENZYME IMMUNOASSAY (CEIA)
Eastern equine encephalitis IgM
St Louis encephalitis IgM
LaCrosse encephalitis IgM
West Nile virus IgM Ab

CAT SCRATCH DISEASE SEROLOGY
Bartonella quintana
Bartonella henselae

CHLAMYDIA-GONORRHEA AMPLIFIED MOLECULAR ASSAY (AMA)
Neisseria gonorrhoeae
Chlamydia trachomatis

CRYPTOSPORIDIUM/GIARDIA DIRECT FLUORESCENCE ANTIGEN (DFA)
Cryptosporidium DFA
Giardia DFA

HANTAVIRUS IgM AND IgG
Hantavirus IgG
Hantavirus IgM

HEPATITIS B IMMUNE STATUS
Hepatitis B core antibody
Hepatitis B surface antibody

HEPATITIS B SERODIAGNOSIS
Hepatitis B surface antigen
Hepatitis B core antibody
Hepatitis B surface antibody

LYME DISEASE
Lyme Disease Western blot IgM
Lyme Disease Western blot IgG

MEASLES IMMUNOGLOBULINS
Measles IgM
Measles IgG

Mumps Immunoglobulins
Mumps IgM
Mumps IgG

Mycobacterium Acid Fast Bacterium (AFB)
Mycobacteriology smear
Mycobacteriology culture direct

Mycoplasma pneumoniae Enzyme Immunoassay (EIA)
Mycoplasma pneumoniae IgM
Mycoplasma pneumoniae IgG

Parvovirus B19
Parvovirus B19 IgG
Parvovirus B19 IgM

Prenatal Screen Panel
ABO group
Rh type
Blood factor antibody
VDRL
Hepatitis B surface antigen
Rubella IgG

Prenatal Screen Panel, Basic Plus HIV
Add: HIV prenatal

Prenatal Screen Panel, Basic Plus HIV/Toxoplasma
Add: HIV prenatal
Toxoplasma IgM serology
Toxoplasma IgG serology

Prenatal Screen Panel, Basic Plus Toxoplasma
Add: Toxoplasma IgM Serology Prenatal
Toxoplasma IgG Serology Prenatal

Q Fever Antibody
Q Fever phase 1
Q Fever phase 2

Rickettsia Antibody
*Rickettsia a*ntibody Rocky Mountain spotted fever
Rickettsia antibody typhus

RUBELLA ANTIBODY
Rubella IgM
Rubella IgG

TOXOPLASMA ANTIBODY
Toxoplasma IgM
Toxoplasma IgG

VARICELLA ZOSTER Antibody
Varicella zoster IgM
Varicella zoster IgG

Sample Immunodiagnostic

Appendix 8

Common Lab Tests

Usage of various terms, both formal and what might appear to be slang, depend upon rules of institution. Combinations of test components under a particular name also depend on institution or laboratory. For example, a chemistry panel at one hospital might routinely include glucose while at another that is an advanced or extra test. Units of measure also vary by institution, method, professionals' preference and units of measure should be transcribed as dictated.

(See Tables following for selected range of values and units of measure.)

LAB TEST NAME	MAY BE HEARD AS	VALUES (SAMPLE)
BLOOD TESTS		
Complete Blood Count	*CBC, hemogram, blood count*	
Red blood cell count (rarely dictated)	*RBC, red cells*	4.2 to 6.2 (million)
White blood cell count	*WBC, white cells*	4.1 to 10.9 (thousand)
White blood cell differential	*diff, differential leukocyte count, peripheral differential, white blood cell morphology, WBC differential*	% or plain #
granulocyte	*polymorphonuclear leukocyte*	
neutrophils	*segs, polys, PMNs*	% or plain #
immature neutrophils	*bands*	% increase = "left shift"
eosinophils	*eos*	% or #
basophils	*basos*	% or #
agranulocyte	*mononuclear leukocytes*	
lymphocytes	lymphs	
monocytes	*monos*	
Hemoglobin (first H of H&H)	*Hb, Hgb*	12.0–18.0
Hematocrit (second H of H&H)	*crit, Hct, packed cell volume, PCV*	38–54

NOTE: Ratio of normal hemoglobin and hematocrit approximately 1:3

Platelets	*thrombocytes*	130 to 400 (thousand)
Reticulocytes	*retic*	%

LAB TEST NAME	MAY BE HEARD AS	VALUES (SAMPLE)
Red blood cell indices		
mean corpuscular volume	*MCV*	80–99
mean corpuscular hemoglobin	*MCH*	27–31
mean corpuscular hemoglobin concentration MCHC		33–37
red cell distribution width	*RDW*	% or #
Blood smear	*morphology, peripheral smear*	descriptive
white blood cell smear		
granulocytes		
neutrophils	*segmented neutrophils*	**abnormalities:** *segs, polys or PMN bands, immature neutrophils: percentage increase = "left shift." toxic granulation, vacuolization, Döhle bodies Auer bodies (Auer Rod), hypersegmentation, Pelger-Huët nucleus, Alder-Reilly granules, Chédiak-Higashi malformations*
eosinophils, basophils		may include same abnormalities
agranulocytes		
lymphocytes (T-cell and B-cells cannot be identified under microscope):		
		abnormalities: Reactive, hairy cell
monocytes		
red blood cell smear		**abnormalities:** *sickle cell, tear-drop, elliptocyte, spherocyte, target cell, Mexican hat cell, ovalocyte*

(continued)

LAB TEST NAME	MAY BE HEARD AS	VALUES (SAMPLE)
<u>Blood Testing</u>		
Electrolytes	*lytes, electrolyte panel*	
sodium	*Na*	136–1445
potassium	*K*	3.5–5.1
chloride	*Cl*	98–107
bicarbonate	*CO2, bicarb, carbon dioxide, HCO3*	22–29
Anion gap (calculated value)		
(Na − (Cl + HCO3))		7–16
((Na + K) − (Cl + HCO3))		10–20

NOTE: Serum is electrically neutral and total anions and total cations must be equal.

Na+ and K+ are the major reported cations.

Cl- and HCO3- are the major reported anions.

There are *unmeasured anions*, resulting in normal net excess in serum of about 17 mEq/L. If the anion gap exceeds 17 mEq/L, indicates increase in *unmeasured anion.*

INCREASED anion gap of concern in: metabolic acidosis such as lactic acidosis; uremia; ketosis; toxin ingestion, such as methanol and salicylates

DECREASED anion gap: laboratory error; abnormal proteins such as multiple myeloma or polyclonal gammopathy; hypoproteinemia.

Kidney Function Tests (Note: sometimes dictated to sound like part of electrolytes. See below for proper format)

blood urea nitrogen	*BUN, urea nitrogen*	6–20
creatinine		0.6–1.3

LAB TEST NAME	MAY BE HEARD AS	VALUES (SAMPLE)
Liver Function Tests		
alkaline phosphatase	*alk phos, ALP*	38–126
alanine amino transferase	*ALT, SGPT, transaminases*	10–40
aspartate amino transferase	*AST, SGOT, transaminases*	10–59
bilirubin	*bili*	
total bilirubin (blood component)	*t-bili, unconjugated*	0.2–1.2
direct bilirubin (liver component)	*direct bili, conjugated bili*	0.0–0.4
indirect bilirubin		calculated value, total minus direct

(NOTE: Special values of bilirubin for neonates and infants, see tables)

Lipid Panel (separate or part of liver function test or chemistry panel)

	lipids lipid profile, lipoprotein analysis, cholesterol test	
total cholesterol		Adult desirable less than 200
HDL cholesterol		Adult desirable greater than 40
LDL cholesterol		Adult desirable less than 130
triglycerides		less than 150
Arterial Blood Gas	*blood gas*	
pH		7.35 to 7.45
PO2		83 to 108
PCO2		32 to 48
bicarbonate	*CO2, HCO3*	22 to 26
oxygen saturation	*sats, O2 sat, SaO2*	95 to 100%

LAB TEST NAME	MAY BE HEARD AS	VALUES (SAMPLE)

CHEMISTRY PANELS (METABOLIC PROFILE)

If CBC, electrolytes, and kidney function tests are all performed, they are usually done in combination and called a CHEMISTRY PANEL. Adding liver function tests and others is called a COMPREHENSIVE chemistry panel, or other terms as indicated. Please refer to tables for range of values for additional components.

LAB TEST NAME	MAY BE HEARD AS
Chemistry Panel	*chem panel, met profile, basic metabolic panel, BMP, chemistries, SMA, SMAC*
Screening ChemistryPanel	*chem 6, chem 7, SMA 6, SMA 7, SMAC 6, SMAC 7 (sometimes has 8 values)*
components: **electrolytes** plus **kidney function test**	
(also add) glucose	*blood glucose, blood sugar, sugars*
May state fasting or nonfasting	
Comprehensive chemistry panel	*chem panel, metabolic panel, SMA 12, SMA 20, SMAC 12, SMAC 20*
Screening chemistry panel plus *liver function tests, lipid panel* and may include any of the following:	
albumin	
total protein	
calcium	*Ca*
can also include:	
phosphorus	*P*
creatinine clearance	*CrCl*
total serum protein	
lactic acid	
uric acid	
magnesium	*Mg*
tests of pancreas function (amylase and lipase)	

LAB TEST NAME	MAY BE HEARD AS	VALUES (SAMPLE)
Cardiac Enzymes	AMI panel	
creatine kinase MB isoenzyme	*serum CK-MB*	0 to 7
troponin-I, cardiac, serum		less than 0.04 (undetectable)
CPK	*CK, serum; CPK; creatine phosphokinase, total, serum; TCK*	10–105
Coagulation Studies	*coags, DIC panel*	
partial thromboplastin time, activated	*aPTT, PTT*	greater than 35 sec
prothrombin time	*PT, pro-time*	less than 20 sec
prothrombin time/ international normalized ratio	PT-INR	birth–6 mo: 1.0–1.6 ± 6 mo–adult 0.9– 1.2

NOTE: Therapeutic values for patients on Coumadin or heparin therapy institution, age, and diagnosis-specific

Iron Studies		
iron	*Fe*	50–175
total iron binding capacity	*TIBC*	50–425
ferritin		10–322
Miscellaneous Blood Tests		
blood alcohol	*EtOH*	values per institution
serum pregnancy test	*beta-hCG*	positive or negative
T3		0.8 to 2.7
free T4		5 to 12
TSH		0.4 to 4.2

Blood Values

TEST	CONVENTIONAL UNITS	SI UNITS
acetone, serum		
Qualitative	Negative	Negative
Quantitative	0.3–2.0 mg/dL	0.05–0.34 mmol/L
acid hemolysis test (Ham test)	<5% lysis	<0.05 lysed fraction
adrenocorticotropin (ACTH), plasma		
8 am	<120 pg/mL	<26 pmol/L
Midnight (supine)	<10 pg/mL	<2.2 pmol/L
alanine aminotransferase (ALT, SGPT), serum		
Male	13–40 U/L (37°C)	0.22–0.68 μkat/L (37°C)
Female	10–28 U/L (37°C)	0.17–0.48 μkat/L (37°C)
albumin, serum		
Adult	3.5–5.2 g/dL	35–52 g/L
>60 y	3.2–4.6 g/dL	32–46 g/L
	Avg. of 0.3 g/dL higher in upright individuals	Avg. of × g/dL higher in upright individuals
aldolase, serum	1.0–7.5 U/L (30°C)	0.02–0.13 μkat/L (30°C)
aldosterone, serum		
Supine	3–16 ng/dL	0.08–0.44 nmol/L
Standing	7–30 ng/dL	0.19–0.83 nmol/L
ammonia, plasma	9–33 μmol/L	9–33 μmol/L
amylase, serum	27–131 U/L	0.46–2.23 μkat/L
amylase:creatine clearance ratio	1–4%	0.01–0.04
androstenedione, serum		
Male	75–205 ng/dL	2.6–7.2 nmol/L
Female	85–275 ng/dL	3.0–9.6 nmol/L
anion gap		
$(Na - (Cl + HCO3))$	7–16 mEq/L	7–16 mmol/L
$((Na + K) - (Cl\ 1\ HCO3))$	10–20 mEq/L	10–20 mmol/L
alpha 1 antitrypsin, serum	78–200 mg/dL	0.78–2.00 g/L
apolipoprotein A1		
Male	94–178 mg/dL	0.94–1.78 g/L
Female	101–199 mg/dL	1.01–1.99 g/L

TEST	CONVENTIONAL UNITS	SI UNITS
apolipoprotein B		
Male	63–133 mg/dL	0.63–1.33 g/L
Female	60–126 mg/dL	0.60–1.26 g/L
arsenic, whole blood	0.2–2.3 μg/dL	0.03–0.31 μmol/L
Chronic poisoning	10–50 μg/dL	1.33–6.65 μmol/L
Acute poisoning	60–930 μg/dL	7.98–124 μmol/L
ascorbic acid, plasma	0.4–1.5 mg/dL	23–85 μmol/L
aspartate aminotransferase (AST, SGOT), serum	10–59 U/L (37°C)	0.17–1.00 22 to 13 kat/L (37°C)
base excess, blood	–2 to +3 mmol/L	–2 to +3 mmol/L
bicarbonate, serum (venous) (bicarb, CO2, HCO3)	22–29 mmol/L	22–29 mmol/L
bilirubin, direct		
Birth–death	0.0–0.4 mg/dL	
bilirubin, total		
Birth–1 day	1.0–6.0 mg/dL	
1–2 days	6.0–7.5 mg/dL	
2–5 days	4.0–13.5 mg/dL	
5 days–death	0.2–1.2 mg/dL	
bilirubin, total, neonatal		
Birth–1 day	1.0–6.0 g/dL	
1–2 days	6.0–7.5 g/dL	
2–5 days	4.0– 13.5 g/dL	
5 days–1 month	0.0–1.8 g/dL	
1 month–death	0.0–1.8 g/dL	
CA 125, serum	<35 U/mL	<35 kU/L
CA 15–3, serum	<30 U/mL	<30 kU/L
CA 19–9, serum	<37 U/mL	<37 kU/L
calcitonin, serum or plasma		
Male	≤100 pg/mL	≤100 ng/L
Female	≤30 pg/mL	≤30 ng/L
calcium, serum	8.6–10.0 mg/dL (Slightly higher in children)	2.15–2.50 mmol/L (Slightly higher in children)
calcium, ionized, serum	4.64–5.28 mg/dl	1.16–1.32 mmol/L
carbon dioxide (PCO2)	Male 35–48 mmHg	4.66–6.38 kPa

Blood Values (continued)

TEST	CONVENTIONAL UNITS	SI UNITS
carbon dioxide, blood, arterial (ABG)	Female 32–45 mmHg	4.26–5.99 kPa
CO2, bicarb, HCO3- (electrolytes)	See bicarbonate, serum	See bicarbonate, serum
carboxyhemoglobin (HbCO, carbon monoxide, hemiglobin)		
Nonsmokers	0.5–1.5% total Hb	0.005–0.015 HbCO fraction
Smokers		
1–2 packs/d	4–5% total Hb	0.04–0.05 HbCO fraction
>2 packs/d	8–9% total Hb	0.08–0.09 HbCO fraction
Toxic	>20% total Hb	>0.20 HbCO fraction
Lethal	>50% total Hb	>0.50 HbCO fraction
carotene, serum	10–85 μg/dL	0.19–1.58 μmol/L
catecholamines, plasma		
Dopamine	<30 pg/mL	<196 pmol/L
Epinephrine	<140 pg/mL	<764 pmol/L
Norepinephrine	<1700 pg/mL	<10,047 pmol/L
carcinoembryonic antigen (CEA), serum		
Nonsmokers	<5.0 ng/mL	<5.0 μg/L
CBC, blood cell counts, adult	BLOOD Cell Counts	
RBC Male	$4.7–6.1 \times 10^6/\mu L$	$4.7–6.1 \times 10^{12}/L$
Female	$4.2–5.4 \times 10^6/\mu L$	$4.2–5.4 \times 10^{12}/L$
WBC		
Total	$4.8–10.8 \times 10^3/\mu L$	$4.8–10.8 \times 10^6/L$
WBC Differential	Percentage	Absolute
Myelocytes	0	0/μL
Neutrophils		
Bands	3–5	150–400/μL
		$150–400 \times 10^6/L$
Segmented	54–62	3000–5800/μL
		$3000–5800 \times 10^6/L$

TEST	CONVENTIONAL UNITS	SI UNITS
Lymphocytes	20.5–51.1	$1.2–3.4 \times 10^3/\mu L$
		$1.2–3.4 \times 109/L$
Monocytes	1.7–9.3	$0.11–0.59 \times 10^3/\mu L$
		$0.11–0.59 \times 10^9/L$
Granulocytes	42.2–75.2	$1.4–6.5 \times 10^3/\mu L$
		$1.4–6.5 \times 10^9/L$
Eosinophils		$0.07 \times 10^3/\mu L$
		$0.07 \times 10^9/L$
Basophils		$0–0.2 \times 10^3/\mu L$
		$0–0.2 \times 10^9/L$
Platelets	$130–400 \times 10^3/\mu L$	$130–400 \times 10^9/L$
Reticulocytes	0.5–1.5% RBCs	0.005–0.015 of RBCs
	24,000–84.000/μL	$24–84 \times 10^9/L$
ceruloplasmin, serum	20–60 mg/dL	0.2–6.0 g/L
chloride (Cl)		
Serum or plasma	98–107 mmol/L	98–107 mmol/L
cholesterol, serum		
Adult desirable	<200 mg/dL	<5.2 mmol/L
borderline	200–239 mg/dL	5.2–6.2 mmol/L
high risk	≤240 mg/dL	≤6.2 mmol/L
cholinesterase, serum	4.9–11.9 U/mL	4.9–11.9 kU/L
chorionic gonadotropin, intact (hCG)		
Serum or plasma		
Male and nonpregnant female	<5.0 mIU/mL	<5.0 IU/L
Pregnant female	Varies with gestational age	
coagulation tests (coags, clotting studies)		
Antithrombin III (synthetic substrate)	80–120% of normal	0.8–1.2 of normal
Bleeding time (Duke)	0–6 min	0–6 min
Bleeding time (Ivy)	1–6 min	1–6 min
Bleeding time (template)	2.3–9.5 min	2.3–9.5 min
Clot retraction, qualitative	50–100% in 2 h	0.5–1.0/2 h

Blood Values (continued)

TEST	CONVENTIONAL UNITS	SI UNITS
coagulation time (Lee-White)	5–15 min (glass tubes)	5–15 min (glass tubes)
cold hemolysin test (Donath-Landsteiner)	No hemolysis	No hemolysis
complement components		
Total hemolytic complement activity, plasma (EDTA)	75–160 U/mL	75–160 kU/L
Total complement decay rate	10–20%	Fraction decay rate: 0.10–0.20
(functional), plasma	Deficiency: >50%	>0.50
C1q, serum	14.9–22.1 mg/dL	149–221 mg/L
C1r, serum	2.5–10.0 mg/dL	25–100 mg/L
C1s(C1 esterase), serum	5.0–10.0 mg/dL	50–100 mg/L
C2, serum	1.6–3.6 mg/dL	16–36 mg/L
C3, serum	90–180 mg/dL	0.9–1.8 g/L
C4, serum	10–40 mg/dL	0.1–0.4 g/L
C5, serum	5.5–11.3 mg/dL	55–113 mg/L
C6, serum	17.9–23.9 mg/dL	179–239 mg/L
C7, serum	2.7–7.4 mg/dL	27–74 mg/L
C8, serum	4.9–10.6 mg/dL	49–106 mg/L
C9, serum	3.3–9.5 mg/dL	33–95 mg/L
Coombs test		
Direct	Negative	Negative
Indirect	Negative	Negative
copper (Cu), Serum		
Male	70–140 µg/dL	11–22 µmol/L
Female	80–155 µg/dL	13–24 µmol/L
RBC indices (corpuscular values)		
(values are for adults; in children values vary with age)		
Mean corpuscular hemoglobin (MCH)	27–31 pg	0.42–0.48 fmol
Mean corpuscular hemoglobin concentration (MCHC)	33–37 g/dL	330–370 g/L
Mean corpuscular volume (MCV)	Male 80–94 μ^3	80–94 fL

TEST	CONVENTIONAL UNITS	SI UNITS
cortisol, serum		
Plasma		
8 am	5–23 μg/dL	138–635 nmol/L
4 pm	3–16 μg/dL	83–441 nmol/L
10 pm	<50% of 8 AM value	<0.5 of 8 AM value
creatine kinase (CK), serum		
Male	15–105 U/L (30°C)	0.26–1.79 μkat/L (30°C)
Female	10–80 U/L (30°C)	0.17–1.36 μkat/L (30°C)
Note: Strenuous exercise or intramuscular injections may cause transient elevation of CK.		
creatine kinase MB isoenzyme (CK-MB), serum	0–7 ng/mL	0–7 μg/l
creatinine		
Serum or plasma, adult		
Male	0.7–1.3 mg/dL	62–115 μmmol/L
Female	0.6–1.1 mg/dL	53–97 μmol/L
cryoglobulins, serum	0	0
cyanide		
Serum		
Nonsmokers	0.004 mg/L	0.15 μmol/L
Smokers	0.006 mg/L	0.23 μmol/L
Nitroprusside therapy	0.01–0.06 mg/L	0.38–2.30 μmol/L
Toxic	>0.1 mg/L	>3.84 μmol/L
Whole blood		
Nonsmokers	0.016 mg/L	0.61 μmol/L
Smokers	0.041 mg/L	1.57 μmol/L
Nitroprusside therapy	0.05–0.5 mg/L	1.92–19.20 μmol/L
Toxic	>1 mg/L	>38.40 μmol/L
cyclic AMP (cAMP)		
Plasma		
Male	4.6–8.6 ng/mL	14–26 nmol/L
Female	4.3–7.6 ng/mL	13–23 nmol/L
C-peptide, serum	0.78–1.89 ng/mL	0.26–0.62 nmol/L

Blood Values (continued)

TEST	CONVENTIONAL UNITS	SI UNITS
C-reactive protein (CRP), serum	<0.5 mg/dL	<5 mg/L
dehydroepiandrosterone (DHEA) serum		
Male	180–1250 ng/dL	6.2–43.3 nmol/L
Female	130–980 ng/dL	4.5–34.0 nmol/L
dehydroepiandrosterone sulfate, DHEAS, serum or plasma		
Male	59–452 μg/dL	1.6–12.2 μmol/L
Female		
Premenopausal	12–379 μg/dL	0.8–10.2 μmol/L
Postmenopausal	30–260 μg/dL	0.8–7.1 μmol/L
glucose (fasting)		
Blood	65–95 mg/dL	3.5–5.3 mmol/L
Plasma or serum	74–106 mg/dL	4.1–5.9 mmol/L
glucose, 2 h postprandial, serum	<120 mg/dL	<6.7 mmol/L
glucose-6-phosphate dehydrogenase, G6PD	12.1 ± 2.1 U/g Hb (SD)	0.78 ± 0.13 mU/mol Hb
in RBC, whole blood	351 ± 60.6 U/1012 RBC	0.35 ± 0.06 nU/RBC
gamma glutamyltrans-ferase (GGT), serum		
Males	2–30 U/L (37°C)	0.03–0.51 μkat/L (37°C)
Females	1–24 U/L (37°C)	0.02–0.41 μkat/L (37°C)
glycated hemoglobin (hemoglobin A1C), whole blood	4.2%–5.9%	0.042–0.059
growth hormone, serum		
Male	<5 ng/mL	<5 μg/L
Female	<10 ng/mL	<10 μg/L
haptoglobin, serum	30–200 mg/dL	0.3–2.0 g/L
HDL-lipid panel		
cholesterol, HDL	>40 mg/dL	
cholesterol, LDL (calculated)		
optimal	<100 mg/dL	
near optimal	100–129 mg/dL	

TEST	CONVENTIONAL UNITS	SI UNITS
borderline high	130–159 mg/dL	
high	>160 mg/dL	
cholesterol, total		
0–1 y	50–120 mg/dL	
1–2 y	70–190 mg/dL	
2–16 y	120–220 mg/dL	
>16 y	0–199 mg/dL	
desirable	<200 mg/dL	
borderline	200–239 mg/dL	
high	>240 mg/dL	
triglycerides		
desirable	<150 mg/dL	
borderline high	150–199 mg/dL	
high	>200 mg/dL	
hematocrit (Hct)		
Males	42–52%	0.42–0.52
Females	37–47%	0.37–0.47
Newborns	53–65%	0.53–0.65
Children (varies with age)	30–43%	0.30–0.43
hemoglobin (Hb)		
Males	14.0–18.0 g/dL	2.17–2.79 mmol/L
Females	12.0–16.0 g/dL	1.86–2.48 mmol/L
Newborn	17.0–23.0 g/dL	2.64–3.57 mmol/L
Children (varies with age)	11.2–16.5 g/dL	1.74–2.56 mmol/L
hemoglobin, fetal	≤1 y old: <2% of total Hb	≤1 y old: <0.02% of total Hb
hemoglobin, plasma	<3 mg/dL	<0.47 mmol/L
hemoglobin electrophoresis, whole blood		
HbA		>0.95 Hb fraction
HbA2	1.5–3.7%	0.015–0.37 Hb fraction
HbF	<2%	<0.02 Hb fraction
beta hydroxybutyric acids, serum, plasma	0.21–2.81 mg/dL	20–270 μmol/L

Blood Values (continued)

TEST	CONVENTIONAL UNITS	SI UNITS
immunoglobulins (Ig), serum		
IgG	700–1600 mg/dL	7–16 g/L
IgA	70–400 mg/dL	0.7–4.0 g/L
IgM	40–230 mg/dL	0.42.3 g/L
IgD	0–8 mg/dL	0–80 mg/L
IgE	3–423 mg/dL	3–423 kIU/L
insulin (Fe) plasma (fasting)	2–25 μU/mL	13–174 pmol/L
iron, serum		
Males	65–175 μg/dL	11.6–31.3 μmol/L
Females	50–170 μg/dL	9.0–30.4 μmol/L
iron binding capacity, total (TBIC), serum	250–425 μg/dL	44.8–71.6 μmol/L
iron saturation, serum		
Male	20–50%	0.2–0.5
Female	15–50%	0.15–0.5
L-lactate		
Plasma		
Venous	4.5–19.8 mg/dL	0.5–2.2 mmol/L
Arterial	4.5–14.4 mg/dL	0.5–1.6 mmol/L
Whole blood, at bed rest		
Venous	8.1–15.3 mg/dL	0.9–1.7 mmol/L
Arterial	<11.3 mg/dL	<1.3 mmol/L
lactate dehydrogenase (LDH)		
Total (L→P), 37°C, serum		
Newborn	290–775 U/L	4.9–13.2 μkat/L
Neonate	545–2000 U/L	9.3–34 μkat/L
Infant	180–430 U/L	3.1–7.3 μkat/L
Child	110–295 U/L	1.9–5 μkat/L
Adult	100–190 U/L	1.7–3.2 μkat/L
>60 y	110–210 U/L	1.9–3.6 μkat/L
LDL-cholesterol (LDL-C), serum or plasma		
Adult desirable	<130 mg/dL	<3.37 mmol/L
borderline	130–159 mg/dL	3.37–4.12 mmol/L
high risk	≤160 mg/dL	≤4.13 mmol/L

TEST	CONVENTIONAL UNITS	SI UNITS
lead (Pb)		
Whole blood	<25 μg/dL	<1.2 μmol/L
lipase, serum	23–300 U/L (37°C)	0.39–5.1 μkat/L (37°C)
luteinizing hormone (LH), serum or plasma		
Male	1.24–7.8 mIU/mL	1.24–7.8 IU/L
Female		
Follicular phase	1.68–15.0 mIU/mL	1.68–15.0 IU/L
Midcycle peak	21.9–56.6 mIU/mL	21.9–56.6 IU/L
Luteal phase	0.61–16.3 mIU/mL	0.61–16.3 IU/L
Postmenopausal	14.2–52.5 mIU/mL	14.2–52.3 IU/L
magnesium, serum	1.3–2.1 mEq/L	0.65–1.07 mmol/L
magnesium, serum	1.6–2.6 mg/dL	16–26 mg/L
mercury (Hg)		
Whole blood	0.6–59 μg/L	<0.29 μmol/L
Toxic	>150 μg/d	>0.75 μmol/d
methemoglobin, (MetHb), whole blood	0.06–0.24 g/dL or	9.3–37.2 μmol/L or
osmolality, serum	275–295 mOsm/kg serum water	275–295 mmol/kg serum water
osmotic fragility of RBC	Begins in 0.45–0.39% NaCl	Begins in 77–67 mmol/L NaCl
oxygen (O2) blood, capacity	16–24 vol% (varies with hemoglobin)	7.14–10.7 mmol/L (varies with hemoglobin)
O2 Content		
Arterial	15–23 vol%	6.69–10.3 mmol/L
Venous	10–16 vol%	4.46–7.14 mmol/L
O2 Saturation		
Arterial and capillary	95–98% of capacity	0.95–0.98 of capacity
Venous	60–85% of capacity	0.60–0.85 of capacity
O2 tension (partial pressure)		
PO2 arterial and capillary	83–108 mmHg	11.1–14.4 kPa
Venous	35–45 mmHg	4.6–6.0 kPa
P50 (blood O2 pressure at which (Hb) is half saturated with O2)	25–29 mmHg (adjusted to pH 7.4)	3.33–3.86 kPa

Blood Values (continued)

TEST	CONVENTIONAL UNITS	SI UNITS
partial thromboplastin time activated (APTT)	<35 sec	<35 sec
pH		
Blood, arterial	7.35–7.45	7.35–7.45
phenylalanine, serum	0.8–1.8 mg/dL	48–109 μmol/L
phosphatase, alkaline (alkphos), total, serum	38–126 U/L (37°C)	0.65–2.14 μkat/L
phosphate, inorganic, serum		
Adults	2.7–4.5 mg/dL	0.87–1.45 mmol/L
Children	4.5–5.5 mg/dL	1.45–1.78 mmol/L
phospholipids, serum	125–275 mg/dL	1.25–2.75 g/L
potassium (K), plasma		
Males	3.5–4.5 mmol/L	3.5–4.5 mmol/L
Females	3.4–4.4 mmol/L	3.4–4.4 mmol/L
potassium (K), serum		
Premature		
Cord	5.0–10.2 mmol/L	5.0–10.2 mmol/L
48 h	3.0–6.0 mmol/L	3.0–6.0 mmol/L
Newborn cord	5.6–12.0 mmol/L	5.6–12.0 mmol/L
Newborn	3.7–5.9 mmol/L	3.7–5.9 mmol/L
Infant	4.1–5.3 mmol/L	4.1–5.3 mmol/L
Child	3.4–4.7 mmol/L	3.4–4.7 mmol/L
Adult	3.5–5.1 mmol/L	3.5–5.1 mmol/L
prealbumin (transthyretin), serum	10–40 mg/dL	100–400 mg/L
progesterone, serum		
Adult		
Male	13–97 ng/dL	0.4–3.1 nmol/L
Female		
Follicular phase	15–70 ng/dL	0.5–2.2 nmol/L
Luteal phase	200–2500 ng/dL	6.4–79.5 nmol/L
Pregnancy	Varies with gestational week	
prolactin, serum		
Males	2.5–15.0 ng/mL	2.5–15.0 μg/L
Females	2.5–19.0 ng/mL	2.5–19.0 μg/L

TEST	CONVENTIONAL UNITS	SI UNITS
prostate-specific antigen (PSA), serum		
Male	<4.0 ng/mL	<4.0 μg/L
protein, serum		
Total	6.4–8.3 g/dL	64–83 g/L
Albumin	3.9–5.1 g/dL	39–51 g/L
Globulin		
alpha1	0.2–0.4 g/dL	2–4 g/L
alpha2	0.4–0.8 g/dL	4–8 g/L
beta	0.5–1.0 g/dL	5–10 g/L
gamma	0.6–1.3 g/dL	6–13 g/L
prothrombin, consumption	>20 sec	>20 sec
prothrombin time-international normalized ratio (PT-INR)		
INR: birth–6 mo	1.0–1.6	
INR: ± mo–adult	0.9–1.2	
protoporphyrin, total, whole blood	<60 μg/dL	<600 μmg/L
pyruvate, blood	0.3–0.9 mg/dL	34–103 μmol/L
sedimentation rate, erythrocyte (ESR, sed rate)		
Westergren		
Male: 0–50 y	0–15 mm/h	
Male: ≤50 y	0–20 mm/h	
Female: 0–50 y	0–20 mm/h	
Female: ≤50 y	0–30 mm/h	
Wintrobe		
Males	<10 mm/h	
Females	<20 mm/h	
Critical value	>75 mm/h	

Blood Values (continued)

TEST	CONVENTIONAL UNITS	SI UNITS
sodium (Na)		
Serum or plasma		
Premature		
Cord	116–140 mmol/L	116–140 mmol/L
48 h	128–148 mmol/L	128–148 mmol/L
Newborn, cord	126–166 mmol/L	126–166 mmol/L
Newborn	133–146 mmol/L	133–146 mmol/L
Infant	139–146 mmol/L	139–146 mmol/L
Child	138–145 mmol/L	138–145 mmol/L
Adult	136–145 mmol/L	136–145 mmol/L
Normal	10–40 mmol/L	10–40 mmol/L
Cystic fibrosis	70–190 mmol/L	70–190 mmol/L
testosterone, serum		
Male	280–1100 ng/dL	0.52–38.17 nmol/L
Female	15–70 ng/dL	0.52–2.43 nmol/L
Pregnancy	3–4 × normal	3–4 × normal
Postmenopausal	8–35 ng/dL	0.28–1.22 nmol/L
thyroid-stimulating hormone (TSH), serum	0.4–4.2 µU/mL	0.4–4.2 mU/L
thyroxine (T4) serum	5–12 µg/dL (varies with age, higher in children and pregnant women)	65–155 nmol/L (varies with age, higher in children and pregnant women)
thyroxine, free, (free T4), serum	0.8–2.7 ng/dL	10.3–35 pmol/L
thyroxine binding globulin (TBG), serum	1.2–3.0 mg/dL	12–30 mg/L
transferrin, serum		
Newborn	130–275 mg/dL	1.30–2.75 g/L
Adult	212–360 mg/dL	2.12–3.60 g/L
>60 yr	190–375 mg/dL	1.9–3.75 g/L
triglycerides, serum, fasting		
Desirable	<250 mg/dL	<2.83 mmol/L
Borderline high	250–500 mg/dL	2.83–5.67 mmol/L
Hypertriglyceridemia	>500 mg/dL	>5.65 mmol/L
triiodothyronine, total (T3) serum	100–200 ng/dL	1.54–3.8 nmol/L

TEST	CONVENTIONAL UNITS	SI UNITS
troponin-I, cardiac, serum	undetectable	undetectable
troponin-T, cardiac, serum	undetectable	undetectable
urea nitrogen, (BUN) serum	6–20 mg/dL	2.1–7.1 mmol urea/L
urea nitrogen/creatinine ratio, (BUN:Cr) serum	12:1 to 20:1	48–80 urea/creatinine mole ratio
uric acid		
Serum, enzymatic		
Male	4.5–8.0 mg/dL	0.27–0.47 mmol/L
Female	2.5–6.2 mg/dL	0.15–0.37 mmol/L
Child	2.0–5.5 mg/dL	0.12–0.32 mmol/L
viscosity, serum	1.00–1.24 cP	1.00–1.24 cP

URINE TESTS	SYNONYMS/DESCRIPTION	QUANTITY/DESCRIPTION
Urine analysis (routine)	*urine, urinalysis, dip, macroscopic*	
color (not mentioned unless abnormal)	*red, brown, orange, green black*	
odor (not mentioned unless abnormal)	*fruity, fetid, maple syrup*	
appearance	*clear, slightly hazy, hazy, slightly cloudy, cloudy, turbid*	
specific gravity		one point ten transcribed 1.010 ten-twenty transcribed 1.020
pH (not mentioned unless abnormal)		4.8–7.5 (normal range)
protein (albumin)		negative, trace
glucose		normal, (or multiples of 50)
bilirubin		negative, 1+, 2+, 3+
urobilinogen		0.1 to 0.8 (at 2 hours)
ketones		trace, 1+, 2+, 3+
leukocyte esterase	*leukesterase, leukoesterase*	small, moderate, large, negative
nitrite		positive, negative
blood (not mentioned unless abnormal)	*gross blood*	negative, trace, small, large
Microscopic		
RBCs per high-power field (HPF)		few, many, 0-3 normal, too numerous to count (TNTC)
WBCs per high-power field (HPF)		few, many, 3-5 normal, too numerous to count (TNTC)
epithelial cells per low-power field (LPF)	*squamous epithelial, epi*	rare, few, many
casts (not mentioned unless abnormal)	*hyaline, granular, cellular cast, red cell cast white cell cast, epithelial cell cast, coarsely granular, finely granular, fatty, waxy*	negative, few, many

URINE TESTS	SYNONYMS/DESCRIPTION	QUANTITY/DESCRIPTION
crystals (not mentioned unless abnormal)		few, many, 1+, 2+, 3+
yeast cells (not mentioned unless abnormal)		rare, few, many, 1+, 2+, 3+
parasites (not mentioned unless abnormal)		rare, few, many, 1+, 2+, 3+
bacteria (not mentioned unless abnormal)		trace, few, many, 1+, 2+, 3+

Normal urinalysis, proper format:
Urinalysis revealed specific gravity of 1.010, negative protein, negative nitrites, negative leukocyte esterase. Microscopic showed 0-3 RBCs, 3-5 WBCs, few squamous epithelial cells.

Abnormal urinalysis, as dictated (bold terms need to be replaced with formal terms):

Urine dipped negative for ketones, spec grav of **ten-twenty**, 2+ protein, positive **nitrates**, positive **leukesterase**, large blood, white cells **TNTC**, red cells 500, many bacteria.

Abnormal urinalysis, as transcribed:
Dip urinalysis revealed negative ketones, specific gravity of 1.020, 2+ protein, positive nitrites, positive leukocyte esterase, large blood Microscopic showed white cells too numerous to count, 500 red cells, many bacteria.

Urine Toxicology Screen (abnormal values test and institution dependent)
amphetamine
barbiturates
benzodiazepine
cocaine
heroin/opiates/morphine
marijuana
methadone
methamphetamine
phencyclidine (PCP)

Urine Test Values

TEST	CONVENTIONAL UNITS	SI UNITS
acetone, urine		
qualitative	Negative	Negative
albumin, urine		
qualitative	Negative	Negative
quantitative	50–80 mg/24 h	50–80 mg/24 h
aldosterone, urine		
alpha-aminolevulinic acid, urine	1.3–7.0 mg/24 h	10–53 μmol/24 h
amylase, urine		
cadmium, urine, 24 h	1–17 U/h	0.017–0.29 μkat/h
calcium, urine	<15 μg/d	<0.13 μmol/d
low calcium diet		
usual diet, trough	50–150 mg/24 h	1.25–3.75 mmol/24 h
catecholamines, urine	100–300 mg/24 h	2.50–7.50 mmol/24 h
dopamine		
epinephrine	65–400 μg/24 h	425–2610 nmol/24 h
norepinephrine	0–20 μg/24 h	0–109 nmol/24
chloride, urine, 24 h	15–80 μg/24 h	89–473 nmol/24
values vary greatly with Cl intake		
infant	2–10 mmol/24 h	2–10 mmol/24 h
child	15–40 nmol/24 h	15–40 mmol/24 h
adult	110–250 mmol/24 h	110–250 mmol/24 h
chorionic gonadotropin, intact, urine, qualitative		
male and nonpregnant female	Negative	Negative
pregnant female	Positive	Positive
copper, urine	3–35 μg/24 h	0.05–0.55 μmol/24 h
cortisol, free urine	<50 μg/24 h	<138 mmol/24 h
creatinine, urine		
male	14–26 mg/kg body	124–230 μmol/kg body
female	11–20 mg/kg body weight/24 h	97–177 μmol/kg body weight/24 h

TEST	CONVENTIONAL UNITS	SI UNITS
creatinine clearance, serum or plasma and urine		
male	94–140 mL/min/1.73 m^2	0.91–1.35 mL/s/m^2
female	72–110 mL/min/1.73 m^2	0.69–1.06 mL/s/m^2
cyclic AMP, urine, 24 h	0.3–3.6 mg/d	100–723 mmol/d or
	or 0.29–2.1 mg/g creatinine	100–723 mmol/mol creatinine
cystine or cysteine, urine, qualitative	Negative	Negative
hemoglobin and myoglobin, urine, qualitative	Negative	Negative
homogentisic acid, urine, qualitative	Negative	Negative
17-hydroxycorticosteroids, urine		
males	3–10 mg/24 h	8.3–27.6 μmol/24 h (as cortisol)
females	2–8 mg/24 h	5.5–22 μmol/24 h (as cortisol)
5-hydroxylindoleacetic acid, urine		
qualitative	Negative	Negative
quantitative	2–7 mg/24 h	10.4–36.6 μmol/24 h
17-ketosteroids, urine		
males	10–25 mg/24 h	38–87 μmol/24 h
females	6–14 mg/24 h (decreases with age)	21–52 μmol/24 h (decreases with age)
L-lactate, urine, 24 h	496–1982 mg/d	5.5–22 mmol/d
lead, urine, 24 h	<80 μg/d	<0.39 μmol/d
magnesium, urine	6.0–10.0 mEq/24 h	3.0–5.0 mmol/24 h
mercury, urine, 24 h	<20 μg/d	<0.01 μmol/d
toxic	>150 μg/d	>0.75 μmol/d
metanephrines, total, urine	0.1–1.6 mg/24 h	0.5–8.1 μmol/24 h
osmolality, urine	50–1200 mOsm/kg water	50–1200 mmol/kg water
ratio, urine:serum	1.0–3.0, 3.0–4.7 after 12 h fluid restriction	1.0–3.0, 3.0–4.7 after 12 h fluid restriction
pH, urine	4.6–8.0 (depends on diet)	Same

Common Lab Tests

Urine Test Values (continued)

TEST	CONVENTIONAL UNITS	SI UNITS
penosulfonphthalein excretion (PSP), urine	28–51% in 15 min	0.28–0.51 in 15 min
	13–24% in 30 min	0.13–0.24 in 30 min
	9–17% in 60 min	0.09–0.17 in 60 min
	3–10% in 2 h	0.03–0.10 in 2 h
	(After injection of 1 mL PSP IV)	(After injection of 1 mL PSP IV)
phosphorus, urine	0.4–1.3 g/24 h	12.9–42 mmol/24 h
porphobilinogen, urine		
qualitative	Negative	Negative
quantitative	<2.0 mg/24 h	<9 μmol/24 h
porphyrins, urine		
coproporphyrin	34–230 μg/24 h	52–351 nmol/ 24 h
uroporphyrin	27–52 μg/24 h	32–63 nmol/ 24 h
potassium		
urine, 24 h	25–125 mmol/d; varies with diet	25–125 mmol/d; varies with diet
protein, urine		
qualitative	Negative	Negative
quantitative	50–80 mg/24 h (at rest)	50–80 mg/24 h (at rest)
sodium, urine, 24 h	40–220 mEq/d (diet dependent)	40–220 mmol/d (diet dependent)
specific gravity, urine	1.002–1.030	1.002–1.030
thiocyanate, urine		
nonsmoker	1–4 mg/d	17–69 μmol/d
smoker	7–17mg/d	120–292 μmol/d
uric acid, urine	250–750 mg/24 h (with normal diet)	1.48–4.43 mmol/24 h (with normal diet)
urobilinogen, urine	0.1–0.8 Ehrlich unit/2 h	0.1–0.8 EU/2 h
vanillylmandelic acid (VMA), urine (4-hydroxy-3-methoxymandelic acid)	1.4–6.5 mg/24 h	7–33 μmol/d

Other Values

TEST	CONVENTIONAL UNITS	SI UNITS
albumin, cerebrospinal fluid	10–30 mg/dL	100–300 mg/dL
bone marrow, differential cell count, adult		
undifferentiated cells	0–1%	0–0.01
myeloblast	0–2%	0–0.02
promyelocyte	0–4%	0–0.04
myelocytes		
neutrophilic	5–20%	0.05–0.20
eosinophilic	0–3%	0–0.03
basophilic	0–1%	0–0.01
metamyelocytes and bands		
neutrophilic	5–35%	0.05–0.35
eosinophilic	0–5%	0–0.05
basophilic	0–1%	0–0.01
segmented neutrophils	5–15%	0.05–0.15
pronormoblast	0–1.5%	0–0.015
basophilic normoblast	0–5%	0–0.05
polychromatophilic normoblast	5–30%	0.05–0.30
orthochromatic normoblast	5–10%	0.05–0.10
lymphocytes	10–20%	0.10–0.20
plasma cells	0–2%	0–0.02
monocytes	0–5%	0–0.05
chloride, sweat		
normal	5–35 mmol/L	5–35 mmol/L
cystic fibrosis	60–200 mmol/L	60–200 mmol/L
chloride, cerebrospinal fluid	118–332 mmol/L (20 mmol/L higher than serum)	118–332 mmol/L (20 mmol/L higher than serum)
fat, fecal, 72 h		
infant, breast-fed	<1 g/d	
pediatrics (0–6 y)	<2 g/d	
adults	<7 g/d	
adult (fat-free diet)	<4 g/d	

TEST	CONVENTIONAL UNITS	SI UNITS
lecithin:sphingomyelin ratio (L:S), amniotic fluid	2.0–5.0 indicates probable fetal lung	2.0–5.0 indicates probable fetal lung
	maturity; >3.5 in diabetic patients	maturity; >3.5 in diabetic patients
occult blood, feces, random	Negative (<2 mL blood/150 g stool/d)	Negative (<13.3 mL blood/kg stool/d)
phosphatidylglycerol (PG), amniotic fluid		
fetal lung immaturity	Absent	Same
fetal lung maturity	Present	Same
potassium, premature, cord	5.0–10.2 mmol/L	5.0–10.2 mmol/L
potassium, newborn, cord	5.6–12.0 mmol/L	5.6–12.0 mmol/L
potassium, cerebrospinal fluid	70% of plasma level or 2.5–3.2 mmol/L; rises with plasma hyperosmolality	0.70 of plasma level; rises with plasma hyperosmolality
protein, cerebrospinal fluid, total	8–32 mg/dL	80–320 mg/dL
sodium, premature, cord	116–140 mmol/L	116–140 mmol/L
sodium, premature, cord, 48 h	128–148 mmol/L	128–148 mmol/L
sodium, newborn, cord	126–166 mmol/L	126–166 mmol/L
sodium, sweat		
normal	10–40 mmol/L	10–40 mmol/L
cystic fibrosis	70–190 mmol/L	70–190 mmol/L

Dictation Samples

AMI PANEL
CPK was 1291, myoglobin was 171, troponin-I was 48, and CPK-MB was 50.59.

ARTERIAL BLOOD GAS
ABG showed a pH of 7.19, a PCO_2 of 65 and a PO_2 of 45, bicarbonate of 24, and an oxygen saturation of 90%.

CBC WITH DIFFERENTIAL
Initial CBC showed a white blood cell count of 3800, hemoglobin of 13.2, hematocrit of 37.2, MCV of 86, and platelets of 224,000 with 63% segmented neutrophils, 28% lymphocytes, 4% monocytes, 4% eosinophils, and 2% basophils.

CHEM-7
On admission, sodium was 137, potassium was 4.4, chloride was 96, CO_2 was 29, glucose was 110, BUN was 30, and creatinine was 1.2.

CHOLESTEROL PROFILE
Total cholesterol was 223 with an HDL of 51, triglycerides of 87, LDL of 155, and cholesterol/HDL ratio of 4.4.

ELECTROLYTE RESULTS
Sodium was 137, potassium was 4.4, chloride was 96, bicarbonate was 29.

KIDNEY FUNCTION TESTS
BUN was 30, and creatinine was 1.2.

LIVER FUNCTION TESTS
Liver function tests showed an SGOT of 61, alkaline phosphatase of 40, SGPT of 138, bilirubin of 9.

THYROID FUNCTION TESTS
The patient's T_3 was 147, free T_4 was 7, and TSH was 1.2.

Drugs of Abuse, Toxicology, and Therapeutic Drug Levels

The following drugs and substances can be identified in various body fluids by rapid screens and more formal chemistry, immunoassay, GCMS, and other procedures. Normal or allowable levels depend on region, type of test, and other complex variables. This list is provided for name reference only.

DRUGS OF ABUSE
chloral hydrate
ethchlorvynol
phenolphthalein
salicylic acid
senna

CLASSES OF DRUGS
cannabinoids
cocaine metabolites
methadone
amphetamines
  amphetamine
  methamphetamine
  methylenedioxyamphetamine (MDA)
  methylenedioxymethamphetamine
    (MDMA)
barbiturates
  amobarbital
  butabarbital
  butalbital
  pentobarbital
  phenobarbital
  secobarbital

benzodiazepines
  alprazolam
  bromazepam
  chlordiazepoxide
  clonazepam
  diazepam
  flunitrazepam
  flurazepam
  lorazepam
  midazolam
  nitrazepam
  oxazepam
  temazepam
  triazolam
opiates
  codeine
  hydrocodone
  morphine
  hydromorphone

INDIVIDUAL SUBSTANCES IDENTIFIED IN LABORATORY (list not intended to be exhaustive). These include medications, naturally occurring substances, poison, drugs of abuse. Generic names only.

acetaminophen	amoxapine	benzoylecgonine
amantadine	amphetamine	benztropine
amitriptyline	anileridine	benzydamine
amobarbital	benzocaine	biperiden

bromazepam
brompheniramine
bupivacaine
bupropion
buspirone
butacaine
butalbital
butorphanol
caffeine
canrenone
carbamazepine
carisoprodol
chlordiazepoxide
chlorophenylpiperazine
chloroquine
chlorpromazine
citalopram
clobazam
clomipramine
clonazepam
clonidine
clozapine
cocaethylene
cocaine
codeine
cotinine
cyclobenzaprine
desethylchloroquine
desipramine
dextromethorphan
diacetylmorphine
diazepam
diclofenac
diethylpropion
diltiazem
diphenhydramine
dilantin
disopyramide
doxepin
doxylamine
ecgonine methyl ester
EDDP
emetine
enalapril

ephedrine/pseudoephedrine
erythromycin
ethosuximide
fluconazole
flunitrazepam
flurazepam
fenfluramine
fenoprofen
fentanyl
fluoxetine
guaifenesin
heroin
hydrocodone
hydrocortisone
hydromorphone
hydroxyzine
ibuprofen
imipramine
indomethacin
ketamine
labetalol
lamotrigine
lidocaine
loratidine
lorazepam
loxapine
maprotiline
MDA
MDMA
meclizine
meclofenamic acid
mefenamic acid
methadone
methamphetamine
methaqualone
metronidazole
meperidine
mephobarbital
mepivacaine
meprobamate
methocarbamol
methotrimeprazine
methylphenidate
methylprednisolone

methyprylon
metoclopramide
metoprolol
mexiletine
midazolam
mirtazepine
moclobemide
6-monoacetylmorphine
morphine
naltrexone
naproxen
nefazodone
nevirapine
nicotine
nitrazepam
nizatidine
nordiazepam
nortriptyline
olanzapine
ondansetron
orphenadrine
oxazepam
oxybenzone
oxycodone
paroxetine
pentazocine
pentobarbital
pentoxyphylline
perphenazine
pethidine
phencyclidine
pheniramine
phenmetrazine
phenobarbital
phentermine
phenylpropanolamine
phenyltolaxamine
phenytoin
prednisolone
primidone
procainamide
procyclidine
procaine
prochlorperazine

Appendix 9

promethazine
propoxyphene
propranolol
psilocin
pseudoephedrine
pyrilamine
quetiapine
quinapril
quinidine
quinine
ranitidine
rofecoxib
ropivacaine
secobarbital
seroquel

sertraline
sildenafil
starnoc
strychnine
theophylline
thiopental
thioridazine
thymol
tolbutamide
topiramate
tramadol
tranylcypromine
trazodone
triamterene
triazolam

trihexyphenidyl
trimeprazine
trimethoprim
trimipramine
tripelennamine
tripolidine
valproate
venlafaxine
verapamil
xylometazoline
zaleplon
zimelidine
zolpidem
zopiclone

2-ethylidene-1,5-dimethyl3,3-diphenylpyrrolidine (EDDP)

Drug Values

TEST	CONVENTIONAL UNITS	SI UNITS
acetaminophen, serum or plasma		
therapeutic	10–30 μg/mL	66–199 μmol/L
toxic	>200 μg/ml	>1324 μmol/L
amikacin, serum or plasma		
therapeutic		
peak	25–35 μg/mL	43–60 μmol/L
trough		
less severe infection	1–4 μg/mL	1.7–6.8 μmol/L
life-threatening infection	4–8 μg/mL	6.8–13.7 μmol/L
toxic		
peak	>35–40 μg/mL	>60–68 μmol/L
trough	>10–15 μg/mL	>17–26 μmol/L
amitriptyline, serum or plasma		
trough (≤12 h after dose)		
therapeutic	80–250 ng/mL	289–903 nmol/L
toxic	>500 ng/mL	>1805 nmol/L
arsenic		
whole blood	0.2–2.3 μg/dL	0.03–0.31 μmol/L
chronic poisoning	10–50 μg/dL	1.33–6.65 μmol/L
acute poisoning	60–930 μg/dL	7.98–124 μmol/L
urine, 24 h	5–50 μg/d	0.07–0.67 μmol/d
ascorbic acid, plasma	0.4–1.5 mg/dL	23–85 μmol/L
cadmium, whole blood	0.1–0.5 μg/dL	8.9–44.5 nmol/L
toxic	10–300 μg/dL	0.89–26.70 μmol/L
cadmium, urine, 24 h	<15 μg/d	<0.13 μmol/d
carbamazepine, serum or plasma, trough		
therapeutic	4–12 μg/mL	17–51 μmol/L
toxic	>15 μg/mL	>63 μmol/L
carotene, serum	10–85 μg/dL	0.19–1.58 μmol/L
chloramphenicol, serum or plasma, trough		
therapeutic	10–25 μg/mL	31–77 μmol/L
toxic	>25 μg/mL	>77 μmol/L

Drugs of Abuse & Toxicology

A81

TEST	CONVENTIONAL UNITS	SI UNITS
clonazepam, serum or plasma, trough		
therapeutic	15–60 ng/mL	48–190 nmol/L
toxic	>80 ng/mL	>254 nmol/L
	weight/24 h	weight/24 h
female	11–20 mg/kg body	97–177 μmol/kg body
	weight/24 h	weight/24 h
cyanide, serum		
nonsmokers	0.004 mg/L	0.15 μmol/L
smokers	0.006 mg/L	0.23 μmol/L
nitroprusside therapy	0.01–0.06 mg/L	0.38–2.30 μmol/L
toxic	>0.1 mg/L	>3.84 μmol/L
cyanide, whole blood		
nonsmokers	0.016 mg/L	0.61 μmol/L
smokers	0.041 mg/L	1.57 μmol/L
nitroprusside therapy	0.05–0.5 mg/L	1.92–19.20 μmol/L
toxic	>1 mg/L	>38.40 μmol/L
cyclosporine, whole blood, therapeutic, trough	100–200 ng/mL	83–166 nmol/L
desipramine, serum or plasma, trough		
12 h after last dose		
therapeutic	75–300 ng/mL	281–1125 nmol/L
toxic	>400 ng/mL	>1500 nmol/L
diazepam, serum or plasma, trough		
therapeutic	100–1000 ng/mL	0.35–3.51 μmol/L
toxic	>5000 ng/mL	>17.55 μmol/L
dibucaine inhibition	79–84%	0.79–0.84
digitoxin, serum or plasma, 7.8 h after dose		
therapeutic	20–35 ng/mL	26–46 nmol/L
toxic	>45 ng/mL	>59 nmol/L

TEST	CONVENTIONAL UNITS	SI UNITS
digoxin, serum or plasma, ≥12 h after dose		
therapeutic		
congestive heart failure	0.8–1.5 ng/mL	1.0–1.9 nmol/L
arrhythmias	1.5–2.0 ng/mL	1.9–2.6 nmol/L
toxic		
adult	>2.5 ng/mL	>3.2 nmol/L
child	>3.0 ng/mL	>3.8 nmol/L
disopyramide, serum or plasma, trough		
therapeutic arrhythmias		
atrial	2.8–3.2 μg/mL	8.3–9.4 μmol/L
aentricular	3.3–7.5 μg/mL	9.7–22 μmol/L
toxic	> 7 μg/mL	20.7 μmol/L
doxepin, serum or plasma, trough (=12 h after dose)		
therapeutic	150–250 ng/mL	537–895 nmol/L
toxic	>500 ng/mL	>1790 nmol/L
ethanol, EtOH, (alcohol), whole blood or serum		
depression of CNS	>100 mg/dL	>21.7 mmol/L
fatalities reported	>400 mg/dL	>86.8 mmol/L
ethosuximide, serum or plasma, trough		
therapeutic	40–100 μg/mL	283–708 μmol/L
toxic	>150 μg/mL	1062 μmol/L
fluoride		
plasma	0.01–0.2 μg/mL	0.5–10.5 μmol/L
urine	0.2–3.2 μg/mL	10.5–168 μmol/L
urine, occupational exposure	<8 μg/mL	<421 μmol/L
fluoride inhibition	58–64%	0.58–0.64
gentamicin, serum or plasma		
therapeutic		
peak		
less severe infection	5–8 μg/mL	10.4–16.7 μmol/L
severe infection	8–10 μg/mL	16.7–20.9 μmol/L

TEST	CONVENTIONAL UNITS	SI UNITS
trough		
less severe infection	<1 µg/mL	<2.1 µmol/L
moderate infection	<2 µg/mL	<4.2 µmol/L
severe infection	<2–4 µg/mL	<4.2–8.4 µmol/L
toxic		
peak	>10–12 µg/mL	>21–25 µmol/L
trough	>2–4 µg/mL	>4.2–8.4 µmol/L
imipramine, serum or plasma, trough ≥12 h after dose		
therapeutic	150–250 ng/mL	536–893 nmol/L
toxic	>500 ng/mL	>1785 nmol/L
lead		
whole blood	<25 µg/dL	<1.2 µmol/L
urine, 24 h	<80 µg/d	<0.39 µmol/d
lidocaine, serum or plasma, 45 minutes after bolus		
therapeutic	1.5–6.0 µg/mL	6.4–26 µmol/L
toxic		
CNS, cardiovascular depression	6–8 µg/mL	26–34.2 µmol/L
seizures, obtundation, decreased cardiac output	>8 µg/mL	>34.2 µmol/L
lithium, serum or plasma, 12 h after last dose		
therapeutic	0.6–1.2 mmol/L	0.6–1.2 mmol/L
toxic	>2 mmol/L	>2 mmol/L
lorazepam, serum or plasma therapeutic	50–240 ng/mL	156–746 nmol/L
mercury		
whole blood	0.6–59 µg/L	<0.29 µmol/L
urine, 24 h	<20 µg/d	<0.01 µmol/d
toxic	>150 µg/d	>0.75 µmol/d

TEST	CONVENTIONAL UNITS	SI UNITS
methotrexate, serum or plasma		
therapeutic	Variable	Variable
toxic		
1–2 wk after low-dose therapy	≥0.02 μmol/L	≥0.02 μmol/L
post-IV infusion 24 h	≥5 μmol/L	≥5 μmol/L
48 h	≥0.5 μmol/L	≥0.5 μmol/L
72 h	≥0.05 μmol/L	≥0.05 μmol/L
nortriptyline, serum or plasma, trough, ≥12 h after dose		
therapeutic	50–150 ng/mL	190–570 nmol/L
toxic	>500 ng/mL	>1900 nmol/L
N-acetylprocainamide, serum or plasma trough		
therapeutic	5–30 μg/mL	18–108 μmol/L
toxic	>40 μg/mL	>144 μmol/L
oxazepam, serum or plasma, therapeutic	0.2–1.4 μg/mL	0.70–4.9 μmol/L
pentobarbital, serum or plasma, trough		
therapeutic		
hypnotic	1.5 μg/mL	4–22 μmol/L
therapeutic coma	20–50 μg/mL	88–221 μmol/L
toxic	>10 μg/mL	>44 μmol/L
phenacetin, plasma		
therapeutic	1.30 μg/mL	6–167 μmol/L
toxic	50–250 μg/mL	279–1395 μmol/L
phenobarbital, serum or plasma, trough		
therapeutic	15–40 μg/mL	65–172 μmol/L
toxic		
slowness, ataxia, nystagmus	35–80 μg/mL	151–345 μmol/L
coma with reflexes	65–117 μg/mL	280–504 μmol/L
coma without reflexes	>100 μg/mL	>430 μmol/L

Drugs of Abuse & Toxicology

TEST	CONVENTIONAL UNITS	SI UNITS
phenytoin, serum or plasma, trough		
therapeutic	10–20 μg/mL	40–79 μmol/L
toxic	>20 μg/mL	>79 μmol/L
phosphatase, acid, prostatic, serum, RIA	<3.0 ng/mL	<3.0 μg/L
primidone, serum or plasma, trough		
therapeutic	5–12 μg/mL	23–55 μmol/L
toxic	>15 μg/mL	>69 μmol/L
procainamide, serum or plasma, trough		
therapeutic	4–10 μg/mL	17–42 μmol/L
toxic (also consider effect of metabolite NAPA)	>10–12 μg/mL	>42–51 μmol/L
propoxyphene, plasma		
therapeutic	0.1–0.4 μg/mL	0.3–1.2 μmol/L
toxic	>0.5 μg/mL	>1.5 μmol/L
propranolol, serum or plasma, trough		
therapeutic	50–100 ng/mL	193–386 nmol/L
quinidine, serum or plasma, trough		
therapeutic	2–5 μg/mL	6–15 μmol/L
toxic	>6 μg/mL	>18 μmol/L
salicylates, serum or plasma, trough		
therapeutic	150–300 μg/mL	1.09–2.17 mmol/L
toxic	>500 μg/mL	>3.62 mmol/L
theophylline, serum or plasma		
therapeutic		
bronchodilator	8–20 μg/mL	44–111 μmol/L
prem. apnea	6–13 μg/mL	33–72 μmol/L
toxic	>20 μg/mL	>110 μmol/L

TEST	CONVENTIONAL UNITS	SI UNITS
thiocyanate, serum or plasma		
nonsmoker	1–4 µg/mL	17–69 µmol/L
smoker	3–12 µg/mL	52–206 µmol/L
therapeutic after nitroprusside infusion	6–29 µg/mL	103–499 µmol/L
urine		
nonsmoker	1–4 mg/d	17–69 µmol/d
smoker	7–17 mg/d	120–292 µmol/d
thiopental, serum or plasma, trough		
hypnotic	1.0–5–0 µg/mL	4.1–20.7 µmol/L
coma	30–100 µg/mL	124–413 µmol/L
anesthesia	7–130 µg/mL	29–536 µmol/L
toxic concentration	>10 µg/mL	>41 µmol/L
tobramycin, serum or plasma		
therapeutic		
peak		
less severe infection	5–8 µg/mL	11–17 µmol/L
severe infection	8–10 µg/mL	17–21 µmol/L
trough		
less severe infection	<1 µg/mL	<2 µmol/L
moderate infection	<2 µg/mL	<4 µmol/L
severe infection	<2–4 µg/mL	<4–9 µmol/L
toxic		
peak	>10–12 µg/mL	>21–26 µmol/L
trough	>2–4 µg/mL	>4–9 µmol/L
	0.5–4.0 EU/d	0.5–4.0 EU/d
valproic acid, serum or plasma, trough		
therapeutic	50–100 µg/mL	347–693 µmol/L
toxic	>100 µg/mL	>693 µmol/L

TEST	CONVENTIONAL UNITS	SI UNITS
vancomycin, serum or plasma		
therapeutic		
peak	20–40 µg/mL	14–28 µmol/L
trough	5–10 µg/mL	3–7 µmol/L
toxic	>80–100 µg/mL	>55–69 µmol/L
vitamin A, serum	30–80 µg/dL	1.05–2.8 µmol/L
vitamin B12, serum	110–800 pg/mL	81–590 pmol/L
vitamin E, serum		
normal	5–18 µg/mL	12–42 µmol/L
therapeutic	30–50 µg/mL	69.6–116 µmol/L
zinc, serum	70–120 µg/dL	10.7–18.4 µmol/L

Common Pathology Report Terms & Guidelines

pathologist: a physician who practices, evaluates, or supervises diagnostic tests, using materials removed from living or dead patients, and functions as a laboratory consultant to clinicians, or who conducts experiments or other investigations to determine the causes or nature of disease changes.

pathology: the medical science, and specialty practice, concerned with all aspects of disease but with special reference to the essential nature, causes and development of abnormal conditions, as well as the structural and functional changes that result from the disease processes.

Pathology Report Common Heading Terms

comment: often incorporated into the body of the report or the diagnosis; may include information regarding technique and procedures used, pending studies, additional tests ordered, and physicians notified of results.

diagnosis (also clinical diagnosis or findings): sometimes postmortem, a determination made from an anatomic and/or histologic study of the specimens presented.

gross description (also gross examination): describes the specimen as viewed by the pathologist without magnification; description may be given by section; dye or ink may be used to mark margins; metric measurements used.

indication (also clinical history, clinical information): the basis for a diagnostic test.

microscopic description (also microscopic examination): describes what is seen when the sample is viewed under the microscope.

specimen (also sample): a small part, or sample, of any substance or material obtained for testing; describes what was submitted for pathological analysis; tissue, fluid, smear, etc.

Pathology Report Common Order for Heading Terms

pathology report, including surgical
indication (or clinical history)
diagnosis or findings (also may be placed near end of report)
specimen/sample
gross description
microscopic description
comment

Autopsy reports may include terminology and headings not found in other types of pathology reports. An example of common heading terms and their sequence is shown below.

autopsy report
manner of death
cause of death
findings
laboratory results
general appearance
identification
external examination
   clothing and valuables
   head and neck
   trunk
   extremities
   scars, tattoos, nevi, and incidental findings
   injuries
internal examination
procedures and specimens
   toxicology
   photography
   trace evidence
   chemistry and cultures
   firearms/weapons examination
   x-rays
   microscopic examination
comments/conclusion

Biopsy Techniques

Specimens or samples submitted for pathologic examination are often obtained through biopsy.

aspiration biopsy: any method in which the specimen for biopsy is removed by aspirating it through an appropriate needle or trocar that pierces the skin, or the external surface of an organ, and into the underlying tissue to be examined. Syn: needle biopsy.

brush biopsy: obtained by abrading the surface of a lesion with a brush to obtain cells and tissue for microscopic examination.

chorionic villus biopsy: transcervical or transabdominal sampling of the chorionic villi for genetic analysis.

endoscopic biopsy: biopsy obtained by instruments passed through an endoscope or obtained by a needle introduced under endoscopic guidance.

excision biopsy: excision of tissue for gross and microscopic examination in such a manner that the entire lesion is removed.

fine needle biopsy: the aspiration and removal of tissue or suspensions of cells through a small needle.

incision biopsy: removal of only a part of a lesion by incising into it.

needle biopsy: Syn: aspiration biopsy.

open biopsy: surgical incision or excision of the region from which the biopsy is taken.

punch biopsy: any method that removes a small cylindrical specimen for biopsy by means of a special instrument that pierces the organ directly or through the skin or a small incision in the skin. Syn: trephine biopsy.

sentinal node biopsy: biopsy preceded by injection of a dye or radioisotope proximal to a tumor to identify for excision the primary node draining the area; used to determine the extent of spread of a malignancy.

shave biopsy: a biopsy technique performed with a surgical blade or a razor blade; used for lesions that are elevated above the skin level or confined to the epidermis and upper dermis, or to protrusions of lesions from internal sites.

sponge biopsy: abrasion of a lesion with a suitable sponge.

trephine biopsy: Syn: punch biopsy.

wedge biopsy: excision of a cuneiform specimen.

Sample Reports

APPENDIX

SPECIMEN: Appendix.

GROSS DESCRIPTION: The specimen consists of a 6.4 × 3.6×3.2-cm vermiform appendix with surrounding fat. The appendiceal surface is covered with hemorrhagic, yellow purulent exudate with no obvious area of perforation identified. The appendiceal lumen is 0.6 cm in diameter and filled with a yellow-green purulent exudate. No fecaliths or masses are identified. The surrounding fat is markedly hemorrhagic.

MICROSCOPIC DESCRIPTION: Sections of the appendix reveal the appendiceal lumen to be patent to the tip. The lumen is filled with pus and blood. There is focal ulceration of the mucosa. The mucosa is colonic in type. There is transmural infiltration by polymorphonuclear leukocytes. There is no evidence of perforation. The serosal surface is heavily infiltrated by polymorphonuclear leukocytes and necrotic debris.

DIAGNOSIS: Appendix, acute appendicitis.

AUTOPSY REPORT

MANNER OF DEATH: Homicide.

CAUSE OF DEATH: Exsanguination from multiple stab wounds and incised wounds of head, neck, trunk and upper extremities.

FINDINGS

1. Generalized pallor and evidence of exsanguination.
2. Multiple stab and incised wounds of head, neck, trunk and upper extremities with 1 stab wound penetrating left skull into brain, 3 stab wounds penetrating right back into chest cavity and right lung, another stab wound at lateral right chest penetrating into right lung, and multiple wounds of upper extremities consistent with defensive injuries.
3. Left lower lateral chest wall abrasions and contusions with overlying rib fractures of left ribs 6, 7 and 8.
4. Subarachnoid hemorrhage of right cerebrum underlying one of the large, undermined right scalp incised wounds.
5. A few other minor blunt-force injuries of head and trunk.
6. Slight emphysematous changes of lungs.

LABORATORY RESULTS

1. Blood: Ethanol level of 0.14 g/100 mL. Cocaine present at less than 0.14 g/100 mL; quantity not sufficient for further examination.
2. Urine: Positive for cocaine and cocaine metabolite enzyme multiplied immunoassay test (EMIT) barbiturates screen.
3. Ocular fluid: Ethanol level of 0.14 g/100 mL.

GENERAL APPEARANCE: This is the body of a well-developed, well-nourished adult black male who appears his stated age. Body height is 72 inches, and body weight is 175 pounds. At autopsy, rigor mortis is generalized. Livor mortis is posterior and blanching . The body is cool to touch. Artifacts of decomposition are absent. There is no evidence of medical or postmortem care. There is obvious evidence of sharp-force injury in multiple regions.

IDENTIFICATION: Identification of the decedent was established by circumstances of death and discovery of the body.

EXTERNAL EXAMINATION

CLOTHING AND VALUABLES: Body submitted to the morgue clothed, within a sheet and body bag. The hands are bagged.

The clothing is very bloody, with injuries matching those found on the trunk. Prior to removal of clothing, trace evidence was collected from the body and clothing by the crime scene technician while I was in attendance. See section titled "Trace Evidence" found later in this report. Clothing consisting of white T-shirt, a pair of black slacks, black belt, black socks, and dress shoes. Valuables with the body include a Bic cigarette lighter, key ring containing 3 keys, cellular phone and $22.38 in cash. Valuables are released to brother of decedent. The body is retained by law enforcement.

HEAD AND NECK: Head is of normal shape. Scalp hair is short, dark brown and slightly curled. Head, face, neck and shoulders show no suffusion. Irides are brown. The pupils are equal and round. The sclerae are white. Conjunctivae with no petechiae. No ecchymosis in the periorbital region. Facial hair is present. Nasal and oral cavities show presence of a small amount of bloody mucus. Multiple caries present; oral hygiene is poor. No petechiae in the oral cavity. Neck with normal range of motion and no crepitus or deformities.

TRUNK: Chest is not increased in the anteroposterior dimension. There is dried blood over the xiphoid and sternal regions. No gynecomastia present. No palpable masses or discharge from the nipples. Abdomen is soft and slightly protuberant. There is no discoloration of the external wall. There are no natural abnormalities of the back or buttocks. The anus is moderately dilated with reddish circumferential ecchymosis;

there are no lacerations or scars visible. External genitalia normal for age, with no injuries.

EXTREMITIES: The extremities are symmetrical, without natural deformities. Lower extremities with no peripheral edema and no atrophy. Fingernails and toenails are short and even.

SCARS, TATTOOS, NEVI AND INCIDENTAL FINDINGS: Midline scar, consistent with laparotomy. Scar found on the right hand in the web space between the 1st and 2nd digits. Left ankle with surgical scar on the lateral aspect.

INJURIES: Multiple incised and stab wounds are present on the head, neck, chest, back and upper extremities. The number of wounds is too numerous to count and detail. In general, however, there are 28 or more on the head, 13 or more on the chest and back, and about 45 defensive incised wounds on the right and left hands and forearms. Most of the sharp-force injuries present are incised wounds, and most of the stab wounds are actually nonpenetrating of the body cavities, except as detailed below, and except for the deeper ones at the upper extremities. There are also some blunt-force injuries and some overlying rib fractures as noted below.

Many of the head wounds are irregular with slightly scalloped or curving borders, as discussed below. The forehead, the right face beside the nose, the lips on the right side, the left side of the head and ear, and the right side of the head have multiple incised wounds. At the forehead, the largest is 5 cm in length and is irregular and mostly vertical. Most of the incised wounds are diagonal, slanting from upper left to lower right, and are about 1.7 cm in length each. The longest, at the right face, is 5.3 cm long. Wounds on the lips are superficial. At the left side of the head are several marks, mostly diagonal downward and to the front and also passing along the left side of the forehead and the left side of the face. At the frontoparietal area is a V-shaped incision which appears to be 2 incisions crossing one another. There are also 5 short, jab-type incisions at the low left forehead. These just penetrate the outer table of the skull beneath this area, the largest being 0.3×0.2 cm. Just inferior and posterior to these jab wounds is a definite penetrating stab wound of the skull. At the skin this is diagonal, with the blunt end 0.1 cm to 0.2 cm in thickness, and being at the anteroinferior aspect of the diagonal stab wound, the acute angle at the superior-posterior aspect, and the wound is about 1.7 cm in length. At the skull, this makes a similar triangular-shaped wound, more horizontal over the left sphenoid bone, with a base thickness of 0.1 to 0.2 cm, with a length of 1.6 cm. The most anterior 1-cm aspect of this stab is the actual penetration of the skull. It passes approximately 3.6 cm through the skin and brain, passing into the brain at the inferolateral left frontal lobe, about 2 cm. This stab wound creates a permanent stab cavity 1 cm wide and 2 cm deep in that area. It just enters the tip of the left lateral ventricle and is accompanied by a slight intraventricular hemorrhage and also by a slight contusion of the white matter surrounding the injury.

The inferior border of the left ear has a prominent red band of abrasion and an upside-down, V-shaped vertical incision, 6 cm in length, passing through the center of the abrasion and onto the upper lateral left neck. The longest incision of the left face is 5 cm in length. At the right side of the head are multiple stab wounds varying from 1.1 to 5.7 cm in length and including a curving stab, 6.5 cm long, with undermining in the posterior direction. In front of the right ear is a 9.5-cm curving incision.

At the top of the head, located mostly on the right front side, is another group of incised wounds, the most prominent having slightly scalloped edges and being 2.2 cm long. At the upper lateral left side of the head are 3 wounds, 0.9 cm between each wound and parallel, each curving slightly and having slightly scalloped edges with the scalloping especially at the left, and with overlying, perpendicular, parallel, pale, reddish-purple abrasion and contusion lines over a total area of 2×3 cm.

Beginning at the middle of the upper right sternocleidomastoid muscle, the right posterolateral and posterior neck have deep, muscular incised wounds actually representing about 3 total cuts. The leftmost aspect has a 1-cm superficial cut, while the major cut passing over to the right posterolateral region is 13.5 cm in length. A separate 2-cm incision overlies the right posterolateral aspect of this incision and combines with the incision for an additional 9 cm, terminating at the right sternocleidomastoid muscle. More inferiorly, the right sternocleidomastoid muscle also has a smaller incision.

The head also has some blunt-force injuries, although these may be ragged incised wounds from a dull object. The back of the head has 5 parallel diagonal (upper left to lower right) lacerations with visible tissue bridging. The uppermost 2 wounds are the most superficial and may actually be incisions. They measure 1.5 cm long and 4.2 cm long, respectively. The lowest 2 are mostly on the left side and are 2.7 and 1.7 cm long respectively, and they have prominent abrasions and contusions around the edges. The back of the right ear also has a reddish-purple and reddish-black abrasion and contusion. The nasal bridge and tip of the nose have some abrasions and contusions. The left scalp above the ear has a linear vertical abrasion. The vertex of the head has a 2.3×0.6-cm irregular abrasion.

Inside the head, the right parietotemporal region of the cerebrum has a focal area of increased subarachnoid hemorrhage. Other than the stab wound at the left frontal lobe, the brain has no contusions, lacerations, subdural hematoma or other injuries. This does lie beneath the larger curving 6.5-cm incised wound discussed earlier. The spinal cord is not examined.

At the left midclavicular region of the upper left chest are some small skip-like abrasions. The midregion of the right clavicle of the upper chest also has a small area of abrasion. At the right parasternal chest is a 5-cm stab wound. The inferior border is slightly curved and has some slight contusions with slightly undulating edges at the inferior one fourth of the stab wound. The upper edge of the stab wound at the skin is squared off, 0.3 cm wide. The stab passes through the sternum in a roughly diagonal fashion with a blunt upper right edge and acute lower left edge, passing into the chest at the right 3rd intercostal space anteriorly. It passes posteriorly, slightly downward and to the right, and it just catches the outer edge of the right lung at the junction of the right upper and right middle lobes. The stab stops in the lung for a total of about 5 cm. Otherwise, the anterior chest has no stab wounds. Laterally, the right upper chest has a 1.7-cm stab wound, horizontal in orientation, with the posterior aspect acute and the anterior aspect blunt. This passes into the right posterolateral chest via the 3rd right intercostal space with no visible entry into the lung and with a depth of the stab greater than or equal to 6 cm.

The lateral left chest at the lower half has several irregular areas of mottled abrasions and contusions without pattern, the 2 largest being 3×0.3 cm and 1×1 cm. These overlie the fractures of the ribs with accompanying slight intercostal space contusion, mainly at the left lateral 6th rib, the left posterolateral 7th rib, and the left posterolateral 8th rib. The 7th rib has a parietal pleural perforation and the greatest amount of hemorrhage from contusion. These are injuries caused by blunt force. At the back, there are multiple shallow stabs and jab-type wounds along with some tiny superficial abrasions or incisions, all less than or equal to 0.3 cm. At the left upper shoulder posteriorly are 2 of the more prominent superficial stab wounds not passing into the chest, the upper right lateral wound being diagonally oriented and 2 cm long, and the more medial wound being 1.5 cm long and oriented horizontally. At the center of the back, slightly more on the right side of the spine than the left, are 7 parallel diagonal stabs. These all have roughly the same appearance on the skin, although their upper and lower edges are less distinct than other stab wounds on the body.

Of these wounds, 3 are chosen for representative measurements. The uppermost right stab of this group is 1.8 cm long and appears to have the blunt edge downward with a V-shaped acute edge superiorly. Bringing the 2 edges of the wound together creates almost a double V, although the inferior aspect is more of a shallow V than is the upper V. The inferiormost right wound in this group is 1.5 cm long and has a prominent inferior V with an acute superior edge. Bringing the 2 sides together creates no V at the top at all but instead makes the inferior V more prominent. The uppermost left wound of this group is 1.8 cm long and has a prominent upper blunt edge and an inferior acute edge. This wound, when the edges are brought together, is a simple slit. Three of the 4 stabs at the right side of this group penetrate the chest, with 1 stab wound going through the 6th posterior right intercostal space, one going through the 7th posterior right intercostal space, and 1 going through the 9th posterior right intercostal space. These go into the right chest cavity with only 1 injury penetrating the right lung for a total depth of greater than or equal to 5 cm. The 2 stab wounds to the left of the spine pass downward, medially and to the front, but they stop at the left lamina and left lateral side of the spinous processes of the back bone with a short overall distance for the stab of about 1.8 cm without penetration of the chest cavity.

As mentioned earlier, the upper extremities have multiple sharp-force injuries. At the anterior distal right wrist are several abrasions and lacerations with slight reddish-purple contusions, the longest 4.3×0.4 cm, and the most prominent being 1×1.5 cm. These are less clearly defined as incised wounds, although they may be from an irregular object. At the back of the right triceps area, almost exposing the bone, is a bloodless 19.5-cm gaping and deeply incised wound. The lateral proximal right shoulder and proximal arm have 3 incisions, the longest more distal and 1.6 cm long, with an irregular distal border suggestive of an acute angle and with a proximal border squared off and 0.2 to 0.3 cm in width. The back of the right forearm has some small abrasions and some small incised wounds toward the wrist. The distal right biceps area, just above the antecubital fossa, has 1 small incised wound.

The left distal forearm has a large gaping incised wound of 3×5 cm in surface area passing through the tendons. Just proximal to this is a 5×4-cm area of dried blood with abrasions and superficial incisions. Just proximal to that and more medial are 2 thin parallel linear abrasions.

The backs of the hands have multiple avulsed and oblique incisions and lacerations, mostly incisions, ranging from 1.5 to 3.2 cm in length. In addition, the back of the right hand has a larger gaping wound that is 5.3×3 cm in length, and the right wounds and the left dorsal wrist wounds have superimposed purple contusions. On the medial edge of the right thumb is a 1.3-cm incised wound which continues onto the thumb pad itself. At the palmar surface of the left hand are approximately 78 oblique incised wounds, the longest being 3.5 cm and having scalloped edges, another being 2.5 cm long and the others varying. The hands do have clumps of straight, long, possibly blond hairs adherent, especially at the left palm. These are collected.

Overall, most of the incised wounds of the trunk suggest a single-edged, thin blade; however, a double-edged blade cannot be excluded. Many of the head wounds, as well as the hand and forearm injuries, suggest a scalloped edge or scalloped object, and the multiple injuries of the hands and forearms are consistent with defensive injuries.

Internally, there is almost no blood present in the heart and great vessels and tissues due to exsanguination from all of these multiple wounds. X-rays of the head and neck and also the chest and upper abdomen show no obvious fractures or foreign bodies. The internal structures of the neck, including the carotid arteries, show no injuries except for the large neck injury passing into the muscle, as mentioned above. The heart and liver have no injuries. See above for stabs of right lung, stab of brain, left rib fractures and right brain subarachnoid hemorrhage.

INTERNAL EXAMINATION: In general, internal artifacts and injuries have been described above and will not be further detailed in this section.

The body cavities are opened in the standard autopsy fashion. The organs are present in their usual anatomic locations and relationships. Little blood is present in the pleural cavities, and there are some slight adhesions at the left upper lobe of the lung. There is no evidence of empyema, purulent exudate or acute inflammation of the serous cavities. There is no tissue discoloration suggestive for carbon monoxide intoxication or jaundice. There is a slight smell suggestive of alcoholic beverages within the body.

The gallbladder contains the usual bile. The stomach contains 30 mL of grayish mucoid fluid with curdled, small, soft, whitish lumps of mostly digested, unrecognizable food. There is no evidence of drug residue in the stomach. The vermiform appendix is present. The urinary bladder contains clear urine. In general, atherosclerosis is very mild. The heart has no evidence of infarction or scarring. The lungs have bullous emphysematous changes to a slight degree, mostly at the upper lobes. The right lung also has the stab wounds mentioned earlier. The liver appears pale but not fatty. The spleen, pancreas, kidneys, heart, adrenals, thyroid, pituitary, prostate and bladder are otherwise unremarkable. The testes show no contusions. The penis is circumcised.

Routine organ weights are as follows: heart, 365 g; right lung, 520 g; left lung, 570 g; liver, 1580 g; spleen, 80 g; pancreas, 165 g; right kidney, 150 g; left kidney, 170 g; brain, 1450 g.

PROCEDURES AND SPECIMENS

TOXICOLOGY: Blood, bile, urine, ocular fluid, nasal swabs.

PHOTOGRAPHY: Slide identification pictures, 35-mm. Instant-print photos are also taken of the scene and of many of the injuries.

TRACE EVIDENCE: Trace materials on tape from right shoulder and chest. Possible small glass fragment from left upper chest. Trace materials on tape from left shoulder, neck, chest. Glass fragments from back. Possible glass fragments from chest. Hairs adherent to right and left sleeves of shirt. Hairs adherent to left hand. One hair from inside oral cavity. Clippings from right fingernails and left fingernails. Adherent hairs from right hand. Purple-topped and red-topped tubes of blood are also collected and sent to the lab.

CHEMISTRY AND CULTURES: None.

FIREARMS EXAMINATION: None performed.

X-RAYS: See section titled "Injuries."

MICROSCOPIC EXAMINATION: Representative sections of major organ systems have been obtained and routinely processed onto glass slides for histologic examination. These have been reviewed.

The liver, heart and kidney are not remarkable aside from some moderately advanced autolysis, especially at the kidney. The lungs show diffuse moderate emphysematous changes, including septal fibrosis and an increased number of macrophages, along with congestion. The cerebrum shows acute petechial hemorrhages at the directed section from the stab-wound area, but otherwise the cerebrum is not remarkable. The anoderm shows no contusion, but it does have dilated submucosal vessels without significant inflammation or scarring. There are no additional significant findings.

BONE MARROW ASPIRATE, BIOPSY, AND PERIPHERAL BLOOD SMEAR

INDICATIONS: Acute promyelocytic anemia. Biopsy taken recently revealed no morphologic evidence of residual disease.

PROCEDURE PERFORMED: Bone marrow biopsy.

GROSS EXAMINATION: The specimen labeled "left bone marrow biopsy" is received in Bouin's solution and consists of 1 elongated, cylindrical, tan-brown fragment of bony material that measures 1.5×0.3×0.4 cm. The specimen is submitted entirely between sponges in a single cassette following decalcification.

PERIPHERAL BLOOD SMEAR: Red blood cells are normochromic and range from microcytic to normocytic. There is occasional polychromasia. A few scattered teardrop forms are identified. Platelets are normal in number with occasional large and hypogranular forms. White blood cells are normal in number, with a normal absolute number of neutrophils. White blood cells are predominantly normal-appearing, segmented neutrophils, with fewer numbers of lymphocytes and monocytes.

BONE MARROW ASPIRATE: The bone marrow aspirate is adequate. Megakaryocytes are present in slightly higher than normal numbers but with normal morphology . The myeloid/erythroid (M:E) ratio is 2:1 to 3:1. Myeloid precursors are normal in number with a left shift, without a relative increase in the number of promyelocytes or blasts. Erythroid precursors are present in normal numbers, also with a slight shift to the left. Iron stores are present within histiocytes; no ringed sideroblasts are identified.

BONE MARROW BIOPSY: The bone marrow biopsy is mildly hypercellular for age, approximately 70%. Megakaryocytes are present in normal numbers and morphology. The M:E ratio is 3:1. Myeloid and erythroid precursors are normal in number and fully mature. The myeloid precursors have a slight left shift. There are no excess blasts. There is an area of fibrosis that appears to be associated with subcortical bone.

COMMENT: The bone marrow aspirate and biopsy reveal left-shifted myelogenesis and erythrogenesis. There is no relative increase in the number of promyelocytes or blasts. Since morphology is limited in distinguishing normal myelogenesis from residual disease, correlation with cytogenetic and/or molecular studies is recommended.

DIAGNOSIS: Bone marrow aspirate, biopsy and peripheral blood smear. Mildly hypercellular marrow with left-shifted myeloid and erythroid maturation.

BREAST CARCINOMA AND OVARIAN TISSUE ANALYSIS

SPECIMENS

1. Right tube and ovary.

2. Left tube and ovary.
3. Right breast and right axillary nodes.
4. Left breast.

GROSS EXAMINATION: Specimen #1, right tube and ovary, received in formalin. Specimen consists of a 3×1-cm fallopian tube segment with a well-healed surgical stump. There is a 4×2.3×2.2-cm ovary with a ruptured capsular surface, gray-pink in color. Cut section of the specimen shows a hemorrhagic corpus luteal cyst and an adjacent edematous ovarian stroma.

Specimen #2, left tube and ovary, also received in formalin. Specimen consists of a 2.8×1-cm fallopian tube stump, including the fimbriated end, with an adjacent 1.5×0.6-cm thin-walled cyst. The ovary is attached, size being 2.5×2×1.5 cm. Ovary has an intact pale-yellow capsule that shows corpus luteal cyst on cut section.

The right side specimen, specimen #3, consists of right breast and right axillary nodes taken from a modified radical mastectomy. The breast weighs 300 g with a 6-cm axillary tail. There is a tan skin ellipse overlying the specimen, 10×5 cm in size. The specimen has a centrally placed everted nipple, and areola with multinodular appearance. Deep surgical margin is inked. Cut section shows lobules of yellow, soft adipose tissue with thin, rubbery, white fibrous bands in the specimen. In the midportion of the breast tissue, 2 cm above the deep resection margin and 2 cm below the skin surface, is a palpable mass, 3×2×2 cm in size. On cut section this mass shows a granular cut surface, tan-gray in color. Other masses are not identified in the specimen. The axillary tail is thin. Enlarged lymph nodes are not readily palpable or identified on gross examination.

Specimen #4 is tissue from the left side. This is from a modified radical mastectomy of the left breast. The breast weighs 280 g. The fatty breast tissue is lobulated and 15×14×6 cm in size. It has an axillary portion that is triangular in shape, measuring 7×5×2 cm. On the superior surface is an ellipse of skin, 7×3.5 cm, with a normal-appearing everted nipple. The deep surgical surface is covered by a white, fibrous membrane with some strands of skeletal muscle present. The breast tissue is sectioned in serial fashion and shows 85% lobulated homogenous fat with fibrous septa and a few areas of dense fibrous tissue beneath the areola. There are no large areas of cysts, tumor nodules or fibrosis. Section of the axillary tail reveals no lymph nodes on gross examination.

MICROSCOPIC EXAMINATION: Section of the left and right fallopian tubes is unremarkable. Both ovaries show benign corpus luteal cysts.

Sections of the right nipple show no evidence of Paget disease or dermal lymphatic tumor spread. Sections of the tumor mid breast show poorly differentiated infiltrating ductal carcinoma with an area of necrosis in the center. The tumor extends into the adjacent adipose tissue. The tumor is not identified at the inked surgical margin. Extensive intraductal component is not identified. The tumor is composed of infiltrating trabecular sheets and nests of moderately pleomorphic oval epithelial cells which contain a large oval to angulated nucleus with coarsely clumped nuclear chromatin and a moderate amount of eosinophilic cytoplasm. There are 4 to 5 mitotic figures seen per high-power field. Sections of adjacent breast tissue show fibrocystic changes and duct ectasia with cyst formation. Axillary lymph nodes, 3 in total, show no evidence of metastasis.

Sections of the left nipple show no evidence of Paget disease or dermal lymphatic tumor spread. Sections of subareolar breast tissue show benign intraductal papilloma. There are mild, nonproliferative, fibrocystic changes of the breast tissue with stromal fibrosis and duct ectasia with small cyst formation. Atypical hyperplasia is not identified, nor is in situ and invasive malignancy.

Diagnoses

1. Right ovary and fallopian tube. Hemorrhagic corpus luteal cyst. Unremarkable fallopian tube.
2. Left ovary and fallopian tube. Benign physiologic cysts and ovary. Unremarkable fallopian tube.
3. Right breast and axillary lymph nodes from modified radical mastectomy.
   a. Infiltrating ductal carcinoma Bloom-Richardson grade 3.
      1. Tumor $3 \times 2 \times 2$ cm in size.
      2. No evidence of tumor extension to deep surgical margins.
      3. Axillary lymph nodes (3 total) show no evidence of metastasis.
      4. No evidence of Paget disease or dermal lymphatic tumor spread.
      5. Pending hormone receptor and DNA analysis.
   b. Mild fibrocystic changes present.
4. Left breast, modified radical mastectomy.
   a. Benign intraductal papilloma.
   b. No evidence of Paget disease or dermal lymphatic tumor spread.
   c. Mild, nonproliferative changes, fibrocystic in nature, without atypia.

Hormone Receptor Analysis: Immunoperoxidase stains for estrogen and progesterone receptors are applied to the paraffin-embedded tissue with good positive and negative internal and external controls. Tumor cells from the right breast tumor show estrogen receptor negative (0% staining of tumor nuclei, histochemical score 0); progesterone receptor negative (0% staining of tumor cells).

BREAST CARCINOMA

Specimens

1. Left breast wide excisional biopsy.
2. Axillary dissection.

Clinical History: The patient is a 36-year-old female who was found to have left breast calcifications on mammography. Stereotactic core biopsy revealed malignancy.

CLINICAL DIAGNOSIS: Stage 1 left breast carcinoma.

GROSS DESCRIPTION: The specimen was received fresh in 2 containers, each labeled with the patient's name and medical record number.

The first container is further labeled "left breast wide excision" and consists of a piece of fibroadipose tissue with a small skin ellipse extending off the medial side of the specimen. A diagram is submitted with the specimen to indicate size and dimension of the specimen. A short suture is present on the superior specimen with a long suture on the lateral. The entire specimen measures 3.5×5.5 cm and skin ellipse measures 2.75×0.5 cm. The specimen is white, rubbery and irregular in shape. There are areas of fibrosis in the inferomedial and deep areas of the specimen. A firm area, measuring 1.5×2.5 cm, is present in the center of the specimen. The specimen is serially sectioned and submitted in its entirety in a cassette with slides labeled "A1 through A10."

The second container is further labeled "axillary tissue" and contains a fresh specimen of fibrofatty tissue measuring 4.5×3.5 cm in aggregate. Contained within the tissue are 12 lymph nodes, the largest of which measures 1.4 cm.

Each lymph node is bisected and placed into a cassette labeled "B1 through B12."

MICROSCOPIC DESCRIPTION: Slides A3 and A4 consist of a portion of breast tissue containing infiltrating ductal carcinoma of the breast. There are infiltrating nests of malignant cells in which there is glandular formation. The cells demonstrate a moderate degree of nuclear pleomorphism with some cells having central nucleoli; however, the mitotic rate is less than 1 per 10 high-power fields. Overall the carcinoma is grade 2. Areas of ductal carcinoma in situ are demonstrated adjacent to the carcinoma. Histologically the tumor is 2.5 mm from the margin. No lymphatic invasion is evident.

The second specimen demonstrates 3 lymph nodes positive for carcinoma with no evidence of extranodal extension.

DIAGNOSES

1. Infiltrating ductal carcinoma of the left breast, grade 2.
2. Foci of ductal carcinoma in situ.
3. Tumor is 2.5 mm from the margin.
4. Fibrocystic disease of the breast.
5. Metastatic carcinoma in 3/12 lymph nodes.

TUMOR MARKERS

1. The tumor is estrogen receptor positive.
2. The tumor is HER-2/neu negative.

FEMORAL HEAD

SPECIMEN: Specimen labeled "right femoral head."

CLINICAL INFORMATION: Severe arthritic changes, right hip.

GROSS DESCRIPTION: The specimen is submitted in formalin. It consists of a femoral head with attached segment of femoral neck. Total weight is 152 g, and specimen measures 6.8×5.3×4.8 cm. The articular surface of the femoral head is coarsely granular, markedly irregular and focally devoid of cartilaginous covering. Marginal osteophytes are also identified. Fragments of congested, hyperplastic synovium are attached to the femoral head. Multiple irregular fragments of hyperplastic-appearing synovium, adipose tissue, striated muscle and minute bone fragments are also submitted in the same container. These fragments together measure 3.7×3.3×2.8 cm. Representative soft tissue is submitted in a single cassette. The bone is set aside for decalcification and subsequent sectioning.

MICROSCOPIC DESCRIPTION: Sections of synovial tissue and fibrocartilage show focal degenerative changes with chronic inflammation. The bony tissues from the surface of the hip joint show marked irregularities with areas of severe bony eburnation.

DIAGNOSIS: Bony tissues from right hip revealing severe degenerative arthritis.

GALLBLADDER

SPECIMEN SUBMITTED: Gallbladder and stones.

CLINICAL INFORMATION: Chronic cholecystitis and cholelithiasis; rule out common duct stone.

OPERATIVE PROCEDURE: Cholecystectomy with cholangiogram and common bile duct exploration.

GROSS DESCRIPTION: The specimen consists of a partly opened gallbladder with attached segment of cystic duct. The gallbladder measures 7.5 cm in length and 3 cm in fundus diameter. The serosal surface is yellow-pink, smooth and glistening. The wall is resilient and up to 4.5 mm in thickness. The lumen and the specimen container have approximately 40 yellow-black angulated calculi measuring from 0.6 to 1.2 cm in maximum diameter. The mucosal surface of the gallbladder is finely to focally moderately reticulated. No nodules are identified. The attached segment of cystic duct measures 1.5 cm in length and 0.5 cm in internal diameter. No calculus is present within the cystic duct. Representative tissue is submitted in a single cassette.

MICROSCOPIC DESCRIPTION: A representative section of the gallbladder demonstrates intact mucosal surface. Focally, the mucosal surface is denuded of epithelial lining. The epithelium is well differentiated, tall columnar in type and reveals no significant atypia. Small to moderate numbers of chronic inflammatory cells are scattered throughout the gallbladder wall. The serosa is edematous and congested. A representative section of the cystic duct also reveals mild chronic inflammation. There is no evidence of malignancy.

DIAGNOSIS: Gallbladder and segment of cystic duct, chronic cholecystitis with cholelithiasis.

SPONTANEOUS ABORTION

SPECIMEN: Products of conception.

CLINICAL HISTORY: Spontaneous abortion at approximately 9 weeks' gestation.

GROSS DESCRIPTION: Tissue consistent with products of conception.

MICROSCOPIC DESCRIPTION: Sections reveal decidua and immature placental tissue. The placental villi are large and poorly vascularized. There is hemorrhage in the decidua associated with infiltrate of intact and karyorrhectic polymorphonuclear leukocytes. The nodular embryo is loosely organized membranous tissue.

DIAGNOSES

1. Products of conception, necrotic decidua and immature placental tissue identified.
2. Nodular embryo identified.

SQUAMOUS CELL CARCINOMA OF LEFT FLOOR OF MOUTH

DIAGNOSIS: Left floor of mouth carcinoma.

GROSS DESCRIPTION: A 3-part specimen is received fresh. Specimen #1 is labeled "? metastatic tumor in jugular vein lymph nodes." This specimen consists of an elliptical fragment of light, whitish-tan tissue that is approximately 0.3×0.2×0.2 cm in size. Specimen is examined by frozen section technique. Diagnosis is ganglion. Remainder of this specimen is submitted as frozen section control #1.

The 2nd part is labeled "resection of floor of mouth, continuous with tongue and mandible, plus left radical neck dissection." As received in the frozen section room, this specimen consists of an identifiable left radical neck dissection and also the entire left ascending ramus of the mandible, the posterior three fourths of the left mandible proper, the left lateral portion of the tongue, and the submental and submaxillary salivary glands. The main lesion is identified on the left side of the floor of the mouth.

There is a lesion that is crater-like, measuring approximately 1.2×0.5 cm in greatest dimension. With the assistants, this specimen is properly oriented. There are 2 areas of interest defined. The initial area of interest is the anterior tongue margin. The 2nd area of interest is the medial tongue margin. Fragments from each of these areas are examined by the frozen section technique. The diagnosis on frozen section #2 (anterior tongue margin) is noted as "no tumor seen." The diagnosis on frozen section #3 (medial tongue margin) is noted as "no tumor seen."

Two additional areas of special interest are also identified. The 1st of these is that portion of the left radical neck dissection which was nearest to the carotid artery. A fragment of tissue is excised from this area and submitted for sectioning labeled "CM." The 2nd area of interest is that portion of the left radical neck dissection bordering the anterior aspect of the vertebral column. A fragment of tissue is excised from this area and submitted for sectioning labeled "VM."

After having photographed the specimen in several positions, it is blocked further. A section is taken through the main tumor mass and submitted for sectioning labeled "T Post." Attention is directed to the left radical neck dissection proper. This part of the specimen is divided into the appropriate 5 levels. Each level is examined for lymph nodes, which are dissected free and submitted in their entirety for sectioning. The remainder of the specimen is saved.

The 3rd and final part of the specimen, labeled "anterior margin of inferior mandible," consists of an irregular fragment of fibrous connective and skeletal muscular tissues and measures approximately $1 \times 0.5 \times 0.2$ cm. The specimen is submitted in its entirety for sectioning on 3 levels.

MICROSCOPIC DESCRIPTION: Examination of frozen section control #1 confirms the original frozen section diagnosis of ganglion. Microscopic examination of frozen section control #2 confirms the original frozen section diagnosis of no tumor seen. Microscopic examination of frozen section control #3 confirms the original frozen section diagnosis of no tumor seen.

Microscopic examination of 2nd part of the specimen reveals foci of moderately well-differentiated squamous cell carcinoma in the floor of the left side of the mouth. The residual tumor is surrounded by large amounts of dense, fibrous connective tissue. Microscopic examination of the section labeled CM, which represents the carotid margin, reveals squamous cell carcinoma that extends to within 0.1 cm of the surgical margin.

Microscopic examination of the section labeled VM, representing the vertebral margin, reveals no evidence of tumor in this location. Microscopic examination of the tissue in level 1 reveals a section of fibrotic and atrophic submaxillary salivary gland. There is also a single lymph node in level 1, being negative for metastatic tumor. Microscopic examination of the tissue in level 2 reveals sections of 11 lymph nodes. None of these lymph nodes contain squamous cell carcinoma. Microscopic examination of the tissue in level 4 reveals sections of 6 lymph nodes. These lymph node sections do not contain metastatic tumor. Microscopic examination of the tissue in level 5 reveals a single lymph node, negative for metastatic tumor.

DIAGNOSES

1. Left floor of mouth squamous cell carcinoma.
2. Squamous cell carcinoma in the extranodal connective tissue of neck, level 3.
3. No pathologic diagnosis in 19 cervical lymph nodes submitted.

STOMACH CARCINOMA

INDICATIONS: Patient with history of gastric ulcer of long duration.

DIAGNOSIS: Carcinoma of stomach.

PROCEDURE PERFORMED: Vagotomy and subtotal gastrectomy.

GROSS DESCRIPTION: Three specimens are received.
Specimen #1 consists of a portion of the stomach, measuring $13 \times 7 \times 2.5$ cm. There is a portion of mesentery attached to the lesser curvature. There is a firm, indurated area in the wall of the lesser curvature. The serosal surface is smooth, glistening and slightly hemorrhagic. On opening the specimen, a penetrating, well-circumscribed ulcer, 1 cm in diameter, is found in the wall of the lesser curvature. This ulcer penetrates to a depth of 1 cm. The ulcer is 3 cm from the proximal portion of the specimen and 4.5 cm from the distal portion. The edges of the ulcer are heaped up and firm, but the surrounding mucosa does not appear to be involved. The rugae or folds radiate toward the center of the ulcer from the superior side. The mucosa of the distal portion of the stomach is smooth.

Specimen #2 consists of a portion of the left anterior vagus. The specimen consists of a piece of pale, gray-white, soft tissue measuring 0.8 cm in length. The entire specimen is submitted for examination.

Specimen #3 is labeled "right posterior vagus" and consists of a piece of soft, gray-white tissue measuring 2 cm in length and 0.4 cm in diameter. The entire specimen is submitted for examination.

MICROSCOPIC EXAMINATION: Microscopic examination reveals a ragged ulcer penetrating to within 5 mm of the serosal surface. The ulcer is surrounded by dense connective tissue and chronic inflammatory infiltrate. The edges are not heaped up; however, several sections of the ulcer reveal malignant changes. The tumor is superficial and composed of poorly formed glands and sheets of malignant cells. The cells are pleomorphic and contain small amounts of eosinophilic cytoplasm. The nuclei are either pyknotic or large with prominent nucleoli and clumped chromatin. Mitoses are rare. The tumor itself does not extend below the mucosa, but a single nest of malignant cells is seen in a submucosal lymphatic space. The surgical margins are free of tumor. There are 4 perigastric lymph nodes. These show no evidence of metastatic spread. There are 2 segments of the large peripheral nerve.

DIAGNOSES

1. Superficial, spreading carcinoma, rising in the margin of a gastric ulcer that is chronic in nature. The surgical margins appear free of tumor.
2. Four perigastric lymph nodes reveal no evidence of metastatic disease.

TONSILS AND ADENOIDS

SPECIMENS

1. Left and right tonsils.
2. Adenoidal tissue.

CLINICAL INFORMATION: Chronic tonsillitis and adenoiditis.

GROSS DESCRIPTION: Tonsillar and adenoidal tissue without gross evidence of hemorrhage.

MICROSCOPIC DESCRIPTION: Sections of the tonsils show they are lined on the surface by nonkeratinizing stratified squamous epithelium. Within the tonsillar crypts are varying degrees of keratinization. There are aggregates of fibrillary bacteria present. There is prominent transepithelial migration of chronic inflammatory cells. The subjacent lymphoid tissue contains prominent and reactive-appearing germinal centers. The subepithelial parafollicular lymphoid tissue is heavily infiltrated by plasma cells.

The adenoid tissue is lined by disordered respiratory epithelium in some areas and in other areas by metaplastic squamous epithelium. There is prominent transepithelial migration of chronic inflammatory cells. Focal areas of epithelial keratinization are seen. The subjacent lymphoid tissue contains prominent and reactive-appearing germinal centers. The subepithelial parafollicular lymphoid tissue is heavily infiltrated with plasma cells.

DIAGNOSES: Chronic follicular tonsillitis. Chronic follicular adenoiditis.

TRANSITIONAL CELL CARCINOMA OF BLADDER

INDICATIONS: Multiple transurethral resection of bladder tumor resections for grade 2 transitional cell cancer.

PREOPERATIVE DIAGNOSIS: Bladder carcinoma; question of scalene lymph node metastasis.

POSTOPERATIVE DIAGNOSIS: Bladder carcinoma.

PROCEDURE PERFORMED: Bladder biopsy and left scalene lymph nodes.

SPECIMENS

1. Bladder tumor.
2. Left scalene lymph node.

GROSS DESCRIPTION: The specimen is received at the lab in 2 parts; #1 labeled "biopsy bladder tumor," and #2 as "scalene node, left." Specimen #1 consists of several fragments of tissue, gray-brown in color. Tissue fragments appear slightly hemorrhagic. These are submitted in their entirety for processing. Specimen #2 consists of multiple fragments of tissue, fatty and yellow in color. This tissue ranges in size from 0.2 cm to 1 cm in diameter. These tissue fragments are submitted in entirety for processing as well.

MICROSCOPIC EXAMINATION: This bladder specimen contains areas of transitional cell carcinoma; no areas of invasion can be identified. There is inflammation, acute and chronic, noted together with some necrosis. The section is examined in 6 levels. The scalene lymph node specimen contains normal nodal tissue with reactive germinal centers.

DIAGNOSES

1. Grade 2 papillary transitional cell carcinoma of bladder.
2. Inflammation, acute and chronic, of bladder, most consistent with recent biopsy procedure.
3. No pathologic diagnosis of left scalene lymph node.

Common Terms by Procedure

Appendix

acute appendicitis
appendiceal lumen
appendiceal surface
appendix
fecalith
focal ulceration
hemorrhagic
mass
mucosa
necrotic debris
perforation
perforation
polymorphonuclear leukocytes
purulent exudate
serosal surface
transmural infiltration
vermiform appendix

Autopsy Report

abdomen
abrasion
acute inflammation
adherent hair
adrenal
anatomic location and relationship
anoderm
antecubital fossa
anteroposterior dimension
anus
artifact of decomposition
atherosclerosis
atrophy
autolysis
barbiturate screen
biceps
bile
bladder
blanching
bloody mucus
blunt-force injury

body bag
body cavity
brain
bullous emphysematous change
buttocks
carotid artery
cerebrum
chest cavity
chest wall abrasion
clavicle
cocaine metabolite
congestion
conjunctiva
contusion
crepitus
curving border
curving incision
decedent
defensive incised wound
defensive injury
digit
dorsal wrist wound
drug residue
ecchymosis
emphysematous change
enzyme multiplied immunoassay test
  (EMIT)
ethanol
exsanguination
external genitalia
forearm
fracture
frontal
gallbladder
glass slide
gynecomastia
head
heart
histologic examination
homicide

incised wound
infarction
instant-print photo
intercostal space
internal artifact
internal structure of neck
intraventricular hemorrhage
iris
jab-type wound
kidney
laceration
liver
livor mortis
lower extremity
lung
macrophage
midclavicular region
middle lobe
mottled abrasion
mucoid fluid
nasal bridge
nasal cavity
nasal swab
natural deformity
neck
nipple
ocular fluid
oral cavity
organ weight
pallor
pancreas
parasternal chest
parietal pleural perforation
parietotemporal region
penis
periorbital region
peripheral edema
petechia
petechial hemorrhage
pituitary
pleural cavity
postmortem
prostate
protuberant

pupil
purple-topped tube
red-topped tube
rib fracture
rigor mortis
scalloped border
scalloped edge
scalp
scar
sclera
septal fibrosis
serous cavity
sharp-force injury
shoulder
skull
slide identification picture
sphenoid bone
spinal cord
spinous process
spleen
stab cavity
stab wound
sternal region
sternocleidomastoid muscle
sternum
subarachnoid hemorrhage
subdural hematoma
suffusion
surgical scar
thumb pad
thyroid
tissue bridging
trace evidence
trace material
triceps
trunk
upper extremity
upper lobe
urinary bladder
ventricle
vermiform appendix
vertex
web space
white matter

xiphoid region

Bone Marrow Aspirate, Biopsy, and Peripheral Blood Smear

absolute number
acute promyelocytic anemia
biopsy
blast
bone marrow aspirate
bone marrow biopsy
bony material
Bouin's solution
cytogenetic study
decalcification
erythrogenesis
erythroid maturation
erythroid precursor
excess blast
fibrosis
histiocyte
hypercellular marrow
hypogranular form
iron store
left shift
left-shifted myelogenesis
lymphocyte
megakaryocyte
microcytic
molecular study
monocyte
morphologic evidence
morphology
myelogenesis
myeloid precursor
myeloid/erythroid (M:E) ratio
neutrophil
normochromic
normocytic
peripheral blood smear
platelet
polychromasia
promyelocyte
red blood cell

residual disease
ringed sideroblast
segmented neutrophil
sponge
subcortical bone
teardrop form
white blood cell

Breast Carcinoma and Ovarian Tissue Analysis

adipose tissue
angulated nucleus
areola
atypia
atypical hyperplasia
axillary lymph node
axillary node
axillary tail
Bloom-Richardson grade
breast tissue
capsular surface
corpus luteal cyst
cut section
cyst formation
deep resection margin
deep surgical margin
dermal lymphatic tumor spread
DNA analysis
duct ectasia
edematous ovarian stroma
enlarged lymph node
eosinophilic cytoplasm
epithelial cell
estrogen receptor
everted nipple
fallopian tube
fallopian tube segment
fallopian tube stump
fatty breast tissue
fibrocystic change
fibrosis
fibrous band
fibrous septum

fibrous tissue
fimbriated end
formalin
granular cut surface
gross examination
hemorrhagic corpus luteal cyst
high-power field
histochemical score
homogenous fat
hormone receptor
immunoperoxidase stain
in situ malignancy
infiltrating ductal carcinoma
inked surgical margin
intraductal component
intraductal papilloma
invasive malignancy
lobulated homogenous fat
lobule
lymphatic tumor
metastasis
microscopic examination
mitotic figure
modified radical mastectomy
multinodular appearance
necrosis
nipple
nuclear chromatin
ovarian stroma
ovary
Paget disease
palpable mass
paraffin-embedded tissue
poorly differentiated infiltrating ductal
    carcinoma
progesterone receptor
resection margin
ruptured capsular surface
serial fashion
skeletal muscle
skin ellipse
soft adipose tissue
stromal fibrosis
subareolar breast tissue

surgical margin
surgical stump
thin-walled cyst
trabecular sheet
tumor cell
tumor extension
tumor nodule
tumor nucleus

Breast Carcinoma

axillary dissection
axillary tissue
breast
breast carcinoma
calcification
ductal carcinoma in situ
estrogen receptor
excisional biopsy
extranodal extension
fibroadipose tissue
fibrocystic disease
fibrofatty tissue
fibrosis
glandular formation
HER-2/neu
infiltrating ductal carcinoma
lymph node
lymphatic invasion
malignancy
malignant cell
mammography
metastatic carcinoma
mitotic rate
nuclear pleomorphism
nucleolus
skin ellipse
stereotactic core biopsy

Femoral Head

adipose tissue
arthritic change
articular surface
bone fragment
bony eburnation
bony tissue

cartilaginous covering
chronic inflammation
decalcification
degenerative arthritis
degenerative change
femoral head
femoral neck
fibrocartilage
formalin
hip joint
hyperplastic synovium
osteophyte
soft tissue
striated muscle
synovial tissue

Gallbladder

atypia
calculus
cholangiogram
cholecystectomy
cholecystitis
cholelithiasis
chronic inflammation
chronic inflammatory cell
common bile duct
common duct stone
cystic duct
epithelial lining
epithelium
fundus
gallbladder
gallbladder wall
lumen
malignancy
mucosal surface
nodule
serosa
serosal surface
stone

Spontaneous Abortion

decidua
hemorrhage

immature placental tissue
infiltrate
karyorrhectic polymorphonuclear
    leukocyte
membranous tissue
necrotic decidua
nodular embryo
placental tissue
placental villus
products of conception
spontaneous abortion

Squamous Cell Carcinoma of Left Floor of Mouth

anterior margin
ascending ramus of mandible
atrophic submaxillary salivary gland
carotid artery
carotid margin
dissection
elliptical fragment
extranodal connective tissue
fibrous connective tissue
floor of mouth
floor of mouth carcinoma
frozen section
frozen section technique
ganglion
jugular vein lymph nodes
lymph node
mandible
mandible proper
metastatic tumor
moderately well-differentiated
    squamous cell carcinoma
mouth carcinoma
radical neck dissection
ramus
residual tumor
skeletal muscular tissue
squamous cell carcinoma
submaxillary salivary glands

submental salivary gland
surgical margin
tongue
tongue margin
tumor mass
vertebral column
vertebral margin
well-differentiated squamous cell
   carcinoma

Stomach Carcinoma

carcinoma
carcinoma of stomach
chromatin
chronic inflammatory infiltrate
clumped chromatin
connective tissue
eosinophilic cytoplasm
gastric ulcer
hemorrhagic
lesser curvature
malignant cell
malignant change
mesentery
metastatic spread
mitosis
mucosa
nucleolus
nucleus
penetrating ulcer
perigastric lymph node
peripheral nerve
pleomorphic
pyknotic
ragged ulcer
ruga
serosal surface
sheet of malignant cells
soft tissue
spreading carcinoma
stomach
submucosal lymphatic space
subtotal gastrectomy

surgical margin
tumor
ulcer
vagotomy
vagus
well-circumscribed ulcer

Tonsils and Adenoids

adenoid tissue
adenoiditis
chronic adenoiditis
chronic follicular adenoiditis
chronic follicular tonsillitis
chronic inflammatory cells
disordered respiratory epithelium
fibrillary bacteria
germinal center
hemorrhage
keratinization
lymphoid tissue
metaplastic squamous epithelium
nonkeratinizing stratified squamous
   epithelium
plasma cell
subepithelial parafollicular lymphoid
   tissue
tonsil
tonsillar crypt
tonsillar tissue
tonsillitis
transepithelial migration

Transitional Cell Carcinoma of Bladder

biopsy
bladder
carcinoma
germinal center
inflammatory reaction
lymph node metastasis
marked inflammatory reaction
necrosis
nodal tissue

papillary transitional cell carcinoma of
   bladder
scalene lymph node
tissue fragment

transitional cell cancer
transitional cell carcinoma
transurethral resection of bladder tumor
tumor

Classification by System Including Grades & Stages

The following guidelines generally follow AHDI (Association for Healthcare Documentation Integrity) Book of Style current recommendations. Alternative methods may be acceptable and vary according to dictator or facility preference. This list is not all-inclusive but representative by system.

With classifying, staging and grading, the range of numbers and/or letters from low to high generally indicates degree of severity or advancement of the disease or condition from least severe to most severe; 1 is less advanced than 2, and 5 is more severe than 3, etc.; I is less advanced than II, and V is more severe than III, A is less severe than D, and C is more advanced than B, etc. Exceptions to this rule are noted.

CANCER

stage: Use roman numerals, capital letters and arabic numerals as shown. Do not capitalize stage.
stage I, stage II, stage III, stage IV, stage IA, stage IB, stage IIA, stage IVC, stage IB3, stage IIA2, etc.

grade: Use arabic numerals. Do not capitalize grade.
grade 1, grade 2, grade, 3, grade 4

Aster-Coller: Colon cancer staging. Use uppercase letters A, B, C, D to indicate stage. A is least advanced, and D indicates extensive disease with nodal involvement. Use arabic numerals to further define.
Aster-Coller A1, Aster-Coller D2, etc.

Breslow: Melanoma (skin) thickness classification system. Use arabic numerals. Thinnest is 1, and thickest is 3.
1, 2, 3

Broders index: Malignant tumor classification. Use arabic numerals.
grade 1, 2, 3, 4 or Broders grade 1, Broders grade 2, etc.

CIN: See OB/GYN.

Clark level: Malignant melanoma of skin (epidermis) classification system. Use roman numerals.
Clark level I, Clark level II, Clark level III, Clark level IV

Dukes classification: Colon or rectal adenocarcinoma. Use uppercase letters.
Dukes A, Dukes B, Dukes C, Dukes D

Durie-Salmon: Multiple myeloma classification system. Use roman numerals and uppercase letters.
I, II, IIIA, IIIB.

Edmondson-Steiner: Hepatocellular carcinoma grading system. Use roman numerals. Grade I, grade II, grade III, grade IV

Enneking: Musculoskeletal tumor staging system. Use roman numerals and uppercase letters.
IA, IIIB, etc.

FAB: Acute nonlymphoid leukemia French-American-British classification system. Use letter M with arabic numerals and uppercase letters.
M1, M2, M3, M4, M5, M6, M4E, M5A, M5B, etc.

FIGO: Gynecologic malignancy Federation International de Gynecologie et Obstetrique staging system. Use roman numerals and lowercase letters for subdivisions.
stage I, stage II, stage III, stage IV, stage Ia, stage IIIb, etc.

Gleason score: Prostate adenocarcinoma tumor grading system. Use arabic numerals. Score is calculated by adding dominant and secondary pattern grade numbers.
Gleason score 3, Gleason score 7, and grade 1, grade 2, grade 3, grade 4, grade 5, etc.

Goseki: Gastric carcinoma grading system. Use roman numerals.
Goseki grade I, Goseki grade II, Goseki grade III, Goseki grade IV

Haggitt: Colorectal adenocarcinoma classification system. Use arabic numerals.
Haggitt level 1, Haggitt level 2, level 3, level 4

International Staging System (INSS): Lung cancer. Use roman numerals and uppercase letters.
IA, IIA, IIIB, etc.

International Staging System (INSS): Neuroblastoma. Use arabic numerals and uppercase letters.
1-4S

Jass: Colorectal carcinoma grading system. Use roman numerals.
grade I, grade II, grade III, grade IV

Jewett-Marshall: Bladder carcinoma classification system. Use uppercase letters O, A, B, C, D, for best to worst prognosis respectively, and arabic numerals.
class A, class B1, class D4, etc.

Karnofsky scale: Malignant neoplasms rating system. Use arabic numerals. Normal level to worst prognosis is represented by 10, 20, 30, 40, 50, 60, 70, 80, 90, 100.

Lugano: Gastric lymphoma staging system. Use roman numerals and uppercase letters. stage I, state II, stage III, stage IV, stage IIE, stage IIIA, etc.

Robson: Renal cell carcinoma staging system Use roman numerals. stage I, stage II, stage III, stage IV

Rye: Hodgkin disease classification system. Use zero and roman numerals. class 0, class I, class I, class II, class III, class IV

Skinner: Testicular carcinoma staging system. Use uppercase letters. stage A, stage B, stage C

TNM: Malignant tumors staging system. Accepted by the International Union Against Cancer and the American Joint Committee on Cancer. Staging criteria may vary by cancer type.

T – tumor
N – node
M – distant metastasis
X – cannot be evaluated
0 (zero) – no evidence
G – histologic grade
H – host performance
L – lymphatic invasion
R – residual tumor
S – invasion of sclerae
Tis – carcinoma in situ
V – venous invasion

Further categorized using arabic numerals 0,1, 2, 3, 4.

No commas used in staging sequences, and spacing as shown below.
T1 N0 MX
T3 N4 M1
Tis N0 M0

prefixes
a – autopsy
c – clinical
p – pathological
r – retreatment

y or yp – during or following
multinodal therapy
aT2
cT4 cN3 cM1
pT1 or pT2 pN3
rT0
yT1 yN0 yM0

suffixes
Use (m) to denote multiple primary tumors. It is used with T only. Lowercase letters
a, b, c, d, etc. used to further classify and are dependent on type of carcinoma.
T3(m), T4(m), T1a, T2c

Van Nuys Criteria: Breast cancer ductal carcinoma in situ (DCIS) scoring system.
Use arabic numerals.
Van Nuys score 1, Van Nuys score 2, etc.

Whitmore-Jewett: Prostate carcinoma staging system. Use uppercase letters.
stage A, stage B, stage C, stage D

CARDIOLOGY
heart murmur
grade– use arabic numerals; grade 1, grade 2, grade 3, grade 4, grade 5, grade 6
grade and scale – grade 2/6 or grade 2 over 6; grade 3.5/6 or grade 3.5 over 6
murmur grade 3/6 to 4/6 or 3 to 4 over 6

Do not use hyphens when transcribing heart murmur grades.

leads
standard bipolar leads– lead I, lead II, lead III
augmented limb leads – aVR, aVL, aVF
precordial leads – V1, V2, V3, V4, V5, V6, (may subscript numeral)
right – add R; V1R, V5R, etc.
ensiform cartilage leads – add E; VE (may subscript E)
3rd interspace leads – use 3; 3V1, 3V3, 3V5, etc. (may subscript last numeral)
esophageal leads – use E and arabic numerals; E20, E25, etc. (may subscript
numeral)
Do not use a hyphen in lead sequences. Use V1 through V4, V1 through V3, etc.

NYHA classification: Cardiac failure classification. Use roman numerals.
class I, class II, class III, class IV

TIMI: Thrombolysis in myocardial infarction grading system. Use arabic numerals.
grade 1, grade 2, grade 3

Classification by System

CRANIAL NERVES: See NEUROLOGY.

DERMATOLOGY
Breslow: See CANCER.

burns: Use ordinals to indicate burn depth.
1st degree, 2nd degree, 3rd degree, 4th degree
When used as an adjective, avoid using hyphens.
2nd degree burn, 4th degree burn, etc.

decubitus ulcers: Use roman numerals.
stage I, stage II, stage III, stage IV

DIABETES: Use arabic numerals for types.
type 1, type 2 (type 1.5 is used in some facilities)
Use uppercase letters to classify gestational diabetes.
class A, class B, class C, class D, class E, class F

HEMATOLOGY
coagulation factor: Use roman numerals.
factor I, factor II, factor III, etc.

MULTIPLE SCLEROSIS
Kurtzke score: Multiple sclerosis evaluation scoring system. Use arabic numerals 1-10. Kurtzke score 2, Kurtzke score 5, Kurtzke score 7, etc.

NEUROLOGIC
cranial nerves: Use roman numerals or arabic numerals.
cranial nerves 2 through 12, or cranial nerves II through XII

Hunt and Hess: Subarachnoid hemorrhage assessment scale. Use arabic numerals.
grade 1, grade 2, grade 3, grade 4

Rancho Los Amigos scale: Cognitive functioning scale. Use roman numerals I through X. I is unresponsive, and X is fully responsive and functional.
level I, level II, level III, level IV, level V, etc.

OB/GYN
Bethesda system: (partial listing for example purposes only): Cervical cytology.
May be used with CIN, below.
ASC: Atypical squamous cells.
ASC-US: ASC of undetermined significance.
ASC-H: ASC, cannot exclude high-grade squamous intraepithelial lesion.
HSIL: High-grade squamous intraepithelial lesion.
LSIL: Low-grade squamous intraepithelial lesion.
AGC: Atypical glandular cells.

CIN: Cervical intraepithelial neoplasia classification system. Use arabic numerals. grade 1, grade, 2, grade 3 and hyphenate
CIN-1, CIN-2, CIN-3

FIGO staging: See CANCER.

Papanicolaou (Pap): Cervical cytology classification. Use roman numerals. class I, class II, class, III, class IV

ORTHOPEDIC

Catterall hip score: Epiphysial osteonecrosis of the upper end of the femur (Legg-Perthes disease, Legg-Calvé-Perthes disease, Legg disease) scoring system. Use roman numerals.
Catterall I, Catterall II, Catterall III, Catterall IV

fractures
Garden: Femoral neck fracture classification. Use arabic numerals.
Garden stage 1, Garden stage II, Garden stage III

LeFort: Facial fracture classification. Use roman numerals
LeFort I, LeFort, II, LeFort III

Mayo: Olecranon fracture classification. Use roman numerals I, II, III with capital letters A, B, C.
Mayo IA, Mayo IIIB, etc.

Neer-Horowitz: Proximal humeral physeal fracture classification. Use roman numerals. Neer-Horowitz I, Neer-Horowitz II, Neer-Horowitz III, Neer-Horowitz IV

Outerbridge scale: Patellar chondromalacia rating. Use arabic numerals. grade 1, grade 2, grade 3, grade 4

Salter: Epiphyseal fracture classification. Use roman numerals.
Salter I, Salter II, Salter III, Salter IV

Salter-Harris: Epiphysial plate injury classification. Use roman numerals.
Salter-Harris type I, Salter-Harris type II, Salter-Harris type III, Salter-Harris type IV, Salter-Harris type V

Schatzker: Tibial plateau fracture classification. Use roman numerals.
Schatzker type I, Schatzker type II, Schatzker type III, Schatzker type IV, Schatzker type V, Schatzker type VI

stress fracture: Use zero and roman numerals.
grade 0 (no fracture), grade I, grade II, grade III, grade IV

mobilization grade: Use arabic numerals.
grade 1, grade 2, grade 3, grade 4, grade 5

Neer staging: Shoulder impingement classification. Use roman numerals.
Neer I, Neer II, Neer III

vertebra
C – cervical spine
T – thoracic spine (syn. D – dorsal spine)
L – lumbar spine
S – sacral spine

Use arabic numerals to indicate vertebra number. Do not use a space between the letter and numeral.
C1, C2, T1, T3, L4, S1, etc.
To list vertebra, repeat letters.
L1, L2, L3, etc.
A hyphen represents a space between vertebrae. Depending on facility preference, the letter may or may not be repeated.
C2-C3 or C2-3; T5-T6 or T5-6; S1-S2 or S1-2; S3-S4 or S3-4; L5-S1, etc.

RESPIRATORY
Mallampati-Samsoon: Airway classification for anesthesiology. Use roman numerals. class I, class II, class III, class IV

VERTEBRA: See ORTHOPEDIC.